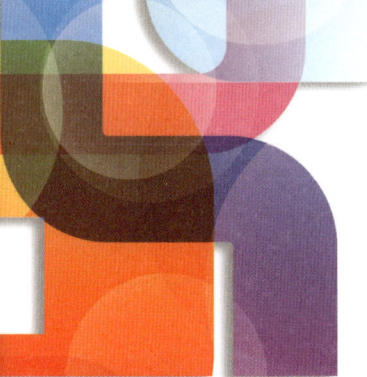

CONTENTS

UNIT 1
Nursing Data Collection, Documentation, and Analysis

1. Nurse's Role in Health Assessment: Collecting and Analyzing Data   1
2. Collecting Subjective Data: The Interview and Health History   12
3. Collecting Objective Data: The Physical Examination   31
4. Validating and Documenting Data   44
5. Thinking Critically to Analyze Data and Make Informed Nursing Judgments   60

UNIT 2
Integrative Holistic Nursing Assessment

6. Assessing Mental Status Including Risk for Substance Abuse   69
7. Assessing Psychosocial, Cognitive, and Moral Development   98
8. Assessing General Health Status and Vital Signs   121
9. Assessing Pain: The Fifth Vital Sign   142
10. Assessing for Violence   161
11. Assessing Culture   181
12. Assessing Spirituality and Religious Practices   202
13. Assessing Nutritional Status   217

UNIT 3
Nursing Assessment of Physical Systems

14. Assessing Skin, Hair, and Nails   247
15. Assessing Head and Neck   280
16. Assessing Eyes   304
17. Assessing Ears   338
18. Assessing Mouth, Throat, Nose, and Sinuses   357
19. Assessing Thorax and Lungs   381
20. Assessing Breasts and Lymphatic System   409
21. Assessing Heart and Neck Vessels   431
22. Assessing Peripheral Vascular System   463
23. Assessing Abdomen   492
24. Assessing Musculoskeletal System   528
25. Assessing Neurologic System   567
26. Assessing Male Genitalia and Rectum   605
27. Assessing Female Genitalia, Anus, and Rectum   637
28. Pulling It All Together: Integrated Head-To-Toe Assessment   672

UNIT 4
Nursing Assessment of Special Groups

29. Assessing Childbearing Women   691
30. Assessing Newborns and Infants   722
31. Assessing Children and Adolescents   761
32. Assessing Older Adults   813
33. Assessing Families   853
34. Assessing Communities   869

APPENDICES

A. Nursing History Guide   887
B. Physical Assessment Guide   889
C. NANDA Approved Nursing Diagnoses 2015–2017   894
D. Selected Collaborative Problems   897

Glossary   899

Index   905

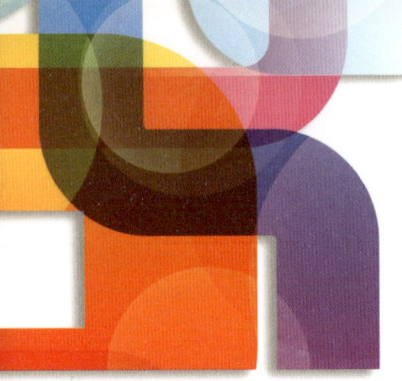

ORGANIZATION OF THE ASSESSMENT CHAPTERS

Assessment chapters walk students through the entire assessment process, from an anatomy and physiology review to data collection to analysis. Each assessment chapter includes the following organization:

LEARNING OBJECTIVES
Each chapter begins with a list of Learning Objectives to give the reader an overview of what will be presented and learned in the chapter.

CONTINUING CASE STUDY
Each chapter introduces a client with a health concern related to the chapter content. The COLDSPA mnemonic is applied as the nurse explores the health concern, a physical assessment of the client is demonstrated, proper documentation technique is applied, diagnostic reasoning is applied, and appropriate nursing conclusions are determined.

STRUCTURE AND FUNCTION
Reviews key anatomy and physiology, which provide the knowledge base the nurse draws on to complete the assessment.

HEALTH ASSESSMENT
Provides in-depth assessment parameters, including nursing health history, physical assessment, and validation and documentation of the data. This approach helps students understand the "Whys" behind the "Whats," promoting critical thinking.

COLLECTING SUBJECTIVE DATA: THE NURSING HEALTH HISTORY
Presents information in two columns: *Questions* that the student will ask the client and *Rationales* explaining why the questions are important. Clinical tips and cultural considerations are included to help highlight critical content.

COLLECTING OBJECTIVE DATA: THE PHYSICAL EXAMINATION
Introduces ways to prepare the client for the examination, including lists of all equipment needed and key points to remember during the assessment. Physical examination procedures are fully illustrated in a step-by-step fashion across three columns: *Assessment Procedure* (explains and illustrates exactly how to perform specific aspects of the examination), *Normal Findings,* and *Abnormal Findings.* Clinical tips, older adult considerations, and cultural considerations are included to help highlight critical content. Also included, where relevant, are the differences between basic examinations and examinations performed only by advanced practice nurses.

VALIDATING AND DOCUMENTING FINDINGS
Includes documentation reminders that are incorporated into the continuing case study.

DIAGNOSTIC REASONING
Provides common nursing diagnoses (health promotion, risk, and actual) and possible collaborative problems related to the specific body system. Students are taught diagnostic reasoning skills to reach possible conclusions.

REPORTING OF DATA USING SBAR
Describes the use and advantages of the SBAR method for reporting findings: Situation, Background, Assessment, Recommendation.

EVIDENCE-BASED HEALTH PROMOTION AND DISEASE PREVENTION
Includes health promotion and disease prevention information for one or more conditions common to the body system covered in the chapter.

DISPLAYS OF ABNORMAL FINDINGS
Includes fully illustrated common abnormal findings, helping students to identify important distinctions.

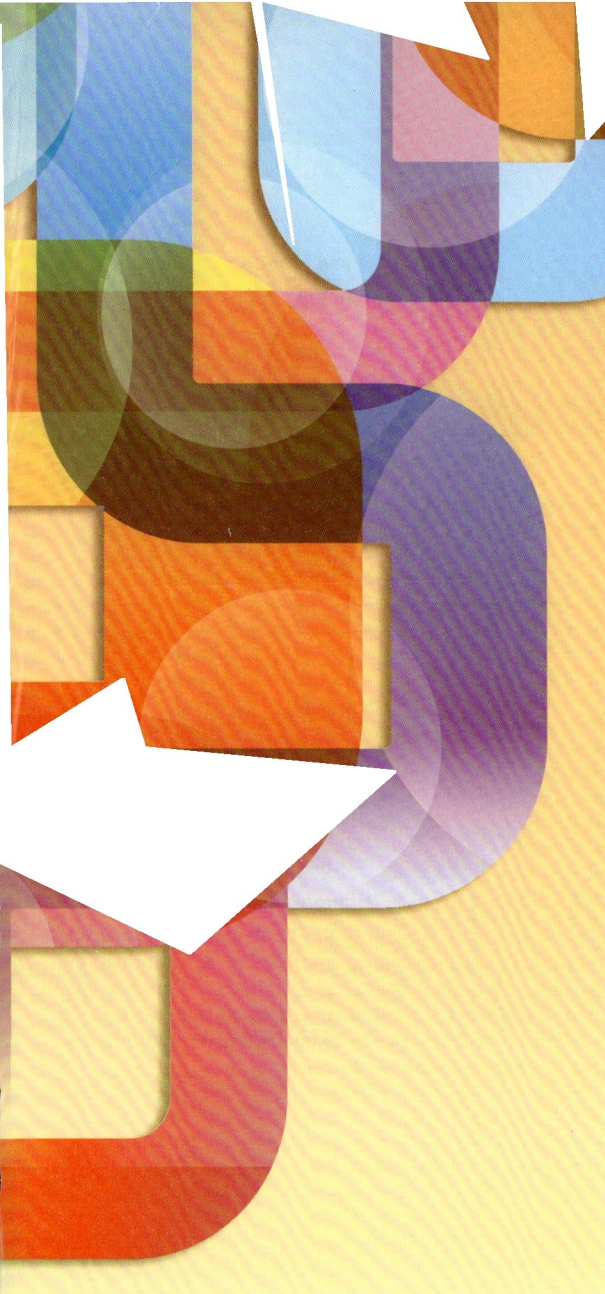

HEALTH ASSESSMENT IN NURSING

6TH EDITION

Janet R. Weber, RN, EdD
Professor Emeritus
Department of Nursing
Southeast Missouri State University
Cape Girardeau, Missouri

Jane H. Kelley, RN, PhD
Retired Professor
School of Nursing
Indiana Wesleyan University
Louisville, Kentucky

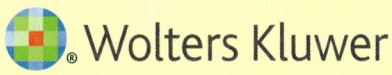 Wolters Kluwer

Philadelphia • Baltimore • New York • London
Buenos Aires • Hong Kong • Sydney • Tokyo

Executive Editor: Kelley Squazzo
Senior Development Editor: Meredith Brittain
Manager, Books Editorial Coordinator Group: Annette Ferran
Production Project Manager: Marian Bellus
Editorial Assistant: Leo Gray
Design Coordinator: Terry Mallon
Manufacturing Coordinator: Karin Duffield
Prepress Vendor: Aptara, Inc.

6th edition

Copyright © 2018 Wolters Kluwer Health.

Copyright © 2014, 2010 Wolters Kluwer Health | Lippincott Williams & Wilkins. Copyright © 2007, 2003 by Lippincott Williams & Wilkins. Copyright © 1998 by Lippincott-Raven Publishers. All rights reserved. This book is protected by copyright. No part of this book may be reproduced or transmitted in any form or by any means, including as photocopies or scanned-in or other electronic copies, or utilized by any information storage and retrieval system without written permission from the copyright owner, except for brief quotations embodied in critical articles and reviews. Materials appearing in this book prepared by individuals as part of their official duties as U.S. government employees are not covered by the above-mentioned copyright. To request permission, please contact Lippincott Williams & Wilkins at Two Commerce Square, 2001 Market Street, Philadelphia, PA 19103, via email at permissions@lww.com, or via our website at lww.com (products and services).

Not authorised for sale in United States, Canada, Australia, New Zealand, Puerto Rico, and U.S. Virgin Islands.

Library of Congress Cataloging-in-Publication Data

Names: Weber, Janet, author. | Kelley, Jane, 1944- author.
Title: Health assessment in nursing / Janet R. Weber, Jane H. Kelley.
Description: Sixth edition. | Philadelphia : Wolters Kluwer, [2018] |
  Includes bibliographical references and index.
Identifiers: LCCN 2017020452 | ISBN 9781496344380
Subjects: | MESH: Nursing Assessment–methods
Classification: LCC RT48 | NLM WY 100.4 | DDC 610.73–dc23
  LC record available at https://lccn.loc.gov/2017020452

This work is provided "as is," and the publisher disclaims any and all warranties, express or implied, including any warranties as to accuracy, comprehensiveness, or currency of the content of this work.

This work is no substitute for individual patient assessment based upon healthcare professionals' examination of each patient and consideration of, among other things, age, weight, gender, current or prior medical conditions, medication history, laboratory data and other factors unique to the patient. The publisher does not provide medical advice or guidance and this work is merely a reference tool. Healthcare professionals, and not the publisher, are solely responsible for the use of this work including all medical judgments and for any resulting diagnosis and treatments.

Given continuous, rapid advances in medical science and health information, independent professional verification of medical diagnoses, indications, appropriate pharmaceutical selections and dosages, and treatment options should be made and healthcare professionals should consult a variety of sources. When prescribing medication, healthcare professionals are advised to consult the product information sheet (the manufacturer's package insert) accompanying each drug to verify, among other things, conditions of use, warnings and side effects and identify any changes in dosage schedule or contraindications, particularly if the medication to be administered is new, infrequently used or has a narrow therapeutic range. To the maximum extent permitted under applicable law, no responsibility is assumed by the publisher for any injury and/or damage to persons or property, as a matter of products liability, negligence law or otherwise, or from any reference to or use by any person of this work.

LWW.com

*My husband, sons, grandsons, mother, father, and grandmothers
who have inspired me by their wisdom and encouragement*
JANET

*My husband, mother, father, and grandmother, each of
whom helped me to see the world through new eyes*
JANE

*But there's no vocabulary
For love within a family, love that's lived in
But not looked at, love within the light of which
All else is seen, the love within which
All other love finds speech. This love is silent.*
FROM *THE ELDER STATESMAN*, T. S. ELIOT (1888–1964)

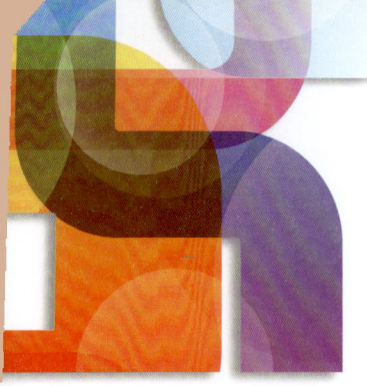

CONTRIBUTORS

Contributors to the 6th Edition

Bobbi Palmer, APRN, MSN, FNP-BC
FNP Program Director
Southeast Missouri State University
Cape Girardeau, Missouri
CASE STUDIES

Michelle Tanz, DNP, APRN, FNP-BC
Assistant Professor
Southeast Missouri State University
Cape Girardeau, Missouri
CHAPTER 8

For a list of the contributors to the Instructor Resources accompanying this book, please visit http://thepoint.lww.com/Weber 6e.

Contributors to the 5th Edition

Shirley Ashburn, RN, BSN, MS
Professor of Nursing
Cypress College
Cypress, California
CHAPTER 7

Jill Cash, MSN, APN
Family Nurse Practitioner
Southern Illinois Rheumatology
Herrin, Illinois
CHAPTERS 29, 30, 31

Kathy Casteel, APRN, MSN, FNP-BC
Family Nurse Practitioner
Columbia, Missouri
CHAPTER 14

Bobbi Palmer, APRN, MSN, FNP-BC
FNP Program Director
Southeast Missouri State University
Cape Girardeau, Missouri
CASE STUDIES

Ann D. Sprengel, RN, EdD
Professor
Director of Undergraduate Studies
Department of Nursing
Southeast Missouri State University
Cape Girardeau, Missouri
CHAPTERS 13, 22

Michelle Tanz, APRN, FNP-BC
Instructor
Southeast Missouri State University
Cape Girardeau, Missouri
CHAPTER 8

Lisa Waggoner, DNP, APN, FNP-BC
Assistant Professor
Arkansas State University
Jonesboro, Arkansas
CHAPTERS 26, 27

Madonna Weiss, APRN, MSN, FNP-BC
Instructor
Southeast Missouri State University
Cape Girardeau, Missouri
CASE STUDIES AND CONSULTANT FOR PHOTO SHOOT

Cathy Young, RN, DNSc, FNP-BC
Coordinator of FNP Track
Arkansas State University
Jonesboro, Arkansas
CHAPTER 10

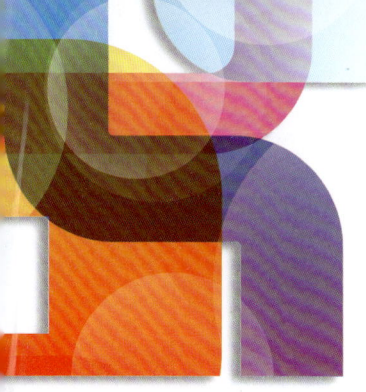

REVIEWERS

Cheryl Alberternst, MSN, RN
Instructor
Southeast Missouri State University
Cape Girardeau, Missouri

James Bockeloh, DNP, FNP-BC
Clinical Assistant Professor
University of Wisconsin – Milwaukee
Milwaukee, Wisconsin

Theresa Capriotti, DO, MSN, RN, CRNP
Clinical Associate Professor
Villanova University
Villanova, Pennsylvania

Darlene Clark, MS, RN
Senior Lecturer in Nursing
Pennsylvania State University
State College, Pennsylvania

Susan Davidson, EdD, APN, NP-C
Professor
University of Tennessee at Chattanooga
Chattanooga, Tennessee

Anne Eby, MN, APRN, FNP-C, CNE
Lecturer RN-BSN Program
Frostburg State University
Frostburg, Maryland

Hobie Feagai, EdD, MSN, FNP-BC, APRN-Rx
Professor
Hawaii Pacific University
Honolulu, Hawaii

Nicholas E. Frusciante, RN, MSN
Professor Nursing Alumnus CCRN
Luzerne County Community College
Nanticoke, Pennsylvania

Tish Gill, RN, MSN, DNP
Assistant Professor
Temple University
Philadelphia, Pennsylvania

Regina Hanchak, RN, MS
Professor
Erie Community College
Williamsville, New York

Kelli Hand, DNP, RN
Assistant Professor
University of Tennessee at Chattanooga
Chattanooga, Tennessee

Kimberly Heien, RN, MSN/Ed, PHN
Clinical Instructor
University of Texas at Arlington
Arlington, Texas

Gabrielle Hennrich-Frye, RN, BSN
Case manager
Pyramid Home Health
Missouri

Sondell Hickson, DNP, APN, ACNS-BC, FNP-BC
Associate Professor
Austin Peay State University
Clarksville, Tennessee

Casey Hill, MSN, RN-BC, CEN, CPS-T

Susan Lindner, MSN, RNC-OB
Clinical Assistant Professor
Virginia Commonwealth University
Richmond, Virginia

Amy Luckowski, PhD, RN, CCRN, CNE
Assistant Professor
Neumann University
Aston Township, Pennsylvania

Shirley MacNeill, MSN, RN, CNE
ADN Program Coordinator
Lamar State College – Port Arthur
Port Arthur, Texas

Tonia Mailow, DNP, RN
Assistant Professor of Nursing
Murray State University
Murray, Kentucky

Jessica Pastor, MSN, ACNP-BC, TNCC, SANE-A
Nursing instructor
Wayne State University
Detroit, Michigan

A. Christy Seckman, DNP, MSN/FNP, RN
Associate Professor
Goldfarb School of Nursing at Barnes-Jewish College
St. Louis, Missouri

Joyce Shanty, PhD, RN
Associate Professor
Indiana University of Pennsylvania
Indiana, Pennsylvania

Jennifer Wheeler, MSN/Ed, RN
Assistant Professor
Jackson College
Jackson, Michigan

Tracy Wilson, MSN, FNP-BC
Instructor
Belmont University
Nashville, Tennessee

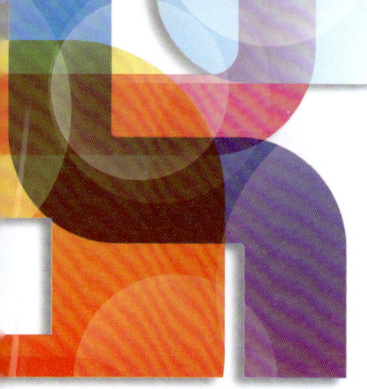

PREFACE

With the sixth edition of *Health Assessment in Nursing*, we continue to strive to help students learn accurate interviewing and physical assessment skills to practice safe, effective nursing care in today's ever-changing health care environment. As nurses provide care in a variety of settings—preventative, acute and chronic long-term care agencies—they need to be more prepared than ever before to perform accurate, timely health assessments based on evidence-based knowledge. No matter where a nurse practices, two components are essential for accurate collection of client data: a comprehensive knowledge base and expert nursing assessment skills. With that in mind, we have filled these pages with in-depth, accurate information, illustrations, and abnormal findings photos, and additional assessment tools to help students develop skills to collect both subjective and objective data. In addition to nursing assessment skills, today's nurses need expert critical thinking skills to analyze the data they collect to detect client problems and make informed nursing judgments—whether these are client problems treated independently by nurses, collaborative problems treated in cooperation with other health care practitioners, or medical problems that require a referral to other health care professionals for further evaluation and treatment.

Highlights of the Sixth Edition

Updating of all content in Units I through IV to include **the latest evidence-based practices and assessment guidelines.**

Culture continues to be a primary focus of this text because of its significance to assessment. It is emphasized throughout the text with the below icon, and a separate chapter (Chapter 11) introduces cultural concepts and their importance in relation to nursing assessment and critical thinking to make informed decisions.

Lifespan, a vitally important topic in today's health care environment, is presented in special individual chapters in Unit 4 that provide comprehensive explanations of the differences inherent in assessing **childbearing women, infants, children through adolescents, and elderly clients.** These chapters explain and illustrate the uniqueness of these differences in regard to body structures and functions, interview techniques, growth and development, and physical examination techniques.

Because of the growing number of elderly clients, chapters in Unit 3 include information on how to adapt the assessment process of each body system for older clients. This unit also describes how some physical changes are actually normal adaptations to aging rather than abnormal health findings. This information is highlighted with the following icon:

Family and Community, highlighted in Chapters 33 and 34, contain the theories of family function, family communication styles, nursing interview techniques for families, internal and external family structuring, and family development stages and tasks. These chapters also explore the types of communities families and individuals live in and how those communities enhance health or present a barrier to effective, healthful functioning. Chapter 10 assists students in assessing the presence of violence in families.

Features of the Sixth Edition

- **New! Routine versus Focused Assessment Charts** differentiate routine screening assessment skills, used by most nurses in any situation, from focused specialty assessment skills, used more by advanced practice nurses or nurses with expertise in highly specialized areas.

General Routine Screening or Focused Specialty Assessment

Assessing the client's visual acuity and eye is always a concern to the nurse. This information may already be documented in the client's record or obtained from the client's history. However, the nurse needs to know all parts of the eye examination to be able to fully understand the status of the client's eyes and vision. In the acute care setting the nurse typically assesses the client's gross vision, peripheral vision, external eye structures, and pupillary response. However, in school settings the school nurse may need to use the Snellen Chart to more accurately assess for visual loss in the child. In the home setting it may be necessary to do the additional visual and eye tests to determine the need for further assessment by the primary care provider and to detect early signs of more serious eye conditions (e.g., increased intracranial pressure). Assessment of the internal eye in intensive care settings is important to check for optic disc swelling due to intracranial swelling or in specialized settings to further assess for glaucoma. See the chart below for a general overview.

General Routine Screening	Focused Specialty Assessment
• Test distant visual acuity.	• Perform corneal light reflex test.
• Test near visual acuity.	• Perform cover test.
• Test visual fields for gross peripheral vision.	• Perform the cardinal fields of gazetest.
• Inspect the eyelids and eyelashes.	• Inspect the palpebral conjunctiva.
• Observe the position and alignment of the eyeball in the eye socket.	• Palpate the lacrimal apparatus.
• Inspect the bulbar conjunctiva and sclera.	• Inspect the cornea and lens.
• Inspect the lacrimal apparatus.	• Assess accommodation of pupils.
• Inspect the iris and pupil.	• Use ophthalmoscope to inspect the optic disc, retinalvessels and background, fovea and macula, and anterior chamber.
• Assess pupillary reaction to light.	

- **New! Boxes highlighting Interdisciplinary Verbal Communication of Assessment Findings Using SBAR** utilize the Situation, Background, Assessment, Recommendation framework to report accurate findings of the case

vii

Interdisciplinary Verbal Communication of Assessment Findings Using SBAR

SITUATION: Susan Jones, a 24-year-old Caucasian woman, came to the clinic holding her right eye that she accidently poked with her key. She reports constant pain as a 4 on scale of 1–10 that is relieved somewhat with keeping eye shut. Reports blurry vision with watery eye.

BACKGROUND: She reports no past problems with eyes or vision, no history of eye surgery or treatment. Her father has glaucoma. She denies exposure to harmful substances. Wears sunglasses about 80% of the time when in the sun. Takes occasional Tylenol for headache, but takes no other medications. Last eye examination was 2 years ago revealing "perfect" vision.

ASSESSMENT: Visual acuity in the left eye is 20/20. Visual acuity of the right eye is 20/30. Client is squinting and blinking repeatedly during the examination. Peripheral vision is intact. Corneal light reflex is symmetric. Extraocular movements smooth and symmetric, with no nystagmus. Eyelids without abnormal widening or ptosis. No redness, discharge, or crusting noted on lid margins. No abnormalities are noted on uninjured left eye. The injured right eye conjunctiva is pink, smooth, and moist. Sclera has dilated vessels and tearing profusely. Right palpebral conjunctiva reveals no foreign body or edema. No swelling or redness noted over the lacrimal gland bilaterally. Puncta visible, without swelling or redness bilaterally. No drainage with nasolacrimal duct palpation bilaterally. Right cornea is transparent, with an area of roughness noted; it is moist with no opacity. Irises are round, flat, and brown in color. Pupils are round, reactive to light and accommodation; 4 mm in size bilaterally. Pupils converge symmetrically. Red reflex is present bilaterally. Right eye: no internal eye structures visualized. Left eye: some internal eye vessels visualized; unable to visualize other internal eye structures.

RECOMMENDATION: Client has acute right eye pain due to the car key being stuck into right eye. She needs to be further assessed by her primary health care provider because of her risk for infection and/or corneal ulceration due to trauma from foreign object.

- **New! Unfolding Patient Stories**, written by the National League for Nursing, are an engaging way to begin meaningful conversations in the classroom. These vignettes, which appear at the end of the first chapter of each unit, feature patients from Wolters Kluwer's *vSim for Nursing | Health Assessment* (co-developed by Laerdal Medical) and DocuCare products; however, each Unfolding Patient Story in the book stands alone, not requiring purchase of these products. For your convenience, a list of these case studies, along with their location in the book, appears in the "Case Studies in This Book" section later in this front matter.

Unfolding Patient Stories: Rashid Ahmed • Part 1

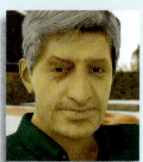

Rashid Ahmed, a 50-year-old male, is admitted to the medical unit with bacterial gastroenteritis. Upon arrival to the unit, the nurse begins the admission assessment. What interviewing techniques can be used by the nurse to establish trust and obtain accurate and thorough information for planning his care? (Rashid Ahmed's story continues in Chapter 6.)

Care for Rashid and other patients in a realistic virtual environment: *vSim for Nursing* (thepoint.lww.com/vSimHealthAssessment). Practice documenting these patients' care in DocuCare (thepoint.lww.com/DocuCareEHR).

- **New! Concept Mastery Alerts** clarify fundamental nursing concepts to improve the reader's understanding of potentially confusing topics, as identified by Misconception Alerts in Lippincott's Adaptive Learning Powered by prepU.

 Concept Mastery Alert

The first step in preparation for an interview with a client that may concern family violence is for the nurse to examine his or her own feelings and determine if there are any beliefs or biases that may interfere with the nurse's ability to "hear" what the client is saying.

- **Evidence-Based Health Promotion and Disease Prevention boxes**—which contain Healthy People 2020 goals, Risk Assessment, and Client Education sections—are an excellent resource for students to use to teach the client ways to reduce risk factors.

18-1 EVIDENCE-BASED HEALTH PROMOTION AND DISEASE PREVENTION: OROPHARYNGEAL CANCER

INTRODUCTION
The fact that the oral cavity and oropharynx, along with other parts of the head and neck, contribute to the ability to chew, swallow, breathe, and talk, oropharyngeal cancer can have significant effects on well-being. American society of Clinical Oncology (ASCO, 2015) lists the following information on oropharyngeal cancer: Two of the most common types of cancer in this anatomical region are cancer of the oral cavity (mouth and tongue) and cancer of the oropharynx (the middle of the throat, from the tonsils to the tip of the larynx); more than 90% of oral and oropharyngeal cancers are squamous cell carcinoma. This year, an estimated 45,780 adults (32,670 men and 13,110 women) in the United States will be diagnosed with oral or oropharyngeal cancer and 8,650 (6,010 men and 2,640 women) will die from the diseases. Rates of oral and oropharyngeal cancer are more than twice as high in men compared with women. If diagnosed at an early stage, the 5-year survival rate is 83%. Cancer of the oral cavity ranks as the eighth most common cancer among men and is increasing, probably because of infection with the human papillomavirus (HPV).

HEALTHY PEOPLE 2020 GOAL
Healthy People 2020 (2015a) includes oral cancers within the category of oral health. Objectives are more comprehensive than simply preventing cancers.

GOAL
Prevent and control oral and craniofacial diseases, conditions, and injuries, and improve access to preventive services and dental care.

OBJECTIVES
Objectives in this topic area address a number of areas for public health improvement for adult dental health, including the need to:
- Increase awareness of the importance of oral health to overall health and well-being.
- Increase accessibility and adoption of effective preventive interventions.
- Increase accessibility and use of oral health care resources.
- Reduce disparities in access to effective preventive and dental treatment services.
- Specific to oral cancers: Increase the proportion of oral and pharyngeal cancers detected at the earliest stage by 10%.

SCREENING
The effectiveness of screening for oropharyngeal cancer is debated. The U.S. Preventive Services Task Force (USPSTF, 2015) concluded that the evidence is insufficient to recommend for or against routinely screening adults for oral cancer. However, due to the significant gains in survival when these cancers are diagnosed at an early stage, the ACS (2015a) and the National Cancer Institute (2016) recommend routine dental screenings, also including a mouth and throat screening. The National Cancer Institute (NCI, 2016) noted that the correlation between screening and mortality has not been established. Regular screening, especially at routine dental examinations, is beneficial, especially for those who are at higher risk, such as those who use tobacco, drink alcohol frequently, have had previous oral cancers, or have had heavy sun exposure. Many organizations agree with routine screening, especially in light of HPV as a cause, which makes individuals at risk somewhat hard to identify. Although dentists are often the first line of assessment, many people do not see dentists; thus, nurses can provide this assessment.

RISK ASSESSMENT
Risk factors for oropharyngeal cancer as listed by the ACS (2015b) are:
- Using tobacco products (including cigarettes, cigars, pipes, and smokeless and chewing tobacco, with pipe smoking being a significant risk factor)
- Heavy alcohol use
- Drinking alcohol and smoking together
- Being infected with a certain types of human papillomavirus (HPV)
- Being exposed to sunlight (lip cancer only)
- Being male (twice as common in men versus women)
- Age over 55
- Fair skin
- Poor oral hygiene
- Poor diet/nutrition: low in fruits and vegetables
- Chewing betel quid (betel nuts and lime wrapped in betel leaves), or chewing *gutka* (a mixture of betel quid and tobacco), both often used in South and Southeast Asia (CDC, 2016)
- Weakened immune system
- Graft-versus-host disease
- Genetic syndromes such as Fanconi anemia, dyskeratosis congenita
- Lichen planus (skin disease with an itchy rash, which can affect mouth and throat lining and is most noted in older people)
- Two controversial potential risks are use of mouthwash with high alcohol content and irritation from dentures

CLIENT EDUCATION
Teach Clients
- Avoid smoking cigarettes or using oral tobacco, or get assistance to stop if smoking or chewing currently.
- Avoid excessive alcohol use, especially if you smoke.
- Avoid chewing betel nuts.
- Avoid infection with HPV, which can be transmitted through oral sex or contact with others who are infected, or seek medical assistance if infection suspected.
- Avoid excessive sun exposure (or tanning booth exposure) to lips. Use adequate sunscreen if unable to avoid sun.
- Eat a diet rich in fruits, vegetables, vitamin A, and generally well rounded.
- Practice regular oral hygiene, using a soft tooth brush, dental floss at least two times per day, and have routine dental care.
- If you have a weakened immune system, take extra precautions to avoid risks for oral cancer.
- Avoid use of mouthwash with high alcohol content
- If wearing dentures, have them checked for good fit with no irritation to gums.

Preface   ix

- **Case Studies**, threaded throughout each chapter, teach students how to apply to a particular client the **COLDSPA** mnemonic, with interview questions, physical assessment, and analysis of data. For your convenience, a list of these case studies, along with their location in the book, appears in the "Case Studies in This Book" section later in this front matter.

CASE STUDY

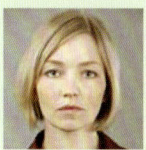 Ms. D is a 32-year-old woman who presents to the outpatient clinic with her husband and two children. She states, "My chest hurts and I cannot breathe easily." She also reports that she is "having difficulty talking." When asked about her injuries, she has poor eye contact and looks away or toward her husband. Her husband interrupts his wife frequently, preventing Ms. D from answering interview questions. The client's two children, a boy and a girl, cling to their mother.

- **Assessment Guides** have been updated and new ones added to help students learn about essential equipment and techniques needed for the client assessment.

ASSESSMENT GUIDE 3-1   How to Use the Stethoscope

The stethoscope is used to listen for (auscultate) body sounds that cannot ordinarily be heard without amplification (e.g., lung sounds, bruits, bowel sounds, and so forth). To use a stethoscope, follow these guidelines:
1. Place the earpieces into the outer ear canal. They should fit snugly but comfortably to promote effective sound transmission. The earpieces are connected to binaurals (metal tubing), which connect to rubber or plastic tubing. The rubber or plastic tubing should be flexible and no more than 12 in long to prevent the sound from diminishing.
2. Angle the binaurals down toward your nose. This will ensure that sounds are transmitted to your eardrums.
3. Use the diaphragm of the stethoscope to detect high-pitched sounds. The diaphragm should be at least 1.5 in wide for adults and smaller for children. Hold the diaphragm firmly against the body part being auscultated.
4. Use the bell of the stethoscope to detect low-pitched sounds. The bell should be at least 1 in wide. Hold the bell lightly against the body part being auscultated.

Some Do's and Don'ts
1. Warm the diaphragm or the bell of the stethoscope before placing it on the client's skin.
2. Explain what you are listening for and answer any questions the client has. This will help alleviate anxiety.
3. Do not apply too much pressure when using the bell—too much pressure will cause the bell to work like the diaphragm.
4. Avoid listening through clothing, which may obscure or alter sounds.

- Updated **Assessment Tools** contain questionnaires for students to use during client interviews.

ASSESSMENT TOOL 10-1   Hurt, Insult, Threaten, Scream (HITS)

Respond to the following four questions to assess frequency of abuse.
1. How often does your partner physically hurt you?
2. How often does your partner insult or talk down to you?
3. How often does your partner threaten you with physical harm?
4. How often does your partner scream or curse at you?

Copyright © 2003 by Kevin Sherin, MD, MPH.

- **Safety Tips** alert students to key information to ensure safe practice.

- **Clinical Tips** help highlight critical content necessary for a thorough assessment.
- **Older Adult Considerations** and **Cultural Considerations** call attention to vital considerations for special populations.

The Teaching-Learning Package

The sixth edition of *Health Assessment in Nursing* provides a robust teaching–learning package, including resources for both students and instructors.

Instructor Resources Available on thePoint

Tools to assist you with bringing health assessment to life are available upon adoption of this text at http://thePoint.lww.com/Weber6e. Resources include:
- Test Generator Questions
- Discussion Topics and Answers
- Image Bank
- PowerPoint Presentations with i-clicker questions and answers
- Assignments and Answers
- Guided Lecture Notes
- Case Studies and Answers
- Full Text Online
- Syllabi
- QSEN Map
- Pre-Lecture Quizzes and Answers
- Strategies for Effective Teaching
- LMS Course Cartridges

Student Resources Available on thePoint

An exciting set of free resources is available to help students review material and become even more familiar with vital concepts. Students can access all these resources at http://thePoint.lww.com/Weber6e using the codes printed in the front of their textbooks.
- Journal Articles
- NCLEX-Style Chapter Review Questions
- Concepts in Action Animations
- Heart and Breath Sounds
- Watch and Learn video clips
- Algorithms
- Spanish-English Audio Glossary
- Assessment Instruments
- Nursing Professional Roles and Responsibilities
- Learning Objectives and Self-Reflection Activity

A Fully Integrated Course Experience

We are pleased to offer an expanded suite of digital solutions and ancillaries to support instructors and students using *Health Assessment in Nursing*, Sixth Edition. To learn more about any solution, please contact your local Wolters Kluwer representative.

Lippincott CoursePoint+

Lippincott CoursePoint+ is an integrated digital learning solution designed for the way students learn. It is the only nursing education solution that integrates:

- **Leading content in context:** Content provided in the context of the student learning path engages students and encourages interaction and learning on a deeper level.
- **Powerful tools to maximize class performance:** Course-specific tools, such as adaptive learning powered by prepU, provide a personalized learning experience for every student.
- **Real-time data to measure students' progress:** Student performance data provided in an intuitive display lets you quickly spot which students are having difficulty or which concepts the class as a whole is struggling to grasp.
- **Preparation for practice:** Integrated virtual simulation and evidence-based resources improve student competence, confidence, and success in transitioning to practice.
  - *vSim for Nursing:* Co-developed by Laerdal Medical and Wolters Kluwer, *vSim for Nursing* simulates real nursing scenarios and allows students to interact with virtual patients in a safe, online environment.
  - *Lippincott Advisor for Education:* With over 8,500 entries covering the latest evidence-based content and drug information, *Lippincott Advisor for Education* provides students with the most up-to-date information possible, while giving them valuable experience with the same point-of-care content they will encounter in practice.
- **Training services and personalized support:** To ensure your success, our dedicated educational consultants and training coaches will provide expert guidance every step of the way.

Simulation and Other Resources

- **vSim for Nursing | Health Assessment, a virtual simulation platform** (available via thePoint): Co-developed by Laerdal Medical and Wolters Kluwer, *vSim for Nursing | Health Assessment* includes 10 health assessment patient scenarios. *vSim for Nursing | Health Assessment* helps students develop clinical competence and decision-making skills as they interact with virtual patients in a safe, realistic environment. *vSim for Nursing* records and assesses student decisions throughout the simulation, then provides a personalized feedback log highlighting areas needing improvement.
- **Lippincott DocuCare** (available via thePoint): Lippincott DocuCare combines web-based electronic health record simulation software with clinical case scenarios. Lippincott DocuCare's nonlinear solution works well in the classroom, simulation lab, and clinical practice.

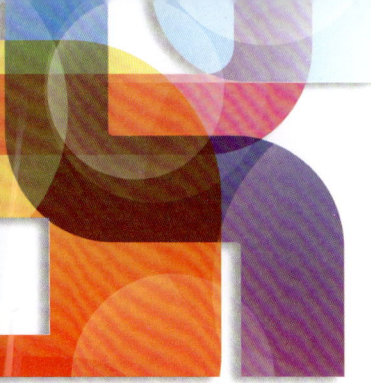

ACKNOWLEDGMENTS

With love, appreciation, and many thanks, we would like to acknowledge the following people for their help in making the sixth edition of *Health Assessment in Nursing* a reality.

JW

- To Jane, coauthor and faithful life-long friend, for your research skills and cultural expertise
- To Bill, my husband, for your love, patience, and continuous support on an ongoing project
- To Joe, my son, for reminding me to put more effort into making things clearer
- To Wes, my son, for his insights into the importance of accurate assessments
- To Eli, my first grandson, for energizing me by your simple innocence and humor
- To my mom, for your wisdom on how to keep life simple

JK

- To Janet, precious friend, loyal colleague, and primary author, for encouraging my participation and for making the challenge a delightful experience
- To Arthur, my husband, for his sense of humor, creative outlook, and encouragement over the years
- To my mother, for inspiring me with an eagerness to learn

JW and JK

- To Kelley Squazzo, Executive Editor, and Leo Gray, Editorial Assistant, for your continuing support and encouragement
- To Annette Ferran, Manager, Books Editorial Coordinator Group; Meredith Brittain, Senior Development Editor; and Marian Bellus, Production Project Manager, for all of your coordination efforts in keeping the project on plan and on track
- To our colleagues and contributors, who have shared their expertise
- To Gabrielle Hennrich-Frye, RN, who reviewed the page proofs for this edition with her keen eye, perfection, and careful reading of every word
- To our students, who gave us insights to improve this edition
- To our friends, for their hope, encouragement, and enthusiasm
- To Tom Mondeau, Mark Hill, Dr. Stanley Sides, Dr. Richard Martin, Dr. Michael Bennett, Curt Casteel, and Dr. Terri Woods, for your wonderful photography

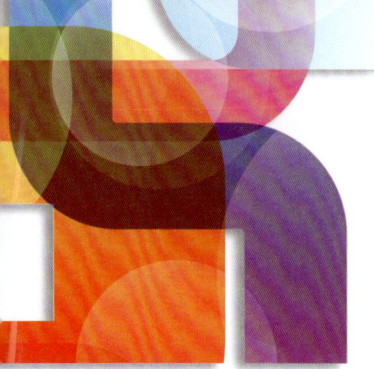

CONTENTS

UNIT 1
Nursing Data Collection, Documentation, and Analysis

1 Nurse's Role in Health Assessment: Collecting and Analyzing Data 1
- **Introduction to Health Assessment in Nursing 1**
- **The Nurse's Role in Health Assessment 2**
- **Assessment: Step 1 of the Nursing Process 3**
  - Focus of Health Assessment in Nursing 4
  - Framework for Health Assessment in Nursing 4
  - Using Evidence to Promote Health and Prevent Disease 5
  - Types of Health Assessment 5
    - Initial Comprehensive Assessment 5
    - Ongoing or Partial Assessment 6
    - Focused or Problem-Oriented Assessment 6
    - Emergency Assessment 6
  - Steps of Health Assessment 7
  - Preparing for the Assessment 7
  - Collecting Subjective Data 7
  - Collecting Objective Data 8
  - Validating Assessment Data 8
  - Documenting Data 8
- **Analysis of Assessment Data/Nursing Diagnosis: Step 2 of the Nursing Process 8**
  - Process of Data Analysis 9
- **Factors Affecting Health Assessment 10**
- **Summary 10**

2 Collecting Subjective Data: The Interview and Health History 12
- **Interviewing 12**
  - Phases of the Interview 12
    - Preintroductory Phase 13
    - Introductory Phase 13
    - Working Phase 13
    - Summary and Closing Phase 14
  - Communication During the Interview 14
    - Nonverbal Communication 14
    - Verbal Communication 16
  - Special Considerations During the Interview 16
    - Gerontologic Variations in Communication 16
    - Cultural Variations in Communication 17
    - Emotional Variations in Communication 17
- **Complete Health History 18**
  - Biographical Data 18
  - Reason(s) for Seeking Health Care 19
  - History of Present Health Concern 21
  - Personal Health History 21
  - Family Health History 23
  - Review of Systems for Current Health Problems 23
  - Lifestyle and Health Practices Profile 25
    - Description of Typical Day 25
    - Nutrition and Weight Management 25
    - Activity Level and Exercise 26
    - Sleep and Rest 26
    - Substance Use 26

  - Self-Concept and Self-Care Responsibilities 28
  - Social Activities 28
  - Relationships 28
  - Values and Belief System 28
  - Education and Work 29
  - Stress Levels and Coping Styles 29
  - Environment 29
- **Summary 30**

3 Collecting Objective Data: The Physical Examination 31
- **Equipment 31**
- **Preparing for the Examination 31**
  - Preparing the Physical Setting 33
  - Preparing Oneself 33
  - Approaching and Preparing the Client 36
  - Physical Examination Techniques 37
    - Inspection 37
    - Palpation 37
    - Percussion 40
    - Auscultation 42
- **Summary 43**

4 Validating and Documenting Data 44
- **Validating Data 44**
  - Purpose of Validation 44
  - Data Requiring Validation 44
  - Methods of Validation 44
  - Identification of Areas for Which Data Are Missing 45
- **Documenting Data 45**
  - Purpose of Documentation 45
  - Information Requiring Documentation 48
    - Subjective Data 48
    - Objective Data 50
  - Guidelines for Documentation 50
  - Assessment Forms Used for Documentation 51
    - Initial Assessment Form 51
    - Frequent or Ongoing Assessment Form 51
    - Focused or Specialty Area Assessment Form 56
- **Verbal Communication of Data 58**
- **Summary 58**

5 Thinking Critically to Analyze Data and Make Informed Nursing Judgments 60
- **Analysis of Data Throughout** *Health Assessment in Nursing* **60**
- **Analysis of Data and Critical Thinking—Step Two of the Nursing Process 61**
  - The Diagnostic Reasoning Process 61
  - Step One—Identify Strengths and Abnormal Data 61
  - Step Two—Cluster Data 62
  - Step Three—Draw Inferences 62
  - Step Four—Propose Possible Nursing Diagnoses 63
  - Step Five—Check for Defining Characteristics 64
  - Step Six—Confirm or Rule out Diagnoses 64
  - Step Seven—Document Conclusions 65
    - Actual Nursing Diagnoses 65
    - Wellness or Health Promotion Nursing Diagnoses 65

xiii

Risk Nursing Diagnoses 66
Syndrome Nursing Diagnoses 66
Collaborative Problems and Referrals 66
Developing Diagnostic Reasoning Expertise and Avoiding Pitfalls 66
Summary 66

UNIT 2
Integrative Holistic Nursing Assessment

6 Assessing Mental Status Including Risk for Substance Abuse 69
Conceptual Foundations 70
Factors Affecting Mental Health 70
Mental Disorders 70
Substance Abuse 70
Health Assessment 71
Collecting Subjective Data: The Nursing Health History 71
Collecting Objective Data: Physical Examination 82
Preparing the Client 82
Equipment 82
Validating and Documenting Findings 94
Analysis of Data: Diagnostic Reasoning 95
Selected Nursing Diagnoses 95
Health Promotion Diagnoses 95
Risk Diagnoses 95
Actual Diagnoses 95
Selected Collaborative Problems 95
Medical Problems 96

7 Assessing Psychosocial, Cognitive, and Moral Development 98
Growth and Development 98
Freud Theory of Psychosexual Development 98
Freud's Major Concepts and Terms 98
Freud's Stages of Psychosexual Development 99
Erikson Theory of Psychosocial Development 100
Erikson's Major Concepts and Terms 100
Erikson's Stages of Psychosocial Development 102
Piaget Theory of Cognitive Development 102
Piaget's Major Concepts and Terms 102
Piaget's Stages of Cognitive Development 102
Kohlberg Theory of Moral Development 102
Kohlberg's Major Concepts and Terms 104
Kohlberg's Stages of Moral Development 104
Health Assessment 104
Collecting Subjective Data: The Nursing Health History 104
Assessing Developmental Level: Psychosocial Status 109
Preparing the Client 109
Validating and Documenting Findings 117
Analysis of Data: Diagnostic Reasoning 119
Selected Nursing Diagnoses 119
Health Promotion Diagnoses 119
Risk Diagnoses 119
Actual Diagnoses 119

8 Assessing General Health Status and Vital Signs 121
Structure and Function 121
Overall Impression of the Client 121
Vital Signs 122
Temperature 122
Pulse 122
Respirations 122
Blood Pressure 122
Pain 124
Health Assessment 124
Collecting Subjective Data: The Nursing Health History 124
Collecting Objective Data: Physical Examination 126
Preparing the Client 126
Equipment 126
Physical Assessment 127
Validating and Documenting Findings 137
Analysis of Data: Diagnostic Reasoning 138
Selected Nursing Diagnoses 138
Health Promotion Diagnoses 138
Risk Diagnoses 138
Actual Diagnoses 138
Selected Collaborative Problems 138
Medical Problems 138

9 Assessing Pain: The Fifth Vital Sign 142
Conceptual Foundations 142
Pathophysiology 142
Physiologic Responses to Pain 143
Classification 144
The Seven Dimensions of Pain 147
Psychosocial Factors Affecting Pain Perception and Assessment 147
Developmental Level 148
Culture 148
Health Assessment 149
Collecting Subjective Data: The Nursing Health History 149
Preparing the Client 150
Pain Assessment Tools 150
Collecting Objective Data: Physical Examination 156
Physical Assessment 156
Validating and Documenting Findings 157
Analysis of Data: Diagnostic Reasoning 158
Selected Nursing Diagnoses 158
Health Promotion Diagnoses 158
Risk Diagnoses 158
Actual Diagnoses 158
Selected Collaborative Problems 158
Medical Problems 158

10 Assessing for Violence 161
Conceptual Foundations 161
Theories of Family Violence 161
Types of Family Violence 162
Physical Abuse 162
Psychological Abuse 162
Economic Abuse 162
Sexual Abuse 162
Categories of Family Violence 163
Intimate Partner Violence 163
Child Abuse 163
Elder Mistreatment 164
Other Types of Violence 164
School Violence (Bullying and Punking) 164
Hate Crimes in the United States 165
Human Trafficking 165
War Crimes 166
Nursing Assessment of Family Violence 167
Preparing Yourself for the Examination 168
Collecting Subjective Data 169
Interview Techniques 169
Collecting Objective Data: Physical Examination 173
Preparing the Client 173
Equipment 174
Physical Assessment 174
Validating and Documenting Findings 177
Analysis of Data: Diagnostic Reasoning 178
Selected Nursing Diagnoses 178
Health Promotion Diagnoses 178
Risk Diagnoses 178
Actual Diagnoses 178
Selected Collaborative Problems 178
Medical Problems 178

11 Assessing Culture 181
Conceptual Foundations 181
Why Nurses Need to Know about Culture 182
Concepts and Terms Related to Culture 182

Cultural Competence 182
  Contexts for Assessment 183
  Race 183
  National Standards for Care 184
Cultural Assessment 184
  Purposes and Scope of Assessment 184
  Factors Affecting Approach to Providers 186
  Communication 186
    Time 186
    Space 186
    Eye Contact and Face Positioning 187
    Body Language and Hand Gestures 187
    Silence 187
    Touch 187
  Factors Affecting Disease, Illness, Health State 187
    Health Care Beliefs 187
    Diet and Nutrition 193
    Spirituality 193
    Biologic Variations 194
    Geographical and Ethnic Disease Variation 195
Heritage Assessment Versus Cultural Assessment 197
Summary 197

12 Assessing Spirituality and Religious Practices 202
Conceptual Foundations 202
  Terms Related to Spirituality 203
  The Relationship Between Spirituality, Religion, and Health 203
    Impact of Religion and Spirituality on Health 204
    Incorporating Religion and Spirituality into Care 205
  Self-Understanding of Spirituality 208
Spiritual Assessment 208
  Approach 208
  Techniques 208
    Nonformal 208
    Formal 209
    Sample Format 209
  Validating and Documenting Findings 214
Analysis of Data: Diagnostic Reasoning 215
  Selected Nursing Diagnoses 215
    Health Promotion Diagnoses 215
    Risk Diagnoses 215
    Actual Diagnoses 215
  Selected Collaborative Problems 215
  Medical Problems 215

13 Assessing Nutritional Status 217
Foundations 217
  Nutrition 217
  Hydration 218
  Food Safety 219
Nutritional Research and Guidelines 219
  Controversies 219
    Low Carbohydrate/High Protein/Fat versus Low Fat Diets 219
    Anti-Inflammatory Diet 220
    Low Glycemic Index Diet 221
    Canada's Guideline Controversy 221
  Optimal Nutrition, Malnutrition, Overnutrition 221
    Optimal Nutrition 221
    Malnutrition 221
    Overnutrition 222
  Optimal Hydration 222
    Dehydration 222
    Overhydration 222
Health Assessment 222
  Components of a Nutritional Assessment 222
  Nutritional Screening Tools 225
  Collecting Subjective Data: The Nursing Health History 227
  Collecting Objective Data: Physical Examination 229
    Preparing the Client 229
    Equipment 230
    Physical Assessment 230
  Laboratory Tests 239
  Validating and Documenting Findings 240
Analysis of Data: Diagnostic Reasoning 240
  Selected Nursing Diagnoses 240
    Health Promotion Diagnoses 240
    Risk Diagnoses 240
    Actual Diagnoses 240
  Selected Collaborative Problems 241
  Medical Problems 242

UNIT 3
Nursing Assessment of Physical Systems

14 Assessing Skin, Hair, and Nails 247
Structure and Function 247
  Skin 247
    Epidermis 247
    Dermis 248
    Subcutaneous Tissue 249
  Hair 249
  Nails 249
Health Assessment 249
  Collecting Subjective Data: The Nursing Health History 249
  Collecting Objective Data: Physical Examination 257
    Preparing the Client 257
    Equipment 257
    Physical Assessment 257
  Validating and Documenting Findings 269
Analysis of Data: Diagnostic Reasoning 269
  Selected Nursing Diagnoses 269
    Health Promotion Diagnoses 269
    Risk Diagnoses 269
    Actual Diagnoses 270
  Selected Collaborative Problems 270
  Medical Problems 270

15 Assessing Head and Neck 280
Structure and Function 280
  The Head 280
    Cranium 280
    Face 280
  The Neck 280
    Muscles and Cervical Vertebrae 281
    Blood Vessels 282
    Thyroid Gland 282
  Lymph Nodes of the Head and Neck 282
Health Assessment 283
  Collecting Subjective Data: The Nursing Health History 283
  Collecting Objective Data: Physical Examination 288
    Preparing the Client 288
    Equipment 289
  Validating and Documenting Findings 297
Analysis of Data: Diagnostic Reasoning 297
  Selected Nursing Diagnoses 297
    Health Promotion Diagnoses 297
    Risk Diagnoses 297
    Actual Diagnoses 298
  Selected Collaborative Problems 298
  Medical Problems 298

16 Assessing Eyes 304
Structure and Function 304
  External Structures of the Eye 304
  Internal Structures of the Eye 305
  Vision 306
    Visual Fields and Visual Pathways 306
    Visual Reflexes 307
Health Assessment 307
  Collecting Subjective Data: The Nursing Health History 307

Collecting Objective Data: Physical Examination   315
   Preparing the Client   315
   Equipment   315
   Physical Assessment   315
Validating and Documenting Findings   327
Analysis of Data: Diagnostic Reasoning   328
   Selected Nursing Diagnoses   328
     Health Promotion Diagnoses   328
     Risk Diagnoses   328
     Actual Diagnoses   328
   Selected Collaborative Problems   328
   Medical Problems   329

17 Assessing Ears   338
Structure and Function   338
   Structures of the Ear   338
     External Ear   338
     Middle Ear   338
     Inner Ear   339
   Hearing   339
Health Assessment   340
   Collecting Subjective Data: The Nursing Health History   340
   Collecting Objective Data: Physical Examination   346
     Preparing the Client   346
     Equipment   346
     Physical Assessment   346
   Validating and Documenting Findings   351
Analysis of Data: Diagnostic Reasoning   353
   Selected Nursing Diagnoses   353
     Health Promotion Diagnoses   353
     Risk Diagnoses   353
     Actual Diagnoses   353
   Selected Collaborative Problems   353
   Medical Problems   353

18 Assessing Mouth, Throat, Nose, and Sinuses   357
Structure and Function   357
   Mouth   357
   Throat   358
   Nose   359
   Sinuses   359
Nursing Assessment   359
   Collecting Subjective Data: The Nursing Health History   359
   Collecting Objective Data: Physical Examination   366
     Preparing the Client   366
     Equipment   366
     Physical Assessment   366
   Validating and Documenting Findings   375
Analysis of Data: Diagnostic Reasoning   375
   Selected Nursing Diagnoses   375
     Health Promotion Diagnoses   375
     Risk Diagnoses   375
     Actual Diagnoses   376
   Selected Collaborative Problems   376
   Medical Problems   376

19 Assessing Thorax and Lungs   381
Structure and Function   381
   Thoracic Cage   381
     Sternum and Clavicles   381
     Ribs and Thoracic Vertebrae   381
     Vertical Reference Lines   382
   Thoracic Cavity   383
     Trachea and Bronchi   383
     Lungs   383
     Pleural Membranes   384
   Mechanics of Breathing   385
Health Assessment   386
   Collecting Subjective Data: The Nursing Health History   386
   Collecting Objective Data: Physical Examination   392
     Preparing the Client   392
     Equipment   392
     Physical Assessment   392
   Validating and Documenting Findings   404
Analysis of Data: Diagnostic Reasoning   405
   Selected Nursing Diagnoses   405
     Health Promotion Diagnoses   405
     Risk Diagnoses   405
     Actual Diagnoses   405
   Selected Collaborative Problems   405
   Medical Problems   405

20 Assessing Breasts and Lymphatic System   409
Structure and Function   409
   External Breast Anatomy   409
   Internal Breast Anatomy   411
   Lymph Nodes   411
Health Assessment   411
   Collecting Subjective Data: The Nursing Health History   411
   Collecting Objective Data: Physical Examination   418
     Preparing the Client   419
     Equipment   419
     Physical Assessment   419
   Validating and Documenting Findings   426
Analysis of Data: Diagnostic Reasoning   426
   Selected Nursing Diagnoses   426
     Health Promotion Diagnoses   427
     Risk Diagnoses   427
     Actual Diagnoses   427
   Selected Collaborative Problems   427
   Medical Problems   427

21 Assessing Heart and Neck Vessels   431
Structure and Function   431
   Heart and Great Vessels   431
     Heart Chambers and Valves   431
     Heart Covering and Walls   433
     Pathways   433
     Electrical Activity   433
     Diastole   434
     Systole   435
     Normal Heart Sounds   435
     Extra Heart Sounds   436
     Murmurs   436
     Stroke Volume   436
     Carotid Artery Pulse   439
     Jugular Venous Pulse and Pressure   439
Health Assessment   439
   Collecting Subjective Data: The Nursing Health History   439
   Collecting Objective Data: Physical Examination   445
     Preparing the Client   445
     Equipment   445
     Physical Assessment   445
   Validating and Documenting Findings   452
Analysis of Data: Diagnostic Reasoning   453
   Selected Nursing Diagnoses   453
     Health Promotion Diagnoses   453
     Risk Diagnoses   453
     Actual Diagnoses   453
   Selective Collaborative Problems   453
   Medical Problems   454

22 Assessing Peripheral Vascular System   463
Structure and Function   463
   Arteries   463
     Major Arteries of the Arm   464
     Major Arteries of the Leg   464
   Veins   464
   Capillaries and Fluid Exchange   466
   Lymphatic System   466
Health Assessment   468
   Collecting Subjective Data: The Nursing Health History   468

Collecting Objective Data: Physical Examination 472
  Preparing the Client 473
  Equipment 473
  Physical Assessment 473
Validating and Documenting Findings 486
Analysis of Data: Diagnostic Reasoning 487
  Selected Nursing Diagnoses 487
    Health Promotion Diagnoses 487
    Risk Diagnoses 487
    Actual Diagnoses 487
  Selected Collaborative Problems 487
  Medical Problems 487

23 Assessing Abdomen 492
Structure and Function 492
  Abdominal Quadrants 492
  Abdominal Wall Muscles 492
  Internal Anatomy 493
    Solid Viscera 494
    Hollow Viscera 495
    Vascular Structures 495
Health Assessment 495
  Collecting Subjective Data: The Nursing Health History 495
  Collecting Objective Data: Physical Examination 502
    Preparing the Client 503
    Equipment 503
    Physical Assessment 503
  Validating and Documenting Findings 520
Analysis of Data: Diagnostic Reasoning 521
  Selected Nursing Diagnoses 521
    Health Promotion Diagnoses 521
    Risk Diagnoses 521
    Actual Diagnoses 521
  Selected Collaborative Problems 522
  Medical Problems 522

24 Assessing Musculoskeletal System 528
Structure and Function 528
  Bones 528
  Skeletal Muscles 528
  Joints 530
Nursing Assessment 534
Collecting Subjective Data: The Nursing Health History 534
  Collecting Objective Data: Physical Examination 539
    Preparing the Client 539
    Equipment 540
    Physical Assessment 540
  Validating and Documenting Findings 559
Analysis of Data: Diagnostic Reasoning 560
  Selected Nursing Diagnoses 560
    Health Promotion Diagnoses 560
    Risk Diagnoses 560
    Actual Diagnoses 560
  Selected Collaborative Problems 561
  Medical Problems 561

25 Assessing Neurologic System 567
Structure and Function 567
  Central Nervous System 567
    Brain 567
    Spinal Cord 569
    Neural Pathways 569
  Peripheral Nervous System 570
    Cranial Nerves 570
    Spinal Nerves 570
    Autonomic Nervous System 572
Health Assessment 572
Collecting Subjective Data: The Nursing Health History 572
  Collecting Objective Data: Physical Examination 576
    Preparing the Client 579
    Equipment 579
    Physical Assessment 579
  Validating and Documenting Findings 597
Analysis of Data: Diagnostic Reasoning 598
  Selected Nursing Diagnoses 598
    Health Promotion Diagnoses 598
    Risk Diagnoses 598
    Actual Diagnoses 598
  Selected Collaborative Problems 599
  Medical Problems 599

26 Assessing Male Genitalia and Rectum 605
Structure and Function 605
  External Genitalia 605
    Penis 605
    Scrotum 606
  Internal Genitalia 606
  Testes 606
    Spermatic Cord 606
  Inguinal Area 606
  Anus and Rectum 607
  Prostate 608
Health Assessment 608
  Collecting Subjective Data: The Nursing Health History 608
  Collecting Objective Data: Physical Examination 616
    Preparing the Client 617
    Equipment 617
    Physical Assessment 617
  Validating and Documenting Findings 626
Analysis of Data: Diagnostic Reasoning 626
  Selected Nursing Diagnoses 626
    Health Promotion Diagnoses 627
    Risk Diagnoses 627
    Actual Diagnoses 627
  Selected Collaborative Problems 627
  Medical Problems 627

27 Assessing Female Genitalia, Anus, and Rectum 637
Structure and Function 637
  External Genitalia 637
  Internal Genitalia 638
  Anus and Rectum 639
Nursing Assessment 639
  Collecting Subjective Data: The Nursing Health History 639
  Collecting Objective Data: Physical Examination 649
    Preparing the Client 650
    Equipment 650
    Physical Assessment 651
  Validating and Documenting Findings 663
Analysis of Data: Diagnostic Reasoning 664
  Selected Nursing Diagnoses 664
    Health Promotion Diagnoses 664
    Risk Diagnoses 664
    Actual Diagnoses 664
  Selected Collaborative Problems 664
  Medical Problems 664

28 Pulling It All Together: Integrated Head-To-Toe Assessment 672
Comprehensive Health Assessment 673
  Preparing the Client 673
  Equipment 673
  Collecting Data 673
    Collecting Subjective Data: The Comprehensive Nursing Health History 673
    Collecting Objective Data: Physical Assessment 676
  Sample Documentation of a Comprehensive Adult Nursing Health History and Physical Assessment 685
  Physical Assessment 687

General Survey 687
Skin, Hair, Nails 687
Head and Neck 687
Eyes 687
Ears 687
Mouth, Throat, Nose, and Sinuses 687
Thorax and Lung 687
Breasts 687
Heart and Neck Vessels 687
Peripheral Vascular 688
Abdomen 688
Musculoskeletal 688
Neurologic 688
Genitalia 688
Anus/Rectum 688
Client's Strengths 688
Nursing Diagnoses 688
Collaborative Problems 688

UNIT 4
Nursing Assessment of Special Groups

29 Assessing Childbearing Women 691
Structure and Function 691
Skin, Hair, and Nails 692
Ears and Hearing 692
Mouth, Throat, Nose, and Sinus 692
Thorax and Lungs 692
Breasts 692
Heart 692
Peripheral Vascular System 692
Abdomen 693
Genitalia 694
Anus and Rectum 694
Musculoskeletal System 695
Neurologic System 695
Health Assessment 697
Collecting Subjective Data: The Nursing Health History 697
Biographical Data 697
Collecting Objective Data: Physical Examination 705
Preparing the Client 705
Equipment 705
Physical Assessment 705
Validating and Documenting Findings 718
Analysis of Data: Diagnostic Reasoning 718
Selected Nursing Diagnoses 718
Health Promotion Diagnoses 719
Risk Diagnoses 719
Actual Diagnoses 719
Selected Collaborative Problems 719
Medical Problems 719

30 Assessing Newborns and Infants 722
Growth and Development 722
Physical Development 722
Skin, Hair, and Nails 722
Head and Neck 723
Eyes 723
Ears 723
Mouth, Throat, Nose, and Sinus 723
Thorax and Lungs 723
Breasts 724
Heart 724
Peripheral Vascular System 724
Abdomen 724
Genitalia 724
Anus, Rectum, and Prostate 724
Musculoskeletal System 724
Neurologic System 724
Motor Development 725
Gross Motor 725
Fine Motor 725
Sensory Perception Development 725
Visual 725
Auditory 726
Olfactory 726
Tactile 726
Cognitive and Language Development (Piaget) 726
Moral Development (Kohlberg) 726
Psychosocial Development (Erikson) 726
Psychosexual Development (Freud)) 727
Normal Infant Nutritional Requirements 727
Normal Infant Sleep Requirements and Patterns 727
Health Assessment 727
Collecting Subjective Data: The Nursing Health History for the Infant 727
Interviewing Parents 727
Collecting Objective Data: Physical Examination 732
Preparing the Infant and Caregiver 732
Equipment 733
Physical Assessment 733
Validating and Documenting Findings 758
Analysis of Data: Diagnostic Reasoning 759
Selected Nursing Diagnoses 759
Health Promotion Diagnoses 759
Risk Diagnoses 759
Actual Diagnoses 759
Selected Collaborative Problems 759
Medical Problems 759

31 Assessing Children and Adolescents 761
Growth and Development 761
Physical Development 761
Skin, Hair, and Nails 761
Head and Neck 761
Eyes 761
Ears 761
Mouth, Nose, Throat, and Sinuses 761
Thorax and Lungs 762
Breasts 762
Heart 762
Abdomen 763
Genitalia 763
Anus and Rectum 764
Musculoskeletal System 764
Neurologic System 765
Growth Patterns 765
Motor Development 765
Toddlers 765
Sensory Perception 767
Toddlers 767
Preschoolers 767
School-Age Children 767
Adolescents 767
Cognitive and Language Development 767
Toddlers 767
Preschoolers 767
School-Age Children 767
Adolescents 768
Moral Development (Kohlberg) 768
Toddler 768
Preschooler 768
School-Age Child 768
Adolescent 768
Psychosocial Development (Erikson) 769
Toddler 769
Preschooler 769
School-Age Child 769
Adolescent 769
Psychosexual Development (Freud) 769
Toddler 770
Preschooler 770
School-Age Child 770
Adolescent 770
Normal Nutritional Requirements 771
Toddlers 771

  Preschoolers 771
  School-Age Children 771
  Adolescents 771
  Nursing History Questions Related to Nutrition 772
 Normal Activity and Exercise 772
 Normal Sleep Requirements and Patterns 772
  Toddlers 772
  Preschoolers 772
  School-Age Children 774
  Adolescents 774
 Socioeconomic Situation 774
 Relationship and Role Development 774
 Self-Esteem and Self-Concept Development 774
 Coping and Stress Management 775
Health Assessment 776
 Collecting Subjective Data: The Nursing Health History 776
 Interviewing 777
  Interviewing Parents 777
  Interviewing Children and Adolescents 777
 Collecting Objective Data: Physical Examination 789
  Preparing the Client 789
  Equipment 789
  Physical Assessment 789
 Validating and Documenting Findings 809
Analysis of Data: Diagnostic Reasoning 811
 Selected Nursing Diagnoses 811
  Health Promotion Diagnoses 811
  Risk Diagnoses 811
  Actual Diagnoses 811
 Selected Collaborative Problems 811
 Medical Problems 811

32   Assessing Older Adults   813
Challenges to Health Assessment of the Older Adult 813
 Loss of Physiologic Reserve 813
  Atypical Presentation of Illness 815
 Collecting Subjective Data: The Nursing Health History 816
  Adapting Interview Techniques 816
  Determining Functional Status 816
  Biographical Data 816
  Assessing Sexuality in Older Adults 817
 Collecting Objective Data: Physical Examination 830
  Preparing the Client 830
  Equipment 830
  Physical Assessment 831
 Validating and Documenting Findings 848
Analysis of Data: Diagnostic Reasoning 848
 Selected Nursing Diagnoses 848
  Health Promotion Diagnosis 848
  Risk Diagnoses 848
  Actual Diagnoses 849
 Selected Collaborative Problems 849
 Medical Problems 849

33   Assessing Families   853
Conceptual Background 853
 Terms Related to Family Assessment 853
 The Relationship Between Families and Illness 854
 Framework of Family Assessment 855
  Family Structure 855
  Family Development 857
  Family Function 857
 Theoretical Concepts of Family Function 857
  Systems Theory 857
  Bowen's Family System Theory 857
  Communication Theory 860
Family Assessment 860
 Technique 860
  Manners 860
  Therapeutic Conversation 861
  Family Genograms and Ecomaps 861
  Commendations 861
 Assessment Procedure 861
 Validating and Documenting Findings 866
Analysis of Data: Diagnostic Reasoning 866
 Selected Nursing Diagnoses 867
  Health Promotion Diagnoses 867
  Risk Diagnoses 867
  Actual Diagnoses 867
 Selected Collaborative Problems 867
 Medical Problems 867

34   Assessing Communities   869
Conceptual Foundations 869
 Definition of Community 869
 Models of Community Assessment 870
Community Assessment 871
 Validating and Documenting Findings 882
Analysis of Data: Diagnostic Reasoning 883
 Selected Nursing Diagnoses 883
  Health Promotion Diagnoses 883
  Risk Diagnoses 883
  Actual Diagnoses 883
 Selected Collaborative Problems 883
 Medical Problems 883

APPENDICES

A   Nursing History Guide   887

B   Physical Assessment Guide   889

C   NANDA Approved Nursing Diagnoses 2015–2017   894

D   Manual of Collaborative Problems   897

Glossary   899

Index   905

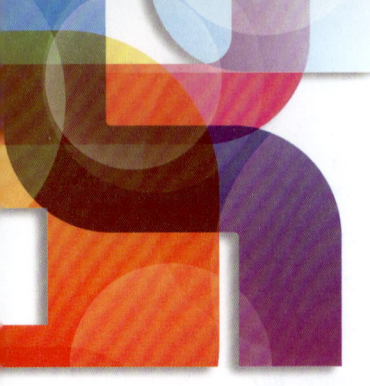

CASE STUDIES IN THIS BOOK

Cases That Unfold Across Units

UNIT 1
Nursing Data Collection, Documentation, and Analysis

Unfolding Patient Stories:
Rashid Ahmed, Part 1   11

Unfolding Patient Stories:
Marvin Hayes, Part 1   11

UNIT 2
Integrative Holistic Nursing Assessment

Unfolding Patient Stories:
Edith Jacobsen, Part 1   96

Unfolding Patient Stories:
Rashid Ahmed, Part 2   96

UNIT 3
Nursing Assessment of Physical Systems

Unfolding Patient Stories:
Kim Johnson, Part 1   278

Unfolding Patient Stories:
Marvin Hayes, Part 2   278

UNIT 4
Nursing Assessment of Special Groups

Unfolding Patient Stories:
Edith Jacobsen, Part 2   720

Unfolding Patient Stories:
Kim Johnson, Part 2   720

Cases That Unfold Within Chapters

CHAPTER 1 Nurse's Role in Health Assessment: Collecting and Analyzing Data
Mrs. Gutierrez, age 52   1, 8, 10

CHAPTER 2 Collecting Subjective Data: The Interview and Health History
Mrs. Gutierrez, age 52   12, 13, 14, 19, 21, 22, 23, 25, 29

CHAPTER 3 Collecting Objective Data: The Physical Examination
Mrs. Gutierrez, age 52   31, 33, 36, 37

CHAPTER 4 Validating and Documenting Data
Mrs. Gutierrez, age 52   44, 45, 47, 48–50, 56–57

CHAPTER 5 Thinking Critically to Analyze Data and Make Informed Nursing Judgments
Mrs. Gutierrez, age 52   60, 61–62, 63, 64, 65, 66

CHAPTER 6 Assessing Mental Status Including Risk for Substance Abuse
Mrs. Jane Wilson, age 61   70, 81–82, 94–95, 96

CHAPTER 7 Assessing Psychosocial, Cognitive, and Moral Development
Mrs. Como-Williams, age 51   98, 108–109, 117–118, 119

CHAPTER 8 Assessing General Health Status and Vital Signs
Mr. Thomas Anthony, age 34   121, 126, 137–138

CHAPTER 9 Assessing Pain: The Fifth Vital Sign
Mr. Leonard Blair, age 55   142, 155–156, 157–159

CHAPTER 10 Assessing for Violence
Ms. D, age 32   161, 172–173, 176–178, 179

Case Studies in This Book

CHAPTER 11 Assessing Culture
Mrs. Samar Al Sayah, age 56 181, 185, 186, 187, 193

CHAPTER 12 Assessing Spirituality and Religious Practices
Mrs. Lindsay Baird, age 40 202, 214–215

CHAPTER 13 Assessing Nutritional Status
Ms. Helen Jones, age 78 217, 229, 240, 242

CHAPTER 14 Assessing Skin, Hair, and Nails
Mrs. Mary Michaelson, age 29 247, 256, 268–269, 270

CHAPTER 15 Assessing Head and Neck
Mrs. Margy Kase, age 22 280, 286, 297, 298

CHAPTER 16 Assessing Eyes
Mrs. Susan Jones, age 24 304, 311, 327–328, 329

CHAPTER 17 Assessing Ears
Mrs. Andrea Lopez, age 47 338, 345, 351, 352, 353

CHAPTER 18 Assessing Mouth, Throat, Nose, and Sinuses
Mr. Jonathan Miller, age 22 357, 365, 374, 375, 376

CHAPTER 19 Assessing Thorax and Lungs
Mr. George Burney, age 67 381, 391–392, 403–405, 406

CHAPTER 20 Assessing Breasts and Lymphatic System
Mrs. Nicole Barnes, age 31 409, 418, 426, 427

CHAPTER 21 Assessing Heart and Neck Vessels
Mr. Malcolm Winchester, age 45 431, 444, 452–453, 454

CHAPTER 22 Assessing Peripheral Vascular System
Mr. Henry Lee, age 46 463, 472, 486–487

CHAPTER 23 Assessing Abdomen
Mrs. Nikki Chen, age 32 492, 502, 520–521, 522

CHAPTER 24 Assessing Musculoskeletal System
Mrs. Frances Funstead, age 55 528, 538–539, 559, 560, 561

CHAPTER 25 Assessing Neurologic System
Mrs. Linda Hutchison, age 49 567, 576, 596, 597–598, 599

CHAPTER 26 Assessing Male Genitalia and Rectum
Mr. Carl Weeks, age 52 605, 616, 626, 627

CHAPTER 27 Assessing Female Genitalia, Anus, and Rectum
Mrs. Melinda Carlisle, age 22 637, 649, 663–664, 665

CHAPTER 28 Pulling It All Together: Integrated Head-To-Toe Assessment
Mrs. Susan Lewis, age 65 672, 685–687

CHAPTER 29 Assessing Childbearing Women
Mrs. Mary Farrow, age 29 691, 704–705, 718, 719

CHAPTER 30 Assessing Newborns and Infants
Kaitlin, age 4 722, 732, 758–759, 760

CHAPTER 31 Assessing Children and Adolescents
Carsen, age 13 761, 787–788, 810, 811

CHAPTER 32 Assessing Older Adults
Mrs. Doris Miller, age 82 813, 829–830, 848, 849–850

CHAPTER 33 Assessing Families
Ross family 853, 865, 866, 867

CHAPTER 34 Assessing Communities
Maple Grove 869, 881–884

UNIT 1

Nursing Data Collection, Documentation, and Analysis

1 NURSE'S ROLE IN HEALTH ASSESSMENT: COLLECTING AND ANALYZING DATA

Learning Objectives

1. Discuss how nursing assessment skills are needed for every situation the nurse encounters.
2. Differentiate between a holistic nursing assessment and a physical medical assessment.
3. Describe which phases of the nursing process involve assessment by the nurse.
4. List and describe the steps of the nursing process, explaining how some steps overlap and may have to be repeated many times when caring for a client.
5. Describe the steps of the "analysis phase" of the nursing process.
6. Compare and contrast the four basic types of nursing assessment: (a) initial comprehensive, (b) ongoing or partial, (c) focused/problem oriented, (d) emergency.
7. Explain how the nurse's role in assessment has changed over the past century.
8. Describe what the nurse's role in assessment may be 25 years from now.

CASE STUDY

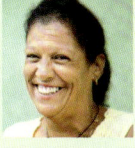

Mrs. Gutierrez, age 52, arrives at the clinic for diabetic teaching. She appears distracted and sad, uninterested in the teaching. She is unable to focus, and paces back and forth in the clinic, wringing her hands. The nurse suspects that Mrs. Gutierrez is upset by her diagnosis of diabetes.

As a professional nurse, you will constantly observe situations and collect information to make nursing judgments. This occurs no matter what the setting: hospital, clinic, home, community, or long-term care. You conduct many informal assessments every day. For example, when you get up in the morning, you check the weather and determine what would be the most appropriate clothing to wear. You assess whether you are hungry. Do you need a light or heavy breakfast? When will you be able to eat next? You may even assess the physical condition of your skin. Do you need moisturizing lotion? What are your family members doing today? Are there special events occurring in your community? You will use this information to assess yourself and determine actions that will influence your comfort and success for the remainder of the day. Likewise, the professional nursing assessments you make on a client, family, or community determine nursing interventions that directly or indirectly influence their health status.

INTRODUCTION TO HEALTH ASSESSMENT IN NURSING

The American Nurses Association publication, *Nursing: Scope and Standards of Nursing Practice* (American Nurses Association

1

[ANA], 2010), defines nursing as "the protection, promotion, and optimization of health and abilities, prevention of illness and injury, alleviation of suffering through the diagnosis and treatment of human responses and advocacy in the care of individuals, families, communities, and populations." Emphasis is placed on "diagnosis and treatment of human responses" based on "accurate client assessments," including how effective nursing interventions are "to promote health and prevent illness and injury." *Nursing: Scope and Standards of Practice* states as Standard 1 that "The registered nurse collects comprehensive data pertinent to the patient's health or situation" (ANA, p. 21). To accomplish this pertinent and comprehensive data collection, the nurse:

- Collects data in a systematic and ongoing process
- Involves the patient, family, other health care providers, and environment, as appropriate, in holistic data collection
- Prioritizes data collection activities based on the patient's immediate condition, or anticipated needs of the patient or situation
- Uses appropriate evidence-based assessment techniques and instruments in collecting pertinent data
- Uses analytical models and problem-solving tools
- Synthesizes available data, information, and knowledge relevant to the situation to identify patterns and variances
- Documents relevant data in a retrievable format (ANA, 2010, p. 21)

Standard 2 states, "The registered nurse analyzes the assessment data to determine the diagnoses or issues. To accomplish this, the registered nurse:

- Derives the diagnosis or issues based on assessment data
- Validates the diagnoses or issues with the client, family, and other health care providers when possible and appropriate
- Documents diagnoses or issues in a manner that facilitates the determination of the expected outcomes and plan (ANA, 2010, p. 22)

THE NURSE'S ROLE IN HEALTH ASSESSMENT

The nurse's role in health assessment has changed significantly over the years (see Box 1-1). In the 21st century, the nurse's role in assessment continues to expand, becoming more crucial than ever. The role of the nurse in assessment and diagnosis is more prevalent today than ever before in the history of nursing. Nurses from numerous countries are expanding their assessment and nursing diagnosis skills (Birks et al., 2013; Institute for Healthcare Improvement, 2015; Partners

---

BOX 1-1 EVOLUTION OF THE NURSE'S ROLE IN HEALTH ASSESSMENT

Physical assessment has been an integral part of nursing since the days of Florence Nightingale.

LATE 1800s–EARLY 1900s

- Nurses relied on their natural senses; the client's face and body would be observed for "changes in color, temperature, muscle strength, use of limbs, body output, and degrees of nutrition, and hydration" (Nightingale, 1992).
- Palpation was used to measure pulse rate and quality and to locate the fundus of the puerperal woman (Fitzsimmons & Gallagher, 1978).
- Examples of independent nursing practice using inspection, palpation, and auscultation have been recorded in nursing journals since 1901. Some examples reported in the *American Journal of Nursing* (1901–1938) include gastrointestinal palpation, testing eighth cranial nerve function, and examination of children in school systems.

1930–1949

- The *American Journal of Public Health* documents routine client and home inspection by public health nurses in the 1930s.
- This role of case finding, prevention of communicable diseases, and routine use of assessment skills in poor inner city areas were performed through the Frontier Nursing Service and the Red Cross (Fitzsimmons & Gallagher, 1978).

1950–1969

Nurses were hired to conduct pre-employment health stories and physical examinations for major companies, such as New York Telephone, from 1953 through 1960 (Bews & Baillie, 1969; Cipolla & Collings, 1971).

1970–1989

- The early 1970s prompted nurses to develop an active role in the provision of primary health services and expanded the professional nurse role in conducting health histories and physical and psychological assessments (Holzemer, Barkauskas, & Ohlson, 1980; Lysaught, 1970).
- Joint statements of the American Nurses Association and the American Academy of Pediatrics agreed that in-depth client assessments and on-the-spot diagnostic judgments would enhance the productivity of nurses and the health care of clients (Bullough, 1976; Fagin & Goodwin, 1972).
- Acute care nurses in the 1980s employed the "primary care" method of delivery of care. Each nurse was autonomous in making comprehensive initial assessments from which individualized plans of care were established.

1990–PRESENT

- Over the last 20 years, the movement of health care from the acute care setting to the community and the proliferation of baccalaureate and graduate education solidified the nurses' role in holistic assessment.
- Downsizing, budget cuts, and restructuring were the priorities of the 1990s. In turn, there was a demand for documentation of client assessments by all health care providers to justify health care services.
- In the 1990s, critical pathways or care maps guided the client's progression, with each stage based on specific protocols that the nurse was responsible for assessing and validating.
- Advanced practice nurses have been increasingly used in the hospital as clinical nurse specialists and in the community as nurse practitioners.
- While state legislators and the American Medical Association struggled with issues of reimbursement and prescriptive services by nurses, government and societal recognition of the need for greater cost accountability in the health care industry launched the advent of diagnosis-related groups (DRGs) and promotion of health care coverage plans such as health maintenance organizations (HMOs) and preferred provider organizations (PPOs).

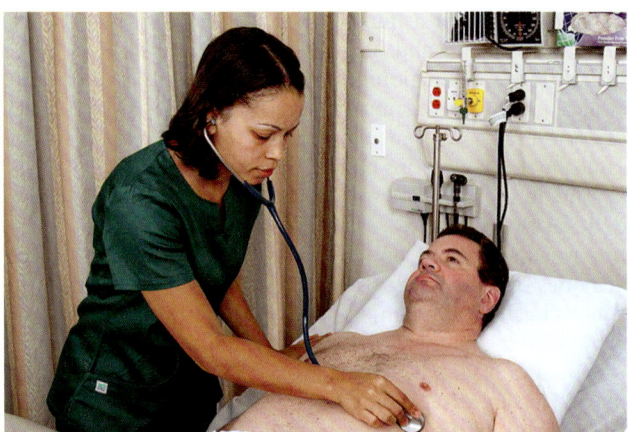

FIGURE 1-1 The acute care nurse performs a focused assessment, then incorporates assessment findings with a multidisciplinary team to develop a comprehensive plan of care.

in Health, 2015; Slåtten, Hatlevik, & Fagerström, 2014). The rapidly evolving roles of nursing (e.g., forensic nursing, nursing informatics) require extensive focused assessments and the development of related nursing diagnoses. Current focus on managed care and internal case management has had a dramatic impact on the assessment role of the nurse. The acute care nurse performs a focused assessment, and then incorporates assessment findings with a multidisciplinary team to develop a comprehensive plan of care (Fig. 1-1). Critical care outreach nurses need enhanced assessment skills to safely assess critically ill clients who are outside the structured intensive care environment (Leach & Mayo, 2013). Ambulatory care nurses assess and screen clients to determine the need for physician referrals. Home health nurses make independent nursing diagnoses and referrals for collaborative problems as needed. Public health nurses assess the needs of communities, school nurses monitor the growth and health of children, and hospice nurses assess the needs of the terminally ill clients and their families. In all settings, the nurse increasingly documents and retrieves assessment data through sophisticated computerized information systems (Cowen & Moorhead, 2014). Nursing health assessment courses with informatics content are becoming the norm in baccalaureate programs.

In a report entitled "The Future of Nursing: Leading Change, Advancing Health," the Institute of Medicine (2010) has proposed an expansion of the roles and responsibilities of nurses in a way that will "bring nurses into the health care system as empowered, full partners with other health professionals, including physicians" (Eastman, 2010). As the scope and environment for nursing assessment diversify, nurses must be prepared to assess populations of clients not only across the continuum of health but also by way of telecommunication systems with online data retrieval and documentation capabilities.

Picture the nurse assessing a client who has "poor circulation." While in the client's home, the nurse can refresh his or her knowledge of the differences between arterial and venous occlusions, using a "point-of-need" learning file accessed over the Internet. Also immediately available are the agency's policies, procedures, and care maps. Digital pictures of the client's legs can be forwarded to the off-site nurse practitioner or physician for analysis. These networks have already been prototyped and will allow nurses to transmit and receive information by video cameras attached to portable computers or television sets in the client's home. The nurse can then discuss and demonstrate assessments with other health care professionals as clearly and quickly as if they were in the same room. Assessment data and findings can be documented over the Internet or in computerized medical records, some small enough to fit into a laboratory coat pocket and many activated by the nurse's voice.

The future will see increased specialization and diversity of assessment skills for nurses. While client acuity increases and technology advances, bedside nurses are challenged to make in-depth physiologic and psychosocial assessments while correlating clinical data from multiple technical monitoring devices. Bedside computers increasingly access individual client data as well as informational libraries and clinical resources (Dykes & Collins, 2013). The communication of health assessment and clinical data will span a myriad of electronic interactivities and research possibilities. Health care networks already comprise a large hospital or medical center with referrals from smaller community hospitals; subacute, rehabilitation, and extended care units; health maintenance organizations (HMOs); and home health services. These structures provide diverse settings and levels of care in which nurses will assess clients and facilitate their progress. New delivery systems such as "integrated clinical practice" for surgical care may require the nurse to assess and follow a client from the preoperative visit to a multidisciplinary outpatient clinic and even into the home by way of remote technology.

There is tremendous growth of the nursing role in the managed care environment. The most marketable nurses will continue to be those with strong assessment and client teaching abilities as well as those who are technologically savvy. The following factors will continue to promote opportunities for nurses with advanced assessment skills:

- Rising educational costs and increased focus on primary care that affect the numbers and availability of medical students
- Increasing complexity of acute care
- Growing aging population with complex comorbidities
- Expanding health care needs of single parents
- Increasing impact of children and the homeless on communities
- Intensifying mental health issues
- Expanding health service networks
- Increasing reimbursement for health promotion and preventive care services
- Limited number of medical students pursuing practice in primary care settings
- Aging of the baby boomer generation

ASSESSMENT: STEP 1 OF THE NURSING PROCESS

Assessment is the first and most critical phase of the nursing process. If data collection is inadequate or inaccurate, incorrect nursing judgments may be made that adversely affect the remaining phases of the process: diagnosis, planning, implementation, and evaluation (Table 1-1). Although the assessment phase of the nursing process precedes the other phases in the formal nursing process, be aware that assessment is ongoing and continuous throughout all phases of the nursing process. Health assessment is more than just gathering information about the health status of the client. It is analyzing and

TABLE 1-1	Phases of the Nursing Process	
Phase	Title	Description
I	Assessment	Collecting subjective and objective data
II	Diagnosis	Analyzing subjective and objective data to make a professional nursing judgment (nursing diagnosis, collaborative problem, or referral)
III	Planning	Determining outcome criteria and developing a plan
IV	Implementation	Carrying out the plan
V	Evaluation	Assessing whether outcome criteria have been met and revising the plan as necessary

synthesizing that data, making judgments about the effectiveness of nursing interventions, and evaluating client care outcomes (AACN, 2008). The nursing process should be thought of as circular, not linear (Fig. 1-2).

Focus of Health Assessment in Nursing

Virtually every health care professional performs assessments to make professional judgments related to clients. A comprehensive health assessment consists of both a health history and physical examination. However, the purpose of a nursing health history and physical examination differs greatly from that of a medical or other type of health care assessment (e.g., dietary assessment or examination for physical therapy).

The purpose of a nursing health assessment is to collect holistic subjective and objective data to determine a client's overall level of functioning in order to make a professional clinical judgment. The nurse collects physiologic, psychological, sociocultural, developmental, and spiritual data *about* the client. Thus the nurse performs holistic data collection.

The mind, body, and spirit are considered to be interdependent factors that affect a person's level of health. The nurse, in particular, focuses on how the client's health status affects activities of daily living (ADL) and how those ADL affect the client's health. For example, a client with asthma may have to avoid extreme temperatures and may not be able to enjoy recreational camping. Walking to work in a smoggy environment may adversely affect this person's asthma.

In addition, the nurse assesses how clients interact within their family and community, and how the clients' health status affects the family and community. For example, a diabetic client may not be able to eat the same foods that the rest of the family enjoys. If this client develops complications of diabetes and has an amputation, the client may not be able to carry out the family responsibility of maintaining the yard. The client may no longer be able to work in the community as a bus driver. The nurse also assesses how family and community affect the individual client's health status. A supportive, creative family may find alternative ways of cooking tasteful foods that are healthy for the entire family. The community may or may not have a diabetic support group for the client and the family.

In contrast, the physician performing a medical assessment focuses primarily on the client's physiologic status. Less focus may be placed on psychological, sociocultural, or spiritual well-being. Similarly, a physical therapist would focus primarily on the client's musculoskeletal system and the effects on ability to perform ADL.

Framework for Health Assessment in Nursing

The framework used to collect nursing health assessment data differs from that used by other professionals. A nursing framework helps to organize information and promotes the collection of holistic data. This, in turn, provides clues that help to determine human responses.

Because there are so many nursing health assessment frameworks available for organizing data, using one assessment framework would limit the use of this text and ignore many other valid nursing assessment framework methods. Therefore, the objective of this textbook is to provide the reader with the essential information necessary to perform a comprehensive nursing health assessment. Readers can take the information in this book and adapt it to the nursing assessment framework of their choice. The book is organized around a head-to-toe assessment of body parts and systems. In each chapter, the nursing health history is organized according to a "generic" nursing history framework, which is an abbreviated version of the complete nursing health history detailed in Chapter 21. The questions asked in each physical system's chapter focus on that particular body system and are broken down into four sections:

- History of present health concern
- Personal health history
- Family history
- Lifestyle and health practices

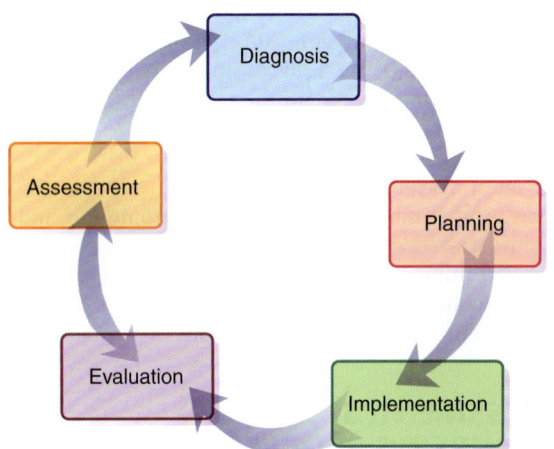

FIGURE 1-2 Each step of the nursing process depends on the accuracy of the preceding step. The steps overlap because you may have to move more quickly for some problems than others. While *Evaluation* involves examining all the previous steps, it especially focuses on achieving desired outcomes. The arrow between *Assessment* and *Evaluation* goes in both directions because assessment and evaluation are ongoing processes as well as separate phases. When the outcomes are not as anticipated, the nurse needs to revisit (reassess) all the steps, collect new data, and formulate adjustments to the plan of care. (Based on information from Alfaro, R. (2014). *Applying nursing process: A tool for critical thinking* (8th ed.). Philadelphia: Lippincott Williams & Wilkins.)

Following the health history and health promotion sections (see the Using Evidence to Promote Health and Prevent Disease section), the physical assessment section provides the procedure, normal findings, and abnormal findings for each step of examining a particular body part or system. The collected data based on the client's answers to the questions asked in the nursing history, along with the objective data gathered during the physical assessment, enable the nurse to make informed judgments about the client, including nursing diagnoses, collaborative problems, referrals, and the need for client teaching. Thus the end result of a nursing assessment is the formulation of nursing diagnoses (health promotion, risk, or actual) that require nursing care, the identification of collaborative problems that require interdisciplinary care, the identification of medical problems that require immediate referral, or client teaching for health promotion.

Using Evidence to Promote Health and Prevent Disease

In order to participate in health promotion and disease prevention, the nurse needs knowledge of physiology as well as factors affecting a client's risk of developing a disease and factors affecting client behavior.

There are many models used to analyze health promotion and disease prevention. Two of the major models are the Health Belief Model (Rosenstock, 1966; revised by Becker & Rosenstock, 1987) and the Health Promotion Model (Pender, 1982; revised, Pender, 1996). The Health Belief Model is based on three concepts: the existence of sufficient motivation; the belief that one is susceptible or vulnerable to a serious problem; and the belief that change following a health recommendation would be beneficial to the individual at a level of acceptable cost (Sturt, n.d., p. 9).

In Pender's Health Promotion Model, there are three focuses of the model: individual characteristics and experiences, behavior-specific cognitions and affect, and behavioral outcomes (Health Promotion Model, 2012). The model proposes that each person has unique characteristics and experiences that affect subsequent actions. Furthermore,
- The set of variables for behavioral-specific knowledge and affect have important motivational significance.
- These variables can be modified through nursing actions.
- Health promoting behavior is the desired behavioral outcome and is the end point in the Health Promotion Model.
- Health promoting behaviors should result in improved health, enhanced functional ability and better quality of life at all stages of development.
- The final behavioral demand is also influenced by the immediate competing demand and preferences, which can derail intended health promoting actions.

Assumptions of the model are:
- Individuals seek to actively regulate their own behavior.
- Individuals in all their biopsychosocial complexity interact with the environment, progressively transforming the environment and being transformed over time.
- Health professionals constitute a part of the interpersonal environment, which exerts influence on persons throughout their life span.
- Self-initiated reconfiguration of person–environment interaction patterns is essential to behavior change.

All of the factors, accompanied by immediate competing demands and preferences, bring about the health promoting behavior (Current Nursing, 2012).

Healthy People 2020 is a model developed by the U.S. Department of Health and Human Services (DHHS) aiming to increase the life span and improve the quality of health for all Americans. The progress toward this goal is evaluated every 10 years, resulting in the development of new goals. Specific outcomes are developed for 10 leading "indicators." Many tools are available for nurses to use to screen clients for health risks through the National Center for Chronic Disease Prevention and Health Promotion. Screening tools for risks are also available through organizations such as the American Cancer Society (ACS), American Heart Association (AHA), American Diabetic Association (ADA), Centers for Disease Control and Prevention (CDC), and the American Academy of Ophthalmology (AAO), among others. These are referred to in related chapters.

Another resource for the nurse to consider is the U.S. Preventive Services Task Force (USPSTF), which determines risk versus benefit in screenings. According to its website, the USPSTF "is an independent panel of non-Federal experts in prevention and evidence-based medicine and is composed of primary care providers (such as internists, pediatricians, family physicians, gynecologists/obstetricians, nurses, and health behavior specialists)," that "conducts scientific evidence reviews of a broad range of clinical preventive health care services (such as screening, counseling, and preventive medications) and develops recommendations for primary care clinicians and health systems." These recommendations are published in the form of "Recommendation Statements."

Types of Health Assessment

The four basic types of assessment are:
- Initial comprehensive assessment
- Ongoing or partial assessment
- Focused or problem-oriented assessment
- Emergency assessment

Each assessment type varies according to the amount and type of data collected.

Initial Comprehensive Assessment

An initial comprehensive assessment involves collection of subjective data about the client's perception of his or her health of all body parts or systems, past health history, family history, and lifestyle and health practices (which include information related to the client's overall functioning) as well as objective data gathered during a step-by-step physical examination.

The nurse typically collects subjective data and objective data in many settings (hospital, community, clinic, or home). Depending on the setting, other members of the health care team may also participate in various parts of the data collection. For example, in a hospital setting the physician usually performs a total physical examination when the client is admitted (if this was not previously done in the physician's office). In this setting, the nurse continues to assess the client as needed to monitor progress and client outcomes. A physical therapist may perform a musculoskeletal examination, as in the case of a stroke patient, and a dietitian may take anthropometric measurements in addition to doing a subjective nutritional assessment. In a community clinic, a nurse practitioner

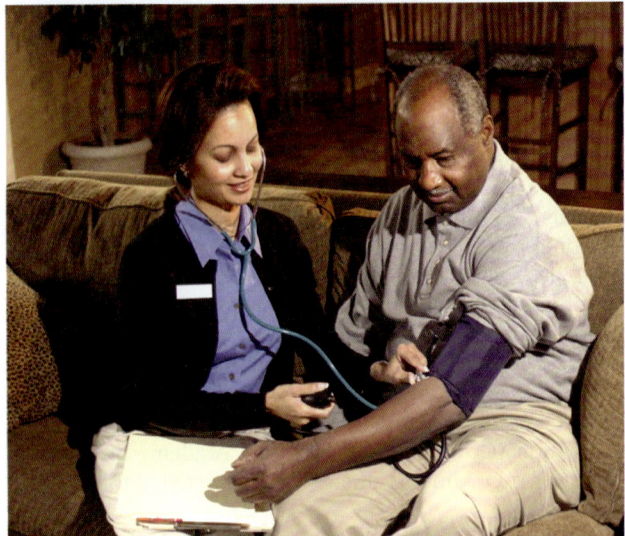

FIGURE 1-3 Assessment is an important part of any home health visit.

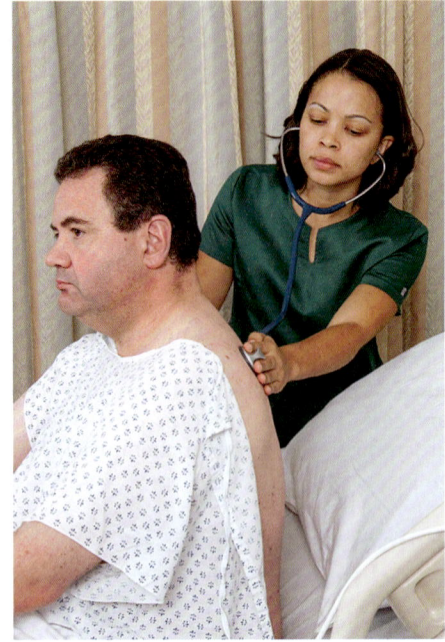

FIGURE 1-4 Nurse listens to client's lung sounds to determine any changes from the baseline data.

may perform the entire physical examination. In the home setting, the nurse is usually responsible for performing most of the physical examination (Fig. 1-3).

Regardless of who collects the data, a total health assessment (subjective and objective data regarding functional health and body systems) is needed when the client first enters a health care system and periodically thereafter to establish baseline data against which future health status changes can be measured and compared. Frequency of comprehensive assessments depends on the client's age, risk factors, health status, health promotion practices, and lifestyle.

Ongoing or Partial Assessment

An ongoing or partial assessment of the client consists of data collection that occurs after the comprehensive database is established. This consists of a minioverview of the client's body systems and holistic health patterns as a follow up on health status. Any problems that were initially detected in the client's body system or holistic health patterns are reassessed to determine any changes (deterioration or improvement) from the baseline data (Fig. 1-4). In addition, a brief reassessment of the client's body systems and holistic health patterns is performed to detect any new problems. This type of assessment is usually performed whenever and wherever the nurse or another health care professional has an encounter with the client, whether in the hospital, community, or home setting. The frequency of this type of assessment is determined by the acuity of the client.

For example, a partial assessment of a client admitted to the hospital with lung cancer requires frequent assessment of respiratory rate, oxygen saturation, lung sounds, skin color, and capillary refill. A total assessment of skin would be performed less frequently, with the nurse focusing on the color and temperature of the extremities to determine level of oxygenation.

Focused or Problem-Oriented Assessment

A focused or problem-oriented assessment does not replace the comprehensive health assessment. It is performed when a comprehensive database exists for a client who comes to the health care agency with a specific health concern. A focused assessment consists of a thorough assessment of a particular client problem and does not address areas not related to the problem. For example, if your client, John P., tells you that he has ear pain, you would ask him questions about the character and location of pain, onset, relieving and aggravating factors, and associated symptoms. However, asking questions about his sexual functioning or his normal bowel habits would be unnecessary and inappropriate. The physical examination should focus on his ears, nose, mouth, and throat. At this time, it would not be appropriate to perform a comprehensive assessment by repeating all system examinations such as the heart and neck vessel or abdominal assessment.

Emergency Assessment

An emergency assessment is a very rapid assessment performed in life-threatening situations (Fig. 1-5). In such situations

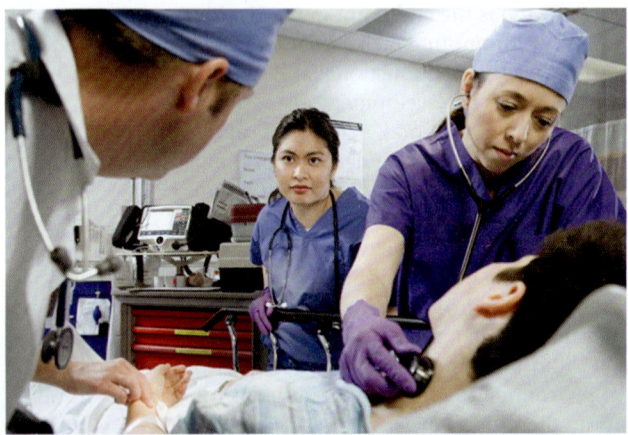

FIGURE 1-5 Assessment of the carotid pulse is vital in an emergency assessment.

(choking, cardiac arrest, drowning), an immediate assessment is needed to provide prompt treatment. An example of an emergency assessment is the evaluation of the client's airway, breathing, and circulation (known as the ABCs) when cardiac arrest is suspected. The major and only concern during this type of assessment is to determine the status of the client's life-sustaining physical functions.

Steps of Health Assessment

The assessment phase of the nursing process has four major steps:
- Collection of subjective data
- Collection of objective data
- Validation of data
- Documentation of data

Although there are four steps, they tend to overlap and you may perform two or three steps concurrently. For example, you may ask your client, Jane Q., if she has dry skin while you are inspecting the condition of the skin. If she answers "no," but you notice that the skin on her hands is very dry, validation with the client may be performed at this point.

Each part of assessment is discussed briefly in the following sections. However, Chapters 2, 3, and 4 provide an in-depth explanation of each of the four assessment steps. In addition, the four steps of the assessment process format are carried throughout this text. All of the physical assessment chapters contain the following sections: collecting subjective data, collecting objective data, and a combined validation and documentation section.

Preparing for the Assessment

Before actually meeting the client and beginning the nursing health assessment, there are several things the nurse should do to prepare. It is helpful to review the client's medical record, if available (Fig. 1-6). Knowing the client's basic biographical data (age, sex, religion, educational level, and occupation) is useful. The medical record provides information about chronic diseases, medications, allergies, and so on, and gives clues to how a present illness may impact the client's ADL. An awareness of the client's previous and current health status provides valuable information to guide your interactions with the client. This information can also be from the medical record, from other health care team members, and from significant others (client's family).

After reviewing the record or discussing the client's status with others, remember to keep an open mind and to avoid premature judgments that may alter your ability to collect accurate data. For example, do not assume that a 30-year-old female client who happens to be a nurse knows everything regarding hospital routine and medical care or that a 60-year-old male client with diabetes mellitus needs client teaching regarding diet. Validate information with the client and be prepared to collect additional data.

Also use this time to educate yourself about the client's diagnoses or tests performed. The client may have a medical diagnosis that you have never heard of or that you have not dealt with in the past. You may review the record, find that the client had a special blood test yielding abnormal results, and realize that you are not familiar with this test. At that time, you should consult the necessary resources (laboratory manual, textbook, or electronic reference resource, such as a smartphone application) to learn about the test and the implications of its findings.

Once you have gathered basic data about the client, take a minute to reflect on your own feelings regarding your initial encounter with the client. For example, the client may be a 22 year old with a drug addiction. If you are 22 years old and a very health-conscious person who does not drink, smoke, use illegal drugs, or drink caffeine, you need to take time to examine your own feelings in order to avoid biases, judgment, and the possibility of projecting those judgments. You must be as objective and open as possible. Other client situations that may require reflection time include those involving sexually transmitted infections, terminal illnesses, amputation, paralysis, early teenage pregnancies, human immunodeficiency virus (HIV) infection or acquired immunodeficiency syndrome (AIDS), abortion, obesity, sexual preference (gay, lesbian, bisexual, transgender), and people with special needs or who are cognitively challenged.

Remember to obtain and organize materials that you will need for the assessment. The materials may be assessment tools such as a guide to interview questions or forms on which to record data collected during the health history interview and physical examination. Most primary care settings use electronic health records (EHRs) for recording data. Also, gather any equipment (e.g., stethoscope, thermometer, otoscope) necessary to perform a nursing health assessment.

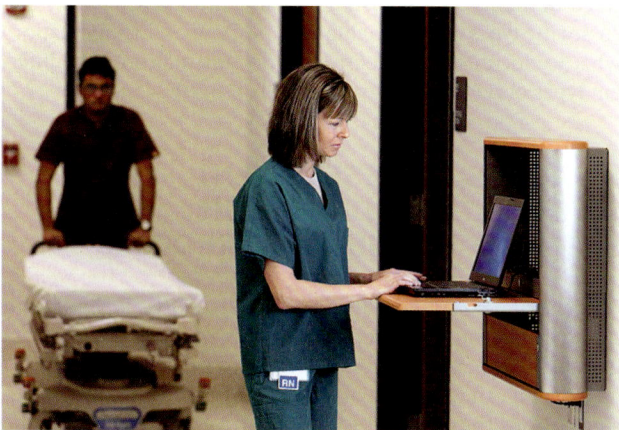

FIGURE 1-6 Reviewing the client's medical record is an important part of preparing for the assessment.

Collecting Subjective Data

Subjective data are sensations or symptoms (e.g., pain, hunger), feelings (e.g., happiness, sadness), perceptions, desires, preferences, beliefs, ideas, values, and personal information that can be elicited and verified only by the client (Fig. 1-7). To elicit accurate subjective data, learn to use effective interviewing skills with a variety of clients in different settings. The major areas of subjective data include:
- Biographical information (name, age, religion, occupation)
- History of present health concern: physical symptoms related to each body part or system (e.g., eyes and ears, abdomen)
- Personal health history
- Family history

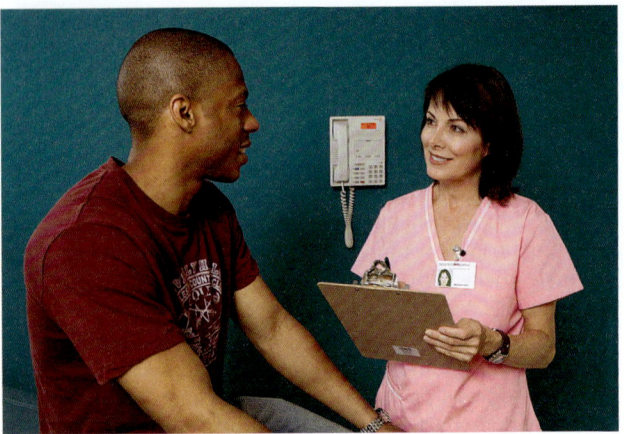

FIGURE 1-7 A comfortable, relaxed atmosphere and an attentive interviewer are essential for a successful clinical interview.

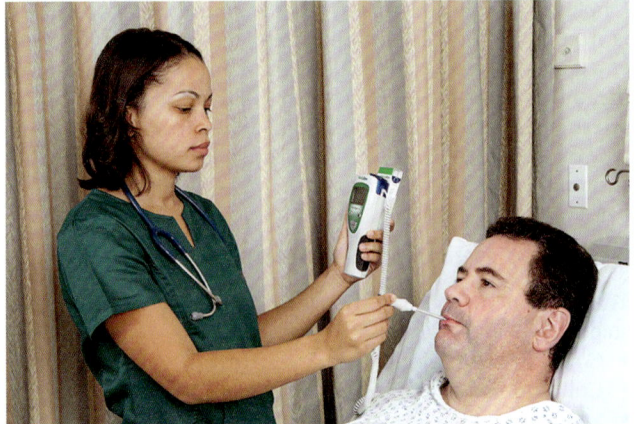

FIGURE 1-8 The nurse directly observes objective data by taking the client's temperature.

- Health and lifestyle practices (e.g., health practices that put the client at risk, nutrition, activity, relationships, cultural beliefs or practices, family structure and function, community environment)
- Review of systems

> **CASE STUDY**
>
>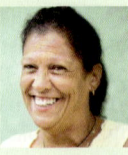
>
> As the assessment progresses, the nurse learns through the interview with Mrs. Gutierrez that she has no appetite and no energy. She feels as though she wants to stay in bed all day. She misses her sisters in Mexico, and cannot do her normal housekeeping or cooking. The nurse thinks that Mrs. Gutierrez is probably suffering from depression. But when the nurse asks Mrs. Gutierrez what she believes is causing her lack of appetite and low energy, Mrs. Gutierrez says she was shocked when her husband was hit by a car. He could not work for a month.

The skills of interviewing and the complete health history are discussed in Chapter 2.

Collecting Objective Data

The examiner directly observes objective data (Fig. 1-8). These data include:
- Physical characteristics (e.g., skin color, posture)
- Body functions (e.g., heart rate, respiratory rate)
- Appearance (e.g., dress and hygiene)
- Behavior (e.g., mood, affect)
- Measurements (e.g., blood pressure, temperature, height, weight)
- Results of laboratory testing (e.g., platelet count, x-ray findings)

This type of data is obtained by general observation and by using the four physical examination techniques: inspection, palpation, percussion, and auscultation. Another source of objective data is the client's medical/health record, which is the document that contains information about what other health care professionals (i.e., nurses, physicians, physical therapists, dietitians, social workers) observed about the client. Objective data may also be observations noted by the family or significant others about the client. See Table 1-2 for a comparison of objective and subjective data.

Validating Assessment Data

Validation of assessment data is a crucial part of assessment that often occurs along with collection of subjective and objective data. It serves to ensure that the assessment process is not ended before all relevant data have been collected, and helps to prevent documentation of inaccurate data. What types of assessment data should be validated, the different ways to validate data, and identifying areas where data are missing are all parts of the process. Validation of data is discussed in detail in Chapter 4 (Fig. 1-9).

Documenting Data

Documentation of assessment data is an important step of assessment because it forms the database for the entire nursing process and provides data for all other members of the health care team. Thorough and accurate documentation is vital to ensure that valid conclusions are made when the data are analyzed in the second step of the nursing process. Chapter 4 discusses the types of documentation, purpose of documentation, what to document, guidelines for documentation, and different types of documentation forms (Fig. 1-10).

ANALYSIS OF ASSESSMENT DATA/NURSING DIAGNOSIS: STEP 2 OF THE NURSING PROCESS

Analysis of data (often called nursing diagnosis) is the second phase of the nursing process. Analysis of the collected data goes hand in hand with the rationale for performing a nursing assessment. The purpose of assessment is to arrive at conclusions about the client's health. To arrive at conclusions, the nurse must analyze the assessment data. Indeed, nurses often begin to analyze the data in their minds while performing

TABLE 1-2 Comparing Subjective and Objective Data

	Subjective	Objective
Description	Data elicited and verified by the client	Data directly or indirectly observed through measurement
Sources	Client	Observations and physical assessment findings of the nurse or other health care professionals
	Client record	Documentation of assessments made in client record
	Other health care professionals	Observations made by the client's family or significant others
Methods used to obtain data	Client interview	Observation and physical examination
Skills needed to obtain data	Interview and therapeutic—communication skills	Inspection
	Caring ability and empathy	Palpation
	Listening skills	Percussion
		Auscultation
Examples	"I have a headache."	Respirations 16 per minute
	"It frightens me."	BP 180/100, apical pulse 80 and irregular
	"I am not hungry."	X-ray film reveals fractured pelvis

assessment. To achieve the goal or anticipated outcome of the assessment, the nurse makes sure that the data collected are as accurate and thorough as possible.

During this phase, you analyze and synthesize data to determine whether the data reveal a nursing concern (nursing diagnosis), a collaborative concern (collaborative problem), or a concern that needs to be referred to another discipline (referral).

A nursing diagnosis is defined by the North American Nursing Diagnosis Association as "a clinical judgment concerning a human response to health conditions/life processes, or a vulnerability for that response, by an individual, family, group, or community. A nursing diagnosis provides the basis for selecting nursing interventions to achieve outcomes for which the nurse is accountable" (NANDA International, 2016, p. 24). Collaborative problems are defined as certain "physiological complications that nurses monitor to detect their onset or changes in status" (Carpenito, 2017). Nurses manage collaborative problems by implementing both physician- and nurse-prescribed interventions to reduce further complications. Referrals occur because nurses assess the "whole" (physical, psychological, social, cultural, and spiritual) client, often identifying problems that require the assistance of other health care professionals. Chapter 5 provides information about nursing diagnoses, collaborative problems, and referrals.

Concept Mastery Alert

Data analysis is the phase in which the nurse examines and groups the data collected to make nursing judgments. The end result of this data analysis portion of the nursing process is formulation of nursing diagnoses, collaborative problems, and/or referrals.

Process of Data Analysis

To arrive at nursing diagnoses, collaborative problems, or referral, you must go through the steps of data analysis. This process requires diagnostic reasoning skills, often called critical thinking. The process can be divided into seven major steps:
- Identify abnormal data and strengths.
- Cluster the data.
- Draw inferences and identify problems.

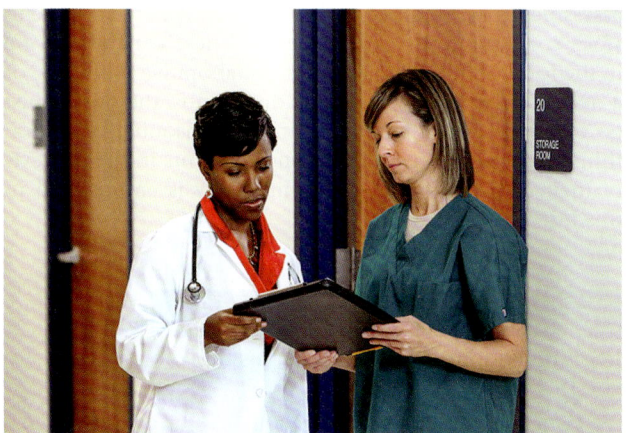

FIGURE 1-9 Validating data with another health care provider is a crucial part of assessment.

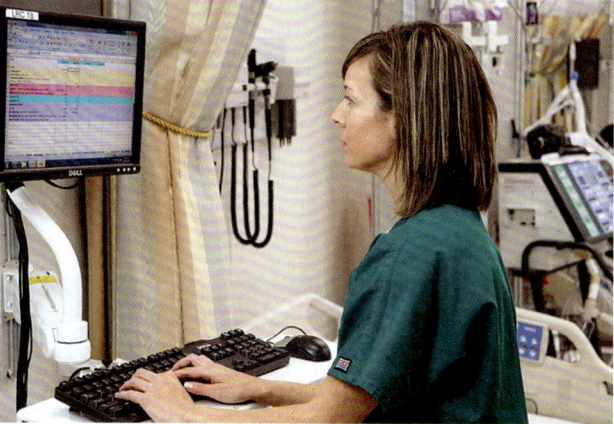

FIGURE 1-10 Accurate documentation is vital to ensure that valid conclusions are made.

- Propose possible nursing diagnoses.
- Check for defining characteristics of those diagnoses.
- Confirm or rule out nursing diagnoses.
- Document conclusions.

Each of these steps is explained in detail in Chapter 5. In addition, each assessment chapter in this text contains a section called "Analysis of Data," which uses these steps to analyze the assessment data presented in a specific client case study related to chapter content.

FACTORS AFFECTING HEALTH ASSESSMENT

In the past, health assessment focused solely on the individual client. But there is a need to place individuals in the contexts that affect their health. Culture, family, and community may all affect a client's health status. When you look at a client, you need to consider these contexts and assess how they may be affecting the client's health. The reverse is also true; the person's family, community, and even spirituality are affected by his or her health status, even if only in subtle ways. Understanding or being aware of the client in context is essential to performing an effective health assessment. Remember, though, that you must be aware of any perceived notions you have about the client's cultural, spiritual, community, or family context.

CASE STUDY

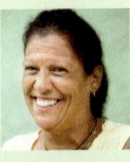

Consider Mrs. Gutierrez, introduced at the beginning of the chapter, to help illustrate the reason for seeing the client in context. The nurse continues to listen to Mrs. Gutierrez and learns that she is also suffering from "susto." Mrs. Gutierrez states that a few days in bed will help her recover her soul and her health. The nurse decides to reschedule the diabetic teaching for a later time and provide only essential information to Mrs. Gutierrez at this visit.

Many systems are operating to create the context in which the client exists and functions. The nurse sees an individual client, but accurate interpretation of what the nurse sees depends on perceiving the client in context. Culture, family, and community operate as systems interacting to form the context.

A health assessment textbook for nurses focuses on providing a solid baseline for determining normal versus abnormal data gathered in a health history and physical assessment. This text must be supported by knowledge or concurrent instruction in medical–surgical and psychosocial nursing and, of course, anatomy and physiology. In this text, we can provide only a review of key concepts of these subjects.

As with anatomy and physiology, medical–surgical nursing, and psychosocial nursing content, a health assessment textbook can only provide key concepts related to culture, family, spirituality, and community. Many texts on transcultural nursing, family nursing, family therapy, social work, community nursing, and spiritual care exist to provide the knowledge base, concurrent instruction, or resources needed for exhaustive information. This assessment text emphasizes the need to consider the client in context for best practice in health assessment. For basic concepts of cultural, spiritual, family, and community assessment, see Chapters 11, 12, 33, and 34.

SUMMARY

Nursing health assessment differs in purpose, framework, and end result from all other types of professional health care assessments. The role of the nurse in health assessment has expanded drastically from the days of Florence Nightingale, when the nurse used the senses of sight, touch, and hearing to assess clients. Today, communication and physical assessment techniques are used independently by nurses to arrive at professional clinical judgments concerning the client's health. In addition, advances in technology have expanded the role of assessment and the development of managed care has increased the necessity of assessment skills. Expert clinical assessment and informatics skills are absolute necessities for the future as nurses from all countries continue to expand their roles in all health care settings.

Assessment is the first and most critical step of the nursing process, and accuracy of assessment data affects all other phases of the nursing process. Health assessment can be divided into four steps: collecting subjective data, collecting objective data, validation of data, and documentation of data. There are four types of nursing assessment: initial comprehensive, ongoing or partial, focused or problem oriented, and emergency.

It is difficult to discuss nursing assessment without taking the process one step further. Data analysis is the second step of the nursing process and the end result of nursing assessment. The purpose of data analysis is to reach conclusions concerning the client's health. These conclusions are in the form of nursing diagnoses, collaborative problems, or a need for referral. To arrive at conclusions, the nurse must go through seven steps of diagnostic reasoning or critical thinking. Maintaining a focus on the clients in the contexts of their culture, family, and community is emphasized in this text.

Want to know more?

A wide variety of resources to enhance your learning and understanding of this book are available on thePoint. Visit thePoint to access:

NCLEX-Style Student Review Questions
Watch and Learn Videos
Concepts in Action Animations
And more!

Unfolding Patient Stories: Rashid Ahmed • Part 1

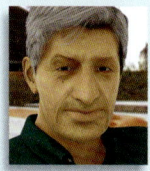

Rashid Ahmed, a 50-year-old male, is admitted to the medical unit with bacterial gastroenteritis. Upon arrival to the unit, the nurse begins the admission assessment. What interviewing techniques can be used by the nurse to establish trust and obtain accurate and thorough information for planning his care? (Rashid Ahmed's story continues in Chapter 6.)

Care for Rashid and other patients in a realistic virtual environment: **vSim** *for Nursing* (thepoint.lww.com/vSimHealthAssessment). Practice documenting these patients' care in DocuCare (thepoint.lww.com/DocuCareEHR).

Unfolding Patient Stories: Marvin Hayes • Part 1

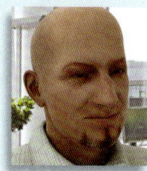

Marvin Hayes is 43 years old and underwent a laparoscopic abdominoperineal resection with a permanent colostomy for rectal cancer. When collecting assessment data, how does the nurse determine that there is a problem—for example, postoperative bleeding? How does the nurse decide when to call the provider with the concern of bleeding? (Marvin Hayes' story continues in Chapter 14.)

Care for Marvin and other patients in a realistic virtual environment: **vSim** *for Nursing* (thepoint.lww.com/vSimHealthAssessment). Practice documenting these patients' care in DocuCare (thepoint.lww.com/DocuCareEHR).

References and Selected Readings

Alfaro-LeFevre, R. (2014). *Applying the nursing process: A tool for critical thinking* (8th ed.). Philadelphia, PA: Lippincott Williams & Wilkins.

American Association of Colleges of Nursing. (2008). *The essentials of baccalaureate education for professional nursing practice.* Available at http://www.aacn.nche.edu/education-resources/BaccEssentials08.pdf

American Nurses Association (ANA). (2010). *Nursing: Scope and standards of practice.* Silver Springs, MD: Author.

Becker, M. H., & Rosenstock, I. M. (1987). Comparing social learning theory and the health belief model. In E. B. Ward (Ed.): *Advances in health education and promotion.* Greenwich, CT: JAI Press.

Bews, D. C., & Baillie, J. H. (1969). Pre-placement health screening by nurses. *American Journal of Public Health and the Nation's Health, 59*(12), 2178–2184.

Birks, M., Cant, R., James, A., Chung, C., & Davis, J. (2013). The use of physical assessment skills by registered nurses in Australia: Issues for nursing education. *Collegian, 20*(1), 27–33. Available at http://www.ncbi.nlm.nih.gov/pubmed/23678781[PubMed]

Bullough, B. (1976). Influences on role expansion. *American Journal of Nursing, 76*(9), 1476–1481.

Carpenito, L. J. (2017). *Nursing diagnosis: Application to clinical practice* (15th ed.). Philadelphia, PA: Lippincott Williams & Wilkins.

Cipolla, J. A., & Collings, G. H., Jr. (1971). Nurse clinicians in industry. *American Journal of Nursing, 71*(8), 1530–1534.

Cowen, P. S., & Moorhead, S. (2014). *Current issues in nursing.* St. Louis, MO: Mosby Elsevier.

Current Nursing. (2012). Health promotion model. Available at http://nursingplanet.com/health_promotion_model.html

Dykes, P. C., & Collins, S. A. (2013). Building linkages between nursing care and improved patient outcomes: The role of health information technology. *The Online Journal of Issues in Nursing, 18*(3, Manuscript 4). Available at http://www.nursingworld.org/Nursing-Care-and-Improved-Outcomes.html

Eastman, P. (2010). New Institute of Medicine report calls for transformation of nursing, increased empowerment and responsibility. *Oncology Times, 32*(20), 42–43.

Fagin, C. M., & Goodwin, B. (1972). Baccalaureate preparation for primary care. *Nursing Outlook, 20*(4), 240–244.

Fitzsimmons, V., & Gallagher, L. P. (1978). Physical assessment skills: A historical perspective. *Nursing Forum, 17*(4), 345–355.

Health Promotion Model. (2012). Available at http://nursingplanet.com/health_promotion_model.html

Holzemer, W. L., Barkauskas, V. H., & Ohlson, V. M. (1980). A program evaluation of four workshops designed to prepare nurse faculty in health assessment. *Journal of Nursing Education, 4*(19), 7–18.

Institute for Healthcare Improvement. (2015). Reinventing nursing education. Available at http://www.ihi.org/resources/Pages/ImprovementStories/ReinventingNursingEducation.aspx

Institute of Medicine (IOM). (2010). The future of nursing: Leading change, advancing health. Available at http://www.nationalacademies.org/hmd/Reports/2010/The-Future-of-Nursing-Leading-Change-Advancing-Health.aspx

Leach, L. S. & Mayo, A. M. (2013). Rapid response teams: Qualitative analysis of their effectiveness. *American Journal of Critical Care, 22*(3), 198–210. Available at http://www.aacn.org/wd/Cetests/media/A13223.pdf

Lysaught, J. (1970). *An abstract for action.* New York: McGraw-Hill.

NANDA International. (2016). Glossary of terms. Available at http://www.nanda.org/nanda-international-glossary-of-terms.html

Nightingale, F. (1992). Role expansion of role extension: Some conceptual differences. *Nursing Forum, 9*(4), 380–390.

Partners in Health. (2015). Empowering nurses to improve care in Haiti. Available at http://www.pih.org/blog/empowering-nurses-to-improve-care-in-haiti

Pender, N. (1982). *Health promotion in nursing practice.* Norwalk, CT: Appleton-Century-Crofts.

Pender, N. (1996). *Health promotion in nursing practice* (3rd ed.). Stamford, CT: Appleton & Lange.

Rosenstock, I. M. (1966). Why people use health services. *Milbank Memorial Fund Quarterly, 44*(3), 94–127.

Slåtten, K., Hatlevik, O., & Fagerström, L. (2014). Validation of a new instrument for self-assessment of nurses' core competencies in palliative care. *Nursing Research and Practice, 2014.* http://dx.doi.org/10.1155/2014/615498

Sturt, G. (n.d.). Theories of health behavior. Available at http://homepage.ntlworld.com/gary.sturt/health/healat2.htm

Tastan, S., Linch, G. C., Keenan, G. M., Stifter, J., McKinney, D., Fahey, L., et al. (2014). Evidence for the existing American Nurses Association-recognized standardized nursing terminologies: A systematic review. *International Journal of Nursing Studies, 51*(8), 1160–1170. Available at http://dx.doi.org/10.1016/j.ijnurstu.2013.12.004

2 COLLECTING SUBJECTIVE DATA: THE INTERVIEW AND HEALTH HISTORY

Learning Objectives

1. Discuss the purpose for each of the four phases of a client interview.
2. Describe effective verbal and nonverbal communication techniques to collect subjective client data.
3. Explain types of communication to avoid in the client interview.
4. Describe ways to adapt the interview for the older client.
5. Describe ways to adapt the interview for the client with emotional issues.
6. Discuss the ways that ethnicity can affect communication patterns.
7. Identify the major categories of a complete client health history.
8. Describe how to use a genogram to illustrate a client's family health history.
9. Describe the process for performing a review of systems.
10. Describe questions to ask to assess the client's lifestyle and health practices.
11. Explain how a nurse would use the "COLDSPA" mnemonic to analyze a client symptom.

CASE STUDY

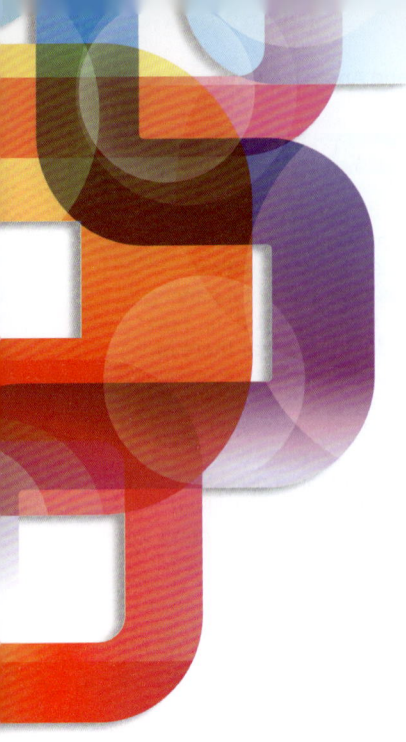

Mrs. Gutierrez, age 52, was introduced in Chapter 1. Recall that she arrived at the clinic for diabetic teaching but appeared distracted and sad, uninterested in the teaching. She was unable to focus, pacing back and forth in the clinic wringing her hands. The nurse suspected that Mrs. Gutierrez was upset by her diagnosis of diabetes. However, during the interview, the nurse learned additional information that changed her thoughts about the client. In this chapter you will learn how to use the nursing interview to collect additional data to better understand what is really happening with Mrs. Gutierrez.

Collecting subjective data is an integral part of interviewing the client to obtain a nursing health history. Subjective data consist of:
- Sensations or symptoms
- Feelings
- Perceptions
- Desires
- Preferences
- Beliefs
- Ideas
- Values
- Personal information

These types of data can be elicited and verified only by the client. Subjective data provide clues to possible physiologic, psychologic, and sociologic problems. They also provide the nurse with information that may reveal a client's risk for a problem as well as areas of strengths for the client.

The information is obtained through interviewing. Therefore, effective interviewing skills are vital for accurate and thorough collection of subjective data.

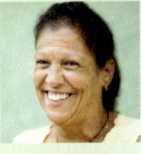 ## INTERVIEWING

Obtaining a valid nursing health history requires professional, interpersonal, and interviewing skills. The nursing interview is a communication process that has two focuses:
- Establishing rapport and a trusting relationship with the client to elicit accurate and meaningful information (Fig. 2-1).
- Gathering information on the client's developmental, psychological, physiologic, sociocultural, and spiritual status to identify deviations that can be treated with nursing and collaborative interventions or strengths that can be enhanced through nurse–client collaboration.

Phases of the Interview

The nursing interview has four basic phases: preintroductory, introductory, working, and summary/closing phases. These

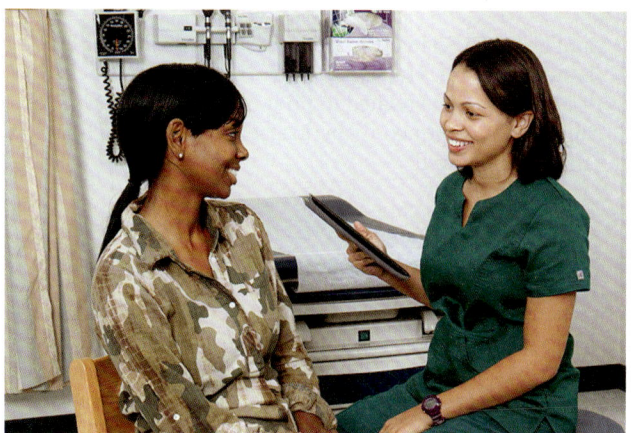
FIGURE 2-1 Establishing rapport with the client is important for effectively collecting data.

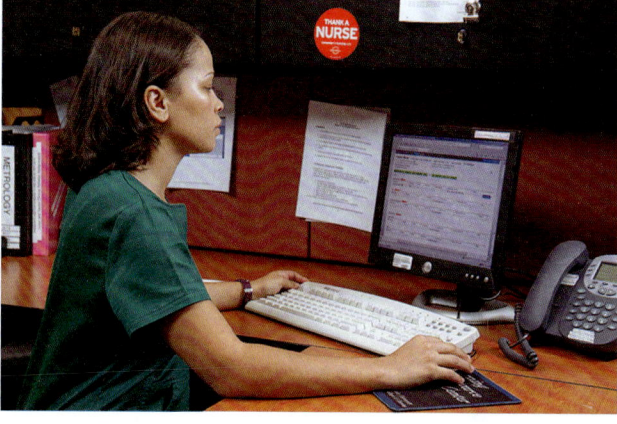
FIGURE 2-2 Nurse reviewing electronic health record (EHR).

phases are briefly explained by describing the roles of the nurse and client during each one.

Preintroductory Phase

The nurse reviews the medical record before meeting with the client (Fig. 2-2). Knowing some of the client's already documented biographical information may assist the nurse with conducting the interview. If the client has been in the system for some time, the record may reveal additional information. For example, it may indicate that the client has difficulty hearing in one ear. This information will ensure that the nurse conducts the interview on the side on which the client hears best. The record may also reveal the client's past health history and reason for seeking health care. However, there may not be a medical record established in some instances. The nurse will then need to rely on interviewing skills to elicit valid and reliable data from the client and the client's family or significant other.

CASE STUDY

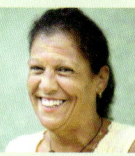
The nurse reviewed Mrs. Gutierrez's medical report sent by her physician and learned that she had her physician refer her to the clinic to obtain diabetic supplies and for diabetic teaching. The report states that she does not routinely monitor and record her blood sugar. Her weight 6 weeks ago was 185 lb.

Introductory Phase

After introducing herself to the client, the nurse explains the purpose of the interview, discusses the types of questions that will be asked, explains the reason for taking notes, and assures the client that confidential information will remain confidential. It is important to understand the HIPAA (Health Insurance Portability and Accountability Act) guidelines enacted by the U.S. Department of Health and Human Services (www.hhs.gov) to ensure confidentiality of client information. The nurse makes sure that the client is comfortable (physically and emotionally) and has privacy. Conducting the interview at eye level with the client demonstrates respect and places the nurse and the client at equal levels. At this point in the interview, it is also essential for nurses to develop trust and rapport, which are essential to promote full disclosure of information. The nurse can begin this process by conveying a sense of priority and interest in the client. Developing rapport depends heavily on verbal and nonverbal communication on the part of the nurse. These types of communication are discussed later in the chapter.

CASE STUDY

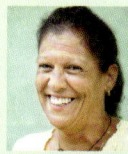
The nurse introduces herself to Mrs. Gutierrez and explains that she will be asking questions in order to better assist her with control of her diabetes. The nurse then sits down with Mrs. Gutierrez at eye level, explaining and ensuring confidentiality of information that will be shared. At that point the nurse asks her if she has any questions, to verify that the client is following and understanding the interview process. The nurse observes and listens to Mrs. Gutierrez to determine her level of comprehending and speaking English.

Concept Mastery Alert

Although the nurse should be at eye level with the client during the interview, it is not necessary to maintain constant eye contact with a client. That may actually cause the client to be uncomfortable. It is important for the nurse to document during the interview and assessment process, which requires the nurse to look away from the client, at times, and toward the documentation form or computer screen.

Working Phase

During this phase, the nurse elicits the client's comments about major biographical data, reasons for seeking care, history of present health concern, past health history, family history, review of body systems (ROS) for current health problems, lifestyle and health practices, and developmental level. The nurse then listens, observes cues, and uses critical thinking skills to interpret and validate information received from the client. The nurse and client collaborate to identify the client's problems and goals. The facilitating approach may be free-flowing or more structured with specific questions, depending on the time available and the type of data needed.

CASE STUDY

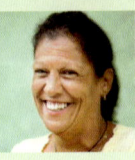

Once the nurse verifies that Mrs. Gutierrez speaks and comprehends English, the nurse then enters the working phase with Mrs. Gutierrez, asking questions about her biographical data, reasons for seeking care, history of present health concern, past health history, family history, ROS for current health problems, lifestyle and health practices, and developmental level. The nurse asks Mrs. Gutierrez what her beliefs are regarding what may be causing her conditions and if she believes she may be experiencing "susto" related to her husband's accident 1 month ago.[1]

Summary and Closing Phase

During the summary and closing, the nurse summarizes information obtained during the working phase and validates problems and goals with the client (see Chapter 4). She also identifies and discusses possible plans to resolve the problem (nursing diagnoses and collaborative problems) with the client (see Chapter 5). Finally, the nurse makes sure to ask if anything else concerns the client and if there are any further questions.

CASE STUDY

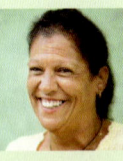

The nurse reviews the data she has gathered from Mrs. Gutierrez and reflects on it. She shares with Mrs. Gutierrez that she thinks her insomnia may be related to stress and anxiety associated with her husband's accident and work setbacks. She outlines a plan for Mrs. Gutierrez to return to see her primary physician for her anxiety, to modify her diet and caffeine intake, and to engage in a daily exercise walking routine. After discussing ways to fully relax before going to sleep, Mrs. Gutierrez agrees to try a bedtime routine of warm milk and enjoyable reading materials. The nurse concludes that the client has insomnia and anorexia related to anxiety associated with her husband's accident. Her collaborative problem may be risk for hypoglycemia related to poor intake at this time. The nurse has postponed diabetic teaching until the client's anxiety is reduced.

Communication During the Interview

The client interview involves two types of communication—nonverbal and verbal. Several special techniques and certain general considerations will improve both types of communication as well as promote an effective and productive interview.

Nonverbal Communication

Nonverbal communication is as important as verbal communication. Your appearance, demeanor, posture, facial expressions, and attitude strongly influence how the client perceives the questions you ask. Facilitate eye level contact. Never overlook the importance of communication or take it for granted.

Appearance

First take care to ensure that your appearance is professional. The client is expecting to see a health professional; therefore, you should look the part. Wear comfortable, neat clothes and a laboratory coat or a uniform. Be sure that your nametag, including credentials, is clearly visible. Your hair should be neat and pulled back if long. Fingernails should be short and neat; jewelry should be minimal.

Demeanor

Your demeanor should also be professional. When you enter a room to interview a client, display poise. Focus on the client and the upcoming interview and assessment. Do not enter the room laughing loudly, yelling to a coworker, or muttering under your breath. This appears unprofessional to the client and will have an effect on the entire interview process. Greet the client calmly, by name and not with references such as honey, sweetie, or sugar. Focus your full attention on the client. Do not be overwhelmingly friendly or "touchy"; many clients are uncomfortable with this type of behavior. It is best to maintain a professional distance.

Facial Expression

Facial expressions are often an overlooked aspect of communication. Because facial expressions often show what you are truly thinking (regardless of what you are saying), monitor them closely. No matter what you think about a client or what kind of day you are having, keep your expression neutral and friendly. If your face shows anger or anxiety, the client will sense it and may think it is directed toward him or her. If you cannot effectively hide your emotions, you may want to explain briefly that you are angry or upset about a personal situation. Admitting this to the client may also help in developing a trusting relationship and genuine rapport.

Displaying a neutral expression does not mean that your face lacks expression. It means using the right expression at the right time. If the client looks upset, you should appear and be understanding and concerned. Conversely, smiling when the client is on the verge of tears will cause the client to believe that you do not care about his or her problem.

---

[1] Susto: a condition mostly associated with Latin America, perceived to be a disease that results from a fright; often thought to be a spirit attack; symptoms are thought to include nervousness, anorexia, insomnia, listlessness, fever, depression, and diarrhea; may be considered a variation on panic attack and distinct from anxiety and depressive disorders (Razzouuk, Nogueira, & Mari Jde J, 2011).

Attitude

One of the most important nonverbal skills to develop as a health care professional is a nonjudgmental attitude. All clients should be accepted, regardless of beliefs, ethnicity, lifestyle, and health care practices. Do not act as though you feel superior to the client or appear shocked, disgusted, or surprised at what you are told. These attitudes will cause the client to feel uncomfortable about opening up to you, and important data concerning his or her health status could be withheld.

Being nonjudgmental involves not "preaching" or imposing your own sense of ethics or morality on the client. Focus on health care and how you can best help the client to achieve the highest possible level of health. For example, if you are interviewing a client who smokes, avoid lecturing condescendingly about the dangers of smoking. Also, avoid telling the client that he or she is foolish and avoid projecting an attitude of disgust. This will only harm the nurse–client relationship and will do nothing to improve the client's health. The client is, no doubt, already aware of the dangers of smoking. Forcing guilt on the client is unhelpful. Accept the client, be understanding of the habit, and work together to improve the client's health. This does not mean you should not encourage the client to quit; it means that how you approach the situation makes a difference. Let the client know you understand that it is hard to quit smoking, support efforts to quit, and offer suggestions on the latest methods available to help kick the smoking habit, such as the Five A's of Behavior Change: Ask, Advise, Assess, Assist, Arrange (AHRQ, 2012).

Silence

Another nonverbal technique to use during the interview process is silence. Periods of silence allow you and the client to reflect and organize thoughts, which facilitate more accurate reporting and data collection.

Listening

Listening is the most important skill to learn and develop fully in order to collect complete and valid data from your client. To listen effectively, you need to maintain good eye contact, smile or display an open, appropriate facial expression, and maintain an open body position (open arms and hands, and lean forward). Avoid preconceived ideas or biases about your client. To listen effectively, you must keep an open mind. Avoid crossing your arms, sitting back, tilting your head away from the client, thinking about other things, looking blank or inattentive, or engaging with an electronic device instead of the client. Becoming an effective listener takes concentration and practice.

In addition, several nonverbal affects or attitudes may hinder effective communication. They may promote discomfort or distrust. Box 2-1 describes communication to avoid.

BOX 2-1 COMMUNICATION TO AVOID

NONVERBAL COMMUNICATION TO AVOID

Excessive or Insufficient Eye Contact

Avoid extremes in eye contact. Some clients feel very uncomfortable with too much eye contact; others believe that you are hiding something from them if you do not look them in the eye. Therefore, it is best to use a moderate amount of eye contact. For example, establish eye contact when the client is speaking to you but look down at your notes from time to time. A client's cultural background often determines how he feels about eye contact (see Cultural Variations in Communication section for more information).

Distraction and Distance

Avoid being occupied with something else while you are asking questions during the interview. This behavior makes the client believe that the interview may be unimportant to you. Avoid appearing mentally distant as well. The client will sense your distance and will be less likely to answer your questions thoroughly. Also try to avoid physical distance exceeding 2–3 ft during the interview. Rapport and trust are established when clients sense that your focus and concern are solely on them and their health. Physical distance may portray a noncaring attitude or a desire to avoid close contact.

Standing

Avoid standing while the client is seated during the interview. Standing puts you and the client at different levels. You may be perceived as the superior, making the client feel inferior. Care of the client's health should be an equal partnership between the health care provider and the client. If the client is made to feel inferior, he or she will not feel empowered to be an equal partner and the potential for optimal health may be lost. In addition, vital information may not be revealed if the client believes that the interviewer is untrustworthy, judgmental, or disinterested.

VERBAL COMMUNICATION TO AVOID

Biased or Leading Questions

Avoid using biased or leading questions. These cause the client to provide answers that may not be true. The way you phrase a question may actually lead the client to think you want her to answer in a certain way. For example, if you ask "You don't feel bad, do you?" the client may conclude that you do not think she should feel bad and will answer "no" even if this is not true.

Rushing Through the Interview

Avoid rushing the client. If you ask questions on top of questions, several things may occur. First, the client may answer "no" to a series of closed-ended questions when he or she would have answered "yes" to one of the questions if it was asked individually. This may occur because the client did not hear the individual question clearly or because the answers to most were "no" and the client forgot about the "yes" answer in the midst of the others. With this type of interview technique, the client may believe that his individual situation is of little concern to the nurse. Taking time with clients shows that you are concerned about their health and helps them to open up. Finally, rushing someone through the interview process undoubtedly causes important information to be left out of the health history. A client will usually sense that you are rushed and may try to help hurry the interview by providing abbreviated or incomplete answers to questions.

Reading the Questions

Avoid reading questions from the history form. This deflects attention from the client and results in an impersonal interview process. As a result, the client may feel ill at ease opening up to formatted questions.

Verbal Communication

Effective verbal communication is essential to a client interview. The goal of the interview process is to elicit as much data about the client's health status as possible. Several types of questions and techniques to use during the interview are discussed in the following sections.

Open-Ended Questions

Open-ended questions are used to elicit the client's feelings and perceptions. They typically begin with the words "how" or "what." An example of this type of question is: "How have you been feeling lately?" These types of questions are important because they require more than a one-word response from the client and, therefore, encourage description. Asking open-ended questions may help to reveal significant data about the client's health status.

The following example shows how open-ended questions work. Imagine yourself interviewing an elderly male client who is at the primary care provider's office because of diabetic complications. He mentions casually to you, "Today is the 2-month anniversary of my wife's death from cancer." Failure to follow up with an open-ended question such as "How does this make you feel?" may result in the loss of important data that could provide clues to the client's current state of health.

Closed-Ended Questions

Use closed-ended questions to obtain facts and to focus on specific information. The client can respond with one or two words. Closed-ended questions typically begin with the words "when" or "did." An example of this type of question is: "When did your headache start?" Closed-ended questions are useful in keeping the interview on course. They can also be used to clarify or obtain more accurate information about issues disclosed in response to open-ended questions. For example, in response to the open-ended question "How have you been feeling lately?" the client says, "Well, I've been feeling really sick to my stomach and I don't feel like eating because of it." You may be able to follow up and learn more about the client's symptom with a closed-ended question such as "When did the nausea start?"

Laundry List

Another way to ask questions is to provide the client with a list of words to choose from in describing symptoms, conditions, or feelings. This laundry list approach helps you to obtain specific answers and reduces the likelihood of the client perceiving or providing an expected answer. For example, "Is the pain severe, dull, sharp, mild, cutting, or piercing?" "Does the pain occur once every year, day, month, or hour?" Repeat choices as necessary.

Rephrasing

Rephrasing information the client has provided is an effective way to communicate during the interview. This technique helps you to clarify information the client has stated; it also enables you and the client to reflect on what was said. For example, your client, Mr. G., tells you that he has been really tired and nauseated for 2 months and that he is scared because he fears that he has some horrible disease. You might rephrase the information by saying, "You are thinking that you have a serious illness?"

Well-Placed Phrases

The nurse can encourage client verbalization by using well-placed phrases. For example, if the client is in the middle of explaining a symptom or feeling and believes that you are not paying attention, you may fail to get all the necessary information. Listen closely to the client during his or her description and use phrases such as "uh-huh," "yes," or "I agree" to encourage the client to continue.

Inferring

Inferring information from what the client tells you and what you observe in the client's behavior may elicit more data or verify existing data. Be careful not to lead the client to answers that are not true (see the Verbal Communication to Avoid section in Box 2-1 for more information). An example of inferring information follows: your client, Mrs. J., tells you that she has bad pain. You ask where the pain is, and she says, "My stomach." You notice the client has a hand on the right side of her lower abdomen and seems to favor her entire right side. You say, "It seems you have more difficulty with the right side of your stomach" (use the word "stomach" because that is the term the client used to describe the abdomen). This technique, if used properly, helps to elicit the most accurate data possible from the client.

Providing Information

Another important thing to do throughout the interview is to provide the client with information as questions and concerns arise. Make sure that you answer every question as thoroughly as you can. If you do not know the answer, explain that you will find out. The more clients know about their own health, the more likely they are to become equal participants in caring for their health. As with nonverbal communication, several verbal techniques may hinder effective communication and should be avoided (see Box 2-1).

Special Considerations During the Interview

Three variations in communication must be considered as you interview clients: gerontologic, cultural, and emotional. These variations affect the nonverbal and verbal techniques you use during the interview. Imagine, for example, that you are interviewing an 82-year-old woman and you ask her to describe how she has been feeling. She does not answer you and she looks confused. This older client may have some hearing loss. In such a case, you may need to modify the verbal technique of asking open-ended questions by following the guidelines provided in the next section.

Gerontologic Variations in Communication

Age affects and commonly slows all body systems to varying degrees. However, normal aspects of aging do not necessarily equate with a health problem, so it is important not to approach an interview with an elderly client assuming that there is a health problem. Older clients have the potential to be as healthy as younger clients. When interviewing an older client, you must first assess hearing acuity. Hearing loss occurs normally with age, and undetected hearing loss is often misinterpreted as mental slowness or confusion. If you detect hearing loss, speak slowly, face the client at all times during the interview, and position yourself so that you are speaking on the side of the client that has the ear with better acuity. Do not yell at the client. Positioning yourself facing the client allows a client who reads lips to better understand.

Older clients may have more health concerns than younger clients and may seek health care more often. Many times, older adult clients with health problems feel vulnerable and scared. They need to believe that they can trust you before they will open up to you about what is bothering them. Thus, establishing and maintaining trust, privacy, and partnership with the older client is particularly important (Fig. 2-3). Older clients may feel as though their health complaints are ignored or not taken seriously, causing them to withhold information. It is often disturbing to older clients that their health problems may be discussed openly among many health care providers and family members. Assure your older adult clients that you are concerned, that you see them as equal partners in health care, and that what is discussed will be between you, their health care provider, and them.

Speak clearly and use straightforward language during the interview with the older adult client. Ask questions in simple terms. Avoid medical jargon and modern slang. However, do not talk down to the client. Being older does not mean that the client is slower mentally. Showing respect is very important. However, if the older client is mentally confused or forgetful, it is important to have a significant other (e.g., spouse, child, close friend) present during the interview to provide or clarify the data.

Cultural Variations in Communication

Ethnic/cultural variations in communication and self-disclosure styles may significantly affect the information obtained (Andrews & Boyle, 2015; Giger, 2013; Hepp, 2015; Muñoz & Luckmann, 2005; Nambudiri & Nambudiri, 2013). Be aware of possible variations in your communication style and the client's. If misunderstanding or difficulty in communicating is evident, seek help from an expert, what some professionals call a "culture broker." This is someone who is thoroughly familiar not only with the client's language, culture, and related health care practices but also with the health care setting and system of the dominant culture. Frequently noted variations in communication styles include:

- Reluctance to reveal personal information to strangers for various culturally based reasons.
- Variation in willingness to openly express emotional distress or pain.
- Variation in ability to receive information (listen).
- Variation in meaning conveyed by language. For example, a client who does not speak the predominant language may not know what a certain medical term or phrase means and, therefore, will not know how to answer your question. Use of slang with nonnative speakers is discouraged as well. Keep in mind that it is hard enough to learn proper language, let alone the idiom vernacular. The nonnative speaker will likely have no idea what you are trying to convey.
- Variation in use and meaning of nonverbal communication: eye contact, stance, gestures, demeanor. For example, direct eye contact may be perceived as rude, aggressive, or immodest by some cultures but lack of eye contact may be perceived as evasive, insecure, or inattentive by other cultures. A slightly bowed stance may indicate respect in some groups; size of personal space affects one's comfortable interpersonal distance; touch may be perceived as comforting or threatening depending on cultural background.
- Variation in disease/illness perception: culture-specific syndromes or disorders are accepted by some groups (e.g., in Latin America, *susto* is an illness caused by a sudden shock or fright).
- Variation in past, present, or future time orientation (e.g., the dominant US culture is future oriented; other cultures may focus more on the past or present).
- Variation in the family's role in the decision-making process: a person other than the client or the client's parent may be the major decision maker regarding appointments, treatments, or follow-up care for the client.

You may have to interview a client who does not speak your language. To perform the best interview possible, it is necessary to use an interpreter (Box 2-2). Possibly the best interpreter would be a culture expert (or culture broker). Consider the relationship of the interpreter to the client. If the interpreter is the client's child or a person of a different sex, age, or social status, interpretation may be impaired. Also keep in mind that communication through use of pictures may be helpful when working with some clients.

Emotional Variations in Communication

Not every client you encounter will be calm, friendly, and eager to participate in the interview process. Clients' emotions vary for a number of reasons. They may be scared or anxious about their health or about disclosing personal information, angry that they are sick or about having to have an examination, depressed about their health or other life events, or they may have an ulterior motive for having an assessment performed (they are trying to avoid work/school). Clients may

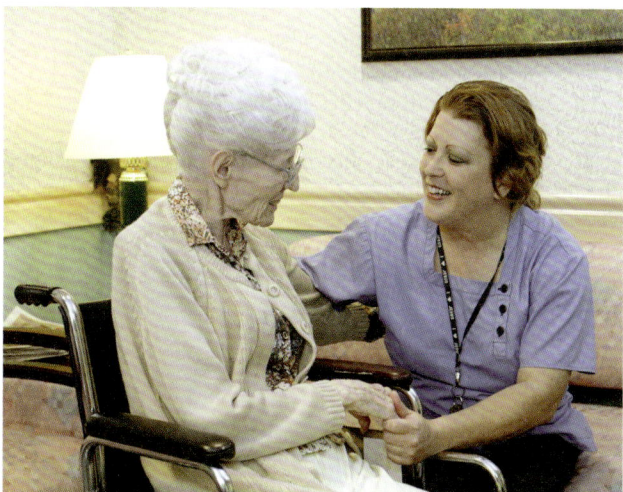

FIGURE 2-3 Establish and maintain trust, privacy, and partnership with older adults to set the tone for effectively collecting data and sharing concerns.

BOX 2-2 TIPS FOR WORKING WITH INTERPRETERS

- **Help the interpreter adapt language to the client's level of speech and comprehension.** Technical terms, and idioms used in health care and in certain cultures are not readily understood by everyone.
- **Help the interpreter adapt communication for clients who cannot communicate clearly.** If the client does not respond directly to questions, it may be the effect of nervousness or medication, or simply the inability to respond clearly. Keep questions simple and direct, and ask "Do you understand?" to clarify.
- **Help the interpreter to be aware of cultural language differences.** Ask clients how they refer to certain bodily functions. If a client's answer does not seem logical, ask if he or she understands the question. Ask clients to describe in their own words what they think is the cause of their symptoms, and clarify the meaning of any terms that could be ambiguous or misunderstood.
- **Help the interpreter to be aware of other potential areas of cultural variation.** Mistrust, embarrassment, and shame may prevent the client from revealing personal information. Family members may try to interpret for the client, but they may be unreliable interpreters and may not remain impartial. Some behaviors common in one culture may cause offense in another. Also, folk beliefs in one culture may differ greatly from those of another culture, or from the health care system norms.
- **Help the interpreter recognize that memory problems and physical distractions may elicit incorrect or insufficient information.**
- **Help the interpreter recognize other potential barriers to communication, such as emotions, interference from relatives, and the barrier of an interpreter between the client and the nurse.**
- **Prior to the interview:**
  - Make sure to allow extra time for interpreting to take place.
  - Clarify the above points with the interpreter concerning any cultural, emotional, or linguistic issues that may arise during the interview.
  - Determine the proper form of address and correct pronunciation of the client's name.
  - Determine with the interpreter whether simultaneous or consecutive mode of interpretation is to be used.
  - Encourage the interpreter to let you know any communication problems if they arise.
- **During the interview:**
  - Introduce yourself and the interpreter to the client.
  - Sit and look directly at the client, not at the interpreter, when asking questions or talking with the client.
  - Watch the client's face throughout the interview for reactions and ask "Do you understand? Do you have questions?"
  - Avoid technical jargon or colorful language.
  - Summarize at the end of the interview and ask the client for any decisions, recommendations, or if any further explanations or clarifications are needed.

Adapted from Mikkelson, H. (2015). The art of working with interpreters: A manual for health care professionals. Available at http://www.acebo.com/pages/the-art-of-working-with-interpreters-a-manual-for-health-care-professionals

---

also have some sensitive issues with which they are grappling and may turn to you for help. Some helpful ways to deal with various clients with problematic emotions and behaviors are discussed in Box 2-3.

COMPLETE HEALTH HISTORY

The health history is an excellent way to begin the assessment process because it provides the foundation for identifying nursing problems and provides a focus for the physical examination. The importance of the health history lies in its ability to provide information that will assist the examiner in identifying areas of strength and limitation in the individual's lifestyle and current health status. Data from the health history also provide the examiner with specific cues to health problems that are most apparent to the client. At this point, these areas may be more intensely examined during the physical assessment. When a client is having a complete, head-to-toe physical assessment, collection of subjective data usually requires that the nurse take a complete health history. The complete health history is modified or shortened when necessary. For example, if the physical assessment will focus on the heart and neck vessels, the subjective data collection would be limited to the data relevant to the heart and neck vessels.

Taking a health history should begin with an explanation to the client of why the information is being requested, for example, "so that I will be able to plan individualized nursing care with you." This section of the chapter explains the rationale for collecting the data, discusses each portion of the health history, and provides sample questions. The health history has eight sections:

- Biographical data
- Reasons for seeking health care
- History of present health concern
- Personal health history
- Family health history
- ROS for current health problems
- Lifestyle and health practices profile
- Developmental level

The organization for collecting data in this text is a generic nursing framework that can be used as is or adapted to use with any nursing framework. See Assessment Tool 2-1 for a summary of the components of a complete client health history. This can be used as a guide for collecting subjective data from the client.

Biographical Data

Biographical data usually include information that identifies the client, such as name, address, phone number, gender, and who provided the information—the client or significant others. The client's birth date, social security number, medical record number, health insurance information, or similar identifying data may be included in the biographical data section.

BOX 2-3 INTERACTING WITH CLIENTS WITH VARIOUS EMOTIONAL STATES

WHEN INTERACTING WITH AN ANXIOUS CLIENT
- Provide the client with simple, organized information in a structured format.
- Explain who you are, along with your role and purpose.
- Ask simple, concise questions.
- Avoid becoming anxious like the client.
- Do not hurry, and decrease any external stimuli.

WHEN INTERACTING WITH AN ANGRY CLIENT
- Approach this client in a calm, reassuring, in-control manner.
- Allow him to ventilate feelings. However, if the client is out of control, do not argue with or touch the client.
- Obtain help from other health care professionals as needed.
- Avoid arguing and facilitate personal space so that the client does not feel threatened or cornered.
- Never allow the client to position him or herself between you and the door.

WHEN INTERACTING WITH A DEPRESSED CLIENT
- Express interest in and understanding of the client and respond in a neutral manner.
- Do not try to communicate in an upbeat, encouraging manner. This will not help the depressed client.

WHEN INTERACTING WITH A MANIPULATIVE CLIENT
- Provide structure and set limits.
- Differentiate between manipulation and a reasonable request.
- If you are not sure whether you are being manipulated, obtain an objective opinion from other nursing colleagues.

WHEN INTERACTING WITH A SEDUCTIVE CLIENT
- Set firm limits on overt sexual client behavior and avoid responding to subtle seductive behaviors.
- Encourage client to use more appropriate methods of coping in relating to others.
- If the overt sexuality continues, do not interact without a witness.
- Report inappropriate behavior to a supervisor.

WHEN DISCUSSING SENSITIVE ISSUES (E.G., SEXUALITY, DYING, SPIRITUALITY)
- First, be aware of your own thoughts and feelings regarding dying, spirituality, and sexuality; then recognize that these factors may affect the client's health and may need to be discussed with someone.
- Ask simple questions in a nonjudgmental manner.
- Allow time for ventilation of client's feelings as needed.
- If you do not feel comfortable or competent discussing personal, sensitive topics, you may make referrals as appropriate, for example, to a pastoral counselor for spiritual concerns or other specialists as needed.

When students are collecting the information and sharing it with instructors, addresses and phone numbers should be deleted and initials (not names) used to protect the client's privacy. The name of the person providing the information needs to be included to assist in determining its accuracy. The client is considered the primary source and all others (including the client's medical record) are secondary sources. In some cases, the client's immediate family or caregiver may be a more accurate source of information than the client. An example would be an older adult client's wife who has kept the client's medical records for years or the legal guardian of a mentally compromised client. In any event, validation of the information by a secondary source may be helpful.

The process of determining the client's culture, ethnicity, and subculture begins with collecting data about date and place of birth; nationality or ethnicity; marital status; religious or spiritual practices; and primary and secondary languages spoken, written, and read. This information helps the nurse to examine special needs and beliefs that may affect the client or family's health care. A person's primary language is usually the one spoken in the family during early childhood and the one in which the person thinks. However, if the client was educated in another language from kindergarten on, that may be the primary language and the birth language would be secondary.

Gathering information about the client's educational level, occupation, and working status at this point in the health history assists the examiner in tailoring questions to the client's level of understanding. In addition, this information can help to identify possible client strengths and limitations affecting health status. For example, if the client was recently downsized from a high-power, high-salary position, the effects of overwhelming stress may play a large part in his or her health status.

Finally, asking who lives with the client and identifying significant others indicate the availability of potential caregivers and support people for the client. Absence of support people would alert the examiner to the (possible) need for finding external sources of support.

CASE STUDY

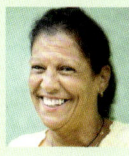

Mrs. Gutierrez, a 52-year-old, married female, has lived in Los Angeles for over half of her life—since she was 20 years old as a homemaker. She was born in Mexico city. Her daughter has dropped her off at the clinic while she runs some errands. Mrs. Gutierrez lives with her husband and three daughters (ages 12, 14, and 17). She has two older sons who are married and live in Mexico. She shares a cell phone and car with her daughter. She completed high school in Mexico. Mrs. Gutierrez's family does not have private health care insurance, due to family income being below Affordable Care Act minimums.

Reason(s) for Seeking Health Care

This category includes two questions: "What is your major health problem or concern at this time?" and "How do you feel about having to seek health care?" The first question assists the

ASSESSMENT TOOL 2-1 Nursing Health History Format Summary (Used for Client Care Plan)

Biographical Data
Name
Address
Phone
Gender
Provider of history (patient or other)
Birth date
Place of birth
Race or ethnic background
Primary and secondary languages (spoken and read)
Marital status
Religious or spiritual practices
Educational level
Occupation
Significant others or support persons (availability)

Reasons for Seeking Health Care
Reason for seeking health care (major health problem or concern)
Feelings about seeking health care (fears and past experiences)

History of Present Health Concern Using COLDSPA
Character (How does it feel, look, smell, sound, etc.?)
Onset (When did it begin; is it better, worse, or the same since it began?)
Location (Where is it? Does it radiate?)
Duration (How long does it last? Does it recur?)
Severity (How bad is it on a scale of 1 [barely noticeable] to 10 [worst pain ever experienced]?)
Pattern (What makes it better? What makes it worse?)
Associated factors (What other symptoms do you have with it? Will you be able to continue doing your work or other activities [leisure or exercise]?)

Past Health History
Problems at birth
Childhood illnesses
Immunizations to date
Adult illnesses (physical, emotional, mental)
Surgeries
Accidents
Prolonged pain or pain patterns
Allergies
Physical, emotional, social, or spiritual weaknesses
Physical, emotional, social, or spiritual strengths

Family Health History
Age of parents (Living? Date of death?)
Parents' illnesses and longevity
Grandparents' illnesses and longevity
Aunts' and uncles' ages and illnesses and longevity
Children's ages and illnesses or handicaps and longevity

Review of Systems for Current Health Problems
Skin, hair, and nails: color, temperature, condition, rashes, lesions, excessive sweating, hair loss, dandruff
Head and neck: headache, stiffness, difficulty swallowing, enlarged lymph nodes, sore throat
Ears: pain, ringing, buzzing, drainage, difficulty hearing, exposure to loud noises, dizziness, drainage
Eyes: pain, infections, impaired vision, redness, tearing, halos, blurring, black spots, flashes, double vision
Mouth, throat, nose, and sinuses: mouth pain, sore throat, lesions, hoarseness, nasal obstruction, sneezing, coughing, snoring, nosebleeds
Thorax and lungs: pain, difficulty breathing, shortness of breath with activities, orthopnea, cough, sputum, hemoptysis, respiratory infections
Breasts and regional lymphatics: pain, lumps, discharge from nipples, dimpling or changes in breast size, swollen and tender lymph nodes in axilla
Heart and neck vessels: chest pain or pressure, palpitations, edema, last blood pressure, last ECG
Peripheral vascular: leg or feet pain, swelling of feet or legs, sores on feet or legs, color of feet and legs
Abdomen: pain, indigestion, difficulty swallowing, nausea and vomiting. Gas, jaundice, hernias
Male genitalia: painful urination, frequency or difficulty starting or maintaining urinary system, blood in urine, sexual problems, penile lesions, penile pain, scrotal swelling, difficulty with erection or ejaculation, exposure to STIs
Female genitalia: pelvic pain, voiding pain, sexual pain, voiding problems (dribbling, incontinence), age of menarche or menopause (date of last menstrual period), pregnancies and types of problems, abortions, STIs, HRT, birth control methods
Anus, rectum, and prostate: pain, with defecation, hemorrhoids, bowel habits, constipation, diarrhea, blood in stool
Musculoskeletal: pain, swelling, redness, stiff joints, strength of extremities, abilities to care for self and work
Neurologic: mood, behavior, depression, anger, headaches, concussions, loss of strength or sensation, coordination, difficulty with speech, memory problems, strange thoughts or actions, difficulty reading or learning

Lifestyle and Health Practices
Description of a typical day (AM to PM)
Nutrition and weight management
24-hour dietary intake (foods and fluids)
Who purchases and prepares meals
Activities on a typical day
Exercise habits and patterns
Sleep and rest habits and patterns
Use of medications and other substances (caffeine, nicotine, alcohol, recreational drugs)
Self-concept
Self-care responsibilities
Social activities for fun and relaxation
Social activities contributing to society
Relationships with family, significant others, and pets
Values, religious affiliation, spirituality
Past, current, and future plans for education
Type of work, level of job satisfaction, work stressors
Finances
Stressors in life, coping strategies used
Residency, type of environment, neighborhood, environmental risks

Developmental Level (See Chapter 7)
Using the Questions in Chapter 7 to Determine Client's Developmental Level
Young adult: intimacy versus isolation
Middlescent: generativity versus stagnation
Older adult: ego integrity versus despair

client in focusing on the most significant health concern and answers the nurse's question, "Why are you here?" or "How can I help you?" Primary care providers call this the client's chief complaint (CC), but a more holistic approach for phrasing the question may draw out concerns that reach beyond a physical complaint and may address stress or lifestyle changes.

The second question, "How do you feel about having to seek health care?" encourages the client to discuss fears or other feelings about having to see a health care provider. For example, a woman visiting a primary care provider states her major health concern: "I found a lump in my breast." This woman may be able to respond to the second question by voicing fears that she has been reluctant to share with her significant others. This question may also draw out descriptions of previous experiences—both positive and negative—with other health care providers.

CASE STUDY

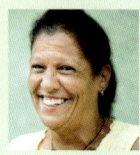

Mrs. Gutierrez states that she has come to the clinic "because my doctor told me I needed diabetic teaching." However, her concern is: "I cannot eat or sleep and I just want to be able to eat and sleep again."

History of Present Health Concern

This section of the health history takes into account several aspects of the health problem and asks questions whose answers can provide a detailed description of the concern. First, encourage the client to explain the health problem or symptom in as much detail as possible by focusing on the onset, progression, and duration of the problem; signs and symptoms and related problems; and what the client perceives as causing the problem. You may also ask the client to evaluate what makes the problem worse, what makes it better, which treatments have been tried, what effect the problem has had on daily life or lifestyle, what expectations are held regarding recovery, and what is the client's ability to provide self-care.

Because there are many characteristics to be explored for each symptom, a memory helper—known as a mnemonic—can help the nurse to complete the assessment of the sign, symptom, or health concern. Many mnemonics have been developed for this purpose (e.g., PQRST, COLDSPAR, COLDSTER, LOCSTAAM). The mnemonic used in this text is COLDSPA, which is designed to help the nurse explore symptoms, signs, or health concerns (see Box 2-4).

The client's answers to the questions provide the nurse with a great deal of information about the client's problem and especially how it affects lifestyle and activities of daily living (ADLs). This helps the nurse to evaluate the client's insight into the problem and the client's plans for managing it. The nurse can also begin to postulate nursing diagnoses from this initial information.

Problems or symptoms particular to body parts or systems are covered in the Nursing History to Collecting Subjective Data: The Nursing Health History section under "History of Present Health Concern" in the physical assessment chapters. Each identified symptom must be described for clear understanding of probable cause and significance.

CASE STUDY

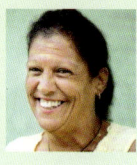

The nurse further explores Mrs. Gutierrez's symptoms of loss of appetite and inability to sleep using COLDSPA.

COLDSPA	Clients Responses for Insomnia and Anorexia
Character: Describe the nature of your inability to sleep. Describe your current appetite by telling me what you eat in a normal day.	I only sleep for 4–5 hours a night. Once I fall asleep, about 10 PM, I wake up about 2 AM and cannot go back to sleep. I do not take naps during the day. I eat cereal in the morning but am not able to eat much the rest of the day. I eat less than one half of what I used to eat. I still try to cook but I only eat one bite of a tamale and maybe a bite or two of beans or rice. I used to bake a lot but no longer have the energy to bake.
Onset	2 months ago, right after my husband was in a car wreck
Location	Nonapplicable
Duration	2 months
Severity	I am so tired in the daytime that I just lay in bed, but I do not sleep. My stomach always feels full and I know I am not eating as I should.
Pattern: What makes it better or worse?	I have tried taking Excedrin PM over the counter (OTC) but it just makes me feel more drowsy all day. My daughter has tried baking me cookies and I eat those sometimes.
Associated factors	Experiencing "susto" and states "My clothes no longer fit and are very loose. I worry a lot as to how we will pay our bills now that my husband has lost his job and we do not have health insurance. I am sometimes nauseated when I cannot eat. The other day I began crying over nothing. I just feel sad all the time."

Personal Health History

This portion of the health history focuses on questions related to the client's personal history, from the earliest beginnings to the present. Ask the client about any childhood illnesses and immunizations to date. Adult illnesses (physical, emotional, and mental) are then explored. Ask the client to recall past surgeries or accidents. Ask the client to describe any prolonged episodes of pain or pain patterns he or she has experienced. Inquire about any allergies (food, medicine, pollens, other) and use of prescription and OTC medications.

BOX 2-4 COMPONENTS OF THE COLDSPA SYMPTOM ANALYSIS MNEMONIC

The COLDSPA example here provides a sample application of the COLDSPA mnemonic adapted to analyze back pain.

Mnemonic	Question
Character	Describe the sign or symptom (feeling, appearance, sound, smell, or taste if applicable). "What does the pain feel like?"
Onset	When did it begin? "When did this pain start?"
Location	Where is it? Does it radiate? Does it occur anywhere else? "Where does it hurt the most? Does it radiate or go to any other part of your body?"
Duration	How long does it last? Does it recur? "How long does the pain last? Does it come and go or is it constant?"
Severity	How bad is it? How much does it bother you? "How intense is the pain? Rate it on a scale of 1–10."
Pattern	What makes it better or worse? "What makes your back pain worse or better? Are there any treatments you've tried that relieve the pain?"
Associated factors/How it affects the client	What other symptoms occur with it? How does it affect you? "What do you think caused it to start? Do you have any other problems that seem related to your back pain? How does this pain affect your life and daily activities?"

These questions elicit data about the client's health history related to his or her strengths and weaknesses. The information gained from these questions assists the nurse in identifying risk factors that stem from previous health problems. Risk factors may relate to the client or to significant others.

Information covered in this section includes questions about birth, growth, development, childhood diseases, immunizations, allergies, medication use, previous health problems, hospitalizations, surgeries, pregnancies, births, previous accidents, injuries, pain experiences, and emotional or psychiatric problems. Sample questions include:

- "Can you tell me how your mother described your birth? Were there any problems? As far as you know, did you progress normally as you grew to adulthood? Were there any problems that your family told you about or that you experienced?"
- "What diseases did you have as a child, such as measles or mumps? What immunizations did you get and are you up to date now?" (Visit www.cdc.gov/vaccines for the latest information on recommended immunizations.)
- "Do you have any chronic illnesses? If so, when were they diagnosed? How are they treated? How satisfied have you been with the treatment?"
- "What illnesses or allergies have you had? How were the illnesses treated?"
- "What medications have you used in the recent past and currently, both those that your doctor prescribed and those you can buy OTC at a drug or grocery store? For what purpose did you take the medication? How much (dose) and how often did you take the medication? Do you take any medications not prescribed for you but prescribed for a family member/friend or purchased on the street?"
- "Have you ever been pregnant and/or delivered a baby? How many times have you been pregnant/delivered?"
- "Have you ever been hospitalized or had surgery? If so, when? What were you hospitalized for or what type of surgery did you have? Was the surgery at an outpatient facility? Were there any complications?"
- "Have you experienced any accidents or injuries? Please describe them."
- "Have you experienced pain in any part of your body? Please describe the pain."
- "Have you ever been diagnosed with/treated for emotional or mental problems? If so, please describe their nature and any treatment received. Describe your level of satisfaction with the treatment."

How clients frame their previous health concerns suggests how they feel about themselves and is an indication of their sense of responsibility for their own health. For example, a client who has been obese for years may blame himself for developing diabetes and fail to comply with his diet, whereas another client may be very willing to share with a support group the treatment of her diabetes and success with an insulin pump. Some clients are very forthcoming about their past health status; others are not. It is helpful to have a series of alternative questions for less responsive clients and for those who may not understand what is being asked.

CASE STUDY

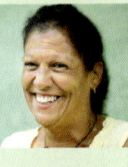

Mrs. Gutierrez does not have an accurate record of childhood health history but received updated immunizations when she came to the United States at 20 years of age. She denies previous surgeries and injuries. No known allergies to food, insects, drugs, and the environment. Does not take any prescribed medications but does "occasionally" use OTC Excedrin PM for sleep and Tylenol for headaches. Says she has been taking Excedrin PM about 3 times a week for the last 2 months. Had five pregnancies and experienced gestational diabetes during her last pregnancy. All five children are still alive. Was diagnosed with type 2 diabetes a month ago.

Family Health History

As researchers discover an increasing number of health problems that seem to run in families and that are genetically based, the family health history assumes greater importance. In addition to genetic predisposition, it is also helpful to be aware of other health problems that may have affected the client by virtue of having grown up in the family and being exposed to these problems. For example, a gene predisposing a person to smoking has not yet been discovered but a family with smoking members can affect other members in at least two ways. First, second-hand smoke can compromise the physical health of nonsmoking members; second, the smoker may serve as a negative role model for children, inducing them to take up the habit as well. Another example is obesity; recognizing it in the family history can alert the nurse to a potential risk factor.

The family history should include as many genetic relatives as the client can recall. Include maternal and paternal grandparents, aunts and uncles on both sides, parents, siblings, and the client's children. Such thoroughness usually identifies those diseases that may skip a generation, such as autosomal recessive disorders. Include the client's spouse but indicate that there is no genetic link. Identifying the spouse's health problems could explain disorders in the client's children not indicated in the client's family history.

Drawing a genogram (Fig. 2-4) helps to organize and illustrate the client's family history. Use a standard format so that others can easily understand the information. Also provide a key to the symbols used. Usually, female relatives are indicated by a circle and male relatives by a square. A deceased relative is noted by marking an X in the circle or square and listing the age at death and cause of death. Identify all relatives, living or dead, by age and provide a brief list of diseases or conditions. If the relative has no problems, the letters "A/W" (alive and well) should be placed next to the age. Straight vertical and horizontal lines are used to show relationships. A horizontal dotted line can be used to indicate the client's spouse; a vertical dotted line can be used to indicate adoption. A sample genogram is illustrated in Figure 2-4.

After the diagrammatic family history, prepare a brief summary of the kinds of health problems present in the family. For example, the client in the genogram depicted in Figure 2-4 has longevity, obesity, heart disease, hypertension (HTN), arthritis, thyroid disorders, type 1 or type 2 diabetes, alcoholism, smoking, myopia, learning disability, hyperactivity disorder, and cancer (one relative) on his maternal side. On the client's paternal side are obesity, heart disease, hypercholesterolemia, back problems, arthritis, myopia, and cancer. The paternal history is not as extensive as the maternal history because the client's father was adopted. In addition, the client's sister is obese and has Graves disease and hypercholesterolemia. His wife has arthritis; his children are both A/W.

CASE STUDY

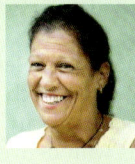

Mrs. Gutierrez has little knowledge of her family history as she was abandoned by her parents as an infant and was adopted. Thus a family genogram as illustrated in Figure 2-4 is not feasible with this client.

Review of Systems for Current Health Problems

In the review of systems (or review of body systems, ROS), each body system is addressed and the client is asked specific questions to elicit further details of current health problems or problems from the recent past that may still affect the client or that are recurring. Care must be taken in this section to include only the client's subjective information and not the examiner's observations. There is a tendency, especially with more experienced nurses, to fill up the spaces with observations such as "erythema of the right eye" or "several vesicles on the client's upper extremities."

During the ROS, document the client's descriptions of her health status for each body system and note the client's denial of signs, symptoms, diseases, or problems that the nurse asks about but are not experienced by the client. For example, under the area "Head and Neck," the client may respond that there are no problems but on questioning from the nurse about headaches, stiffness, pain, or cracking in the neck with motion, swelling in the neck, difficulty swallowing, sore throat, enlarged lymph nodes, and so on, the client may suddenly remember that he did have a sore throat a week ago that he self-treated with zinc lozenges. This information might not have emerged without specific questions. Also, if the lone entry "no problems" is entered on the health history form, other health care professionals reviewing the history cannot ascertain what specific questions had been asked, if any.

The questions about problems and signs or symptoms of disorders should be asked in terms that the client understands, but findings should be recorded in standard medical terminology. If the client is determined to have a limited vocabulary, the nurse may need to ask questions in several different ways and use very basic lay terminology. If the client is well educated and seems familiar with medical terminology, the nurse should not insult her by talking at a much lower level. The most obvious information to collect for each body part or system is presented in the following list. See the physical assessment chapters for in-depth questions and rationales for each body part or system.

- *Skin, hair, and nails:* skin color, temperature, condition, excessive sweating, rashes, lesions, balding, dandruff, condition of nails
- *Head and neck:* headache, swelling, stiffness of neck, difficulty swallowing, sore throat, enlarged lymph nodes
- *Eyes:* vision, eye infections, redness, excessive tearing, halos around lights, blurring, loss of side vision, moving black spots/specks in visual fields, flashing lights, double vision, and eye pain
- *Ears:* hearing, ringing or buzzing, earaches, drainage from ears, dizziness, exposure to loud noises
- *Mouth, throat, nose, and sinuses:* condition of teeth and gums; sore throats; mouth lesions; hoarseness; rhinorrhea; nasal obstruction; frequent colds; sneezing or itching of eyes, ears, nose, or throat; nose bleeds; snoring
- *Thorax and lungs:* difficulty breathing, wheezing, pain, shortness of breath during routine activity, orthopnea, cough or sputum, hemoptysis, respiratory infections
- *Breasts and regional lymphatics:* lumps or discharge from nipples, dimpling or changes in breast size, swollen or tender lymph nodes in axilla

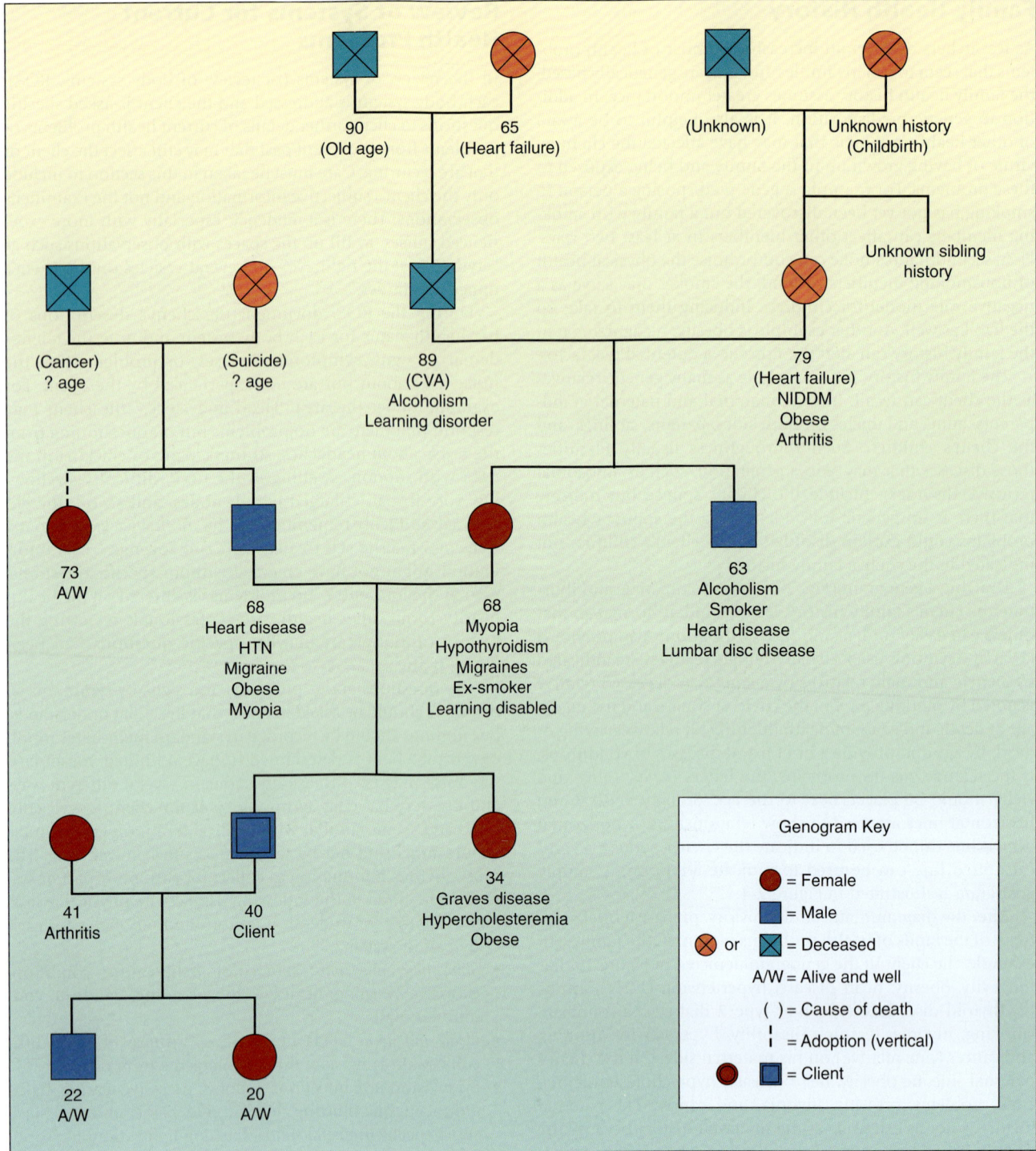

FIGURE 2-4 Genogram of a 40-year-old male client.

- *Heart and neck vessels:* last blood pressure, electrocardiogram (ECG) tracing or findings, chest pain or pressure, palpitations, edema
- *Peripheral vascular:* swelling, or edema, of legs and feet; pain; cramping; sores on legs; color or texture changes on the legs or feet
- *Abdomen:* indigestion, difficulty swallowing, nausea, vomiting, abdominal pain, gas, jaundice, hernias
- *Male genitalia:* excessive or painful urination, frequency or difficulty starting and maintaining urinary stream, leaking of urine, blood noted in urine, sexual problems, perineal lesions, penile drainage, pain or swelling in scrotum, difficulty achieving an erection and/or difficulty ejaculating, exposure to sexually transmitted infections (STIs)
- *Female genitalia:* sexual problems; STIs; voiding problems (e.g., dribbling, incontinence); reproductive data such as age at menarche, menstruation (length and regularity of cycle), pregnancies, and type of or problems with delivery, abortions, pelvic pain, contraception, menopause (date or

year of last menstrual period), and use of hormone replacement therapy (HRT)
- *Anus, rectum, and prostate:* bowel habits, pain with defecation, hemorrhoids, blood in stool, constipation, diarrhea
- *Musculoskeletal:* swelling, redness, pain, stiffness of joints, ability to perform ADLs, muscle strength
- *Neurologic:* general mood, behavior, depression, anger, concussions, headaches, loss of strength or sensation, coordination, difficulty speaking, memory problems, strange thoughts and/or actions, difficulty learning

Anus, rectum, and prostate: reports a daily bowel movement of well-formed brown stool. Denies tenesmus, hemorrhoids, hematochezia, melena, constipation, diarrhea.
Musculoskeletal: denies swelling, redness, pain, and stiffness of joints. Is able to perform ADLs without difficulty.
Neurologic: describes sadness and being tearful at times. Denies depression, anger, and suicidal thoughts. Denies concussions, headaches, loss of strength or sensation, lack of coordination, difficulty speaking, memory problems, strange thoughts and/or actions, or difficulty learning.

CASE STUDY

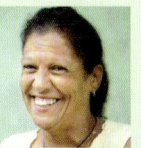

Review of systems for Mrs. Gutierrez:

Skin, hair, and nails: denies problems with skin, hair, or nails. Denies alopecia, dandruff, oiliness, thin nails, brittle nails, clubbing nails, dry skin, onychomycosis, lesions, changes in moles, rashes, and so on.
Head and neck: denies headaches, swelling, stiffness of neck, difficulty swallowing, sore throat, enlarged lymph nodes.
Eyes: wears glasses for reading, denies eye infections, redness, excessive tearing, halos around lights, blurring, loss of side vision, moving black spots/specks in visual fields, flashing lights, double vision, and eye pain.
Ears: denies loss of hearing, ringing or buzzing, earaches, drainage from ears, dizziness, exposure to loud noises.
Mouth, throat, nose, and sinuses: reports missing upper molars, denies bleeding of gums or other dental problems, sore throats; mouth lesions; hoarseness; rhinorrhea; nasal obstruction; frequent colds; sneezing or itching of eyes, ears, nose, or throat; nose bleeds; snoring.
Thorax and lungs: denies difficulty breathing, wheezing, pain, shortness of breath during routine activity, orthopnea, cough or sputum, hemoptysis, respiratory infections.
Breasts and regional lymphatics: denies lumps or discharge from nipples, dimpling or changes in breast size, swollen or tender lymph nodes in axilla.
Heart and neck vessels: reports last blood pressure was 130/84, denies chest pain or pressure, palpitations, edema.
Peripheral vascular: denies swelling, or edema, of legs and feet; pain; cramping; sores on legs; color or texture changes on the legs or feet.
Abdomen: describes anorexia and abdominal fullness. Denies difficulty swallowing, nausea, vomiting, gas, jaundice, hernias.
Female genitalia: Denies sexual problems; STIs; denies urgency, frequency, incontinence, dysuria, hematuria, changes in urinary stream, polyuria, nocturia, oliguria, and hesitancy; age 13 at menarche, menopause at age 51; 5 pregnancies (gravida 5, para 5, aborto 0). Gestational diabetes with last child. Denies abortions, pelvic pain, use of contraception, or use of HRT.

Lifestyle and Health Practices Profile

This is a very important section of the health history because it deals with the client's human responses, which include nutritional habits, activity and exercise patterns, sleep and rest patterns, self-concept and self-care activities, social and community activities, relationships, values and beliefs system, education and work, stress level and coping style, and environment.

Here clients describe how they are managing their lives, their awareness of healthy versus toxic living patterns, and the strengths and supports they have or use. When assessing this area, use open-ended questions to promote a dialog with the client. Follow up with specific questions to guide the discussion and clarify the information as necessary. Be sure to pay special attention to the cues the client may provide that point to possibly more significant content. Take brief notes so that pertinent data are not lost and so there can be follow up if some information needs clarification or expansion. If clients give permission and it does not seem to cause anxiety or inhibition, using a recording device frees the nurse from the need to write while clients talk.

In this section, each area is discussed briefly, then followed by a few sample questions. These questions elicit data in the client's health history related to his or her strengths and weaknesses. The client's strengths may be social (e.g., active in community services), emotional (e.g., expresses feeling openly), or spiritual (often turns to faith for support). The data may also point to trends of unhealthy behaviors such as smoking or lack of physical activity.

Description of Typical Day

This information is necessary to elicit an overview of how the client sees his usual pattern of daily activity. The questions you ask should be vague enough to allow the client to provide the orientation from which the day is viewed, for example, "Please tell me what an average or typical day is for you. Start with awakening in the morning and continue until bedtime." Encourage the client to discuss a usual day, which, for most people, includes work or school. If the client gives minimal information, additional specific questions may be asked to elicit more details.

Nutrition and Weight Management

Ask the client to recall what consists of an average 24-hour intake with emphasis on what foods are eaten and in what amounts. Also ask about snacks, fluid intake, and other substances consumed. Depending on the client, you may want to ask who buys and prepares the food as well as when and where meals are eaten. These questions uncover food habits that are health promoting as well as those that are less desirable. The client's answers about food intake should be compared with the various guidelines described in Chapter 13. MyPlate, developed by the U.S. Department of Agriculture, is designed to teach people what types and amounts of food to eat to ensure a balanced diet, promote health, and prevent disease (ChooseMyPlate, n.d.). Consider reviewing the food pyramid with the client and explaining what a serving size is.

Sample questions include:
- "What do you usually eat during a typical day? Please tell me the kinds of foods you prefer, how often you eat throughout the day, and how much you eat."
- "Do you eat out at restaurants frequently?"
- "Do you eat only when hungry? Do you eat because of boredom, habit, anxiety, depression?"
- "Who buys and prepares the food you eat?"
- "Where do you eat your meals?"
- "How much and what types of fluids do you drink?"

Activity Level and Exercise

Next, assess how active the client is during an average week either at work or at home. Inquire about regular exercise. Some clients believe that if they do heavy physical work at their job, they do not need additional exercise. Make it a point to distinguish between activities done when working, which may be stressful and fatiguing, and exercise, which is designed to reduce stress and strengthen the individual. Compare the client's answers with the current exercise regimen recommended for adults of 150 minutes per week, with muscle strengthening activities on 2 or more days a week (CDC, 2015). Explain to the client that regular exercise reduces the risk of heart disease, strengthens heart and lungs, reduces stress, and manages weight.

Sample questions include:
- "What is your daily pattern of activity?"
- "Do you follow a regular exercise plan? What types of exercise do you do?"
- "Are there any reasons why you cannot follow a moderately strenuous exercise program?"
- "What do you do for leisure and recreation?"
- "Do your leisure and recreational activities include exercise?"

Sleep and Rest

Inquire whether the client feels he is getting enough sleep and rest. Questions should focus on specific sleep patterns, such as how many hours a night the person sleeps, interruptions, whether the client feels rested, problems in sleeping (e.g., insomnia), rituals the client uses to promote sleep, and concerns the client may have regarding sleep habits. Some of this information may have already been presented by the client, but it is useful to gather data in a more systematic and thorough manner at this time. Inquiries about sleep can bring out problems, such as anxiety, which manifests as sleeplessness, or inadequate sleep time, which can predispose the client to accidents. Compare the client's answers with the normal sleep requirement for adults, which is usually between 5 and 8 hours a night. Keep in mind that sleep requirements vary depending on age, health, and stress levels.

Sample questions include:
- "Tell me about your sleeping patterns."
- "Do you have trouble falling asleep or staying asleep?"
- "How much sleep do you get each night?"
- "Do you feel rested when you awaken?"
- "Do you nap during the day? How often and for how long?"
- "What do you do to help you fall asleep?"

See Evidence-Based Health Promotion and Disease Prevention 2-1 and Box 2-5 for more detailed discussions of sleep and insomnia (in addition, see National Center for Complementary and Integrative Health, 2014; National Sleep Foundation, 2014; Rettner, 2015).

Substance Use

The information gathered about substance use provides the nurse with data concerning lifestyle and a client's self-care ability. Substance use can affect the client's health and cause loss of function or impaired senses. In addition, certain substances can increase the client's risk for disease. Also, because many people use vitamins or a variety of herbal supplements, it is important to ask which ones and how often. These supplements and prescription medications may interact (e.g., garlic decreases coagulation and interacts with warfarin [Coumadin]).

Sample questions include:
- "How much beer, wine, or other alcohol do you drink on average?"

BOX 2-5 STANFORD SLEEPINESS SCALE

This is a quick way to assess how alert you are feeling. During the day when you go about your business, ideally you would want a rating of "1." Take into account that most people have two peak times of alertness daily, at about 9 AM and 9 PM. Alertness wanes to its lowest point at around 3 PM, and after that begins to build again. Rate your alertness at different times during the day. If your score is greater than "3" during a time when you should feel alert, you may have a serious sleep debt and require more sleep.

DEGREE OF SLEEPINESS SCALE RATING

Feeling active, vital, alert, or wide awake	1
Functioning at high levels, but not at peak; able to concentrate	2
Awake, but relaxed; responsive but not fully alert	3
Somewhat foggy, let down	4
Foggy; losing interest in remaining awake; slowed down	5
Sleepy, woozy, fighting sleep; prefer to lie down	6
No longer fighting sleep, sleep onset soon; having dream-like thoughts	7
Asleep	X

Stanford Sleepiness Scale. Available at http://chicagosleepapneasnoring.com/test-your-sleepiness/stanford-sleepiness-scale

2-1 EVIDENCE-BASED HEALTH PROMOTION AND DISEASE PREVENTION: INSOMNIA

INTRODUCTION

The National Center for Complementary and Alternative Medicine (Wickwire, 2014) reported that insomnia and sleep disorders affect millions of people, and studies estimate the related cost to be between $30 and $107 billion yearly plus high levels of lost productivity. Of more than 80 sleep disorders, insomnia is one of the more common. Insomnia is a term that is used in many ways in the lay and medical literature. In the clinical guideline for managing adult insomnia, Schutte-Rodin et al. (2008) defined insomnia as "the subjective perception of difficulty with sleep initiation, duration, consolidation, or quality that occurs despite adequate opportunity for sleep, and that results in some form of daytime impairment." The American Sleep Association (2015) says that insomnia exists when a person has trouble falling or staying asleep. Insomnia can be acute or chronic, and primary or secondary. Criteria for chronic insomnia include episodes occurring at least 3 times per week over a minimum period of 1 month. Secondary insomnia, the most common form, results as a symptom or side effect of another condition, such as pain, anxiety, depression, illness (including lung and heart), or substance intake (caffeine, tobacco, alcohol), or of other sleep disorders, including restless leg syndrome, poor sleep environment, or change in sleep routine.

According to Healthy People 2020 (HealthyPeople.gov, 2014), the many areas of well-being for which adequate sleep is necessary include fighting off infection, preventing diabetes by supporting sugar metabolism, working and performing effectively and safely at school and at work. In addition, Healthy People 2020 notes that sleep timing and duration have effects on endocrine, metabolic, and neurologic functions, and chronic short sleep has been associated with heart disease, HTN, obesity, diabetes, and all-cause mortality.

Heffron (2014) reported that 10% of US adults have chronic insomnia, and up to 35% experience brief insomnia symptoms. Separate analysis remains to be done on the precise categories of sleep disorders identified in the *International Classification of Sleep Disorders—Third Edition (ICSD-3)* (American Academy of Sleep Medicine, 2014). These categories include: insomnia, sleep-related breathing disorders, central disorders of hypersomnolence, circadian rhythm sleep–wake disorders, parasomnias, and sleep-related movement disorders.

HEALTHY PEOPLE 2020 GOAL

Healthy People 2020 have placed sleep health as a new category in their topics and objectives, with an update in 2014. The foci of the topic for major sleep disorders are sleep apnea and insomnia, as well as all sleep disorders that affect well-being.

Goal

Increase public knowledge of how adequate sleep and treatment of sleep disorders improve health, productivity, wellness, quality of life, and safety on roads and in the workplace.

Objectives

- Increase the proportion of persons with symptoms of obstructive sleep apnea who seek medical evaluation.
- Reduce the rate of vehicular crashes per 100 million miles traveled that are due to drowsy driving.
- Increase the proportion of students in grades 9 through 12 who get sufficient sleep.
- Increase the proportion of adults who get sufficient sleep.

SCREENING

There are many screening tools that can be used in a primary care or in-patient setting. In addition, there are medical examinations that can be done at sleep clinics to evaluate sleep breathing and brain patterns. An easy way to evaluate sleep is the Sleep Self-Assessment Quiz found online at http://www.talkaboutsleep.com/sleep-self-assessment-quiz/

RISK ASSESSMENT

There are many risk factors that can lead to insomnia. Frequently noted are:
- Gender (especially female, due to hormone changes)
- Age (older than 60; older adults have more difficulty in falling asleep and staying asleep; amount of sleep needed does not decrease with age)
- Mental health and psychiatric disorders
- Stress and anxiety (especially causing hypervigilance and hyperarousal)
- Depression
- Pain medications, decongestants, and antihistamines, which cause frequent urination
- Medications for weight loss, heart, thyroid, HTN, asthma, depression, and birth control
- Stimulants (coffee, tea, soft drinks, energy drinks, and others)
- Alcohol (prevents deeper stages of sleep)
- Medical conditions
- Chronic pain and chronic low back pain
- Breathing difficulties
- Arthritis
- Diabetes
- Cardiovascular disease
- Cancer
- Frequent urination
- Gastroesophageal reflux disease (GERD)
- Sleep disorders (sleep apnea, restless leg syndrome)
- Obesity
- Environmental changes (shift work, long distance travel/jet lag)
- Sleep habits (no bedtime routine or stimulating activities before bed, heavy meal before bed)

(Healthline, 2014; Mayo Clinic, 2014; National Sleep Foundation, 2014; Sleepdex, n.d.)

CLIENT EDUCATION

- Establish a regular sleep schedule; maintain a regular bed and wake time schedule, including weekends.
- Establish a regular, relaxing bedtime routine such as soaking in a hot bath or hot tub and then reading a book or listening to soothing music.
- Create a sleep-conducive environment that is dark, quiet, comfortable, and cool.
- Sleep on a comfortable mattress and pillows.
- Use your bedroom only for sleep and sex.
- Finish eating at least 2–3 hours before your regular bedtime.
- Exercise regularly; complete exercise at least a few hours before bedtime.
- Avoid caffeine (coffee, tea, sodas), nicotine, and alcohol (drinking alcohol does not aid sleep because it prevents deep sleep).
- Use OTC sleep medications with caution, and only for short periods.
- Seek medical advice for prescription sleep medications and only use them short term.
- Seek cognitive-behavioral therapies for long-term benefits.
- Avoid napping during the day.

Explain to clients that caution should be used with complementary and alternative medicine (CAM) approaches for insomnia. Some personal research is needed before implementing some of these therapies, especially herbs. Research studies are just beginning to be completed on many of these, and early results are mixed. CAM therapies for insomnia include:
- Herbs, aromatherapy, chamomile tea, and herbal supplements such as valerian, as well as kava and various "sleep formula" products (Kava has shown a possible side effect of liver dysfunction.)
- Melatonin and related dietary supplements
- Acupuncture, music therapy, and relaxation techniques (these therapies have some supportive findings)

- "Do you drink coffee or other beverages containing caffeine (e.g., cola)? If so, how much and how often?"
- "Do you now or have you ever smoked cigarettes or used any other form of nicotine? How long have you been smoking/did you smoke? How many packs per week? Tell me about any efforts to quit."
- "Have you ever taken any medication *not prescribed* by your health care provider? If so, when, what type, how much, and why?"
- "Have you ever used, or do you now use, recreational drugs? Describe any usage."
- "Do you take vitamins or herbal supplements? If so, what?"

Self-Concept and Self-Care Responsibilities

This includes assessment of how the client views herself and investigation of all behaviors that a person does to promote her health. Examples of subjects to be addressed include sexual responsibility; basic hygiene practices; regularity of health care checkups (i.e., dental, visual, medical); breast/testicular self-examination; and accident prevention and hazard protection (e.g., seat belts, smoke alarms, and sunscreen).

You can correlate answers to questions in this area with health promotion activities discussed previously and with risk factors from the family history. This will help to point out client strengths and needs for health maintenance. Questions to the client can be open ended but the client may need prompting to cover all areas.

Sample questions include:
- "What do you see as your talents or special abilities?"
- "How do you feel about yourself? About your appearance?"
- "Can you tell me what activities you do to keep yourself safe, healthy, or to prevent disease?"
- "Do you practice safe sex?"
- "How do you keep your home safe?"
- "Do you drive safely?"
- "How often do you have medical checkups or screenings?"
- "How often do you see the dentist or have your eyes (vision) examined?"

Social Activities

Questions about social activities help the nurse to discover what outlets the client has for support and relaxation and if the client is involved in the community beyond family and work. Information in this area also helps to determine the client's current level of social development. Sample questions include:
- "What do you do for fun and relaxation?"
- "With whom do you socialize most frequently?"
- "Are you involved in any community activities?"
- "How do you feel about your community?"
- "Do you think that you have enough time to socialize?"
- "What do you see as your contribution to society?"

Relationships

Ask clients to describe the composition of the family into which they were born and about past and current relationships with these family members. In this way, you can assess problems and potential support from the client's family of origin. In addition, similar information should be sought about the client's current family (Fig. 2-5). If the client does not have any family by blood or marriage, then information should be gathered about any significant others (including pets) who may constitute the client's "family."

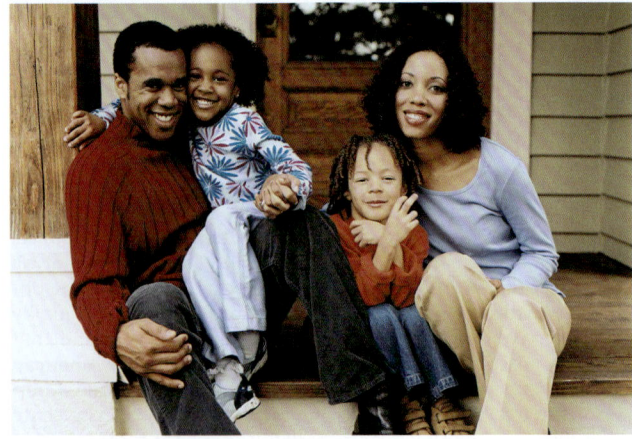

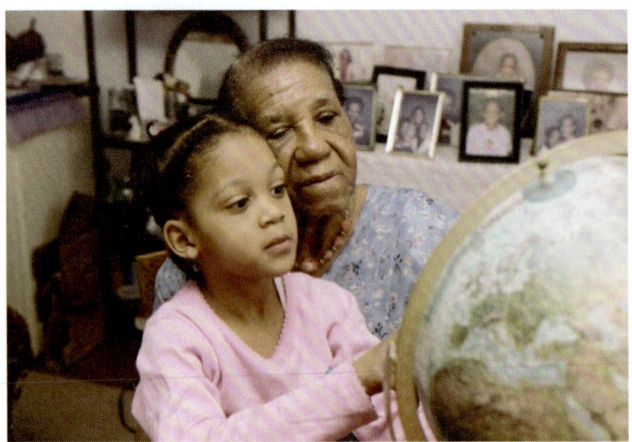

FIGURE 2-5 Discussing family relationships is a key way to assess support systems.

Sample questions include:
- "Who is (are) the most important person(s) in your life? Describe your relationship with that person."
- "What was it like growing up in your family?"
- "What is your relationship like with your spouse?"
- "What is your relationship like with your children?"
- "Describe any relationships you have with significant others."
- "Do you get along with your in-laws?"
- "Are you close to your extended family?"
- "Do you have any pets?"
- "What is your role in your family? Is it an important role?"
- "Are you satisfied with your current sexual relationships? Have there been any recent changes?"

Values and Belief System

Assess the client's values. In addition, discuss the client's philosophical, religious, and spiritual beliefs. Some clients may not be comfortable discussing values or beliefs. Their feelings should be respected. However, the data can help to identify important problems or strengths.

Sample questions include:
- "What is most important to you in life?"
- "What do you hope to accomplish in your life?"
- "Do you have a religious affiliation? Is this important to you?"
- "Is a relationship with God (or another higher power) an important part of your life?"
- "What gives you strength and hope?"

Education and Work

Questions about education and work help to identify areas of stress and satisfaction in the client's life. If the client does not perceive that he has enough education or his work is not what he enjoys, he may need assistance or support to make changes. Sometimes discussing this area will help the client feel good about what he has accomplished and promote his sense of life satisfaction. Questions should bring out data about the kind and amount of education the client has, whether the client enjoyed school, whether he perceives his education as satisfactory or whether there were problems, and what plans the client may have for further education, either formal or informal. Similar questions should be asked about work history.

Sample questions include:
- "Tell me about your experiences in school or about your education."
- "Are you satisfied with the level of education you have? Do you have future educational plans?"
- "What can you tell me about your work? What are your responsibilities at work?"
- "Do you enjoy your work?"
- "How do you feel about your coworkers?"
- "What kind of stress do you have that is work related? Any major problems?"
- "Who is the main provider of financial support in your family?"
- "Does your current income meet your needs?"

Stress Levels and Coping Styles

To investigate the amount of stress clients perceive they are under and how they cope with it, ask questions that address what events cause stress for the client and how they usually respond. In addition, find out what the client does to relieve stress and whether these behaviors or activities can be construed as adaptive or maladaptive. To avoid denial responses, nondirective questions or observations regarding previous information provided by the client may be an easy way to get the client to discuss this subject.

Sample questions include:
- "What types of things make you angry?"
- "How would you describe your stress level?"
- "How do you manage anger or stress?"
- "What do you see as the greatest stressors in your life?"
- "Where do you usually turn for help in a time of crisis?"

Environment

Ask questions regarding the client's environment to assess health hazards unique to the client's living situation and lifestyle. Look for physical, chemical, or psychological situations that may put the client at risk. These may be found in the client's neighborhood, home, work, or recreational environment. They may be controllable or uncontrollable.

Sample questions include:
- "What risks are you aware of in your environment such as in your home, neighborhood, on the job, or any other activities in which you participate?"
- "What types of precautions do you take, if any, when playing contact sports, using harsh chemicals or paint, or operating machinery?"
- "Do you believe you are ever in danger of becoming a victim of violence? Explain."

CASE STUDY

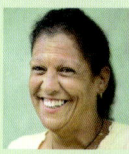

Mrs. Gutierrez reports that she gets up at 6 AM every day, does laundry, housework, and begins to prepare meals for the day. She enjoys working outside but has not been able to do so as much as she did since her husband's accident. She used to attend the 7 AM Sunday mass service at her church, but has not done so recently. She talks with her sisters in Mexico once a week. Bedtime is usually after the news, at 10:30 PM.

Twenty-four hour dietary recall:
- *Breakfast*: small (4 oz) bowl of oatmeal with milk and sugar
- *Lunch*: plain tortilla with a glass of milk
- *Supper*: a few bites of chicken and rice with a glass of water. Currently, her daughter does all the grocery shopping that she used to do. Client does not typically eat at restaurants.

When feeling well, client does all housework and gardening by herself. Denies any participation in a regular aerobic exercise routine. She likes to attend the dinners at church and Bingo on Friday nights. Denies any hobbies for leisure.

Falls asleep about 10 PM, wakes up about 2 AM and cannot go back to sleep. Does not nap during the day. Has difficulty staying asleep. Feels tired all day long. Used to sleep all night without a problem, but has had continued problems getting to sleep and staying asleep since husband's accident 2 months ago.

Does not drink alcohol. Used to drink 3–4 cups of coffee a day, but has stopped in order to help her sleep. Denies use of tobacco products, recreational drugs, or complementary and alternative medications.

She describes her talent as being a good mother and housekeeper. "I used to be pretty, but I have gained so much weight and do not feel like taking care of myself. My husband and I used to have a good relationship, but we do not spend much time with each other over the last 5 years or so. I do not drive, my daughter takes me where I need to go." Sees a primary care provider yearly and goes to the eye doctor whenever her prescription needs to be changed (unable to give an estimate of how often).

Reports "frequent feelings of loneliness." She cannot describe how often but indicates a general sense of loneliness with her siblings and parents living so far away in Mexico. "I worry a lot, especially when my husband had the accident and cannot work. We were planning a trip to Mexico to see my family and now we cannot go because we do not have enough money. I used to pray when I worried but that does not seem to help anymore. His accident was such a shock to me!"

Client lives in a three-bedroom home with city water, hot water heater, electricity, and a gas stove, but she says the electricity bill is so high that they often avoid using any source of heat or cooling. She denies smoke detectors or CO detectors. States that there are often neighborhood fights outside, but she and her husband do not get involved. Feels fairly safe, but worries about the neighborhood sometimes. She denies guns or ammunition in house. States medications are kept in kitchen cabinet. Says car has seatbelts but often they are not used in her community or by her and her husband.

SUMMARY

Collecting subjective data is a key step of nursing health assessment. Subjective data consist of information elicited and verified only by the client. Interviewing is the means by which subjective data are gathered. Two types of communication are useful for interviewing: nonverbal and verbal. Variations in communication—such as gerontologic, cultural, and emotional variations—may be encountered during the client interview.

The complete health history is performed to collect as much subjective data about a client as possible. It consists of eight sections: biographical data, reasons for seeking health care, history of present health concern, personal health history, family health history, ROS for current health problems, lifestyle and health practices, and developmental level.

Want to know more?

A wide variety of resources to enhance your learning and understanding of this book are available on thePoint. Visit thePoint to access:

NCLEX-Style Student Review Questions
Watch and Learn Videos
Concepts in Action Animations
And more!

References and Selected Readings

Agency for Healthcare Research & Quality (AHRQ). (2012). Five major steps to intervention: The five A's. Available at http://www.ahrq.gov/professionals/clinicians-providers/guidelines-recommendations/tobacco/5steps.html

American Academy of Sleep Medicine. (2014). International classification of sleep disorders—third edition (ICSD-3) online version. Available at http://www.aasmnet.org/store/product.aspx?pid=849

American Sleep Association. (2015). About insomnia. Available at https://www.sleepassociation.org/patients-general-public/insomnia/insomnia/

Andrews, M., & Boyle, J. (2015). *Transcultural concepts in nursing care* (7th ed.). Philadelphia, PA: Wolters Kluwer/Lippincott Williams & Wilkins.

Centers for Disease Control & Prevention (CDC). (2015). How much physical activity do you need? Available at http://www.cdc.gov/physicalactivity/basics/index.htm

Giger, J. (2013). *Transcultural nursing: Assessment and intervention* (6th ed.). St. Louis, MO: Mosby-Year Book.

Healthline. (2014). Insomnia: Causes and risk factors Available at http://www.healthline.com/health/insomnia-causes#Overview1

HealthyPeople.gov. (2014). Sleep health. Available at https://www.healthypeople.gov/2020/topics-objectives/topic/sleep-health

Heffron, T. (2014). Insomnia Awareness Day facts and stats. Available at http://www.sleepeducation.com/news/2014/03/10/insomnia-awareness-day-facts-and-stats

Hepp, A. (2015). *Transcultural communication.* Hoboken, NJ: Wiley-Blackwell.

Mayo Clinic. (2014). Insomnia: Risk factors. Available at http://www.mayoclinic.org/diseases-conditions/insomnia/basics/risk-factors/con-20024293

Muñoz, C., & Luckmann, J. (2005). *Transcultural communication in health care* (2nd ed.). Albany, NY: Thomson-Delmar.

Nambudiri, N., & Nambudiri, V. E. (2013). "What brings you in today?" *Journal of ParticipativeMedicine,* 5. Available at http://www.medscape.com/viewarticle/810475

National Center for Complementary and Integrative Health (NCCIH). (2014). Sleep disorders and complementary health approaches. Available at https://nccih.nih.gov/health/providers/digest/sleep-disorders

National Sleep Foundation. (2014). Insomnia. Available at http://sleepfoundation.org/insomnia/home

Razzouk, D., Noguiera, B., & Mari Jde, J. (2011). The contribution of Latin American and Caribbean countries on culture bound syndromes studies for the ICD-10 revision: Key findings from a working in progress. *Revista Brasileira Psiquiatria. 33* Suppl 1, S5–S20.

Rettner, R. (2015). Insomnia: Symptoms, treatment & prevention. Available at http://www.livescience.com/34756-sleep-disorder-insomnia.html

Schutte-Rodin, S., Broch, L., Buysee, D., Dorsey, C., & Sateia, M. (2008). Clinical guideline for the evaluation and management of chronic insomnia in adults. *Journal of clinical sleep medicine, 4*(5), 487–504. Available at http://www.aasmnet.org/Resources/clinicalguidelines/040515.pdf

Sleepdex. (n.d.). Stress and its connection to insomnia. Available at http://www.sleepdex.org/stress.htm

U.S. Department of Agriculture (USDA). (n.d.). ChooseMyPlate. Available at http://www.choosemyplate.gov/

Wickwire, E. (2014). Financial costs of insomnia. Available at http://www.sleepreviewmag.com/2014/12/financial-costs-insomnia/

3 COLLECTING OBJECTIVE DATA: THE PHYSICAL EXAMINATION

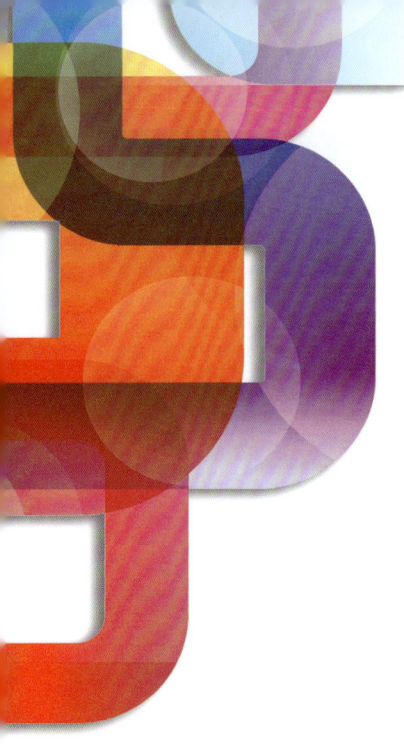

Learning Objectives

1. Explain how to prepare oneself, the physical environment, and the client for a physical examination.
2. Survey the various pieces of equipment needed to perform a physical examination.
3. Describe various client positions used for different parts of the physical examination.
4. Demonstrate correct inspection, palpation, percussion, and auscultation examination techniques.
5. Differentiate between light, deep, and bimanual palpation.
6. Describe the purpose of direct, indirect, and blunt percussion.
7. Discuss the purpose of the bell and diaphragm of the stethoscope.

CASE STUDY

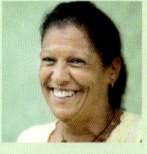

After establishing a working relationship with Mrs. Gutierrez through the patient interview described in Chapter 2, the nurse prepares to perform a physical assessment to collect objective data on Mrs. Gutierrez. The information collected in the interview warrants that a physical assessment is necessary. These additional data will help determine Mrs. Gutierrez's nursing diagnoses, collaborative problems, and whether a referral to a primary caregiver is necessary.

A complete nursing assessment includes both the collection of subjective data (discussed in Chapter 2) and the collection of objective data. Objective data include information about the client that the nurse directly observes during interaction with the client and information elicited through physical assessment (examination) techniques.

To become proficient with physical assessment skills, the nurse must have basic knowledge in three areas:
- Types and operation of equipment needed for the particular examination (e.g., penlight, sphygmomanometer, otoscope, tuning fork, stethoscope)
- Preparation of the setting, oneself, and the client for the physical assessment
- Performance of the four assessment techniques: inspection, palpation, percussion, and auscultation

EQUIPMENT

Each part of the physical examination requires specific pieces of equipment. Table 3-1 lists equipment necessary for each part of the examination and describes the general purpose of each piece of equipment. More detailed descriptions of each piece of equipment and the procedures for using them are provided in the chapters on the body systems where each item is used. For example, technique for using an ophthalmoscope is included in the eye assessment chapter. However, because the stethoscope is used during the assessment of many body systems, this chapter includes a description of it and guidelines on how to use it.

Prior to the examination, collect the necessary equipment and place it in the area where the examination will be performed. This promotes organization and prevents the nurse from leaving the client to search for a piece of equipment.

CASE STUDY

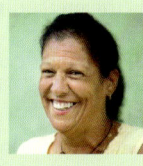

The nurse gathers all of the equipment needed for the physical assessment to use with Mrs. Gutierrez.

PREPARING FOR THE EXAMINATION

How well you prepare the physical setting, yourself, and the client can affect the quality of the data you elicit. As an

31

TABLE 3-1 Equipment Needed for Physical Examination

Examination	Equipment	Purpose
All examinations	Gloves and gown	Protect examiner in any part of the examination when the examiner may have contact with blood, body fluids, secretions, excretions, and contaminated items, or when disease-causing agents could be transmitted to or from the client
Vital signs	Sphygmomanometer	Measure diastolic and systolic blood pressure. Stethoscope to auscultate blood sounds when measuring blood pressure
	Thermometer (oral, rectal, tympanic)	Measure body temperature
	Watch with second hand	Take heart rate, pulse rate
	Pain rating scale	Determine perceived pain level
Nutritional status examination	Skinfold calipers	Measure skinfold thickness of subcutaneous tissue
	Flexible tape measure	Measure midarm circumference
	Skin-marking pen	Mark measurements
	Platform scale with height attachment	Measure height and weight
Skin, hair, and nail examination	Examination light, penlight	Provide adequate lighting
	Mirror	Client's self-examination of the skin
	Metric ruler	Measure size of skin lesions
	Magnifying glass	Enlarge visibility of lesion
	Wood's light	Test for fungus
	Braden Scale for predicting Pressure sore risk	Predict one's risk to develop pressure sore
	Pressure Ulcer Scale for Healing (PUSH)	Determine the degree of healing of a pressure ulcer
Head and neck examination	Stethoscope	Auscultate the thyroid
	Small cup of water	Help client swallow during examination of the thyroid gland
Eye examination	Penlight	Test pupillary constriction
	Snellen E chart	Test distant vision
	Newspaper	Test near vision
	Opaque card	Test for strabismus
	Ophthalmoscope	View the red reflex and to examine the retina of the eye
Ear examination	Tuning fork	Test for bone and air conduction of sound
	Otoscope	View the ear canal and tympanic membrane
Mouth, throat, nose, and sinus examination	Penlight	Provide light to view the mouth and the throat and to transilluminate the sinuses
	4 × 4-in small gauze pad	Grasp tongue to examine mouth
	Tongue depressor	Depress tongue to view throat, check looseness of teeth, view cheeks, and check strength of tongue
	Otoscope with wide-tip attachment	View the internal nose
Thoracic and lung examination	Stethoscope (diaphragm)	Auscultate breath sounds
	Metric ruler and skin-marking pen	Measure diaphragmatic excursion
Heart and neck vessel examination	Stethoscope (bell and diaphragm)	Auscultate heart sounds
	Two metric rulers	Measure jugular venous pressure
Peripheral vascular examination	Sphygmomanometer and stethoscope	Measure blood pressure and auscultate vascular sounds
	Flexible metric measuring tape	Measure size of extremities for edema
	Tuning fork	Detect vibratory sensation
	Doppler ultrasound device and conductivity gel	Detect pressure and weak pulses not easily heard with a stethoscope
Abdominal examination	Stethoscope	Detect bowel sounds
	Flexible metric measuring tape and skin-marking pen	Measure size and mark the area of percussion of organs
	Two small pillows	Place under knees and head to promote relaxation of abdomen
Musculoskeletal examination	Flexible metric measuring tape	Measure size of extremities
	Goniometer	Measure degree of flexion and extension of joints

Examination	Equipment	Purpose
Neurologic examination	Cotton-tipped applicators and substances to smell and taste	Test taste smell perception
	Same equipment as for eye examination (see above)	Test vision and extraocular movements and papillary response
	Objects to feel, such as a coin or key	Test for stereognosis (ability to recognize objects by touch)
	Reflex (percussion) hammer	Test deep tendon reflexes
	Cotton ball and paper clip	Test for light, sharp, and dull touch and two-point discrimination
	Tongue depressor	Test for rise of uvula and gag reflex
	Tuning fork	Test for vibratory sensation
Male genitalia and rectum examination	Gloves and water-soluble lubricant	Promote comfort for client
	Penlight	Scrotal illumination
	Specimen card	Detect occult blood
Female genitalia and rectum examination	Vaginal speculum and water-soluble lubricant	Inspect cervix through dilatation of the vaginal canal
	Bifid spatula, endocervical broom	Obtain endocervical swab and cervical scrape and vaginal pool sample
	Large swabs	Vaginal examination
	Liquid Pap medium	Pap smear
	Specimen card	Detect occult blood

examiner, you must make sure that you have prepared for all three aspects before beginning an examination. Practicing with a friend, relative, or classmate will help you to achieve proficiency in all three aspects of preparation.

Preparing the Physical Setting

The physical examination may take place in a variety of settings such as a hospital room, outpatient clinic, physician's office, school health office, employee health office, or a client's home. It is important that the nurse strive to ensure that the examination setting meets the following conditions:

- Comfortable, warm room temperature: Provide a warm blanket if the room temperature cannot be adjusted.
- Private area free of interruptions from others: Close the door or pull the curtains if possible.
- Quiet area free of distractions: Turn off the radio, television, or other noisy equipment.
- Adequate lighting: It is best to use sunlight (when available). However, good overhead lighting is sufficient. A portable lamp is helpful for illuminating the skin and for viewing shadows or contours.
- Firm examination table or bed at a height that prevents stooping: A roll-up stool may be useful when it is necessary for the examiner to sit for parts of the assessment.
- A bedside table/tray to hold the equipment needed for the examination.

CASE STUDY

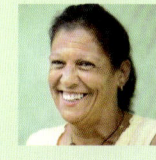 The nurse provides privacy and asks Mrs. Gutierrez to empty her bladder and put on an examination gown.

 ## Preparing Oneself

As a beginning examiner, it is helpful to assess your own feelings and anxieties before examining the client. Anxiety is easily conveyed to the client, who may already feel uneasy and self-conscious about the examination. Achieve self confidence in performing a physical assessment by practicing the techniques on a classmate, friend, or relative. Encourage your "pretend client" to simulate the client role as closely as possible. It is also important to perform some of your practice assessments with an experienced instructor or practitioner who can give you helpful hints and feedback on your technique.

Another important aspect of preparing yourself for the physical assessment examination is preventing the transmission of infectious agents. In 2007, the Centers for Disease Control and Prevention (CDC) and the Hospital Infection Control Practices Advisory Committee (HICPAC) updated Standard Precautions to be followed by all health care workers caring for clients (CDC & HICPAC, 2007). These Standard Precautions, shown in Box 3-1, are a modified combination of the original Universal Precautions and Body Substance Isolation Guidelines and are updated each year as necessary. The specific precaution or combination of precautions varies with the care to be provided. The CDC has superseded these general guidelines when care is provided for Ebola virus disease (see CDC, 2015, February 15 for details). For example, performing venipuncture requires only gloves, but intubation requires gloves, gown, and face shield, mask, or goggles. General principles to keep in mind while performing a physical assessment include the following:

- Wash your hands before beginning the examination, immediately after accidental direct contact with blood or other body fluids, and after completing the physical examination or after removing gloves. If possible, wash your hands in the examining room in front of the client. This assures your client that you are concerned about his or her safety. Review Box 3-1 for recommended hand hygiene practices.

BOX 3-1 CENTERS FOR DISEASE CONTROL AND PREVENTION (CDC) AND HEALTHCARE INFECTION CONTROL PRACTICES ADVISORY COMMITTEE (HICPAC) ISOLATION PRECAUTION GUIDELINES

STANDARD PRECAUTIONS

Assume that every person is potentially infected or colonized with an organism that could be transmitted in the health care setting, and apply the following infection control practices during the delivery of health care.

Hand Hygiene

- During the delivery of health care, avoid unnecessary touching of surfaces in close proximity to the patient to prevent both contamination of clean hands from environmental surfaces and transmission of pathogens from contaminated hands to surfaces.
- When hands are visibly dirty, contaminated with proteinaceous material, or visibly soiled with blood or body fluids, wash hands with either a nonantimicrobial soap and water or an antimicrobial soap and water.
- If hands are not visibly soiled, or after removing visible material with nonantimicrobial soap and water, decontaminate hands in the clinical situations described later. The preferred method of hand decontamination is with an alcohol-based hand rub. Alternatively, hands may be washed with an antimicrobial soap and water. Frequent use of alcohol-based hand rub immediately following hand washing with nonantimicrobial soap may increase the frequency of dermatitis.
- Perform hand hygiene
  - Before having direct contact with patients
  - After contact with blood, body fluids or excretions, mucous membranes, nonintact skin, or wound dressings
  - After contact with a patient's intact skin (e.g., when taking a pulse or blood pressure or lifting a patient)
  - If hands will be moving from a contaminated body site to a clean body site during patient care
  - After contact with inanimate objects (including medical equipment) in the immediate vicinity of the patient
  - After removing gloves
- Wash hands with nonantimicrobial soap and water or with antimicrobial soap and water if contact with spores (e.g., *Clostridium difficile* or *Bacillus anthracis*) is likely to have occurred. The physical action of washing and rinsing hands under such circumstances is recommended because alcohols, chlorhexidine, iodophors, and other antiseptic agents have poor activity against spores.
- Do not wear artificial fingernails or extenders if duties include direct contact with patients at high risk for infection and associated adverse outcomes (e.g., those in intensive care units [ICUs] or operating rooms).
- Develop an organizational policy on the wearing of non-natural nails by health care personnel who have direct contact with patients outside of the groups specified in the preceding text.

Personal Protective Equipment (PPE)

- Observe the following principles of use:
  - Wear PPE (gloves, gown, mouth/nose/eye protection) when the nature of the anticipated patient interaction indicates that contact with blood or body fluids may occur.
  - Prevent contamination of clothing and skin during the process of removing PPE.
  - Before leaving the patient's room or cubicle, remove and discard PPE.

Gloves

- Wear gloves when it can be reasonably anticipated that contact with blood or other potentially infectious materials, mucous membranes, nonintact skin, or potentially contaminated intact skin (e.g., of a patient incontinent of stool or urine) could occur.
- Wear gloves with fit and durability appropriate to the task.
- Wear disposable medical examination gloves for providing direct patient care.
- Wear disposable medical examination gloves or reusable utility gloves for cleaning the environment or medical equipment.
- Remove gloves after contact with a patient and/or the surrounding environment (including medical equipment) using proper technique to prevent hand contamination. Do not wear the same pair of gloves for the care of more than one patient. Do not wash gloves for the purpose of reuse since this practice has been associated with transmission of pathogens.
- Change gloves during patient care if the hands will move from a contaminated body site (e.g., perineal area) to a clean body site (e.g., face).

Gowns

- Wear a gown that is appropriate to the task to protect skin and prevent soiling or contamination of clothing during procedures and patient care activities when contact with blood, body fluids, secretions, or excretions is anticipated.
- Wear a gown for direct patient contact if the patient has uncontained secretions or excretions.
- Remove gown and perform hand hygiene before leaving the patient's environment.
- Do not reuse gowns, even for repeated contacts with the same patient.
- Routine donning of gowns upon entrance into a high-risk unit (e.g., ICU, neonatal intensive care unit [NICU], or hematopoietic stem cell transplant [HSCT] unit) is not indicated.

Mouth, Nose, Eye Protection

- Use PPE to protect the mucous membranes of the eyes, nose, and mouth during procedures and patient care activities that are likely to generate splashes or sprays of blood, body fluids, secretions, and excretions. Select masks, goggles, face shields, and combinations of each according to the need anticipated by the task performed.
- During aerosol-generating procedures (e.g., bronchoscopy, suctioning of the respiratory tract [if not using in-line suction catheters], endotracheal intubation) in patients who are not suspected of being infected with an agent for which respiratory protection is otherwise recommended (e.g., *Mycobacterium tuberculosis*, severe acute respiratory syndrome [SARS], or hemorrhagic fever viruses), wear one of the following: a face shield that fully covers the front and sides of the face, a mask with attached shield, or a mask and goggles (in addition to gloves and gown).

Respiratory Hygiene/Cough Etiquette

- Educate health care personnel on the importance of source control measures to contain respiratory secretions to prevent droplet and fomite transmission of respiratory pathogens, especially during seasonal outbreaks of viral respiratory tract infections (e.g., influenza, respiratory syncytial virus [RSV], adenovirus, parainfluenza virus) in communities.
- Implement the following measures to contain respiratory secretions in patients and accompanying individuals

who have signs and symptoms of a respiratory infection, beginning at the point of initial encounter in a health care setting (e.g., triage, reception and waiting areas in emergency departments, outpatient clinics, and physician offices).
- Post signs at entrances and in strategic places (e.g., elevators, cafeterias) within ambulatory and inpatient settings with instructions to patients and other persons with symptoms of a respiratory infection to cover their mouths/noses when coughing or sneezing, to use and dispose of tissues, and to perform hand hygiene after hands have been in contact with respiratory secretions.
- Provide tissues and no-touch receptacles (e.g., pedal-operated lid or open, plastic-lined waste basket) for disposal of tissues.
- Provide resources and instructions for performing hand hygiene in or near waiting areas in ambulatory and inpatient settings; provide conveniently located dispensers of alcohol-based hand rubs and, where sinks are available, supplies for hand washing.
- During periods of increased prevalence of respiratory infections in the community (e.g., as indicated by increased school absenteeism or increased number of patients seeking care for a respiratory infection), offer masks to coughing patients and other symptomatic persons (e.g., persons who accompany ill patients) upon entry into the facility or medical office and encourage them to maintain special separation, ideally a distance of at least 3 feet, from others in common waiting areas. Some facilities may find it logistically easier to institute this recommendation year-round as a standard of practice.

Patient Placement
- Include the potential for transmission of infectious agents in patient placement decisions. Place patients who pose a risk for transmission to others (e.g., uncontained secretions, excretions, or wound drainage; infants with suspected viral respiratory or gastrointestinal infections) in a single-patient room when available.
- Determine patient placement based on the following principles:
  - Route(s) of transmission of the known or suspected infectious agent
  - Risk factors for transmission in the infected patient
  - Risk factors for adverse outcomes resulting from a health care–associated infection in other patients in the area or room being considered for patient placement
  - Availability of single-patient rooms
  - Patient options for room sharing (e.g., cohorting patients with the same infection)

Patient Care Equipment and Instruments/Devices
- Establish policies and procedures for containing, transporting, and handling patient care equipment and instruments/devices that may be contaminated with blood or body fluids.
- Remove organic material from critical and semicritical instrument/devices using recommended cleaning agents before high-level disinfection and sterilization to enable effective disinfection and sterilization processes.
- Wear PPE (e.g., gloves, gown), according to the level of anticipated contamination, when handling patient care equipment and instruments/devices that are visibly soiled or may have been in contact with blood or body fluids.

Care of the Environment
- Establish policies and procedures for routine and targeted cleaning of environmental surfaces as indicated by the level of patient contact and degree of soiling.
- Clean and disinfect surfaces that are likely to be contaminated with pathogens, including those that are in close proximity to the patient (e.g., bedrails, overbed tables) and frequently touched surfaces in the patient care environment (e.g., door knobs, surfaces in and surrounding toilets in patients' rooms) on a more frequent schedule compared to that for other surfaces (e.g., horizontal surfaces in waiting rooms).
- Use Environmental Protection Agency (EPA)-registered disinfectants that have microbicidal (i.e., killing) activity against the pathogens most likely to contaminate the patient care environment, in accordance with the manufacturer's instructions.
- Review the efficacy of in-use disinfectants when evidence of continuing transmission of an infectious agent (e.g., rotavirus, *C. difficile*, norovirus) may indicate resistance to the in-use product and change to a more effective disinfectant as indicated.
- In facilities that provide health care to pediatric patients or have waiting areas with children's play toys (e.g., obstetric/gynecology offices and clinics), establish policies and procedures for cleaning and disinfecting toys at regular intervals. Use the following principles in developing this policy and procedures:
  - Select toys that can be easily cleaned and disinfected.
  - Do not permit use of stuffed furry toys if they will be shared.
  - Clean and disinfect large stationary toys (e.g., climbing equipment) at least weekly and whenever visibly soiled.
  - If toys are likely to be mouthed, rinse with water after disinfection; alternatively, wash in a dishwasher.
  - When a toy requires cleaning and disinfection, do so immediately or store in a designated labeled container separate from toys that are clean and ready for use.
- Include multiuse electronic equipment in policies and procedures for preventing contamination and for cleaning and disinfecting, especially those items that are used by patients, those used during delivery of patient care, and mobile devices that are moved in and out of patient rooms frequently (e.g., daily).
- No recommendation for use of removable protective covers or washable keyboards (*unresolved issue*).

Textiles and Laundry
- Handle used textiles and fabrics with minimum agitation to avoid contamination of air, surfaces, and persons.
- If laundry chutes are used, ensure that they are properly designed, maintained, and used in a manner to minimize dispersion of aerosols from contaminated laundry.

Safe Injection Practices
The following recommendations apply to the use of needles, cannulas that replace needles, and, where applicable, intravenous delivery systems:
- Use aseptic technique to avoid contamination of sterile injection equipment.
- Do not administer medications from a syringe to multiple patients, even if the needle or cannula on the syringe is changed. Needles, cannulas, and syringes are sterile, single-use items; they should not be reused for another patient or used to access a medication or solution that might be intended for a subsequent patient.

Continued on following page

BOX 3-1 CENTERS FOR DISEASE CONTROL AND PREVENTION (CDC) AND HEALTHCARE INFECTION CONTROL PRACTICES ADVISORY COMMITTEE (HICPAC) ISOLATION PRECAUTION GUIDELINES (Continued)

- Use fluid infusion and administration sets (i.e., intravenous bags, tubing, and connectors) for one patient only and dispose appropriately after use. Consider a syringe or needle/cannula contaminated once it has been used to enter or connect to a patient's intravenous infusion bag or administration set.
- Use single-dose vials for parenteral medications whenever possible.
- Do not administer medications from single-dose vials or ampules to multiple patients or combine leftover contents for later use.
- If multidose vials must be used, both the needle or the cannula and syringe used to access the multidose vial must be sterile.
- Do not keep multidose vials in the immediate patient treatment area and store in accordance with the manufacturer's recommendations; discard if sterility is compromised or questionable.
- Do not use bags or bottles of intravenous solution as a common source of supply for multiple patients.

Infection Control Practices for Special Lumbar Puncture Procedures

- Wear a surgical mask when placing a catheter or injecting material into the spinal canal or subdural space (i.e., during myelograms, lumbar puncture, and spinal or epidural anesthesia).

Worker Safety

- Adhere to federal and state requirements for protection of health care personnel from exposure to blood-borne pathogens.

Siegel, J. D., Rhinehart, E., Jackson, M., Chiarello, L., and the Healthcare Infection Control Practices Advisory Committee. (2007). Guidelines for isolation precautions: Preventing transmission of infectious agents in healthcare settings. Available at http://www.cdc.gov/ncidod/dhqp/pdf/isolation2007.pdf

---

- Always wear gloves if there is a chance that you will come in direct contact with blood or other body fluids. In addition, wear gloves if you have an open cut or skin abrasion, if the client has an open or weeping cut, if you are collecting body fluids (e.g., blood, sputum, wound drainage, urine, or stools) for a specimen, if you are handling contaminated surfaces (e.g., linen, tongue blades, vaginal speculum), and when you are performing an examination of the mouth, an open wound, genitalia, vagina, or rectum. Change gloves when moving from a contaminated to a clean body site, and between patients.
- If a pin or other sharp object is used to assess sensory perception, discard the pin and use a new one for your next client.
- Wear a mask and protective eye goggles if you are performing an examination in which you are likely to be splashed with blood or other body fluid droplets (e.g., if you are performing an oral examination on a client who has a chronic productive cough).

Concept Mastery Alert

The most important reason for wearing gloves is to prevent the nurse's hands from being a vehicle of transmission from one patient to another. This is why the nurse wears gloves while caring for one patient and then removes the gloves and performs hand hygiene before entering another patient's room. Gloves are intended to prevent exposure.

CASE STUDY

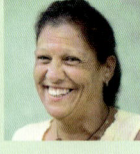 The nurse reviews the data on Mrs. Gutierrez and reviews her knowledge of diabetes, anorexia, and insomnia to explore possible physical findings that may be correlated with these conditions.

Approaching and Preparing the Client

Establish the nurse–client relationship during the client interview before the physical examination takes place. This is important because it helps alleviate any tension or anxiety that the client is experiencing. At the end of the interview, explain to the client that the physical assessment will follow and describe what the examination will involve. For example, you might say to a client, "Mr. Smith, based on the information you have given me, I believe that a complete physical examination should be performed so I can better assess your health status. This will require you to remove your clothing and to put on this gown. You may leave on your underwear until it is time to perform the genital examination."

Respect the client's desires and requests related to the physical examination. Some client requests may be simple, such as asking to have a family member or friend present during the examination. Another request may involve not wanting certain parts of the examination (e.g., breast, genitalia) to be performed. In this situation, you should explain to the client the importance of the examination and the risk of missing important information if any part of the examination is omitted. Ultimately, however, whether to have the examination is the client's decision. Some health care providers ask the client to sign a consent form before a physical examination, especially in situations where a vaginal or rectal examination will be performed.

If a urine specimen is necessary, explain to the client the purpose of a urine sample and the procedure for giving a sample; provide him or her with a container to use. If a urine sample is not necessary, ask the client to urinate before the examination to promote an easier and more comfortable examination of the abdomen and genital areas. Ask the client to undress and put on an examination gown. Allow him or her to keep on underwear until just before the genital examination to promote comfort and privacy. Leave the room while the client changes into the gown and knock before reentering the room to ensure the client's privacy.

Begin the examination with the less intrusive procedures such as measuring the client's temperature, pulse, blood pressure, height, and weight. These nonthreatening/nonintrusive procedures allow the client to feel more comfortable with you and help ease the client's anxiety about the examination. Throughout the examination, continue to explain what procedure you are performing and why you are performing it. This helps ease your client's anxiety. It is usually helpful to integrate health teaching and health promotion during the examination (e.g., breast self-examination technique during the breast examination).

Approach the client from the right-hand side of the examination table or bed because most examination techniques are performed with the examiner's right hand (even if the examiner is left-handed). You may ask the client to change positions frequently, depending on the part of the examination being performed. Prepare the client for these changes at the beginning of the examination by explaining that these position changes are necessary to ensure a thorough examination of each body part and system. Many clients need assistance getting into the required position. Box 3-2 illustrates various positions and provides guidelines for using them during the examination. Box 3-3 provides considerations for older adult clients.

CASE STUDY

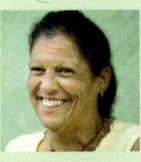

The nurse explains to Mrs. Gutierrez that a physical examination of her mental status, hair, skin, nails, head, neck, eyes, ears, mouth, nose, throat, sinuses, thorax, lungs, heart, peripheral vascular system, abdomen, and musculoskeletal and neurologic systems will be necessary to better assess her diabetes, anorexia, and insomnia. As she goes through the examination using the techniques of inspection, palpation, percussion, and auscultation, the nurse explains why she is performing each part of the examination. See physical assessment findings documented in Chapter 4.

Physical Examination Techniques

Four basic techniques must be mastered before you can perform a thorough and complete assessment of the client. These techniques are *inspection, palpation, percussion,* and *auscultation*. This chapter provides descriptions of each technique along with guidelines on how to perform the basic technique. Using each technique for assessing specific body systems is described in the appropriate chapter. After performing each of the four assessment techniques, examiners should ask themselves questions that will facilitate analysis of the data and determine areas for which more data may be needed. These questions include:
- Did I inspect, palpate, percuss, or auscultate any deviations from the normal findings? (Normal findings are listed in the second column of the Physical Assessment sections in the body systems chapters.)
- If there is a deviation, is it a normal physical, gerontologic, or cultural finding; an abnormal adult finding; or an abnormal physical, gerontologic, or cultural finding? (Normal gerontologic and cultural findings are in the second column of the Physical Assessment sections in the body systems

chapters. Abnormal adult, gerontologic, and cultural findings can be found in the third column of the Physical Assessment sections.)
- Based on my findings, do I need to ask the client more questions to validate or obtain more information about my inspection, palpation, percussion, or auscultation findings?
- Based on my observations and data, do I need to focus my physical assessment on other related body systems?
- Should I validate my inspection, palpation, percussion, or auscultation findings with my instructor or another practitioner?
- Should I refer the client and data findings to a primary care provider?

These questions help ensure that data are complete and accurate, which will help facilitate analysis.

Inspection

Inspection involves using the senses of vision, smell, and hearing to observe and detect any normal or abnormal findings. This technique is used from the moment that you meet the client and continues throughout the examination. Inspection precedes palpation, percussion, and auscultation because the latter techniques can potentially alter the appearance of what is being inspected. Although most of the inspection involves the use of the senses only, a few body systems require the use of special equipment (e.g., ophthalmoscope for the eye inspection, otoscope for the ear inspection).

Use the following guidelines as you practice the technique of inspection:
- Make sure the room is a comfortable temperature. A too cold or too hot room can alter the normal behavior of the client and the appearance of the client's skin.
- Use good lighting, preferably sunlight. Fluorescent lights can alter the true color of the skin. In addition, abnormalities may be overlooked with dim lighting.
- Look and observe before touching. Touch can alter appearance and distract you from a complete, focused observation.
- Completely expose the body part you are inspecting while draping the rest of the client as appropriate.
- Note the following characteristics while inspecting the client: color, patterns, size, location, consistency, symmetry, movement, behavior, odors, or sounds.
- Compare the appearance of symmetric body parts (e.g., eyes, ears, arms, hands) or both sides of any individual body part.

Palpation

Palpation consists of using parts of the hand to touch and feel for the following characteristics:
- Texture (rough/smooth)
- Temperature (warm/cold)
- Moisture (dry/wet)
- Mobility (fixed/movable/still/vibrating)
- Consistency (soft/hard/fluid filled)
- Strength of pulses (strong/weak/thready/bounding)
- Size (small/medium/large)
- Shape (well defined/irregular)
- Degree of tenderness

Three different parts of the hand—the fingerpads, ulnar/palmar surface, and dorsal surface—are used during palpation. Each part of the hand is particularly sensitive to certain characteristics. Determine which characteristic you are trying

BOX 3-2 POSITIONING THE CLIENT

SITTING POSITION

The client should sit upright on the side of the examination table. In the home or office setting, the client can sit on the edge of a chair or bed. This position is good for evaluating the head, neck, lungs, chest, back, breasts, axillae, heart, vital signs, and upper extremities. This position is also useful because it permits full expansion of the lungs and it allows the examiner to assess symmetry of upper body parts. Some clients may be too weak to sit up for the entire examination. They may need to lie down, face up (supine position), and rest throughout the examination. Other clients may be unable to tolerate the position for any length of time. An alternative position is for the client to lie down with head elevated.

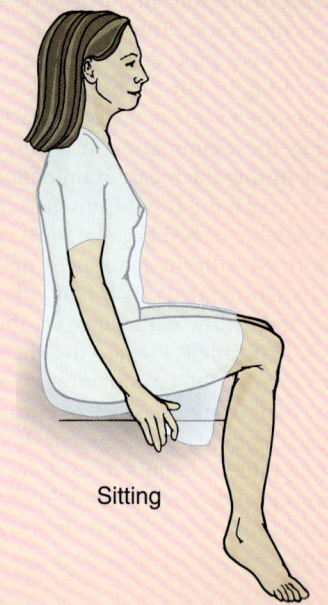
Sitting

SUPINE POSITION

Ask the client to lie down with the legs together on the examination table (or bed if in a home setting). A small pillow may be placed under the head to promote comfort. If the client has trouble breathing, the head of the bed may need to be raised. This position allows the abdominal muscles to relax and provides easy access to peripheral pulse sites. Areas assessed with the client in this position may include head, neck, chest, breasts, axillae, abdomen, heart, lungs, and all extremities.

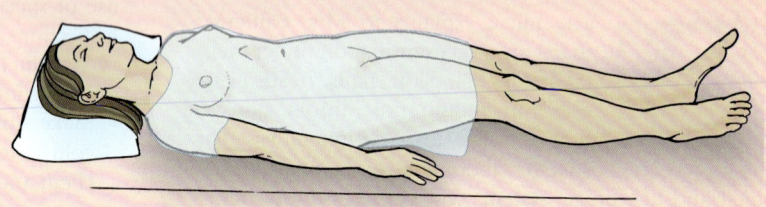
Supine

DORSAL RECUMBENT POSITION

The client lies down on the examination table or bed with the knees bent, the legs separated, and the feet flat on the table or the bed. This position may be more comfortable than the supine position for clients with pain in the back or the abdomen. Areas that may be assessed with the client in this position include head, neck, chest, axillae, lungs, heart, extremities, breasts, and peripheral pulses. The abdomen should not be assessed because the abdominal muscles are contracted in this position.

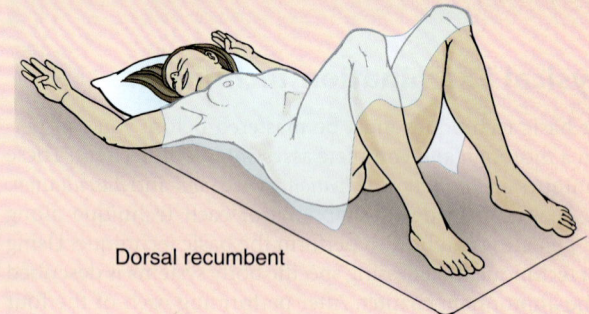
Dorsal recumbent

SIMS' POSITION

The client lies on the right or left side with the lower arm placed behind the body and the upper arm flexed at the shoulder and the elbow. The lower leg is slightly flexed at the knee while the upper leg is flexed at a sharper angle and pulled forward. This position is useful for assessing the rectal and vaginal areas. The client may need some assistance getting into this position. Clients with joint problems and elderly clients may have some difficulty assuming and maintaining this position.

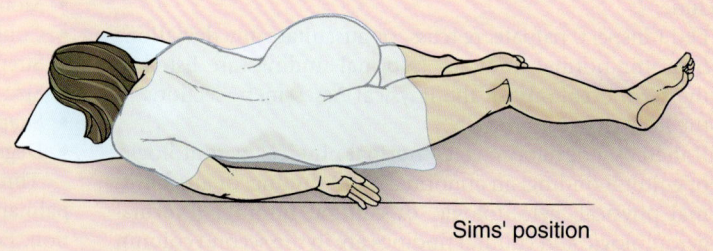
Sims' position

STANDING POSITION

The client stands still in a normal, comfortable, resting posture. This position allows the examiner to assess posture, balance, and gait. This position is also used for examining the male genitalia.

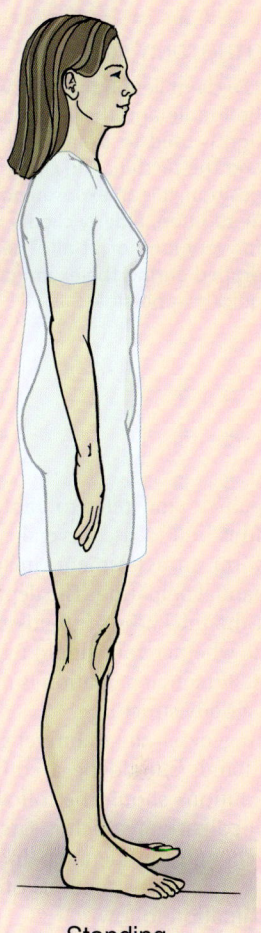
Standing

PRONE POSITION

The client lies down on the abdomen with the head to the side. The prone position is used primarily to assess the hip joint. The back can also be assessed with the client in this position. Clients with cardiac and respiratory problems cannot tolerate this position.

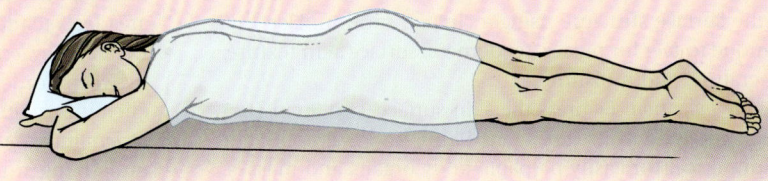
Prone

KNEE–CHEST POSITION

The client kneels on the examination table with the weight of the body supported by the chest and the knees. A 90-degree angle should exist between the body and the hips. The arms are placed above the head, with the head turned to one side. A small pillow may be used to provide comfort. The knee–chest position is useful for examining the rectum. This position may be embarrassing and uncomfortable for the client; therefore, the client should be kept in the position for as limited a time as possible. Elderly clients and clients with respiratory and cardiac problems may be unable to tolerate this position.

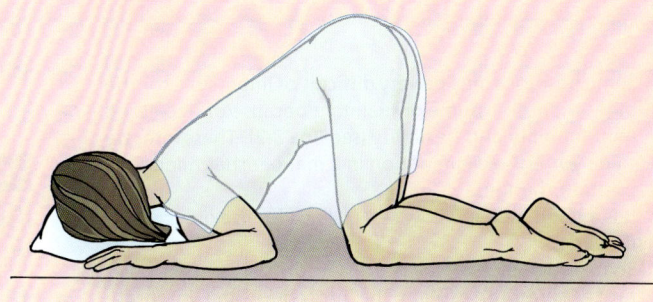
Knee-chest

Continued on following page

BOX 3-2 POSITIONING THE CLIENT (Continued)

LITHOTOMY POSITION

The client lies on the back with the hips at the edge of the examination table and the feet supported by stirrups. The lithotomy position is used to examine the female genitalia, reproductive tracts, and the rectum. The client may require assistance getting into this position. It is an exposed position, and clients may feel embarrassed. In addition, elderly clients may not be able to assume this position for very long or at all. Therefore, it is best to keep the client well draped during the examination and to perform the examination as quickly as possible.

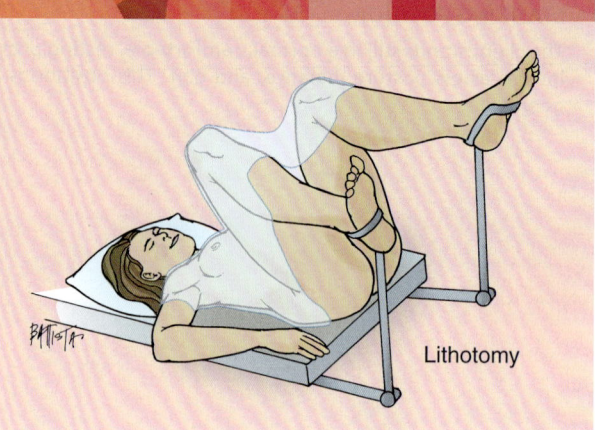

Lithotomy

---

to palpate and refer to Table 3-2 to find which part of the hand is best to use. Several types of palpation can be used to perform an assessment, including light, moderate, deep, or bimanual palpation. The depth of the structure being palpated and the thickness of the tissue overlying that structure determine whether you should use light, moderate, or deep palpation. Bimanual palpation is the use of both hands to hold and feel a body structure.

In general, the examiner's fingernails should be short and the hands should be a comfortable temperature. Standard precautions should be followed if applicable. Proceed from light palpation, which is safest and the most comfortable for the client, to moderate palpation, and finally to deep palpation. Specific instructions on how to perform the four types of palpation follow:

- *Light palpation:* To perform light palpation (Fig. 3-1), place your dominant hand lightly on the surface of the structure. There should be very little or no depression (less than 1 cm). Feel the surface structure using a circular motion. Use this technique to feel for pulses, tenderness, surface skin texture, temperature, and moisture.
- *Moderate palpation:* Depress the skin surface 1 to 2 cm (0.5 to 0.75 in) with your dominant hand, and use a circular motion to feel for easily palpable body organs and masses. Note the size, consistency, and mobility of structures you palpate.
- *Deep palpation:* Place your dominant hand on the skin surface and your nondominant hand on top of your dominant hand to apply pressure (Fig. 3-2). This should result in a surface depression between 2.5 and 5 cm (1 and 2 in). This allows you to feel very deep organs or structures that are covered by thick muscle.
- *Bimanual palpation:* Use two hands, placing one on each side of the body part (e.g., uterus, breasts, spleen) being palpated (Fig. 3-3). Use one hand to apply pressure and the other hand to feel the structure. Note the size, shape, consistency, and mobility of the structures you palpate.

Percussion

Percussion involves tapping body parts to produce sound waves. These sound waves or vibrations enable the examiner to assess underlying structures. Percussion has several different assessment uses, including:

- *Eliciting pain:* Percussion helps detect inflamed underlying structures. If an inflamed area is percussed, the client's physical response may indicate or the client will report that the area feels tender, sore, or painful.
- *Determining location, size, and shape:* Percussion note changes between borders of an organ and its neighboring organ can elicit information about location, size, and shape.
- *Determining density:* Percussion helps determine whether an underlying structure is filled with air or fluid or is a solid structure.
- *Detecting abnormal masses:* Percussion can detect superficial abnormal structures or masses. Percussion vibrations penetrate approximately 5 cm deep. Deep masses do not produce any change in the normal percussion vibrations.
- *Eliciting reflexes:* Deep tendon reflexes are elicited using the percussion hammer.

The three types of percussion are *direct*, *blunt*, and *indirect*. Direct percussion (Fig. 3-4) is the direct tapping of a body part

BOX 3-3 GENERAL CONSIDERATIONS FOR EXAMINING OLDER ADULTS

- Some positions may be very difficult or impossible for the older client to assume or maintain because of decreased joint mobility and flexibility (see Box 3-2). Therefore, try to perform the examination in a manner that minimizes position changes.
- It is a good idea to allow rest periods for the older adult, if needed.
- Some older clients may process information at a slower rate. Therefore, explain the procedure and integrate teaching in a clear and slow manner.

See Chapter 32 for physical examination of the frail elderly client.

TABLE 3-2 Parts of Hand to Use When Palpating

Hand Part	Sensitive To
Fingerpads	Fine discriminations: pulses, texture, size, consistency, shape, crepitus
Ulnar or palmar surface	Vibrations, thrills, fremitus
Dorsal (back) surface	Temperature

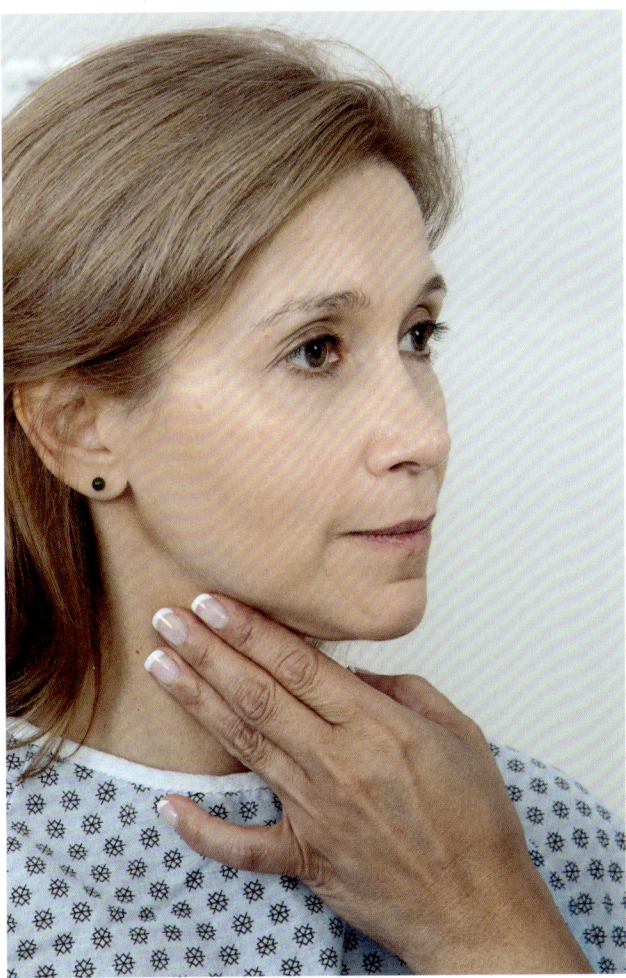

FIGURE 3-1 Light palpation.

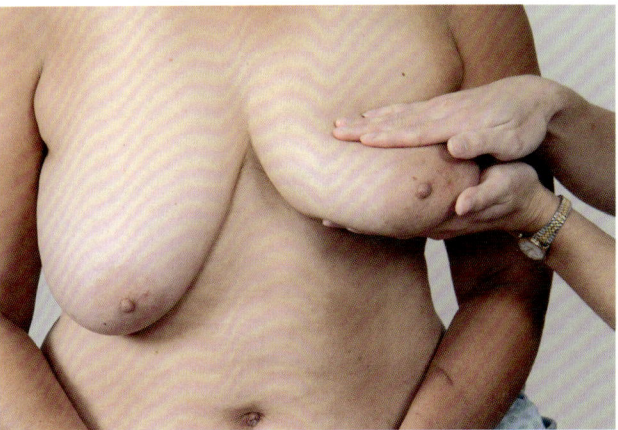

FIGURE 3-3 Bimanual palpation of the breast.

sound of the tone becomes quieter. Solid tissue produces a soft tone, fluid produces a louder tone, and air produces an even louder tone. These tones are referred to as percussion notes and are classified according to origin, quality, intensity, and pitch (Table 3-3).

The following techniques help develop proficiency in the technique of indirect percussion:

- Place the middle finger of your nondominant hand on the body part you are going to percuss.

with one or two fingertips to elicit possible tenderness (e.g., tenderness over the sinuses). Blunt percussion (Fig. 3-5) is used to detect tenderness over organs (e.g., kidneys) by placing one hand flat on the body surface and using the fist of the other hand to strike the back of the hand flat on the body surface. Indirect or mediate percussion (Fig. 3-6) is the most commonly used method of percussion. The tapping done with this type of percussion produces a sound or tone that varies with the density of underlying structures. As density increases, the

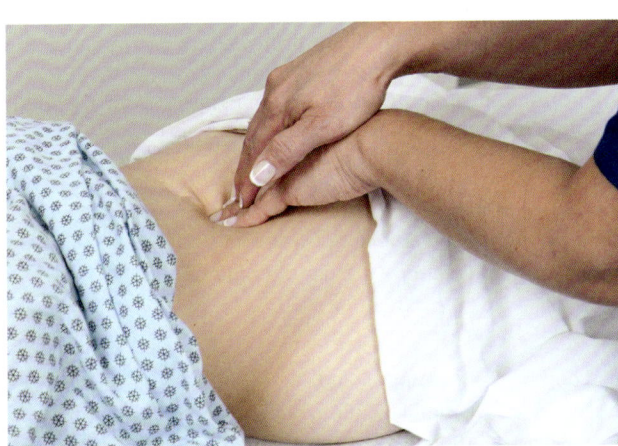

FIGURE 3-2 Deep palpation.

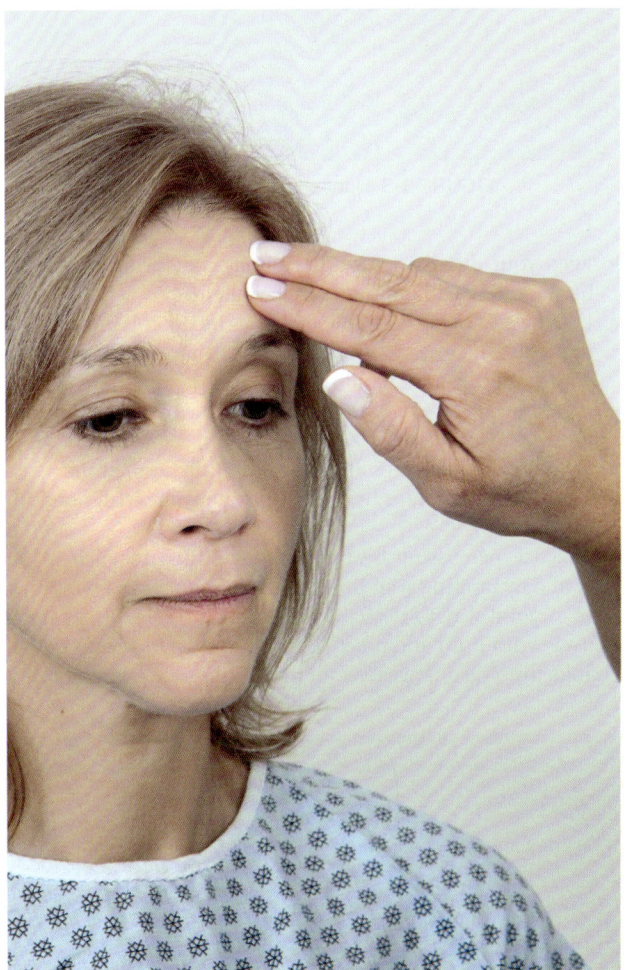

FIGURE 3-4 Direct percussion of sinuses.

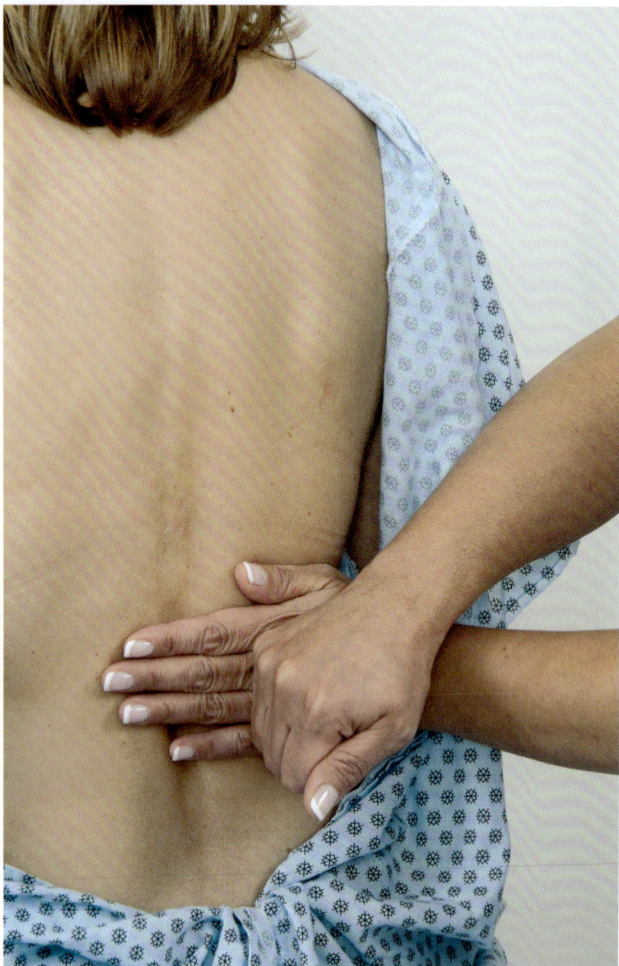

FIGURE 3-5 Blunt percussion of kidneys.

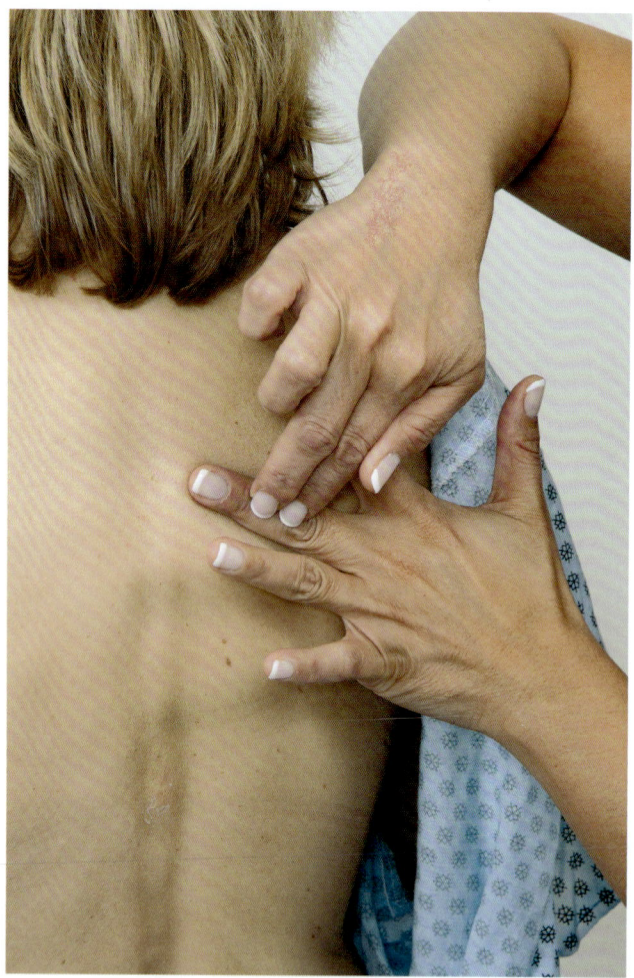

FIGURE 3-6 Indirect or mediate percussion of lungs.

- Keep your other fingers off the body part being percussed because they will damp the tone you elicit.
- Use the pad of your middle finger of the other hand (ensure that this fingernail is short) to strike the middle finger of your nondominant hand that is placed on the body part.
- Withdraw your finger immediately to avoid damping the tone.
- Deliver two quick taps and listen carefully to the tone.
- Use quick, sharp taps by quickly flexing your wrist, not your forearm.

Practice percussing by tapping your thigh to elicit a flat tone and by tapping your puffed-out cheek to elicit a tympanic tone. A good way to detect changes in tone is to fill a carton halfway with fluid and practice percussing on it. The tone will change from resonance over air to a duller tone over the fluid.

Auscultation

Auscultation is a type of assessment technique that requires the use of a stethoscope to listen for heart sounds, movement of blood through the cardiovascular system, movement of the bowel, and movement of air through the respiratory tract. A stethoscope is used because these body sounds are not audible to the human ear. The sounds detected using auscultation are classified according to the intensity (loud or soft), pitch (high or low), duration (length), and quality (musical, crackling, raspy) of the sound (see Assessment Guide 3-1).

These guidelines should be followed as you practice the technique of auscultation:
- Eliminate distracting or competing noises from the environment (e.g., radio, television, machinery).

TABLE 3-3 Sounds (Tones) Elicited by Percussion

Sound	Intensity	Pitch	Length	Quality	Example of Origin
Resonance (heard over part air and part solid)	Loud	Low	Long	Hollow	Normal lung
Hyperresonance (heard over mostly air)	Very loud	Low	Long	Booming	Lung with emphysema
Tympany (heard over air)	Loud	High	Moderate	Drumlike	Puffed-out cheek, gastric bubble
Dullness (heard over more solid tissue)	Medium	Medium	Moderate	Thud-like	Diaphragm, pleural effusion, liver
Flatness (heard over very dense tissue)	Soft	High	Short	Flat	Muscle, bone, sternum, thigh

ASSESSMENT GUIDE 3-1 How to Use the Stethoscope

The stethoscope is used to listen for (auscultate) body sounds that cannot ordinarily be heard without amplification (e.g., lung sounds, bruits, bowel sounds, and so forth). To use a stethoscope, follow these guidelines:

1. Place the earpieces into the outer ear canal. They should fit snugly but comfortably to promote effective sound transmission. The earpieces are connected to binaurals (metal tubing), which connect to rubber or plastic tubing. The rubber or plastic tubing should be flexible and no more than 12 in long to prevent the sound from diminishing.
2. Angle the binaurals down toward your nose. This will ensure that sounds are transmitted to your eardrums.
3. Use the diaphragm of the stethoscope to detect high-pitched sounds. The diaphragm should be at least 1.5 in wide for adults and smaller for children. Hold the diaphragm firmly against the body part being auscultated.
4. Use the bell of the stethoscope to detect low-pitched sounds. The bell should be at least 1 in wide. Hold the bell lightly against the body part being auscultated.

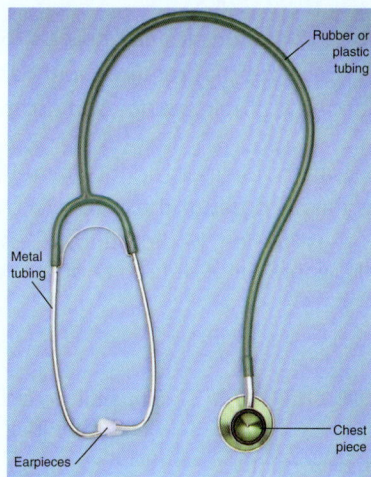

Some Do's and Don'ts
1. Warm the diaphragm or the bell of the stethoscope before placing it on the client's skin.
2. Explain what you are listening for and answer any questions the client has. This will help alleviate anxiety.
3. Do not apply too much pressure when using the bell—too much pressure will cause the bell to work like the diaphragm.
4. Avoid listening through clothing, which may obscure or alter sounds.

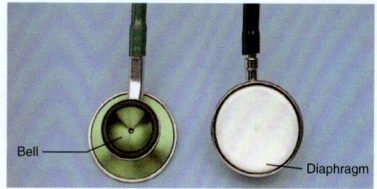

- Expose the body part you are going to auscultate. Do not auscultate through the client's clothing or gown. Rubbing against the clothing obscures the body sounds.
- Use the diaphragm of the stethoscope to listen for high-pitched sounds, such as normal heart sounds, breath sounds, and bowel sounds, and press the diaphragm firmly on the body part being auscultated.
- Use the bell of the stethoscope to listen for low-pitched sounds such as abnormal heart sounds and bruits (abnormal loud, blowing, or murmuring sounds). Hold the bell lightly on the body part being auscultated.

SUMMARY

Collecting objective data is essential for a complete nursing assessment. The nurse must have knowledge of and skill in three basic areas to become proficient in collecting objective data: necessary equipment and how to use it; preparing the setting, oneself, and the client for the examination; and how to perform the four basic assessment techniques. Collecting objective data requires a great deal of practice to become proficient. Proficiency is needed because how the data are collected can affect the accuracy of the information elicited.

Want to know more?
A wide variety of resources to enhance your learning and understanding of this book are available on thePoint. Visit thePoint to access:

NCLEX-Style Student Review Questions   Concepts in Action Animations
Watch and Learn Videos   And more!

References and Selected Readings

Centers for Disease Control and Prevention (CDC). (2015, February 15). Infection prevention and control recommendations for hospitalized patients under investigation (PUIs) for Ebola virus disease (EVD) in U.S. hospitals. Available at http://www.cdc.gov/vhf/ebola/healthcare-us/hospitals/infection-control.html

Centers for Disease Control and Prevention (CDC) & the Hospital Infection Control Practices Advisory Committee (HICPAC). (2007). *Guidelines for isolation precautions: Preventing transmission of infectious agents in healthcare settings 2007. Part III. A. Standard precautions*. Atlanta, GA: CDC. Available at http://www.cdc.gov/hicpac/2007IP/2007isolationPrecautions.html

4 VALIDATING AND DOCUMENTING DATA

Learning Objectives

1. Describe the significance and process for validation of client data.
2. Discuss situations that require client data to be rechecked or verified.
3. Describe the multiple purposes of accurate and timely documentation of client data.
4. Identify safe guidelines for documentation of client data.
5. Discuss the purposes of the client electronic health record (EHR).
6. Use SBAR (situation, background, assessment, and recommendation) method to verbally report client data to another health care provider.

CASE STUDY

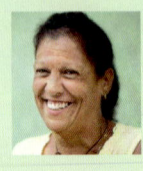

You met Mrs. Gutierrez in Chapter 1 and learned how the nurse interviewed her in Chapter 2 to obtain additional data. In this chapter, you will learn how the nurse validates, documents, and communicates data gathered from Mrs. Gutierrez.

Although validation, documentation, and communication of data often occur concurrently with collection of subjective and objective assessment data, looking at each step separately can help emphasize each step's importance in nursing assessment.

VALIDATING DATA

Purpose of Validation

Validation of data is the process of confirming or verifying that the subjective and objective data you have collected are reliable and accurate. The steps of validation include deciding whether the data require validation, determining ways to validate the data, and identifying areas for which data are missing. Failure to validate data may result in premature closure of the assessment or collection of inaccurate data. Errors during assessment cause the nurse's judgments to be made on unreliable data, which results in diagnostic errors during the second part of the nursing process—analysis of data (determining nursing diagnoses, collaborative problems, and referrals). Thus validation of the data collected during assessment of the client is crucial to the first step of the nursing process.

Data Requiring Validation

Not every piece of data you collect must be verified. For example, you would not need to verify or repeat the client's pulse, temperature, or blood pressure unless certain conditions exist. Conditions that require data to be rechecked and validated include:

- Discrepancies or gaps between the subjective and objective data. For example, a male client tells you that he is very happy despite learning that he has terminal cancer.
- Discrepancies or gaps between what the client says at one time versus another time. For example, your female client says that she has never had surgery, but later in the interview, she mentions that her appendix was removed at a military hospital when she was in the Navy.
- Findings that are highly abnormal and/or inconsistent with other findings. For example, the following are inconsistent with each other: the client has a temperature of 104°F, is resting comfortably, and her skin is warm to the touch and not flushed.

Methods of Validation

There are several ways to validate your data:

- Recheck your own data through a repeat assessment. For example, take the client's temperature again with a different thermometer.
- Clarify data with the client by asking additional questions. For example, if a client is holding his abdomen, the nurse may assume that he is having abdominal pain, when actually the client is very upset about his diagnosis and is feeling nauseated.
- Verify the data with another health care professional. For example, ask a more experienced nurse to listen to the abnormal heart sounds you think you have just heard.
- Compare your objective findings with your subjective findings to uncover discrepancies. For example, if the client states that she "never gets any time in the sun," yet has dark, wrinkled, suntanned skin, you need to validate the client's perception of never getting any time in the sun by asking exactly how much time is spent working, sitting, or doing other activities outdoors. Also, ask what the client wears when engaging in outdoor activities.

> ### CASE STUDY
>
>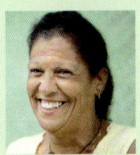
> Mrs. Gutierrez told the nurse that she had a fever for the last 2 days. The nurse would need to take her temperature again to confirm whether she still had a fever. The nurse would also need to ask her if she took any medication for the fever that may mask it at this time.

Identification of Areas for Which Data Are Missing

Once you establish an initial database, you can identify areas for which more data are needed. You may have overlooked certain questions. In addition, as data are examined in a grouped format, you may realize that additional information is needed. For example, if an adult client weighs only 98 lb, you would explore further to see if the client recently lost weight or this has been the usual weight for an extended time. If a client tells you that he lives alone, you may need to identify the existence of a support system, his degree of social involvement with others, and his ability to function independently.

> ### CASE STUDY
>
>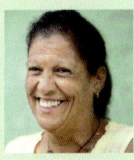
> The nurse would want to weigh Mrs. Gutierrez and call her primary care provider's office to ask for her weight at her last visit, since she said that her clothes are loose and no longer fit. This would also provide additional data to assess how severe her anorexic state was at this time.

DOCUMENTING DATA

In addition to validation, documentation of assessment data is another crucial part of the first step in the nursing process. The significance of this aspect of assessment is addressed specifically by various state nurse practice acts, accreditation and/or reimbursement agencies (e.g., Joint Commission on Accreditation of Healthcare Organizations [TJC], Medicare, Medicaid), professional organizations (local, state, and national), and institutional agencies (acute, transitional, long-term, and home care). TJC, for example, has specific standards that address documentation for assessments.

Health care institutions have developed assessment and documentation policies and procedures that provide not only the criteria for documenting but also assistance in completing the forms. The categories of information within the electronic health record (EHR) are designed to ensure that the nurse gathers pertinent information needed to meet the standards and guidelines of the specific institutions mentioned previously and to develop a plan of care for the client.

Purpose of Documentation

The primary reason for documentation of assessment data is to promote effective communication among multidisciplinary health team members to facilitate safe and efficient client care. Documented assessment data provide the health care team with a database that becomes the foundation for care of the client. It helps identify health problems, formulate nursing diagnoses, and plan immediate and ongoing interventions. If the nursing diagnosis is made without supporting assessment data, incorrect conclusions and interventions may result. The initial and ongoing assessment documentation database also establishes a way to communicate with the multidisciplinary team members.

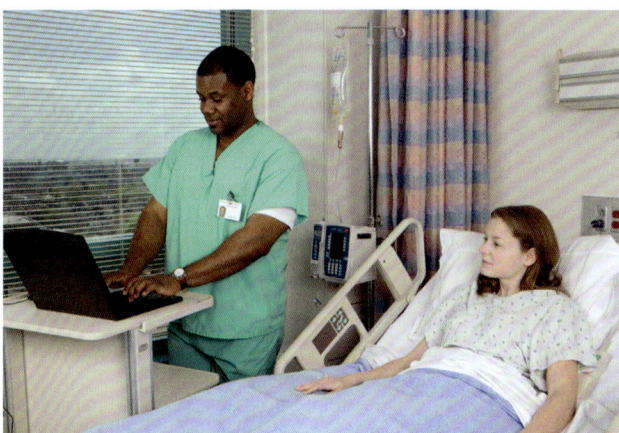

FIGURE 4-1 Nurse using bedside computer.

With the advent of computer-based documentation systems, these databases can link to other documents and health care departments, eliminating repetition of similar data collection by other health team members. The use of EHRs has improved diagnostic and clinical outcomes, reduced errors, and improved patient safety (Health IT, 2014) (Fig. 4-1). Nurses need to be involved in the selection of comprehensive and systematic nursing databases that streamline data collection and organization and yet maintain a concise record that satisfies legal standards (Wood, 2014). Box 4-1 describes the many other purposes that assessment documentation serves.

> *Concept Mastery Alert*
>
> The purposes of documentation are to provide a legal record of a client's care and to form a foundation for that client's care while in the health care facility. Standards for client care are developed through research over time, which demonstrate the most evidence-based method for caring for a client.

On February 17, 2009, the Health Information Technology for Economic and Clinical Health (HITECH) Act was signed into law as part of the American Recovery and Reinvestment Act of 2009 to promote the adoption and meaningful use of health information technology (HIT). Since this Act was adopted, there has been a slow but steady use of EHRs by health care agencies and primary health care providers. To encourage the use of EHRs, Medicare and Medicaid began to offer federal incentive payments of $2 million or more to health care providers and hospitals to use EHR technologies. In addition, penalties will be applied for providers unable to demonstrate meaningful use of EHRs by 2015.

BOX 4-1 PURPOSES OF ASSESSMENT DOCUMENTATION

- Provides a chronological source of client assessment data and a progressive record of assessment findings that outline the client's course of care.
- Ensures that information about the client and the family is easily accessible to members of the health care team; provides a vehicle for communication; and prevents fragmentation, repetition, and delays in carrying out the plan of care.
- Establishes a basis for screening or validating proposed diagnoses.
- Acts as a source of information to help diagnose new problems.
- Offers a basis for determining the educational needs of the client, family, and significant others.
- Provides a basis for determining eligibility for care and reimbursement. Careful recording of data can support financial reimbursement or gain additional reimbursement for transitional or skilled care needed by the client.
- Constitutes a permanent legal record of the care that was or was not given to the client.
- Forms a component of client acuity system or client classification systems. Numeric values may be assigned to various levels of care to help determine the staffing mix for the unit.
- Provides access to significant epidemiologic data for future investigations and research and educational endeavors.
- Promotes compliance with legal, accreditation, reimbursement, and professional standard requirements.

The two terms electronic health records (EHRs) and electronic medical records (EMRs) are often used in place of each other. However, they represent two different forms of electronic documentation. The term EMR (Fig. 4-2), which existed before the term EHR, referred to medical records supplied by physicians who made medical diagnoses and prescribed treatments. The more recent term EHR (Fig. 4-3) is more commonly used, as it refers to the more comprehensive health status of the client and not only the medical status. Thus, the EHR may be used by a variety of health care providers, not just physicians. EHRs focus on the total health (emotional, physical, social, spiritual) of the client and are designed to reach out *beyond* the health organization that originally obtains the client data. These records share data with other health care providers, such as dietitians, physical therapists, laboratories, and other specialists, to promote collaboration of all those

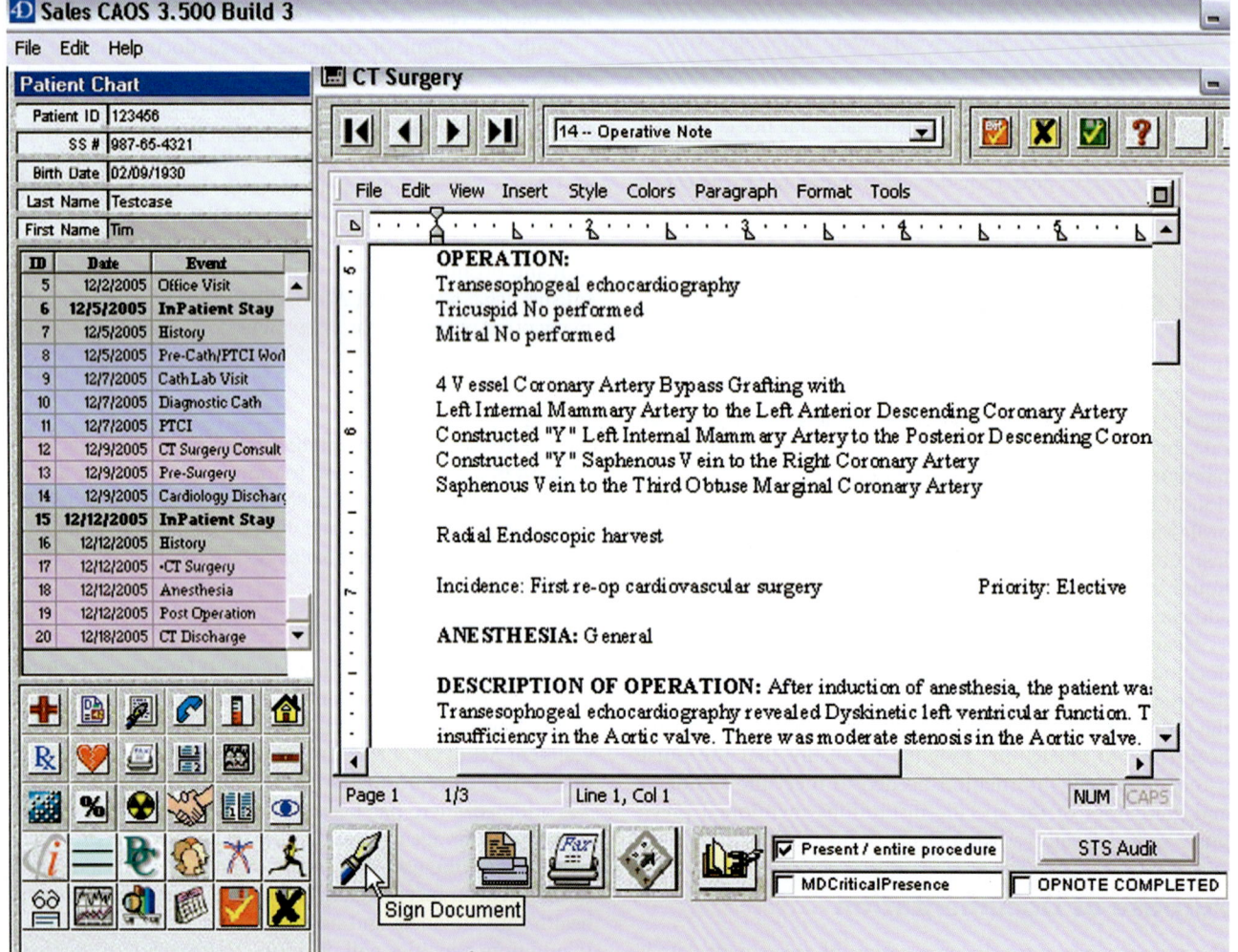

FIGURE 4-2 Electronic medical record.

FIGURE 4-3 Example of electronic health record screen.

involved in the client's care. Thus, EHRs provide nationwide access to client information compiled from data collected by a variety of health care providers.

As a result of the HITECH Act passage, EHRs are rapidly becoming part of the daily practice of the bedside nurse for documenting client data (American Sentinel University, 2013). Meaningful use of the EHR implies that electronic documentation will improve the quality, safety, and efficiency of client care while reducing disparities (see Fig. 4-3). It also means that patients and their families will be actively engaged in their care and treatment through electronic communication. Thus, coordination of client care should improve. Both privacy and security protection for personal health information must be ensured for all clients. Last but not least, the health data of populations will be able to be accessed for research purposes to improve client care.

A study of 16,362 nurses working at 316 hospitals across the United States revealed that nurses who used EHR systems had fewer reports of unfavorable client safety issues, medication errors, and low quality of care. These nurses also had a 14% decrease in reporting that data were missing or lost when clients were transferred between units (Kutney-Lee & Kelly, 2011). The use of EHRs may allow for more comprehensive reports and discharge summaries to other health care providers by facilitating seamless transitions for clients throughout the health care continuum.

Lavin et al. (2015) recognize the positive and negative aspects of use of the EHR by nurses. They describe benefits to client care and the difficulties nurses experience in mastering the complex systems currently in place. These authors urge nurses to report their concerns to those responsible for improving the EHRs and to continue to develop their own documentation and informatics skills.

CASE STUDY

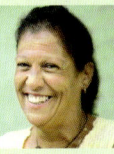

You may recall that Mrs. Gutierrez's husband, 60 years old, was in a car accident 2 months ago. When this occurred, the nurses in the emergency department (ED) were alerted before he arrived at the hospital about his injuries, the name of his primary health care provider, his Medicaid status, his blood type, and that he was currently taking these prescribed drugs: warfarin, metoprolol, lisinopril, and metformin. Both a health care smart card and an EHR were used to transfer these data to the nurses at the hospital. The nurses were able to have the medications ordered from the pharmacy and equipment needed for prompt treatment of Mr. Gutierrez when he arrived at the ED.

Information Requiring Documentation

Every institution is unique when it comes to documenting assessments. However, two key elements need to be included in every documentation: nursing history and physical assessment, also known as subjective and objective data. Most data collection starts with subjective data and ends with objective data.

As discussed in previous chapters, subjective data consist of the information that the client or significant others tell the nurse, and objective data are what the nurse observes through inspection, palpation, percussion, or auscultation. **It is important to remember to document only what the client tells you and what you observe—not what you interpret or infer from the data.** Interpretation or inference takes place during the analysis phase of the nursing process (see Chapter 5).

Subjective Data

Subjective data typically consist of biographical data, present health concern(s) and symptoms (or the client's reason for seeking care), personal health history, family history, and lifestyle and health practices information:

- Biographical data typically consist of the client's name, age, occupation, ethnicity, and support systems or resources.
- The present health concern review is recorded in statements that reflect the client's current symptoms. Statements should begin, "Client (or significant other) states...." Describe items as accurately and descriptively as possible. For example, if a client complains of difficulty breathing, report how the client describes the problem, when the problem started, what started it, how long it occurred, and what makes the breathing better or worse. Use a memory tool, such as COLDSPA, described in Chapter 2, to further explore every symptom reported by the client. This information provides the health care team members with details that help in diagnosis and clinical problem solving. Sometimes, you may need to record the absence of specific signs and symptoms (e.g., no vomiting, diarrhea, or constipation).
- Personal health history data tell the nurse about events that happened before the client's admission to the health care facility or the current encounter with the client. The data may be about previous hospitalizations, surgeries, treatment programs, acute illness, chronic illnesses, injuries, allergies, and medication (prescribed or over the counter) use. Be sure to include all pertinent information, for example, dates of hospitalization. Also be sure to include all data, even negative history (e.g., "client denies prior surgeries").
- Family history data include information about the client's biologic family (e.g., family history of diseases or behaviors that may be genetic or familial). A genogram may be helpful in recording family history (see Chapter 2).
- Lifestyle and health practices information includes details about risk behaviors, such as poor nutrition (excess or deficit), excess sun exposure, past or present smoking, alcohol use, illicit drug use, unprotected sex, and *lack of* exercise, sleep, and recreation, and leisure activities. Additional data collected include environmental factors that may affect health; social and psychological factors that may affect the client's health; client and family health education needs; and family and other relationships. Be sure to be comprehensive, yet succinct.

CASE STUDY

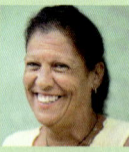

Mrs. Gutierrez, a 52-year-old female, was born in Mexico City and moved to Los Angeles when she was 20 years old. She has been a homemaker all of her adult life. Her daughter has dropped her off at the clinic while she runs some errands. She lives with her husband and three daughters (aged 12, 14, and 17 years). She has two older sons who are married and live in Mexico. She shares a cell phone and car with her oldest daughter. She completed high school in Mexico. Mrs. Gutierrez's family does not have private health care insurance.

Mrs. Gutierrez states that she has come to the clinic "because her doctor told her she needed diabetic teaching." However, her concern is: "I cannot eat or sleep and I just want to be able to eat and sleep again."

Mrs. Gutierrez's symptoms of loss of appetite and inability to sleep were further explored using COLDSPA.

COLDSPA	Client's Responses for Insomnia and Anorexia
Character: Describe the nature of your inability to sleep. Describe your current appetite by telling me what you eat in a normal day.	"I only sleep for 4–5 hours a night. Once I fall asleep about 10 PM, I wake up about 2 AM or 3 AM, and cannot go back to sleep. I do not take naps during the day. I eat cereal in the morning but am not able to eat much the rest of the day. I eat less than one half of what I use to eat. I still try to cook but find it hard to stay focused. I only eat one bite of a tamale and maybe a bite or two of beans or rice."
Onset	"Two months ago right after my husband was in a car wreck."
Location	Nonapplicable
Duration	Two months
Severity	"I am so tired in the daytime that I have let my housework pile up. Sometimes I just lay in bed but I do not sleep. I know I should be eating but I do not feel hungry and food is not appetizing to me."
Pattern: What makes it better or worse?	"I have tried taking Excedrin PM but it makes me feel more drowsy all day. I only drink a cup of coffee in the morning and stopped drinking tea in the afternoon. My daughter has tried to fix my favorite foods, but I still cannot eat."

COLDSPA	Client's Responses for Insomnia and Anorexia
Associated factors	Experiencing "susto" and states "My clothes no longer fit and are very loose. I worry a lot as to how we will pay our bills now that my husband has lost his job and we do not have health insurance. The other day I began crying over nothing. I just feel sad all the time."

After exploring Mrs. Gutierrez's loss of appetite and inability to sleep using COLDSPA, the nurse continues with the health history. Mrs. Gutierrez does not have an accurate record of childhood medical history but received updated immunizations when she came to the United States at 20 years of age. No past surgeries or injuries. No known allergies. Does not take any prescribed medications but does occasionally use over-the-counter Excedrin PM for sleep and Tylenol for headaches. Has been taking Excedrin PM now for 2 months. Gravida 5, para 5, aborta 0. Gestational diabetes during her last pregnancy. Was diagnosed with type 2 diabetes mellitus a month ago.

Mrs. Gutierrez has little knowledge of her family history, as she was abandoned by her parents as an infant and later adopted.

The review of systems for Mrs. Gutierrez is as follows:

Skin, hair, and nails: Denies problems with skin, hair, or nails. Denies alopecia, dandruff, oiliness, thin nails, brittle nails, clubbing nails, dry skin, onychomycosis, lesions, changes in moles, rashes, and so on.

Head and neck: Denies headaches, swelling, stiffness of neck, difficulty swallowing, sore throat, enlarged lymph nodes.

Eyes: Wears glasses for reading, denies eye infections, redness, excessive tearing, halos around lights, blurring, loss of side vision, moving black spots/specks in visual fields, flashing lights, double vision, and eye pain.

Ears: Denies loss of hearing, ringing or buzzing, earaches, drainage from ears, dizziness, exposure to loud noises.

Mouth, throat, nose, and sinuses: Reports missing upper molars, denies bleeding of gums or other dental problems, sore throats; mouth lesions; hoarseness; rhinorrhea; nasal obstruction; frequent colds; sneezing or itching of eyes, ears, nose, or throat; nose bleeds; snoring.

Thorax and lungs: Denies difficulty breathing, wheezing, pain, shortness of breath during routine activity, orthopnea, cough or sputum, hemoptysis, respiratory infections.

Breasts and regional lymphatics: Denies lumps or discharge from nipples, dimpling or changes in breast size, swollen or tender lymph nodes in axilla.

Heart and neck vessels: Reports last blood pressure was 130/84, denies chest pain or pressure, palpitations, edema.

Peripheral vascular: Denies swelling, or edema, of legs and feet; pain; cramping; sores on legs; color or texture changes on the legs or feet.

Abdomen: Describes anorexia and abdominal fullness. Denies difficulty swallowing, nausea, vomiting, gas, jaundice, hernias.

Female genitalia: Denies sexual problems; STIs; denies urgency, frequency, incontinence, dysuria, hematuria, changes in urinary stream, polyuria, nocturia, oliguria, and hesitancy; menarche at the age of 13 years, menopause at the age of 51 years; five pregnancies (Gravida 5, Para 5, aborto 0). Gestational diabetes with last child. Denies abortions, pelvic pain, use of contraception, or use of hormone replacement therapy (HRT).

Anus, rectum, and prostate: Reports a daily bowel movement of well-formed brown stool. Denies tenesmus, hemorrhoids, hematochezia, melena, constipation, diarrhea.

Musculoskeletal: Denies swelling, redness, pain, and stiffness of joints. Is able to perform ADLs without difficulty.

Neurologic: Describes sadness and being tearful at times. Denies depression, anger, and suicidal thoughts. Denies concussions, headaches, loss of strength or sensation, lack of coordination, difficulty speaking, memory problems, strange thoughts and/or actions, or difficulty learning.

Lifestyle and Health Practices Profile

Mrs. Gutierrez reports that she gets up at 6 AM every day, does laundry and housework, and begins to prepare meals for the day. She enjoys working outside but has not been able to do so as much as she did since her husband's accident. She used to attend the 7:00 AM Sunday mass service at her church but has not done so recently. She talks with her sisters in Mexico once a week. Bedtime is usually after the news, at 10:30 PM.

Twenty-four hour dietary recall:

Breakfast: Small (4 oz) bowl of oatmeal with milk and sugar

Lunch: Plain tortilla with a glass of milk

Supper: A few bites of chicken and rice with a glass of water. Currently, her daughter does all the grocery shopping that she used to do. Client does not typically eat at restaurants.

When feeling well, client does all housework and gardening by herself. Denies any participation in a regular aerobic exercise routine. She likes to attend the dinners at church and bingo on Friday nights. Denies any hobbies for leisure.

Falls asleep about 10 PM, wakes up about 2 AM and cannot go back to sleep. Does not nap during the day. Has difficulty staying asleep. Feels tired all day long. Used to sleep all night without a problem but has had continued problems getting to sleep and staying asleep since husband's accident 2 months ago.

Does not drink alcohol. Used to drinks 3 to 4 cups of coffee a day but has stopped in order to help her sleep. Denies the use of tobacco products, recreational drugs, or complementary and alternative medications.

She describes her talent as being a good mother and housekeeper. "I used to be pretty, but do not feel like taking care of myself. My husband and I used to have a good relationship, but we do not spend much time with each other anymore. I do not drive; my daughter takes me where I need to go." Sees a primary care provider yearly and goes to the eye doctor whenever her prescription needs to be changed (unable to give an estimate of how often).

Reports frequent feelings of loneliness. She cannot describe how often but indicates a general sense of loneliness with her siblings and parents living so far away in Mexico. "I worry a lot, especially since my husband had

> the accident and cannot work. We were planning a trip to Mexico to see my family and now we cannot go because we do not have enough money. I used to pray when I worried but that does not seem to help anymore. His accident was such a shock to me!"
>
> Client lives in a three-bedroom home with city water, hot water heater, electricity, and a gas stove, but she says that the electricity bill is so high that they often avoid using any source of heat or cooling. She denies smoke detectors or CO detectors. States that there are often neighborhood fights outside, but she and her husband do not get involved. Feels fairly safe but worries about the neighborhood sometimes. She denies guns or ammunition in house. States medications are kept in kitchen cabinet. Says car has seat belts but often they are not used in her community or by her and her husband.

Objective Data

After you complete the nursing history, the physical examination begins. This examination includes inspection, palpation, percussion, and auscultation. These data help further define the client's problems, establish baseline data for ongoing assessments, and validate the subjective data obtained during the nursing history interview. A variety of systematic approaches may be used: head-to-toe, major body systems, functional health patterns, or human response patterns.

No matter which approach is used, general rules apply:

- Make notes as you perform the assessments and document as concisely as possible.
- Avoid documenting with general nondescriptive or nonmeasurable terms such as normal, abnormal, good, fair, satisfactory, or poor.
- Instead, use specific descriptive and measurable terms (e.g., 3 in in diameter, red excoriated edges, with purulent yellow drainage) about what you inspected, palpated, percussed, and auscultated.

Guidelines for Documentation

The way that nursing assessments are recorded varies among practice settings. However, several general guidelines apply to all settings with both written notes and electronic documentation methods. They include:

- *Keep confidential all documented information in the client record.* Most agencies require nurses to complete the Health Insurance Portability and Accountability Act (HIPAA, 1996) training to ensure that the use, disclosure of, and requests for protected information are used only for intended purposes and kept to a minimum. Clients must also be educated on their rights in relation to HIPAA.
- *Document legibly or print neatly in nonerasable ink.* Errors in documentation are usually corrected by drawing one line through the entry, writing "error," and initialing the entry. Never obliterate the error with white paint or tape, an eraser, or a marking pen. Keep in mind that the health record is a legal document.
- *Use correct grammar and spelling.* **Use only abbreviations that are acceptable and approved by the institution.** Avoid slang, jargon, or labels unless they are direct quotes.
- *Avoid wordiness that creates redundancy.* For example, do not record: "Auscultated gurgly bowel sounds in right upper, right lower, left upper, and left lower abdominal quadrants. Heard 36 gurgles per minute." Instead record: "Bowel sounds present in all quadrants at 36/minute."
- *Use phrases instead of sentences to record data.* For example, avoid recording: "The client's lung sounds were clear both in the right and left lungs." Instead record: "Bilateral lung sounds clear."
- *Record data findings, not how they were obtained.* For example, do not record: "Client was interviewed for past history of high blood pressure, and blood pressure was taken." Instead record: "Has 3-year history of hypertension treated with medication. BP sitting right arm 140/86, left arm 136/86."
- *Write entries objectively without making premature judgments or diagnoses.* Use quotation marks to identify clearly the client's responses. For example, record: "Client crying in room, refuses to talk, husband has gone home" instead of "Client depressed due to fear of breast biopsy report and not getting along well with husband." Avoid making inferences and diagnostic statements until you have collected and validated all data with client and family.
- *Record the client's understanding and perception of problems.* For example, record: "Client expresses concern regarding being discharged soon after gallbladder surgery because of inability to rest at home with six children."
- *Avoid recording the word "normal" for normal findings.* For example, do not record: "Liver palpation normal." Instead record: "Liver span 10 cm in right MCL and 4 cm in MSL." No tenderness on palpation. "Also avoid using the terms *good, fair, poor, sometimes, occasional, frequently, recently,* or *some.* Instead, use specific quantitative or qualitative descriptive terms. In some health care settings, however, only abnormal findings are documented if the policy is to chart by exception only. In that case, no normal findings would be documented in any format.
- *Record complete information and details for all client symptoms or experiences.* For example, do not record: "Client has pain in lower back." Instead record: "Client reports aching-burning pain in lower back for 2 weeks. Pain worsens after standing for several hours. Rest and ibuprofen used to take edge off pain. No radiation of pain. Rates pain as 7 on scale of 1 to 10."
- *Include additional assessment content when applicable.* For example, include information about the caregiver or last physician contact.
- *Support objective data with specific observations obtained during the physical examination.* For example, when describing the emotional status of the client as depressed, follow it with a description of the ways depression is demonstrated such as "dressed in dirty clothing, avoids eye contact, unkempt appearance, and slumped shoulders."

See Table 4-1 for examples of vague versus clear, concise documentation.

TABLE 4-1 Examples of Vague Versus Clear and Concise Documentation of Data

Vague Documentation	Clear and Concise Documentation
Source and reliability of information: Client	Client awake, alert, and oriented to person, place, time, and events. Initiates and maintains conversation. Asks and answers questions that are appropriate.
Memory intact	Recent and remote memory intact.
Vital signs good	Temperature: 98.6 degrees F; Pulse 66 regular Respirations 18, Blood pressure: 160/88
Skin color normal	Skin pink with consistent pigmentation
Appetite good	Reports no change in appetite (list 24-hour diet recall on a typical day)
Swelling of ankles	Pitting edema 3+ of both ankles that lasts 10 seconds
Hears poorly	"My wife says I always turn the radio and TV up too loud so I guess I am hard of hearing"
Heart rate regular	Heart regular rate and rhythm: S1 and S2 present; S1 loudest at the apex, S2 loudest at base; no S3, S4, murmur, rub, or gallop
Chest sounds clear	Anterior, posterior, and bilateral chest sounds clear to auscultation
Normal bowel sounds	5–20 bowel sounds per minute, active bowel sounds in all 4 quadrants.
Voids a lot	Polyuria, urinary output (UOP) = 3,000 mL/day

Assessment Forms Used for Documentation

Standardized assessment forms have been developed to ensure that content in documentation and assessment data meets regulatory requirements and provides a thorough database. The type of assessment form used for documentation varies according to the health care institution. In fact, a variety of assessment forms may even be used within an institution. Typically, however, three types of assessment forms are used to document data: an initial assessment form, frequent or ongoing assessment forms, and focused or specialized assessment forms.

Initial Assessment Form

An initial assessment form is called a nursing admission or admission database. Four types of frequently used initial assessment documentation forms are known as open-ended, cued or checklist, integrated cued checklist, and nursing minimum data set (NMDS) forms. Box 4-2 describes each type of initial assessment form. In addition, Figure 4-4 is an example of the cued or checklist admission documentation form used in an acute care setting.

Frequent or Ongoing Assessment Form

Various institutions have created flowcharts that help staff to record and retrieve data for frequent reassessments. Examples of two types of flowcharts are the frequent vital signs sheet, which allows for vital signs to be recorded in a graphic format that promotes easy visualization of abnormalities, and the assessment flowchart, which allows for rapid comparison of recorded assessment data from one time period to the next (Fig. 4-5).

Progress notes (Fig. 4-6) may be used to document unusual events, responses, significant observations, or interactions whose data are inappropriate for flow records. Flow sheets

---

BOX 4-2 FEATURES OF TYPES OF INITIAL ASSESSMENT DOCUMENTATION FORMS

OPEN-ENDED FORMS (TRADITIONAL FORM)
- Calls for narrative description of problem and listing of topics.
- Provides lines for comments.
- Individualizes information.
- Provides "total picture," including specific complaints and symptoms in the client's own words.
- Increases risk of failing to ask a pertinent question because questions are not standardized.
- Requires a lot of time to complete the database.

CUED OR CHECKLIST FORMS
- Standardizes data collection.
- Lists (categorizes) information that alerts the nurse to specific problems or symptoms assessed for each client (see Fig. 4-1).
- Usually includes a comment section after each category to allow for individualization.
- Prevents missed questions.
- Promotes easy, rapid documentation.
- Makes documentation somewhat like data entry because it requires nurse to place check marks in boxes instead of writing narrative.
- Poses chance that a significant piece of data may be missed because the checklist does not include the area of concern.

INTEGRATED CUED CHECKLIST
- Combines assessment data with identified nursing diagnoses.
- Helps cluster data, focuses on nursing diagnoses, assists in validating nursing diagnosis labels, and combines assessment with problem listing in one form.
- Promotes use by different levels of caregivers, resulting in enhanced communication among the disciplines.

NURSING MINIMUM DATA SET
- Comprises format commonly used in long-term care facilities.
- Has a cued format that prompts nurse for specific criteria; usually computerized.
- Includes specialized information, such as cognitive patterns, communication (hearing and vision) patterns, physical function and structural patterns, activity patterns, restorative care, and the like.
- Meets the needs of multiple data users in the health care system.
- Establishes comparability of nursing data across clinical populations, settings, geographic areas, and time.

SOUTHEAST MISSOURI HOSPITAL — ADULT ADMISSION HEALTH HISTORY

NAME:
SEX:
PHYS: DOB: AGE:
Account #:
Med Rec #:

Unless the nurse asks you to, you do NOT need to complete this again if the last admission was after Feb 1, 2001.
Unable to take history   ☐ Patient confused/unresponsive
☐ Patient not accompanied by family/significant other(s)   ☐ History taken from previous medical record

YES NO **HEALTH MANAGEMENT**   COMMENTS
Patient lives: ☐ Home ☐ Other_____
☐ ☐ Live alone
    Primary support person:_____
☐ ☐ Receives home care services
☐ ☐ Metal or foreign objects in body
    (i.e., shrapnel, metal slivers) _____
☐ ☐ Mechanical devices on or implanted
    in the body_____
☐ ☐ Have you ever smoked?
    packs per day____#years____date quit____
☐ ☐ Drink alcohol? Drinks per day
☐ ☐ Used/uses recreational drugs

NUTRITION/ METABOLIC
☐ ☐ Special diet/restrictions at home
☐ ☐ Undesired weight loss
☐ ☐ Undesired weight gain
☐ ☐ Recent loss of appetite
☐ ☐ Difficulty eating/swallowing
    ☐ onset during the last 7 days
☐ ☐ Recent vomiting (more than 3 days)
☐ ☐ Stomach/intestinal problems
    (i.e., hiatus hernia, severe heartburn, reflux, etc)
☐ ☐ Feeding tube   Company: _____

METABOLIC
☐ ☐ Have you ever had cancer
☐ ☐ Medication pump Company: _____
☐ ☐ Diabetes—for how long:
☐ ☐ Thyroid problems

RESPIRATORY/ CIRCULATORY
☐ ☐ Recent cold, flu, sore throat
☐ ☐ Asthma or emphysema
☐ ☐ Pneumonia/bronchitis
☐ ☐ COPD
☐ ☐ Shortness of breath
☐ ☐ Taking breathing treatments
☐ ☐ Uses oxygen Company:
☐ ☐ Sleep apnea
☐ ☐ Uses CPAP or other device Company:

CARDIOVASCULAR
☐ ☐ CHF (congestive heart failure)
☐ ☐ Chest pain or heart attack
☐ ☐ Pacemaker
☐ ☐ Mitral valve prolapse
☐ ☐ Heart murmur
☐ ☐ Rheumatic fever
☐ ☐ High blood pressure
☐ ☐ Circulatory trouble

ELIMINATION
☐ ☐ Kidney or urinary problems
☐ ☐ Bladder/voiding problems
☐ ☐ Uses a catheter
☐ ☐ Has an ostomy

SEXUALITY/REPRODUCTIVE
Female:
    Number of pregnancies
    Number of live births
    Date of last menstrual period
☐ ☐ Is there a chance you are
    pregnant

YES NO **HEMATOLOGY**
☐ ☐ Bleeding/bruising tendency
☐ ☐ Ever had blood transfusions
☐ ☐ Ever had severe anemia
☐ ☐ Ever had blood clots

ACTIVITY/EXERCISE
☐ ☐ Needs help with self care
    ☐ onset during last 7 days
☐ ☐ Problems with walking
    ☐ onset during last 7 days
☐ ☐ Arm/leg weakness/paralysis
    ☐ onset during last 7 days
☐ ☐ Bone/joint problems or arthritis
☐ ☐ Back or neck problems
☐ ☐ Recent fracture or surgical procedure
    involving the arms, legs or spine:
    Use of special equipment
☐ ☐ Walker   ☐ Brought with patient
               Company obtained from:
☐ ☐ Wheelchair ☐ Brought with patient
               Company obtained from:
☐ ☐ Cane   ☐ Brought with patient
               Company obtained from:
☐ ☐ Crutches ☐ Brought with patient
               Company obtained from:
☐ ☐ Other   ☐ Brought with patient
               Company obtained from:

COGNITIVE/PERCEPTUAL
☐ ☐ Stroke
☐ ☐ Memory loss or confusion
☐ ☐ Difficulty speaking or communicating
    ☐ onset during last 7 days
☐ ☐ Fainting spells or dizziness
☐ ☐ Convulsions, seizures, or epilepsy
☐ ☐ Nervous or mental disorders
☐ ☐ Eye problems or glaucoma
☐ ☐ Hearing problems
☐ ☐ Claustrophobia—If yes, how bad:

EDUCATION
☐ ☐ Is there anything you would like to learn about your
    condition? Explain:
Education needs for the following departments:
Patient educators   Receives ☐ Needs ☐
Cardiac rehab   Receives ☐ Needs ☐
Nutrition services Receives ☐ Needs ☐
Respiratory ther.   Receives ☐ Needs ☐
Pulmonary rehab   Receives ☐ Needs ☐

VALUE/BELIEF
☐ ☐ Is there anything in your religious or cultural belief
    that affects the care we provide or how we treat you?
    Explain: _____

☐ ☐ Would you like hospital chaplain to visit?

INFECTIOUS DISEASE
☐ ☐ Confirmed HIV positive
☐ ☐ Ever had hepatitis
    What type:_____   Year _____
☐ ☐ Ever had MRSA   Year _____
☐ ☐ Ever had VRE   Year _____
☐ ☐ Ever had tuberculosis (TB) Year _____
☐ ☐ Ever had chicken pox   ☐ Vaccine
☐ ☐ Had contact with chicken pox 10–21 days ago?

FIGURE 4-4 Printout of computerized admission form. (Used with permission from Southeast Missouri Hospital, Cape Girardeau, MO.)

| SOUTHEAST MISSOURI HOSPITAL | ADULT ADMISSION HEALTH HISTORY | NAME:
SEX:
PHYS: | Account #:
Med Rec #:
DOB: AGE: |

Previous surgeries: (type, date, and facility)

Allergic to latex: ☐ Yes ☐ No Symptoms

Food allergies:	Symptoms

Medication allergies:	Symptoms

Other allergies:	Symptoms

FIGURE 4-4 (*Continued*)

PATIENT ASSESSMENT FLOWSHEET

INITIALS/SIGNATURE _____
_____
_____
_____

Addressograph

Date _____

INITIAL ASSESSMENT	2300-0700 TIME/INITIALS _____	0700-1500 TIME/INITIALS _____	1500-2300 TIME/INITIALS _____
NUTRITION/ METABOLIC	SKIN: ☐ Dry ☐ Intact ☐ Warm ☐ Cold ☐ Other _____ Turgor: _____ ☐ N/V _____ TUBES: (feeding) _____ IV: Date Of Insertion: ____ SITE: _____ FLUIDS: _____ WOUNDS/DRSGS: _____	SKIN: ☐ Dry ☐ Intact ☐ Warm ☐ Cold ☐ Other _____ Turgor: _____ ☐ N/V _____ TUBES: (feeding) _____ IV: Date Of Insertion: ____ SITE: _____ FLUIDS: _____ WOUNDS/DRSGS: _____	SKIN: ☐ Dry ☐ Intact ☐ Warm ☐ Cold ☐ Other _____ Turgor: _____ ☐ N/V _____ TUBES: (feeding) _____ IV: Date Of Insertion: ____ SITE: _____ FLUIDS: _____ WOUNDS/DRSGS: _____

RESPIRATORY/ CIRCULATORY	BREATH SOUNDS: _____
	
	RESPIRATIONS: _____
	
	OXYGEN: _____
	PULSE OX: _____
	☐ Cough _____
	☐ Sputum _____
	APICAL PULSE: _____
	☐ Regular ☐ Irregular
	TELEMETRY: _____
	
	NAILBED COLOR: ☐ Pink
	☐ Pale ☐ Blue
	PEDAL PULSES: R ☐— ☐+
	                              L ☐— ☐+
	EDEMA: R ☐— ☐+
	                              L ☐— ☐+
	CALF R ☐— ☐+
	TENDERNESS: L ☐— ☐+
		BREATH SOUNDS: _____
		
		RESPIRATIONS: _____
		
		OXYGEN: _____
		PULSE OX: _____
		☐ Cough _____
		☐ Sputum _____
		APICAL PULSE: _____
		☐ Regular ☐ Irregular
		TELEMETRY: _____
		
		NAILBED COLOR: ☐ Pink
		☐ Pale ☐ Blue
		PEDAL PULSES: R ☐— ☐+
		                              L ☐— ☐+
		EDEMA: R ☐— ☐+
		                              L ☐— ☐+
		CALF R ☐— ☐+
		TENDERNESS: L ☐— ☐+
			BREATH SOUNDS: _____
			
			RESPIRATIONS: _____
			
			OXYGEN: _____
			PULSE OX: _____
			☐ Cough _____
			☐ Sputum _____
			APICAL PULSE: _____
			☐ Regular ☐ Irregular
			TELEMETRY: _____
			
			NAILBED COLOR: ☐ Pink
			☐ Pale ☐ Blue
			PEDAL PULSES: R ☐— ☐+
			                              L ☐— ☐+
			EDEMA: R ☐— ☐+
			                              L ☐— ☐+
			CALF R ☐— ☐+
			TENDERNESS: L ☐— ☐+

FIGURE 4-5 Assessment flow sheet. Form is used when computerized form is unavailable. (Used with permission from Southeast Missouri Hospital, Cape Girardeau, MO.)

	PATIENT ASSESSMENT FLOWSHEET, Page 2		
Addressograph	Date _____		
INITIAL ASSESSMENT	2300-0700 TIME/INITIALS _____	0700-1500 TIME/INITIALS _____	1500-2300 TIME/INITIALS _____
ELIMINATION	ABDOMEN: ☐ Soft ☐ Firm ☐ Nondistended ☐ Distended BOWEL SOUNDS: ☐ Normoactive ☐ Hyperactive ☐ Hypoactive ☐ Absent LBM: _____ TUBES: _____	ABDOMEN: ☐ Soft ☐ Firm ☐ Nondistended ☐ Distended BOWEL SOUNDS: ☐ Normoactive ☐ Hyperactive ☐ Hypoactive ☐ Absent LBM: _____ TUBES: _____	ABDOMEN: ☐ Soft ☐ Firm ☐ Nondistended ☐ Distended BOWEL SOUNDS: ☐ Normoactive ☐ Hyperactive ☐ Hypoactive ☐ Absent LBM: _____ TUBES: _____
ACTIVITY/ EXERCISE	MAE: ☐ Full ☐ Impaired _____ Fall Prevention _____	MAE: ☐ Full ☐ Impaired _____ Fall Prevention _____	MAE: ☐ Full ☐ Impaired _____ Fall Prevention _____
COGNITIVE/ PERCEPTUAL	LOC: ☐ Alert ☐ Lethargic ☐ Unresponsive ORIENTATION: ☐ Person ☐ Place ☐ Time ☐ Pain _____	LOC: ☐ Alert ☐ Lethargic ☐ Unresponsive ORIENTATION: ☐ Person ☐ Place ☐ Time ☐ Pain _____	LOC: ☐ Alert ☐ Lethargic ☐ Unresponsive ORIENTATION: ☐ Person ☐ Place ☐ Time ☐ Pain _____
PLAN OF CARE	Discussed Plan of Care with: ☐ Patient ☐ Family/Significant Other(s)	Discussed Plan of Care with: ☐ Patient ☐ Family/Significant Other(s)	Discussed Plan of Care with: ☐ Patient ☐ Family/Significant Other(s)
CARE PER STANDARD			
ONGOING PATIENT TEACHING (Time and Initial each entry)	☐ Video ☐ Handout/Booklet _____ ☐ Verbal - See Nurses Notes _____ ☐ Pt/Family Response: _____	☐ Video ☐ Handout/Booklet _____ ☐ Verbal - See Nurses Notes _____ ☐ Pt/Family Response: _____	☐ Video ☐ Handout/Booklet _____ ☐ Verbal - See Nurses Notes _____ ☐ Pt/Family Response: _____
EDUCATIONAL (To be completed on Admission and PRN)	Motivation: ☐ Appears Interested ☐ Seems Uninterested ☐ Denies Need for Education Factors Affecting Teaching: _____	Motivation: ☐ Appears Interested ☐ Seems Uninterested ☐ Denies Need for Education Factors Affecting Teaching: _____	Motivation: ☐ Appears Interested ☐ Seems Uninterested ☐ Denies Need for Education Factors Affecting Teaching: _____

FIGURE 4-5 (*Continued*)

11/28/2013 Client dyspneic and tachypneic with respiratory rate of 32 breaths/min. Color is ruddy. Chest barrel shaped. Tactile fremitus diminished bilaterally. Hyperresonance bilateral. Chest expansion and diaphragmatic excursion decreased. Nonproductive, frequent cough. Diminished breath sounds with expiratory wheezes and prolonged expiratory phase. Clients states, "I feel like I can't catch my breath."

FIGURE 4-6 Documentation of assessment findings on a narrative progress note.

streamline the documentation process and prevent needless repetition of data. Emphasis is placed on quality, not quantity, of documentation.

Focused or Specialty Area Assessment Form

Some institutions may use assessment forms that are focused on one major area of the body for clients who have a particular problem. Examples include cardiovascular or neurologic assessment documentation forms. In addition, forms may be customized. For example, a form may be used as a screening tool to assess specific concerns or risks such as falling or skin problems. These forms are usually abbreviated versions of admission data sheets, with specific assessment data related to the purpose of the assessment (Fig. 4-7).

CASE STUDY

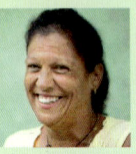

The nurse does a focused assessment on Mrs. Gutierrez focusing on her diabetes, anorexia, and insomnia. Her physical assessment findings follow:

General Survey
Ht: 5 ft 1 in; Wt: 175 lb; Radial pulse: 68; Resp: 18; B/P: R arm—132/76, L arm—128/72; Temp: 98.6. Client alert and cooperative. Sitting comfortably on table with arms at sides. Dress is neat and clean. Walks steadily, with posture erect.

Mental Status Examination: Pleasant and friendly. Appropriately dressed for weather with matching colors and patterns. Clothes neat and clean. Facial expressions symmetrical and correlate with mood and topic discussed. Speech clear and appropriate. Tearful as she discusses her husband and his accident. Carefully chooses words to convey feelings and ideas. Oriented to person, place, time, and events. Remains attentive and able to focus on examination during entire interaction. Unable to recall what was consumed at breakfast and lunch. Able to recall birthday and anniversary dates. General information questions answered correctly 100% of the time. Vocabulary suitable to educational level. Explains proverb accurately. Is able to identify similarities 5 seconds after being asked. Answers judgment questions in realistic manner.

Skin, Hair, and Nails
Skin: Light brown, warm, and dry to touch. Skinfold returns to place after 1 second when lifted over clavicle. No evidence of vascular or purpuric lesions.
Hair: Straight, clean, black with white and gray streaks, thick and supple in texture. No scalp lesions or flaking. No hair noted on axilla or on chest, back, or face.
Nails: Fingernails short in length and thickness, clear. No clubbing or Beau lines.

Head and Neck
Head symmetrically rounded, neck nontender with full ROM. Neck symmetric without masses, scars, pulsations. Lymph nodes nonpalpable. Trachea in midline. Thyroid nonpalpable.

Eyes
Eyes 2 cm apart without protrusion. Eyebrows thick with equal distribution. Lids light brown without ptosis, edema, or lesions, and freely closeable bilaterally. Lacrimal apparatus nonedematous. Sclera white without increased vascularity or lesions noted. Palpebral and bulbar conjunctiva slightly reddened without lesions noted. Iris uniformly brown. PERRLA, EOMs intact bilaterally.

Ears
Auricles without deformity, lumps, or lesions. Auricles and mastoid processes nontender. Bilateral auditory canals clear. Tympanic membranes pearly gray bilaterally with visible landmarks. Hearing intact with Whisper test bilaterally. Weber test: Vibrations heard equally well in both ears with no lateralization to either side. Rinne test: Air conduction is heard longer than bone conduction in both ears (AC > BC).

Mouth, Throat, Nose, and Sinuses
Lips moist, no lesions or ulcerations. Buccal mucosa pink and moist with patchy areas of dark pigment on ventral surface of tongue, gums, and floor of mouth. No ulcers or nodules. Gums pink and moist without inflammation, bleeding, or discoloration. Hard and soft palates smooth without lesions or masses. Tongue midline when protruded, no lesions, or masses. No lesions, discolorations, or ulcerations on floor of mouth, oral mucosa, or gums. Uvula in midline and elevates on phonation. External structure of nose without deformity, asymmetry, or inflammation. Nares patent. Turbinates and middle meatus pale pink, without swelling, exudate, lesions, or bleeding. Nasal septum midline without bleeding, perforation, or deviation. Frontal and maxillary sinuses nontender.

Thorax and Lung
Skin light brown without scars, pulsations, or lesions. No hair noted. Thorax expands evenly bilaterally without retractions or bulging. Respirations even, unlabored, and regular. No tenderness, crepitus, or masses. Tactile fremitus equal and symmetric bilaterally. Vesicular breath sounds heard throughout. No crackles, wheezes, or friction rubs.

Heart and Neck Vessels
No pulsations visible. No heaves, lifts, or vibrations. Apical impulse: 5th ICS to LMCL. Clear, brief heart sounds throughout. S1, S2 present. No S3, S4, gallops, murmurs, or rubs.

Abdomen
Abdomen rounded, symmetric without masses, lesions, pulsations, or peristalsis noted. Abdomen free of hair, bruising, and increased vasculature. Umbilicus in midline, without herniation, swelling, or discoloration. Bowel sounds low pitched and gurgling at 16/min × 4 quads. Aortic, renal, and iliac arteries auscultated without bruit. No venous hums or friction rubs auscultated over liver or spleen. Tympany percussed throughout. No tenderness or masses noted with light and deep palpation. Liver and spleen nonpalpable. Liver span is 10 cm in MCL. Aorta 3 cm with strong regular pulse.

Peripheral Vascular

Upper Extremities: Equal in size and symmetry bilaterally; light brown; warm and dry to touch without edema, bruising, or lesions. Radial pulses = in rate and 2+ bilaterally. Brachial pulses equal and 2+ bilaterally.

Lower Extremities: Legs symmetric. Skin intact, light brown; warm and dry to touch without edema, bruising, lesions, or increased vascularity. Femoral pulses 2+ and equal without bruits. Dorsalis pedal and posterior tibial pulses 1+ and equal. No edema palpable.

Musculoskeletal

Posture erect: Gait steady, smooth, and coordinated with even base. Full ROM of cervical and lumbar spine. Full ROM of upper and lower extremities. Strength 5/5 of upper and lower extremities.

Neurologic

Cranial Nerve Examination: Cranial nerves II through XII grossly intact.

Motor and Cerebellar Examination: Muscle tone firm at rest, abdominal muscles slightly relaxed. Muscle size adequate for age. No fasciculations or involuntary movements noted. Gross and fine motor movements intact. Romberg: Minimal swaying. Tandem walk: Steady. No involuntary movements noted.

Sensory Status Examination: Superficial light and deep touch sensation intact on arms, hands, fingers, legs, feet, and toes. Position sense of toes and fingers intact bilaterally. Stereognosis and graphesthesia intact.

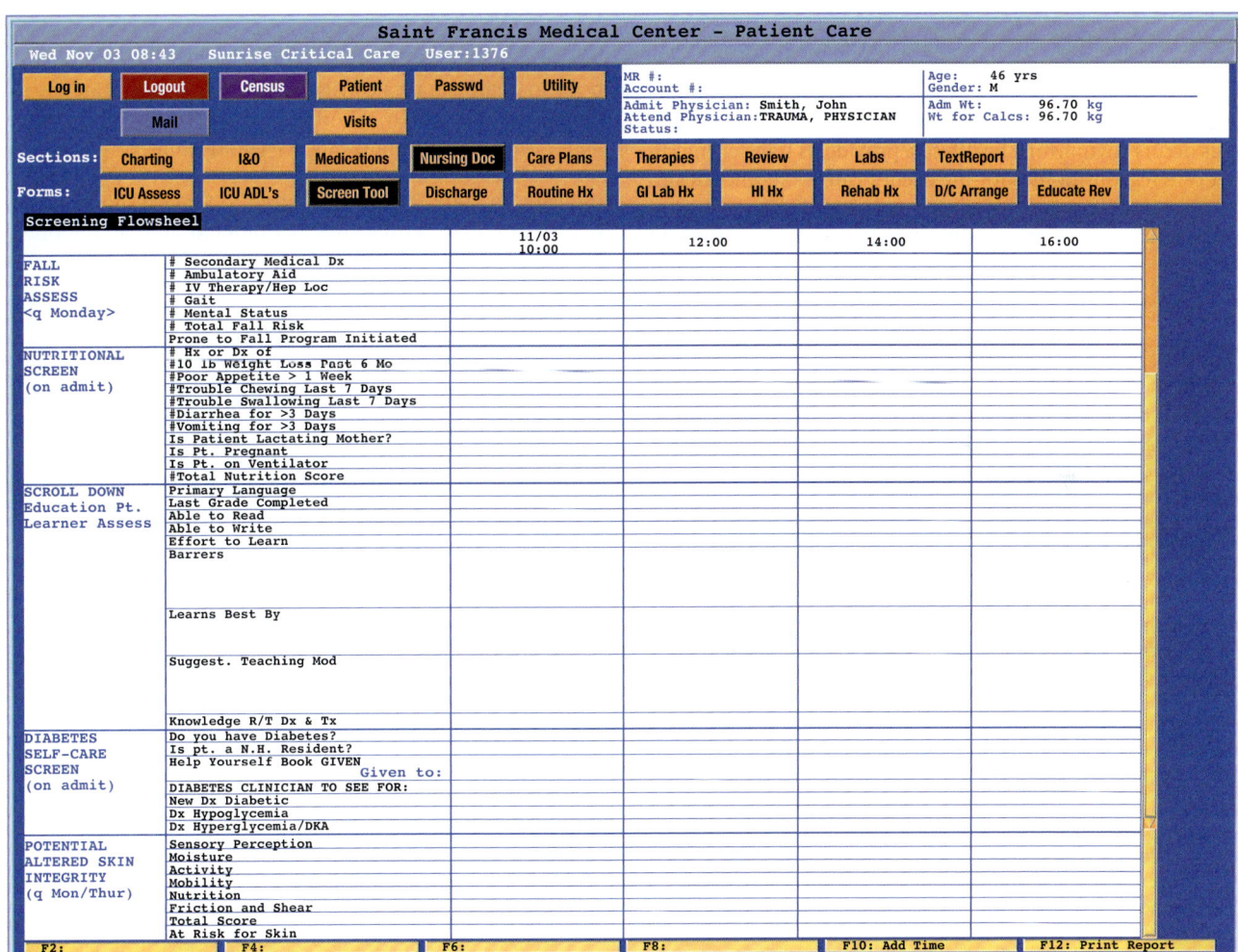

FIGURE 4-7 Portions of a computerized screening flow sheet. The full assessment document includes cells for systemic findings as well as functional data, such as nutrition, activities of daily living, and client education needs. (Used with permission from Saint Francis Medical Center, Cape Girardeau, MO.)

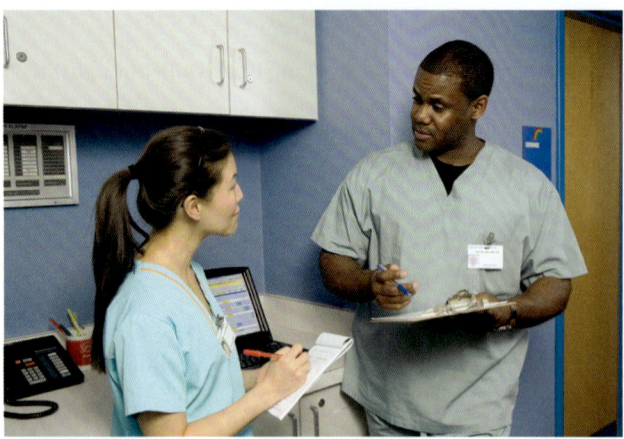

FIGURE 4-8 It is important to report assessment findings verbally in an effective manner to other health care workers.

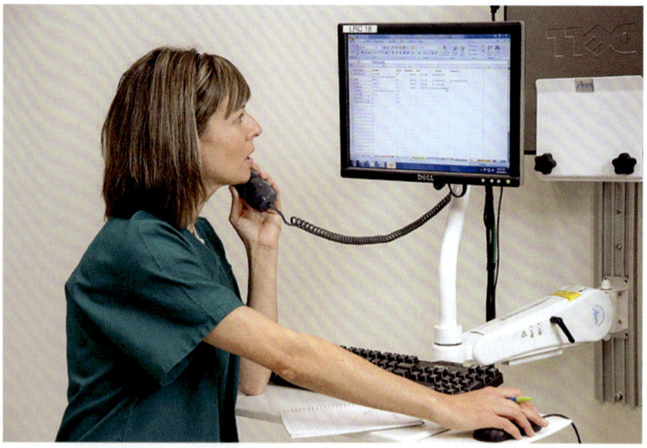

FIGURE 4-9 When reporting over a telephone, ask the receiver to read back what he or she heard you report and document the phone call with time, receiver, sender, and information shared.

VERBAL COMMUNICATION OF DATA

Nurses are often in situations in which they are required to verbally share their subjective and objective assessment findings. They must be able to report assessment findings verbally in an effective manner to other health care workers (Fig. 4-8). This occurs anytime one health care provider is transferring client care responsibilities for the client's care to another health care provider. This is referred to as a "handoff." This handoff may occur when the agency shift changes, nurses leave the unit for a break or meal, a client is transferred to another unit or facility, and when a client leaves his or her unit for a test or procedure.

The SBAR (Situation, Background, Assessment, Recommendation) model of communication will be used throughout this book to demonstrate a consistent way to communicate assessment data. Originally, SBAR was developed by the United States Navy as a communication technique that could be used on nuclear submarines and was later used by the aviation industry. In 2002, it was introduced to rapid response teams (RRTs) at Kaiser Permanente in Colorado and later adopted by many other health care organizations. It is one of the most common handover mnemonic models used in health care. The Joint Commission recognizes it as a best practice for standardized communication among health care providers. SBAR, described in Box 4-3, has been found to improve quality and patient safety outcomes when used by health team members to communicate or hand off client information (Beckett & Kipnis, 2009). The more people are involved in a handoff of information, the greater the risk of a communication error. To prevent data communication errors, it is important to:

- Use a standardized method of data communication such as SBAR (see Box 4-3).
- Communicate face to face with good eye contact.
- Allow time for the receiver to ask questions.
- Provide documentation of the data you are sharing.
- Validate what the receiver has heard by questioning or asking him or her to summarize your report.
- When reporting over a telephone (Fig. 4-9), ask the receiver to read back what he or she heard you report and document the phone call with time, receiver, sender, and information shared.

BOX 4-3 SBAR (SITUATION, BACKGROUND, ASSESSMENT, AND RECOMMENDATION)

Situation: State concisely why you need to communicate the client data that you have assessed (example: Mary Lorno, 18 years of age, is experiencing a sudden onset of periumbilical pain).

Background: Describe the events that led up to the current situation (example: Client first noticed periumbilical pain at 10:30 AM. She denies any precipitating factors).

Assessment: State the subjective and objective data you have collected (example: *Subjective:* Client rated pain as 7–8 on a scale of 0 to 10 at onset and now rates the pain as 3–4 on scale of 0 to 10. She denies nausea, vomiting, and diarrhea. She voices anorexia. Eating and drinking exacerbates the pain and lying in a knee–chest position diminishes pain. Describes the pain as "stabbing." *Objective:* Client is awake, alert, and oriented. She makes and maintains conversation. Does not appear to be in acute distress. T—98.7, P—72, R—16, BP—112/64. Color pink. Skin warm and dry. Mucous membranes moist. Abdomen flat without visible pulsations. Bowel sounds present and hypoactive. Abdomen tympanic upon percussion. Abdomen is soft. Light palpation reveals minimal tenderness in RLQ. Deep palpation reveals minimal tenderness in RLQ. Rovsing sign is negative. Obturator sign is negative. No rebound tenderness noted.)

Recommendation: Suggest what you believe needs to be done for the client based on your assessment findings (Example: Suggest that the primary care provider come to further assess the client and intervene).

SUMMARY

Validation, documentation, and verbal communication of data are three crucial aspects of nursing health assessment. Nurses need to concentrate on learning how to perform these three skills steps of assessment thoroughly and accurately.

Validation of data verifies the assessment data that you have gathered from the client. It consists of determining which data require validation, implementing techniques to validate, and identifying areas that require further assessment data.

Documentation of data is the act of recording the client assessment findings. Nurses first need to understand the purpose of documentation, next learn which information to document, then be aware of and follow the individual documentation guidelines of their particular health care facility. In addition, it is important for nurses to be familiar with the different documentation forms used in the health care agency in which they practice.

Finally, nurses need to know how to verbally communicate assessment findings in a clear and concise manner to other health care providers.

> **Want to know more?**
>
> A wide variety of resources to enhance your learning and understanding of this book are available on thePoint. Visit thePoint to access:
>
> NCLEX-Style Student Review Questions
> Watch and Learn Videos
> Concepts in Action Animations
> And more!

References and Selected Readings

American Sentinel University. (2013). EHR integration and meaningful use. Available at http://www.americansentinel.edu/blog/2013/01/03/ehr-integration-and-meaningful-use-a-nursing-perspective/

Beckett, C., & Kipnis, G. (2009). Collaborative communication: Integrating SBAR to improve quality/patient safety outcomes. *Journal for Healthcare Quality, 31*(5), 19–28. Available at http://onlinelibrary.wiley.com/doi/10.1111/j.1945-1474.2009.00043.x/full

Health IT. (2014). Benefits of EHRs. Available at www.healthit.gov/providers-professional/improved-diagnostics-patient-outcomes

Health Information Technology for Economic and Clinical Health (HITECH) Act. (2009). Available at http://www.apapracticecentral.org/advocacy/technology/hitech-act.aspx

Health Insurance Portability and Accountability Act (HIPAA). (1996). Available at https://aspe.hhs.gov/report/health-insurance-portability-and-accountability-act-1996

Kutney-Lee, A., & Kelly, D. (2011). The effect of hospital electronic health record adoption on nurse-assessed quality of care and patient safety. *Journal of Nursing Administration, 41*(11), 466–472.

Lavin, M., Harper, E., & Barr, N. (2015, April 14). Health information technology: Patient safety and professional nursing care documentation in acute care settings. *OJIN: The Online Journal of Issues in Nursing, 20*(2). Available at http://www.nursingworld.org/MainMenuCategories/ANAMarketplace/ANAPeriodicals/OJIN/TableofContents/Vol-20-2015/No2-May-2015/Articles-Previous-Topics/Technology-Safety-and-Professional-Care-Documentation.html#Cipriano

Wood, D. (2014). Nurses' vital role in EMR upgrades creating opportunities. Available at www.nursezone.com/Nursing-News-Events/more-news/Nurses-Vital-Role-in-EMR-Upgrades-Creating-Opportunities_42142.aspx

5 THINKING CRITICALLY TO ANALYZE DATA AND MAKE INFORMED NURSING JUDGMENTS

Learning Objectives

1. Describe how the nurse uses critical thinking to formulate clinical judgments.
2. Assess your grown critical thinking skills.
3. Discuss the characteristics of critical thinking.
4. Explain the seven distinct steps described in this textbook to perform a data analysis.
5. Define nursing diagnoses (wellness, risk, and actual) with examples of each.
6. Define collaborative problem with examples.
7. Explain why experienced nurses are better able to formulate accurate nursing judgments as compared with novice nurses.
8. Describe ways to avoid the common "Pitfalls" and ways to increase the accuracy of one's diagnostic reasoning skills.

CASE STUDY

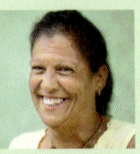

You met Mrs. Gutierrez in Chapter 1. Recall that she arrived at the clinic for diabetic teaching but appeared distracted and sad, uninterested in the teaching. She was unable to focus, pacing back and forth in the clinic and wringing her hands. The nurse suspected that Mrs. Gutierrez was upset by her diagnosis of diabetes. However, through the interview, the nurse learned additional information that changed her thoughts about the client.

You learned how the nurse collected subjective and objective data from Mrs. Gutierrez in Chapters 2 and 3. In Chapter 4, you learned how the nurse validated, documented, and communicated data gathered from Mrs. Gutierrez. In this chapter, you will learn how to analyze the subjective and objective data.

Data analysis is often referred to as the diagnostic phase or clinical reasoning phase because the end result or purpose is the identification of a nursing diagnosis (health promotion, wellness, actual, or risk), collaborative problem, or need for referral to another health care professional. Critical thinking is the way in which the nurse processes information using knowledge, past experiences, intuition, and cognitive abilities to formulate conclusions or diagnoses.

ANALYSIS OF DATA THROUGHOUT HEALTH ASSESSMENT IN NURSING

The purpose of assessing a client's health status is to analyze the subjective and objective data collected. In the clinical assessment chapters of this textbook, *Analysis of Data* sections have been developed to help the reader visualize, understand, and practice analyzing data (diagnostic reasoning).

The *Analysis of Data* section includes health promotion diagnoses, risk diagnoses, actual diagnoses, collaborative problems, and referrals to health care providers for possible medical problems. A list of possible nursing diagnoses and collaborative problems is presented to familiarize the reader with some potential conclusions seen with a particular body part or system. They also serve as a reference for the case study in each chapter. Lists of nursing diagnoses and collaborative problems can also be found in the appendices of this textbook.

The case study that is introduced at the beginning of each chapter ends with possible nursing diagnoses, collaborative problems, and referrals for the particular client who was assessed throughout the chapter. An algorithm depicting the process of diagnostic reasoning for the particular client case in each chapter is available on thePoint. This algorithm illustrates the seven key steps of data analysis. It is designed to help the reader use critical thinking to analyze client data.

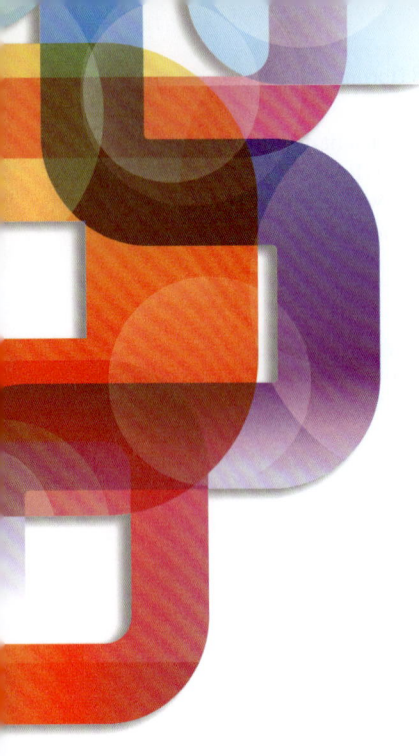

ANALYSIS OF DATA AND CRITICAL THINKING—STEP TWO OF THE NURSING PROCESS

As the second step of the nursing process, data analysis can be challenging because the nurse is required to use diagnostic reasoning skills to interpret data accurately. Diagnostic reasoning is a form of critical thinking. Due to the complex nature of nursing as both a science and an art, the nurse must think critically—in a rational, self-directed, intelligent, and purposeful manner.

The nurse must develop several characteristics to think critically (Box 5-1). Ask yourself the following questions to determine your critical thinking skills:
- Do you reserve your final opinion or judgment until you have collected more or all of the information?
- Do you support your opinion or comments with supporting data, sound rationale, and literature?
- Do you explore and consider other alternatives before making a decision?
- Can you distinguish between a fact, opinion, cue, or inference?
- Do you ask your client for more information or clarification when you do not understand?
- Do you validate your information and judgments with experts in the field?
- Do you use your past knowledge and experiences to analyze data?
- Do you try to avoid biases or preconceived ways of thinking?
- Do you try to learn from past mistakes in your judgments?
- Are you open to the fact that you may not always be right?

If you answered "yes" to most of these questions, you have already started to develop a critical thinking mindset. If you need practice, many books (some with practice exercises) are available on how to think critically as a nurse. Such books can help the nurse to learn and continue to develop critical thinking skills.

The Diagnostic Reasoning Process

Before you begin analyzing data, make sure you have accurately performed the steps of the assessment phase of the nursing process (collection and organization of assessment data, validation of data, and documentation of data). This information will have a profound effect on the conclusions you reach in the analysis step of the nursing process.

If you are confident of your work during the assessment phase, you are ready to analyze your data—the diagnostic phase of the nursing process. This phase consists of the following essential components: grouping and organizing data, validating data and comparing the data with norms, clustering data to make inferences, generating possible hypotheses regarding the client's problems, formulating a professional clinical judgment, and validating the judgment with the client. These basic components have been organized in various ways to break the process of diagnostic reasoning into easily understood steps. Regardless of how the information is organized or the title of the steps, diagnostic reasoning always consists of these components.

This text presents seven distinct steps to provide a clear, concise explanation of how to perform data analysis. Each step is described in detail and is followed by a case study to illustrate how each step works when analyzing data for a client. These seven steps are used throughout this text in the Analysis of Data sections of the assessment chapters.

Step One—Identify Strengths and Abnormal Data

Identifying client strengths and abnormal findings requires the nurse to have and use a knowledge base of anatomy and physiology, psychology, and sociology. In addition, the nurse should compare collected assessment data with findings in reliable charts and references that provide standards and values for physical and psychological norms (i.e., height, nutritional requirements, growth and development). In addition, the nurse should have a basic knowledge of risk factors for the client. Risk factors are based on client data such as gender, age, ethnic background, genetic predisposition, family history, lifestyle, health practices, and occupation. Therefore, the nurse needs to have access to both the data supplied by the client and the known risk factors for specific diseases or disorders.

The nurse's knowledge of anatomy and physiology, psychology, and sociology; use of reference materials; and attention to risk factors helps to identify strengths, risks, and abnormal findings. Remember to analyze both subjective and objective data when identifying strengths and abnormal findings.

> **CLINICAL TIP**
> Identified strengths are used in formulating health promotion diagnoses and to minimize potential and/or actual weaknesses. Identified potential weaknesses are used in formulating risk diagnoses, and actual weaknesses/abnormal findings are used in formulating actual nursing diagnoses.

BOX 5-1 ESSENTIAL ELEMENTS OF CRITICAL THINKING

- Keep an open mind.
- Use rationale to support opinions or decisions.
- Reflect on thoughts before reaching a conclusion.
- Use past clinical experiences to build knowledge.
- Acquire an adequate knowledge base that continues to build.
- Be aware of the interactions of others.
- Be aware of the environment.

CASE STUDY

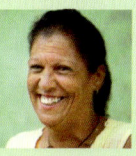

Using Mrs. Gutierrez's case, you may identify the following:

Identified Strengths and Abnormal Data: Subjective
- "Cannot eat or sleep"
- "I only sleep for 4 to 5 hours a night. Once I fall asleep, about 10 PM, I wake up about 2 AM and cannot go back to sleep right away. I do not take naps during the day. I am so tired in the daytime that I just lie in bed but I do not sleep."

- "I eat cereal in the morning but I am not able to eat much the rest of the day. I eat less than one half of what I used to eat. I still try to cook but I only eat one bite of a tamale and maybe a bite or two of beans or rice. I used to bake a lot but no longer have the energy to bake. My stomach always feels full and I know I am not eating as I should. My daughter has tried baking me cookies and I eat those sometimes. I am sometimes nauseated when I cannot eat."
- Symptoms started "two months ago, right after my husband was in a car wreck."
- States has had "susto" since her husband's accident.
- "I have tried taking Excedrin PM over the counter but it just makes me feel more drowsy all day."
- "My clothes no longer fit and are very loose."
- "I worry a lot as to how we will pay our bills now that my husband has lost his job and we do not have health insurance."
- "The other day I began crying over nothing. I just feel sad all the time."
- Has husband and three daughters living at home, two older sons in Mexico.
- Daughter shares car and now shops and helps her mother.
- When feeling well, client says she does all housework and gardening by herself.
- States lacks health insurance.
- States has gained so much weight over last few years and was pretty before. Now has lost weight and clothes hang on her, but still overweight.
- States lives in a three-bedroom house in neighborhood that is not really safe.

Identified Strengths and Abnormal Data: Objective
- Tearful when speaking of husband's accident
- No health insurance
- Lives in a relatively unsafe neighborhood
- All physical systems otherwise within normal limits

Step Two—Cluster Data

During step two, the nurse looks at the identified strengths and abnormal findings for cues that are related. Cluster both abnormal cues and strength cues.

While clustering the data, you may find that certain cues support a problem but that more data are needed to support the determination of that problem. For example, a client may have a nonproductive cough with labored respirations at a rate of 24 per minute; however, you have gathered no data on the status of breath sounds. In such a situation, you would need to assess the client's breath sounds to formulate an appropriate nursing diagnosis or collaborative problem.

CASE STUDY

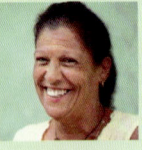

Using the sample case of Mrs. Gutierrez, one identified cue cluster would be:
- "Cannot sleep"
- "I only sleep for 4–5 hours a night. Once I fall asleep, about 10 PM, I wake up about 2 AM and cannot go back to sleep right away. I do not take naps during the day. I am so tired in the daytime that I just lay in bed but I do not sleep."
- Symptoms started "two months ago, right after my husband was in a car wreck."
- States has had "susto" since her husband's accident.
- "I have tried taking Excedrin PM over the counter but it just makes me feel more drowsy all day."
- "I worry a lot as to how we will pay our bills now that my husband has lost his job and we do not have health insurance."
- "The other day I began crying over nothing. I just feel sad all the time."
- Tearful when speaking of husband's accident.
- Short-term memory deficient, long-term memory intact.

Step Three—Draw Inferences

Step three requires the nurse to document inferences (hunches or assumptions) about each cue cluster. For example, based on the cue cluster presented in step two—rash on face, neck, chest, and back; patchy alopecia; "so ugly"—you would write down what you think these data are saying and determine whether it is something that the nurse can treat independently. Your inference about this data cluster might be: "Changes in physical appearance are affecting self-perception." This is something for which the nurse would intervene and treat independently. Therefore, the nurse would move to step four: analysis of data to formulate a nursing diagnosis.

However, if the inference you draw from a cue cluster suggests the need for both medical and nursing interventions to resolve the problem, you would attempt to identify collaborative problems. Collaborative problems are defined as "certain physiological complications that nurses monitor to detect their onset or changes in status; nurses manage collaborative problems using physician-prescribed and nursing-prescribed interventions to minimize the complications of events" (Carpenito, 2017). Collaborative problems are equivalent in importance to nursing diagnoses but represent the interdependent or collaborative role of nursing. A list of collaborative problems is given in Appendix D. Figure 5-1 illustrates how to differentiate between nursing diagnoses and collaborative problems.

Another purpose of step three is the referral of identified problems for which the nurse cannot prescribe definitive treatment. Referring can be defined as connecting clients with other professionals and resources. For example, if the collaborative problem for which the nurse is monitoring occurs, an immediate referral to the client's health care provider is necessary for implementing medical treatment. Another example may be a diabetic client who is experiencing difficulty understanding a diabetic diet. Although the nurse has knowledge in this area, referral to a dietitian can provide the client with updated information and allow the nurse more time to deal with client problems within the nursing domain. Another important reason for referral is the identification or suspicion of a medical problem. In such cases, a referral must be considered.

5 Thinking Critically to Analyze Data and Make Informed Nursing Judgments 63

Step Four—Propose Possible Nursing Diagnoses

If resolution of the situation requires primarily nursing interventions, you would hypothesize and generate possible nursing diagnoses. The nursing diagnoses may be wellness, or health promotion diagnoses; risk diagnoses; or actual diagnoses; and syndrome diagnoses (NANDA, 2014).

A wellness diagnosis, or a health promotion nursing diagnosis, indicates that the client (individual, family, community) has the motivation to increase well-being and enhance health behaviors. There are occasions when clients are ready to improve their current health state, which may be a healthy state or an unhealthy state. When such an opportunity exists, the nurse can support the client's movement toward greater health and wellness by identifying "readiness for enhanced" as the diagnostic label (e.g., readiness for enhanced sleep pattern).

A risk diagnosis indicates the client does not currently have the problem but is vulnerable to developing it (e.g., risk for impaired skin integrity related to immobility, poor nutrition, and incontinence).

An actual nursing diagnosis indicates that the client is currently experiencing the stated problem or has a dysfunctional pattern (e.g., impaired skin integrity: reddened area on right buttocks). Table 5-1 provides a comparison of wellness, risk, and actual nursing diagnoses. Appendix C provides a list of common nursing diagnoses.

On occasion, a syndrome diagnosis is appropriate. When a cluster of nursing diagnoses is related in a way that they occur together, a syndrome diagnosis is made.

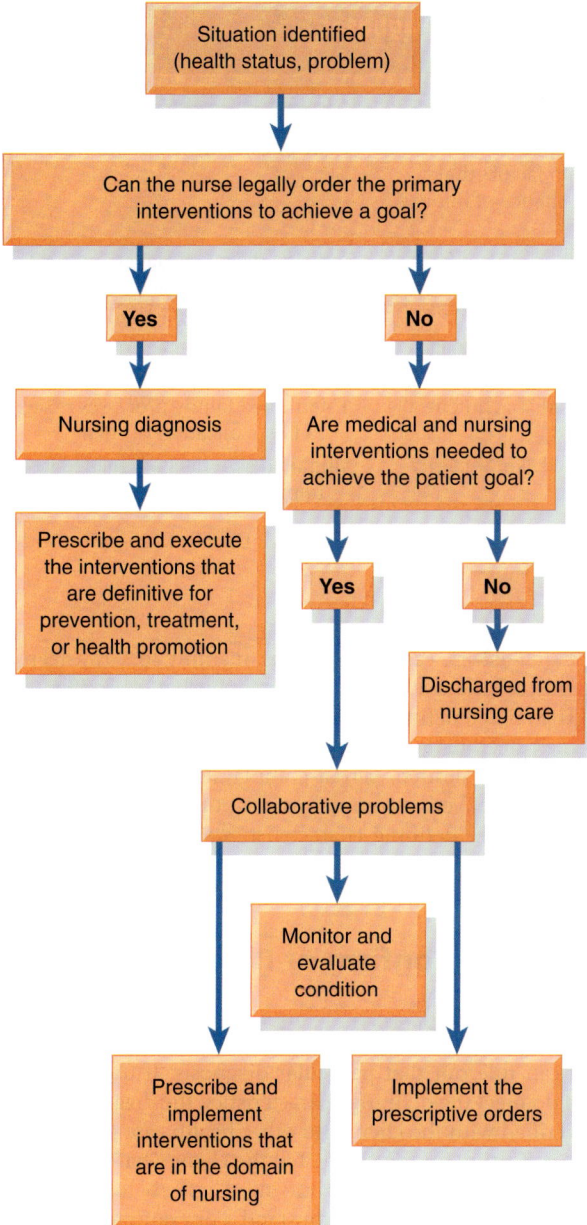

FIGURE 5-1 Differentiating nursing diagnoses and collaborative problems. (Redrawn from Carpenito, L. J. (2017). Nursing diagnosis: Application to clinical practice (15th ed.). Philadelphia, PA: Wolters Kluwer.)

The referral process differs from health care setting to health care setting. To save time and to provide high-quality care for the client, make sure you are familiar with the referral process/policy used in your health care setting.

CASE STUDY

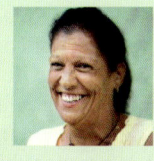

Inferences drawn from the case study of Mrs. Gutierrez:
Sleep deficit and emotional stress from husband's accident.

CASE STUDY

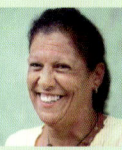

Using the case of Mrs. Gutierrez, the cue cluster from step two was determined to be:
- "Cannot sleep"
- "I only sleep for 4–5 hours a night. Once I fall asleep, about 10 PM, I wake up about 2 AM and cannot go back to sleep right away. I do not take naps during the day. I am so tired in the daytime that I just lay in bed but I do not sleep."
- Symptoms started "two months ago, right after my husband was in a car wreck."
- States has had "susto" since her husband's accident.
- "I have tried taking Excedrin PM over the counter but it just makes me feel more drowsy all day."
- "I worry a lot as to how we will pay our bills now that my husband has lost his job and we do not have health insurance."
- "The other day I began crying over nothing. I just feel sad all the time."
- Tearful when speaking of husband's accident.
- Short-term memory deficient, long-term memory intact.

A possible nursing diagnosis based on these inferences is:
- Disturbed sleep pattern related to prolonged time to fall asleep, early awakenings, inability to stay asleep, "susto" and associated worry after husband's accident.

TABLE 5-1 Comparison of Health Promotion, Risk, and Actual Nursing Diagnoses (described by NANDA-I, 2014)

	Health Promotion Diagnoses	Risk Diagnoses	Actual Diagnoses
Client status	Client verbalizes desire to increase well-being and actualize human health potential.	Vulnerability, especially as a result of exposure to factors that increase the chance of injury or loss.	State of existing health problems
Format for stating	Readiness for enhanced … or stated as problem such as: Diversional activity deficit, sedentary lifestyle	"Risk for …"	Nursing diagnostic label and "related to" clause
Examples	Readiness for enhanced communication	Risk for disturbed body image	Disturbed body image related to hand wound that is not healing
	Readiness for enhanced health management	Risk for impaired attachment	Interrupted family processes related to hospitalization of client
	Readiness for enhanced diversional activity	Risk for impaired skin integrity	Impaired skin integrity related to immobility

From Nursing Diagnoses: Definitions and Classifications 2015–2017. Copyright © 2014, by NANDA International. Used by arrangement with John Wiley & Sons Limited.

Step Five—Check for Defining Characteristics

At this point in analyzing the data, the nurse must check for defining characteristics for the data clusters and hypothesized diagnoses in order to choose the most accurate diagnoses and delete those diagnoses that are not valid or accurate for the client. This step is often difficult because diagnostic labels overlap, making it hard to identify the most appropriate diagnosis. For example, the diagnostic categories of impaired gas exchange, ineffective airway clearance, and ineffective breathing patterns all reflect respiratory problems but each is used to describe a very different human response pattern and set of defining characteristics.

NANDA-I's definition for defining characteristics is "Observable cues/inferences that cluster as manifestations of a problem-focused, health-promotion diagnosis or syndrome" (NANDA-I, 2015).

Reference texts such as North American Nursing Diagnosis Association (NANDA) *Nursing Diagnoses: Definitions and Classifications 2015–2017* can assist the nurse in determining when and when not to use each nursing diagnostic category (NANDA, 2014). It assists with ruling out invalid diagnoses and selecting valid diagnoses. Thus both the definitions of the diagnoses and defining characteristics should be compared with the client's data (cues) to make sure the correct diagnoses are chosen. For an example of how to check for defining characteristics, consider the nursing diagnosis hypothesized in step four. Defining characteristics, as defined by NANDA-I, 2016), are "observable cues/inferences that cluster as manifestations of a problem-focused, health-promotion diagnosis or syndrome. This does not only imply those things that the nurse can see, but things that are seen, heard (e.g., the patient/family tells us), touched or smelled".

CASE STUDY

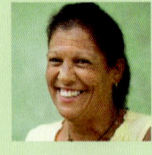

The nurse now determines if the data collected from Mrs. Gutierrez meet defining characteristics of the identified nursing diagnosis: "Disturbed sleep pattern related to prolonged time to fall asleep, early awakenings, inability to stay asleep, "susto," and associated worry after husband's accident." The related defining characteristics (prolonged awakenings, sleep maintenance insomnia, awakening earlier or later than desired, verbal complaints of difficulty falling asleep, verbal complaints of not feeling well rested) meet these defining characteristics associated with the diagnosis.

Step Six—Confirm or Rule out Diagnoses

If the cue cluster data do not meet the defining characteristics, you can rule out that particular diagnosis. If the cue cluster data do meet the defining characteristics, the diagnosis should be verified with the client and other health care professionals who are caring for the client. Tell the client what you perceive the diagnosis to be. Often nursing diagnosis terminology is difficult for the client to understand. For example, you would not report that you believe the client has impaired nutrition: less than body requirements. Instead you might say that you believe current nutritional intake is not adequate to promote healing of body tissues. Then you would ask the client if this seems to be an accurate statement of the problem. When the client is not cognitively impaired, it is important to promote patient understanding of the problem so that mutual goal setting can be promoted. If the client is not in a coherent state of mind to help validate the problem, consult with family members or significant others, or even other health care professionals.

Validation is also important with the client who has a collaborative problem or who requires a referral. If the client has a collaborative problem, you need to inform the client about which signs you are monitoring. For example, you explain that you will be monitoring blood pressure and level of consciousness every 30 minutes for the next several hours. It is also important to collaborate with the client regarding referrals to determine what is needed to resolve the problem and to discuss possible resources to help the client. When possible, provide the client with a list of possible resources (including availability and cost). Help the client to make the contact as necessary. Then follow up to determine if the referral was made and if the client was connected to the appropriate resources.

CASE STUDY

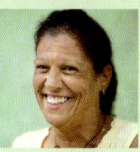

Using the sample case of Mrs. Gutierrez, we have identified the nursing diagnosis: disturbed sleep pattern related to prolonged time to fall asleep, early awakenings, inability to stay asleep, "susto," and associated worry after her husband's accident. You accept the diagnosis because it meets defining characteristics and is validated by the client.

Step Seven—Document Conclusions

Be sure to document all of your professional observations and the data that support the diagnoses, collaborative problems, and referrals. Documentation of data collection before analysis is described in Chapter 4. Guidelines for correctly documenting nursing diagnoses, collaborative problems, and referrals are described in the sections that follow.

Nursing diagnostic statements are often documented and worded in different formats depending on the agency's documentation policy and procedures. However for the purposes of this book the NANDA-International formats for actual, wellness or health promotion, risk, and syndrome nursing diagnoses will be used and are described in the following sections. In addition, the major conclusions of a nursing assessment are compared in Table 5-2.

Actual Nursing Diagnoses

The most useful format for an actual nursing diagnosis is:
- NANDA-label (for problem) + related to (r/t) + etiology + as manifested by (AMB) + defining characteristics
- *Example:* Fatigue r/t an increase in job demands and personal stress AMB client's statements of feeling exhausted all of the time and inability to perform usual work and home responsibilities (e.g., cooking, cleaning).

Shorter formats are often used to describe client problems. However, this format provides all of the necessary information and provides the reader with the clearest and most accurate description of the client's problem.

Wellness or Health Promotion Nursing Diagnoses

Health promotion diagnoses represent those situations in which the client may or may not have a problem but now desires to attain a higher level of health. In other words, the client wishes to increase his or her well-being and actualize human potential. This type of diagnosis is worded "readiness for enhanced…." It indicates an opportunity to make greater, to increase the quality of, or to attain the most desired level of function in the area of the diagnostic category. When documenting these diagnoses, it is best to use the following format:
- Readiness for enhanced + nursing diagnosis problem-oriented diagnostic label + r/t + statement of desire to improve etiology

TABLE 5-2 Major Conclusions of Assessment

	Health Promotion Nursing Diagnosis	Actual Problem Nursing Diagnosis	Risk Nursing Diagnosis	Collaborative Problem	Problem for Referral
Who identifies the concern?	Nurse	Nurse	Nurse	Nurse or other provider	Nurse or other provider
Who deals with the concern?	Nurse (independent practice)	Nurse (independent practice)	Nurse (independent practice)	Nurse (independent practice)	Other provider
What content knowledge is needed?	Nursing science Sciences Basic studies	Nursing science Sciences Basic studies	Nursing science Sciences Basic studies	Nursing science Sciences Basic studies Domain of other providers	Nursing science Sciences Basic studies Domain of other providers
What minimum work experience is needed?	Average	Average	Better than average	Average	Average
What does first part of conclusion statement look like?	Readiness for enhanced …	Taxonomy label or other descriptive label	Usually taxonomy label of "Risk for …"	Risk for complication (RC)	N/A
Are related factors included?	Yes (but not mandatory)	Yes, unless unknown	Yes (mandatory)	Sometimes	N/A
What might complete statement look like?	Readiness for enhanced health management r/t expressed desire to establish exercise routine	Ineffective family coping r/t lack of knowledge, new baby in family, and husband's loss of job	Risk for impaired skin integrity r/t immobility, incontinence, and fragile skin	RC: Blood product side effects	Unsafe housing (referral is necessary)

r/t, related to; RC, risk for complication.

- *Example:* Readiness for enhanced sleep pattern r/t expressed desire to learn ways to stay asleep throughout night.

Health promotion diagnoses other than those for which NANDA has labels may be formulated by using the following format:

- Readiness for enhanced + NANDA problem-oriented diagnostic label minus the modifiers + r/t + etiology + AMB + symptoms (defining characteristics)
- *Example:* Readiness for enhanced parenting r/t expressed desire to improve parenting AMB parent's verbalized concern to continue effective parenting skills during child's illness.

Risk Nursing Diagnoses

A risk diagnosis describes a situation in which the client is vulnerable to an actual diagnosis that will most likely occur if the nurse does not intervene. In this case, the client does not manifest any symptoms or defining characteristics, thus a shorter statement is sufficient:

- Risk for + diagnostic label + r/t + etiology
- *Example:* Risk for Infection r/t presence of dirty knife wound, leukopenia, and lack of client knowledge of how to adequately care for the wound.

Syndrome Nursing Diagnoses

Syndrome diagnoses are clinical judgments that describe a specific cluster of nursing diagnoses that occur together and have similar nursing interventions to resolve the situation. NANDA-I has listed a number of syndrome nursing diagnoses as actual or risk diagnoses. These include: disuse syndrome, frail elderly syndrome, pain syndrome, posttrauma syndrome, rape trauma syndrome, relocation stress syndrome, sudden infant death syndrome (NANDA-I, 2014).

Collaborative Problems and Referrals

Collaborative problems (as described by Carpenito, 2017) should be documented as risk for complications (or RC): _____ (what the problem is). Nursing goals for collaborative problems should also be documented as which parameters the nurse must monitor and how often they should be monitored. In addition, the nurse needs to indicate when the health care provider should be notified and identify nursing interventions to help prevent the complication from occurring, as well as nursing interventions to be initiated if a change occurs. If a referral is indicated, document the problem (or suspected problem), the need for immediate referral, and to whom the client is being referred.

CASE STUDY

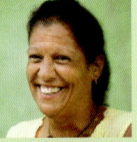

Using the sample case of Mrs. Gutierrez, the cue cluster we have identified, the nurse would document the following conclusion:
- Disturbed sleep pattern r/t prolonged time to fall asleep, early awakenings, inability to stay asleep, "susto," and associated worry after husband's accident.

Developing Diagnostic Reasoning Expertise and Avoiding Pitfalls

A diagnosis is considered to be highly accurate if the diagnosis is as precise as possible and is supported by highly relevant cues (defining characteristics) (Lunney, 2009). Developing expertise in making professional judgments comes with accumulation of both knowledge and experience. One does not become an expert diagnostician overnight. It is a process that develops with time and practice. A beginning nurse attempts to make accurate diagnoses but, because of a lack of knowledge and experience, often finds that he or she has made diagnostic errors. Experts have an advantage because they know when exceptions can be applied to the rules that the novice is accustomed to using and applying. Beginning nurses tend to see things as right or wrong, whereas experts realize there are shades of gray or areas between right and wrong. Novices also tend to focus on details and may miss the big picture, whereas experts have a broader perspective in examining situations.

Although beginning nurses lack the depth of knowledge and expertise that expert nurses have, they can still learn to increase their diagnostic accuracy by becoming aware of, and avoiding, the several pitfalls of diagnosing. These pitfalls decrease the reliability of cues and decrease diagnostic accuracy. There are two sets of pitfalls: those that occur during the assessment phase and those that occur during the analysis of data phase.

The first set of pitfalls is discussed in detail in Chapter 4. They include too many or too few data, unreliable or invalid data, and an insufficient number of cues available to support the diagnoses.

The second set of pitfalls occurs during the analysis phase. Cues may be clustered yet unrelated to each other. For example, a client may be very quiet and appear depressed. A nurse may assume the client is grieving because her husband died a year ago but the client may just be fatigued because of all the diagnostic tests she has just undergone.

Another common error is quickly diagnosing a client without hypothesizing several diagnoses. For example, a nurse may assume that a readmitted diabetic client with hyperglycemia has deficient knowledge concerning the recommended diabetic diet. However, further exploration of data reveals that the client has low self-esteem and feelings of powerlessness and hopelessness in controlling a labile blood glucose level. The nurse's goal is to avoid making diagnoses too quickly without taking sufficient time to process the data.

Another pitfall to avoid is incorrectly wording the diagnostic statement. This leads to an inaccurate picture of the client for others caring for him. Finally, do not overlook consideration of the client's cultural background when analyzing data. Clients from other cultures may be misdiagnosed because the defining characteristics and labels for specific diagnoses do not accurately describe the human responses in their culture. Therefore, it is essential to look closely at cultural norms and responses for clients from various cultures.

SUMMARY

Analysis of data is the second step of the nursing process. It is often called the diagnostic phase because the purpose of this phase is identification of nursing diagnoses, collaborative problems, or need for referral to another health care professional. The thought process required for data analysis is called diagnostic reasoning—a form of critical thinking. Therefore, it is important to develop the characteristics of critical thinking in order to analyze the data as accurately as possible.

Seven key steps for data analysis have been developed that clearly explain how to analyze assessment data. These steps include:

1. Identify abnormal data and strengths.
2. Cluster data.
3. Draw inferences.
4. Propose possible nursing diagnoses.
5. Check for presence of defining characteristics.
6. Confirm or rule out nursing diagnoses.
7. Document conclusions.

Keep in mind that developing expertise in formulating nursing diagnoses requires much knowledge and experience. However, the novice nurse can learn to increase diagnostic accuracy by becoming aware of, and avoiding, the pitfalls of diagnosing. Because analysis of data is so closely linked to assessment, a special section addressing analysis of data is included in each body part or system assessment chapter.

> **Want to know more?**
> A wide variety of resources to enhance your learning and understanding of this book are available on thePoint. Visit thePoint to access:
> NCLEX-Style Student Review Questions
> Watch and Learn Videos
> Concepts in Action Animations
> And more!

References and Selected Readings

Carpenito-Moyet, L. J. (2017). *Nursing diagnosis: Applications to clinical practice* (15th ed.). Philadelphia, PA: Lippincott Williams & Wilkins.

Lunney, M. (2009). *Critical thinking to achieve positive health outcomes: Nursing case studies and analyses.* Ames, Iowa: John Wiley & Sons.

NANDA International Inc. (NANDA-I). (2014). Nursing diagnoses: Definitions and classification, 2015–2017. Herdman, T. H. (Ed.). Oxford: Wiley-Blackwell.

NANDA-I. (2016). Glossary of terms. Available at http://www.nanda.org/nanda-international-glossary-of-terms.html

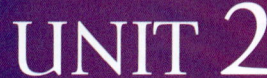

UNIT 2
Integrative Holistic Nursing Assessment

6   ASSESSING MENTAL STATUS INCLUDING RISK FOR SUBSTANCE ABUSE

Learning Objectives

1. Discuss how both mental health and mental disorders affect your mental status.
2. Describe risk factors for mental disorders and substance abuse across various cultures.
3. Interview and assess a client's mental status history and risk for substance abuse.
4. Differentiate between skills needed for general routine screening and skills needed for focused specialty assessment of mental status and risk for substance abuse.
5. Use the Saint Louis University Mental Status (SLUMS) Examination tool to assess cognitive function.
6. Use the Glasgow Coma Scale to assess one's level of consciousness (response to stimuli) when at high risk for deterioration of the nervous system.
7. Explain when and how to use the CAGE Self-Assessment tool to assess alcohol dependence.
8. Use the Alcohol Use Disorders Identification Text (AUDIT): Interview Version, to assess a client for alcohol abuse.
9. Describe the seven warning signs of Alzheimer disease.
10. Use the Confusion Assessment Method (CAM) to assess a client for confusion.
11. Use the Quick Inventory of Depressive Symptomatology (Self-Report) to assess for indications of depression in a client.
12. Use the modified SAD Person's Suicide Risk tool to assess a client's suicide risk.
13. Differentiate between normal and abnormal findings of a mental health status and substance abuse assessment.
14. Analyze client's mental status and substance abuse risk assessment data to formulate valid nursing diagnoses, collaborative problems, and/or referrals.
15. Communicate interview and assessment findings through clear concise documentation and verbal reports.

CASE STUDY

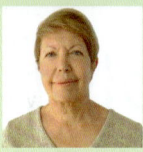

Jane Wilson, a 61-year-old Caucasian female, comes to the local family clinic. Her husband, Steve, accompanies her. When asked about the reason for her visit, she states, "I'm very nervous and not thinking straight."

Mrs. Wilson reports difficulty sleeping, loss of appetite, and a general feeling of anxiety. She says that she has excessively been "worrying over little things." She is fearful of someone breaking into her house and often checks and rechecks the locks despite her husband's reassurance that the doors are locked. She states, "I'm afraid I am losing my mind." Mrs. Wilson's case will be discussed throughout this chapter.

CONCEPTUAL FOUNDATIONS

Mental status refers to a client's level of cognitive functioning (thinking, knowledge, problem solving) and emotional functioning (feelings, mood, behaviors, stability). One cannot be totally healthy without "mental health." Mental health is an essential part of one's total health and is more than just the absence of mental disabilities or disorders. The World Health Organization (WHO, 2014) states: "Health is a state of complete physical, mental and social well-being and not merely the absence of disease or infirmity." WHO further defines mental health as "a state of well-being in which an individual realizes his or her own abilities, can cope with the normal stresses of life, can work productively and is able to make a contribution to his or her community."

A healthy mental status is needed to think clearly, respond appropriately, and function effectively in all activities of daily living (ADLs). It is reflected in one's appearance, behaviors, speech, thought patterns, decisions, and in one's ability to function in an effective manner in relationships in home, work, social, and recreational settings. One's mental health may vary from day to day depending on a variety of factors.

Factors Affecting Mental Health

There are several factors that may influence the client's mental health or put him or her at risk for impaired mental health. These include:
- Economic and social factors, such as rapid changes, stressful work conditions, and isolation
- Unhealthy lifestyle choices, such as sedentary lifestyle or substance abuse
- Exposure to violence, such as being a victim of child abuse
- Personality factors such as poor decision-making skills, low self-concept, poor self-control
- Spiritual factors (see Chapter 12)
- Cultural factors (see Chapter 11)
- Changes or impairments in the structure and function of the neurologic system: for example, cerebral abnormalities often disturb the client's intellectual ability, communication ability, or emotional behaviors (see Chapter 25)
- Psychosocial developmental level and issues (see Chapter 7)

Mental Disorders

The National Institute of Mental Health (NIMH) reports that in 2013, 18.5% of US adults suffered from some form of mental illness (NIMH, 2013) (Fig. 6-1). The *Diagnostic and Statistical Manual of Mental Disorders* (*DSM*) is published by the American Psychiatric Association and is widely used for defining mental disorders and identifying symptoms. The *DSM-5* definition for a mental disorder is a disorder that has the following features (American Psychiatric Association, 2012):

A. A behavioral or psychological syndrome or pattern that occurs in an individual
B. That reflects an underlying psychobiologic dysfunction
C. The consequences of which are clinically significant distress (e.g., a painful symptom) or disability (i.e., impairment in one or more important areas of functioning)
D. Must not be merely an expectable response to common stressors and losses (e.g., the loss of a loved one) or a culturally sanctioned response to a particular event (e.g., trance states in religious rituals)
E. That is not primarily a result of social deviance or conflicts with society

Mental disorders may affect other body systems when prompt assessment and intervention is delayed. For example, clients with depression may have decreased or loss of appetite and over time may develop nutritional deficiencies that affect the gastrointestinal system as well as other body systems.

Substance Abuse

The World Health Organization (WHO) describes substance abuse as the "harmful or hazardous use of psychoactive substances, including alcohol and illicit drugs." This abuse can

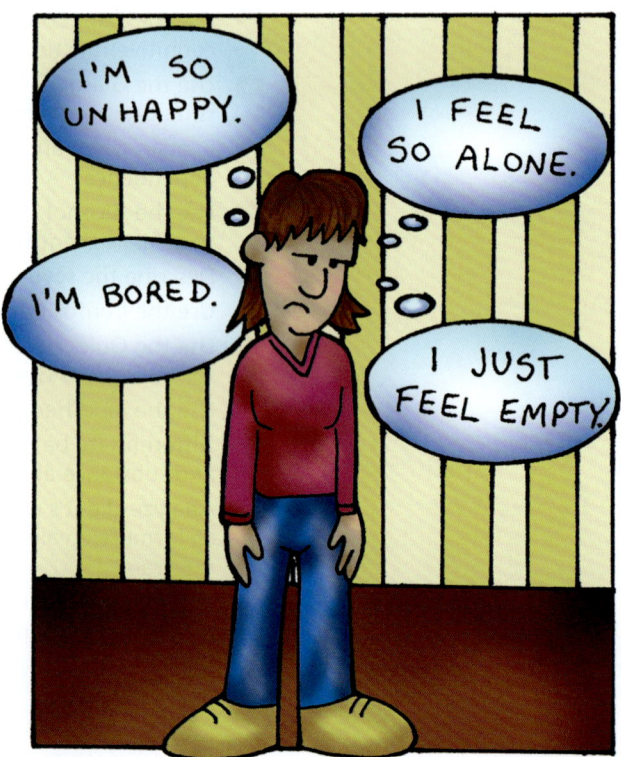

FIGURE 6-1 Unstable, unhappy affect of borderline personality disorder.

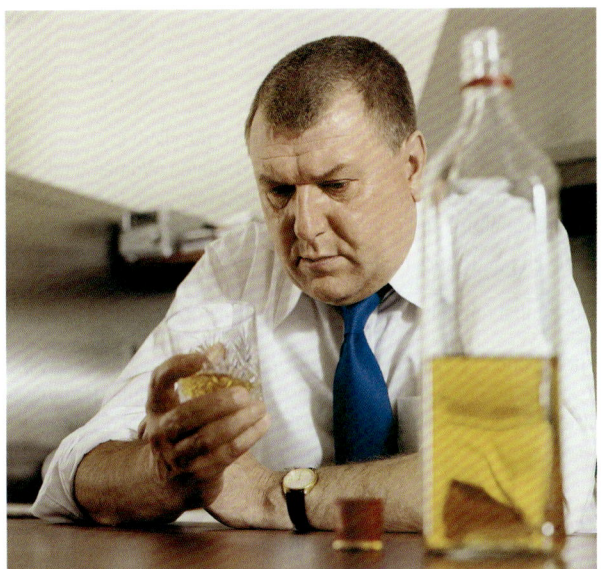

FIGURE 6-2 Many people drink alcohol excessively, use illegal ("street") drugs, or abuse legally prescribed drugs to deal with stress. This is called substance abuse. Although substance abuse may provide short-term relief from the pressures of daily life, in the long run, it is not an effective coping mechanism.

CLINICAL TIP
It is best to validate client responses by asking additional questions, verifying data with another health care professional, or comparing objective with subjective findings before completing the entire assessment. If the nurse finds out that the client's thought processes, perceptions, or level of orientation are impaired, another means of obtaining necessary subjective data must be identified.

lead to a dependence syndrome, which manifests itself in a cluster of behavioral, cognitive, and physiologic phenomena that develop after repeated substance use. The person has a strong desire to take the drug, difficulty controlling its use, and the need to continue its use despite harmful consequences. The abuse may become the person's priority in life, resulting in avoidance of responsibilities and leading to a physical withdrawal state (WHO, 2015).

The 2013 National Survey on Drug Use and Health revealed that an estimated 24.6 million individuals aged 12 years or older were current illicit drug users in 2013. More than 60 million individuals aged 12 years or older were past month binge drinkers, including 1.6 million adolescents (Substance Abuse and Mental Health Services Administration [SAMHSA], 2013) (Fig. 6-2).

HEALTH ASSESSMENT

Collecting Subjective Data: The Nursing Health History

Assessment of mental status is accomplished by interviewing the client and observing his or her behaviors. Important verbal and behavioral clues about mental status can be assessed from the very outset and throughout the entire duration of your interaction with the client.

Before asking questions to determine the client's mental status, explain the purpose of this part of the examination. Explain that some questions you ask may sound silly or irrelevant, but they will help determine how certain thought processes and ADLs are affecting the client's current health status. For example, it is only through in-depth questioning that the examiner may be able to tell that the client is having difficulty with concentration, which may be due to an excessively stressful life situation or a neurologic problem. Tell clients that they may refuse to answer any questions with which they are uncomfortable. Ensure confidentiality and respect for all that the clients share with you.

Keep in mind that problems with other body systems may affect mental status. For example, a client with a low blood sugar may report anxiety and other mental status changes. Regardless of the source of the problem, the client's total lifestyle and level of functioning may be affected. Because of the subjective nature of mental status, an in-depth nursing history is necessary to detect problems in this area affecting the client's ADLs. For example, precise questioning during the interview may elicit that the client is having difficulty concentrating or remembering.

Clients who are experiencing symptoms such as memory loss or confusion may fear that they have a serious condition such as a brain tumor or Alzheimer disease. They may also fear a loss of control, independence, and role performance. Be sensitive to these fears and concerns because the client may decline to share important information with you if these concerns are not addressed. It is important for the nurse to assess the client's mental status within the context of the client's own culture. Often, clients prefer to have a physiologic problem rather than a mental disorder because of a cultural belief that mental health problems may signify weakness or lack of self-control. Mental health problems often affect the client's self-image and self-concept in a negative manner.

While interviewing the client, you may encounter a variety of emotions expressed by the client. For example, clients may be very anxious about their health problem or angry that they are having a health problem. In addition, you may have to discuss sensitive issues such as sexuality, dying, or spirituality. Therefore, there are many interviewing skills you will need to develop to effectively complete a psychosocial history. For guidelines, see Chapter 2, Box 2-3: "Interacting With Clients With Various Emotional States."

Biographical Data

QUESTION	RATIONALE
What is your name, address, and telephone number?	These answers will provide baseline data about the client's level of consciousness, memory, speech patterns, articulation, or speech defects. Inability to answer these questions may indicate a cognitive/neurologic defect.

Continued on following page

Biographical Data (Continued)

QUESTION	RATIONALE
How old are you? What is your date of birth? Note if the client is male or female. With which gender do you identify?	This information helps determine a reference point with which the client's psychosocial developmental level and appearance can be compared. Women tend to have a higher incidence of depression and anxiety, whereas men tend to have a higher incidence of substance abuse and psychosocial disorders. Apparent male or female characteristics may not reflect a person's gender identity.
What is your marital status?	Either healthy or dysfunctional relationships will affect one's mental health status.
What is your educational level and where are you employed?	Clients from higher socioeconomic levels tend to participate in more healthy lifestyles. They are less likely to smoke and more likely to exercise and eat healthfully. Healthy lifestyles may influence one's ability to more effectively cope with mental disorders.

History of Present Health Concern

QUESTION	RATIONALE
What is your most urgent health concern at this time? Why are you seeking health care?	This information will help the examiner determine the client's perspective and ability to prioritize the reality of symptoms related to the current health status.
Are you experiencing any other health problems? Do you have headaches? Describe. Do you ever have trouble breathing or have heart palpitations? Do you have insomnia? Do you have irritability or mood swings? Do you suffer from fatigue? Do you have suicidal thoughts?	Tension headaches may be seen in clients experiencing stressful situations. See Abnormal Findings 15-1 for a differentiation of types of headaches. Clients with anxiety disorders may hyperventilate or have palpitations. The sleep–wake cycle may be reversed in delirium. Decreased sleep and a tendency to awaken early are seen with depression. Rapid mood swings, anxiety, and fearfulness are seen in delirium. Agitation or a flat affect are seen in dementia, whereas sadness, apathy, irritability, and anxiety are seen in depression. Fatigue is often seen in depression. Suicide is between the 8th and 10th leading cause of death in the United States (Rockett & Caine, 2015). Persons at highest risk are those aged 45 years and older (followed by those from age 15 to 24 years, with only a small risk for those younger than 14 years) and white males (followed by Native American and Alaska Native males living in the Western United States), with Montana leading (American Foundation for Suicide Prevention, 2015). Risk for suicide may be seen with or without a psychiatric diagnosis. Sometimes clients with suicidal/homicidal thoughts are reluctant to talk or may even appear despondent. It is important for the client to understand that the nurse is ready to listen and comfortable with discussing any concerns in this area.
Do you have thoughts of wanting to hurt or kill anyone?	Signs of violent behavior include loud aggressive speech, aggressive actions, tense posture, pacing, throwing objects, hitting the wall, pounding fists, or hitting self. Consider any angry client potentially violent and take action to protect yourself and others.

Personal Health History

QUESTION	RATIONALE
Have you ever received medical treatment or hospitalization for a mental health problem or received any type of counseling services? Please explain.	Some clients may have had a positive or a negative past experience with mental health care services or counseling that may influence their decision to seek help in this area again. A past hospitalization for mental health may indicate a more serious problem than if the client received outpatient services. Some mental health disorders may recur or symptoms may intensify. Clients who have depression early in life have a twofold increased risk for dementia (Bowers, 2014).
Have you ever had any type of head injury, meningitis, encephalitis, or stroke? What changes did you notice as a result of these?	These conditions can affect the developmental level and the mental status of the client. Changes in behavior, communication patterns, and sleep habits, as well as other physical changes, may occur with these conditions.
Have you ever served on active duty in the armed forces? Explain.	Posttraumatic syndrome may be seen in veterans who experienced traumatic conditions in military combat.

Family History

QUESTION	RATIONALE
Is there a history of mental health problems (anxiety, depression, bipolar disorder, schizophrenia) or Alzheimer disease in your family? How were they treated? Was the treatment effective?	Some psychiatric disorders may have a genetic or familial connection such as anxiety, depression, bipolar disorder and/or schizophrenia, or Alzheimer disease. Effectiveness of past family treatments may give direction for future treatments for this client.

Lifestyle and Health Practices

QUESTION	RATIONALE
Describe a typical day. Does your present health concern affect your activities of daily living? Describe your energy level.	Neurologic and mental illnesses can alter one's responses to activities of daily living (ADLs). Clients with dementia or Alzheimer disease may have trouble performing ADLs (see Evidence-Based Practice 6-1). Anxious clients may be restless, while depressed clients may feel fatigued. Clients with eating disorders may exercise excessively. Obsessive–compulsive working habits may cause fatigue leading to impairment of one's mental health.
Describe your usual eating habits over a 24-hour period.	Poor appetite may be seen with depression, eating disorders, and substance abuse. A decrease in weight may be seen with eating disorders, early dementia, and anxiety.
Describe your daily bowel elimination patterns.	Irritable bowel syndrome or peptic ulcer disease may be associated with psychological disorders.
Describe your sleep patterns.	Insomnia is often seen in depression, anxiety disorders, bipolar disorder, and substance abuse. Hypersomnolence may also be a symptom of depression.
Describe any exercise regimens.	Depression may be seen in those with sedentary lifestyles. Excessive exercise may accompany eating disorders and obsessive–compulsive disorder.
Do you drink caffeinated beverages? If so, how many per day?	Caffeine is a psychostimulant with the potential to increase stress (Lande, 2011). In healthy people, caffeine promotes cognitive arousal and fights fatigue. However, caffeine can produce symptomatic distress in a small subset of the population. A person in this subset is at high risk if he or she consumes enough caffeine, is vulnerable to caffeine, and/or has a pre-existing medical or psychiatric condition (especially mood disorders) that is aggravated by mild psychostimulant use (Arria & O'Brien, 2011; Butt & Sultan, 2011).
	It has become common for young people to overdose on energy drinks, which can be an especially serious issue in itself but more so if combined with alcohol intake (Pomeranz et al., 2013).
Do you take any prescribed or over-the-counter medications?	Use of these substances may alter one's level of consciousness, decrease response times, and cause changes in mood and temperament. Inappropriate use of any of these substances may indicate substance abuse problems.
Do you drink alcohol? Is so, what type, how much, and how often? Use the SBIRT (Screening, Brief Intervention, and Referral to Treatment) (SAMSA-HRSA, 2011) tool to identify, reduce, and prevent problematic use, abuse, and dependence on alcohol and illicit drugs. This is the most current recommended tool to use when substance abuse is suspected. The tool is designed for use by physicians, other health workers, and mental health professionals and can be used with clients 12 years of age and older.	Excessive drinking over an extended period can lead to certain types of cancer, liver damage, immune system disorders, and brain damage. It can also aggravate some conditions such as osteoporosis, diabetes, high blood pressure, and ulcers. Drinking in some older adults may cause symptoms of forgetfulness or confusion, which could be mistaken for signs of Alzheimer disease. Sometimes clients try to self-medicate a mental health disorder that has not been diagnosed with drugs or alcohol, especially when they have not been able to afford treatment. The SBIRT tool can be used to assess the client's risk for substance abuse, teach the client about the risks, and make appropriate referrals for treatment.

Continued on following page

Lifestyle and Health Practices (Continued)

QUESTION	RATIONALE
An app describing use of this tool can be found online (search on the key term "SBIRT app"). The CAGE Self-Assessment (see Ewing, 1984) has also been found to be an efficient screening test to detect alcohol dependence in trauma center populations. It is recommended that CAGE be used with alcohol testing to identify at-risk clients (Soderstrom et al., 1997). The AUDIT questionnaire (see Assessment Tool 6-1) may also be used to assess alcohol-related disorders by asking the client questions and then calculating a score.	**CULTURAL CONSIDERATIONS** Substance abuse, violence, HIV risk, depressive symptoms, and socioeconomic conditions are directly linked to health disparities among Latinas (Gonzalez-Guarda et al., 2012).
Do you use recreational drugs such as marijuana, tranquilizers, barbiturates, crack, or cocaine, methamphetamine? If so, how much do you use and how often?	Cognition, mood, behavior changes may be noted with recreational drug use. Some recreational drugs increase risk taking and risky behavior. Some clients may view and use marijuana as a natural herb or alternative medical substance to treat headaches or anxiety and not as a recreational drug. Marijuana use is now legal in many states. Evidence-Based Practice 6-2 discusses substance abuse.
Have you been exposed to any environmental toxins such as pesticides, herbicides, occupational chemicals?	Cognition may be altered with toxin exposure.
What religious affiliations do you have? What religious activities are important to you? What religiously affiliated practices do you participate in on a regular basis?	Certain religious beliefs can affect the client's ability to cope in a positive or negative manner. Extreme, rigid religious practices may be a source of stress and anxiety for some clients. Yet, the evidence tends to support the belief that a strong religious affiliation provides comfort to many individuals (Hamilton et al., 2013).
How do you feel about yourself and your relationship with others? Use the PHQ-2 (Maurer, 2012) to screen for depression during a routine client interview) Use the PHQ-9 (Maurer, 2012) to further assess a client who indicates depression using the PHQ-2. The client can perform a self-assessment for risk factors for depression using the Quick Inventory of Depressive Symptomatology (Self-Report) (see Box 6-1). **OLDER ADULT CONSIDERATIONS** Use Geriatric Depression Scale if depression is suspected in the older client (see Chapter 32). Read the questions to the client if the client cannot read.	Clients with a low self-concept may be depressed or suffer from eating disorders or have substance abuse problems, such as being suicidal or homicidal. Clients with psychological problems often have difficulty maintaining effective meaningful relationships. Using a PHQ-2 threshold score of 2 or higher rather than 3 or higher results in more depressed patients being correctly identified. A PHQ-9 score of 10 or higher appears to detect more depressed patients than the originally described PHQ-9 scoring for major depression (Arroll et al., 2010).
Describe your support systems and how you are using them at this time.	This may help determine the availability and effectiveness of the client's support systems. It also provides information for referrals and possible use of social services.
What do you perceive as your role in your family or relationship with your significant other? Whom do you care for on a daily basis (e.g., children, family member who is ill or disabled, frail elderly parent, relative, or friend)?	Mental health problems often interfere with one's role in families and relationships. In turn, stressful relationships or roles may interfere with one's mental health. Excessive family demands may also impair one's coping mechanisms. Living with others (spouse, children, or parents) with mental health disorders can impair one's own mental health and coping abilities. Clients who are living with others who have serious mental illness are vulnerable to depression, which needs to be detected early (Zauszniewski et al., 2010). Caregiver burden can be a significant problem for more than 43 million individuals providing care for midlife and older adults (Adelman et al, 2014). Those who care for the frail elderly often experience anxiety and depression.

QUESTION	RATIONALE
Describe current stressors in your life (e.g., loss of family member, financial difficulties, lack of transportation, change in role at home or at work, enrollment in school or continuing education, inability to speak English language, inability to read or write).	Ineffective or lack of grieving may impair one's mental status and ability to make good judgments. Loneliness and/or dysfunctional family relationships are often a source of mental stress. Loss of or inadequate financial resources may also impair mental health. Inability to seek counseling or to seek needed mental health treatment adds to current mental health stressors.
How do you feel about the future? Have you ever had thoughts of hurting yourself or doing away with yourself? Have you ever had thoughts of hurting yourself? Use the Columbia Suicide Severity Rating Scale (C-SSRS) for clients to assess for suicide risk (Posner, 2008). The C-SSRS is currently the only approved scale that meets the FDA Draft Guidance for Prospective Assessment of Suicidal Ideation and Behavior. https://www.ert.com/suicide-risk/c-ssrs/?gclid=CP76t LPVkMkCFQasaQodMroOtw	It is important to assess for suicidal thoughts and risk. Clients who are suicidal may share past attempts of suicide, share a plan for suicide, verbalize worthlessness about self, and joke about death frequently. Assess for common risk factors (see Assessment Guide 6-1). Additional risk factors include family history of suicide, suicide attempts, psychiatric disorders, family history of child abuse or violence, isolation, barriers to accessing mental health treatment, loss (relational, social, work, or financial). Clients undergoing hemodialysis often have depression and suicidal ideation (Andrade et al., 2015). This tool may assist practitioners to take liability precautions for legal protection by asking and documenting that the questions were asked and the responses received.

6-1 EVIDENCE-BASED HEALTH PROMOTION AND DISEASE PREVENTION: DEMENTIA AND ALZHEIMER DISEASE

INTRODUCTION

Normal aging has common forms of decline that are often mistaken for dementia or resemble dementia. These include slower thinking, problem solving, learning, and recall; decreased attention and concentration; more distractedness; and need for hints to jog memory. It is important to differentiate dementia from common cognitive changes that occur with age.

According to Healthy People 2020, dementia is not a disease but a set of symptoms associated with the loss of cognitive functioning—thinking, remembering, and reasoning—to such an extent that it interferes with a person's daily life. The cognitive changes occur because of brain diseases or trauma and can have a rapid or a gradual onset. Memory loss is a common symptom of dementia, although memory loss by itself does not mean a person has dementia.

Alzheimer disease, the most common cause of dementia of the elderly, results from gradual destruction of brain nerve cells and a shrinking brain. The Alzheimer's Association describes three states of Alzheimer disease: Stage 1, preclinical, Stage 2, mild cognitive impairment, and Stage 3, dementia of Alzheimer disease (Alzheimer's Association, 2015a).

Symptoms resemble general dementia symptoms but in the various stages may include loss of recent memory, depression, anxiety, personality changes, unpredictable quirks or behaviors, confusion, aggression, agitation, suspicion, wandering, trouble sleeping, inability to recognize family members, and problems with language, calculation, and abstract thinking. Inability to manage a budget is a common symptom. Gradually worsening ability to remember new information is a key symptom.

General symptoms of dementia include (Alzheimer's Association, 2014):
- Memory loss that disrupts daily life
- Challenges in planning or solving problems
- Difficulty completing familiar tasks at home, at work, or at leisure
- Confusion with time or place
- Trouble understanding visual images or spatial relationships
- New problems with words in speaking or writing
- Misplacing things and losing the ability to retrace steps
- Decreased or poor judgment
- Withdrawal from work or social activities
- Changes in mood or personality

The difference between Alzheimer disease and typical age-related changes is illustrated in the following table:

Signs of Alzheimer Disease	Typical Age-Related Changes
Poor judgment and decision making	Making a bad decision once in a while
Inability to manage a budget	Missing a monthly payment
Losing track of the date or the season	Forgetting which day it is and remembering later
Difficulty having a conversation	Sometimes forgetting which word to use
Misplacing things and being unable to retrace steps to find them	Losing things from time to time

From Alzheimer's Association. (2014). Know the 10 signs. Available at http://www.alz.org/national/documents/10warningsigns.pdf

Alzheimer disease is the sixth leading cause of death among adults aged 18 years and older. As the population is aging, the numbers are predicted to double by 2050 unless more effective methods for treating and preventing Alzheimer disease are found (Alzheimer's Association, 2015a).

HEALTHY PEOPLE 2020 GOAL

Reduce the morbidity due to associated costs with and maintain or enhance the quality of life for persons with dementia, including Alzheimer disease (Healthy People 2020, 2014a).

Continued on following page

6-1 EVIDENCE-BASED HEALTH PROMOTION AND DISEASE PREVENTION: DEMENTIA AND ALZHEIMER DISEASE (Continued)

SCREENING

As of 2014, the U.S. Preventive Services Task Force Summary of Recommendations on Screening for Dementia concluded that "the current evidence is insufficient to assess the balance of benefits and harms of screening for cognitive impairment."

Other researchers and organizations recommend screening. One way of screening is the Everyday Cognition questionnaire. The shortened form of the ECog Scale (ECog-12) is an informant-rated questionnaire designed to detect cognitive and functional decline. Items included in the ECog-12 (Farias et al., 2011, p. 10):

- Remembering the location of objects
- Remembering the current date or day of the week
- Communicating thoughts in a conversation
- Understanding spoken directions or instructions
- Reading a map and helping with directions when someone else is driving
- Finding the way around a familiar house or building
- Anticipating weather changes and planning accordingly
- Thinking ahead
- Keeping living and work space organized
- Balancing the checkbook/account without error
- Doing two things at once (e.g., cooking and talking on the phone at the same time)

RISK ASSESSMENT

Assess for the Following Risk Factors (Alzheimer's Association, 2015)

- Increasing age, especially 65 years of age or older
- Genetic predisposition and family history
- Mild cognitive impairment
- Latino or African American descent due to higher vascular disease rates
- Diseases that predispose a client to vascular complications (such as diabetes, high blood pressure, and high cholesterol)
- Head trauma (traumatic brain injury)
- Smoking
- Hormone therapy, starting therapy later in life (starting therapy at menopause may be protective, but risk increases when started later in life (Shao et al., 2012)
- Not maintaining healthy aging behaviors, including keeping weight within recommended guidelines, avoiding tobacco use and excess alcohol intake, active social and cognitive engagement, and exercising both body and mind
- Fewer years of formal education

CLIENT EDUCATION

Teach Clients (and Their Families)

Resources for caregivers and ways to prevent or delay onset of Alzheimer disease (Alzheimer's Association, 2015b):

- Actively participate in four healthy behaviors, physical health and exercise, diet and nutrition, cognitive activity, and social engagement, which can help keep your body and brain healthy and potentially reduce your risk of cognitive decline.
- Keep a Helpline phone number available for questions re: Alzheimer disease.
- Use Alzheimer's Association resources.
- Engage client in mentally challenging activities (e.g., card and board games [which also fulfill a social function when done with others], jigsaw puzzles, reading, crossword puzzles, sudoku, brain teasers, and activities that require both physical and mental exertion such as yard work, cooking, and playing with pets) (Health communities.com, 2011).
- Help client engage in healthy aging behaviors, including maintaining healthy weight, avoiding tobacco use and excess alcohol intake, staying socially connected, and exercising both body and mind.
- Help client avoid activities that have a risk of head trauma.
- Ask a physician about initiating hormonal therapy, beginning the therapy at menopause rather than later in life.
- Help client maintain a heart healthy diet and exercise program.

ASSESSMENT TOOL 6-1   The Alcohol Use Disorders Identification Test (AUDIT): Interview Version

Instructions: Read questions as written. Record answers carefully. Begin the AUDIT by saying "Now I am going to ask you some questions about your use of alcoholic beverages during this past year." Explain what is meant by "alcoholic beverages" by using local examples of beer, wine, vodka, etc. Code answers in terms of "standard drinks." Place the correct answer number in the box at the right.

Questions

1. **How often do you have a drink containing alcohol?** ☐
   (0) Never
   (1) 1 Monthly or less
   (2) 2 to 4 times a month
   (3) 2 to 3 times a week
   (4) 4 or more times a week
   If the score for Question 1 is 0, skip to Question 9.

2. **How many drinks containing alcohol do you have on a typical day when you are drinking?** ☐
   (0) 1 or 2
   (1) 3 or 4
   (2) 5 or 6
   (3) 7, 8, or 9
   (4) 10 or more

ASSESSMENT TOOL 6-1 The Alcohol Use Disorders Identification Test (AUDIT): Interview Version (Continued)

3. **How often do you have six or more drinks on one occasion?** ☐
   - (0) Never
   - (1) Less than monthly
   - (2) Monthly
   - (3) Weekly
   - (4) Daily or almost daily

   Skip to Questions 9 and 10 if total score for Questions 2 and 3 is 0.

4. **How often during the last year have you found that you were not able to stop drinking once you had started?** ☐
   - a(0) Never
   - (1) Less than monthly
   - (2) Monthly
   - (3) Weekly
   - (4) Daily or almost daily

5. **How often during the last year have you failed to do what was normally expected from you because of drinking?** ☐
   - (0) Never
   - (1) Less than monthly
   - (2) Monthly
   - (3) Weekly
   - (4) Daily or almost daily

6. **How often during the last year have you needed a first drink in the morning to get yourself going after a heavy drinking session the night before?** ☐
   - (0) Never
   - (1) Less than monthly
   - (2) Monthly
   - (3) Weekly
   - (4) Daily or almost daily

7. **How often during the last year have you had a feeling of guilt or remorse after drinking?** ☐
   - (0) Never
   - (1) Less than monthly
   - (2) Monthly
   - (3) Weekly
   - (4) Daily or almost daily

8. **How often during the last year have you been unable to remember what happened the night before because you had been drinking?** ☐
   - (0) Never
   - (1) Less than monthly
   - (2) Monthly
   - (3) Weekly
   - (4) Daily or almost daily

9. **Have you or someone else been injured as a result of your drinking?** ☐
   - (0) No
   - (2) Yes, but not in the last year
   - (4) Yes, during the last year

10. **Has a relative or friend or a doctor or another health worker been concerned about your drinking or suggested you cut down?** ☐
    - (0) No
    - (2) Yes, but not in the last year
    - (4) Yes, during the last year

    Total Score: ☐

Scoring: The AUDIT is easy to score. Each of the questions has a set of responses to choose from, and each response has a score ranging from 0 to 4. The interviewer enters the score (the number within parentheses) corresponding to the patient's response into the box beside each question. All the response scores should then be added and recorded in the box labeled "Total."

Total scores of 8 or more are recommended as indicators of hazardous and harmful alcohol use, as well as possible alcohol dependence. (A cutoff score of 10 will provide greater specificity but at the expense of sensitivity.) Since the effects of alcohol vary with average body weight and differences in metabolism, establishing the cutoff point for all women and men older than 65 years one point lower at a score of 7 will increase sensitivity for these population groups.

Selection of the cutoff point should be influenced by national and cultural standards and by clinician judgment, which also determine recommended maximum consumption allowances. Technically speaking, higher scores simply indicate greater likelihood of hazardous and harmful drinking. However, such scores may also reflect greater severity of alcohol problems and dependence, as well as a greater need for more intensive treatment.

More detailed interpretation of a patient's total score may be obtained by determining on which questions points were scored. In general, a score of 1 or more on Question 2 or Question 3 indicates consumption at a hazardous level. Points scored above 0 on Questions 4 to 6 (especially weekly or daily symptoms) imply the presence or incipience of alcohol dependence.

Points scored on Questions 7 to 10 indicate that alcohol-related harm is already being experienced. The total score, consumption level, signs of dependence, and present harm all should play a role in determining how to manage a patient. The final two questions should also be reviewed to determine whether patients give evidence of a past problem (i.e., "yes, but not in the past year"). Even in the absence of current hazardous drinking, positive responses on these items should be used to discuss the need for vigilance by the patient.

6-2 EVIDENCE-BASED HEALTH PROMOTION AND DISEASE PREVENTION: SUBSTANCE ABUSE

INTRODUCTION

As defined in the Healthy People 2020 report (Healthy People 2020, 2014b), substance abuse is "a set of related conditions associated with the consumption of mind- and behavior-altering substances that have negative behavioral and health outcomes." The National Institute on Drug Abuse (NIDA, 2015) report lists the most abused drugs, which include alcohol and tobacco, cocaine and heroin, hallucinogens, methamphetamine, and many others medically prescribed, over-the-counter, or illegal. Causes for substance abuse are suspected to be a combination of environmental (such as family context, peer behaviors, etc.) and genetic predisposition (NIDA, 2010a).

Two groups of individuals are of particular interest in substance abuse study: Adolescents, who—in addition to alcohol, marijuana, and other illegal substances—are using an increasing amount of prescription drugs, especially from their parents' medicine cabinets, in the belief that these are less harmful than street drugs; and military personnel serving in Iraq and Afghanistan, who are under great strain from combat environments, which often cause mental and family problems and even lead to cases of suicide. Healthy People 2020 reports that "Data from the Substance Abuse and Mental Health Services Administration (SAMHSA, 2013) National Survey on Drug Use and Health indicates that from 2004 to 2006, 7.1% of veterans (an estimated 1.8 million people) had a substance use disorder in the past year" (Health People 2020, 2014b).

Data from the 2014 National Survey on Drug Use and Health (SAMHSA, 2015) found that there were approximately 21.5 million Americans aged 12 years and older who had a substance abuse problem in the last year. The effects of substance abuse on individuals, families, and communities are substantial and cumulative. According to Healthy People 2020, these problems include teenage pregnancy, HIV/AIDS, other STIs, domestic violence, child abuse, motor vehicle accidents, interpersonal violence of fights, crime, homicide, and suicide (Healthy People 2020, 2014b).

HEALTHY PEOPLE 2020 GOAL

Reduce substance abuse to protect the health, safety, and quality of life for all, especially children.

SCREENING

The efficacy of initial screening in a clinic setting is debated, but most organizations recommend use of a simple screening tool to identify those at risk for substance abuse. In 1990, an Institute of Medicine report recommended "that patients in all medical settings be screened for the full spectrum of problems that can accompany alcohol use and, when necessary, be offered brief intervention or referral to treatment services," and questions should be asked on at least an annual basis (National Institute on Alcohol Abuse and Alcoholism [NIAAA], 2005).

The NIAAA describes major screening tools. Tools for use in primary care vary from one simple question to more standardized questionnaires, such as the Michigan Alcoholism Screening Test (MAST) and the Alcohol Use Disorders Identification Test (AUDIT). Also, the CAGE questionnaire is a short, four-question tool (Ewing, 1984). The AUDIT has been found to be especially useful for screening women and minorities.

The NIAAA (2005) notes that screening is not diagnosis. Also, the level of screening is dependent on client characteristics, such as medical or psychiatric problems, as well as the time available with the client.

The U.S. Preventive Services Task Force (USPSTF) has recommendations for screening for both alcohol misuse and illicit drug use. The USPSTF (2013) recommends screening and behavioral counseling interventions to reduce alcohol misuse by adults—including pregnant women—in primary care settings but concludes that the evidence is insufficient to recommend for or against screening and behavioral counseling interventions to prevent or reduce alcohol misuse by adolescents in primary care settings. For illicit drug use screening, the USPSTF (2008) concluded that the current evidence is insufficient to assess the balance of benefits and harms of screening adolescents, adults, and pregnant women for illicit drug use.

RISK ASSESSMENT

The NIDA (2010a) cautions that having risk factors for substance abuse does not mean that a person will ultimately abuse drugs. Many factors affect the person's risk, both to increase the chances for abuse and to reduce the changes through protective factors. The NIDA cautions the health care professional doing the risk assessment to remember that most people who are at risk do not start using drugs or become addicted.

A difficulty in assessing substance abuse risk is that the risks change over different ages and developmental levels. The importance of a particular risk is associated with age and development. The NIDA suggests assessing for the following risk factors:

- A history of early aggressive behavior
- Lack of parental supervision
- A history of substance abuse
- Drug availability
- Poverty

In addition, the NIDA Recommends Assessing for Protective Factors

- Self-control
- Parental monitoring
- Academic competence
- Antidrug use policies at school
- Strong neighborhood attachment

The NIDA (2010b, p. 1) emphasized that the strategic goal of prevention is to prevent the initiation of drug use and the escalation to addiction in those who have already initiated use.

CLIENT EDUCATION

Teach Clients

Teaching should be adjusted according to the developmental level of the client.

Teach the Family

- Be aware of early aggressive behavior and seek professional assistance from behavioral counselors, if necessary.
- Provide support and supervision to young children and adolescents, including developing a close relationship by learning to listen versus criticizing, becoming involved in the child's/adolescent's activities.
- Discuss substance abuse issues with the young person.
- Avoid allowing easy access to family members' prescription drugs.

- Convey a belief that substance abuse is damaging to all people, not just young people.
- Avoid serving as a role model for substance abuse (seek professional help or group help for personal addictions).
- Seek help for young people who abuse substances (prescription drugs, alcohol, other addictive drugs, including marijuana).
- Help to establish a strong community attachment base (including family, community, and school) as support for the young person.
- Note slipping academic performance as an indicator for substance abuse and follow up on this or other behavioral or mood changes.
- Monitor young person's behaviors for signs of substance abuse.

Teach Young Clients
- To reach out to parents and friends who are not substance abusers if tempted to experiment or if dependence becomes noticeable to you or to your friends
- That drugs can alter the way a person behaves and feels
- To express your feelings constructively and show respect for the feelings of others
- To seek ways to increase your personal confidence and self-esteem
- To value your body and recognize your individuality
- About the physical and emotional effects of alcohol and other substances on the body and personality
- About the physical and emotional differences between people and how to accept them
- Responsible attitudes toward medicines and health professionals
- Ways that substances can get into the body
- A responsible attitude toward the social use of alcohol (where laws allow it)
- Critical responses to the advertising of medicines and other health supplements
- To recognize situations in which choices can be made and to identify the consequences of your choices
- To follow simple safety instructions and know when and how to get help from adults and others, such as police or ambulance services

---

BOX 6-1 QUICK INVENTORY OF DEPRESSIVE SYMPTOMATOLOGY (SELF-REPORT)

PLEASE CHECKMARK THE ONE RESPONSE TO EACH ITEM THAT IS MOST APPROPRIATE TO HOW YOU HAVE BEEN FEELING OVER THE PAST 7 DAYS.

1. **Falling asleep:**
   - ☐ 0 I never took longer than 30 minutes to fall asleep.
   - ☐ 1 I took at least 30 minutes to fall asleep, less than half the time (3 days or less out of the past 7 days).
   - ☐ 2 I took at least 30 minutes to fall asleep, more than half the time (4 days or more out of the past 7 days).
   - ☐ 3 I took more than 60 minutes to fall asleep, more than half the time (4 days or more out of the past 7 days).

2. **Sleep during the night:**
   - ☐ 0 I didn't wake up at night.
   - ☐ 1 I had a restless, light sleep, briefly waking up a few times each night.
   - ☐ 2 I woke up at least once a night, but I got back to sleep easily.
   - ☐ 3 I woke up more than once a night and stayed awake for 20 minutes or more, more than half the time (4 days or more out of the past 7 days).

3. **Waking up too early:**
   - ☐ 0 Most of the time, I woke up no more than 30 minutes before my scheduled time.
   - ☐ 1 More than half the time (4 days or more out of the past 7 days), I woke up more than 30 minutes before my scheduled time.
   - ☐ 2 I almost always woke up at least 1 hour or so before my scheduled time, but I got back to sleep eventually.
   - ☐ 3 I woke up at least 1 hour before my scheduled time and couldn't get back to sleep.

4. **Sleeping too much:**
   - ☐ 0 I slept no longer than 7–8 hours/night, without napping during the day.
   - ☐ 1 I slept no longer than 10 hours in a 24-hour period including naps.
   - ☐ 2 I slept no longer than 12 hours in a 24-hour period including naps.
   - ☐ 3 I slept longer than 12 hours in a 24-hour period including naps.

5. **Feeling sad:**
   - ☐ 0 I didn't feel sad.
   - ☐ 1 I felt sad less than half the time (3 days or less out of the past 7 days).
   - ☐ 2 I felt sad more than half the time (4 days or more out of the past 7 days).
   - ☐ 3 I felt sad nearly all of the time.

Please complete either 6 or 7 (not both)

6. **Decreased appetite:**
   - ☐ 0 There was no change in my usual appetite.
   - ☐ 1 I ate somewhat less often or smaller amounts of food than usual.
   - ☐ 2 I ate much less than usual and only by forcing myself to eat.
   - ☐ 3 I rarely ate within a 24-hour period and only by really forcing myself to eat or when others persuaded me to eat.

7. **Increased appetite:**
   - ☐ 0 There was no change in my usual appetite.
   - ☐ 1 I felt a need to eat more frequently than usual.
   - ☐ 2 I regularly ate more often and/or greater amounts of food than usual.
   - ☐ 3 I felt driven to overeat both at mealtime and between meals.

Continued on following page

BOX 6-1 QUICK INVENTORY OF DEPRESSIVE SYMPTOMATOLOGY (SELF-REPORT) (Continued)

Please complete either 8 or 9 (not both)

8. **Decreased weight (within the last 14 days)**
   - ☐ 0 My weight has not changed.
   - ☐ 1 I feel as if I've had a slight weight loss.
   - ☐ 2 I've lost 2 lb (about 1 kg) or more.
   - ☐ 3 I've lost 5 lb (about 2 kg) or more.

9. **Increased weight (within the last 14 days):**
   - ☐ 0 My weight has not changed.
   - ☐ 1 I feel as if I've had a slight weight gain.
   - ☐ 2 I've gained 2 lb (about 1 kg) or more.
   - ☐ 3 I've gained 5 lb (about 2 kg) or more.

10. **Concentration/decision making:**
    - ☐ 0 There was no change in my usual ability to concentrate or make decisions.
    - ☐ 1 I occasionally felt indecisive or found that my attention wandered.
    - ☐ 2 Most of the time, I found it hard to focus or to make decisions.
    - ☐ 3 I couldn't concentrate well enough to read or I couldn't make even minor decisions.

11. **Perception of myself:**
    - ☐ 0 I saw myself as equally worthwhile and deserving as other people.
    - ☐ 1 I put the blame on myself more than usual.
    - ☐ 2 For the most part, I believed that I caused problems for others.
    - ☐ 3 I thought almost constantly about major and minor defects in myself.

12. **Thoughts of my own death or suicide:**
    - ☐ 0 I didn't think of suicide or death.
    - ☐ 1 I felt that life was empty or wondered if it was worth living.
    - ☐ 2 I thought of suicide or death several times for several minutes over the past 7 days.
    - ☐ 3 I thought of suicide or death several times a day in some detail, or I made specific plans for suicide or actually tried to take my life.

13. **General interest:**
    - ☐ 0 There was no change from usual in how interested I was in other people or activities.
    - ☐ 1 I noticed that I was less interested in other people or activities.
    - ☐ 2 I found I had interest in only one or two of the activities I used to do.
    - ☐ 3 I had virtually no interest in the activities I used to do.

14. **Energy level:**
    - ☐ 0 There was no change in my usual level of energy.
    - ☐ 1 I got tired more easily than usual.
    - ☐ 2 I had to make a big effort to start or finish my usual daily activities (e.g., shopping, homework, cooking, or going to work).
    - ☐ 3 I really couldn't carry out most of my usual daily activities because I just didn't have the energy.

15. **Feeling more sluggish than usual:**
    - ☐ 0 I thought, spoke, and moved at my usual pace.
    - ☐ 1 I found that my thinking was more sluggish than usual or my voice sounded dull or flat.
    - ☐ 2 It took me several seconds to respond to most questions and I was sure my thinking was more sluggish than usual.
    - ☐ 3 I was often unable to respond to questions without forcing myself.

16. **Feeling restless (agitated, not relaxed, fidgety):**
    - ☐ 0 I didn't feel restless.
    - ☐ 1 I was often fidgety, wringing my hands, or needed to change my sitting position.
    - ☐ 2 I had sudden urges to move about and was quite restless.
    - ☐ 3 At times, I was unable to stay seated and needed to pace around.

PLEASE CHECKMARK THE ONE RESPONSE TO EACH ITEM THAT IS MOST APPROPRIATE TO HOW YOU HAVE BEEN FEELING OVER THE PAST 7 DAYS.

QUICK INVENTORY OF DEPRESSIVE SYMPTOMATOLOGY (SCORE SHEET)
NOTE: THIS SECTION IS TO BE COMPLETED BY THE STUDY PERSONNEL ONLY.

_____ Enter the highest score on any 1 of the 4 sleep items (1–4)
_____ Item 5
_____ Enter the highest score on any 1 of the appetite/weight items (6–9)
_____ Item 10
_____ Item 11
_____ Item 12
_____ Item 13
_____ Item 14
_____ Enter the highest score on either of the 2 psychomotor items (15 and 16)
_____ Total score (range: 0–27)

Interpretation of Scores
- 0–5 = No risk of depression
- 6–10 = Mild
- 11–15 = Moderate
- 16–20 = Severe
- 21–27 = Very Severe

Rush et al, *Biol Psychiatry* (2003) 54: 573–583.

© UT Southwestern Medical Center, Dallas, Texas.

ASSESSMENT GUIDE 6-1   Modified SAD PERSONS Suicide Risk Assessment

This assessment guide can be used to assess the likelihood of a suicide attempt. Consider risk factors within the context of the clinical presentation. Some professionals recommend that scoring not be used, but the examiner should look at the risk factors and respond accordingly.

Risk Factors
- Sex
- Age
- Depression
- Previous attempt
- Ethanol abuse
- Rational thinking loss
- Social supports lacking
- Organized plan
- No spouse
- Sickness

Adapted from Patterson, W. M., Dohn, H. H., Bird J., et al. (1983). Evaluation of suicidal patients: The SAD PERSONS scale. Psychosomatics, 24(4), 343–345, 348–349.

Recall the case study introduced at the beginning of the chapter. The nurse uses COLDSPA to explore Mrs. Wilson's presenting concerns and obtains a health history.

CASE STUDY

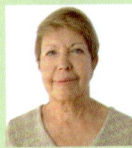

The nurse interviews Mrs. Wilson using specific probing questions. The client reports, "I'm very nervous and not thinking straight. I'm afraid I am losing my mind." Mrs. Wilson also reports that she is "worrying over little things." She does have stress at work and believes that her symptoms are related to that; however, her memory is continuing to decline despite attempts to "de-stress." Concentration is difficult at home and at work. The nurse explores this health concern using the COLDSPA mnemonic.

Mnemonic	Question	Data Provided
Character	Describe the sign or symptom.	"I cannot remember names of friends. I should know and sometimes cannot remember where I put things or where I am going next."
Onset	When did it begin?	"Three months ago. I thought it was stress, but it is getting worse."
Location	Where does it occur?	"I forget people's names at work and at church. I misplace things at work and home all the time."
Duration	How long does it last? Does it recur?	"I often have to ask people their name because I just cannot recall. Sometimes it takes me 5 to 10 minutes to remember what I started to do next."
Severity	How bad is it? How much does it bother you?	"I cannot get things done as fast as I used to because I am always forgetting what I intended to do and where I put things. I get so frustrated; I just want to give up."
Pattern	What makes it better or worse?	"Sometimes it is better in the morning if I get a good night's sleep, but gets worse as the day goes on." However, the client reports increasing episodes of insomnia.
Associated factors/How it Affects the client	What other symptoms occur with it? How does it affect you?	"I have trouble getting my secretarial work done on time and I am afraid I am going to overlook or lose something important and lose my job." She reports increasing episodes of insomnia, tiredness, difficulty concentrating, and decreased appetite.

After exploring the client's main concern of loss of memory, the nurse continues with past health history, family history, and lifestyle practices.

Mrs. Wilson denies previous treatment or hospitalization for mental health reasons. She denies any history of meningitis, encephalitis, head injury, or stroke. The client reports occasional headaches (every 1–2 months) relieved with a dose of acetaminophen. Mrs. Wilson denies chest pain, palpitations, and shortness of breath.

The nurse explores Mrs. Wilson's family history. Her family history is significant for Alzheimer disease, coronary artery disease, and colon cancer. Her mother died at the age of 82 years due to colon cancer. Her father died at the age of 47 years due to accident. Her maternal grandmother died at the age of 76 years due to Alzheimer disease and "heart trouble," and her maternal grandfather died at the age of 80 years due to "heart attack." She does not know her paternal grandparents' medical history.

The nurse asks Mrs. Wilson to describe her typical day during the work week. She awakens at 6 AM, showers, fixes her hair and makeup, and dresses for work. She leaves for work at 7:30 AM (approximate 3-mile drive). She eats lunch at her desk at 11:30 AM. Mrs. Wilson returns home at 4:00 PM. She watches TV or naps for approximately 30 minutes and then prepares a small supper for her husband. She prepares for bedtime at 8:00 PM. She reports that she falls asleep in 1 to 2 hours if "I am lucky." Most nights she lies in bed for hours before going to sleep. Her 24-hour diet recall over the last 2 months typically consists of breakfast—one cup black coffee, one slice buttered toast; lunch—half peanut butter and jelly sandwich and 32 oz diet Coke; and dinner—"picked at" chicken breast and mashed potatoes, half glass 2% milk (4 oz). Mrs. Wilson states that she has lost approximately 10 lb in the last month due to lack of appetite. She reports an erratic bowel pattern with episodes of constipation alternating with diarrhea. Last bowel movement was 3 days ago, described as hard in consistency and brown in color. Also reports "bloating" and "gas," especially after eating.

Current medications include:
- Acetaminophen: One to two 325-mg tablets every 4 hours as needed for headache/pain twice a month
- Multivitamin: 1 daily
- Correctol: 1 to 2 tablets once every 2 weeks for constipation
- Imodium AD: One to two times a year for diarrhea

Mrs. Wilson reports no known drug, food, environmental, or insect allergies.

When asked, she denies any use of recreational drugs, alcohol, or tobacco products and exposure to secondhand smoke or toxins. Her caffeine intake consists of one cup of coffee and 32 oz of diet cola daily.

Mrs. Wilson faithfully attends a local Catholic church with her husband and has a close relationship with women in her church group. She explains that her participation in church activities has declined over the past 2 to 3 months due to increased fatigue and embarrassment about memory difficulties.

The nurse explores her self-concept. Mrs. Wilson reports that her self-esteem is "not what it used to be." In fact, her usual confidence in abilities at home and work has declined, and she is worried that others have noticed that she is "not up to par." She states that her clothes do not fit well due to weight loss and that she does not "have the energy to care." She denies crying episodes but cannot control worrying about things that usually were not problematic. She reports an overall sense of sadness. Mrs. Wilson denies any suicidal thoughts or ideations.

Support for Mrs. Wilson is provided by her husband and children, who have been worried about her recently. No appointments have been made regarding counseling, psychiatric evaluation, or intervention.

She reports a good relationship with her husband, a retired high school mathematics teacher, and describes him as "caring and patient." Mrs. Wilson has three grown children and four grandchildren who live within 20 miles of her home and visit often. She describes her role as a wife, mother, grandmother, and coworker as stressful due to increasing nervousness, worry, and fatigue. She states, "I can't keep up the way I used to. I'm afraid everyone thinks I'm crazy."

Mrs. Wilson denies any financial or relationship problems. She reports work stress due to increased workload recently and admits to having difficulty "keeping up" with work assignments while having to answer the phone and take messages. She states that she sometimes forgets about messages, which is causing some of her coworkers to become aggravated.

Collecting Objective Data: Physical Examination

Sometimes the mental status examination is performed with a complete neurologic assessment (see Chapter 25). Of the neurologic assessments, the mental status examination assesses the highest level of cerebral integration. Many find assessing mental status at the very beginning of the head-to-toe examination advantageous, as it provides clues regarding the validity of the subjective information provided by the client throughout the examination.

A comprehensive mental status examination is lengthy and involves great care on the part of the examiner to put the client at ease. There are several parts of the examination, which include assessment of the client's level of consciousness, posture, gait, body movements, dress, grooming, hygiene, facial expressions, behavior and affect, speech, mood, feelings, expressions, thought processes, perceptions, and cognitive abilities. Cognitive abilities include orientation, concentration, recent and remote memory, abstract reasoning, judgment, visual perception, and constructional ability.

Preparing the Client

Some of the questions you will be asking when collecting both subjective and objective data may seem silly or may embarrass the client. For example, the client will be asked to explain the meaning of a proverb, such as "a stitch in time saves nine." He or she will also be asked to name the day of the week and explain where he or she is at the time of the examination. With practice, you will learn how to infer this information by observing the client's responses to other questions during the examination, negating the need for direct questioning.

Equipment
- Pencil and paper
- Glasgow Coma Scale
- PHQ-2 to screen for depression during a routine client interview
- PHQ-9 to further assess for client who indicates depression using the PHQ 2
- Depression Questionnaire
- Columbia Suicide Severity Rating Scale (CSSRS)
- SAD PERSONS Suicide Risk Assessment
- Saint Louis University Mental Status (SLUMS) Assessment
- Confusion Assessment Method (CAM)
- SBIRT (Screening, Brief Intervention, and Referral to Treatment)
- CAGE Questionnaire
- The Alcohol Use Disorders Identification Test (AUDIT)

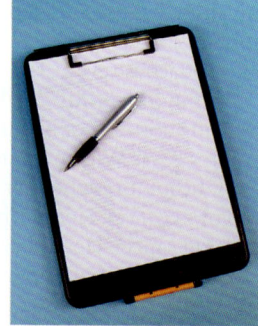

General Routine Screening Versus Focused Specialty Assessment

The nurse completes all of the general screening for all patients as indicated in the box below. Much of this assessment can be accomplished when the nurse first meets the client and observes how the client communicates, interacts, and processes information. Most often, the nurse does not perform a total mental status and substance abuse assessment as would a neurologist, psychiatrist, or a nurse practitioner employed in a mental health clinic. Yet, it is essential that all nurses know how to conduct a complete mental status examination and a risk for substance abuse assessment to clearly understand and communicate mental status findings. The nurse routinely evaluates the client's mental status by assessing level of consciousness; orientation to person, time, place, and events; posture; gait; behavior; affect; dress, grooming, and hygiene; facial expression; speech; mood; feelings; expressions; thought processes and perceptions; concentration; and recent and remote memory.

If a mental status abnormality is noted, further assessment is warranted. More in-depth assessments would include the ability to think abstractly and make appropriate judgments or decisions. If a client seems confused or reports inability to recall short-term or long-term information, the SLUMS tool can help identify signs of dementia. The Glasgow Coma Scale is useful for clients who are unresponsive or are not responding to questions. Clients who indicate that they are experiencing difficulty with life, or other symptoms of anxiety or depression (such as headache, fatigue, insomnia, hypochondriasis, back ache, nausea, abdominal pain, constipation, or diarrhea), may require further assessment for anxiety and/or depression using the PHQ-2, followed by the PHQ-9 if depression is indicated, or the Depression Questionnaire. If a risk for suicide is detected, the Columbia Suicide Severity Rating Scale or the SAD Persons Suicide Risk Tool would be appropriate. For clients concerned about their alcohol intake, the SBIRT, AUDIT, or the CAGE Self-Assessment tool may be used.

General Routine Screening
- Observe the client's level of consciousness.
- Observe posture, gait, and body movements
- Observe behavior and affect
- Ask the client: Do you drink alcohol? What type, how much, and how often?
- Do you use illicit drugs? Type, how much and how often?
- Observe dress and grooming
- Observe facial expressions
- Assess speech
- Observe mood, feelings, and expressions.
- Observe thought processes and perceptions. Identify possibly self-injurious or suicidal tendencies
- Assess orientation
- Assess concentration
- Assess recent and remote memory

Focused Specialty Assessment
- Use the Glasgow Coma Scale (GCS) for clients who have experienced a traumatic brain injury
- Use the PHQ-9 (Maurer, 2012) to further assess a client who indicates depression using the PHQ
- Use Quick Inventory of Depressive Symptomatology (Self-Report) Box 6-2 to determine whether the client is at risk for depression
- Use the Columbia Suicide Severity Rating Scale (CSSRS) for clients to assess for suicide risk
- Use the SBIRT (Screening, Brief Intervention, and Referral to Treatment) (SAMSA-HRSA, 2011) tool to identify, reduce, and prevent problematic use, abuse, and dependence on alcohol and illicit drugs.
- Use the CAGE Self-Assessment (Ewing, 1984) to detect alcohol dependence in trauma center populations.
- Use the AUDIT questionnaire (Tool 6-1) to assess alcohol-related disorders
- Use Geriatric Depression Scale (Chapter 32) if you suspect depression in the older client.
- Use Assessment Guide 6-1, the SAD PERSONS Suicide Risk Assessment, to determine the risk factors
- Assess abstract reasoning
- Use the SLUMS Dementia/Alzheimer's Test Examination (Assessment Tool 6-3)
- Assess judgment ability
- Assess visual, perceptual, and constructional ability.
- To distinguish delirium from other types of cognitive impairment, use the Confusion Assessment Method (CAM) Assessment Tool 6-4

PHYSICAL ASSESSMENT

Assessment Procedure	Normal Findings	Abnormal Findings
LEVEL OF CONSCIOUSNESS AND MENTAL STATUS		

 OLDER ADULT CONSIDERATIONS
When assessing the mental status of an older client, be sure first to check vision and hearing before assuming that the client has a mental problem.

Observe the client's level of consciousness. Ask the client his or her name, address, and phone number. Ask the client to identify where you currently are (e.g., hospital, clinic), the day, and the approximate time of day (Fig. 6-3).

Client is alert and oriented to person, place, time and events. Responds to your questions and interacts appropriately.

Makes and maintains eye contact and conversation. Asks and answers questions appropriately.

Client is not alert to person, place, day or time; does not make or maintain eye contact; does not respond appropriately.

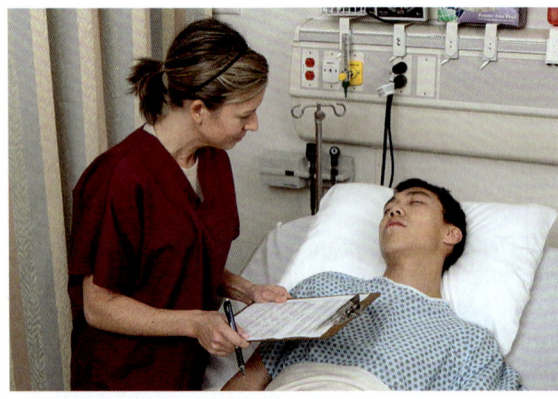

FIGURE 6-3 Assessing level of consciousness.

If the client does not respond appropriately, call the client's name and note the response. If the client does not respond, call the name louder. If necessary, shake the client gently. If the client still does not respond, apply a painful stimulus.

 CLINICAL TIP
When assessing level of consciousness, always begin with the least noxious stimulus: verbal, tactile, to painful.

Client is alert and awake, with eyes open and looking at examiner. Client responds appropriately.

OLDER ADULT CONSIDERATIONS
Although the older client's response and ability to process information may be slower, he or she is normally alert and oriented.

Abnormal Findings 6-1 describes abnormal levels of consciousness. Client with lesions of the corticospinal tract draws hands up to chest (*decorticate* or abnormal flexor posture) when stimulated (Fig. 6-4).

Client with lesions of the diencephalon, midbrain, or pons extends arms and legs, arches neck, and rotates hands and arms internally (*decerebrate* or abnormal extensor posture) when stimulated (Fig. 6-5).

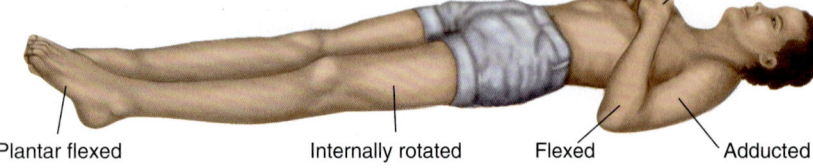

FIGURE 6-4 Decorticate posture.

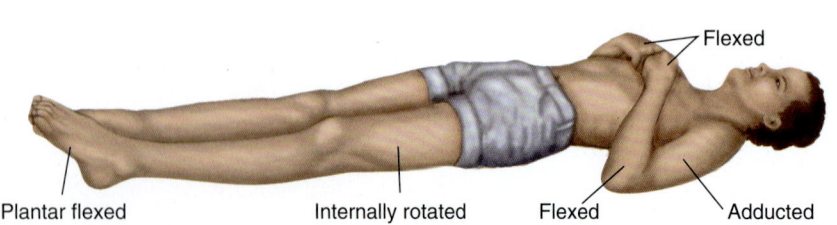

FIGURE 6-5 Decerebrate posture.

Assessment Procedure	Normal Findings	Abnormal Findings
Use the Glasgow Coma Scale (GCS) for clients who have experienced a traumatic brain injury (see Assessment Tool 6-2). **◎ CLINICAL TIP** The GCS cannot be used to assess a verbal score in intubated or aphasic clients; however, it is still the most widely used scoring system for intensive care unit (ICU) comatose patients (Fischer et al., 2010).	GCS score of 15 indicates an optimal level of consciousness.	GCS score of less than 15 indicates some impairment in the level of consciousness. A score of 3, the lowest possible score, indicates deep coma.
Observe posture, gait, and body movements.	The client is relaxed, with shoulders and back erect when standing or sitting. Gait is rhythmic and coordinated, with arms swinging at sides.	Slumped posture may reflect feelings of powerlessness or hopelessness characteristic of depression or organic brain disease. Bizarre body movements and behavior may be noted in schizophrenia or may be a side effect of drug therapy or other activity. Tense or anxious clients may elevate their shoulders toward their ears and hold the entire body stiffly. **OLDER ADULT CONSIDERATIONS** In the older adult, purposeless movements, wandering, aggressiveness, or withdrawal may indicate neurologic deficits.
Observe behavior and affect.	Client is cooperative and purposeful in his or her interactions with others. Affect is appropriate for the client's situation. Mild to moderate anxiety may be seen in a client who is apprehensive about having a health assessment performed.	Uncooperative, bizarre behavior may be seen in the angry, mentally ill, or violent client. Anxious clients are often fidgety and restless. Some degree of anxiety is often seen in ill clients. Apathy or crying may be seen with depression. Incongruent behavior may be seen in clients who are in denial of problems or illness. Prolonged, euphoric laughing is typical of mania.
Observe dress and grooming. Keep the examination setting and the reason for the assessment in mind as you note the client's degree of cleanliness and attire. For example, if the client arrives directly from home, he or she may be neater than if he or she comes to the assessment from the workplace. **◎ CLINICAL TIP** Be careful not to make premature judgments regarding the client's dress. Styles and clothing fads (e.g., torn jeans, oversized clothing, baggy pants), developmental level, and socioeconomic level impact an individual's mode of dress.	Dress is appropriate for occasion and weather. Dress varies considerably from person to person, depending on individual preference. There may be several normal dress variations depending on the client's developmental level, age, socioeconomic level, and culture or subculture. **CULTURAL CONSIDERATIONS** Culture may influence a person's dress (e.g., Indian women may wear saris; Hasidic Jewish men wear black suits and black skull caps). **OLDER ADULT CONSIDERATIONS** Some older adults may wear excess clothing because of slowed metabolism and loss of subcutaneous fat, resulting in cold intolerance.	Unusually meticulous grooming and finicky mannerisms may be seen in obsessive–compulsive disorder. Poor hygiene and inappropriate dress may be seen with organic brain syndrome. Bizarre dress and exaggerated makeup/cosmetics may be seen in schizophrenia or manic disorders. Extreme unilateral neglect may result from a lesion due to a cerebral vascular accident (CVA). Uncoordinated clothing, extremely light clothing, or extremely warm clothing for the weather conditions may be seen on mentally ill, grieving, depressed, or poor clients. This may also be noted in clients with heat or cold intolerances. Extremely loose clothing held up by pins or a belt may suggest recent weight loss. Clients wearing long sleeves in warm weather may be protecting themselves from the sun or covering up needle marks secondary to drug abuse. Soiled clothing may indicate homelessness, vision deficits in older adults, or mental illness.

Continued on following page

PHYSICAL ASSESSMENT (Continued)

Assessment Procedure	Normal Findings	Abnormal Findings
Observe hygiene. Consider normal level of hygiene for the client's developmental level, socioeconomic status, and ethnic/cultural background.	The client is clean and groomed appropriately for occasion. Stains on hands and dirty nails may reflect certain occupations such as mechanic or gardener. **CULTURAL CONSIDERATIONS** Asians and Native Americans have fewer sweat glands and, therefore, less obvious body odor than most Caucasians and black Africans, who have more sweat glands. Additionally, some cultures do not use deodorant products (see Chapter 11 for more information).	A dirty, unshaven, unkempt appearance with a foul body odor may reflect depression, drug abuse, or low socioeconomic level (i.e., homeless client). Poor hygiene may be seen in dementia or other conditions and may indicate a self-care deficit. If others care for the client, poor hygiene may reflect neglect by caregiver or caregiver role strain. Breath odors from smoking or from drinking alcoholic beverages may be noted.
Observe facial expressions, eye contact, and affect.	Client maintains eye contact, smiles, and frowns appropriately. **CULTURAL CONSIDERATIONS** Eye contact and facial expressions such as smiling differ in some cultures. Eye contact is often related to status or gender (who initiates eye contact with whom), and smiling often does not imply agreement with the speaker or friendliness. See Chapter 11 for more details.	Reduced eye contact is seen in depression or apathy. Extreme facial expressions of happiness, anger, or fright may be seen in anxious clients. Clients with Parkinson disease may have a mask-like, expressionless face. Staring watchfulness appears in metabolic disorders and anxiety. Inappropriate facial expressions (e.g., smiling when expressing sad thoughts) may indicate mental illness. Drooping or gross asymmetry occurs with neurologic disorder or injury (e.g., Bell palsy or stroke).
Assess speech. Note tone, clarity, and pace of speech. ◎ **CLINICAL TIP** Speech is largely influenced by experience, level of education, and culture. First, always assess the client's skill with English or the language being used for the assessment. If the client has difficulty with speech, perform additional tests: • Ask the client to name objects in the room. • Ask the client to read from printed material appropriate for his or her educational level. • Ask the client to write a sentence.	Speech is in a moderate tone, clear, with moderate pace, and culturally appropriate. **OLDER ADULT CONSIDERATIONS** Responses may be slowed, but speech should be clear and moderately paced. Client names familiar objects without difficulty and reads age-appropriate written print. Client writes a coherent sentence with correct spelling and grammar.	Slow, repetitive speech is characteristic of depression or Parkinson disease. Loud, rapid speech may occur in manic phases of bipolar disorder. Disorganized speech, consistent (nonstop) speech, or long periods of silence may indicate mental illness or a neurologic disorder (e.g., dysarthria, dysphasia, speech defect, garbled speech). See Abnormal Findings 6-2 for information about voice and speech problems. Client cannot name objects correctly, read print correctly, or write a basic sentence correctly. Deficits in this area require further neurologic assessment to identify any dysfunction of higher cortical levels.

Assessment Procedure	Normal Findings	Abnormal Findings
Observe mood, feelings, and expressions. Ask client "How are you feeling today?" and "What are your plans for the future?" 🎯 **CLINICAL TIP** Moods and feelings often vary from sadness to joy to anger, depending on the situation and circumstance.	Cooperative or friendly, expresses feelings appropriate to situation, verbalizes positive feelings regarding others and the future, expresses positive coping mechanisms (support groups, exercise, sports, hobbies, counseling).	Flat affect, euphoria, anxiety, fear, ambivalence, irritability, depression, and/or rage are all examples of altered mood expressions. Depression, anxiety, and somatization are common mental disorders seen in at least 5% to 10% of clients (Kroenke et al., 2010). Expression of prolonged negative, gloomy, despairing feelings is noted in depression. Expression of elation and grandiosity, high energy level, and engagement in high-risk but pleasurable activities is seen in manic phases. Excessive worry may be seen in anxiety or obsessive–compulsive disorders. Eccentric moods not appropriate to the situation are seen in schizophrenia.
Use the PHQ-9 (Maurer, 2012) to further assess a client who indicates depression using the PHQ 2.	Using the PHQ-2, a threshold score of less than 2.	Using a PHQ-2 threshold score of 2 or higher rather than 3 or higher resulted in more depressed patients being correctly identified. A PHQ-9 score of 10 or higher appears to detect more depressed patients than the originally described PHQ-9 scoring for major depression (Arroll et al., 2010).
Use Box 6-1: Quick Inventory of Depressive Symptomatology (Self-Report) to determine whether the client is at risk for depression and needs to be referred to a primary care health provider for further evaluation. 🪑 **OLDER ADULT CONSIDERATIONS** See the Geriatric Depression Scale in Chapter 32 if you suspect depression in the older client.	Inventory scores of 0–5 = No risk of depression	Inventory scores of 6–10 = Mild 11–15 = Moderate 16–20 = Severe 21–27 = Very severe
Observe thought processes and perceptions. Observe thought processes for clarity, content, and perception by inquiring about client's thoughts and perceptions expressed. Use statements such as "Tell me more about what you just said" or "Tell me what your understanding is of the current situation or your health."	Client expresses full, free-flowing thoughts; follows directions accurately; expresses realistic perceptions; is easy to understand and makes sense; does not voice suicidal/homicidal thoughts.	Abnormal processes include persistent repetition of ideas, illogical thoughts, interruption of ideas, invention of words, or repetition of phrases, as in schizophrenia; rapid flight of ideas, repetition of ideas, and use of rhymes and punning, as in manic phases of bipolar disorder; continuous, irrational fears, and avoidance of an object or situation, as in phobias; delusion, extreme apprehension; compulsions, obsessions, and illusions are also abnormal (see the glossary for definitions). Confabulation (making up of answers to cover for not knowing) is seen in Korsakoff syndrome. Also seen in cognitive deficits/decline (Alzheimer's and other dementias).
Identify possibly self-injurious or suicidal tendencies in client's thought processes and perceptions by asking, "How do you feel about the future?" or "Have you ever had thoughts of hurting yourself or doing away with yourself?" or "How do others feel about you?" Have you ever thought about hurting yourself or someone else?	Verbalizes positive, healthy thoughts about the future and self. Answers no to all questions related to suicidal ideation, suicidal behaviors, and both suicidal ideation and behavior.	Clients who are suicidal may share past attempts at suicide, give plan for suicide, verbalize worthlessness about self, joke about death frequently. Clients who are depressed or feel hopeless are at higher risk for suicide. Clients who have depression early in life have a twofold increased risk for dementia (Bowers, 2014).

Continued on following page

PHYSICAL ASSESSMENT (Continued)

Assessment Procedure	Normal Findings	Abnormal Findings
If suicidal thoughts seem evident, use the Columbia Suicide Severity Rating Scale (CSSRS) to assess for suicide risk if not used during the interview.		Clients undergoing hemodialysis often have depression and suicidal ideation (Andrade et al., 2015). Suicidal **ideation**: A "yes" answer at any time during treatment to any one of the five suicidal ideation questions (categories 1–5) on the C-SSRS. Suicidal **behavior**: A "yes" answer at any time during treatment to any one of the five suicidal behavior questions (categories 6–10) on the C-SSRS. Suicidal **ideation or behavior**: A "yes" answer at any time during treatment to any one of the 10 suicidal ideation and behavior questions (categories 1–10) on the C-SSRS.
Use Assessment Guide 6-1, the SAD PERSONS Suicide Risk Assessment, to determine the risk factors the client may have that may put him or her at risk for suicide.	No risk factors present on the SAD PERSONS factors.	Evaluate any risk factors on the SAD PERSONS. Suicide is the 10th leading cause of death in the United States for all ages and is four times more prevalent in men. Firearms accounted for 17,352 deaths, suffocation 8,161 deaths, and poisoning 6,358 deaths (CDC, 2015). Women attempt suicide more frequently. Men are more successful. **OLDER ADULT CONSIDERATIONS** Older, single/widowed, Caucasian males are at greatest risk for suicide.

COGNITIVE ABILITIES

Assessment Procedure	Normal Findings	Abnormal Findings
Assess orientation. Ask for the client's name and names of family members (person), the time such as hour, day, date, or season (time), and where the client lives or is now (place) (Fig. 6-6). **CLINICAL TIP** When assessing orientation to person, place, time, and events, remember that orientation to time is usually lost first and orientation to person is usually lost last.	Client is aware of self, others, time, home address, and current location. Client is oriented to person, place, time and events. **OLDER ADULT CONSIDERATIONS** Some older clients may seem confused, especially in a new or acute care setting, but most know who and where they are and the current month and year.	Reduced degree of orientation may be seen with organic brain disorders or psychiatric illness such as withdrawal from chronic alcohol use or schizophrenia. (*Note:* Schizophrenia may be marked by hallucinations—sensory perceptions that occur without external stimuli—as well as disorientation.)

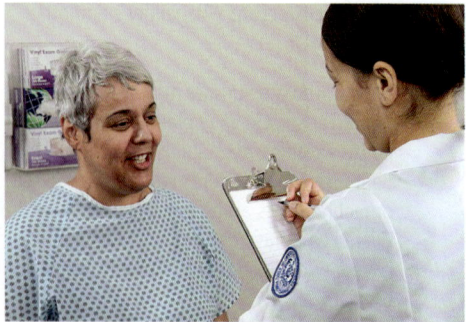

FIGURE 6-6 Assessing orientation by asking the client to identify a family member.

Assessment Procedure	Normal Findings	Abnormal Findings
Assess concentration. Note the client's ability to focus and stay attentive to you during the interview and examination. Give the client directions such as "Please pick up the pencil with your left hand, place it in your right hand, then hand it to me."	Client listens and can follow directions without difficulty. **OLDER ADULT CONSIDERATIONS** Some older clients may like to reminisce and tend to wander somewhat from the topic at hand.	Distraction and inability to focus on task at hand are noted in anxiety, fatigue, attention deficit disorders, and impaired states due to alcohol or drug intoxication.
Assess recent memory. Ask the client "What did you have to eat today?" or "What is the weather like today?"	Recalls recent events without difficulty. **OLDER ADULT CONSIDERATIONS** Some older clients may exhibit hesitation with short-term memory.	Inability to recall recent events is seen in delirium, dementia, depression, and anxiety. **OLDER ADULT CONSIDERATIONS** Although some health care providers are concerned about potential harm from labeling or identifying clients with a dementia diagnosis, Patterson et al. (2017) noted that screening is appropriate for common conditions that carry a high burden of suffering.
Assess remote memory. Ask the client: "When did you get your first job?" or "When is your birthday?" Information on past health history also gives clues as to the client's ability to recall remote events.	Client correctly recalls past events.	Inability to recall past events is seen in cerebral cortex disorders.
Assess use of memory to learn new information. Ask the client to repeat four unrelated words. The words should not rhyme and they cannot have the same meaning (e.g., rose, hammer, automobile, brown). Have the client repeat these words in 5 minutes, again in 10 minutes, and again in 30 minutes.	Client is able to recall words correctly after a 5-, a 10-, and a 30-minute period. **OLDER ADULT CONSIDERATIONS** Clients older than 80 years should recall two to four words after 5 minutes and possibly after 10 and 30 minutes with hints that prompt recall.	Inability to recall words after a delayed period is seen in anxiety, depression, or dementia—Alzheimer's is one type of dementia. See Box 6-2 for seven early warning signs of dementia or cognitive impairment seen in Alzheimer disease.
Assess abstract reasoning. Ask the client to compare objects. For example, "How are an apple and orange the same? How are they different?" Also ask the client to explain a proverb. For example, "A rolling stone gathers no moss" or "A stitch in time saves nine." ◎ **CLINICAL TIP** If clients have limited education, note their ability to joke or use puns, which also requires abstract reasoning.	Client explains similarities and differences between objects and proverbs correctly. The client with limited education can joke and use puns correctly.	Inability to compare and contrast objects correctly or interpret proverbs correctly is seen in schizophrenia, mental retardation, delirium, and dementia.
Assess judgment. Ask the client, "What do you do if you have pain?" or "What would you do if you were driving and a police car was behind you with its lights and siren turned on?"	Answers to questions are based on sound rationale.	Impaired judgment may be seen in organic brain syndrome, emotional disturbances, mental retardation, or schizophrenia.
Assess visual, perceptual, and constructional ability. Ask the client to draw the face of a clock or copy simple figures (Fig. 6-7).	Draws the face of a clock fairly well. Can copy simple figures.	Inability to draw the face of a clock or copy simple figures correctly is seen with mental retardation, dementia, or parietal lobe dysfunction of the cerebral cortex.

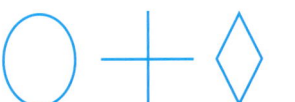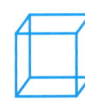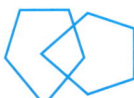

FIGURE 6-7 Figures to be drawn by client.

Continued on following page

COGNITIVE ABILITIES (Continued)

Assessment Procedure	Normal Findings	Abnormal Findings
Use the SLUMS Dementia/Alzheimer Test Examination (Assessment Tool 6-3) if time is limited and a quick measure is needed to evaluate cognitive function. If further assessment is needed to distinguish delirium from other types of cognitive impairment, use the Confusion Assessment Method (CAM; see Assessment Tool 6-4). **◎ CLINICAL TIP** The SLUMS and CAM test level of orientation, memory, speech, and cognitive functions but not mood, feelings, expressions, thought processes, or perceptions.	A score between 27 and 30 for clients with a high school education and a score of 20–30 for clients with less than a high school education is considered normal. **OLDER ADULT CONSIDERATIONS** See differences between signs of Alzheimer disease and typical age-related changes in the table within Evidence-Based Practice 6-1.	For clients with a high school education, a score of 20–27 indicates mild cognitive impairment (MCI) and for clients with less than a high school education, a score of 14–19 indicates MCI. For clients with a high school education, a score of 1–19 indicates dementia and for clients with less than a high school education, a score of 1–14 indicates dementia. Over half a million people in the United States have young-onset dementia and another half million have MCI, a precursor of dementia (Hunt, 2011). A diagnosis of delirium by CAM requires the presence of features 1 and 2 and either 3 or 4 under the CAM Diagnostic Algorithm (see Assessment Tool 6-4). Refer to Table 6-1.

ASSESSMENT TOOL 6-2   Glasgow Coma Scale

The Glasgow Coma Scale is useful for rating one's response to stimuli. The client who scores 10 or lower needs emergency attention. The client with a score of 7 or lower is generally considered to be in a coma.

		Score
Eye opening response	Spontaneous opening	4
	To verbal command	3
	To pain	2
	No response	1
Most appropriate verbal response	Oriented	5
	Confused	4
	Inappropriate words	3
	Incoherent	2
	No response	1
Most integral motor response (arm)	Obeys verbal commands	6
	Localizes pain	5
	Withdraws from pain	4
	Flexion (decorticate rigidity)	3
	Extension (decerebrate rigidity)	2
	No response	1
TOTAL SCORE		3–15

From Teasdale, G., & Jennett, B. (1974). Assessment of coma and impaired consciousness: A practical scale. *The Lancet, 304*(7872), 81–84. Used with permission.

BOX 6-2 SEVEN WARNING SIGNS OF ALZHEIMER DISEASE

1. Asking the same question over and over again
2. Repeating the same story, word for word, again and again
3. Forgetting how to cook, or how to make repairs, or how to play cards—activities that were previously done with ease and regularity
4. Losing one's ability to pay bills or balance one's checkbook
5. Getting lost in familiar surroundings or misplacing household objects
6. Neglecting to bathe, or wearing the same clothes over and over again, while insisting that they have taken a bath or that their clothes are still clean
7. Relying on someone else, such as a spouse, to make decisions or answer questions they previously would have handled themselves (WebMD, 2005–2007)

From the University of South Florida, Suncoast Gerontology Center. Used with permission.

ASSESSMENT TOOL 6-3 SLUMS Mental Status Examination

Saint Louis University

Mental Status (SLUMS) Examination

Name _____   Age _____

Is patient alert? _____   Level of education _____

—/1 ❶ 1. What day of the week is it?
—/1 ❶ 2. What is the year?
—/1 ❶ 3. What state are we in?

4. Please remember these five objects. I will ask you what they are later.
   Apple   Pen   Tie   House   Car

5. You have $100 and you go to the store and buy a dozen apples for $3 and a tricycle for $20.
   ❶   How much did you spend?
—/3 ❷   How much do you have left?

6. Please name as many animals as you can in one minute.
—/3   ⓿ 0–5 animals   ❶ 5–10 animals   ❷ 10–15 animals   ❸ 15+ animals

—/5 ❺ 7. What were the 5 objects I asked you to remember? 1 point for each one correct.

8. I am going to give you a series of numbers and I would like you to give them to me backwards. For example, if I say 42, you would say 24.
—/2   ⓿ 87   ⓿ 649   ⓿ 8537

9. This is a clock face. Please put in the hour markers and the time at ten minutes to eleven o'clock.
   ❷   Hour markers okay
—/4 ❷   Time correct

—/2 ❶ 10. Please place an X in the triangle.

❶ Which of the above figures is largest?

11. I am going to tell you a story. Please listen carefully because afterwards, I'm going to ask you some questions about it.

Jill was a very successful stockbroker. She made a lot of money on the stock market. She then met Jack, a devastatingly handsome man. She married him and had three children. They lived in Chicago. She then stopped work and stayed at home to bring up her children. When they were teenagers, she went back to work. She and Jack lived happily ever after.

❷ What was the female's name?   ❷ What work did she do?
—/8 ❷ When did she go back to work?   ❷ What state did she live in?

Scoring

High School Education		Less than High School Education
27–30	Normal	25–30
21–26	MNCD*	20–24
1–20	Dementia	1–19

*Mild Neurocognitive Disorder

For further information on using the tool, visit http://www.elderguru.com/downloads/SLUMS_instructions.pdf.

ASSESSMENT TOOL 6-4 The Confusion Assessment Method (CAM)

The Confusion Assessment Method (CAM) Instrument

1. [Acute Onset] Is there evidence of an acute change in mental status from the patient's baseline?

2A. [Inattention] Did the patient have difficulty focusing attention, for example, being easily distractible, or having difficulty keeping track of what was being said?

2B. [If present or abnormal] Did this behavior fluctuate during the interview, that is, tend to come and go or increase and decrease in severity?

3. [Disorganized thinking] Was the patient's thinking disorganized or incoherent, such as rambling or irrelevant conversation, unclear or illogical flow of ideas, or unpredictable switching from subject to subject?

4. [Altered level of consciousness] Overall, how would you rate this patient's level of consciousness? (Alert [normal]; Vigilant [hyperalert, overly sensitive to environmental stimuli, startled very easily]; Lethargic [drowsy, easily aroused]; Stupor [difficult to arouse]; Coma [unarousable]; Uncertain)

5. [Disorientation] Was the patient disoriented at any time during the interview, such as thinking that he or she was somewhere other than the hospital, using the wrong bed, or misjudging the time of day?

6. [Memory impairment] Did the patient demonstrate any memory problems during the interview, such as inability to remember events in the hospital or difficulty remembering instructions?

7. [Perceptual disturbances] Did the patient have any evidence of perceptual disturbances, for example, hallucinations, illusions, or misinterpretations (such as thinking something was moving when it was not)?

8A. [Psychomotor agitation] At any time during the interview did the patient have an unusually increased level of motor activity such as restlessness, picking at bedclothes, tapping fingers, or making frequent sudden changes of position?

8B. [Psychomotor retardation] At any time during the interview did the patient have an unusually decreased level of motor activity such as sluggishness, staring into space, staying in one position for a long time, or moving very slowly?

9. [Altered sleep-wake cycle] Did the patient have evidence of disturbance of the sleep-wake cycle, such as excessive daytime sleepiness with insomnia at night?

The Confusion Assessment Method (CAM) Diagnostic Algorithm

Feature 1: *Acute Onset or Fluctuating Course*
This feature is usually obtained from a family member or nurse and is shown by positive responses to the following questions: Is there evidence of an acute change in mental status from the patient's baseline? Did the (abnormal) behavior fluctuate during the day, that is, tend to come and go, or increase and decrease in severity?

Feature 2: *Inattention*
This feature is shown by a positive response to the following question: Did the patient have difficulty focusing attention, for example, being easily distractible, or having difficulty keeping track of what is being said?

Feature 3: *Disorganized Thinking*
This feature is shown by a positive response to the following question: Was the patient's thinking disorganized or incoherent, such as rambling or irrelevant conversation, unclear or illogical flow of ideas, or unpredictable switching from subject to subject?

Feature 4: *Altered Level of Consciousness*
This feature is shown by any answer other than "alert" to the following question: Overall, how would you rate this patient's level of consciousness? (Alert [normal]; Vigilant [hyperalert, overly sensitive to environmental stimuli, startled very easily]; Lethargic [drowsy, easily aroused]; Stupor [difficult to arouse]; Coma [unarousable])

The diagnosis of delirium by CAM requires the presence of features 1 and 2 and either 3 or 4.

The Confusion Assessment Method (CAM) Algorithm: Inouye, S. K., vanDyck, C. H, Alessi, C. A., Balkin, S., Siegal, A. P., & Horwitz, R. I. Clarifying confusion: The confusion assessment method: A new method for detection of delirium. *Ann Intern Med.* 1990;113:941–948. Used with permission.

TABLE 6-1 Summary of Differences Between Dementia and Delirium

	Dementia — Alzheimer Disease (AD)	Dementia — Vascular (Multi-Infarct) Dementia	Delirium
Etiology	Early-onset (familial, genetic [chromosomes 14, 19, 21]) Late-onset sporadic—etiology unknown	Cardiovascular (CV) disease Cerebrovascular disease Hypertension	Drug toxicity and interactions; acute disease; trauma; chronic disease exacerbation Fluid and electrolyte disorders
Risk factors	Advanced age; genetics	Pre-existing CV disease	Pre-existing cognitive impairment
Occurrence	70% of dementias	10–20% of dementias	7–61% among hospitalized people
Onset	Slow	Often abrupt Follows a stroke or transient ischemic attack	Rapid, acute onset A harbinger of acute medical illness
Age of onset	Early-onset AD: 30s–65 years Late-onset AD: 65+ years Most commonly: 85+ years	Most commonly 50–70 years	Any age, although predominantly in older persons
Gender	Males and females equally	Predominantly males	Males and females equally
Course	Chronic, irreversible; progressive, regular, downhill	Chronic, irreversible Fluctuating, stepwise progression	Acute onset Hypoalert—hypoactive Hyperalert—hyperactive Mixed hypo—hyper
Duration	2–20 years	Variable; years	Lasts 1 day to 1 month
Symptom progress	Onset insidious: *Early*—mild and subtle *Middle and late*—intensified Progression to death (infection or malnutrition)	Depends on location of infarct and success of treatment; death attributed to underlying CV disease	Symptoms are fully reversible with adequate treatment; can progress to chronicity or death if underlying condition is ignored
Mood	Depression common	Labile: mood swings	Variable
Speech/language	Speech remains intact until late in disease: *Early*—mild anomia (cannot name objects); deficits progress until speech lacks meaning; echoes and repeats words and sounds; mutism	May have speech deficit/aphasia depending on location of lesion	Fluctuating; often cannot concentrate long enough to speak May be somnolent
Physical signs	*Early*—no motor deficits *Middle*—apraxia (cannot perform purposeful movement) *Late*—Dysarthria (impaired speech) *End stage*—loss of all voluntary activity; positive neurologic signs	According to location of lesion: focal neurologic signs, seizures Commonly exhibits motor deficits	Signs and symptoms of underlying disease
Orientation	Becomes lost in familiar places (topographic disorientation) Has difficulty drawing three-dimensional objects (visual and spatial disorientation) Disorientation to time, place, and person—with disease progression		May fluctuate between lucidity and complete disorientation to time, place, and person
Memory	Loss is an early sign of dementia; loss of recent memory is soon, followed by progressive decline in recent and remote memory		Impaired recent and remote memory; may fluctuate between lucidity and confusion
Personality	Apathy, indifference, irritability: *Early disease*—social behavior intact; hides cognitive deficits *Advanced disease*—disengages from activity and relationships; suspicious; paranoid delusions caused by memory loss; aggressive; catastrophic reactions		Fluctuating; cannot focus attention to converse; alarmed by symptoms (when lucid); hallucinations; paranoid
Functional status, activities of daily living	Poor judgment in everyday activities; has progressive decline in ability to handle money, use telephone, use computer and other electronic devices, function in home and workplace		Impaired
Attention span	Distractible; short attention span		Highly impaired; cannot maintain or shift attention
Psychomotor activity	Wandering, hyperactivity, pacing, restlessness, agitation		Variable; alternates between high agitation, hyperactivity, restlessness, and lethargy
Sleep–wake cycle	Often impaired; wandering and agitation at nighttime		Takes brief naps throughout day and night

Reprinted with permission from Hinkle, J. L., & Cheever, K. H. (2018). *Brunner and Suddarth's textbook of medical surgical nursing* (14th ed.). Philadelphia: Lippincott Williams & Wilkins.

CASE STUDY

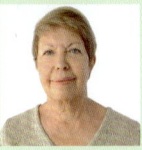

After preparing Mrs. Wilson by explaining the purpose and procedure, the nurse obtains vital signs, height, and weight, and then proceeds with the mental status assessment.

The nurse observes Mrs. Wilson's appearance. She is thin and frail. Her skin is pale, warm, and dry. Mrs. Wilson is clean and appropriately dressed for the season; she is not wearing jewelry or makeup. Her hair is disheveled. The nurse does not note any acute physical distress.

When questioned, Mrs. Wilson is alert and oriented to person, place, time, and events. She makes brief eye contact and often stares at the floor. Her affect is flat, and she frequently wrings her hands. Mrs. Wilson does not initiate conversation and questions must often be repeated due to client's difficulty concentrating. Throughout the examination, she anxiously looks at husband for reassurance. Her speech is clear, although volume is low and responses are brief. She is unable to recall what she ate for dinner last night; however, she remembers her wedding anniversary date and place. The nurse points to objects in the room (clock, waste basket, etc.), and Mrs. Wilson is able to name them. She explains the meaning of the proverb about a stitch in time. When asked how to respond to an emergency at work, she provides a logical answer. She scores 22/30 on the Saint Louis University Mental Status (SLUMS) examination. Mrs. Wilson expresses that she used to find enjoyment and satisfaction in roles as wife, mother, grandmother, school secretary, and church member, but now finds that her memory issues make these roles stressful and agitating.

Validating and Documenting Findings

Validate the mental status assessment data you have collected (by asking additional questions, verifying data with another health care professional, or comparing objective with subjective findings). This is necessary to verify that the data are reliable and accurate. Document the data following the health care facility or agency policy.

CLINICAL TIP
When documenting your assessment findings, it is better to describe the client's response than to label his or her behavior.

CASE STUDY

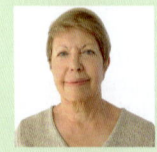

Think back to the case study. The nurse completed the following documentation of her assessment of Mrs. Wilson. **Biographical Data:** JW. Born January 20, 1950. White. Employed as a secretary. Married.

History of Present Health Concern: "I'm very nervous and not thinking straight. I'm afraid I am losing my mind." Often cannot remember names of friends, where she puts things, or what she was about to do. Began 3 months ago. Symptoms sometimes improve in AM if she gets a good night's sleep, but she has bouts of insomnia. She is worried about losing her job.

Past Health History: Denies previous treatment or hospitalization for mental health reasons. Negative history of meningitis, encephalitis, head injury, or stroke. Reports occasional headache, relieved with acetaminophen. Denies chest pain, palpitations, and shortness of breath.

Family History: Positive for Alzheimer disease, coronary artery disease, and colon cancer.

Lifestyle and Health Practices: Typical day: Wakes at 6:00 AM and gets ready for work, goes to work at 7:30 AM, eats lunch at 11:30 AM, returns home at 4:00 PM, watches TV or naps for 30 minutes, makes dinner for husband, goes to bed at 8:00 PM but does not fall asleep for 1 to 2 hours. 24-hour diet recall: Breakfast—one cup black coffee, one slice buttered toast; lunch—half peanut butter and jelly sandwich and 32 oz diet Coke; dinner—"picked at" chicken breast and mashed potatoes, half glass 2% milk. Lost 10 lb recently.

Erratic bowel pattern with episodes of constipation alternating with diarrhea. Reports "bloating" and "gas."

Current meds: acetaminophen, 325 to 650 mg every 4 hours PRN for headache/pain, daily multivitamin, Correctol PRN for constipation, Imodium AD PRN for diarrhea.

No known drug, food, environmental, or insect allergies. Denies any use of recreational drugs, alcohol, or tobacco. Caffeine intake: one cup coffee and a 44-oz diet cola daily.

Attends a local Catholic church; participation declined over the past 2 to 3 months due to increased fatigue and embarrassment about memory difficulties. Self-esteem is "not what it used to be." Confidence in abilities declined. Does not "have the energy to care" that clothes no longer fit. Denies crying episodes but cannot control worrying and overall sadness. Denies any suicidal thoughts or ideations.

Support includes husband (good relationship) and children who have been worried. No inquiries made regarding counseling, psychiatric evaluation, or intervention.

Role as a wife, mother, grandmother, and coworker is stressful due to increasing nervousness, worry, and fatigue. "I can't keep up the way I used to. I'm afraid everyone thinks I'm crazy."

Denies any financial or relationship problems. She reports work stress due to increased workload.

Physical Examination (Objective Data):

Vital signs: Temp, 96.3°F; Pulse, 82; Resp, 18; BP, 100/62. Height: 5'5"; Weight 115 lb.

General Survey: Thin and frail in appearance. Skin pale, warm, and dry. No acute physical distress noted. Alert and oriented to person, place, time, and events.

Mental Status Findings: Clean and appropriately dressed for the season, without jewelry or makeup. Hair disheveled. Makes brief eye contact and often stares at the floor. Affect is flat. Frequently wrings hands. Does not initiate conversation. Questions must often be repeated due to JW's difficulty concentrating. Speech clear; volume is low and responses are brief. Unable to recall what she ate for dinner last night. Able to recall wedding anniversary date and place. Looks at husband frequently for reassurance. Able to name familiar objects in examination room. Explained the meaning of common proverbs. Explained what to do in an emergency situation. Scored 22/30 on the SLUMS examination. Expressed stress handling roles as wife, mother, grandmother, school secretary, and church member.

Interdisciplinary Verbal Communication of Assessment Findings Using SBAR

SITUATION: Today, Mrs. Wilson came to the clinic with concerns of anxiety, fearfulness, anorexia, insomnia, fatigue, inability to concentrate, and "being very nervous and unable to think straight" over the last 3 months.

BACKGROUND: She is a 61-year-old Caucasian female employed as a secretary with a family history of Alzheimer disease. Lost 10 lb, has erratic bowel pattern with episodes of constipation, followed by diarrhea self-treated with Correctol and Imodium once every 2 weeks, and headaches treated with Tylenol. Takes multivitamin daily. Has experienced difficulty recalling peoples' names and other information, which has led to less frequent socialization in church activities, and difficulty "keeping up" at work and with family activities.

ASSESSMENT: Thin and frail (but BMI 19), has brief eye contact and often stares at the floor, flat affect, frequently wrings hands. Does not initiate conversation. Questions must often be repeated due to her difficulty concentrating. Recent memory not intact, remote memory intact. Judgment and reasoning intact. Scored 22/30 on the SLUMS examination. SLUMS: mild neurocognitive disorder. Anxiously looks at husband for reassurance. Able to name familiar objects in examination room. Explained the meaning of common proverbs and what to do in an emergency situation.

RECOMMENDATION: I believe Mrs. Wilson needs a comprehensive physical and psychiatric examination.

ANALYSIS OF DATA: DIAGNOSTIC REASONING

After collecting subjective and objective data pertaining to the mental status examination, identify abnormal findings and client strengths using diagnostic reasoning. Then, cluster the data to reveal any significant patterns or abnormalities. The following sections provide possible conclusions that the nurse may make after assessing a client's mental status and substance use.

Selected Nursing Diagnoses

The following is a list of selected nursing diagnoses that may be identified when analyzing data from assessing mental health.

Health Promotion Diagnoses

- Readiness for enhanced health management related to desire and request to learn more about health promotion
- Readiness for enhanced coping

Risk Diagnoses

- Risk for self-directed violence related to depression, suicidal tendencies, developmental crisis, lack of support systems, loss of significant others, poor coping mechanisms, and behaviors
- Risk for developmental delay related to lack of healthy environmental stimulation and activities
- Risk for powerlessness related to prolonged disability

Actual Diagnoses

- Anxiety related to awareness of increasing memory loss
- Impaired verbal communication related to international language barrier (inability to speak English or accepted dominant language)
- Impaired verbal communication related to hearing loss
- Impaired verbal communication related to inability to clearly express self or understand others (aphasia)
- Impaired verbal communication related to aphasia, psychological impairment, or organic brain disorder
- Acute or chronic confusion related to dementia, head injury, stroke, alcohol or drug abuse
- Impaired memory related to dementia, stroke, head injury, alcohol or drug abuse
- Dressing/grooming self-care deficit related to confusion and lack of resources/support from caregivers
- Disturbed thought processes related to alcohol or drug abuse, psychotic disorder, or organic brain dysfunction
- Social isolation related to inability to relate/communicate effectively with others
- Complicated grieving related to suicide of child and increasing isolation from support systems

Selected Collaborative Problems

After you group the data, it may become apparent that certain collaborative problems emerge. Remember that collaborative problems differ from nursing diagnoses in that they cannot be prevented by nursing interventions. However, these physiologic complications of medical conditions can be detected and monitored by the nurse. In addition, the nurse can use physician- and nurse-prescribed interventions to minimize the complications of these problems. The nurse may also have to refer the client in such situations for further treatment of the problem. Following is a list of collaborative problems that may be identified when obtaining a general impression. These

problems are worded as risk for complications (RC), followed by the problem.
- RC: Stroke
- RC: Increased intracranial pressure (ICP)
- RC: Seizures
- RC: Meningitis
- RC: Depression

Medical Problems

After you group the data, it may become apparent that the client has signs and symptoms that require psychiatric medical diagnosis and treatment. Refer to a primary care provider as necessary.

> ### CASE STUDY
>
>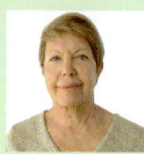
>
> After collecting and analyzing the data for Mrs. Wilson, the nurse determines that the following conclusions are appropriate.
>
> **Nursing Diagnoses Include**
> - Anxiety
>
> **Potential Collaborative Problems Include**
> - RC: Depression. If her anxiety needs pharmacotherapy, it would also be a collaborative problem.
>
> To view an algorithm depicting the process for diagnostic reasoning in this case, go to thePoint.

ABNORMAL FINDINGS 6-1 Abnormal Levels of Consciousness

Lethargy: Client opens eyes, answers questions, and falls back asleep.
Obtunded: Client opens eyes to loud voice, responds slowly with confusion, and seems unaware of environment.
Stupor: Client awakens to vigorous shake or painful stimuli but returns to unresponsive sleep.
Coma: Client remains unresponsive to all stimuli; eyes stay closed.

ABNORMAL FINDINGS 6-2 Sources of Voice and Speech Problems

Dysphonia is voice volume disorder caused by laryngeal disorders or impairment of cranial nerve X (vagus nerve).
Cerebellar dysarthria is irregular, uncoordinated speech caused by multiple sclerosis.
Dysarthria is a defect in muscular control of speech (e.g., slurring) related to lesions of the nervous system, Parkinson disease, or cerebellar disease.
Aphasia is difficulty producing or understanding language, caused by motor lesions in the dominant cerebral hemisphere.
Wernicke aphasia is rapid speech that lacks meaning, caused by a lesion in the posterior superior temporal lobe.
Broca aphasia is slowed speech with difficult articulation, but fairly clear meaning, caused by a lesion in the posterior inferior frontal lobe.

> ### Want to know more?
>
> A wide variety of resources to enhance your learning and understanding of this book are available on thePoint. Visit thePoint to access:
>
> NCLEX-Style Student Review Questions
> Watch and Learn Videos
> Concepts in Action Animations
> And more!

Unfolding Patient Stories: Edith Jacobson • Part 1

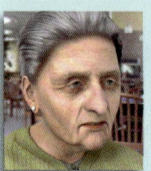

Edith Jacobson is 85 years old and fell at home. She fractured her hip and hit her head. Compare the pain assessment the nurse would perform if Edith is awake and coherent versus drowsy and confused. (Edith Jacobson's story continues in Chapter 29.)
Care for Edith and other patients in a realistic virtual environment: *vSim for Nursing* (thepoint.lww.com/vSimHealthAssessment). Practice documenting these patients' care in DocuCare (thepoint.lww.com/DocuCareEHR).

Unfolding Patient Stories: Rashid Ahmed • Part 2

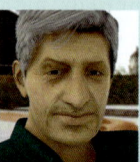

Recall from Chapter 1 **Rashid Ahmed**, who is admitted to the medical unit with bacterial gastroenteritis. During the admission assessment he informs the nurse that he is Muslim. What questions can the nurse ask to identify his religious and spiritual needs during hospitalization? How can the nurse incorporate his Muslim practices into the plan of care?
Care for Rashid and other patients in a realistic virtual environment: *vSim for Nursing* (thepoint.lww.com/vSimHealthAssessment). Practice documenting these patients' care in DocuCare (thepoint.lww.com/DocuCareEHR).

References and Selected Readings

Adelman, R., Tmanova, L., Delgado, D., Dion, S., & Lachs, M. (2014). Caregiver burden: A clinical review. *Journal of the American Medical Association, 311*(10), 1052–1060. doi:10.1001/jama.2014.304. Available at http://jama.jamanetwork.com/article.aspx?articleid=1840211

Alzheimer's Association. (2014). Know the 10 signs. Available at http://www.alz.org/national/documents/10warningsigns.pdf

Alzheimer's Association. (2015a). Alzheimer's disease facts and figures. Available at https://www.alz.org/facts/downloads/facts_figures_2015.pdf

Alzheimer's Association. (2015b). Brain health. Available at http://www.alz.org/we_can_help_brain_health_maintain_your_brain.asp

American Foundation for Suicide Prevention. (2015). Facts and figures. Available at https://www.afsp.org/understanding-suicide/facts-and-figures

American Psychiatric Association (APA). (2012). DSM-5 development: Definition of a mental disorder. Available at http://www.dsm5.org/ProposedRevisions/Pages/proposedrevision.aspx?rid=465

Andrade, S., Sesso, R., & Diniz, D. (2015). Hopelessness, suicide ideation, and depression in chronic kidney disease patients on hemodialysis or transplant recipients. *Jornal Brasileiro de Nefrologia, 37*(1):55–63. doi:10.5935/0101-2800.20150009. Available at http://www.ncbi.nlm.nih.gov/pubmed/25923751

Arria, A. M., & O'Brien, M. C. (2011). The "high" risk of energy drinks. *Journal of the American Medical Association, 305*(6), 600–601.

Arroll, B., Goodyear-Smith, F., Crengle, S., Gunn, J., Kerse, N., Fishman, T.... Hatcher, S. (2010). Validation of PHQ-2 and PHQ-9 to screen for major depression in the primary care population. *Annals of Family Medicine, 8*(4), 348–353. Available at http://www.ncbi.nlm.nih.gov/pmc/articles/PMC2906530/

Bowers, E. S. (2014). Depression as a risk factor for dementia. Available at http://www.everydayhealth.com/news/depression-risk-factor-dementia/

Butt, M. S., & Sultan, M. T. (2011). Coffee and its consumption: Benefits and risks. *Critical Reviews in Food Science Nutrition, 51*(4), 363–373.

Centers for Disease Control and Prevention (CDC). (2015). *Suicide*. Available at http://www.cdc.gov/violenceprevention/pdf/suicide-datasheet-a.PDF

Ewing, J. A. (1984). Detecting alcoholism: The CAGE Questionnaire. *Journal of the American Medical Association, 252*, 1905–1907.

Farias, S. T., Mungas, D., Harvey, D., Simmons, A., Reed, B., & DiCarli, C. (2011). The measurement of everyday cognition (ECog). Development and validation of a short form. *Alzheimer's & Dementia, 7*(6), 593–601. Available at http://www.ncbi.nlm.nih.gov/pmc/articles/PMC3211103/pdf/nihms-283862.pdf

Fischer, M., Rüegg, S., Czaplinski, A., et al. (2010). Inter-rater reliability of the full outline of unresponsiveness score and the Glasgow Coma Scale in critically ill patients: A prospective observational study. *Critical Care, 14*:R64.

Gonzalez-Guarda, R., McCabbe, F., Vermeesch, A., Cianelli, R., Florom-Smith, A., & Peragallo, N. (2012). Cultural phenomena and the syndemic factor: Substance abuse, violence, HIV, and depression among Hispanic women. *Annals of Anthropological Practice, 36*(2), 212–231. Available at https://www.ncbi.nlm.nih.gov/pubmed/24575326

Hamilton, J., Moore, A., Johnson, K., & Koenig, H. (2013). Reading the Bible for guidance, comfort, and strength during stressful life events. *Nursing Research, 62*(3), 178–184. doi:10.1097/NNR.0b013e31828fc816. Available at http://www.ncbi.nlm.nih.gov/pubmed/23636344

Healthy People 2020. (2014a). Dementias, including Alzheimer's disease. Available at http://www.healthypeople.gov/2020/topics-objectives/topic/dementias-including-alzheimers-disease

Healthy People 2020. (2014b). Substance abuse. Available at http://www.healthypeople.gov/2020/topics-objectives/topic/substance-abuse

Hunt, D. (2011). Young-onset dementia: a review of the literature and what it means for clinicians. *Journal of Psychosocial Nursing and Mental Health Services, 49*(4), 28–33. Abstract available at http://www.ncbi.nlm.nih.gov/pubmed/21410087

Kroenke, K., Spitzer, R., Williams, J., & Löwe, B. (2010). The Patient Health Questionnaire Somatic, Anxiety, and Depressive Symptom Scales: A systematic review. *General Hospital Psychiatry, 32*(4), 345–359. Abstract available at http://www.ghpjournal.com/article/S0163-8343(10)00056-3/abstract

Lande, R. G. (2011). Caffeine-related psychiatric disorders. Available at http://emedicine.medscape.com/article/290113-overview

Maurer, D. (2012). Screening for depression. *American Family Physician, 85*(2), 139–144. Available at http://www.aafp.org/afp/2012/0115/p139.html

Mentally challenging activities & delaying dementia. (2011). Available at http://www.healthcommunities.com/dementia/mentally-challenging-activities_jhmwp.shtml

National Institute on Alcohol Abuse and Alcoholism. (2005). Screening for alcohol and alcohol related problems. Alcohol Alert. No. 65. Available at http://pubs.niaaa.nih.gov/publications/aa65/aa65.htm

National Institute on Drug Abuse. (2010a). The science of addiction. Available at http://www.drugabuse.gov/drugs-abuse/commonly-abused-drugs-charts-0

National Institute on Drug Abuse (NIDA). (2010b). 2010 Strategic plan. Available at https://www.drugabuse.gov/about-nida/strategic-plan/2010-strategic-plan

National Institute on Drug Abuse. (2015). Commonly abused drugs. Available at http://www.drugabuse.gov/drugs-abuse/commonly-abused-drugs-charts-0

National Institute of Mental Health. (2013). Any mental illness (AMI) among adults. Available at http://www.nimh.nih.gov/health/statistics/prevalence/any-mental-illness-ami-among-adults.shtml

Patterson, C., Gauthier, S., Bergman, H., Cohen, C., Feightner, J., Feldman, H.,... Hogan, D. (2017). The recognition, assessment and management of dementing disorders. *The Canadian Journal of Neurological Sciences, 28*(Suppl 1), S3–S16.

Pomeranz, J., Munsell, C., & Harris, J. (2013). Energy drinks: An emerging public health hazard for youth. Available at http://www.uconnruddcenter.org/resources/upload/docs/what/law/EnergyDrinks_JPHP_3.13.pdf

Posner, K. (2008). Columbia-Suicide Severity Rating Scale. Available at http://www.integration.samhsa.gov/clinical-practice/Columbia_Suicide_Severity_Rating_Scale.pdf

Rockett, I., & Caine, E. (2015). Self-injury is the eighth leading cause of death in the United States. *JAMA Psychiatry, 72*(11), 1069–1070. doi:10.1001/jamapsychiatry.2015.1418. Available at http://archpsyc.jamanetwork.com/article.aspx?articleid=2436271

Shao, H., Breitner, J., Whitmer, R., Wang, J., Hayden, K., Wengreen, H.,...Zandi, P.; Cache County Investigators. (2012). Hormone therapy and Alzheimer disease dementia: New findings from the Cache County Study. *Neurology, 79*(18), 1846–1852. doi:http://dx.doi.org/10.1212/WL0b013e318271f823

Soderstrom, C., Smith, G., Kufera, J., Dischinger, P., Hebel, J., McDuff, D.,... Read, K. (1997). The accuracy of the CAGE, the Brief Michigan Alcoholism Screening Test, and the Alcohol Use Disorders Identification Test in screening trauma center patients for alcoholism. *Journal of Trauma-Injury Infection & Critical Care, 43*(6), 962–960.

Substance Abuse and Mental Health Services Administration (SAMHSA). (2013). National survey on drug use and health. Available at https://nsduhweb.rti.org/respweb/homepage.cfm

Substance Abuse and Mental Health Services Administration (SAMHSA). (2015). Behavioral health trends in the United States: Results from the 2014 National Survey on Drug Use and Health. Available at http://www.samhsa.gov/data/sites/default/files/NSDUH-FRR1-2014/NSDUH-FRR1-2014.pdf

Substance Abuse and Mental Health Services Administration–Health Resources and Services Administration (SAMHSA-HRSA). (2011). SBIRT: Screening, brief intervention, and referral to treatment. Available at http://www.integration.samhsa.gov/clinical-practice/SBIRT

U.S. Preventive Services Task Force (USPSTF). (2008). Screening for illicit drug use. Available at http://www.uspreventiveservicestaskforce.org/uspstf/uspsdrug.htm

U.S. Preventive Services Task Force (USPSTF). (2013). Final recommendation statement. Alcohol misuse: Screening and behavioral counseling interventions in primary care. Available at https://www.uspreventiveservicestaskforce.org/Page/Document/RecommenationStatementFinal/alcohol-misuse-screning-and-behavioral-counseling-interventions-in-primary-care

World Health Organization (WHO). (2014). Mental health: Strengthening our response. Available at http://www.who.int/mediacentre/factsheets/fs220/en/

World Health Organization (WHO). (2015). Substance abuse. Available at http://www.who.int/topics/substance_abuse/en//

Zauszniewski, J., Bekhet, A., & Suresky, M. J. (2010). Resilience in family members of persons with serious mental illness. Available at http://epublications.marquette.edu/cgi/viewcontent.cgi?article=1078&context=nursing_fac

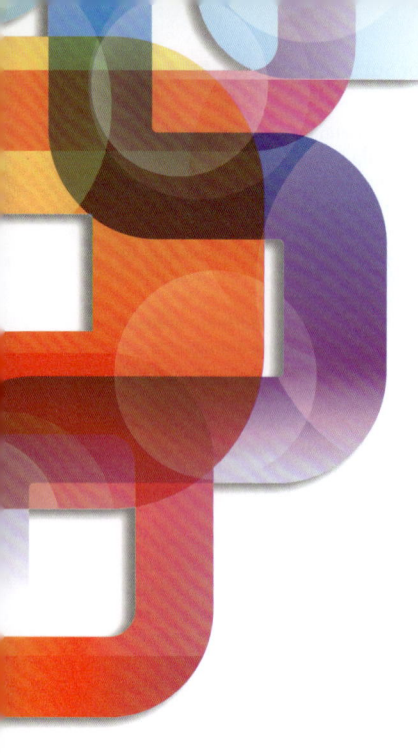

7 ASSESSING PSYCHOSOCIAL, COGNITIVE, AND MORAL DEVELOPMENT

Learning Objectives

1. Describe the following developmental theories: Freud (psychosexual), Erickson, (psychosocial), Piaget (cognitive), and Kohlberg (moral)
2. Interview clients for an accurate history reflecting their psychosocial, cognitive, and moral development.
3. Assess a client's psychosocial, cognitive, and moral development based on subjective and objective data findings.
4. Differentiate between normal and abnormal findings of psychosocial, cognitive, and moral development.
5. Describe findings frequently seen when assessing the older client's psychosocial, cognitive, and moral development.
6. Analyze client subjective and objective data to formulate valid nursing diagnoses, collaborative problems, and/or referrals related to psychosocial, cognitive, and moral development.

CASE STUDY

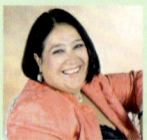

Constance (Connie) Como-Williams is a 51-year-old woman who divorced at 45 years of age and remarried last year. At the age of 21 years, Connie received a bachelor's degree, majoring in education from Purdue University in Indiana. Immediately after graduation, she married her college boyfriend, Joseph Como. Subsequently, she taught first grade at a public elementary school for 2 years. She then gave birth to a daughter, Monica, and decided to postpone her teaching career, becoming a full-time mother and wife. She remained at home raising her daughter. After her divorce, she returned to teaching, second grade. It was during this time that she met and married her second husband, Jeffrey. Mrs. Como-Williams's case will be discussed throughout the chapter.

An overview of the developmental concepts of Sigmund Freud (1856–1939), Erik Erikson (1902–1994), Jean Piaget (1896–1980), and Lawrence Kohlberg (1927–1987) will be presented in this chapter. Having a basic understanding of the significant contributions made by these theorists of the psychosexual, psychosocial, cognitive, and moral development of humans is fundamental to performing a holistic nursing assessment.

This chapter will describe methods for assessing the various developmental levels across the life span using the principles of selected developmental theorists. Combining the developmental information from this chapter with the concepts and content in the remainder of this textbook will provide a holistic approach to assessment.

GROWTH AND DEVELOPMENT

No single theory has been formulated to embrace all aspects of why humans behave, think, or believe the way they do. New theories continue to emerge in an attempt to explain human conduct. The developmental theories presented in this chapter focus on the *growth* (addition of new skills or components) and *development* (refinement, expansion or improvement of existing skills or components) of an individual throughout the life span. Each theorist varies on how to categorize the phases of the life cycle (e.g., infancy, adolescence, adulthood).

Freud Theory of Psychosexual Development

Sigmund Freud (1935), a Viennese physician, developed the first formal theory of personality. He originated the concept of psychoanalysis and believed that personality development was based on understanding the individual life history of a person.

Freud's Major Concepts and Terms

Freud (1935) postulated that the psychological nature of human beings is determined by the result of conflict between biologic drives (*instincts*) and social expectations. He believed that people generally are not aware of the underlying reasons for their behavior. Originally, Freud conceived the concept of *mental qualities,* which influence behavior and occur at three levels of awareness.

The first level, *consciousness,* refers to whatever a person is sensing, thinking about, or experiencing at any given moment. Freud considered this level to be limited, since only a small amount of such thought exists at one time. The second level, *preconsciousness,* involves all of a person's memories and stored knowledge that can be recalled and brought to the *conscious* level. Freud declared the third level, *unconsciousness,* as the largest and most influential. This level corresponds to socially unacceptable sexual desires, shameful impulses, and irrational wishes, as well as anxieties and fears.

Later, Freud revised his theory to include three basic structures in his anatomy of the personality: the *id, ego,* and *super-ego* (Freud, 1949). He believed that these structures could operate within any of the levels of awareness; however, he declared the id to be completely unconscious. According to Freud, the id is the inherited system. Containing the basic motivational drives for such entities as air, water, warmth, and sex, it seeks instant gratification and supplies the psychic energy for the ego and the superego. Freud considered sex to be the most important drive. Defining sex in very broad terms, he stated that it included all pleasurable thoughts and beliefs. He added that the id knows no perception of reality or morality (what is right and wrong). Until the ego begins to develop in very late infancy, the infant performs only at the level of the id.

The ego emerges to act initially as an intermediary between the id and the external world, or reality (Freud, 1949). It includes many processes such as learning, perceptions, memory, problem solving, and decision making. According to Freud, the ego must attempt to postpone or redirect id satisfaction. Since this is a source of much conflict, Freud contended that people make use of a variety of *defense mechanisms* (e.g., denial, rationalization, repression) to protect the ego. Although the ego plays an important role in behavior, it does not possess a concept of morality.

The superego, often referred to as the moral component of personality (or in lay terms, one's "conscience"), provides feedback to the person regarding how closely his or her behavior conforms to the external value system. It strives for perfection, disregards reality, usually operates at the unconscious level, and is an insistent force against the desires of the id. Freud believed that the superego originates in the learned rules of conduct imposed by a person's parents. It emerges during the fifth year of life and in the course of a person's development could be influenced by "later successors and substitutes of his parents such as teachers, admired figures in public life, or high social ideals (Fodor & Gaynor, 1958, p. 150). According to Freud, personality development is predetermined by the end of the preschool years and is complete by the end of adolescence. He defined adult behavior as the result of the interactions among the id, ego, and superego as they relate to a person's experience with the outer world. In some form, the id is always seeking pleasure and avoiding pain. The superego is trying to reconcile the *instincts* of the id while discouraging the expression of undesirable behavior and encouraging correct goals. The ego must decide whether the id or the superego prevails with regard to the conflict or establish a compromise between these two opposing forces.

Freud's Stages of Psychosexual Development

In his 1935 work, Sigmund Freud described how he developed his psychoanalysis as he listened to and attempted to direct the thoughts of his adult patients, who presented with a variety of symptoms (such as paranoia, phobia, or paralysis) that appeared to have no physical basis. He became convinced that their symptoms could be relieved by encouraging them to talk with him about painful events from early childhood. He maintained that how parents manage their child's sexual and aggressive drives is focal to personality development. He thus constructed a theory that people may go through five psychosexual stages of development that could overlap or exist simultaneously. He postulated that as children mature, they invest instinctual, sexual–sensual energy (*libido*) in one biophysical area of the body (*pleasure-seeking* or *erogenous zone*) during each stage. That zone dominates the mode of interaction with oneself and others at that time. He also posited that people who became either *undergratified* or *overgratified* during any of these stages could become *fixated*. Table 7-1 presents a summary of Freud's psychosexual stages of development

TABLE 7-1 Sigmund Freud's Stages of Psychosexual Development

Stage	Approximate Age	Psychosexual Developments
Oral	0–1.5 years	Pleasure derived from the mouth—such as sucking, eating, chewing, biting, and vocalizing—serve to reduce the infant's tension. The *id* controls this stage.
Anal	1.5–3 years	Pleasure involves the elimination of feces. As the *ego* develops, the child decides to expel or retain the bowel movement.
Phallic	3–6 years	Pleasure is derived from the genital region. This can involve exploring and manipulating the genitals of self and others. A child can express curiosity about how a baby is "made" and born. The *superego* emerges from interactions with parents. Parents insist that the child control biologic impulses. *Oedipal* (for males) and *Electra* (for females) complexes appear.
Latency	6–11 years	Abeyance of sexual urges occurs as the child develops more intellectual and social skills. It is a time of school activities, hobbies, sports, and for developing friendships with members of the same sex. The superego continues to develop. Defense mechanisms appear.
Genital	Adolescence	Puberty allows sexual impulses to reappear. Once conflicts with parents are resolved and if no major *fixations* have occurred, the individual will develop heterosexual attachments outside of the family. Romantic love can lead to successful marriage and parenting.

Information from Freud, S. (1935). *A general introduction to psychoanalysis* (English translation of the revised edition by Joan Riviere). New York: Liveright; and Freud, S. (1949). *An outline of psychoanalysis* (authorized translation by James Strachey). New York: W. W. Norton & Company, Inc.

(Freud was not explicit in identifying exact ages in years for each stage).

Erikson Theory of Psychosocial Development

Erik Erikson was a psychoanalyst who adapted and expanded Sigmund Freud's psychosexual theory. Erikson theory has become known as a psychosocial theory, with *psychosocial* being defined as the intrapersonal and interpersonal responses of a person to external events (Schuster & Ashburn, 1992).

Erikson concluded that societal, cultural, and historical factors—as well as biophysical processes and cognitive function—influence personality development (Erikson, 1968). He declared that the ego not only mediates between the id's abrupt impulses and the superego's moral demands but that it can positively affect a person's development as more skills and experience are gained. Unlike Freud, Erikson believed that personality development continues to evolve throughout the life span. Whereas Freud attempted to explain reasons for pathology, Erikson searched for foundations of healthy personality development.

Erikson's Major Concepts and Terms

Erikson is best known for identifying eight stages of the life span through which a person may sequentially develop (Table 7-2) (Fig. 7-1). In his 1963 and 1968 works, Erikson proposed that each stage (or achievement level) has a central

TABLE 7-2 Erik Erikson's Stages of Psychosocial Development

Developmental Level	Central Task	Focal Relationships/Issues	Negative Resolution	Positive Resolution (Basic Virtues)
Infant	Basic trust vs. basic mistrust	Mother, primary caregivers, feeding, *"feeling and being comforted,"* sleeping, teething, *"taking in,"* trusting self, others, and environment	Suspicious, fearful	Drive and hope
Toddler	Autonomy vs. shame and doubt	Parents primary caregivers, toilet training, bodily functions, experimenting with *"holding on and letting go,"* having control without loss of self-esteem	Doubts abilities, feels ashamed for not trying	Self-confidence and willpower
Preschooler	Initiative vs. guilt	Family, play, exploring and discovering, learning how much assertiveness influences others and the environment, developing a sense of moral responsibility	May fear disapproval of own powers	Direction and purpose
School-aged child	Industry vs. inferiority	School, teachers, friends, experiencing physical independence from parents, neighborhood, wishing to accomplish, learning to create and produce, accepting when to stop working on a project, learning to complete a project, learning to cooperate, developing an attitude toward work	May feel sense of failure	Method and competence
Adolescent	Identity vs. role confusion	Peers and groups, experiencing emotional independence from parents, seeking to be the same as others yet unique, planning to actualize abilities and goals, fusing several identities into one	Confused, nonfocused	Devotion and fidelity
Young adult	Intimacy vs. isolation	Friends, lovers, spouses, community, work connections (networking), committing to work relationships, committing to social relationships, committing to intimate relationships	Loneliness, poor relationships	Affiliation and love
Middle-aged adult	Generativity vs. stagnation	Younger generation—often children (whether one's own or those of others), family, community, mentoring others, helping to care for others, discovering new abilities/talents, continuing to create, *"giving back"*	Shallow involvement with the world in general, selfish, little psychosocial growth	Production and care
Older adult	Ego integrity vs. despair[a]	All mankind, reviewing one's life, acceptance of self-uniqueness, acceptance of worth of others, acceptance of death as an entity	Regret, discontent, pessimism	Renunciation and wisdom

[a]Based on his experiences/research and as he continued to live longer, Erikson contemplated extending this phase of generativity and suggested that a ninth stage might be added to his theory. He posited that those who positively resolved generativity could move to a higher level that addressed a *"premonition of immortality"* (i.e., a new sense of self that transcends universe and time).

Information from Erikson, E. H. (1963). *Childhood and society* (2nd ed.). New York: W. W. Norton & Company, Inc.; Erikson, E. H. (1968). *Identity: Youth and crisis*, New York: W. W. Norton & Company, Inc.; Erikson, E. H., Erikson, J. M., & Kivnick, H. Q. (1986). *Vital involvement in old age*. New York: W.W. Norton & Company, Inc.; Erikson, E. H. (1991). Erikson's stages of personality development. In E. H. Erikson. *Children and society*. New York: W. W. Norton & Company, Inc.; and Schuster, C. S., & Ashburn, S. S. (1992). *The process of human development: A holistic approach* (3rd ed.). Philadelphia, PA: J. B. Lippincott Company.

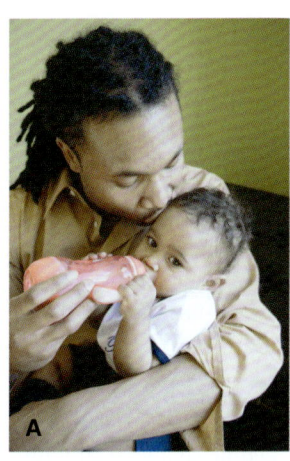
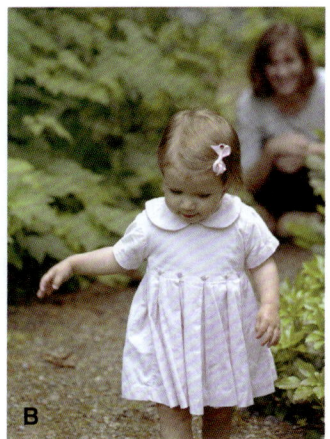
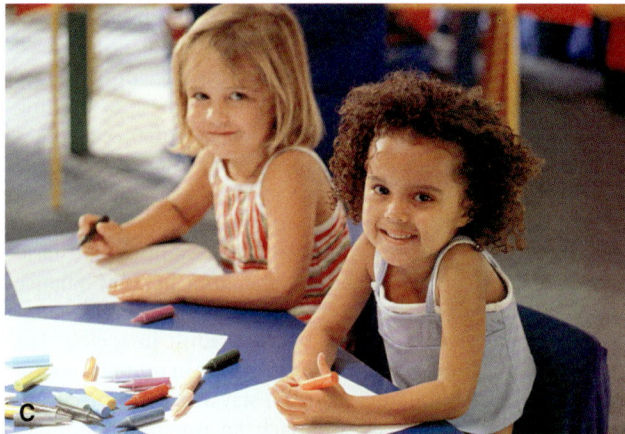
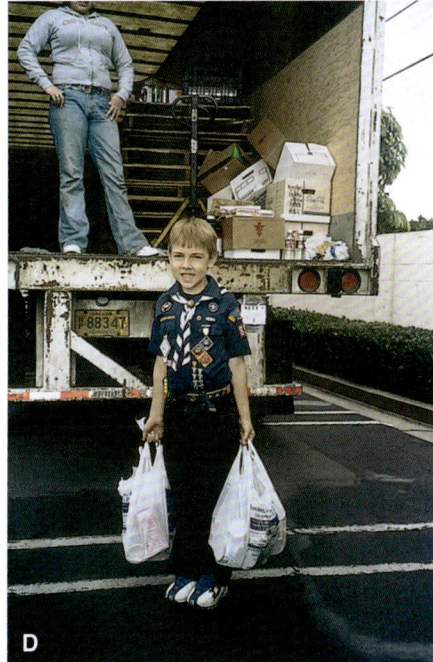
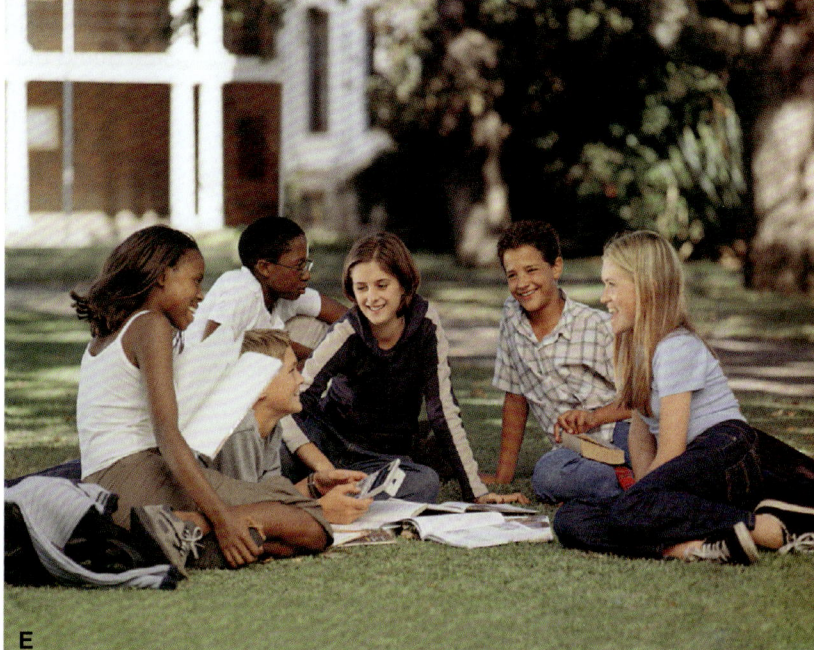
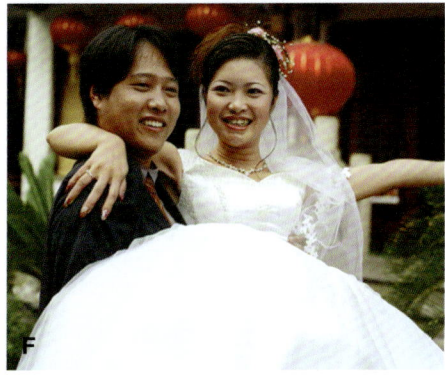
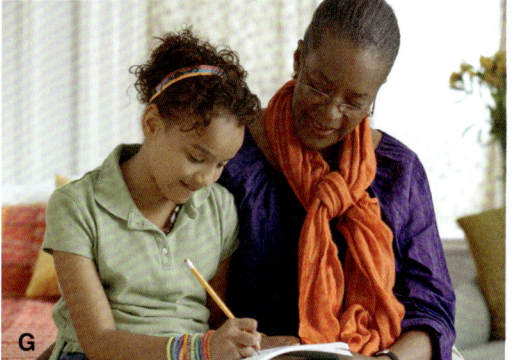
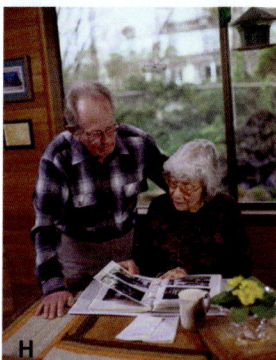

FIGURE 7-1 Erikson's psychosocial model involves eight life stages. **A.** Infants gain trust. **B.** Toddlers develop autonomy. **C.** Preschoolers learn initiative. **D.** School-aged children develop industry. **E.** Adolescents achieve identify. **F.** Young adults achieve intimacy. **G.** Middle-aged adults attain generativity. **H.** Older adults achieve ego identity.

developmental task corresponding to both biophysical maturity and societal expectations. He called these tasks *crises*, dilemmas that are composed of opposing viewpoints (e.g., *basic trust versus basic mistrust*). He viewed these as turning points wherein increased vulnerability and enhanced potential are presented to a person during each stage. Over time, if a person resolves the challenge in favor of the more positive of the two viewpoints (e.g., *basic trust*), then that person has achieved positive resolution of the developmental task. Simultaneously, a person must negotiate a healthy balance between the two concepts in order to move to the next stage and eventually become a well-adjusted adult in society. For example, a person needs some *basic mistrust* in numerous situations throughout the life span (e.g., stay a safe distance from blazing flames, cautiously approach an unfamiliar animal, first look through the peephole before answering the door, ensure that a written contract accompanies a formal agreement). Positive resolution for a crisis in one stage is necessary for positive resolution in the next stage. In addition, Erikson proposed *basic virtues* (vital strengths) that emerge with the positive resolution of each crisis. These outcomes are animating life forces that need to be reaffirmed continuously throughout one's life span (Table 7-2).

If a task is only partially resolved, then a person will experience difficulty in subsequent developmental tasks. Erikson affirmed that such a person must readdress and remediate unmet issues in order to realize psychosocial potential. Some people regress to a previous stage when under stress. However, Erikson believed that the ability to reclaim lost stages is possible.

Erikson's Stages of Psychosocial Development

Erikson did not strictly define chronological boundaries for his stages. He did assign selected developmental levels throughout the life span (Table 7-2), termed *critical periods*, as times when a person possesses criteria to attempt a given developmental task (Erikson, 1963). Each person develops at his or her own rate in accordance with individual potential and experience.

Erikson used several techniques to form his theory, including therapy analysis of people with emotional disturbances as well as observations of people who were assessed to have healthy psychosocial development. He performed anthropological studies of Native Americans and psychohistorical analyses of figures who have profoundly influenced mankind (e.g., Mahatma Gandhi, Adolf Hitler, Maxim Gorky, Martin Luther, and World War II veterans).

Piaget Theory of Cognitive Development

Dr. Jean Piaget (1970) described himself as a genetic epistemologist (one who studies the origins of knowledge). His theory is a description and an explanation of the growth and development of intellectual structures. He focused on *how* a person learns, not *what* the person learns.

Cognition is the process of obtaining understanding about one's world (Schuster & Ashburn, 1992). Piaget acknowledged that interrelationships of physical maturity, social interaction, environmental stimulation, and experience in general were necessary for cognition to occur (Piaget & Inhelder, 1969). His primary focus, however, was the biology of thinking.

Piaget's Major Concepts and Terms

Piaget believed that individual cognitive development occurs as the result of one's organization and adaptation to the perceived environment. To explain his theory, he applied the concepts of *schema* (plural: *schemata*), *assimilation*, *accommodation*, and *equilibration* (equilibrium). A schema is a unit of thought and a classification for a phenomenon, behavior, or event. A schema may consist of a thought, emotional memory, movement of a part of the body, or a sensory experience (such as making use of sight, hearing, taste, smell, or touch). Schemata can be categorized using either *assimilation* or *accommodation*.

Assimilation is an adaptive process whereby a stimulus or information is incorporated into an already existing schema. Another way of saying this is that people change reality into what they already know. Thus, a young child who has only been exposed to a pet cat ("Kitty") sees a dog for the first time and thinks that the new animal is called "Kitty." Accommodation is the creation of a new schema or the modification of an old one to differentiate more accurately a stimulus or a behavior from an existing schema. One changes the self to fit reality. The same young child may meet several other cats and modify "Kitty" to "cat" and eventually, with experience and guidance, meet more dogs and create the idea of "dog." Equilibration is the balance between assimilation and accommodation. When disequilibrium occurs, it provides motivation for the individual to assimilate or accommodate further.

A person who only assimilated stimuli would not be able to detect differences; a person who only accommodated stimuli would not be able to detect similarities. Piaget emphasized that schemata, assimilation, accommodation, and equilibration are all essential for cognitive growth and development.

Piaget's Stages of Cognitive Development

Piaget (1970) postulated that a person may progress through four major stages of intellectual development. He theorized that intellectual development begins the moment a baby is born. He did not believe that absolute ages should be attached to these stages, since individuals progress at their own rate. At each new stage, previous stages of thinking are incorporated and integrated. Piaget acknowledged that a person may, at times, display intellectual behaviors suggestive of more than one developmental level. If a person attains formal operational thinking (Table 7-3), he declared that qualitative changes in thinking cease and quantitative changes in the content and function of thinking may continue.

Kohlberg Theory of Moral Development

Lawrence Kohlberg, a psychologist, expanded Piaget's thoughts on morality; in doing so, he developed a comprehensive theory of moral development. Traditionally, Kohlberg (1981) proposed, individual morality has been viewed as a dynamic process that extends over one's lifetime, primarily involving the affective and cognitive domains in determining what is "right" and "wrong." It has also been frequently associated with those requirements necessary for people to live together and coexist in a group. Dr. Kohlberg was most concerned with examining the *reasoning* a person used to

TABLE 7-3   Jean Piaget's Stages of Cognitive Development

Stage	Approximate Age	Significant Characteristics
Sensorimotor	0–2 years	Thoughts are demonstrated by physical manipulation of objects/stimuli.
Substage 1: Making use of ready-made reflexes (pure *assimilation*)	0–1 month	Pure reflex adaptation (e.g., if lips are touched, baby sucks; if object placed in palm, baby grasps).
Substage 2: Primary circular reactions (*assimilation, accommodation,* and *equilibrium* are now used as individual grows and develops)	1–4 months	Actions centered on infant's body, and endlessly repeated reflex activities become modified and coordinated with each other with experience. Infant repeats behaviors for sensual pleasure (e.g., kicks repetitively, plays with own hands and fingers, sucking for a long time). Early coordination of selected reflexes (e.g., sucking and swallowing) and schema (e.g., hearing and looking at same object).
Substage 3: Secondary circular reactionary	4–8 months	Center of interest is not on own body's action but the environmental consequences of those actions. Behavior becomes *intentional.* Baby repeats behaviors that produce *novel* (i.e., pleasing, interesting) effects on environment (e.g., crying to get caregiver's attention). Increased voluntary coordination of motor skills enabling exploration (e.g., mouthing objects by combining grasping and sucking). Appearance of *cognitive object constancy*—awareness that an object or person is the same regardless of the angle from which it is viewed (e.g., baby will anticipate eating when he sees bottle of formula even if it is upside down and across the room).
Substage 4: Coordination of secondary circular reactions in new situations	8–12 months	Infant consciously uses an action that is a means to an end and solves simple problems (e.g., will reach for a toy and then will use that toy to retrieve another toy originally out of reach). *Object permanence* appears at approximately 8 months. This is the awareness that an object continues to exist even though one is not in direct contact with that object (e.g., when infant sees someone hide a favorite toy under a blanket, he will attempt to retrieve it from under the blanket). Imitates simple behaviors of others.
Substage 5: Tertiary circular reactions	12–18 months	Child now "experiments" (much trial and error) in order to discover new properties of objects and events. Varies approaches to an old situation or applies old approaches to a new problem. Must physically solve a problem to understand cause–effect relationship. Imitates simple novel behaviors.
Substage 6: Invention of new means through mental combinations	18–24 months	Invention of new means can occur without actual physical experimentation. Occasional new means through physical experimentation—still much trial-and-error problem solving. Child begins to *mentally represent* object/events before physically acting (e.g., can solve "detour" problems to go one small distance to another). Engages in early symbolic play. Both immediate and deferred imitation of actions and words noted.
Preoperational Divided into two substages: preconceptual (2–4 years) and intuitive (4–7 years). During the preconceptual substage, the child inconsistently assigns any word to several similar stimuli (e.g., child calls all four-legged mammals by his pet cat's name.) During the intuitive stage, the child begins to realize the ability of a word to truly represent a specific object, event, or action.	2–7 years	Increasing ability to make a mental representation for something not immediately present using language as a major tool. Eventually, the child is able to give reasons for beliefs and rationales for action; however, they remain biased and immature. Magical thought (wishing something will make it so) predominates. The following characteristics (although they go through modification as the child develops from 2 to 7 years of age) serve as some obstacles to "adult logic": • *Fundamental egocentrism*—never thinks that anything is other than the way the child perceives it (e.g., "If I'm going to bed now, every child is going to bed now"). • *Centration*—tends to focus on one aspect of an object or experience (e.g., when asked to compare two rows of like objects, with one row containing six pennies and the other a longer row containing three pennies spaced further apart, would answer that the longer row is "more"). • *Limited transformation*—is not able to comprehend the steps of how an object is changed from one state to another (e.g., could not explain the sequence of events that occurs when an ice cube melts and turns into a puddle of water). • *Action rather than abstraction*—perceives an event as if actually participating in the event again (e.g., when asked about riding in toy car, may imitate turning the steering wheel when child thinks about it). • *Irreversibility*—unable to follow a line of reasoning back to its beginning (e.g., if child is taken on a walk, especially one with a turn, child is unable to retrace steps and return to the original point). • *Transductive reasoning*—thinks specific to specific; if two things are alike in one aspect, child thinks they are alike in all aspects (e.g., child thinks beetle seen on a picnic in the park is the same beetle seen in child's backyard). • *Animism*—believes that inert objects are alive with feelings and can think and function with intent (e.g., child thinks that if vacuum cleaner "eats" the dirt, then it can "eat" him).

Continued on following page

TABLE 7-3	Jean Piaget's Stages of Cognitive Development (Continued)	
Stage	Approximate Age	Significant Characteristics
Concrete Operational	7–11 years	Begins to think and reason logically about objects in the environment. Can mentally perform actions that previously had to be carried out in actuality. Reasoning is limited to concrete objects and events ("what is") and not abstract objects and events ("what might be"). *Inductive* reasoning (specific to general) has begun. Can consider viewpoints of others. Understands and uses time on a clock. Understands days of week, months of year. Best understands years within life experience. Can de-center, understands transformations. Can reverse thoughts. Progressively able to *conserve* (understand that properties of substances will remain the same despite changes made in shape or physical arrangement) numbers, mass, weight, and volume in that order. Begins to understand relationship between distance and speed. Learns to add, subtract, multiply, and divide. Can organize then classify objects. Progressively capable of money management.
Formal Operational	11–15+ years	Develops ability to problem solve both real-world and theoretical situations. Can logically and flexibly think about the past, present, and future. Possesses ability to think about symbols that represent other symbols (e.g., $x = 1$, $y = 2$). Can think abstractly when presented with information in verbal (as opposed to written) form. Able to envision and systematically test many possible combinations in reaching a conclusion. Is able to generate multiple potential solutions while considering the possible positive/negative effects of each solution. Can perform *deductive* reasoning (general to specific). Can hypothesize ("If…then" thinking). Can think about thinking (metacognition).

Information from Piaget, J. (1952). *The origins of intelligence in children* (M. Cook, Trans.). New York: International Universities Press; Piaget, J. (1969). *The language and thought as the child* (M. Gabain, Trans.). New York: Meridian Books; Piaget, J., & Inhelder, B. (1969). *The psychology of the child* (H. Weaver, Trans.). New York: Basic Books, Inc.; Piaget, J. (1981). *The psychology of intelligence* (M. Piercy & D. E. Beryne, Trans.). Totowa, NJ: Littlefield, Adams; Piaget, J. (1982). *Play, dreams and imitation in childhood* (C. Gattengo & F. M. Hodgson, Trans.). New York: Norton; and Schuster, C. S., & Ashburn, S. S. (1992). *The process of human development: A holistic life-span approach* (3rd ed.). Philadelphia, PA: J. B. Lippincott Company.

make a decision, as opposed to the *action* that resulted after that decision was made.

Kohlberg's Major Concepts and Terms

Kohlberg recognized that moral development is influenced by cognitive structures. However, he did not view moral development as parallel to cognitive development. In his later years, he discussed how some components of his theory contained elements of affective or reflective characteristics of people and proclaimed these to be *soft* stages. Those stages that contained only the Piagetian structures were differentiated as *hard* stages (Levine et al., 1985).

Kohlberg viewed *justice* (or fairness) as the goal of moral judgment. He often coauthored, publishing new thoughts regarding the form and content of his theory. This included the addition of several substages to his existing proposed stages of moral development.

Kohlberg's Stages of Moral Development

Kohlberg (Colby et al., 1983) proposed three levels of moral development, best recognized as encompassing six stages (Table 7-4). He believed that few people progress past the second level. Asserting that moral development extends beyond adolescence, he saw moral decisions and reasoning as becoming increasingly differentiated, integrated, and universalized (i.e., independent of culture) at each successive stage of development.

Kohlberg assumed that a person must enter the moral stage hierarchy in an ordered and irreversible sequence. No guarantee was made that a person enters a stage based on biologic age. He further concluded that a person may never attain a higher stage of moral development and thus not ascend this proposed hierarchy of stages. He believed that the process was partially determined by how much a person is challenged with decisions of a higher order.

Kohlberg did not theorize that infants and young toddlers were capable of moral reasoning. He viewed them as being naïve and egocentric.

HEALTH ASSESSMENT

Collecting Subjective Data: The Nursing Health History

Each person can be studied and assessed as a composition of developmental domains (e.g., psychosexual, psychosocial, cognitive, moral) and data collected from more than one type of history (biographical, present health concerns, personal health, family, and lifestyle and health practices). Subjective and objective data are interdependent in defining the needs of the individual person. The following suggested questions could be asked of any adult (young adult, middle-aged adult, or older adult).

TABLE 7-4 Lawrence Kohlberg's Stages of Moral Development[a]

Level	Stage	Average Age	Characteristic Moral Reasoning That May Influence Behavior
Preconventional (premoral)	1. Orientation to punishment and obedience	Preschool through early school age	Finding it difficult to consider two points of view in a moral dilemma, individual ignores—or is unaware of—meaning, value, or intentions of others and instead focuses on fear of authority. Will avoid punishment by obeying caregiver/supervisor commands. The physical consequences of individual actions determine "right" or "wrong." Punishment means action was "wrong."
	2. Orientation to instrumental relativism (individual purpose)	Late preschool through late school age	Slowly becoming aware that people can have different perspectives in a moral dilemma. Individual views "right" action as what satisfies personal needs and believes others act out of self-interest. No true feelings of loyalty, justice, or gratitude. Individual conforms to rules out of self-interest or in relation to what others can do in return. Desires reward for "right" action.
Conventional (maintaining external expectations of others)	3. Orientation to interpersonal concordance (unity and mutuality)	School age through adulthood	Attempting to adhere to perceived norms; desires to maintain approval and affection of friends, relatives, and significant others. Wants to avoid disapproval and be considered a "good person" who is trustworthy, loyal, respectful, and helpful. Capable of viewing a two-person relationship as an impartial observer (beginning to judge the intentions of others—may or may not be correct in doing so).
	4. Orientation to maintenance of social order ("law and order")	Adolescence through adulthood	Attempting to make decisions and behave by strictly conforming to fixed rules and the written law—whether these are of a certain group, family, community, or the nation. "Right" consists of "doing one's duty."
Postconventional (maintaining internal principles of self—Piaget concept of formal operations must be employed at this level)	5. Orientation to social contract legalism	Middlescence through older adulthood (only 10-20% of the dominant American *culture* attain this stage)	Regarding rules and laws as changeable with due process. "Right" is respecting individual rights while emphasizing the needs of the majority. Outside of legal realm, will honor an obligation to another individual or group, even if the action is not necessarily viewed as the correct thing to do by friends, relatives, or numerous others.
	6. Orientation to universal ethical principle	Middlescence through older adulthood (few people either attain or maintain this stage)	Making decisions and behaving based on internalized rules, on conscience instead of social law, and on self-chosen ethical principles that are consistent, comprehensive, and universal. Believes in absolute justice, human equality, reciprocity, and respect for the dignity of every individual person. Is willing to act alone and be punished (or actually die) for belief. Such behavior may be seen in times of crisis.

[a]Shortly before his death, Kohlberg added a seventh stage of moral reasoning: Orientation to self-transcendence and faith. Kohlberg proposed that this stage moved beyond the concept of justice—the goal was to achieve a sense of unity with the cosmos, nature, or God. The person attaining this stage views everyone and everything as being connected; thus, any action of a person affects everyone and everything with any consequences of that person's action ultimately returning to him. According to Garsee and Schuster (1992), the person in stage six may be willing to *die* for his principles whereas the person in stage seven is willing to *live* for his beliefs.

Information from Colby, A., Kolberg, L., Gibbs, J., et al. (1983). A longitudinal study of moral behavior. *Monographs of the Society of Research in Child Development*, 48(1-2), 1-124; Garsee, J. W., & Schuster, C. S. (1992). Moral development. In C. S. Schuster & S. S. Ashburn (Eds.). *The process of human development: A holistic approach*. Philadelphia, PA: J. B. Lippincott Company; Kohlberg, L. (1984). *Essays on moral development*. Vol. 2. San Francisco, CA: Harper & Row; Kohlberg, L. (1981). *The philosophy of moral development*. San Francisco, CA: Harper & Row; Kohlberg, L., & Ryncarz, R. (1990). Beyond justice reasoning: Moral development and consideration of a seventh stage. In C. Alexander & E. Langer (Eds.). *Higher stages of human development* (pp. 191-207). New York: Oxford University Press; Levine, C., Kohlberg, L., & Hewer, A. (1985). The current formulation of Kohlberg's theory and a response to critics. *Human Development*, 28(2), 94-100; and Schuster, C. S., & Ashburn, S. S. (1992). *The process of human development: A holistic life-span approach* (3rd ed.). Philadelphia, PA: J. B. Lippincott Company.

Biographical Data

QUESTION	RATIONALE
How old are you?	It is not always easy to assess a person's age. How a person answers this question assesses sense of hearing, ability to communicate, and level of cognition. Knowing a person's age provides a beginning point for developmental assessment. Although helpful in establishing a baseline for information, biologic age (level of physical growth and development related to physical health and capacity of vital organs) and chronologic age (time since birth) are not indicative of psychosexual, psychosocial, cognitive, or moral development.
Where were you born? How long have you been in this country?	Culture guides what is acceptable behavior for people in a specific group. It influences a person's self-concept and expectations. Cultural influences are largely unconscious (Purnell, 2013).
Tell me about your birthplace and the other places you have lived.	The geographical area(s) in which a person is raised and has lived may influence how the person lives now and can affect values, beliefs, and patterns of behavior.
With what cultural group(s) do you most identify? What is your primary language? When do you speak it? Are you fluent in other languages?	The person who recognizes and respects cultural diversity will be better prepared to provide cultural sensitivity. Language is initially promulgated via culture. Piaget postulated that cultural factors contribute significantly to differences in cognitive development. Freud (1935) and Erikson (1950) acknowledged differences of behavior caused by cultural conditions. Kohlberg (Kohlberg & Gilligan, 1971) noted that cultures teach different beliefs, but that the stage sequence is universal and not affected by cultural difference.
What is your highest level of formal education?	Piaget stated that learning takes place as a result of interaction with the environment and included schooling as an influential variable. He also stated that individual differences in cognitive processes among adults are influenced more by aptitude and experiences such as career and education. Erikson viewed experience with others as a source of knowledge and upheld that the school environment offers an opportunity for psychosocial and cognitive growth. He viewed psychosocial development as dependent on interaction with others, which occurs in classrooms as well as transactions via electronic devices. Kohlberg focused on a person's general development and experience, viewing formal education as one of many factors that significantly affect one's cognitive, psychosocial, and moral growth. He maintained that education can stimulate moral reasoning.
Discuss your history of employment. (If a person states that he or she is retired, inquire from what occupation[s].) How do you presently make a living and maintain your everyday needs?	One's sense of identity, ability to problem-solve, and level of morality may be reflected in choices and patterns of employment. For many retired from formal employment, former career and work are interwoven into sense of identity.

History of Present Health Concerns

QUESTION	RATIONALE
Describe how you are feeling right now. What concerns do you have about your health? Describe any changes you have recently experienced in your health.	Freud assumed that the tensions felt by a person are caused by the needs of the instincts of the id. Piaget discussed how physical structures set broad limits on intellectual functioning. Erikson recognized that biophysical and cognitive processes determine a person's state of being. Kohlberg discussed how a person's feelings, problem-solving abilities, and general outlook on life are affected by one's moral development.
Discuss any concerns you have about your body weight.	Freud proclaimed that people who overeat are orally fixated and that those who deny themselves food are using oral zone control. Erikson discussed how body image contributes to one's sense of identity.
What major stressors are you currently experiencing? How do you cope with stress? When you are having a problem, how do you usually handle it? Does this work? To whom do you turn when you are having a conflict/crisis?	Stress can have physical, emotional, social, cognitive, and/or spiritual consequences for a person. Different types of stresses may occur in different age groups (refer to Normal and Abnormal Findings following Assessment Procedure in the next section). Each person uniquely perceives stress (Selye, 1976).

QUESTION	RATIONALE
Do you have any trouble making decisions? Please give me some examples of recent decisions you have had to make.	Problem-solving skills can increase steadily, often peaking during the middle-age years. As people age, they adopt more simple, judgmental strategies and use preexisting knowledge and experience more than younger adults. Cognitively healthy adults are able to employ Piaget's *formal operations* as well as any of their preceding stages as necessary (some problems do not require abstract reasoning).
Tell me about life changes you have had to make and/or anticipate having to make. How will you make these changes?	A person's choices are affected by several factors: aptitude, intellect, knowledge base, motivation, self-discipline, values, moral development, psychosocial maturity, previous experiences, and available opportunities. Freud suggested that the mature adult must balance two critical themes to find success and happiness: love and work.

Personal Health History

QUESTION	RATIONALE
How would you describe yourself to others? What are your strengths? Weaknesses?	Self-concept (self-image) is important to health and well-being throughout the life span. One's self-concept can facilitate or impede personal growth. Young and middle-aged adulthood issues that affect self-concept include emphasis on fitness, energy, sexuality, and style. Erikson emphasized young adulthood as the time for a person to gain knowledge and acceptance of one's self in order to feel free to know and be known by others. He pronounced productivity, accountability, and commitment to cultivating future generations as goals for middle-aged adults. Eriksonian tasks for older adults embrace realistically reviewing and viewing life, recognizing errors and poor choices, learning from past experiences what strengths one has, acknowledging accomplishments, and developing new wisdom. Freud extolled the importance of adults meeting the role expectations of maturity in order to avoid neuroses. Piaget described the use of formal operations as helpful in anticipating and negotiating the decline in physical and possibly cognitive abilities. Older adults suffer multiple losses and must problem-solve concerning possible increased dependency, decreased choices, and impending death. Death is seen by the formal operational thinker as universal, inevitable, and irreversible. Kohlberg professed that those who have attained his sixth stage of *personal principles* make use of self-evaluation, self-motivation, and self-regulation, meeting expectations of his ego ideal. He believed that the person operating at the *universal principle* stage is aware of his "reason for existence" (Levine et al., 1985, pp. 94–100).
How do you learn best?	Erikson discussed the importance of the "quality of the maternal relationship" as fundamental to the progress through developmental tasks (Erikson, 1963, p. 249). Piaget stated that the infant begins to form organized patterns of activity that are basic to the development of more complex cognitive functioning later (Phillips, 1975, p. 27). Kohlberg did not recognize the period of infancy as a foundation for moral development.
	Each person learns differently. Teaching must relate to the individual person's learning style.
	Adult learners are most interested in learning material that they deem relevant and can be immediately used. Erikson discussed the concept of trust as being a critical element in the teaching process. Piaget maintained that individual differences in education, experience, aptitude, motivation, talents, and interests become significant in shaping the direction of *formal operational thought*. He asserted that any cognitive advancement beyond the acquisition of this form of thinking was quantitative rather than qualitative. Kohlberg believed that a person continues to learn about self and others because identity development can be dynamic and continue throughout the life span (Kohlberg & Ryncarz, 1990).
Have you ever been treated (or are currently being treated) for a psychological or psychiatric problem? If so, please explain whether this treatment helped you deal with (or is currently helping you deal with) problems.	It is important to assess the person's ability to see himself or herself as others do and to fit into the norm for the culture in which he or she lives. Such information may give clues to the person's perception of stressors, use of defense mechanisms, and methods of problem solving.
Are you taking any prescribed medications, herbs, or supplements? Are you currently receiving any medical treatment or therapy?	Any chemical that enters the human body can affect biophysical, psychosexual, psychosocial, or cognitive functioning/development. One's moral development could influence choices regarding adherence to a prescription or prescribed medical treatment or therapy, or taking over-the-counter medications/herbs.

Continued on following page

Personal Health History (Continued)

QUESTION	RATIONALE
Describe any changes you have recently experienced concerning your weight, eating, elimination patterns, and sleep. Please tell me about any allergies or sensitivities you have.	Behavior is an integrated function of all subsystems of the human system. Kohlberg asserted that a person's willingness or ability to stop unhealthy behavior and change life patterns to facilitate a higher level of wellness may be influenced by his or her moral stage of development. Kohlberg also believed that continued practices that negatively affect the self or others might be associated with a *preconventional level* of moral development (such a person may need to perceive positive attention from others to try new behaviors).
Do you have any chronic illnesses (conditions you take medication for every day)? Has your life changed since you were diagnosed (if so, how)?	Chronic illness can affect all domains of a person. Freud discussed the uses of *repression* and *regression* as characteristics/symptoms of neuroses (Freud, 1935). To expand Freud theory, Erikson discussed how the ego "safeguards itself" (Erikson, 1963, p. 193) by using defense mechanisms—healthy as well as unhealthy ones—when coping with stress. Chronic illnesses are stressors.

Family History

QUESTION	RATIONALE
Whom do you consider to be your family?	A family is two or more people who are emotionally connected (Purnell, 2013). Families provide continuity of past, present, and future. A family can share values, beliefs, goals, and identity.
Describe your life growing up as a child.	People's perceptions of their early childhood experiences may affect their adult behavior and attainment of developmental levels in all domains.
Do you have brothers? Sisters? Tell me about them and the relationships you have with them.	Sibling rivalry is often present among brothers and sisters. Freud explained that a child in his earliest years first loves himself only (perceiving various degrees of *hatred* toward brothers/sisters) and may begin to love them later (Freud, 1935). He went on to discuss that brothers/sisters could later be viewed as *love object*s by the same child (Freud, 1935). Erikson discussed *anticipatory rivalry* (Erikson, 1963) against older siblings as well as jealousy directed against *encroachment* by younger brother/sisters. Piaget saw the development of language as a gradual transition from egocentric speech to socialized intercommunication speech, which would involve others, including brothers/sisters. During the adult years, many siblings who had earlier disagreements come to value each other as companions and/or persons of shared heritage. Much has been researched about the effect of birth order on personality development.
Are you aware of any genetic predisposition or characteristic trait or disorder that you inherited?	A person may have inherited a genetic disorder from one parent or both. Freud stated that all of the varying forms of human mental health are to be viewed as an interplay between inherited dispositions and experience (Freud, 1949). Both Erikson and Piaget spoke to the *epigenetic principle* (Erikson, 1968, p. 91; Ginsburg & Opper, 1969, p. 209), which states that anything that grows has a "ground plan," and that from this plan each part arises having its time of special ascendancy, until all parts have arisen to form a functioning whole.

Lifestyle and Health Practices

Because of the unique assessment topic of this chapter, questions related to the client's lifestyle and health practices are addressed in the *Assessing Developmental Level: Psychosexual, Psychosocial, Cognitive, and Moral Development* section on pages 109–117.

CASE STUDY

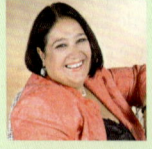

Recall the case study introduced at the beginning of this chapter.

One week following Mrs. Como-Williams's annual physical checkup with her primary physician, the nurse practitioner at the Women's Wellness Center interviews her using specific open-ended questions/comments.

The nurse begins by asking Mrs. Como-Williams why she came for this special appointment. "Oh, please," Mrs. Como-Williams responds with a smile, "just call me Connie. I've been doing a lot of thinking since my check-up last week. I weighed 210 pounds last week and, according to your scales, I'm now 212! It's time I lost weight and kept it off. I was also told that my cholesterol and triglycerides levels are high. This information scares me." Mrs. Como-Williams continues, "It started with my first marriage. I weighed 130 pounds, but quickly gained 10 pounds the first year of marriage. Then I never lost all of the 50 pounds I put on the next year with the birth of my daughter, Monica. I don't think I was less than 180 pounds after that. I haven't stepped on the scale since then, unless I was at the doctor's office."

When asked for the primary reason why she now wishes to lose weight, Mrs. Como-Williams states that she wants "to be healthier" and to "feel less tired." She adds, "I know I could look better . . . for my husband and family ... for my job ... for myself." She explains that she was busy from 8 AM to 5 PM weekdays teaching second graders ("There are twenty-nine of them in the classroom most of the time and so many have family issues"). She shares that she had remarried last year, after being divorced for 5 years. She goes on to say that her second husband also teaches school full time and adds that when they both return from work in the evening, they take care of their 4-year-old granddaughter, Christine: "My daughter Monica dropped out of school, gave birth to Christine, never married, and is currently taking classes to further her education. Monica and Christine live with us. Monica is also working part-time as a waitress. Jeff [husband] picks up Christine from preschool on his way home from work. Monica gets home around 7 PM and we all eat together. Then she plays with Christine and gets her ready for bed. Monica usually studies in the evening after helping me clean up in the kitchen." During the interview, Mrs. Como-Williams reveals that she is afraid her husband will think her unattractive and repulsive due to her being overweight. She realizes that this belief has affected her ability to respond sexually to her husband. She says that she thought at first their infrequent intimacy was related to how tired they are from hard work and family responsibilities but has come to realize that her self-esteem is low because of her fear that her husband will reject her. She says that they are intimate about once a month.

When asked more about her usual daily routine, Mrs. Como-Williams replies, "On weekdays, I'm up at 5:30 in the morning to prepare breakfast for the family. Jeff usually makes the coffee. Monica gets up soon after and gets herself ready for school and Christine ready for preschool." Mrs. Como-Williams pauses and then adds, "I do my best to have a bowel movement during this time but it tends to happen more like every other day. You'd think that as much as I eat, it would be more often. I often feel bloated. Also, the bowel movements I do have tend to be hard and difficult to pass." She continues, "Then Jeff and I are off to work—we drive separately to our respective schools. Monica drives Christine to preschool and then heads to her own classes at the college. I'm at work all day and stay about an hour and a half after the children leave to perform more teaching duties."

The nurse asks Mrs. Como-Williams about her eating habits. She said, "I'm not very good about providing myself or my family with the healthiest foods. I tend to go for what's easiest and most convenient. I know better." She added, "Breakfast is scrambled eggs, microwave bacon strips, toaster pastries, and waffles.... Christine is a picky eater and often eats the colored, sugary cereals. I nibble on everything as I fix it. At school, I tend to eat grilled sandwiches prepared in the cafeteria as well as at least one dessert. Someone is always bringing in cake or cookies to the teachers' lounge and I can't resist. I often end up buying fast food for dinner for all of us ... and I'm so hungry as I drive the half hour home that I eat extras I buy for myself. I know that's not healthy and I need to change. You see, I'm pretty tired after work and don't like to cook after teaching all day. No matter what we eat for dinner, I always have a glass of wine with it. Jeff drinks with dinner, too, but of course Monica and Christine don't. I may as well confess that I usually have a bowl of ice cream before I go to sleep. I like to read in bed and I find the later I stay up, the more I eat. I know that's got to stop. Plus, as it is, I end up only getting about 6 hours of sleep at night if I'm lucky. I get up once during the night to pee."

When asked about how frequently she urinates during the day, she states that she doesn't "have much time to go at work. ... I do go at lunchtime and just try to hold it until the children leave. That can be uncomfortable at times, but then I don't drink much except a soda at lunch. When asked about hormone replacement therapy, she replies, "No. I don't take any replacement hormones." She mentions her hysterectomy 2 years ago for endometriosis and fibroids. Describes hysterectomy as vaginal with tubes and ovaries removed. She reports occasional vaginal dryness but no dyspareunia. She then adds, "Anyway, there are several lifestyle changes that I must make ... and I'm ready to do so with your help."

After the nurse acknowledges Mrs. Como-Williams's last comment, she inquires as to when Mrs. Como-Williams began eating so many sweets and foods high in starch, fat, and salt. "I've always overeaten. Mom said she starting feeding me solid food as a baby much earlier than she did my two older sisters. She said my grandmother told her to feed me more if I cried. We're also Italian ... so ever since I can remember it's been big family gatherings to celebrate with lots of food ... always, among other things, pasta, sausage, cheese, bread and potatoes ... with each birthday, anniversary, holiday, wedding, baby shower, funeral ... you name it. And, of course, rich desserts such as spumoni and tiramisu. The adults always drink wine. I actually have a glass every evening no matter what we're eating for dinner." Mrs. Como-Williams pauses for a few seconds and then states, "You know, we have always been a very close, loving family. I talk to my sisters and mother probably every other day on the phone. Dad passed away a couple years ago ... he suffered a heart attack...." She pauses again and then states, "I never thought about it before. I really do equate food with love."

When asked by the nurse about family history, Mrs. Como-Williams reports that no one was "really overweight" but that her father had "high blood pressure and high cholesterol."

The nurse asks her to describe a typical weekend. "It seems as if there is always a family function for something. Between preparing for that and Monica and cleaning the house and doing the laundry and shopping ... I guess you could call that my form of exercise! Plus I'm standing up and walking around most of the day at work." In response to inquiry about coping with stress, she said that she does not smoke or abuse drugs and had "got away from going to church" but still prays. "I deal with stress more than anything by just eating."

Assessing Developmental Level: Psychosocial Status

Preparing the Client

As with the collection of subjective data in the nursing history, maintain a caring, helping, trusting relationship with the client while assessing his or her developmental level.

General Routine Screening Versus Focused Specialty Assessment

Assessment of a client's developmental level is a lengthy process that occurs over time as the nurse develops a working relationship with the client. During short-term acute care, it is impractical to explore all the questions and areas of a client's developmental level. As the nurse interacts with the client, issues or questions may arise in which the nurse has the prime opportunity to explore additional information to better understand the client. As the nurse gets to know the client more, more information may become available to better assess the client's developmental level. It obviously takes a period of time to get to know the client to obtain more personal data. The nurse uses professional judgment to determine the need and best time to ask various questions presented in this chapter. Nurses in all situations need to know how and when to assess the client's developmental level. There are no questions or assessments in this chapter that would be limited to specialty situations. The depth of the assessment is totally dependent on available time with the client and when clues are presented that require additional more in-depth assessment.

ASSESSMENT PROCEDURE	NORMAL FINDINGS	ABNORMAL FINDINGS
Assessment of Freud's Stages of Psychosexual Development		
Determine the client's psychosocial level by asking the following suggested questions. Does the **young adult**: • Still live with parent(s) at home? • Accept roles and responsibilities at place of residence? • Have experience of growing up in a single-parent home? • Have unresolved issues with parent(s)? • Have a satisfying sexual relationship with a significant other? • Have gainful employment?	Many young adults today still live with parent(s) to continue higher education, become established in a career, or decrease financial hardship (Parker, 2012). Others return home to recover from divorce, obtain support with their children, or regain financial stability. It is important that the young adult assume different roles than those performed during the earlier years of development. Freud emphasized the significance of first maternal and then later paternal influences on the person's ability to fulfill a socially acceptable gender role. Those born from 1965 on (Generation X, Millennials, and Generations Y and Z) are much more accepting of same-gender relationships (Pew Research Center, 2015). Freud declared that it was normal for young people to marry (Fig. 7-1A). Single-parent families were not common during the time of Freud. Many independent people today choose to remain single. Freud believed that healthy young adults should expend their genital energies in a heterosexual relationship and then marriage, followed by parenthood. He believed that reproduction within a heterosexual marriage was a socially acceptable reason to engage in sexual intercourse. His 19th-century values do not correlate with the well-adjusted person who is content with an "alternate life style," including homosexuality. In the 21st century, a healthy sexual relationship includes practicing "safe sex" to decrease the risk of experiencing the high level of anxiety often associated with having an unwanted pregnancy or contracting a sexually transmitted infection. The young adult is more likely to possess a sense of positive self-preservation if he or she can meet some financial expenses. Today's healthy young adult experiences mild anxiety while attempting to balance employment, continued formal education, and relationship/family responsibilities. Many more women are now performing these multiple roles (however, note that Freud affirmed that women should remain in the home as housekeepers, cooks, and primary caregivers).	If the young adult demonstrates extreme dependence on a parent (e.g., assumes no responsibility for household they share), Freud would state that the id, ego, and super ego are not fully developed and that this person's behavior would be influenced by the body organ that dominates his or her mode of interaction. This young adult might make poor relationship choices. According to Freud, this person would experience gender role confusion. The confused young adult often experiences more than mild anxiety (not being able to perceive all relevant aspects of a situation). The unhealthy young adult suffers from low self-esteem. Several defense mechanisms including projection (attributing one's unacceptable or anxiety-provoking feelings, thoughts, impulses, wishes, or characteristics to another person). As with all adults, hallucinations and delusions are unexpected findings. If the young adult does not possess a sense of healthy sexuality, social and emotional isolation may occur. This person has difficulty establishing healthy relationships with others. The young adult who is concerned about finances and does not have a career could experience depression and heightened anxiety. This person may have poor eating habits, have difficulty sleeping, or endure vivid dreams.

ASSESSMENT PROCEDURE	NORMAL FINDINGS	ABNORMAL FINDINGS
Does the **middle-aged adult**: • Demonstrate nervous mannerisms? • Frequently derive pleasure from selected activities? • Cope effectively with stress? • Have a satisfying sexual relationship? • Believe that physical changes of aging have affected any relationships?	The healthy middle-aged adult copes with stress in a socially acceptable manner. All people experience stress throughout the life cycle. Mild anxiety (remaining attentive and alert to relevant stimuli) is normal throughout adulthood and provides motivation. A variety of adaptive defense (coping) mechanisms may be used. Positive coping includes making use of previously successful actions to decrease stress. Healthy middle-aged adults may vent frustration to significant others, effectively communicating in relationships and seeking assistance when needed. Activities meet socially accepted norms. A balance of responsibilities and leisure activities is necessary. Each person experiences "midlife crisis" differently. Those who effectively prioritize issues as they arise create an adaptive midlife transition. Freud might contend that the person who is successfully motivated during this period of life uses repression (involuntary exclusion of anxiety-producing feelings, thoughts, and impulse from awareness) and/or sublimation (substitution of a socially acceptable behavior for an unacceptable sexual or aggressive drive or impulse). Many common stressors include facilitating adolescents to be more emotionally independent, providing assistance/care to aging parents, grieving the loss of a parent/grandparent, and maintaining career/social status occur during the middle-aged years. The healthy middle-aged person, according to Freud, has attained and maintained the genital stage, and he purported that a satisfying sexual relationship was fundamental to a successful marriage. Freud might label the decision to not engage in an extramarital affair as suppression (exclusion of something from consciousness). Freud emphasized the importance of "romance." Current research (Kazer, 2012; Mayo Clinic Staff, 2014) has shown that slowing of the sexual response cycle occurs with age. Healthy middle-aged adults begin to value the quality of their sexual relationship more than the quantity of sexual intercourse. Practicing "safe sex" reduces risks of complications, especially if engaging in an extramarital affair.	Nervous mannerisms could indicate an unhealthy psychosexual state in many stages of the life cycle. For example, Freud might interpret fixation at the oral stage if a person is engaged in at least one of the following behaviors: overreacting, excessive talking, smoking, thumb sucking, and nail biting. Likewise, he would attribute other socially unacceptable behaviors or negative habits as being fixated at one of his other stages (anal, phallic, latency, or genital). Freud discussed fetishes as a way the libido attaches to objects other than a socially acceptable love object. Freud would label the person who engages in an extramarital affair(s) as narcissistic. He would say the same of the person with a body image disturbance related to grieving the loss of a youthful physical appearance. Some unhealthy middle-aged adults refrain from social relationships/outings because they no longer look the same as they did when younger.
Does the **older adult**: • Engage in sexual activity? • Positively cope with loss? • Believe that any changes in cognition have occurred? • Believe that any significant changes have occurred in interests/relationships?	Many older adults enjoy sexual intimacy (Mayo Clinic Staff, 2014). Many older adults make effective use of communication and companionship to have a healthy sense of sexuality (Fig. 7-2). Freud might interpret alternative ways of satisfying sexual needs as compensation (overachievement in one area to offset deficiencies real or imagined, or to overcome failure or frustration in another area).	The unhealthy older adult may avoid relationships and mainstream society in general. Chronic depression is not normal in older adulthood. Freud often interpreted the misplacing of objects as intentional. Current research on effects of stress and

Continued on following page

ASSESSMENT PROCEDURE	NORMAL FINDINGS	ABNORMAL FINDINGS

Assessment of Freud's Stages of Psychosexual Development (Continued)

| | It is not uncommon to occasionally forget (e.g., lose keys, misplace a pen or glasses, not recall a person's name). The older adult makes effective use of previous experiences, self, and others to grieve loss. Experiencing more than one loss does not make a subsequent loss less painful. | symptoms of dementia has not supported this belief (National Institute on Aging, 2015; UCSF Medical Center, 2015). |

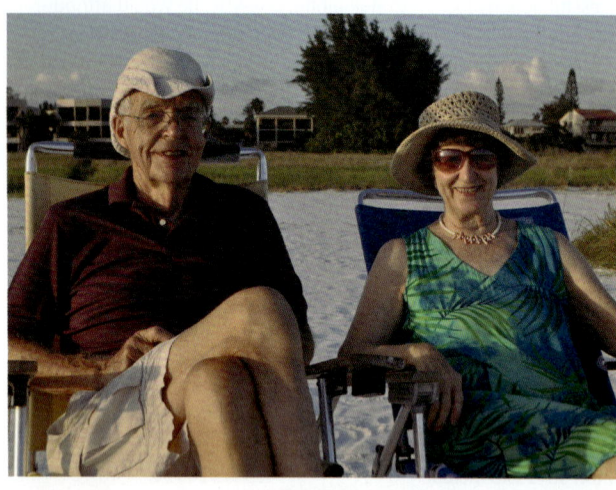

FIGURE 7-2 Stereotypical images of the older adult as narrow-minded, forgetful, sexless, and dependent are untrue for most of the older-adult population. This older couple exhibits the vitality, joy, and spontaneity of a young couple.

Assessment of Erikson's Psychosocial Development

Determine the client's psychosocial developmental level by answering the following questions. If you do not have enough data to answer these questions, you may need to ask the client additional questions or make further observations.

🎯 **CLINICAL TIP**
Erikson's psychosocial developmental stages are based on ego development with distinct conflicts (indicated as "Normal and Abnormal Findings" in this section) across the life span. These stages are a lifelong process and may overlap each other.

Does the **young adult**:
- Accept self—physically, cognitively, and emotionally?
- Have independence from the parental home?
- Express love responsibly, emotionally, and sexually?
- Have close or intimate relationships with a partner?
- Have a social group of friends?
- Have a physiology of living and life?

Intimacy
The young adult should have achieved self-efficacy during adolescence and is now ready to open up and become intimate with others (Fig. 7-3). Although this stage focuses on the desire for a special and permanent love relationship, it also includes the ability to have close, caring relationships with friends of both genders and a variety of ages. Spiritual love also develops during this stage. Having established an identity apart from the childhood family, the young adult is now able to form adult

Isolation
If the young adult cannot express emotion and trust enough to open up to others, social and emotional isolation may occur. Loneliness may cause the young adult to turn to addictive behaviors such as alcoholism, drug abuse, or sexual promiscuity. Some people try to cope with this developmental stage by becoming very spiritual or social, playing an acceptable role, but never fully sharing who they are

ASSESSMENT PROCEDURE	NORMAL FINDINGS	ABNORMAL FINDINGS
• Have a profession or a life's work that provides a means of contribution? • Solve problems of life that accompany independence from the parental home?	friendships with parents and siblings. However, the young adult will always be a son or daughter.	or becoming emotionally involved with others. When adults successfully navigate this stage, they have stable and satisfying relationships with important others.

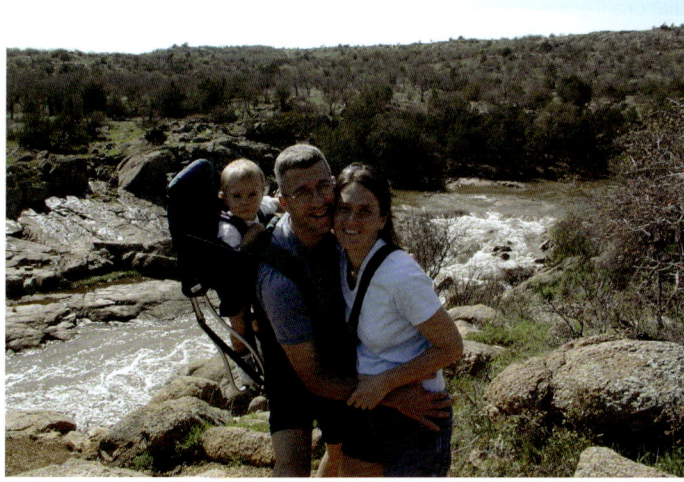

FIGURE 7-3 This young couple has reached Erikson's stage of intimacy. They have developed a loving relationship apart from their original families and have started a family of their own.

Does the **middle-aged adult**: • Have healthful life patterns? • Derive satisfaction from contributing to growth and development of others? • Have an abiding intimacy and long-term relationship with a partner? • Maintain a stable home? • Find pleasure in an established work or profession? • Take pride in self and family accomplishments and contributions? • Contribute to the community to support its growth and development?	**Generativity** During this stage, the middle-aged adult is able to share self with others and establish nurturing relationships. The adult will be able to extend self and possessions to others. Although traditionalists tend to think of generativity in terms of raising their children and guiding their lives, generativity can be realized in several ways, even without having children. Generativity implies mentoring and giving to future generations (Fig. 7-1G, p. 101). This can be accomplished by producing ideas, products, inventions, paintings, writings, books, films, or any other creative endeavors that are then offered to people for unrestricted use. Generativity also includes teaching others, children or adults, mentoring young workers, or providing experience and wisdom to assist a new business to survive and grow. Also implied in this stage is the ability to guide, then let go of one's creations. Successful movement through this stage results in a fuller and more satisfying life and prepares the mature adult for the next stage.	**Stagnation** Without the important step of generativity, the gift is not given and the stage does not come to successful completion. Stagnation occurs when the middle-aged person has not accomplished one or more of the previous developmental tasks and is unable to give to future generations. Sometimes severe losses may result in withdrawal and stagnation. In these cases, the person may have total dependency on work, a favorite child, or even a pet, and be incapable of giving to others. A project may never be finished or schooling never completed because the person cannot let go and move on. Without a creative outlet, a paralyzing stagnation sets in.

Continued on following page

ASSESSMENT PROCEDURE	NORMAL FINDINGS	ABNORMAL FINDINGS

Assessment of Erikson's Psychosocial Development (Continued)

Does the **older adult**:
- Adjust to the changing physical self?
- Recognize changes present as a result of aging, in relationships and activities?
- Maintain relationships with children, grandchildren, and other relatives?
- Continue interests outside of self and home?
- Complete transition from retirement from work to satisfying alternative activities?
- Establish relationships with others who are his or her own age?
- Adjust to deaths of relatives, spouse, and friends?
- Maintain a maximum level of physical functioning through diet, exercise, and personal care?
- Find meaning in past life and face inevitable mortality of self and significant others?
- Integrate philosophical or religious values into self-understanding to promote comfort?
- Review accomplishments and recognize meaningful contributions he or she has made to community and relatives?

Integrity
According to Erikson (1950), a person in this stage looks back and either finds that life was good or despairs because goals were not accomplished. This stage can extend over a long time and include excursions into previous stages to complete unfinished business. Successful movement through this stage does not mean that one day a person wakes up and says, "My life has been good." Rather, it encompasses a series of reminiscences in which the person may be able to see past events in a new and more positive light.

This can be a very rich and rewarding time in a person's life, especially if there are others with whom to share memories and who can assist with reframing life experiences (Fig. 7-1H, p. 101). For some people, resolution and acceptance do not come until the final weeks of life, but this still allows for a peaceful death.

Despair
If the older person cannot feel grateful for his or her life, cannot accept those less desirable aspects as merely part of living, or cannot integrate all of the experiences of life, then the person will spend his or her last days in bitterness and regret and will ultimately die in despair.

Assessment of Piaget's Cognitive Development

Determine the client's cognitive level by asking the following questions: Does the **young adult**:
- Assume responsibility for independent decision making?
- Realistically self-evaluate strengths and weaknesses?
- Identify and explore multiple options and potential outcomes?
- Seek assistance as necessary?
- Place decision into long-range context?
- Make realistic plans for the future?
- Seek career mentors?

Does the **middle-aged adult**:
- Differentiate discrepancies among goals, wishes, and realities?
- Identify factors that give life meaning and continuity?
- Effectively share knowledge and experience with others?
- Separate emotional (affective) issues from the cognitive domain for decision making?

The young adult who has attained formal operational thought continues to use sensorimotor thought and learning. Being alert to both internal and external stimuli assists information processing. Cognitive regression occurs in all individuals throughout the life cycle under conditions of stress. However, it should be regained in a timely manner. Formal operations incorporate deductive reasoning. The young adult can evaluate the validity of reasoning. The person who engages in self-evaluation must be able to make objective judgment. All people learn at their own pace and with their own style. Young adults are interested in learning that which is considered relevant and worthy of use and are capable of making realistic plans for the future.

The middle-aged adult using formal operational thought is capable of readjusting/modifying goals as necessary. Improving active and developing latent interests and talents increases creativity. The healthy middle-aged person provides mentorship to others due to increased problem-solving abilities and experiences (Fig. 7-4). Seeking new information maintains currency and promotes continued self-development and responsibility. This is especially true regarding rapid progress in technology and emphasis on computerization. The older members of generation X (born between 1965 and 1981) wish to learn to advance in their careers and other responsibilities. The "baby boomers" (born between 1946 and 1964) learn to adapt to

The young adult who has not attained formal operations will operate at the stage in which cognitive arrest occurred. This person will have difficulty with abstract thinking when information is presented in written form. This young adult will find it difficult to understand and process the information in some high school and definitely college-level textbooks.

The middle-aged adult who has not attained/maintained formal operational thought experiences difficulty remaining current at work and meeting expectations in all aspects of life in general. This person has not made adequate realistic plans for the future. The middle-aged client who has

ASSESSMENT PROCEDURE	NORMAL FINDINGS	ABNORMAL FINDINGS
• Seek new ways to improve/add to knowledge? • Adapt quickly to change and new knowledge?	fast change. Many of these adults have been called the "sandwich generation" (Schuster & Ashburn, 1992, p. 786; Touhy & Jett, 2012, p. 4) because they try to meet the needs of their teenagers/adult children (who have often returned to live at home and bring grandchildren) as well as caring for aging parents/grandparents. They are attempting to guide young people who are seeking independence while managing older people who are experiencing loss of independence.	not attained formal operational thought may be able to teach other "hands-on" skills that don't require in-depth explanations and rationales.

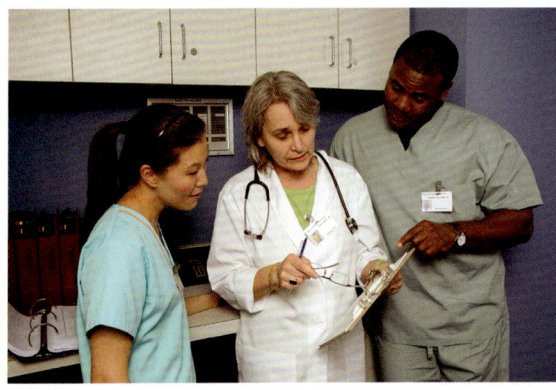

FIGURE 7-4 Middle-aged adults are able to mentor young adults in the workplace because they have increased problem-solving abilities and life experience.

Does the **older adult**: • Maintain maximal independence with activities of daily living? • Look for ways to find satisfaction with life? • Determine realistic plans for the future, including own mortality?	The older adult who uses formal operational thinking continues to share expertise with others (Fig. 7-5). This person can remember events and stories that reflect earlier years, teaching others about history, and the continuities of life. Many older adults prefer gradual transitions as opposed to abrupt change. The older adult, who has seen much change, can demonstrate flexibility. This person is capable of making realistic decisions regarding pacing of activities, planning self-care, making living arrangements, providing for transportation, adhering to medical regimen, and managing finances. "Traditionalists" (born before 1946) value high achievement and are often fiscally conservative; many have survived the rationing necessary during World War II and the Great Depression (that began in 1929). Older adults are capable of gradually transferring social/civic responsibilities to others and solidify the concepts of life and death. It is never too late to acquire new learning. Piaget believed that new learning can occur throughout the adult years.	The older adult who does not possess formal operational thinking eventually profits from assistance from others, especially in obtaining activities of daily living, correctly taking medication, and maintaining the highest level of wellness.

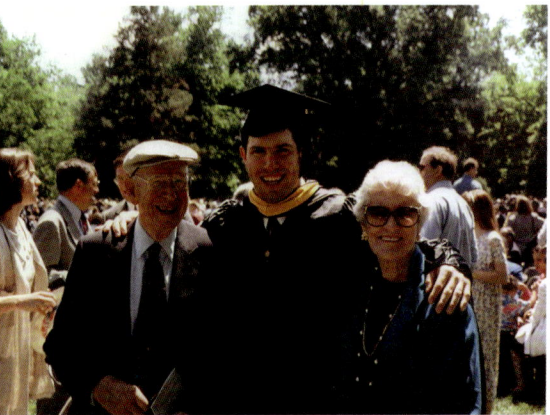

FIGURE 7-5 Older adults proud of their grandson.

Continued on following page

ASSESSMENT PROCEDURE	NORMAL FINDINGS	ABNORMAL FINDINGS

Assessment of Kohlberg's Moral Development

Determine the client's moral level by asking the following questions.

Does the **young adult**:
- State priorities to be considered when making a moral decision?
- Perceive having approval of family?
- Perceive having approval of peers?
- Perceive having approval of supervisor/teachers/authority figures?
- Perceive having approval of significant other?
- Consider self to be a "good person"? Why or why not?
- Have the ability to judge the intentions of others?

According to Kohlberg theory, which was based on male behavior, the young adult who has at least reached Piaget's stage of concrete operations may have attained the conventional level of moral reasoning. As the young adult attempts to take on new roles (adult student, exclusive sexual relationship, vocation, marriage, parent), attempts are made to maintain expectations and rules of the family, group, partnership, or society. This young adult obeys the law because it is respect for authority. Guilt can be a motivator to do the "right" thing. Decisions and behaviors are based on concerns about gaining approval from others. Some young adults who are capable of Piaget's formal operations will vacillate between the conventional and postconventional levels. For example, a young adult may intentionally break the law and join a protest group to stop medical research and experimentation on animals, believing that the principle of being humane to animals justifies the revolt. That same person may, however, exhibit more conventional reasoning when making decisions about "doing one's duty" at work, fulfilling the role of accountable student, and responsibly parenting a child.

The young adult who continues to make decisions and behave solely for self-satisfaction has not attained the conventional level. Continued behavior that negatively affects the comfort zone of others or infringes on the rights of others is not normal (Fig. 7-6). Those persons experiencing extreme stress overload may demonstrate moral regression.

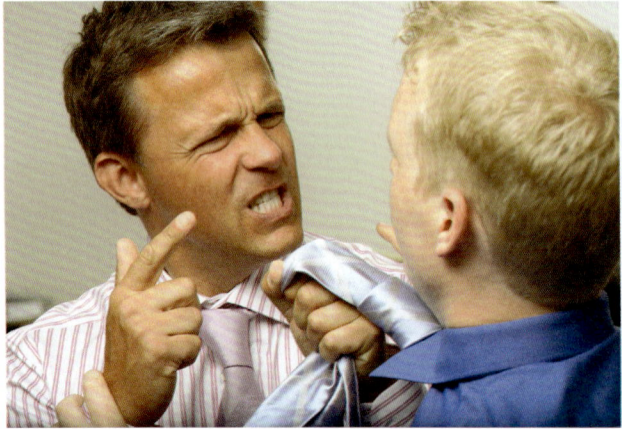

FIGURE 7-6 The young adult who continually exhibits behavior that negatively affects the comfort zone of others or infringes on the rights of others is not normal.

Does the **middle-aged adult**:
- State priorities to be considered when making a moral decision?
- Focus more on law and order or individual rights when making a decision?
- Express willingness to stop unhealthy behavior and change lifestyle patterns to foster a higher level of wellness?

Kohlberg found that although many adults are capable of Piaget's stage of formal operations, few demonstrated the postconventional level of behavior and, if healthy, were more than likely at the conventional level. Kohlberg believed that if a person was capable of formal operations and experienced additional positive personal moral choices, that person could reach a higher level of moral development. Many older middle-aged adults questioned authority and challenged the status quo during their young–adult years. There are many healthy middle-aged people who feel that they have learned from mistakes made earlier during young adulthood.

The person who has consistently used maladaptive coping will not reach the postconventional level. Such a person could regress as far as the premoral (or even amoral) level. This person fears authority and hopes to "not get caught."

ASSESSMENT PROCEDURE	NORMAL FINDINGS	ABNORMAL FINDINGS
Does the **older adult**: • State priorities to be considered when making a moral decision? • View rules and laws as changeable using legal means? • Make decisions consistently on internalized rules and in terms of conscience? • Believe in equality for every person?	Kohlberg believed that very few people attain and maintain the highest stage of the postconventional level. During the fifth stage, the person believes in respect for individuals while still emphasizing that the needs of the majority are more important. During the sixth stage, the person believes in absolute justice for every individual and is willing to make a decision or perform an action risking external punishment. It may be that the older adult perceives more authority, time, and courage to "speak one's mind." Today's senior citizen may have developed belief patterns during a time very different from the 21st century. A few older adults, as they ponder their mortality, may enter Kohlberg's seventh stage. Such people would analyze the "whole picture" and conclude that all organisms are interconnected.	It is difficult to assess anyone as normal or abnormal unless that person is harming self or others. Kohlberg hypothesized that older adults who are still at the preconventional level obey rules to avoid the disapproval of others. Kohlberg believed that older adults at the conventional level adhere to society's rules and laws because they believe that this is what others expect of them.

CASE STUDY

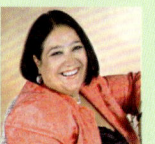

Returning to the case study of Mrs. Como-Williams, the nurse collects objective data to supplement subjective data.

Mrs. Como-Williams is a 51-year-old Caucasian female who was diagnosed 1 week ago by her primary physician as being overweight/borderline obesity. She presents with a clean appearance and no odors. She is dressed appropriately for the season and is wearing makeup.

Her verbal and nonverbal behaviors are congruent. Freud might label her as fixated in the oral stage since she is an excessive talker and an overeater. He would state that she has anxiety about her body weight and lifestyle and is coping with this by talking about it as well as seeking resources to decrease her discomfort. Her first marriage of 25 years resulted in the birth of a daughter. She divorced and subsequently remarried. Freud would determine her to be heterosexual and as having attained the genital stage in some aspects of her life. He would probably view her role of being a woman working out of the home while being a wife, mother, and grandmother as a basis for neurotic behavior.

Mrs. Como-Williams is positively resolving Erikson generativity versus stagnation task. Her behaviors that demonstrate this include "giving back" to the community by teaching second-grade students and counseling their families; providing emotional and financial support for her daughter in order for the daughter to further her career; providing emotional and physical safety, security, and guidance to her preschool-aged granddaughter; actively participating in social gatherings and relationships; and committing to a marital partner after experiencing a divorce. In addition, she expresses a desire to be physically healthier in order to better fulfill these activities. Her area of difficulty in her generativity is the impaired sexual expression related to her body image difficulties.

She is willing to accommodate her lifestyle in order to attain a higher level of wellness. Piaget would interpret her ability to correctly hypothesize about the benefits of a healthier future for herself as well as her family as an example of formal operational thought. Mrs. Como-Williams is willing to seek new information to attain this goal. In doing so, she would be engaged in quantitative learning. She has the opportunity to mentor junior faculty at her place of work.

Since Mrs. Como-Williams makes use of Piaget's formal operational thought, Kohlberg would assess her reasoning to determine whether she had attained the conventional level of moral development. Although she personally desires to look and feel better, she also wishes to have the approval of others. More data need to be collected regarding her reasoning and beliefs to ascertain her current stage of moral development.

Validating and Documenting Findings

Validate the psychosocial assessment data you have collected. This is necessary to verify that the data are reliable and accurate. Document the data following the health care facility or agency policy.

CASE STUDY

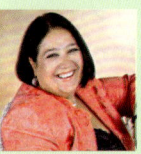

Think back to the case study. The nurse completed the following documentation of her assessment of Mrs. Como-Williams.

Biographical Data: CC-W, 51 years old. Caucasian, with both sets of grandparents being born in Italy.

Reason for Seeking Care: "It's time I lost weight and kept it off … [high] cholesterol and triglyceride levels." Admits her body image as overweight is affecting sexual relations with husband of 1 year. Employed full-time as an elementary (second grade) teacher in a public school. Obtained B.S. in Education from Purdue University in Indiana. Divorced after being married 25 years; has been remarried to second husband for approximately 1 year. Oriented to person, place, time, and event. Behavior appropriate and congruent. Demonstrates Piaget's formal operational thinking in stating that by losing weight she will be healthier, and that by making lifestyle changes her immediate family will be positively affected. Demonstrates Kohlberg's conventional level of moral development by demonstrating empathy for family and students (implying that family would eat nutritious food if she made healthier choices in preparing food and showing concern for second-grade students' issues that affect their ability to learn). Meets most of Erikson generativity versus stagnation stage challenges, other than a developing issue with her sense of body image affecting sexual relations with husband.

History of Present Health Concerns: Presently weighs 212 lb. Height measures 5'4." BMI 36.4 categorizes her as obese. States that she has always overeaten. Total cholesterol = 280 mg/dL. HDL = 90 mg/dL. LDL = 190 mg/dL. Triglycerides = 225 mg/dL. BP = 130/80 (prehypertensive).

Personal Health History: Diagnosed as obese, with hypercholesterolemia and hyperlipidemia last week by primary physician. States that significant weight gain began in her 20s and continued to gain weight with pregnancy during that time. Reports that she has weighed at least 180 lb postpregnancy (Ideal Body Weight with [IBW] = 120 lb). Previous total vaginal hysterectomy with bilateral salpingooophorectomy. Reports occasional "hot flash" at night. Immunizations current. No known allergies to drugs, food, insects, the environment.

Family History: States father, who died of "heart attack," had been diagnosed with hypertension and hypercholesterolemia; two older sisters and mother still living, all alive and well. Denies any family history of obesity. Married to second husband. Client has one daughter from former marriage. Both daughter and preschool-aged granddaughter live with Mr. and Mrs. Williams. Providing emotional and financial support to daughter and granddaughter, sharing responsibilities with her husband, and guiding the education of children are behaviors that exemplify positive resolution of Erikson's stage of generativity.

Lifestyle and Health Practices: Denies tobacco use and medication/supplement use/misuse. Admits to overeating and consuming many high-calorie, carbohydrate-dense, and fatty foods throughout waking hours. Drinks one glass of wine with dinner daily and at social functions. Often gets less than 6 hours of sleep nightly, denies napping. States that cleaning house on the weekend is her "exercise." Works Monday through Friday as full-time school teacher. Married and active participant in family functions on many weekends. Denies strong religious affiliation.

Physical Assessment: 51-year-old Caucasian female. Standing height is 5 ft 4 in: weight without shoes is 212 lb. IBW = 125 lb; BMI is 36.4 (obese).

Laboratory results from last week: hemoglobin = 13 g/dL; hematocrit = 38%; triglycerides = 225 mg/dL; fasting blood glucose = 100 mg/dL; and A1c = 5%. All thyroid panel values were within normal limits. Urine negative for white blood cells, red blood cells, glucose, and ketones.

Temperature 98.8° (tympanic); respirations 18 (regular, moderate depth); pulse 86 (apical, regular); blood pressure 130/80 (left arm). Alert X4. Responds to voice and touch.

Skin: Light olive-toned skin. Warm and dry. Pedal and radial pulses 2+. Slight dryness of skin over elbows and on heels and bottom of feet. Beginning "crow's feet" around lateral canthus of eyes bilaterally. No dryness or excessive tearing of eyes. Slight nasolabial folds noted. Oral and nasal mucous membranes are pink and moist. Natural teeth are intact. Short black hair is graying and dry on ends. All nails are clean, cut short, attached to nail bed. No clubbing noted.

Wears glasses to correct vision to 20/25 in both eyes. PERRLA: right = 3/2; left = 3/2. Peripheral vision to 90 degrees. Whisper test intact at 5 feet bilaterally.

Thyroid nonpalpable.

Moisture and slight redness under breasts and panniculus; no notable odor. Breasts are minimally fibrocystic. Lungs clear bilaterally. Abdomen round and soft; no tenderness reported. Active bowel sounds in all quadrants. Liver not palpable.

Full range of motion in all extremities. Strength 5/5 and equal in all extremities. Gait coordinated and steady. Arms swing in opposition. Capillary refill immediate.

Pelvic and rectal examinations deferred.

Interdisciplinary Verbal Communication of Assessment Findings Using SBAR

SITUATION: Constance (Connie) Como-Williams comes to the Women's Wellness Center 1 week after her physical examination with her primary care physician indicating that she wants to lose weight to be healthier and to look better for her husband, family, and self. She feels unattractive related to her obesity and believes that this has affected her ability to respond sexually to her husband.

BACKGROUND: She is a 51-year-old Caucasian female school teacher who divorced at 45 years of age, remarried last year, and has one daughter from first marriage. Reports that "I'm not very good about providing myself or my family with the healthiest foods." Diet consists of high fats and carbohydrates, claims her Italian heritage has affected her inclination to equate food with love. Reports nightly hot flashes. Does not take any hormone replacement therapy.

ASSESSMENT: Height measures 5 ft 4 in; BMI = 36.4. The number identified previously is obese. States that she has always overeaten. Total cholesterol = 280 mg/dL. HDL = 90 mg/dL.

LDL = 190 mg/dL. Triglycerides = 225 mg/dL. BP = 130/80 (prehypertension).

RECOMMENDATION: It would be helpful for Mrs. Como-Williams to be seen by a dietitian/nutritionist and to assist her with a weight reduction plan. Encourage client to investigate physical fitness programs or trainers. In addition, talking with a counselor to explore her feelings of low self-esteem may assist her to be more successful with her weight loss plan.

ANALYSIS OF DATA: DIAGNOSTIC REASONING

After collecting data pertaining to the patient's developmental level, identify abnormal findings and strengths. Then cluster the data to reveal any significant patterns or abnormalities. These data may be used to make clinical judgments about the status of developmental level in your patient's life.

Selected Nursing Diagnoses

Following is a listing of selected nursing diagnoses (health promotion, risk, or actual) that you may identify when analyzing data for the assessment of developmental (psychosexual, psychosocial, cognitive, moral) levels of the young adult, middle-aged adult, or elderly adult. Please note that an individual, depending on his or her level in any of these domains, could be assessed with one or more of these nursing diagnoses. A person could be at a high level/stage in one domain and at a low level/stage in another domain. Biologic age is irrelevant.

Health Promotion Diagnoses

- Young adult: Readiness for enhanced knowledge, readiness for self-health management, readiness for enhanced relationship, readiness for enhanced parenting
- Middle-aged adult: Readiness for enhanced knowledge, readiness for enhanced self-health management, readiness for enhanced family processes, readiness for enhanced coping, readiness for enhanced family coping, readiness for enhanced community coping
- Older adult: Readiness for enhanced knowledge, readiness for enhanced self-health management, readiness for enhanced relationship, readiness for enhanced religiosity

Risk Diagnoses

- Young adult: Risk for disturbed personal identity, risk for self-directed violence, risk for other-directed violence, risk for isolation, risk for ineffective relationship, risk for impaired parenting, risk for impaired attachment, risk for posttrauma syndrome, risk for loneliness, risk for situational low self-esteem, risk for suicide
- Middle-aged adult: Risk for disturbed personal identity, risk for loneliness, risk for situational low self-esteem, risk for caregiver role strain, risk for posttrauma syndrome, risk for spiritual distress, risk for complicated grieving, risk for suicide
- Older adult: Risk for disturbed personal identity, risk for loneliness, risk for situational low self-esteem, risk for caregiver role strain, risk for powerlessness, risk for hopelessness, risk for posttrauma syndrome, risk for spiritual distress, risk for impaired religiosity, risk for complicated grieving, risk for relocation stress syndrome, risk for suicide

Actual Diagnoses

Again, the reader is reminder that a nursing diagnosis is determined depending on the individual's levels of assessed development. A nursing diagnosis can be labeled as primarily "psychosocial" when the probable etiology is of a psychosocial nature. Many of the following selected nursing diagnoses, while common to the phase under which they are listed, could apply to a person in another phase of the life span.

- Young adult: Anxiety, disturbed body image, parental role conflict, ineffective coping, dysfunctional family processes, fear, ineffective health maintenance, deficient knowledge, sedentary lifestyle, moral distress, imbalanced nutrition (less/more than body requirements), impaired parenting, posttrauma syndrome, risk-prone health behavior, ineffective role performance, chronic low self-esteem, sexual dysfunction, sleep deprivation, social isolation, spiritual distress
- Middle-aged adult: Anxiety, disturbed body image, caregiver role strain, decisional conflict, parental role conflict, defensive coping, deficient knowledge, compromised family coping, fear, anticipatory grieving, moral distress, imbalanced nutrition (less/more than body requirements), posttrauma syndrome, sexual dysfunction, sleep deprivation, social isolation, spiritual distress
- Older adult: Anxiety, disturbed body image, caregiver role strain, decisional conflict, ineffective community coping, deficient diversional activity, fear, impaired home maintenance, interrupted family processes, hopelessness, impaired physical mobility, moral distress, imbalanced nutrition (less/more than body requirements), powerlessness, relocation stress syndrome, disturbed sleep pattern, social isolation, spiritual distress, impaired religiosity

CASE STUDY

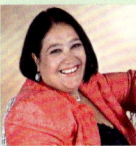

After collecting and analyzing the data for Mrs. Como-Williams, the nurse determines that the following conclusions are appropriate:

Nursing diagnoses include:
- Disturbed body image r/t changes in physical appearance from increasing weight to 212 lb.
- Risk for sexual dysfunction r/t low self-esteem from increasing overweight.
- Obesity related to many years of overeating and limited exercise.

Potential Collaborative Problems are worded as Risk for Complications (RC), followed by the problem. These include:
- RC: Depression
- RC: Type 2 diabetes mellitus
- RC: Coronary heart disease
- RC: Hypertension

Refer to nutritionist, dietary counseling, and follow-up with primary physician. Refer to gynecologist for screening mammogram and pelvic examination.

References and Selected Readings

Colby, A., Kohlberg, L., Gibbs, J., et al. (1983). A longitudinal study of moral behavior. *Monographs of the Society of Research in Child Development, 48*(1–2), 1–124.

Erikson, E. H. (1950). *Childhood and society.* New York: W. W. Norton Company, Inc.

Erikson, E. H. (1963). *Childhood and society* (2nd ed.). New York: W. W. Norton Company, Inc.

Erikson, E. H. (1968). *Identity: Youth and crisis.* New York: W. W. Norton & Company, Inc.

Erikson, E. H., & Erikson, J. M. (1992). *The life cycle completed.* New York: W. W. Norton.

Fodor, N., & Gaynor, F. (Eds). (1958). *Freud: Dictionary of psychoanalysis.* Greenwich, CT: A Fawcett Premier Book.

Freud, S. (1935). *A general introduction to psychoanalysis (authorized English translation of the revised edition by Joan Riviere).* New York: Liveright.

Freud, S. (1949). *An outline of psychoanalysis (authorized translation by James Strachey).* New York: W. W. Norton & Company, Inc.

Garsee, J. W., & Schuster, C. S. (1992). Moral development. In C. S. Schuster, & S. S. Ashburn. (Eds.). *The process of human development: A holistic life-span approach.* Philadelphia, PA: J. B. Lippincott Company.

Gilligan, C. (1984). *In a different voice.* Cambridge, MA: Harvard University Press.

Gilligan, C. (1996). *In a different voice: Psychological theory and women's development.* Cambridge, MA: Harvard University Press.

Ginsburg, H., & Opper, S. (1969). *Piaget's theory of intellectual development: An introduction.* Englewood Cliffs, NJ; Prentice-Hall, Inc.

Kazer, M. (2012). *Sexuality assessment for older adults.* Retrieved at http://consultgerirn.org/uploads/File/trythis/try_this_10.pdf

Kohlberg, L. (1978). The cognitive-developmental approach to moral education. In P. Scharf (Ed.): *Readings in moral education* (pp. 36–51). Minneapolis, MN: Winston Press.

Kohlberg, L. (1981). *The philosophy of moral development.* San Francisco, CA: Harper & Row.

Kohlberg, L., & Gilligan, C. (1971). *The adolescent as a philosopher: The discovery of the self in a postconventional world.* Los Angeles, CA: Daedalus.

Kohlberg, L., & Ryncarz, R. (1990). Beyond justice reasoning: Moral development and consideration of a seventh stage. In C. Alexander, & E. Langer (Eds.). *Higher stages human development* (pp. 191–207), New York: Oxford University Press.

Levine, C., Kohlberg, L., & Hewer, A. (1985). The current formulation of Kohlberg's theory and a response to critics. *Human Development, 28*(2), 94–100.

Mayo Clinic Staff. (2014). *Sexual health and aging: Keep the passion alive.* Retrieved at http://www.mayoclinic.org/healthy-lifestyle/sexual-health/in-depth/sexual-health/art-20046698

National Institute on Aging. (2015). Forgetfulness: Knowing when to ask for help. Retrieved at https://www.nia.nih.gov/health/publication/forgetfulness

Parker, K. (2012). *The boomerang generation: Feeling OK about living with mom and dad.* Retrieved at www.pewsocialtrends.org

Pew Research Center. (2015). *Changing attitudes on gay marriage.* Retrieved at http://www.pewforum.org/2015/07/29/graphics-slideshow-changing-attitudes-on-gay-marriage/

Phillips, J. L., Jr. (1975). *The origins of intellect: Piaget's theory* (2nd ed.). San Francisco, CA: W. H. Freeman & Co.

Piaget, J. (1970). Piaget's theory. In P. H. Mussen (Ed.): *Carmichael's manual of child Psychology* (3rd ed.). New York: Wiley.

Piaget, J., & Inhelder, B. (1969). *The psychology of the child* (H. Weaver, Trans.) (pp. 703–732). New York: Basic Books, Inc.

Purnell, L. D. (2013). *Guide to culturally competent care* (4th ed.). Philadelphia, PA: F.A. Davis.

Schuster, C. S., & Ashburn, S. S. (1992). *The process of human development: A holistic life-span approach* (3rd ed.). Philadelphia, PA: J. B. Lippincott Company.

Selye, H. (1976). *The stress of life (rev.).* New York: McGraw-Hill.

Touhy, T. A., & Jett, K. (2012). *Ebersole and Hess' toward healthy aging: Human needs & nursing response* (8th ed.). St. Louis, MO: Elsevier Mosby.

University of California San Francisco (UCSF) Medical Center. (2015). *Coping strategies for vascular dementia caregivers.* Retrieved at http://www.ucsfhealth.org/education/coping_strategies_for_vascular_dementia_caregivers/

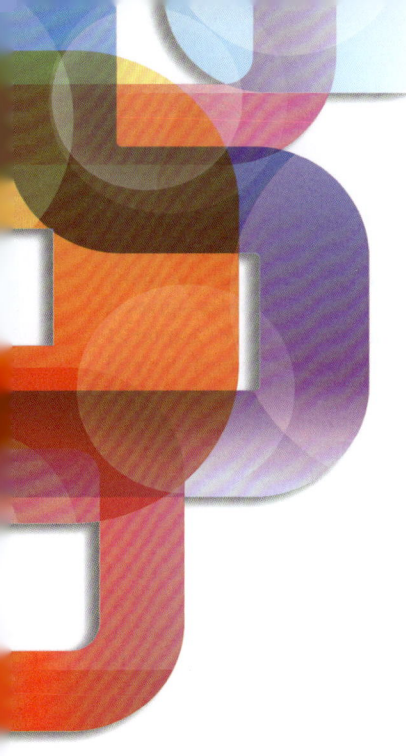

8 ASSESSING GENERAL HEALTH STATUS AND VITAL SIGNS

Learning Objectives

1. Prepare the client for a survey of general health status and vital signs.
2. Interview the client for an accurate survey of his or her general health status and vital signs.
3. Correctly perform an accurate general survey.
4. Assess accurate vital signs.
5. Discuss the assessment of pain as a fifth vital sign.
6. Describe findings often seen when assessing an older client's general health status and vital signs.
7. Differentiate between normal and abnormal findings in the general survey and vital signs.
8. Analyze general survey and vital sign assessment data to formulate valid nursing diagnoses, collaborative problems, and/or referrals.

CASE STUDY

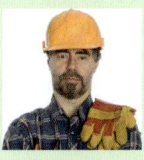

Thomas Anthony is a 34-year-old construction worker who presents to his local urgent care center with complaints of fever and fatigue. When obtaining the intake history, Mr. Anthony reports a rapid heart rate and feeling like his "heart is skipping a beat." He also reports dizziness when going from a sitting to standing position. He is not sure why he is feeling this way, but is concerned because he was unable to go to work today. He cannot afford to miss a day of work. Mr. Anthony's case will be discussed throughout the chapter.

STRUCTURE AND FUNCTION

The general survey is the first part of the physical examination that begins the moment the nurse meets the client. It requires the nurse to use all observational skills while interviewing and interacting with the client. These observations will lead to clues about the health status of the client. The outcome of the general survey provides the nurse with an overall impression of the client's whole being. The general survey includes observation of the client's:

- Physical development and body build
- Gender and sexual development
- Apparent age as compared to reported age
- Skin condition and color
- Dress and hygiene
- Posture and gait
- Level of consciousness
- Behaviors, body movements, and affect
- Facial expression
- Speech
- Vital signs

The client's vital signs (temperature, pulse, respirations, blood pressure, and pain) are the body's indicators of health. Usually when a vital sign (or signs) is abnormal, something is wrong in at least one of the body systems. Traditionally, vital signs have included the client's pulse, respirations, blood pressure, and temperature. Today, "pain" is considered to be the "fifth vital sign" (Lorenz et al., 2009). Pain is inexpensive to assess and does not involve the use of fancy instruments, yet it can be an early predictor of impending disability. For example, early and correct assessment of a client's chest pain may promote early treatment and prevention of complications and the high cost of cardiovascular damage and/or failure. Assessment of pain is presented in Chapter 9.

Overall Impression of the Client

The first time you meet a client, you tend to remember certain obvious characteristics. Forming an overall impression consists of a systematic examination and recording of these general characteristics and impressions of the client. If possible, try to observe the client and environment quickly before interacting with the client. This gives you the opportunity to "see" the client before he or she assumes a social face or behavior and allows you to assess any distress, sadness, or pain before the client, knowingly or unknowingly, may mask it.

When you meet for the first time, observe any significant abnormalities in the client's skin color, dress, hygiene, posture and gait, physical development, body build, apparent age, and gender. If you observe abnormalities, you may need to perform an in-depth assessment of the body area that appears to be affected (e.g., an unusual gait may prompt you to perform a detailed musculoskeletal assessment). You should also generally assess the client's level of consciousness, level of comfort, behavior, body movements, affect, facial expression, speech, and mental acuities. If you detect any abnormalities during your general impression examination, you will need to do an in-depth mental status examination. This examination is described in Chapter 6. Additional preparation involves creating a comfortable, nonthreatening atmosphere to relieve anxiety in the client.

Vital Signs

It is a good idea to begin the "hands-on" physical examination by taking vital signs. This is a common, noninvasive physical assessment procedure that most clients are accustomed to. Vital signs provide data that reflect the status of several body systems, including but not limited to the cardiovascular, neurologic, peripheral vascular, and respiratory systems. Note that activity, talking, gum-chewing, and anxiety affect pulse, respirations, and blood pressure. Allow 5 minutes of rest before beginning to take vital signs.

Temperature

For the body to function at a cellular level, a core body temperature between 36.5°C and 37.7°C (96.0°F and 99.9°F orally) must be maintained. An approximate reading of core body temperature can be taken at various anatomic sites. None of these is completely accurate; they are simply an approximate reflection of the core body temperature.

Several factors may cause normal variations in the core body temperature. Strenuous exercise, stress, and ovulation can raise temperature. Body temperature is lowest early in the morning (4:00 to 6:00 AM) and highest late in the evening (8:00 PM to midnight). Hypothermia (lower than 36.5°C or 96.0°F) may be seen in prolonged exposure to the cold, hypoglycemia, hypothyroidism, or starvation. Hyperthermia (higher than 38.0°C or 100°F) may be seen in viral or bacterial infections, malignancies, trauma, and various blood, endocrine, and immune disorders.

> **OLDER ADULT CONSIDERATIONS**
> In the older adult, temperature may range from 95.0°F to 97.5°F. Therefore, the older client may not have an obviously elevated temperature with an infection or be considered hypothermic below 96°F.

Pulse

A shock wave is produced when the heart contracts and forcefully pumps blood out of the ventricles into the aorta. The shock wave travels along the fibers of the arteries and is commonly called the *arterial* or *peripheral pulse*. The body has many arterial pulse sites. One of them—the radial pulse—gives a good overall picture of the client's health status (see Chapter 21 for more information about additional pulse sites). Several characteristics should be assessed when measuring the radial pulse: rate, rhythm, amplitude and contour, and elasticity.

Amplitude can be quantified as follows:
- 0 Absent
- 1+ Weak, diminished (easy to obliterate)
- 2+ Normal (obliterate with moderate pressure)
- 3+ Bounding (unable to obliterate or requires firm pressure)

If abnormalities are noted during assessment of the radial pulse, perform further assessment. For more information on assessing pulses and abnormal pulse findings, refer to Chapters 21 and 22.

Respirations

The respiratory rate and character are additional clues to the client's overall health status. Observe respirations without alerting the client by watching chest movement while continuing to palpate the radial pulse. Notable characteristics of respiration are rate, rhythm, and depth (see Chapter 18 for more information about respirations).

Blood Pressure

Blood pressure reflects the pressure exerted on the walls of the arteries. This pressure varies with the cardiac cycle, reaching a high point with systole and a low point with diastole (Fig. 8-1). Therefore, blood pressure is a measurement of the pressure of the blood in the arteries when the ventricles are contracted (systolic blood pressure) and when the ventricles are relaxed (diastolic blood pressure). Blood pressure is expressed as the ratio of the systolic pressure over the diastolic pressure. A client's blood pressure is affected by several factors (Box 8-1):
- Cardiac output
- Elasticity of the arteries
- Blood volume
- Blood velocity (heart rate)
- Blood viscosity (thickness)

A client's blood pressure will normally vary throughout the day due to external influences. These include the time of day, caffeine or nicotine intake, exercise, emotions, pain, and temperature. The difference between systolic and diastolic pressure

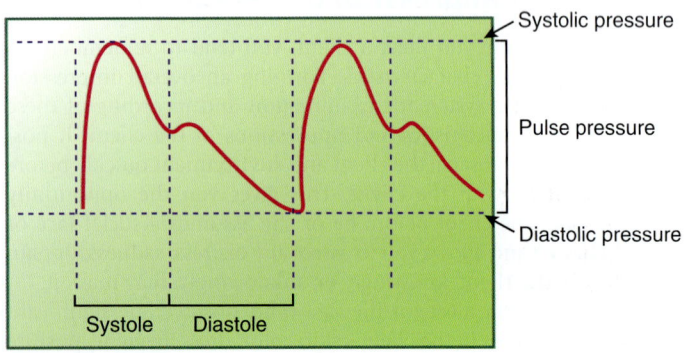

FIGURE 8-1 Blood pressure measurement identifies the amount of pressure in the arteries when the ventricles of the heart contract (systole) and when they relax (diastole).

BOX 8-1   FACTORS CONTRIBUTING TO BLOOD PRESSURE

1. **Cardiac Output.** The more blood the heart pumps, the greater the pressure in the blood vessels. For example, BP increases during exercise.

2. **Peripheral Vascular Resistance.** An increase in resistance in the peripheral vascular system, as happens with people who have circulatory disorders, will increase BP.

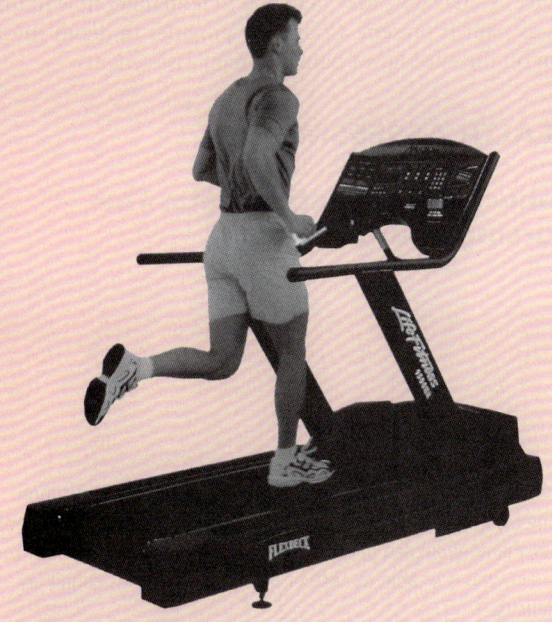

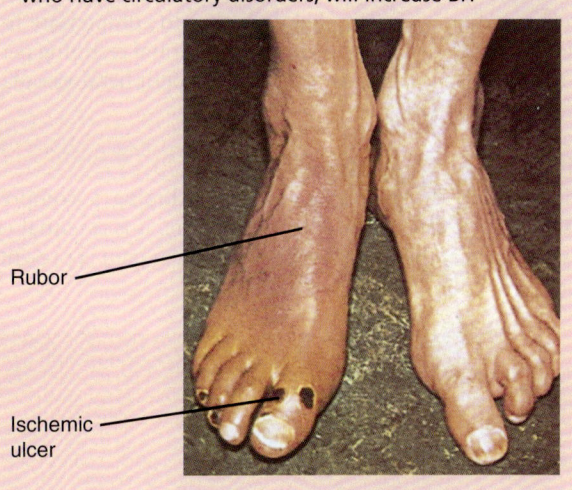

3. **Circulating Blood Volume.** An increase in volume will increase BP. A sudden drop in BP may indicate a sudden blood loss, as with internal bleeding.

4. **Viscosity.** When the blood becomes thicker or more viscous (as with polycythemia), the pressure in the blood vessels will increase.

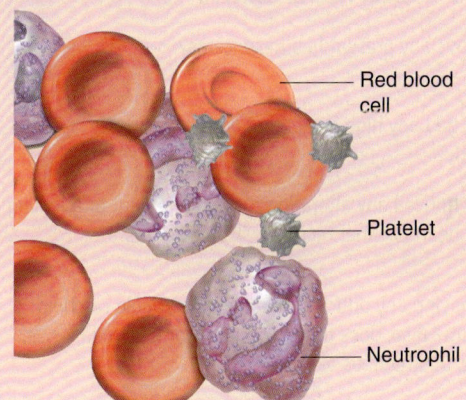

Densely Packed Red Blood Cells

5. **Elasticity of Vessel Walls.** An increase in stiffness of the vessel walls (e.g., atherosclerotic changes) will increase BP.

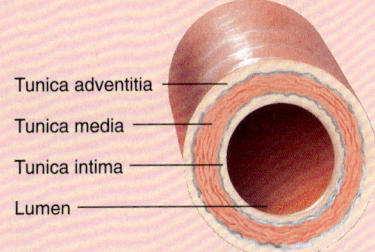
Normal coronary artery

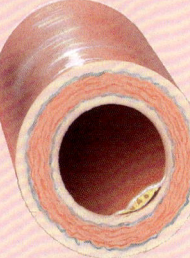
Fatty streak

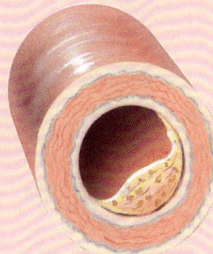
Fibrous plaque

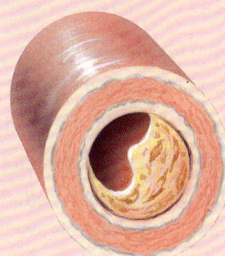
Complicated plaque

is termed the *pulse pressure*. Determine the pulse pressure after measuring the blood pressure because it reflects the stroke volume (the volume of blood ejected with each heartbeat).

Blood pressure may also vary depending on the positions of the body and of the arm. Blood pressure in a normal person who is standing is usually slightly higher to compensate for the effects of gravity. Blood pressure in a normal reclining person is slightly lower because of decreased peripheral vascular resistance.

Pain

Pain screening is very important in developing a comprehensive plan of care for the client. Therefore, it is essential to assess for pain at the initial assessment. When pain is present, identify the location, intensity, quality, duration, and any alleviating or aggravating factors to the client. Pain intensity measurement tools such as a 1 to 10 Likert scale (described in Chapter 9) may be used. Pain quality may be described as "dull," "sharp," "radiating," or "throbbing." The mnemonic device "COLDSPA" may help you to remember how to further assess pain if present. Chapter 9 provides in-depth information on the etiology of pain and pain assessment.

HEALTH ASSESSMENT

Collecting Subjective Data: The Nursing Health History

Initial Health History	
QUESTION	**RATIONALE**
General Survey Questions	
What are your name, address, and telephone number (including cell phone number and email address)?	Answers to these questions provide verifiable and accurate identification data about the client. They also provide baseline information about level of consciousness, memory, speech patterns, articulation, or speech defects. For example, a client who is unable to answer these questions has cognitive/neurologic deficits.
How old are you?	Establishes baseline for comparing appearance and development to chronologic age.
History of Present Health Concern	
Do you have any present health concerns?	This allows the client to voice her concerns and provides a focus for the examination.
Have you had any high fevers that occur often or persistently?	A pattern of elevated temperatures may indicate a chronic infection such as tuberculosis or blood disorder such as leukemia.
Have you noticed any alteration to your heartbeat or a feeling that your heart is either racing or skipping beats?	An alteration in heartbeat felt by a client is called a palpitation and can be caused by various circumstances, including SA node dysfunction, thyroid dysfunction, medication reaction, or alteration in fluid volume.
Are you having any difficulty breathing or trouble catching your breath? If so, does this occur at rest or with mild, moderate, or strenuous exercise?	Difficulty with breathing or dyspnea can be a sign of chronic heart failure (CHF), pneumonia, asthma, bronchitis, chronic obstructive pulmonary disease (COPD), or other chronic lung disease.
Do you have any pain? (If yes, ask the client to describe the pain using the COLDSPA mnemonic.) **Character:** How does it feel (dull, sharp, aching, throbbing)? How does area of pain look (shiny, bumpy, red, swollen, bruised)? **Onset:** When did it begin? **Location:** Where is it? Does it radiate? If so, where? **Duration:** How long does it last? Does it recur? **Severity:** How bad is it (on a scale of 1–10)? **Pattern:** What makes it better? What makes it worse? Have you tried therapies/treatments? Were they effective? **Associated Factors:** What other symptoms occur with it?	Exploring the pain in depth helps the nurse to understand the cause and significance of the pain.
Personal History	
Do you know what your usual blood pressure is?	Knowing blood pressure indicates client is involved in his or her own health care and provides a baseline for comparison.

QUESTION	RATIONALE
When and where did you last have your blood pressure checked?	Answer provides a baseline for comparison, and indicates if client consults professionals for health care, relies on possibly erroneous equipment in public places (e.g., drug stores), or has approved equipment at home that he or she is trained to use.
Are you aware if your heartbeat is unusually fast or slow?	Often a client will know that his or her heart rate frequently runs either high or low, especially if taking certain medications. In addition, well-trained athletes will often have a lower-than-average heart rate due to their level of physical fitness. This is a normal variation in those individuals. Those taking beta blockers may also have a low heart rate.
What medications do you take? Please list prescription and over-the-counter medications, vitamins and minerals, and any herbal supplements taken routinely or on an as-needed basis.	Having a complete list of all medications, vitamins, and herbal supplements is essential in assessing the general status of the client. Many medications have side effects that can alter a client's vital signs and may even affect general appearance. It is important to have the client bring a list from home that contains all the information needed, including names; dosages; route of administration; and time given for all medications, vitamins, and supplements. Ask client to bring actual medication containers if possible.
What allergies do you have to medications, foods, insects, or the environment?	It is important to gather a client's list of allergies in order to provide safe nursing care.
Family History	
Do you have any family history of heart disease, diabetes, thyroid disease, lung disease, high blood pressure, or cancer? Are you aware of any other family history?	Frequently diseases such as heart disease, diabetes, thyroid disease, lung disease, hypertension, or cancer can be hereditary; thus, it is important to ask about them when assessing the general status of your client. Even if there is no personal history of these diseases, the client's family history would put the client at an increased risk of developing such diseases in the future.
Lifestyle and Health Practices	
What is your educational background?	This gives you a basis for communication and understanding your client's level of comprehension.
Are you currently employed? If so, what is your occupation? If not, are you disabled, or are you seeking employment?	An occupation can provide insight into the client's condition and may lead to identification of significant health concerns.
How satisfied are you with your life?	Asking about life satisfaction can help elicit evidence of or potential for psychological problems such as anxiety, depression, or suicidal ideation, as well as information about developmental level.
How often do you seek health care?	This question provides insight into the client's health practices.
Do you use any tobacco products including cigarettes, e-cigarettes, chewing tobacco, snuff, or dip?	Tobacco use causes vasoconstriction of blood vessels, which leads to hypertension and/or peripheral vascular disease. Tobacco use can also cause chronic lung disease and/or cancer. Note that e-cigarettes may cause as much or more harm as regular tobacco cigarettes.
Do you drink alcohol? If so, how much and how often? What type of alcohol do you drink? Do you use any illicit drugs? If so, which one(s) and how often?	Excessive alcohol and/or illicit drug use may indicate poor lifestyle management and may represent psychological illness. These behaviors can also lead to obesity or malnutrition depending on which substance is abused. For example, methamphetamines often cause anorexia and malnutrition while alcoholism can lead to abdominal obesity and malnutrition.
Do you follow any special diet?	Clients with hypertension may follow a low-sodium (low-salt) diet. Other clients with obesity may follow a low-fat, low-cholesterol, low-carbohydrate diet. Clients with diabetes may consume a specific number of carbohydrates each day and not eat concentrated sweets or sugar. There are many different diets available to clients. Some are prescribed, while others are not. It is important to know what dietary restrictions clients have, as these diets directly affect the client's general status.
Do you exercise regularly? What type of exercise do you do and how often?	Exercise status can directly affect the musculature and build of a client. Exercise also may reduce anxiety and depression!

CASE STUDY

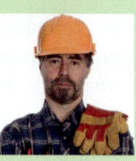

Recall the case study introduced at the beginning of the chapter. The nurse uses COLDSPA to explore Mr. Anthony's presenting concerns and obtains a general survey history.

The nurse interviews Mr. Anthony, using specific probing questions. The client reports a fever. The nurse explores this health concern using the COLDSPA mnemonic.

Mnemonic	Question	Data Provided
Character	Describe the sign or symptom (feeling, appearance, sound, smell, or taste if applicable)	Fever for the past 3 days, not sure how high because I don't own a thermometer. I can tell I was having a fever because I had chills and sweating off and on.
Onset	When did it begin?	Three days ago.
Location	Where is it? Does it radiate? Does it occur anywhere else?	My whole body shakes with chills and then I sweat all over my body.
Duration	How long does it last? Does it recur?	Comes and goes each day. Lasts for several hours, then I sweat and it improves. It recurs about three times daily.
Severity	How bad is it? How much does it bother you?	Varies in severity. It is very bothersome when I have chills because I can't get warm even with a lot of blankets.
Pattern	What makes it better or worse?	It seems to improve after I take two Tylenol extra-strength tablets, but the fever and chills return in about 4 hours. I tried taking a warm bath and it also helped some. I feel worse when I get cold.
Associated factors/How it affects the client	What other symptoms occur with it? How does it affect you?	I feel a lot of fatigue. I'm having trouble getting anything done at home, and I can't work.

After exploring the client's fever, the nurse continues with the present history. Mr. Anthony reports that he has also been experiencing a rapid heart rate, a feeling that his heart is skipping a beat, and dizziness. He denies dyspnea. The nurse notes that Mr. Anthony is dressed in soiled work clothes, is malodorous, diaphoretic, very thin, and appears to be much older than he states. He is unaware of his usual baseline vital signs, including blood pressure, because he has not sought health care in several years. He last checked his blood pressure in Walmart 3 years ago, but he cannot recall the results. Mr. Anthony states that he does not take any routine medications but does take two extra-strength Tylenol tablets, as needed for occasional headache about once a month. His last dose of Tylenol was yesterday at 5:00 PM. He denies any known allergies to medications or insects, but does report that he is allergic to mold. He has a family history of hypertension and diabetes through his father. His mother has a history of breast cancer at the age of 62. His older sister is alive and well with no current health problems. He is not married and has no children. Mr. Anthony is currently employed as a roofer and has been working 12 hours daily in intense heat. He has been avoiding taking trips to the water cooler because he is working on the roof and the water cooler is on the ground. He has a high school diploma and is satisfied with his family life. He has not been seen by a health care provider in over 5 years. He denies any current or former use of any form of tobacco product or any illicit drugs. He does drink one or two beers every night and has for several years. Mr. Anthony denies any special diet or exercise routine but does state that he gets regular exercise when working by hammering, lifting, walking, and climbing.

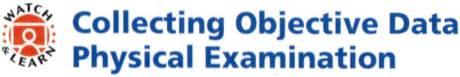

Collecting Objective Data: Physical Examination

Preparing the Client

The general survey begins when the nurse first meets the client. During this time observe the client's posture, movements, and overall appearance. The client should be in a comfortable sitting position in a chair, on the examination table, or on a bed in the home setting. Prepare the client for the general survey examination by explaining its purpose. Then explain that vital signs will be taken.

Equipment

- Thermometer: tympanic thermometer, temporal artery thermometer, electronic oral and/or axillary thermometer, or rectal thermometer
- Protective, disposable covers for type of thermometer used
- Aneroid or mercury sphygmomanometer or electronic blood pressure–measuring equipment

- Stethoscope
- Watch with a second hand, or cell phone with a timer

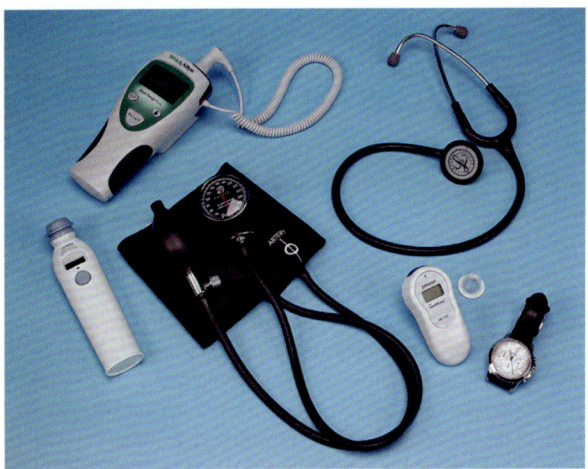

Physical Assessment
- Identify the equipment needed to measure vital signs and the proper use of each piece of equipment.
- If available, use a mobile monitoring system, such as "DINAMAP," which can be taken from room to room to perform multiple vital signs simultaneously. These devices often have a thermometer, electronic sphygmomanometer, oxygenation saturation detector, and pulse monitor (Fig. 8-2).

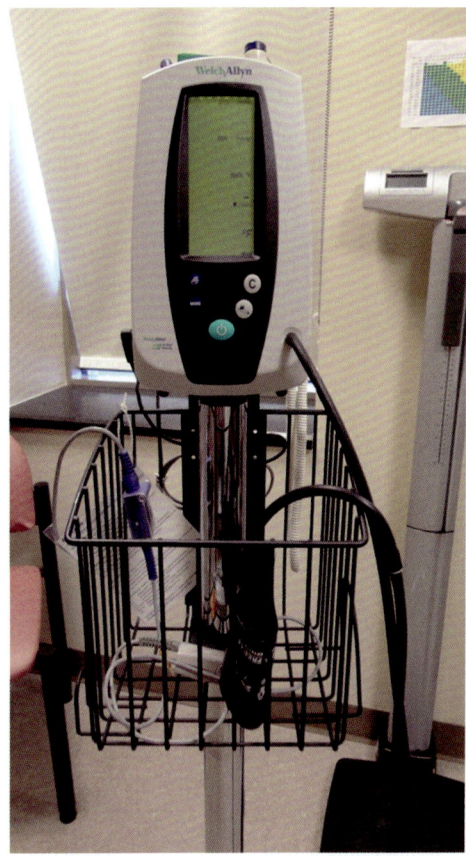

FIGURE 8-2 Mobile monitoring system.

General Routine Screening Versus Focused Specialty Assessment for General Health

Most often the nurse performs a general survey from the moment she first meets the client and continues to collect general survey data throughout the examination. Vital signs may be taken by the nurse or a trained assistant. Tympanic or temporal artery temperature readings are the most common, noninvasive, safe methods used. The nurse observes and gains a general impression while talking and interacting with the client. Some of the general survey data may not be obtained with the first meeting but the nurse will continue to observe the client with each interaction, gaining additional data for a more in-depth general survey. If a nurse observes that the client is in pain, a more in-depth pain assessment needs to occur first to intervene to relieve the pain before continuing the assessment. Pain will often interfere with further accurate assessment if the client is not comfortable. More advanced electronic methods of assessing pulse and blood pressure are often available in acute care settings when it is difficult to assess using manual methods.

General Routine Screening
- Observe physical development, body build, and fat distribution.
- Observe gender and sexual development.
- Compare client's stated age to apparent age and developmental stage.
- Observe posture and gait.
- Measure body temperature.
- Measure pulse rate.
- Measure respirations.
- Measure blood pressure.
- Assess pain.

Focused Specialty Assessment
- Use Doppler to measure pulse and blood pressure when unable to measure by manual methods (see Chapter 22).
- Further assess irregular heart rate (see Chapter 21).

ASSESSMENT PROCEDURE	NORMAL FINDINGS	ABNORMAL FINDINGS
General Impression		
Observe physical development, body build, and fat distribution.	A wide variety of body types fall within a normal range: from small amounts of fat and muscle to larger amounts of fat and muscle. See Chapter 13, Assessing Nutritional Status, for more information.	A lack of subcutaneous fat with prominent bones is a sign of malnutrition (Swartz, 2014). Abundant fatty tissue is seen in obesity (see Abnormal Findings 8-1).
	Body proportions are normal. Arm span (distance between fingertips with arms extended) is approximately equal to height. The distance from the head crown to the symphysis pubis is approximately equal to the distance from the symphysis pubis to the sole of the client's foot.	Decreased height and delayed puberty, with chubbiness, are seen in hypopituitary dwarfism (MedicineNet, 2015). Skeletal malformations with a decrease in height are seen in achondroplastic dwarfism (MedicineNet, 2014). In gigantism, there is increased height and weight with delayed sexual development. Overgrowth of bones in the face, head, hands, and feet with normal height is seen in hyperpituitarism (acromegaly; Mayo Clinic, 2013). Extreme weight loss is seen in anorexia nervosa. Arm span is greater than height, and pubis to sole measurement exceeds pubis to crown measurement in Marfan syndrome (The Marfan Foundation, 2014). Excessive body fat that is evenly distributed is referred to as exogenous obesity. Central body weight gain with excessive cervical obesity (Buffalo hump), also referred to as endogenous obesity, is seen in Cushing syndrome (see Abnormal Findings 8-1).
Observe gender and sexual development.	Sexual development is appropriate for gender and age.	Abnormal findings include delayed puberty, male client with female characteristics, and female client with male characteristics.
Compare client's stated age with apparent age and developmental stage (see Chapter 7).	Client appears to be her stated chronologic age.	Client appears older than actual chronologic age (e.g., due to outdoor manual labor, chronic illness, alcoholism, smoking).
Observe skin condition and color (see Chapter 14). ⊙ **CLINICAL TIP** Keep in mind that underlying red tones from good circulation give a liveliness or healthy glow to all shades of skin color.	Color is even without obvious lesions: light to dark beige-pink in light-skinned client; light tan to dark brown or olive in dark-skinned clients.	Abnormal findings include extreme pallor, flushed skin, or yellow skin in light-skinned client; loss of red tones and ashen gray cyanosis in dark-skinned client. See abnormal skin colors and their significance in Chapter 14.
Observe posture and gait.	Posture is erect and comfortable for age. Gait is rhythmic and coordinated, with arms swinging at side.	Curvatures of the spine (lordosis, scoliosis, or kyphosis) may indicate a musculoskeletal disorder. Stiff, rigid movements are common in arthritis or Parkinson disease (see Chapter 24). Slumped shoulders may signify depression, osteoporosis, kyphosis, compression fracture. Clients with chronic pulmonary obstructive disease tend to lean forward and brace themselves with their tripod or three point position (see Chapter 19 Figure 19-10). **OLDER ADULT CONSIDERATIONS** In older adults, osteoporotic thinning and collapse of the vertebrae secondary to bone loss may result in kyphosis. In older men, gait may be wider based, with arms held outward. Older women tend to have a narrow base and may waddle to compensate for a decreased sense of balance. Steps shorten, with decreased speed and arm swing. Mobility may be decreased, and gait may be rigid.

ASSESSMENT PROCEDURE	NORMAL FINDINGS	ABNORMAL FINDINGS

Vital Signs

MEASURE TEMPERATURE

| | **OLDER ADULT CONSIDERATIONS** Some research has shown that for older adults, normal body temperature values for all routes are consistently lower than values reported in younger populations (Lu, Leasure, & Dai, 2010). | *Concept Mastery Alert* Because geriatric clients often have a body temperature that is lower than is usually seen in children and adults, an older client with a slightly elevated temperature above 96.6–99.5 should be evaluated immediately for a possible infection. |
| **To measure tympanic temperature,** place the probe very gently at the opening of the ear canal for 2–3 seconds until the temperature appears in the digital display (Fig. 8-3). | The tympanic membrane temperature is normally about 0.8°C (1.4°F) higher than the normal oral temperature. Normal tympanic temperature range is 36.7–38.3°C (98.0–100.9°F) | Temperatures below 36.7°C (98.0°F) represent hypothermia and can be a result of prolonged exposure to cold, hypoglycemia, hypothyroidism, starvation, neurologic dysfunction, or shock.

Temperatures above 38.3°C (100.9°F) represent hyperthermia and can indicate bacterial, viral, or fungal infections, an inflammatory process, malignancies, trauma, or various blood, endocrine, and immune disorders. |

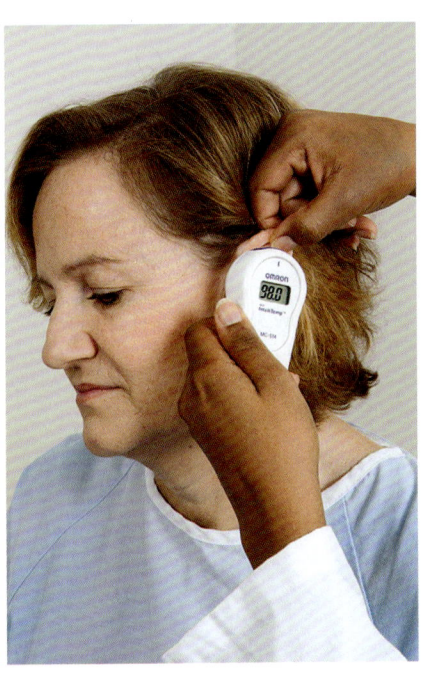

FIGURE 8-3 Taking a tympanic temperature.

> **CLINICAL TIP**
> An electronic tympanic thermometer measures the temperature of the tympanic membrane quickly and safely. It is also a good device for measuring core body temperature because the tympanic membrane is supplied by a tributary of the artery (internal carotid) that supplies the hypothalamus (the body's thermoregulatory center).

Continued on following page

130   UNIT 2 Integrative Holistic Nursing Assessment

ASSESSMENT PROCEDURE	NORMAL FINDINGS	ABNORMAL FINDINGS
Vital Signs (Continued)		
To measure oral temperature, use an electronic thermometer with a disposable protective probe cover. Then place the thermometer under the client's tongue to the right or left of the frenulum deep in the posterior sublingual pocket (Fig. 8-4). Ask the client to close his or her lips around the probe. Hold the probe until you hear a beep. Remove the probe and dispose of its cover by pressing the release button. Electronic thermometers give a digital reading in about 10 seconds or less.	Oral temperature is 35.9–37.5°C (96.6–99.5°F).	Oral temperature is below 35.9°C (96.6°F) or over 37.5°C (99.5°F).

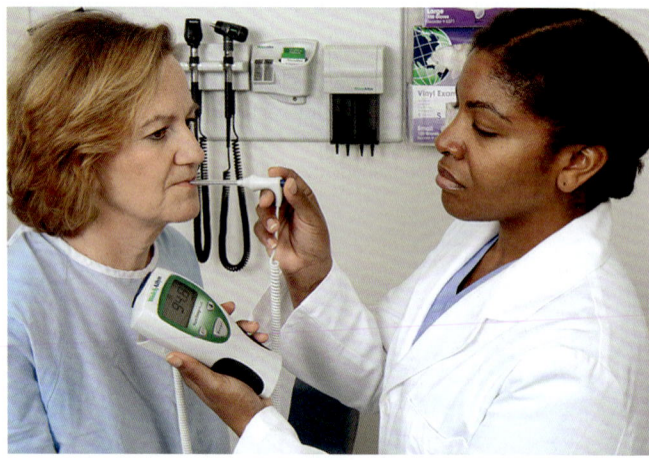

FIGURE 8-4 Taking an oral temperature.

To measure axillary temperature, hold the glass or electronic thermometer under the axilla firmly by having the client hold the arm down and across the chest for 10 minutes (Fig. 8-5).	The axillary temperature is 0.5°C (1°F) lower than the oral temperature. Normal axillary temperature range is 35.4–37.0°C (95.6–98.5°F).	Axillary temperature below 35.4°C (95.6°F) or above 37.0°C (98.5°F).

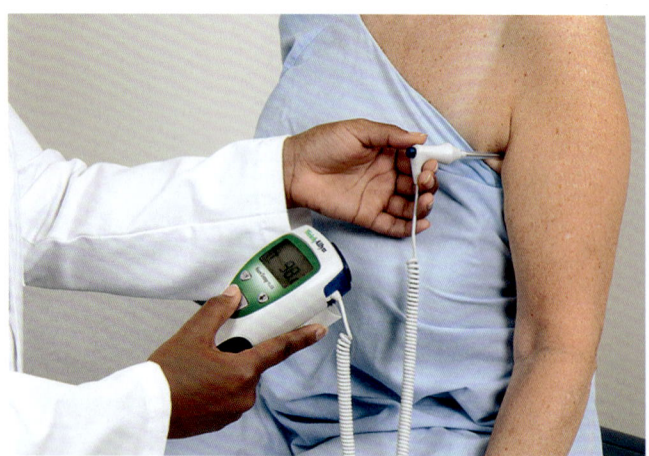

FIGURE 8-5 Taking an axillary temperature.

ASSESSMENT PROCEDURE	NORMAL FINDINGS	ABNORMAL FINDINGS
To measure temporal arterial temperature, remove the protective cap from the thermometer. Place the thermometer over the client's forehead and while pressing the scan button, gently stroke the thermometer across the client's forehead over the temporal artery to a point directly behind the ear (Fig. 8-6). You will hear beeping and a red light will blink to indicate a measurement is taking place. Release the scan button and remove the thermometer from the forehead. Read the temperature on the display.	The temporal artery temperature is approximately 0.4°C (0.8°F) higher than axillary (Haddad et al., 2012). Normal temporal artery temperature range is 36.3–37.9°C (97.4–100.3°F).	Temporal artery temperature below 36.3°C (97.4°F) or above 37.9°C (100.3°F).

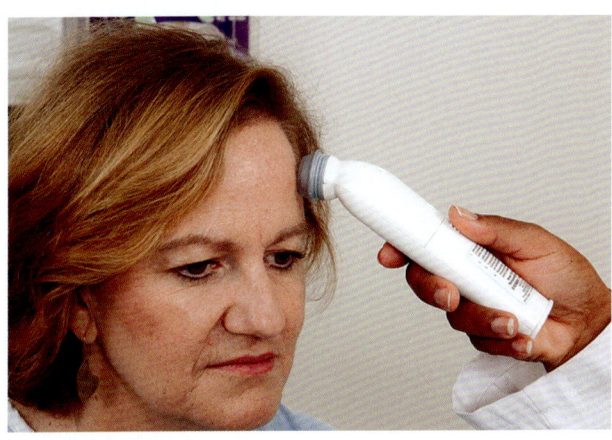

FIGURE 8-6 Taking a temporal artery temperature.

> **CLINICAL TIP**
> A temporal artery thermometry uses a noninvasive device that the operator sweeps from the center of the forehead to a point behind the ear. Temperature measurement takes approximately 6 seconds. The infrared scanner in the device takes multiple readings that result in a calculated value.

To measure rectal temperature, cover the glass thermometer with a disposable, sterile sheath, and lubricate the thermometer. Wear gloves, and insert thermometer 1 in into rectum. Hold a glass thermometer in place for 3 minutes; hold an electronic thermometer in place until the temperature appears in the display window.	The rectal temperature is between 0.4°C and 0.5°C (0.7°F and 1°F) higher than the normal oral temperature. Normal rectal temperature range is 36.3°–37.9°C (97.4–100.3°F).	Rectal temperature below 36.3°C (97.4°F) or above 37.9°C (100.3°F).

> **SAFETY TIP** *Use this route only if other routes are not practical (e.g., client cannot cooperate, is comatose, cannot close mouth, or tympanic thermometer is unavailable. Never force the thermometer into the rectum and never use a rectal thermometer for clients with severe coagulation disorders, recent rectal, anal, vaginal or prostate surgeries, diarrhea, hemorrhoids, colitis, or fecal impaction.*

Continued on following page

ASSESSMENT PROCEDURE	NORMAL FINDINGS	ABNORMAL FINDINGS
Vital Signs (Continued)		
MEASURE PULSE RATE		
Measure the radial pulse rate. Use the pads of your first (index) and second (middle) fingers and lightly palpate the radial artery on the lateral aspect of the client's wrist (Fig. 8-7). Count the number of beats you feel for 15 seconds and multiply by 4 or for 30 seconds and multiply by 2 if the pulse rhythm is regular. Multiply by 2 to get the rate. Count for a full minute if the rhythm is irregular. Then, verify by taking an apical pulse as well.	A pulse rate ranging from 60 to 100 beats/min is normal for adults. Tachycardia may be normal in clients who have just finished strenuous exercise. Bradycardia may be normal in well-conditioned athletes.	**Tachycardia** is a rate greater than 100 beats/min. May occur with fever, certain medications, stress, and other abnormal states, such as cardiac dysrhythmias. **Bradycardia** is a rate less than 60 beats/min. Sitting or standing for long periods may cause the blood to pool and decrease the pulse rate. Heart block or dropped beats can also manifest as bradycardia. Perform cardiac auscultation of the apical pulse if the client exhibits any abnormal findings (see Chapter 21 for more detail).

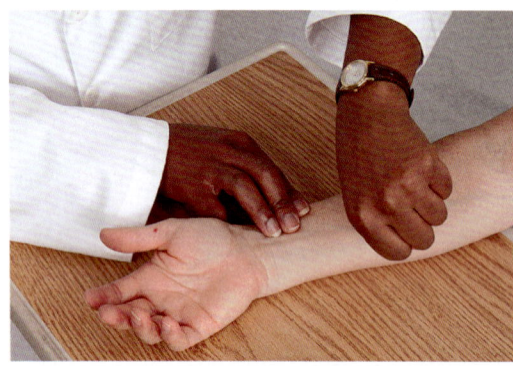

FIGURE 8-7 Timing the radial pulse rate.

Evaluate pulse rhythm. Palpate the pulse with the tips of the first two fingers feeling for each beat. Evaluate beats for regularity (equal length of time between each beat) or irregularity (unequal length of time between beats).	There are regular intervals between beats.	Perform auscultation of the apical pulse if the client exhibits irregular intervals between beats (see Chapter 21). When describing irregular beats, indicate whether they are regularly irregular or irregularly irregular. Regular rhythm is present when there is an equal amount of time between beats. An irregular rhythm may be regularly irregular or irregularly irregular. A regularly irregular pulse would be one that follows a pattern of variation while an irregularly irregular pulse follows no pattern.
Assess pulse amplitude and contour.	Normally, pulsation is equally strong in both wrists. Upstroke is smooth and rapid with a more gradual downstroke.	A bounding or weak and thready pulse is abnormal. Delayed upstroke is also abnormal. Follow up on abnormal amplitude and contour findings by palpating the carotid arteries, which provides the best assessment of amplitude and contour (see Chapter 21).
Palpate arterial elasticity.	Artery feels straight, resilient, and springy. **OLDER ADULT CONSIDERATIONS** The older client's artery may feel more rigid, hard, and bent.	Artery feels rigid.
MEASURE RESPIRATIONS		
Monitor the respiratory rate. Observe the client's chest rise and fall with each breath. Count respirations for 30 seconds and multiply by 2 (refer to Chapter 19 for more information). 🎯 **CLINICAL TIP** If you place the client's arm across the chest while palpating the pulse, you can also count respirations. Do this by keeping your fingers on the client's pulse even after you have finished taking it.	Between 12 and 20 breaths/min is normal. **OLDER ADULT CONSIDERATIONS** In the older adult, the respiratory rate may range from 15 to 22. The rate may increase with a shallower inspiratory phase because vital capacity and inspiratory reserve volume decrease with aging.	Fewer than 12 breaths/min or more than 20 breaths/min is abnormal.

ASSESSMENT PROCEDURE	NORMAL FINDINGS	ABNORMAL FINDINGS
Observe respiratory rhythm.	Rhythm is regular (if irregular, count for 1 full minute).	Rhythm is irregular (see Chapter 19 for more detail).
Observe respiratory depth.	There is equal bilateral chest expansion of 1–2 in.	Unequal, shallow, or extremely deep chest expansion (see Chapter 19 for more detail) and labored or gasping breaths are abnormal.

MEASURE BLOOD PRESSURE

Measure blood pressure. Assessment Guide 8-1 and Table 8-1 provide guidelines. Measure on dominant arm first. Take blood pressure in both arms when recording it for the first time. Take subsequent readings in arm with highest measurement. 🎯 **CLINICAL TIP** Advise client to avoid nicotine and caffeine for 30 minutes prior to measurement. Ask client to empty bladder before evaluating and avoid talking to the client while taking the reading. Each of these prevents elevating blood pressure prior to/during reading (Mayo Clinic, 2015).	Systolic pressure is <120 mmHg. Diastolic pressure is <80 mmHg; varies with individuals. A pressure difference of 10 mmHg between arms is normal.	Tables 8-2 through 8-4 provide blood pressure classifications and recommended follow-up criteria. More than a 10-mmHg pressure difference between arms may indicate coarctation of the aorta or cardiac disease. 🪑 **OLDER ADULT CONSIDERATIONS** More rigid, arteriosclerotic arteries account for higher systolic blood pressure in older adults. Systolic pressure over 140 but diastolic pressure under 90 is called isolated systolic hypertension.
If the client takes antihypertensive medications or has a history of fainting or dizziness, assess for possible orthostatic hypotension. Measure blood pressure and pulse with the client in a standing or sitting position after measuring the blood pressure with the client in a supine position. **SAFETY TIP** *An ill client may not be able to stand; sitting is usually adequate to detect if the client truly has orthostatic hypotension.*	A drop of less than 20 mmHg from recorded sitting position is normal.	A drop of 20 mmHg or more from the recorded sitting blood pressure may indicate orthostatic (postural) hypotension. Pulse will increase to accommodate the drop in blood pressure. Orthostatic hypotension may be related to a decreased baroreceptor sensitivity, fluid volume deficit (e.g., dehydration), or certain medications (i.e., diuretics, antihypertensives). Symptoms of orthostatic hypotension include dizziness, lightheadedness, and falling. Further evaluation and referral to the client's primary care provider are necessary.
Assess the pulse pressure, which is the difference between the systolic and diastolic blood pressure levels. Record findings in mmHg. For example, if the blood pressure was 120/80, then the pulse pressure would be 120 minus 80 or 40 mmHg.	Pulse pressure is 30–50 mmHg. 🪑 **OLDER ADULT CONSIDERATIONS** **Widening of the pulse pressure is seen with aging due to less elastic peripheral arteries.**	A pulse pressure lower than 30 mmHg or higher than 50 mmHg may indicate cardiovascular disease.

ASSESS PAIN

Observe comfort level.	Client assumes a relatively relaxed posture without excessive position shifting. Facial expression is alert and pleasant.	Facial expression indicates discomfort (grimacing, frowning). Client may brace or hold a body part that is painful. Breathing pattern indicates distress (e.g., shortness of breath, shallow, rapid breathing).
Ask the client if he or she has any pain.	No subjective report of pain.	Explore any subjective report of pain using the mnemonic COLDSPA. Refer to Chapter 9 for further assessment of pain.

TABLE 8-1 Identifying Korotkoff Sounds

Phase	Description
I	Phase I is characterized by the first appearance of faint, clear, repetitive tapping sounds that gradually intensify for at least two consecutive beats. This coincides approximately with the resumption of a palpable pulse. The number on the pressure gauge at which you hear the first tapping sound is the systolic pressure.
II	Phase II is characterized as muffled or swishing; these sounds are softer and longer than phase I sounds. They also have the quality of an intermittent murmur. They may temporarily subside, especially in hypertensive people. The loss of the sound during the latter part of phase I and during phase II is called the auscultatory gap. The gap may cover a range of as much as 40 mmHg; failing to recognize this gap may cause serious errors of underestimating systolic pressure or overestimating diastolic pressure.
III	Phase III is characterized by a return of distinct, crisp, and louder sounds as the blood flows relatively freely through an increasingly open artery.
IV	Phase IV is characterized by sounds that are muffled, less distinct, and softer (with a blowing quality).
V	It is characterized by all sounds disappearing completely. The last sound heard before this period of continuous silence is the onset of phase V and is the pressure commonly considered to define the diastolic measurement. (Some clinicians still consider the last sounds of phase IV the first diastolic value.)

> **CLINICAL TIP**
> The American Heart Association recommends that values in phase IV and phase V be recorded when both a change in the sounds and a cessation in the sounds occur.
> These recommendations apply particularly to children under age 13, pregnant women, and clients with high cardiac output or peripheral vasodilation. For example, such a blood pressure would be recorded as 120/80/64.

Adapted from Taylor, C., Lillis, C., Lynn, P., et al. (2015). *Fundamentals of nursing: The art and science of person-centered nursing care* (8th ed.). Philadelphia, PA: Wolters Kluwer Heath | Lippincott Williams & Wilkins.

ASSESSMENT GUIDE 8-1 Measuring Blood Pressure

Preparation
Before measuring the blood pressure, consider the following behavioral and environmental conditions that can affect the reading:
- Room temperature too hot or cold
- Recent exercise
- Alcohol intake
- Nicotine use
- Muscle tension
- Bladder distension
- Background noise
- Talking (either client or nurse)
- Arm position

Steps for Measuring Blood Pressure
1. Assemble your equipment so that the sphygmomanometer, stethoscope, and your pen and recording sheet are within easy reach.

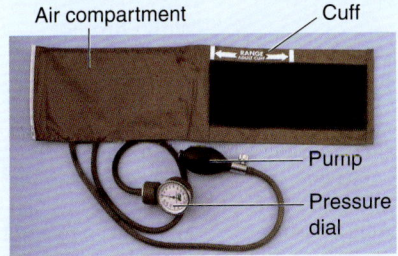

A sphygmomanometer, or blood pressure cuff.

   Assist the client into a comfortable, quiet, restful position for 5–10 minutes. Client may lie down or sit.
2. Remove client's clothing from the arm and palpate the pulsations of the brachial artery. (If the client's sleeve can be pushed up to make room for the cuff, make sure that the clothing is not so constrictive that it would alter a correct pressure reading.)
3. Place the blood pressure cuff so that the midline of the bladder is over the arterial pulsation, and wrap the appropriate-sized cuff smoothly and snugly around the upper arm, 1 in above the antecubital area so that there is enough room to place the bell of the stethoscope. The bladder inside the cuff should encircle 80% of the arm circumference in adults and 100% of the arm circumference in children younger than age 13 years. A cuff that is too small may give a false or abnormally high blood pressure reading. An aneroid or mercury sphygmomanometer can be used; however, many areas have prohibited the use of mercury-containing devices and instead use electronic blood pressure cuffs.
4. Support the client's arm slightly flexed at heart level with the palm up.
5. Put the earpieces of the stethoscope in your ears, then palpate the brachial pulse again and place the stethoscope lightly over this area. Position the mercury gauge on the manometer at eye level.
6. Adjust the screw above the bulb to tighten the valve on the air pump, and make sure that the tubing is not kinked or obstructed.
7. Inflate the cuff by pumping the bulb to about 30 mmHg above the point at which the radial pulse disappears. This will help you avoid missing an auscultatory gap.
8. Deflate the cuff slowly—about 2 mm per second—by turning the valve in the opposite direction while listening for the first of Korotkoff sounds.

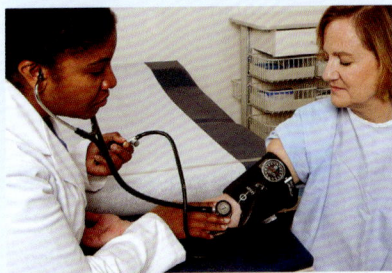

Once the cuff is inflated, the examiner releases the pressure and listens for sounds in the vessels with a stethoscope.

   Read the point, closest to an even number, on the mercury gauge at which you hear the first faint but clear sound. Record this number as the systolic blood pressure. This is phase I of Korotkoff sounds.
9. Next, note the point, closest to an even number, on the mercury gauge at which the sound becomes muffled (phase IV of Korotkoff sounds). Finally, note the point at which the sound subsides completely (phase V of Korotkoff sounds). When both a change in sounds and a cessation of the sounds are heard, record the numbers at which you hear phase I, IV, and V sounds. Otherwise, record the first and last sounds.
10. Deflate the cuff at least another 10 mmHg to make sure you hear no more sounds. Then deflate completely and remove.
11. Record readings to the nearest 2 mmHg.

Cuff Selection Guidelines
The "ideal" cuff should have a bladder length that is 80% and a width that is at least 40% of the arm circumference (a length-to-width ratio of 2:1). A recent study comparing intra-arterial and auscultatory blood pressure concluded that the error is minimized with a cuff of 46% of the arm circumference. The recommended cuff sizes are:
- 12 × 22 cm for arm circumference of 22–26 cm, which is the "small adult" size
- 16 × 30 cm for arm circumference of 27–34 cm, which is the "adult" size
- 16 × 36 cm for arm circumference of 35–44 cm, which is the "large adult" size
- 16 × 42 cm for arm circumference of 45–52 cm, which is the "adult thigh" size

Summary Points for Clinical Blood Pressure Measurement
- The patient should be seated comfortably, with the back supported and the upper arm bared, without constrictive clothing. The legs should not be crossed.
- The arm should be supported at heart level, and the bladder of the cuff should encircle at least 80% of the arm circumference.
- The mercury column should be deflated at 2 to 3 mm per second; the first and last audible sounds should be taken as systolic and diastolic pressure. The column should be read to the nearest 2 mmHg.
- Neither the patient nor the observer should talk during the measurement.

From Vidt, D. (2010). Taking blood pressure: Too important to trust to humans? *Cleveland Clinic Journal of Medicine, 77*(10), 683–688. Used with permission.

TABLE 8-2 Changes in Blood Pressure Classification[a]

JNC 6 Category	SBP/DBP	JNC 7 Category
Optimal	<120/80	Normal
Normal	120–129/80–84	Prehypertension
Borderline	130–139/85–89	Prehypertension
Hypertension	≥140/90	Hypertension
Stage 1	140–159/90–99	Stage 1
Stage 2	160–179/100–109	Stage 2[0]
Stage 3	≥180/110	Stage 2[0]

Sources: The Sixth Report of the Joint National Committee on Prevention, Detection, Evaluation and Treatment of High Blood Pressure (1997). *Archives of Internal Medicine*, 157, 2413–2446; and The Seventh Report of the Joint National Committee on Prevention, Detection, Evaluation and Treatment of High Blood Pressure (2003). *Journal of the American Medical Association*, 289, 2560–2571.

[a]According to Krakoff et al. (2014), a report of the Eighth Joint National Committee on Prevention, Detection, Evaluation, and Treatment of High Blood Pressure has resulted in much controversy due to the recommendation to consider BP of 140 mmHg/90 mmHg as hypertension for those between 60 and 80 years of age, and to begin pharmacological treatment to lower BP at a systolic of 150 mmHg. Among others, Krakoff et al. strongly disagree with the new 2014 recommendation, because the recommended change places high-risk older women, especially African Americans, at unnecessary excessive risk, and would magnify the existing sex and racial/ethnic disparities in cardiovascular disease. Table 8-3 shows the various organizations and recommendations for determining hypertension and for initiating pharmacological treatment. The controversy continues.

TABLE 8-3 Various Recommendations for Diagnosing and Treating Hypertension

SOURCE	Recommended Threshold for Hypertension Diagnosis — Patients <60 Years Old	Patients ≥60 Years Old	Recommended Blood Pressure Treatment Goals — With Diabetes	With Chronic Renal Failure	Elderly Patients >80 Years Old	Recommended Management for Patients with Diabetes — Without Chronic Renal Disease	With Chronic Renal Disease or Proteinuria
ASH/ISH 2014	140 systolic/90 diastolic mmHg	140/90	140/90	140/90 <150/90 is appropriate for >80 years old	<150/90	Angiotensin converting enzyme inhibitor or Angiotensin receptor blocker	Angiotensin converting enzyme inhibitor or Angiotensin receptor blocker
ADA 2013	140/80	140/80	140/80	140/80	Not stated	Angiotensin converting enzyme inhibitor or Angiotensin receptor blocker	Angiotensin converting enzyme inhibitor or Angiotensin receptor blocker
AHA/ACC Go et al. 2013	140/90	140/90	140/90	140/90	Not stated	Thiazide+	Not stated
ESC/ESH 2013	140/90	140/90	140/90	140/90	<150/90	Any class	Angiotensin converting enzyme inhibitor or Angiotensin receptor blocker+
JNC-8P 2013	140/90	150/90	140/90 for <60 years old <150/90 for older patients	140/90 for <60 years old <150/90 for older patients	<150/90	Any class	Angiotensin converting enzyme inhibitor or Angiotensin receptor blocker+
AHA/ACC Elderly 2011	140/90	140/90	<130/80	<130/80	<140–145 if tolerated, avoid low diastolic pressures	Not stated	Angiotensin converting enzyme inhibitor or Angiotensin receptor blocker+
JNC-7 2003	140/90	140/90	<130/80	<130/80	<140/90	Angiotensin converting enzyme inhibitor or Angiotensin receptor blocker+	Angiotensin converting enzyme inhibitor or Angiotensin receptor blocker+

TABLE 8-4 Recommendations for Follow-Up Based on Initial Blood Pressure Measurements for Adults without Acute End-Organ Damage

Initial Blood Pressure, mmHg[a]	Follow-Up Recommended[b]
Normal	Recheck in 2 years
Prehypertension	Recheck in 1 year[c]
Stage 1 hypertension	Confirm within 2 months[c]
Stage 2 hypertension	Evaluate or refer to source of care within 1 month. For those with higher pressures (e.g., >180/110 mmHg), evaluate and treat immediately or within 1 week depending on clinical situation and complications.

[a]If systolic and diastolic categories are different, follow recommendations for shorter time follow-up (e.g., 160/86 mmHg should be evaluated or referred to source of care within 1 month).
[b]Modify the scheduling of follow-up according to reliable information about past BP measurements, other cardiovascular risk factors, or target organ disease.
[c]Provide advice about lifestyle modifications.
From National High Blood Pressure Education Program; National Heart, Lung, and Blood Institute; National Institutes of Health. Available at http://www.nhlbi.nih.gov/files/docs/guidelines/express.pdf.

The chapter case study demonstrates a physical assessment of Mr. Anthony's general status and vital signs.

CASE STUDY

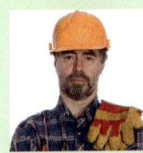

After asking Mr. Anthony to put on a gown and leaving the room while he does so, the nurse returns to perform a physical examination. Mr. Anthony's posture is somewhat slumped. Disheveled, male, dressed in soiled work clothes; however, attire is appropriate for summer season and occupation. Malodorous (from sweat) and diaphoretic. Well-developed body build for age; however, he appears to be much older than he states. There is even distribution of fat and firm muscles. His skin is warm and moist without erythema. Client is alert and cooperative, answering questions with good eye contact. Smiles and laughs appropriately. Speech is fluent, clear, and moderately paced. Thoughts are free flowing. Able to recall events earlier in day (e.g., what he had for breakfast) without difficulty.

Vital Signs: Oral temperature: 101.2°F; radial pulse: 118/min regular, bilateral, equally thready, and weak; respirations: 22/min regular, equal bilateral chest expansion; blood pressure: sitting position—102/52 right arm, 98/48 left arm; standing position—80/40, RA; 78/42, LA.

Validating and Documenting Findings

Validate the assessment data you have collected by asking additional questions, verifying data with another health care professional, or comparing objective with subjective findings. This is necessary to verify that the data are reliable and accurate. Document the assessment data following the health care facility or agency policy.

CASE STUDY

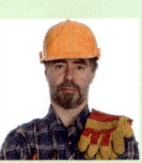

Think back to the case study. The nurse documented the following assessment findings of Mr. Anthony:
Biographic Data: Mr. Anthony states age is 34 years, weight is 160 lb and height is 5 ft 10 in. BMI = 23.0 (Ideal weight).
Reason for Seeking Care: Fever, fatigue, a rapid heart rate and dizziness.
History of Present Health Concern: Over the past 3 days he has been running a fever with chills and sweats, occurring three times a day, lasting for several hours each day. Is unsure of actual temperature as he does not own a thermometer. Fever and chills relieved with two extra-strength Tylenol tablets, but returns in 4 hours. Feels fatigued and is not able to continue with ADL's.
Personal Health History: He is unaware of his usual baseline vital signs including blood pressure because he has not sought health care in several years. He last checked his blood pressure in Walmart 3 years ago, but he cannot recall the results. He does not take any routine medications but does take Tylenol, two extra-strength tablets, as needed for headache. His last dose of Tylenol for fever and chills was just before coming to the clinic. He denies any known allergies to medications or foods, but does report that he is allergic to mold.
Family History: Positive family history for hypertension and diabetes in his father, who died at age 84. His mother has died at age 70 with breast cancer. His older sister is alive and well, with no current health problems. He is not married and has no children.
Lifestyle and Health Practices: He has been working 12 hours daily in intense heat. He has been avoiding taking trips to the water cooler because he is working on the roof and the water cooler is down on the ground. He has a high school diploma and is satisfied with his family life. He has not been seen by a doctor in over 5 years. He denies any current or former use of any form

of tobacco product or any illicit drugs. He does drink one or two beers every night and has for several years. Mr. Anthony denies any special diet or exercise routine but does state that he gets regular exercise when working by hammering, lifting, walking, and climbing.

Physical Examination Findings: Posture is somewhat slumped. Disheveled, male, dressed in soiled work clothes; however, attire is appropriate for summer season and occupation. Malodorous (from sweat) and diaphoretic. Well-developed body build for age; however, he appears to be much older than he states. There is even distribution of fat and firm muscles. His skin is warm and moist without erythema. Client is alert and cooperative, answering questions with good eye contact. Smiles and laughs appropriately. Speech is fluent, clear, and moderately paced. Thoughts are free flowing. Short-term memory intact. Able to recall events earlier in day (e.g., what he had for breakfast) without difficulty.

Vital Signs: Oral temperature: 101.2°F; radial pulse: 118/min regular, bilateral, equally thready and weak; respirations: 22/min regular, equal bilateral chest expansion; blood pressure: sitting position—102/52 right arm, 98/48 left arm; standing position—80/40, RA; 78/42, LA.

ANALYSIS OF DATA: DIAGNOSTIC REASONING

After collecting subjective and objective data pertaining to general survey and vital signs, identify abnormal findings and client strengths using diagnostic reasoning. Then cluster the data to reveal any significant patterns or abnormalities. These data may then be used to make clinical judgments about the client.

The following sections provide possible conclusions that the nurse may make after performing a general survey and vital signs assessment on a client.

Selected Nursing Diagnoses

The following is a listing of selected nursing diagnoses that you may identify when analyzing data for this part of the assessment.

Health Promotion Diagnoses

- Readiness for enhanced health management related to desire and request to learn more about health promotion

Risk Diagnoses

- Risk for imbalanced body temperature related to febrile illness
- Risk for self-directed violence, related to depression, suicidal tendencies, developmental crisis, lack of support systems, loss of significant others, poor coping mechanisms and behaviors
- Risk for falls related to orthostatic hypotension
- Risk for ineffective health maintenance related to knowledge deficit of effects of dehydration

Actual Diagnoses

- Impaired verbal communication related to international language barrier (inability to speak English or accepted dominant language)
- Impaired verbal communication related to hearing loss
- Impaired verbal communication related to inability to clearly express self or understand others (aphasia)
- Impaired walking related to deconditioning (inability to climb stairs) after illness
- Acute pain related to tissue inflammation and injury
- Dressing/grooming self-care deficit related to impaired upper-extremity mobility and lack of resources
- Bathing/hygiene self-care deficit related to inability to wash body parts or inability to obtain water

Selected Collaborative Problems

After you group the data, it may become apparent that certain collaborative problems emerge. Remember that collaborative problems differ from nursing diagnoses in that they cannot be prevented by nursing interventions. However, these physiologic complications of medical conditions can be detected and monitored by the nurse. In addition, the nurse can use physician- and nurse-prescribed interventions to minimize the complications of these problems. The nurse may also have to refer the client in such situations for further treatment of the problem. Following is a list of collaborative problems that may be identified when obtaining a general impression. These problems are worded as Risk for Complications (RC), followed by the problem.

- RC: Hypertension
- RC: Hypotension
- RC: Dysrhythmias
- RC: Hyperthermia
- RC: Hypothermia
- RC: Tachycardia
- RC: Bradycardia
- RC: Dyspnea
- RC: Hypoxemia

Medical Problems

After you group the data, it may become apparent that the client has signs and symptoms that require medical diagnosis and treatment. Refer to a primary care provider as necessary.

For the chapter case study, the nurse uses diagnostic reasoning to analyze the data collected on Mr. Anthony, including general status and vital signs to arrive at the following possible conclusions.

CASE STUDY

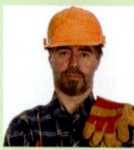

The nurse determines that the following conclusions are appropriate.

Nursing Diagnoses
- Ineffective health maintenance r/t lack of knowledge of dangers of dehydration
- Risk for deficient fluid volume r/t 12-hour daily work in intense heat

Potential Collaborative Problems
- RC: Shock syndrome
- RC: Dysrhythmias
- RC: Hypoxemia

To view an algorithm depicting the process of diagnostic reasoning for this case, go to thePoint.

Interdisciplinary Verbal Communication of Assessment Findings Using SBAR

SITUATION: Thomas Anthony comes to the local urgent care center reporting a rapid heart rate and a feeling that his heart is skipping a beat, dizziness when going from a sitting to standing position, and fever, chills, sweats for 3 days somewhat relieved with Tylenol. Very fatigued. Concerned about being unable to go to work today and effects on his finances.

BACKGROUND: He is a 34-year-old single male, Caucasian construction worker. Unaware of his usual baseline vital signs. Positive family history for hypertension and diabetes through his father. Employed as a roofer working 12 hours daily in intense heat. Avoids trips to the water cooler because he is on roof and water cooler is down on ground. He drinks one or two beers every night for several years. Has not seen doctor in over 5 years.

ASSESSMENT: Weight is 160 lb and height is 5 ft 10 in. BMI = 23. Oral temperature: 101.2°F; radial pulse: 118/min regular, bilateral, equally thready and weak; respirations: 22/min regular, equal bilateral chest expansion; blood pressure: sitting position—102/52 right arm, 98/48 left arm; standing position—80/40, RA; 78/42, LA.

RECOMMENDATION: I believe Mr. Anthony has ineffective health maintenance related to his lack of knowledge of dehydration dangers and is at risk for deficient fluid volume related to his 12-hour daily roofing work in intense heat. He needs to be further evaluated for dehydration, shock, and his reported dysrhythmias.

ABNORMAL FINDINGS 8-1 | **Deviations Related to Physical Development, Body Build, and Fat Distribution**

DWARFISM
These images show the associated decreased height and skeletal malformations.

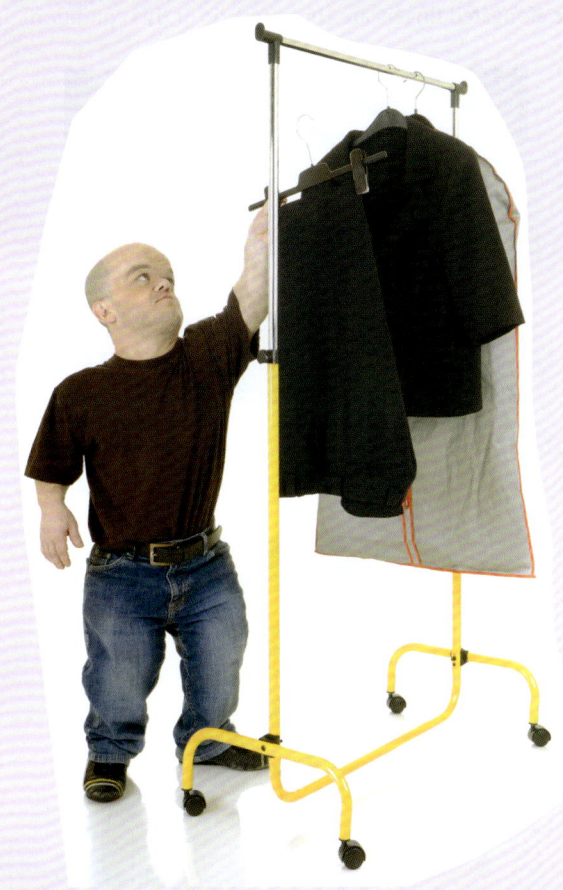

GIGANTISM
Note the disparity in height between the affected person and a person of the same age.

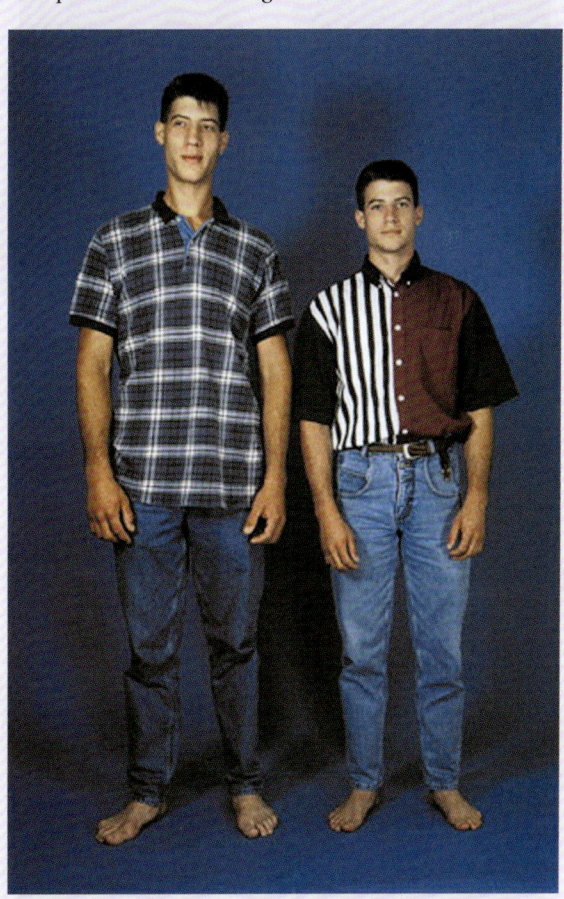

Continued on following page

ABNORMAL FINDINGS 8-1 Deviations Related to Physical Development, Body Build, and Fat Distribution (Continued)

ACROMEGALY
The affected client shows the characteristic overgrowth of bones in the face, head, and hands.

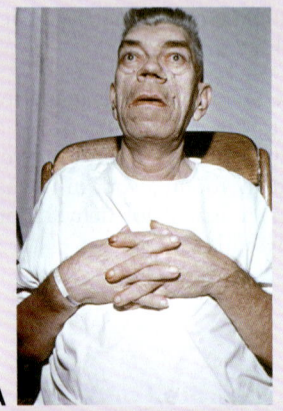
A

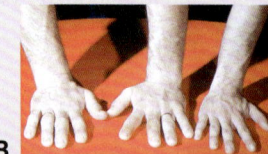
B

ANOREXIA NERVOSA
The client shows the emaciated appearance that follows self-starvation and accompanying extreme weight loss.

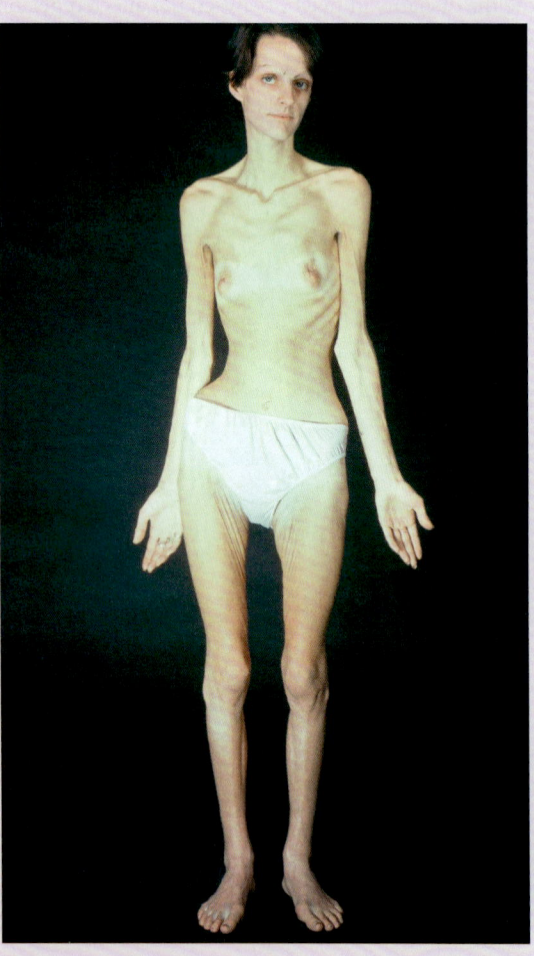

OBESITY
Obesity is defined as having an excessive amount of body fat. It increases the risk of diseases and health problems such as heart disease, diabetes, and high blood pressure (Mayo Clinic, 2012).

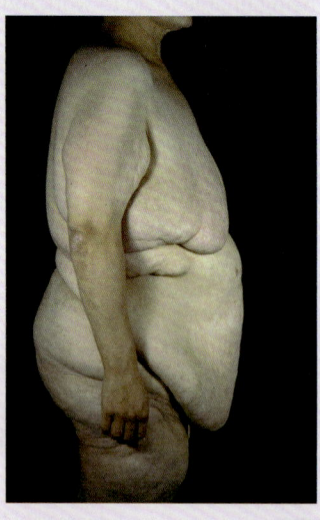

MARFAN SYNDROME
The elongated fingers are characteristic of this condition.

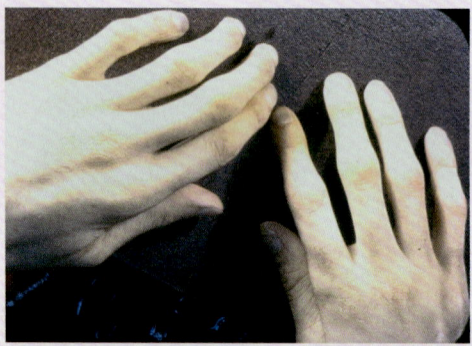

CUSHING SYNDROME
The affected client reflects the centralized weight gain.

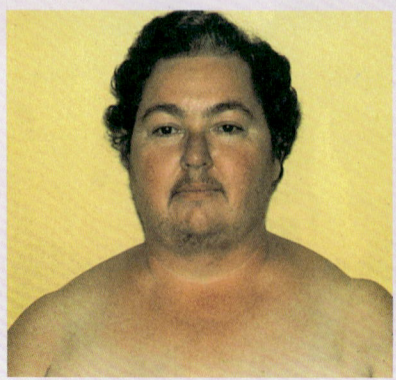

> **Want to know more?**
>
> A wide variety of resources to enhance your learning and understanding of this book are available on thePoint. Visit thePoint to access:
>
> NCLEX-Style Student Review Questions   Concepts in Action Animations
> Watch and Learn Videos   And more!

References and Selected Readings

Haddad, L., Smith, S., Phillips, K., et al. (2012). Comparison of temporal artery and axillary temperatures in healthy newborns. *Journal of Obstetric & Gynecological Neonatal Nursing*, 41(3), 383–388. doi: 10.1111/j.1552-6909.2012.01367.x Available at http://www.ncbi.nlm.nih.gov/pubmed/22834884

Krakoff, L., Gillespie R., Ferdinand, K., et al. (2014). 2014 hypertension recommendations from the Eighth Joint National Committee panel members raise concerns for elderly black and female populations. *Journal of the American College of Cardiology*, 64(4), 394–402. doi: 10.1016/j.jacc.2014.06.014. Available at http://content.onlinejacc.org/article.aspx?articleID=1889491

Lorenz, K. A., Sherbourne, C. D., Shugarman, L. R., et al. (2009). How reliable is pain as the fifth vital sign? *Journal of the American Board of Family Medicine*, 22(3), 291–298. Available at http://jabfm.org/content/22/3/291.full.pdf+html

Lu, S., Leasure, A., & Dai, Y. (2010). A systematic review of body temperature variations in older people. *Journal of Clinical Nursing*, 19(1–2), 4–16. Abstract available at http://www.ncbi.nlm.nih.gov/pubmed/19886869

Mayo Clinic. (2012). Obesity. Available at http://www.mayoclinic.com [search by subject]

Mayo Clinic. (2013). Acromegaly. Available at http://www.mayoclinic.org/diseases-conditions/acromegaly/basics/definition/con-2001921

Mayo Clinic. (2015). Blood pressure test. Available at http://www.mayoclinic.org/tests-procedures/blood-pressure-test/basics/how-you-prepare/prc-20020082

MedicineNet.com. (2014). Achondroplasia. Available at https://www.google.com/webhp?sourceid=chrome-instant&ion=1&espv=2&ie=UTF-8#q=achondroplasi

The Marfan Foundation. (2014). Bones and joints. Available at https://www.marfan.org/about/body-systems/skeleton-and-joints

Medline Plus. (2010). Marfan's syndrome. Available at http://www.nlm.nih.gov/medlineplus/ency/article/000418.htm

Swartz, M. (2014). *Textbook of physical diagnosis: History and examination*. Philadelphia: PA: Elsevier/Saunders.

9 ASSESSING PAIN: THE FIFTH VITAL SIGN

Learning Objectives

1. Explain the pathophysiology of pain.
2. Differentiate between the etiology of acute and chronic pain.
3. Discuss the various physiologic responses to pain.
4. Assess pain as the fifth vital sign.
5. Interview a client for their subjective experience of pain.
6. Perform a physical assessment of a client experiencing pain.
7. Analyze subjective and objective data of a client experiencing pain to formulate valid nursing diagnoses, collaborative problems, and/or referrals.

CASE STUDY

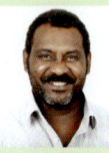

Leonard Blair is an African American, 55-year-old man. He is divorced with two children and works as a financial manager. Two years ago, he experienced dysuria and difficulty starting a stream and went to the clinic, where a PSA among other tests was performed. His PSA was elevated; he was referred for biopsy and was diagnosed with prostate cancer. Mr. Blair underwent prostatectomy followed by cycles of radiation and chemotherapy 1 year ago. For the past 8 to 10 months, he has complained of continuous low back pain and leg pain that becomes worse at night and while walking. Mr. Blair's case will be discussed throughout the chapter.

CONCEPTUAL FOUNDATIONS

The International Association for the Study of Pain (IASP) has defined pain as "an unpleasant sensory and emotional experience, which we primarily associate with tissue damage or describe in terms of such damage" (International Association for the Study of Pain, 2011). The **most important** definition of pain as it is experienced is that by McCaffery and Pasero (1999): "Pain is whatever the person says it is." It is important to remember this definition when assessing and treating pain.

Recent literature has emphasized the importance and undertreatment of pain, and has recommended that pain be considered the fifth vital sign. Some states have passed laws necessitating the adoption of an assessment tool and documenting pain assessment in client records, along with temperature, pulse, heart rate, and blood pressure (see Chapter 8). In addition, the Joint Commission has established standards for pain assessment and management (Box 9-1). Inadequate treatment of acute pain has been shown to result in physiologic, psychological, and emotional distress that can lead to chronic pain (Dunwoody et al., 2008). Healthy People has added a new topic for 2020 that includes pain as it affects "Health-Related Quality of Life and Well-Being." Health-related quality of life (HRQoL) is defined by Healthy People 2020 as "a multidimensional concept that includes domains related to physical, mental, emotional, and social functioning. It goes beyond direct measures of population health, life expectancy, and causes of death, and focuses on the impact health status has on quality of life. A related concept of HRQoL is well-being, which assesses the positive aspects of a person's life, such as positive emotions and life satisfaction." Well-being is a relative state in which a person maximizes his or her physical, mental, and social functioning in the context of supportive environments to live a full, satisfying, and productive life (Healthy People 2020, 2015). The effect of pain on HRQoL and related Healthy People 2020 goals will be included in this topic as it is developed.

By contrast, in its recommendation for or against screening of pain, the US Preventive Services Task Force (USPSTF, 2011) has found insufficient evidence to recommend for or against the routine use of interventions to prevent low back pain in adults in primary care settings.

Pain is a combination of physiologic phenomena but with psychosocial aspects that influence perception of the pain.

Pathophysiology

The pathophysiologic phenomena of pain are associated with the central and peripheral nervous systems. The source of pain stimulates peripheral nerve endings (**nociceptors**), which transmit the sensations to the central nervous system (CNS). They are sensory receptors that detect signals from damaged tissue and chemicals released from the damaged tissue (Dafny, 1997–present). Nociceptors are located at the peripheral ends of both myelinated nerve endings of type A fibers or unmyelinated type C fibers. There are three types that are stimulated by different stimuli: mechanosensitive nociceptors (of A-delta fibers), sensitive to intense mechanical stimulation (e.g., pliers pinching skin); temperature-sensitive (thermosensitive) nociceptors (of A-delta fibers), sensitive to intense heat and cold;

> **BOX 9-1 JOINT COMMISSION STANDARDS FOR PAIN MANAGEMENT**
>
> Joint Commission Standards for Pain Management were revised and published in 2000–2001. The standards require health care providers and organizations to improve pain assessment and management for all patients.
> - Recognize that patients have a right to appropriate pain assessment and management.
> - Screen initially and assess periodically for pain (nature and intensity).
> - Record pain assessment results and follow-up with reassessments.
> - Assess staff for level of knowledge and educate in pain assessment and management as needed.
> - Establish organizational policies and procedures that support appropriate ordering or prescribing of effective pain medications.
> - Educate patients and their families about the importance of effective pain management.
> - Address patient needs for symptom management in the discharge planning process.
> - Collect data to monitor the appropriateness and effectiveness of pain management.
>
> (Modified from Berry, P., & Dahl, J. (2000). The new JCAHO pain standards: Implications for pain management nurses. Pain Management Nursing, 1(1), 3–12.) Updates to the Joint Commission Standards for Pain Management have been made, with the newest ones clarified in a report for those effective January 1 and July 1, 2015 (Joint Commission, 2015).

and polymodal nociceptors (of C fibers), sensitive to noxious stimuli of mechanical, thermal, or chemical nature (Patestas & Gartner, 2006). Some nociceptors may respond to more than one type of stimulus. Nociceptors are distributed in the body, skin, subcutaneous tissue, skeletal muscle, joints, peritoneal surfaces, pleural membranes, dura mater, and blood vessel walls. Note that they are not located in the parenchyma of visceral organs. Physiologic processes involved in pain perception (or nociception) include transduction, transmission, perception, and modulation (Fig. 9-1).

Transduction of pain begins when a mechanical, thermal, or chemical stimulus results in tissue injury or damage stimulating the nociceptors, which are the primary afferent nerves for receiving painful stimuli. Noxious stimuli initiate a painful stimulus that results in an inflammatory process leading to release of cytokines and neuropeptides from circulating leukocytes, platelets, vascular endothelial cells, immune cells, and cells from within the peripheral nervous system. This results in the activation of the primary afferent nociceptors (A-delta and C fibers). Furthermore, the nociceptors themselves release a substance P that enhances nociception, causing vasodilation, increased blood flow, and edema with further release of bradykinin, serotonin from platelets, and histamine from mast cells.

A-delta primary afferent fibers (small-diameter, lightly myelinated fibers) and C fibers (unmyelinated, primary afferent fibers) are classified as nociceptors because they are stimulated by noxious stimuli. A-delta primary afferent fibers transmit fast pain to the spinal cord within 0.1 second, which is felt as a pricking, sharp, or electric-quality sensation and usually is caused by mechanical or thermal stimuli. **C fibers** transmit slow pain within 1 second, which is felt as burning, throbbing, or aching and is caused by mechanical, thermal, or chemical stimuli, usually resulting in tissue damage. By the direct excitation of the primary afferent fibers, the stimulus leads to the activation of the fiber terminals.

The transmission process is initiated by this inflammatory process, resulting in the conduction of an impulse in the primary afferent neurons to the dorsal horn of the spinal cord. There, neurotransmitters are released and concentrated in the substantia gelatinosa (which is thought to host the gating mechanism described in the gate control theory) and bind to specific receptors. The output neurons from the dorsal horn cross the anterior white commissure and ascend the spinal cord in the anterolateral quadrant in ascending pathways (Fig. 9-2).

There are several tracts within the anterolateral quadrant: spinothalamic, spinoreticular, spinomesencephalic, spinotectal, and spinohypothalamic. The anterolateral tracts relay sensations of pain, temperature, nondiscriminative (crude) touch, pressure, and some proprioceptive sensation (Dafny, 1997–present). The pathways for the spinothalamic tract and its anterior and lateral portions are shown in Figure 9-2.

The process of pain **perception** is still poorly understood. Studies have shown that emotional status (depression and anxiety) affects directly the level of pain perceived and thus reported by clients. The hypothalamus and limbic system are responsible for the emotional aspect of pain perception, while the frontal cortex is responsible for the rational interpretation and response to pain.

Modulation of pain is a difficult phenomenon to explain. Modulation changes or inhibits the pain message relay in the spinal cord. The descending modular pain pathways either increase (excite) or inhibit pain transmission. Endogenous neurotransmitters involved with modulating pain include: endogenous opioids, such as endorphins and enkephalins; serotonin; norepinephrine (noradrenaline); gamma-aminobutyric acid (GABA); neurotensin; acetylcholine; and oxytocin (Wood, 2008).

Physiologic Responses to Pain

Pain elicits a stress response in the human body that triggers the sympathetic nervous system, resulting in physiologic responses such as:
- Anxiety, fear, hopelessness, sleeplessness, thoughts of suicide
- Focus on pain, reports of pain, cries and moans, frowns, and facial grimaces
- Decrease in cognitive function, mental confusion, altered temperament, high somatization, and dilated pupils
- Increased heart rate; peripheral, systemic, and coronary vascular resistance; increased blood pressure
- Increased respiratory rate and sputum retention, resulting in infection and atelectasis
- Decreased gastric and intestinal motility
- Decreased urinary output, resulting in urinary retention, fluid overload, depression of all immune responses
- Increased antidiuretic hormone, epinephrine, norepinephrine, aldosterone, glucagons; decreased insulin, testosterone

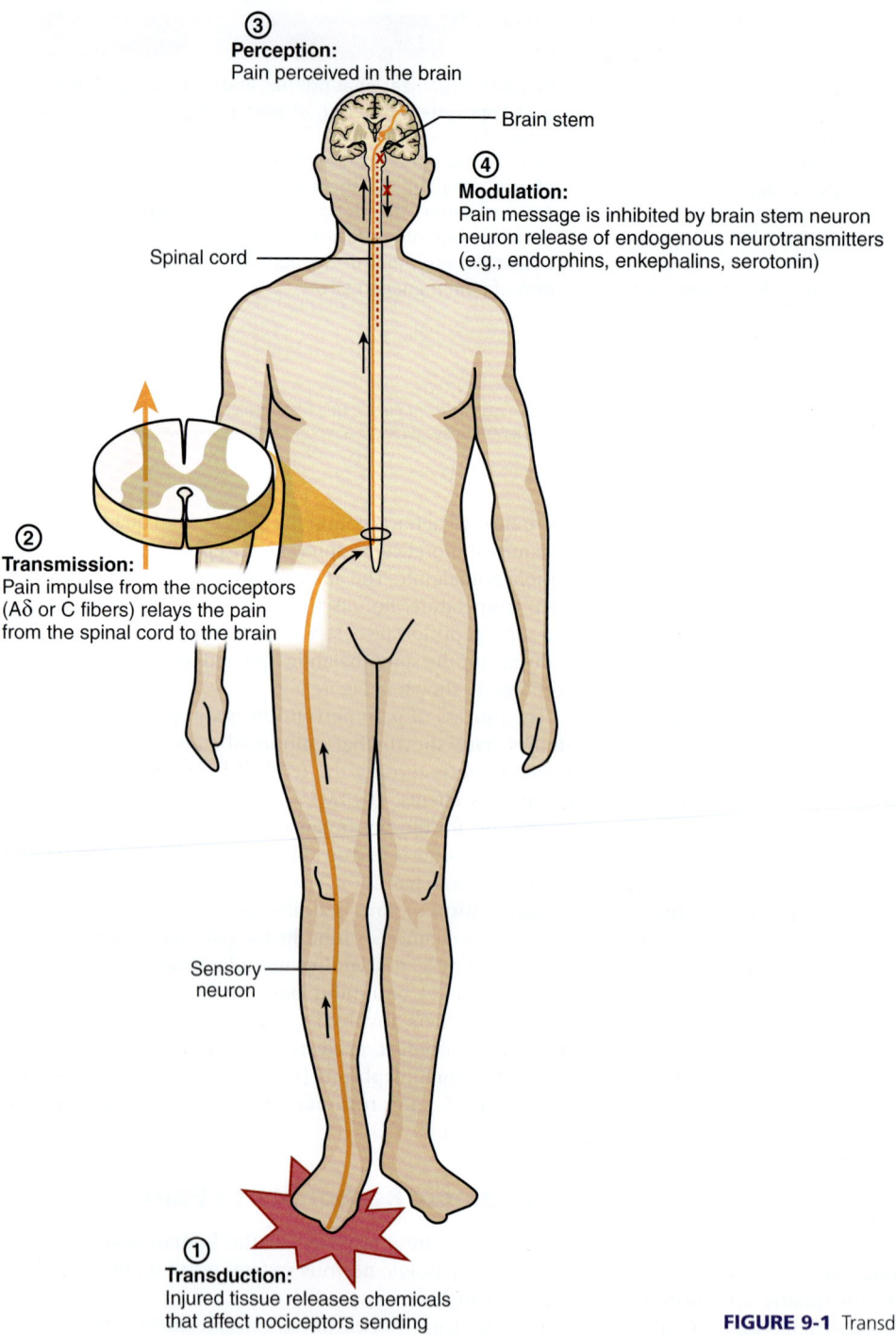

FIGURE 9-1 Transduction, transmission, perception, and modulation of pain.

- Hyperglycemia, glucose intolerance, insulin resistance, protein catabolism
- Muscle spasm, resulting in impaired muscle function and immobility, perspiration

Classification

Classification of pain can assist assessment. Pain is classified in several ways, and these ways may overlap. Causes, etiology, duration, intensity, location, and severity are some of these. Classifications of pain by cause, duration, etiology, and location follow, but a short quick reference for pain classification is seen in Box 9-2.

Classification of pain by cause includes:
- **Nociceptive:** response to noxious insult or injury of tissues such as skin, muscles, visceral organs, joints, tendons, or bones
- **Neuropathic:** pain initiated or caused by a primary lesion or disease in the somatosensory nervous system
- **Inflammatory:** a result of activation and sensitization of the nociceptive pain pathway by a variety of mediators released at a site of tissue inflammation

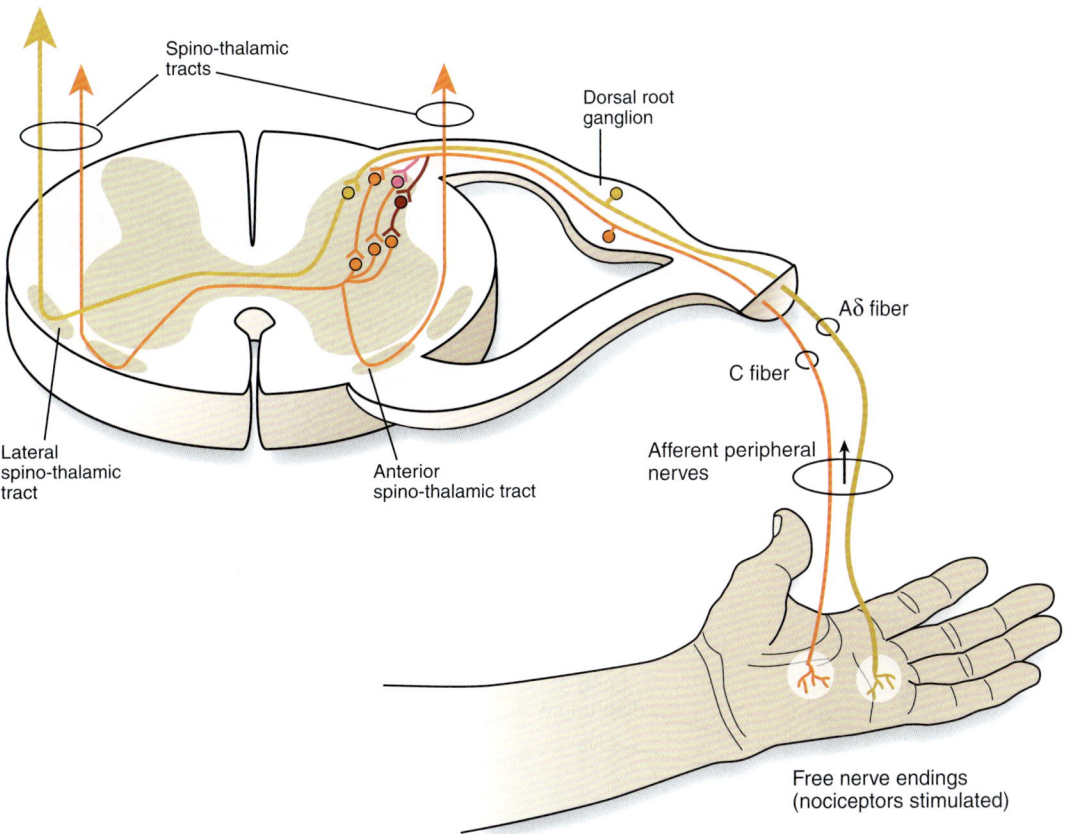

FIGURE 9-2 Pathways for transmitting pain.

Duration and etiology are often classified together to differentiate **acute pain, chronic nonmalignant pain,** and **cancer pain.**
- **Acute pain:** usually associated with a recent injury
- **Chronic nonmalignant pain:** usually associated with a specific cause or injury and described as a constant pain that persists for more than 6 months
- **Cancer pain:** often due to the compression of peripheral nerves or meninges or from the damage to these structures following surgery, chemotherapy, radiation, or tumor growth and infiltration (Box 9-3)
- **Intractable pain:** defined by its high resistance to pain relief

Pain location classifications include:
- **Cutaneous pain** (skin or subcutaneous tissue)
- **Visceral pain** (abdominal cavity, thorax, cranium)
- **Deep somatic pain** (ligaments, tendons, bones, blood vessels, nerves)

Another aspect of pain location is whether it is perceived at the site of the pain stimuli if it is **radiating** (perceived both at the source and extending to other tissues) or **referred** (perceived in body areas away from the pain source; see Fig. 9-3). **Phantom pain** can be perceived in nerves left by a missing, amputated, or paralyzed body part.

(See Board of Regents for the University of Wisconsin, 2010 for further details).

BOX 9-2 CLASSIFICATION OF PAIN

Nociceptive: represents the normal response to noxious insult or injury of tissues such as skin, muscles, visceral organs, joints, tendons, or bones.
- Examples include:
  - Somatic: musculoskeletal (joint pain, myofascial pain), cutaneous; often well localized
  - Visceral: hollow organs and smooth muscle; usually referred

Neuropathic: pain initiated or caused by a primary lesion or disease in the somatosensory nervous system.
- Sensory abnormalities range from deficits perceived as numbness to hypersensitivity (hyperalgesia or allodynia), and to paresthesias such as tingling.
- Examples include, but are not limited to, diabetic neuropathy, postherpetic neuralgia, spinal cord injury pain, phantom limb (postamputation) pain, and poststroke central pain.

Inflammatory: a result of activation and sensitization of the nociceptive pain pathway by a variety of mediators released at a site of tissue inflammation.
- The mediators that have been implicated as key players are proinflammatory cytokines such IL-1-alpha, IL-1-beta, IL-6 and TNF-alpha, chemokines, reactive oxygen species, vasoactive amines, lipids, ATP, acid, and other factors released by infiltrating leukocytes, vascular endothelial cells, or tissue resident mast cells
- Examples include appendicitis, rheumatoid arthritis, inflammatory bowel disease, and herpes zoster.

From University of Wisconsin School of Medicine and Public Health, http://projects.hsl.wisc.edu/GME/PainManagement/session2.4.html

BOX 9-3 CANCER PAIN

Cancer pain is a special category of pain because it may reflect all of the pain types at the same time or at different times during the course of the disease. Cancer pain may be caused by the cancer, its treatment, or its metastasis. Some important facts about cancer pain are as follows:

- It can be acute (sudden and severe) or chronic (lasting more than 3 months).
- Its types include somatic pain, visceral pain, and neuropathic pain.
- It causes breakthrough pain (brief, severe pain that occurs in spite of pain medication) in many clients.
- It depends on many factors, including the type and stage of the cancer.
- It may be triggered by blocked blood vessels or pressure on a nerve from a tumor.
- Side effects of cancer treatments—such as surgery, radiation, and chemotherapy—may include pain.
- About 90% of clients with advanced cancer experience severe pain, which often is undertreated.
- Cancer pain can result from:
  - Blocked blood vessels causing poor circulation
  - Bone fracture from metastasis
  - Infection
  - Inflammation
  - Psychological or emotional problems
  - Side effects from cancer treatments (e.g., chemotherapy, radiation)
  - Tumor exerting pressure on a nerve (Healthcommunities.com, 1998–2008)

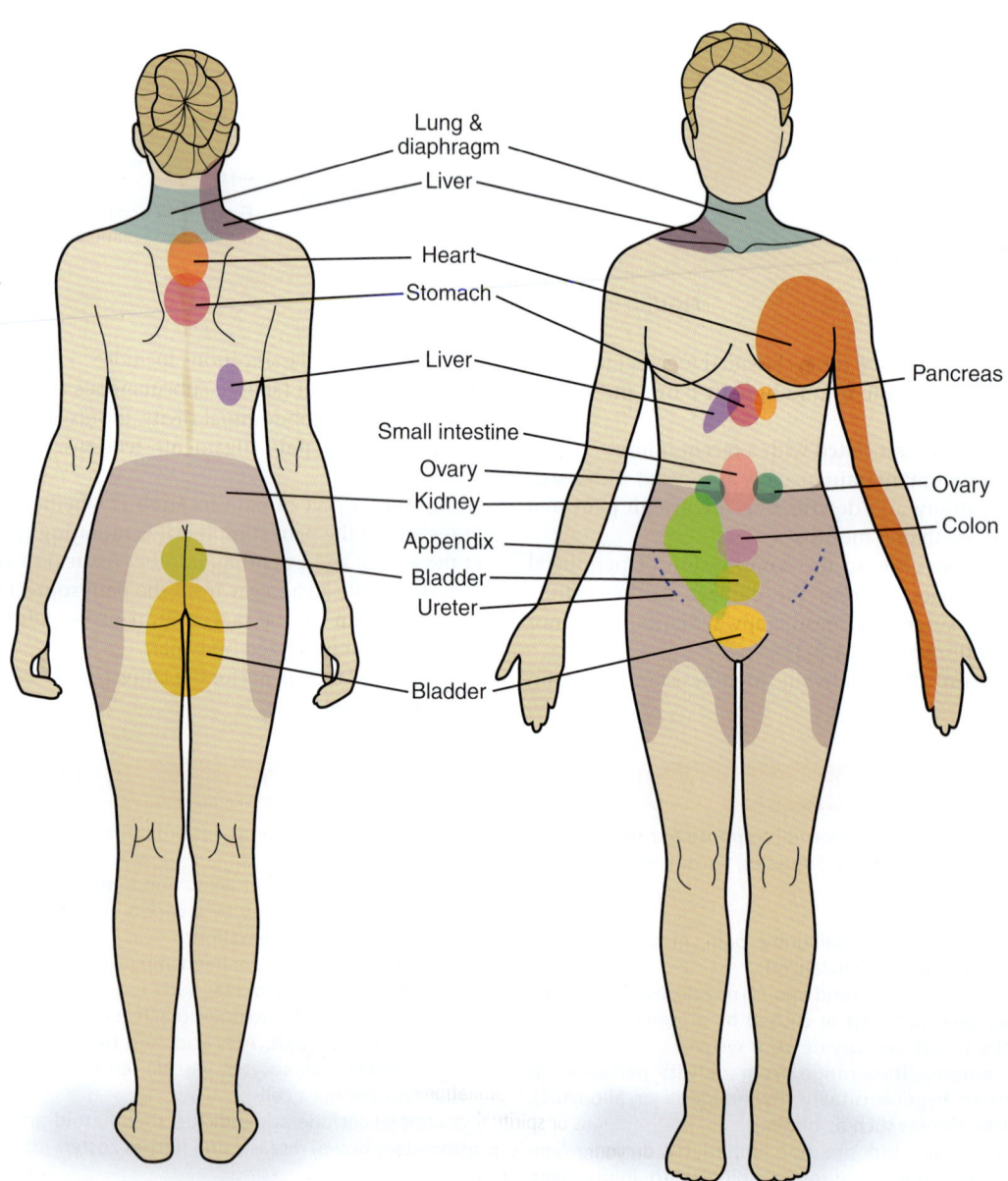

FIGURE 9-3 Areas of referred pain. Posterior view (*left*). Anterior view (*right*).

The Seven Dimensions of Pain

The experience of pain is highly complex. It is more than the physiologic and neurochemical responses. Silkman (2008) describes the multidimensional complexity of pain in seven dimensions: physical, sensory, behavioral, sociocultural, cognitive, affective, and spiritual.

- **Physical dimension** refers to the physiologic effects just described. This dimension includes the patient's perception of the pain and the body's reaction to the stimulus.
- **Sensory dimension** concerns the quality of the pain and how severe the pain is perceived to be. This dimension includes the patient's perception of the pain's location, intensity, and quality.
- **Behavioral dimension** refers to the verbal and nonverbal behaviors that the patient demonstrates in response to the pain.
- **Sociocultural dimension** concerns the influences of the patient's social context and cultural background on the patient's pain experience.
- **Cognitive dimension** concerns "beliefs, attitudes, intentions, and motivations related to the pain and its management" (p. 14). Of course, beliefs, attitudes, intentions, and motivations are affected by all of the dimensions mentioned, but can be associated with the management part of the pain experience, which is dependent on cognition.
- **Affective dimension** concerns feelings, sentiments, and emotions related to the pain experience. The pain can affect the emotions and the emotions can affect the perception of pain.
- **Spiritual dimension** refers to the meaning and purpose that the person "attributes to the pain, self, others, and the divine" (p. 15). For some suggested questions to assess each dimension, see Assessment Guide 9-1.

Psychosocial Factors Affecting Pain Perception and Assessment

Several factors, including **developmental level** or **age** and **culture**, affect pain perception and assessment.

Although psychological factors and culture were thought to account for gender differences in pain perception, more recent research has demonstrated physiologic bases for differences (Bulls et al., 2015; Medical News Today, 2015; WebMD, 2015). Women seem to be more sensitive to pain and have less efficient endogenous pain inhibitory capacity compared with men. The role of estrogen may be the source of this difference, or at least partially so. Estrogen appears to lower tolerance to pain and to lower the pain threshold, while testosterone appears to elevate pain tolerance.

ASSESSMENT GUIDE 9-1 Pain Dimensions: Sample Assessment Questions

Here are examples of questions to ask your client when assessing the seven dimensions of pain.

Dimension	Sample Questions
Physical: effect of anatomic structure and physiologic functioning on the experience of pain	What surgeries or other medical procedures have you had? What medical conditions do you have? What conditions brought you to the hospital or doctor's office in the past?
Sensory: qualitative and quantitative descriptions of pain	Where is the pain located? What does the pain feel like? How would you rate the pain on a scale of 1 to 10, with 10 being the worst pain imaginable? When did the pain begin? How long does the pain usually last?
Behavioral: verbal and nonverbal behaviors associated with pain	I notice that you are _____ (fill in the patient's behavior, such as grimacing). Are you having pain?
Sociocultural: effect of social and cultural backgrounds on the experience of pain	What is your country of origin? Do you have any special cultural or social practices that influence the decisions you make about health care? How do you manage your pain at home?
Cognitive: thoughts, beliefs, attitudes, intentions, and motivations related to the experience of pain	How effective is the pain relief treatment you are currently getting? What is the highest level of education you have completed? What do you do for a living? What do you think is causing your pain? What do you think will relieve it?
Affective: feelings and emotions that result from pain	How does the pain affect your overall mood? Daily life and activities? Social activities and interactions? Personal relationships?
Spiritual: ultimate meaning and purpose attributed to pain, self, others, and the divine	What is your religious affiliation? What religious or spiritual practices and preferences do you have? How do your religious or spiritual beliefs influence your health care decisions? How would you describe the support you receive from friends and loved ones?

Copyright ©2018, HealthCom Media. All rights reserved. *American Nurse Today*, February 2008. www.AmericanNurseToday.com.

Developmental Level

The two extremes of development, pediatric (neonate to later childhood) and geriatric age groups, have characteristics that make pain assessment more difficult. Because pain has both sensory and emotional components, assessment strategies usually use quantitative and qualitative information. The American Pain Society (2008) reports that chronic pain affects 15% to 20% of children. For the population aged 60 and older, 71% to 83% of assisted living or nursing home residents and 64% to 78% of persons between 60 and 89 years of age living in the community experience significant pain (Martinez, 2011). Although debated in the pro- and antiabortion literature, some investigators find that fetuses at 26 weeks of gestation perceive pain, and may feel pain as early as 20 weeks (Doctors on Fetal Pain, 2015).

Not knowing whether fetuses, premature infants, neonates, young children, the elderly, and the cognitively impaired (elderly or others) are feeling pain can lead to gross undertreatment of pain in these groups. The results of undertreated pain in any client can be profound, resulting in both physical and psychological problems that can be avoided if pain is assessed and treated properly. Undertreated pain in children can lead to chronic pain conditions when they become adults. The mnemonic QUESTT was developed by Baker and Wong (1987) and described in Box 9-4.

Banicek (2010) lists tools and behaviors for assessing pain in older adults with and without cognitive impairment. For the older adult without cognitive impairment, three tools are the Visual Analog Scale (VAS), the Numeric Pain Intensity Scale (NPIS), and the categorical rating scale using words such as "none (0)," "mild (1)," "moderate (2)," or "severe (3)." To assess pain in the cognitively impaired older adult, observe behaviors that may indicate pain: facial expressions (frowning, grimacing); vocalization (crying, groaning); change in body language (rocking, guarding); behavioral change (refusing to eat, alteration in usual patterns); physiologic change (blood pressure, heart rate); and physical change (skin tears, pressure areas). The NRS has been shown to be best for older adults with no cognitive impairment, and the Faces Pain Scale-Revised (FPS-R) for cognitively impaired adults (Flaherty, 2008). The elderly people in this study tended to prefer the vertical to the horizontal form of the VAS. This study suggests that clinicians should collaborate with each elderly client to choose a pain intensity scale that is best suited to individual needs and preferences.

BOX 9-4 QUESTT PRINCIPLES FOR PAIN IN CHILDREN

Main points that underlie the mnemonic are that in clinical assessment of pain, regular and systematic assessment is essential; the health care provider should believe the client's or family's report of the pain and should empower everyone by involving all in decision making. The mnemonic is:
- **Question the child.**
- **Use pain-rating scales.**
- **Evaluate behavior and physiologic changes.**
- **Secure parents' involvement.**
- **Take cause of pain into account.**
- **Take action and evaluate results.**

Culture

Pain is a universal human experience, but how people respond to it varies with the meaning placed on pain and the response to pain that is expected in the culture in which the person is raised. There are certain patterns of pain expression that vary across cultures. Pain can have several meanings between different cultures that lead to these different response patterns. Refer to the examples shown in Table 9-1, "Cultural Expressions of Pain." Although these examples of differences in meaning and expression of pain show some of the cultural variations that are important for the nurse assessing for pain, the most important factor is this: Do Not Stereotype! This means that even though there are tendencies for people from a particular cultural background to exhibit certain characteristics, many people of that culture will not. The nurse must assess what the person says about pain, what the person says about asking

TABLE 9-1 Cultural Expressions of Pain

Cultural Group	Pain Expression/Beliefs
Asian and Asian American	• Pain is natural. • Use mind over body; positive thinking. • Pain is honorable. • Pain may be caused by past transgressions and helps to atone and achieve higher spirituality. • Stigma against narcotic use may result in underreporting of pain.
African American	• Pain is a challenge to be fought. • Pain is inevitable and is to be endured. • Pain is stigmatized, resulting in inhibition in expressing pain or seeking help. • Pain may be a punishment from God. • God and prayer will help more than medicine.
Hindu	• Pain must be endured as part of preparing for the next life in the cycle of reincarnation. • Must remain conscious when nearing death to experience the events of dying and perhaps rebirth.
Native American	• Pain is to be endured. • May not ask for medication due to respect for caregivers who should know their needs. • Metaphors and images from nature are used to describe pain (Kaegi, 2004).
Hispanic	• Pain response is often very expressive, especially in women, though pain must be endured to perform gender role duties. Men often are stoic to avoid appearing weak. • Pain is natural, but may be the result of sinful or immoral behavior.
Jewish	• Pain is expressed openly, with much complaining, especially with respect to the effect their pain has on their health or their family. • Pain must be shared, recognized, and validated by others so that the experience is affirmed (Steefel, 2001).

BOX 9-5 BARRIERS TO PAIN ASSESSMENT

Barriers to correct pain assessment may be present and must be assessed as well. Cultural and physiologic differences account for most of these. Consider cultural variation to exist in all patient populations and not just among persons from other countries. Also, gender differences are expressed differently in different cultures. Nurses' and other health care providers' beliefs about pain can also affect the assessment.

BARRIERS BASED ON BELIEFS

- Acknowledging pain is not manly; it is a sign of weakness.
- Pain is a punishment (often thought to be from God) for past mistakes, sins, or behaviors, and must be tolerated.
- Pain indicates that my condition/disease is getting worse, and that I am going to die soon. If I don't acknowledge it, it won't be so bad.
- Pain medications are addictive; cause awful side effects; and make me "dopey," confused, and sleepy or unconscious.
- All people have pain, especially as they age. This is just normal pain and I should not say anything about it.

BARRIERS BASED ON PHYSICAL CONDITIONS

- The disease/illness/injury for which the patient is being treated is not the source of the pain.
- Both the current disease and another disease are causing pain.
- The patient expresses few, if any, pain-related behaviors once accommodated to prolonged chronic pain conditions.

BARRIERS BASED ON HEALTH CARE PROVIDERS' BELIEFS

- Patients who complain of pain frequently are just trying to get more pain medicine or are addicts wanting more narcotics.
- Patients who complain of pain but do not show physical and behavioral signs of pain do not need more pain medication, whether they are chronic pain patients or acute pain patients.
- Old people simply have more pain.
- Confused or demented patients, or very young patients, neonates, and fetuses do not feel pain.
- Patients who are sleeping do not have pain.
- Pain medication causes addiction/respiratory depression/too many side effects.
- Giving as much pain medication as possible at night will make the patients sleep and not disturb the nurses.

---

for pain medication, what the person says about the meaning pain has, how the person behaves when undergoing known-to-be painful procedures, and how the person behaves when others are present or absent. In other words, treat each client as a unique individual, assess each client, respect each client's responses to pain, and treat each client with dignity and consideration.

It is very important for you as a nurse to recognize your own response to pain. How did you respond to pain in your family? What did you think about pain when you were a child? Did your parents respond the same way? What did they teach you about pain? Some are raised to deny pain, since it is just a normal part of life. Others are raised to respond verbally and loudly to pain, since it indicates an invasion of the body and is a sign that something bad has happened or will happen. Are you stoic? Are you vocal and loud, moaning or crying, if pain is intense? Knowing your own response to pain lets you know a little about what you believe about pain. A perception that our responses and beliefs are "normal" and those of others are not can lead to miscommunications between nurses and clients. To be a **culturally competent nurse** caring for clients in pain:

- Be aware of your own cultural and family values.
- Be aware of your personal biases and assumptions about people with different values than yours.
- Be aware and accept cultural differences between yourself and individual clients.
- Be capable of understanding the dynamics of the difference.
- Be able to adapt to diversity (Weissman, Gordon, & Bidar-Sielaff, 2004).

A variety of issues can create barriers to pain assessment (Box 9-5). For an excellent source for interventions to overcome cultural and communication barriers when caring for clients in pain, see *What Color Is Your Pain?* by Louise Kaegi (2004).

HEALTH ASSESSMENT

There are few objective findings on which the assessment of pain can rely. Pain is a subjective phenomenon and thus the main assessment lies in the client's reporting.

Collecting Subjective Data: The Nursing Health History

The client's description of pain is quoted. The exact words used to describe the experienced pain are used to help in the diagnosis and management. A thorough pain assessment includes questions about **location, intensity, quality, pattern, precipitating factors,** and **pain relief,** as well as the effect of the pain on **daily activities,** what **coping strategies** have been used, and **emotional responses** to the pain. Past experience with pain, in addition to past and current therapies, are explored. Note that pain assessment lends itself well to the COLDSPA mnemonic. Review Box 9-6 before assessing the client's subjective experience of pain.

BOX 9-6 TIPS FOR COLLECTING SUBJECTIVE DATA

- Maintain a quiet and calm environment that is comfortable for the patient being interviewed.
- Maintain the client's privacy and ensure confidentiality.
- Ask the questions in an open-ended format.
- Listen carefully to the client's verbal descriptions and quote the terms used.
- Watch for the client's facial expressions and grimaces during the interview.
- DO NOT put words in the client's mouth.
- Ask the client about past experiences with pain.
- Believe the client's expression of pain.

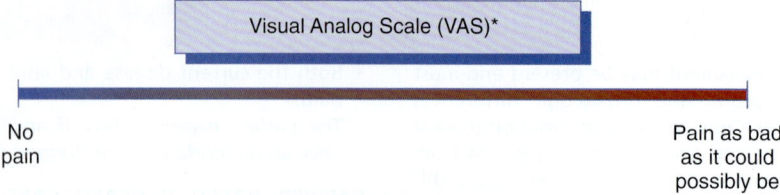

FIGURE 9-4 Visual Analog Scale (VAS). (From Riegel, & Bram (n.d.). Pain assessment. Available at http://www.burnsurvivorsttw.org, with permission. Burn Survivors Throughout The World, Inc. is an international nonprofit organization offering a support team, advocacy, medical referrals, email, and chat room for burn survivors.)

Some clients may be unable to self-report pain. This includes unconscious clients, cognitively impaired clients, elders with dementia, intubated clients, infants, and preverbal toddlers. For nonverbal persons or those with cognitive impairment, it has been recommended that the Hierarchy of Pain Assessment Techniques (McCaffery & Pasero, 1999) be used (Herr et al., 2006;2011). The Hierarchy includes five items:

1. Self-report—always try to get a self-report, but note if unable and go on to the other items.
2. Search for potential causes of pain—pathologic conditions, procedures such as surgery, wound care, positioning, skin invasion by needle or catheter, or other known painful producers or diseases.
3. Observe patient behaviors—many scales reflect pain-related behaviors of different patient types. See Pain Scales listed by Herr and associates and selected ones later in this chapter. Note: Patient behaviors may not accurately reflect pain intensity.
4. Surrogate reporting (family members, parents, caregivers) of pain and behavior/activity changes—Note: Discrepancies may exist between self-report of pain and surrogate reports, and between surrogates and health care providers on judgments of pain and its intensity.
5. Attempt an analgesic trial—a full protocol is recommended. After an analgesic is ordered, the nurse needs to observe for changes in self-report, if any, or in any behaviors.

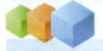 **Concept Mastery Alert**

When assessing pain in a nonresponsive client, the nurse should use the Hierarchy of Pain Assessment Techniques. When self-report is not possible the hierarchy then progresses to assessment of possible causes of pain and then observation of the client's behavior that would indicate pain. If these techniques do not provide the necessary information, the nurse requests information about the client's behavior from family members.

Preparing the Client

In preparation for the interview, clients are seated in a quiet, comfortable, and calm environment with minimal interruption. Explain to the client that the interview will entail questions to clarify the picture of the pain experienced in order to develop the plan of care.

Pain Assessment Tools

There are many assessment tools, some of which are specific to special types of pain. The main issues in choosing the tool are its reliability and its validity. Moreover, the tool must be clear and, therefore, easily understood by the client. It must require little effort from the client and the nurse.

Select one or more pain assessment tools appropriate for the client. There are many pain assessment scales, such as:

- Visual Analog Scale (VAS) (Fig. 9-4)
- Numeric Rating Scale (NRS) (Fig. 9-5)
- Numeric Pain Intensity Scale (NPI)
- Verbal Descriptor Scale (Fig. 9-6)
- Simple Descriptive Pain Intensity Scale
- Graphic Rating Scale
- Verbal Rating Scale
- Faces Pain Scales (FPS, FPS-R; see Chapter 30).

You can look at all of these and other scales at http://www.partnersagainstpain.com/hcp/index.aspx. Most of these scales have been shown to be reliable measures of client pain. The three most popular scales are the NRS, the Verbal Descriptor Scale, and the FPS, although VASs are often mentioned as very simple. The NRS has been shown to be best for older adults with no cognitive impairment, and the (FPS-R) for cognitively impaired adults (Flaherty, 2008).

A pain assessment tool integrating several assessment tools and verbal translation to several languages, known as the Universal Pain Assessment Tool, has been developed (UCLA, n.d.). See Assessment Tool 9-1.

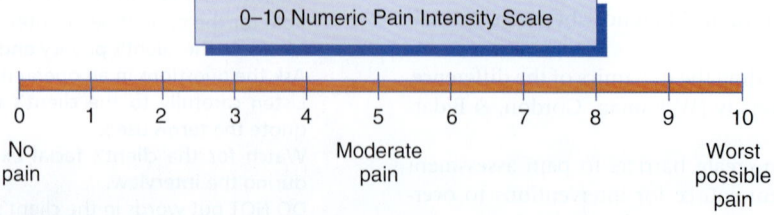

FIGURE 9-5 Numeric Rating Scale (NRS). (From Acute Pain Management: Operative or Medical Procedures and Trauma, Clinical Practice Guideline No. 1. (1992). Agency for Health Care Research and Quality (AHRQ) Publication No. 92–0032; with permission.)

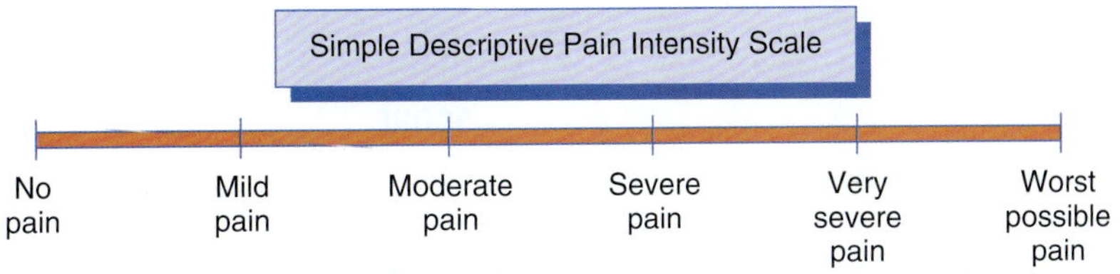

Simple Descriptive Pain Intensity Scale

| No pain | Mild pain | Moderate pain | Severe pain | Very severe pain | Worst possible pain |

FIGURE 9-6 Verbal Descriptor Scale (VDS). (From Acute Pain Management: Operative or Medical Procedures and Trauma, Clinical Practice Guideline No. 1. (1992). Agency for Health Care Research and Quality (AHRQ) Publication No. 92–0032; with permission.)

It is hard to evaluate pain in neonates and infants. Behaviors that indicate pain are used to assess their pain. One tool for such assessment is the N-PASS: Neonatal Pain, Agitation, & Sedation Scale (Hummel & Puchalski, 2000). Another popular tool for assessing pediatric pain is the FLACC Scale (Face, Legs, Activity, Cry, and Consolability); see Assessment Tool 9-2.

Memorial Sloan-Kettering Cancer Center has developed a cancer pain assessment tool that has four parts. This self-assessment tool provides feedback on the type and level of pain as well as the patient's mood and pain relief from pain treatment (Box 9-7).

Three pain assessment tools that serve well for the patient's initial assessment are the Initial Pain Assessment Tool (Assessment Tool 9-3; McCaffery & Pasero, 1999), the Brief Pain Inventory (Short Form; Cleeland, 1992), and for pediatric pain assessment, the Initial Pain Assessment for Pediatric Use Only (Otto, Duncan, & Baker, 1996).

ASSESSMENT TOOL 9-1 Universal Pain Assessment Tool

UNIVERSAL PAIN ASSESSMENT TOOL

This pain assessment tool is intended to help patient care providers assess pain according to individual patient needs. Explain and use 0-10 Scale for patient self-assessment. Use the faces or behavioral observations to interpret expressed pain when patient cannot communicate his/her pain intensity.

0–10 scale: 0 = No pain, 5 = Moderate pain, 10 = Worst possible pain

Wong-Baker Facial Grimace Scale: 0 | 1-2 (MILD) | 3-4 | 5-6 (MODERATE) | 7-8 | 9-10 (SEVERE)

Activity Tolerance Scale	NO PAIN	CAN BE IGNORED	INTERFERES WITH TASKS	INTERFERES WITH CONCENTRATION	INTERFERES WITH BASIC NEEDS	BEDREST REQUIRED
SPANISH	NADA DE DOLOR	UN POQUITO DE DOLOR	UN DOLOR LEVE	DOLOR FUERTE	DOLOR DEMASIADO FUERTE	UN DOLOR INSOPORTABLE
FRENCH	AUCUNE DOULEUR	LÉGÈRE DOULEUR	DOULEUR MODÉRÉE	FORTE DOULEUR	TRÈS FORTE DOULEUR	DOULEUR EXTRÊME
GERMAN	KEINE SCHMERZEN	LEICHTE SCHMERZEN	MÄSSIGE SCHMERZEN	STARKE SCHMERZEN	SEHR STARKE SCHMERZEN	EXTREME SCHMERZEN
JAPANESE	痛みなし	軽い痛み	中程度の痛み	ひどい痛み	非常にひどい痛み	最悪の痛み
TAGALOG	HINDI MASAKIT	KAUNTIG SAKIT	MEDYO MASAKIT	TALAGANG MASAKIT	MASAKIT NA MASAKIT	PINAKAMASAKIT
HINDI	DARD NAHI HAI	BAHUT KAM	HILNE SE TAKLEF HOTI HAI	SOCH NAHIN SAK TE	KUCH NAHIN KAR SAKTE	DARD BAHUT HAI

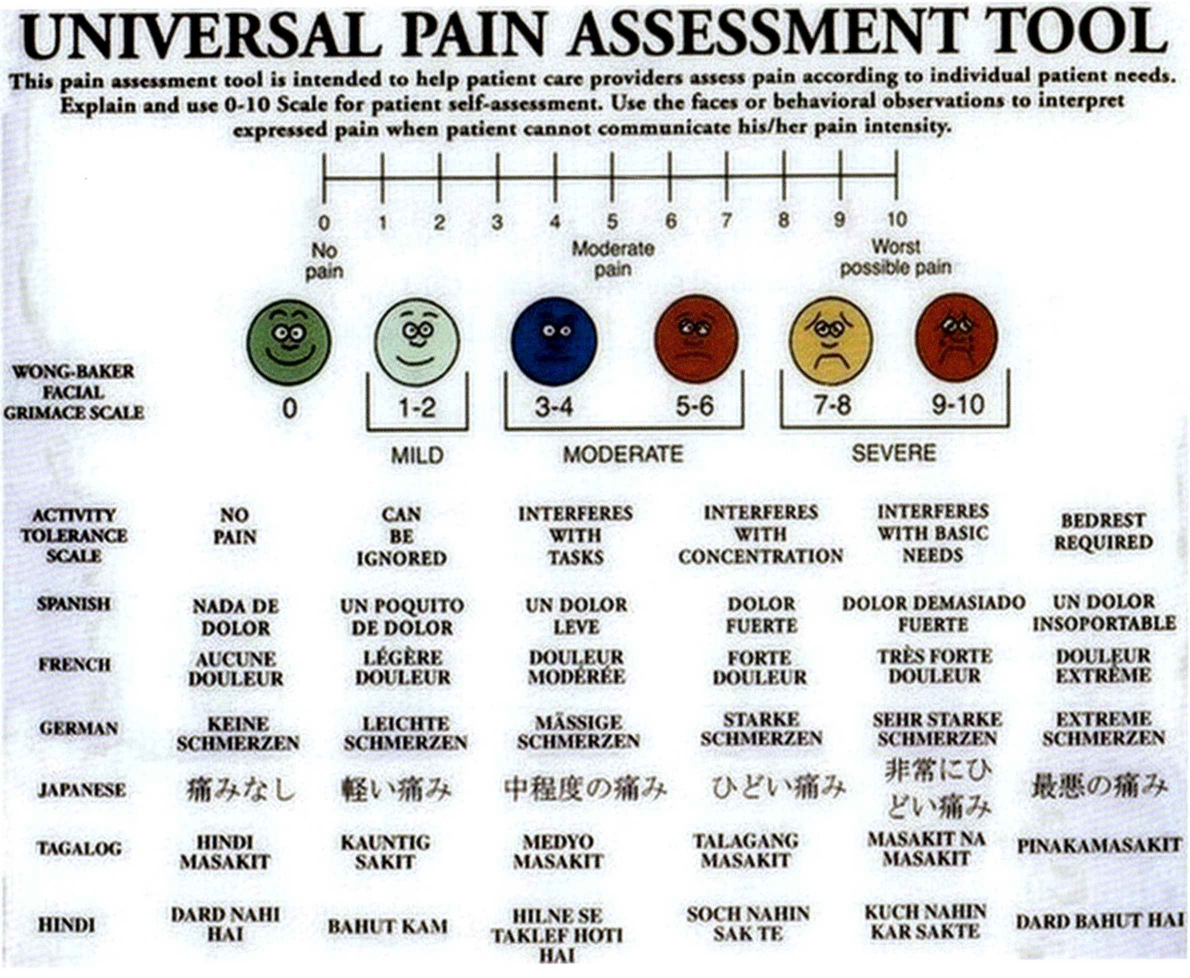

(From: Department of Anesthesiology, David Geffen School of Medicine at UCLA. Available at http://www.anes.ucla.edu/pain/index.htm)

ASSESSMENT TOOL 9-2 Face, Legs, Activity, Cry, Consolability (FLACC) Behavioral Scale

ITEM	SCORE 0	SCORE 1	SCORE 2
FACE	No particular expression or smile.	Occasional grimace, frown, withdrawn, or disinterested.	Frequent to constant frown, clenched jaw, quivering chin.
LEGS	Normal position or relaxed.	Uneasy, restless, tense.	Kicking, or legs drawn up.
ACTIVITY	Lying quietly, normal position, moves easily.	Squirming, shifting back and forth, or tense.	Arched, rigid, or jerking.
CRY	No cry.	Moans, whimpers, or occasional complaint.	Crying steadily, screams or sobs, frequent complaints.
CONSOLABILITY	Content, relaxed.	Reassured by occasional touching, hugging, or being talked to; distractible.	Difficult to console or comfort.

Each of the five categories—(F) Face; (L) Legs; (A) Activity; (C) Cry; and (C) Consolability—is scored from 0 to 2, which results in a total score between 0 and 10.

The revised FLACC can be used for children with cognitive disability.

Procedure:

Patients who are awake: Observe for at least 1–2 minutes. Observe legs and body uncovered. Reposition patient or observe activity; assess body for tenseness and tone. Initiate consoling interventions if needed.

Patients who are asleep: Observe for at least 2 minutes or longer. Observe body and legs uncovered. If possible, reposition the patient. Touch the body and assess for tenseness and tone.

Printed with permission © The Regents of the University of Michigan.

BOX 9-7 SELF-ASSESSMENT: MEMORIAL PAIN ASSESSMENT CARD

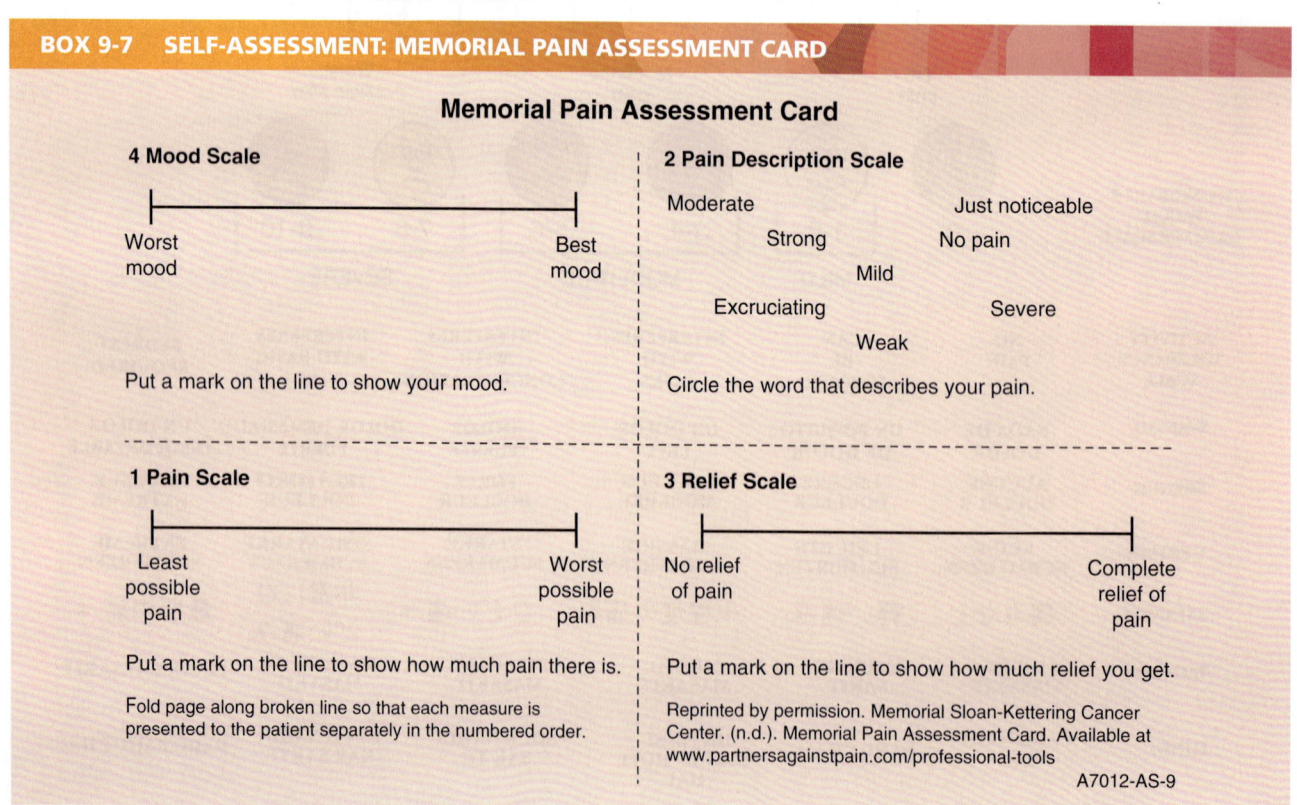

From http://projects.hsl.wisc.edu/GME/PainManagement/session2.4.html

ASSESSMENT TOOL 9-3 McCaffrey Initial Pain Assessment Tool

McCaffrey Initial Pain Assessment Tool

Date _____

Patient's Name _____ Age _____ Room _____

Diagnosis _____ Physician _____

Nurse _____

1. LOCATION: Patient or nurse marks drawing.

2. INTENSITY: Patient rates the pain. Scale used _____
   Present: _____
   Worst pain gets: _____
   Best pain gets: _____
   Acceptable level of pain: _____
3. QUALITY: (Use patient's own words, e.g., prick, ache, burn, throb, pull sharp) _____

4. ONSET, DURATION, VARIATIONS, RHYTHMS: _____

5. MANNER OF EXPRESSING PAIN? _____

6. WHAT RELIEVES THE PAIN? _____

7. WHAT CAUSES OR INCREASES THE PAIN? _____

8. EFFECTS OF PAIN: (Note decreased function, decreased quality of life.)
   Accompanying symptoms (e.g., nausea) _____
   Sleep _____
   Appetite _____
   Physical activity _____
   Relationship with others (e.g., irritability) _____
   Emotions (e.g., anger, suicidal, crying) _____
   Concentration _____
   Other _____
9. OTHER COMMENTS: _____
10. PLAN: _____

May be duplicated for use in clinical practice. From McCaffery M, Pasero C: *Pain: Clinical manual*, p. 60. Copyright ©1999, Mosby, Inc.

History of Present Health Concern

QUESTION	RATIONALE
Are you experiencing pain now or have you in the past 24 hours? If the client answers yes, use the COLDSPA mnemonic to assess the pain.	To establish the presence or absence of perceived pain.
Character. Describe the pain in your own words.	Clients are quoted so that terms used to describe their pain may indicate the type and source. The most common terms used are: throbbing, shooting, stabbing, sharp, cramping, gnawing, hot-burning, aching, heavy, tender, splitting, tiring-exhausting, sickening, fearful, punishing.
Onset. When did the pain start?	The onset of pain provides data on how long the client has had the pain.
Location. Where is it? Does it radiate or spread? Does it occur anywhere else?	The location of pain helps to identify the underlying cause. Radiating or spreading pain helps to identify the source. For example, chest pain radiating to the left arm is most probably of cardiac origin while the pain that is pricking and spreading in the chest muscle area is probably musculoskeletal in origin.
Duration. How long does it last? Does it recur?	This is also to help identify the nature of the pain.
Severity. Ask the client to rate the severity of their pain using the visual analog scale (Fig. 9-1); the Universal Pain Assessment Tool (Assessment Tool 9-1); Self-Assessment: Memorial Pain Assessment Card (Box 9-7)	Using a standardized tool helps to determine how much the pain worsens or improves.
Pattern. Is the pain continuous or intermittent? If intermittent pain, how often do the episodes occur and for how long do they last?	Understanding the course of the pain provides a pattern that may help to determine the source.
Associated factors/How it affects the client. Are there any other concurrent symptoms accompanying the pain?	Accompanying symptoms also help to identify the possible source. For example, right lower quadrant pain associated with nausea, vomiting, and the inability to stand up straight is possibly associated with appendicitis.
What were you doing when the pain first started?	This helps to identify the precipitating factors and what might have exacerbated the pain.
What factors relieve your pain?	Relieving factors help to determine the source and the plan of care.
What factors increase your pain?	Identifying factors that increase pain helps to determine the source and helps in planning to avoid aggravating factors.
Has this pain been treated with any medication, therapy, or surgery (prescribed medications or therapies, complimentary or alternative medications or therapies [CAM])? Have any of these decreased or increased your pain?	This question establishes any current treatment modalities and their effect on the pain. This helps in formulating the future plan of care.
Does this pain have any special meaning to you?	Some cultures view pain as a punishment or view pain as the main symptom to be treated as opposed to treating the underlying disease.
Is there anything you would like to add?	An open-ended question allows the client to mention anything that has been missed or the issues that were not fully addressed by the above questions.

Personal Health History

QUESTION	RATIONALE
Have you had any previous experience with pain?	Past experiences of pain may shed light on the previous history of the client in addition to possible positive or negative expectations of pain therapies.
Have you taken any medications (prescribed, over the counter, or herbal) for pain relief? If so, what medications, what doses, and over what time period?	Types of medications, pattern of use, and doses may provide evidence of effectiveness or potential addiction to pain medications.

Family History

QUESTION	RATIONALE
Does anyone in your family experience pain?	This helps to assess possible family-related perceptions of pain or any past experiences with family members in pain.
How does pain affect your family?	This helps assess the extent that the pain is interfering with the client's family relations.

Lifestyle and Health Practices

QUESTION	RATIONALE
What are your concerns about pain?	Identifying the client's fears and worries helps in prioritizing the plan of care and providing adequate psychological support.
How does your pain interfere with the following? • General activity • Mood/emotions • Concentration • Physical ability • Work • Relations with other people • Sleep • Appetite • Enjoyment of life	These are the main lifestyle factors with which pain interferes. The more that pain interferes with the client's ability to function in his/her daily activities, the more it will reflect on the client's psychological status and, thus, his or her quality of life.

CASE STUDY

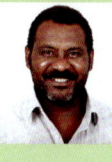

The case study demonstrates a nursing health history related to pain; the following questions and tools provide guidance in conducting the interview. The nurse interviews Mr. Blair regarding his experience of pain associated with his prostate cancer. He reports back and leg pain that worsens at night and when walking. "I sometimes feel that I will fall down while walking and at night I am awakened by stabbing, deep, dull pain in my back that shoots down into my legs. I am not able to sleep at night and during the day I feel tired and unable to proceed with my work, especially meeting my clients."

The nurse explores this health concern using the COLDSPA mnemonic.

Mnemonic	Question	Data Provided
Character	Describe the sign or symptom (feeling, appearance, sound, smell, or taste if applicable). In this case the pain.	"Stabbing, deep, dull low back pain and pain in both legs."
Onset	When did it begin?	"About 8 to 10 months ago"
Location	Where is it? Does it radiate? Does it occur anywhere else?	"In lower back and radiates down both legs"
Duration	How long does it last? Does it recur?	"Continuous, getting worse at night and when walking"
Severity	How bad is it? How much does it bother you now? Using the visual analog scale (Fig. 9-1), ask the client to rate his pain.	On Visual Analog Scale is 7/10. "It bothers me a lot."
Pattern	What makes it better or worse?	"Walking and being in bed at night make it worse. During the day, when I am resting, it is not as bad."
Associated factors/ How it affects the client	What other symptoms occur with it? How does it affect you?	Client had prostatectomy for prostate cancer followed by radiation and chemotherapy ending 1 year ago. I have lost my appetite. The pain "affects everything I do. I am not able to sleep at night and during the day I feel tired and unable to work, especially meeting my clients."

After exploring the basic information on Mr. Blair's pain using the COLDSPA mnemonic, the nurse continues with the client history, using the Joint Commission standards as a guideline. Mr. Blair reports that he is indeed experiencing pain now, even sitting in the examination room. It continues to be located in his lower back, radiating to his legs. Since his surgery for prostate cancer and the following treatments, he has not had lower abdominal discomfort except for occasional bouts of constipation, about once a month, from the pain medications, but usually has had more diarrhea after the radiation than constipation. The pain started a few months after the chemotherapy/radiation. He does not remember exactly when, but states about 8 to 10 months ago, and that it began gradually and soon got to the level it is now. He reports a loss of appetite that is getting worse and has lost 6 kg in the past 3 months. He takes analgesics (Motrin 600 mg every 4 hours) for moderate pain and narcotic analgesics (oxycodone 5 mg every 6 hours) when the pain reaches a 7 out of 10 on the VAS. He is worried that the pain in his back and legs means the cancer has come back.

Collecting Objective Data: Physical Examination

Objective data for pain are collected by observing the client's movement and responses to touch or descriptions of the pain experience. Many of the pain assessment tools incorporate a section to evaluate the objective responses to pain.

Physical Assessment

During examination of the client, remember these key points:

- Choose an assessment tool reliable and valid to the client's culture.
- Explain to the client the purpose of rating the intensity of pain.
- Ensure the client's privacy and confidentiality.
- Respect the client's behavior toward pain and the terms used to express it.
- Understand that different cultures express pain differently and maintain different pain thresholds and expectations.

General Routine Screening or Focused Specialty Assessment for Pain

Since pain is the fifth vital sign, it should be routinely and completely assessed upon first meeting the client in any setting or any situation by any nurse. The nurse needs to be aware of any pain the client is experiencing as it can interfere with the reliability of data collected during the interview and physical examination.

If the client does have pain, the nurse needs to complete an in depth assessment of the client's pain using additional tools as described above in the client interview section (e.g., Visual Analog Scale [Fig. 9-1]; the Universal Pain Assessment Tool [Assessment Tool 9-1]; Self-Assessment: Memorial Pain Assessment Card [Box 9-7]). The McCaffrey Initial Pain Assessment Tool (Assessment Tool 9-3) is very useful to establish an initial baseline of the client's pain experience. If a nonverbal infant, child, or adult needs to be assessed for pain, the FLACC Behavioral Scale (Assessment Tool 9-2) can be useful in focused assessments for pain when the client is awake or asleep.

General Routine Screening
- Observe posture.
- Observe facial expression.
- Inspect joints and muscles.
- Observe skin for scars, lesions, rashes, changes, or discoloration.
- Measure heart rate.
- Measure respiratory rate.
- Measure blood pressure.

Focused Specialty Assessment
- Assess nonverbal client (infant, children to 7 years, adults in intensive care, or other nonverbal conditions) for pain by observing face, legs, activity, cry, and consolability, using Assessment Tool 9-2 (FLACC Behavioral Scale)

ASSESSMENT PROCEDURE	NORMAL FINDINGS	ABNORMAL FINDINGS
General Impression		
INSPECTION		
Observe posture.	Posture is upright when the client is comfortable, attentive, and without excessive changes in position and posture.	Client is slumped, with the shoulders not straight (indicates being disturbed/uncomfortable). Client is inattentive and agitated. Client might be guarding affected area and have tachypnea or guarded respirations.

ASSESSMENT PROCEDURE	NORMAL FINDINGS	ABNORMAL FINDINGS
Observe facial expression.	Client smiles, makes and maintains eye contact and conversation, asks and answers questions appropriately with appropriate facial expressions, and maintains adequate eye contact.	Client's facial expressions indicate distress and discomfort, including frowning, moans, cries, and grimacing. Eye contact is not maintained, indicating discomfort. Nodding up and down or saying, "yeah, yeah," may not indicate a client's positive response to questions, but rather only listening or not wanting to be negative.
Assess face, legs activity, cry, and consolability using Assessment Tool 9-2 (FLACC Behavioral Scale).	A score of "0" indicates no behavioral indication of pain.	Any score greater than "0" indicates some behavioral indication of pain.
Inspect joints and muscles.	Joints without edema, muscles relaxed.	Edema of a joint may indicate injury. Pain may result in muscle tension.
Observe skin for scars, lesions, rashes, changes, or discoloration.	Skin without scars, lesions, rashes, or discoloration. No inconsistency, wounds, or bruising is noted.	Bruising, wounds, or edema may be the result of injuries or infections, which may cause pain.

Vital Signs

INSPECTION

Measure heart rate.	Heart rate ranges from 60 to 100 beats/min.	Increased heart rate may indicate discomfort or pain. A normal heart rate may be present with chronic pain.
Measure respiratory rate.	Respiratory rate ranges from 12 to 20 breaths/min.	Respiratory rate may be increased, and breathing may be irregular and shallow.
Measure blood pressure.	Blood pressure ranges from: Systolic: 100 to 130 mmHg Diastolic: 60 to 80 mmHg.	Increased blood pressure often occurs in severe pain. May be normal in chronic pain.

Note: Refer to physical assessment chapter appropriate to affected body area. Body system assessment will include techniques for assessing for pain, for example, palpating the abdomen for tenderness and performing range of motion test on the joints.

CASE STUDY

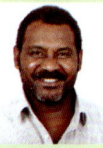

As Mr. Blair enters the room, he limps. He sits on the chair with his shoulders slumped. Mr. Blair changes his position every 2 to 3 minutes, his facial expression is one of frowning and grimacing. He rates his pain on average on the Visual Analog Scale (VAS) to be 7/10. ROM tests of legs: Standing: lifts knees only 20 degrees from straight position when asked to raise knees. Lying: able to lift each leg with knee unbent 15 degrees before pain starts. Lying prone: able to lift each leg only 10 degrees before pain begins.

The nurse collects the following vital signs: Tympanic temperature: 98.8°F, HR = 110 beats/min, RR = 22 breaths/min, BP = 135/85 mmHg.

Validating and Documenting Findings

Validate the pain assessment data you have collected with the client. It is also useful to validate the findings with other caregivers and family members, especially if the client is reluctant to express pain. This is necessary to verify that the data are reliable and accurate. Document the assessment data following the health care facility or agency policy.

CASE STUDY

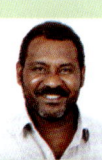

Think back to the case study. The nurse documented the following assessment findings.

Biographical Data: Leonard Blair, 55-year-old, male African American, divorced with two children, financial manager.

General Survey: Awake, alert, and oriented. Asks and answers questions appropriately. Makes and maintains eye contact and conversation.

Reason for Seeking Care: Continuous pain in lower back, radiating to legs: "I sometimes feel that I will fall down while walking and at night I am awakened by stabbing, deep, dull pain in my lower back that spreads to my legs. I am not able to sleep at night and during the day I feel tired and unable to proceed with my work, especially meeting my clients." Takes analgesics for moderate pain, and narcotic analgesics (Motrin 600 mg every 4 hours) and narcotic analgesics (oxycodone 5 mg every 6 hours) for pain 7 to 10 on VAS.

History of Present Health Concern: Continuous low back pain radiating to legs starting after surgery and treatment for prostate cancer; began about 8 to 10 months ago, worsens at night or with walking. Rates pain now at 7/10 of VAS. Loss of appetite and weight loss of 6 kg in the last 3 months. "Walking and being in bed at night make it worse. During the day, when I am resting, it is not as bad." Worried about return of cancer.

Personal Health History: Prostate cancer treated with surgery, radiation, and chemotherapy ending 1 year ago. No other illnesses or surgeries.

Lifestyle and Health Practices: Pain affects entire lifestyle, work, and sleep. Client is very concerned that the pain indicates a return of the cancer.

Physical Examination Findings: Limps into room. Sits with shoulders slumped. Changes position every 2 to 3 minutes. Appears uncomfortable; frowning and grimacing. ROM tests of legs: Standing: lifts knees only 20 degrees from straight position when asked to lift knees. Lying: able to lift each leg with knee unbent 15 degrees before pain starts. Lying prone: able to lift each leg only 10 degrees before pain begins. Vital signs: Tympanic temperature: 98.8 degrees, HR = 110 beats/min, RR = 22 breaths/min, BP = 135/85 mmHg.

ANALYSIS OF DATA: DIAGNOSTIC REASONING

After collecting the assessment data, identify abnormal findings and client strengths using diagnostic reasoning. Then, cluster the data to reveal any significant patterns or abnormalities. The following sections provide possible conclusions that the nurse may make after assessing a client's pain.

Selected Nursing Diagnoses

The following is a list of selected nursing diagnoses that may be identified when analyzing data from a pain assessment.

Health Promotion Diagnoses

- Readiness for enhanced spiritual well-being related to coping with prolonged physical pain
- Readiness for enhanced comfort

Risk Diagnoses

- Risk for activity intolerance related to chronic pain and immobility
- Risk for constipation related to nonsteroidal anti-inflammatory agents or opiates intake or poor eating habits
- Risk for spiritual distress related to anxiety, pain, life change, and chronic illness
- Risk for powerlessness related to chronic pain, health care environment, pain treatment–related regimen

Actual Diagnoses

- Acute pain related to injury agents (biologic, chemical, physical, or psychological)
- Chronic pain related to chronic inflammatory process of rheumatoid arthritis
- Ineffective breathing pattern related to abdominal pain and anxiety
- Fatigue related to stress of handling chronic pain
- Impaired physical mobility related to chronic pain
- Bathing/hygiene self-care deficit related to severe pain (specify)

Selected Collaborative Problems

After grouping the data, certain collaborative problems may become apparent. Remember that collaborative problems differ from nursing diagnoses in that they cannot be prevented by nursing intervention. However, these physiologic complications of medical conditions can be detected and monitored by the nurse. In addition, the nurse can use physician- and nurse-prescribed interventions to minimize the complications of these problems. The nurse may also have to refer the client in such situations for further treatment of the problem. Following is a list of collaborative problems that may be identified when obtaining a general impression. These problems are worded as Risk for Complications (RC), followed by the problem.

- RC: Angina
- RC: Decreased cardiac output
- RC: Endocarditis
- RC: Peripheral vascular insufficiency
- RC: Paralytic ileus/small bowel obstruction
- RC: Sickling crisis
- RC: Peripheral nerve compression
- RC: Corneal ulceration
- RC: Osteoarthritis
- RC: Joint dislocation
- RC: Pathologic fractures
- RC: Renal calculi
- RC: Metastatic cancer
- RC: Peripheral neuropathy

Medical Problems

After grouping the data, the client's signs and symptoms may clearly require medical diagnosis and treatment. Referral to a primary care provider is necessary.

CASE STUDY

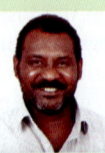

The nurse used diagnostic reasoning to analyze the data collected on Mr. Blair's pain to arrive at the following possible conclusions.

Nursing Diagnoses

- Chronic pain r/t unknown etiology after prostatectomy, radiation, chemotherapy
- Impaired physical mobility r/t chronic pain in lower back radiating to legs
- Sleep deprivation r/t chronic pain exacerbated at night and worry that cancer may have returned
- Anxiety r/t prolonged pain affecting daily activities and worry that cancer may have returned
- Risk for powerlessness r/t chronic pain
- Risk for constipation r/t nonsteroidal anti-inflammatory agents and opiate intake

- Risk for spiritual distress r/t anxiety, pain, life change, and chronic illness

Potential Collaborative Problem
- RC: Prostate cancer metastases

To view an algorithm depicting the process for diagnostic reasoning in this case, go to **thePoint**.

Interdisciplinary Verbal Communication of Assessment Findings Using SBAR

SITUATION: Leonard Blair, 55-year-old African American man, presents with continuous, stabbing, deep, dull low back pain radiating down both legs for last 8 to 10 months. Leg pain worsens at night and while walking. Takes Motrin 600 mg every 4 hours for mild to moderate pain and oxycodone 5 mg every 6 hours for pain of 7 to 10 on Visual Analog Scale. Has lost appetite. Pain affects ability to sleep at night and feels tired and unable to work and meet with his clients. Worried about return of cancer.

BACKGROUND: Financial manager divorced with two children. Diagnosed with prostate cancer and had a prostatectomy followed by radiation and chemotherapy 1 year ago.

ASSESSMENT: Tympanic temperature: 98.8°F, HR = 110 beats/min, RR = 22 breaths/min, BP = 135/85 mmHg, weight loss of 6 kg in the last 3 months. Client limps and has his shoulders slumped, changing position every 2 to 3 minutes, frowning and grimacing. Standing: lifts knees only 20 degrees from straight position when asked to raise knees. Lying: able to lift each leg with knee unbent 15 degrees before pain starts. Lying prone: able to lift each leg only 10 degrees before pain begins.

RECOMMENDATION: Client has chronic pain r/t unknown etiology after prostatectomy, radiation, chemotherapy. He also has impaired physical mobility r/t chronic pain in lower back radiating to legs. He is experiencing sleep deprivation r/t chronic pain exacerbated at night and worry that cancer may have returned. He has anxiety r/t prolonged pain affecting daily activities and worry that cancer may have returned. He needs to be seen by his primary care provider for further assessment and treatment of his pain and possible prostate cancer metastases.

Want to know more?

A wide variety of resources to enhance your learning and understanding of this book are available on **thePoint**. Visit thePoint to access:

NCLEX-Style Student Review Questions
Watch and Learn Videos
Concepts in Action Animations
And more!

References and Selected Readings

Acute pain management: Operative or medical procedures and trauma. (1992, February). *Clinical Practice Guidelines No. 1 (AHCPR Publication No. 92–0032)*. Rockville, MD: Agency for Healthcare Research and Quality.

American Pain Society. (2008). Advocacy. Pediatric chronic pain: A position statement from the American Pain Society. Available at http://www.ampainsoc.org/advocacy/pediatric

Baker, C., & Wong, D. (1987). QUEST: A process of pain assessment in children. *Orthopedic Nursing, 6*(1), 11–21.

Banicek, J. (2010). How to ensure acute pain in older people is appropriately assessed and managed. Available at http://www.nursingtimes.net/how-to-ensure-acute-pain-in-older-people-is-appropriately-assessed-and-managed/5017667.article

Board of Regents for the University of Wisconsin System. (2010). Classification of pain. Available at http://projects.hsl.wisc.edu/GME/PainManagement/session2.4.html

Bulls, H., Freeman, E., Anderson, A., et al. (2015). Sex differences in experimental measures of pain sensitivity and endogenous pain inhibition. *Journal of Pain Research, 8*, 311–320. Doi: 10.2147/JPR.S84607. Available at http://www.ncbi.nlm.nih.gov/pubmed/26170713

Burn Survivors Throughout the World. (n.d.). Visual Analog Scale (VAS). Available at www.burnsurvivorsttw.org

Cleeland, C. (1992). Brief pain inventory short form [BPI SF]. In C. Cleeland, D. Turk, & R. Melzack. *Handbook of pain assessment*. New York, NY: Guildford Press, pp. 367–370, 383–384.

Dafny, N. (1997–2012). Pain principles. In J. H. Byrne (Ed.): *Neuroscience Online* (Chapter 6). Available at http://neuroscience.uth.tmc.edu/s2/chapter06.html

Doctors on Fetal Pain. (2015). Fetal pain: The evidence. Available at http://www.doctorsonfetalpain.com

Dunwoody, C., Krenzischek, D., Pasero, C., et al. (2008). Assessment, physiological monitoring, and consequences of inadequately treated acute pain. *Pain Management Nursing, 9*(1), S11–S21.

Flaherty, E. (2008). Pain assessment for older adults. *American Journal of Nursing, 108*(6), 45–47.

Healthcommunities.com. (1998–2008). Cancer pain. Available at http://www.oncologychannel.com/pain

Healthy People 2020. (2015). Health-related quality of life and well-being. Available at http://www.healthypeople.gov/2020/topics-objectives/topic/health-related-quality-of-life-well-being

Herr, K., Coyne, P., Key, T., et al. (2006). Pain assessment in the nonverbal patient: Position statement with clinical practice recommendations. *Pain Management Nursing, 7*(2), 44–52.

Herr, K., Coyne, P., McCaffery, M., et al. (2011). Pain assessment in the patient unable to self-report: Position statement with clinical practice recommendations. *Pain Management Nursing, 12*(4), 230–250.

Hummel, P., & Puchalski, M. (2000). *N-Pass: Neonatal pain, agitation, & sedation scale*. Chicago, IL: Loyola University Health System. Available at http://www.n-pass.com

International Association for the Study of Pain. (2011). Definition of pain. Available at http://www.iasp-pain.org

Joint Commission on Accreditation of Healthcare Organizations (Joint Commission). (2015). Clarification of the pain management standard. Available at http://www.jointcommission.org/assets/1/18/Clarification_of_the_Pain_Management__Standard.pdf

Kaegi, L. (2004). What color is your pain? Available at http://www.minoritynurse.com/nurse-led-interventions/what-color-your-pain

McCaffery, M., & Pasero, C. (1999). *Pain: Clinical manual* (2nd ed.). St. Louis, MO: Mosby.

Martinez, E. (2011). Pain and age—the older adult. Available at http://painconnection.surtos.com/MyTreatment/MyTreatment_DisparatiesInPain_Age.asp

Medical News Today. (2015, June 30). Gender difference in pain transmission reports new study. Available at http://www.medicalnewstoday.com/articles/296042.php

Memorial Sloan Kettering Cancer Center. (n.d.). Memorial Pain Assessment Card. (n.d.). Available at http://www.partnersagainstpain.com/professional-tools

NANDA International. (2015). *Nursing diagnoses: Definitions & classification 2015–2017*. Philadelphia, PA: NANDA International.

Otto, S., Duncan, S., & Baker, L. (1996). Initial pain assessment for pediatric use only. Distributed by the City of Hope Pain/Palliative Care Resource Center. Available at http://www.cityofhope.org/prc/pain_assessment.asp

Patestas, M., & Gartner, L. P. (2006). Ascending sensory pathways. In M. A. Patestas & L. P. Gartner. *A textbook of neuroanatomy*. Hoboken, NJ: Blackwell Publishing. Available at http://www.blackwellpublishing.com/patestas/chapters/10.pdf

Regents of the University of Wisconsin. (2010). Classification of pain. Available at http://projects.hsl.wisc.edu/GME/PainManagement/session2

Silkman, C. (2008). Assessing the seven dimensions of pain. *American Nurse Today*, 3(2), 12–15.

Steefel, L. (2001). Treat pain in any culture. Available at http://www2.nursingspectrum.com/articles/print.html?AID=5410

Universal Pain Assessment Tool (UCLA). (n.d.). Available at http://www.anes.ucla.edu/pain

U.S. Preventive Services Task Force (USPSTF). (2011). First annual report to Congress on high-priority evidence gaps for clinical preventive services—Appendix C. Available at http://www.uspreventiveservicestaskforce.org/Page/Name/first-annual-report-to-congress-on-high-priority-evidence-gaps-for-clinical-preventive-services—appendix-c

WebMD. (2015). Chronic pain conditions: What is the role of age and gender in pain? Available at http://www.webmd.com/pain-management/chronic-pain-conditions

Weissman, D.E., Gordon, D., & Bidar-Sielaff, S. (2004). Cultural aspects of pain management. *Journal of Palliative Medicine, 7*(5), 715–717.

Wood, S. (2008). Anatomy and physiology of pain. Available at http://www.nursingtimes.net/nursing-practice/1860931.article

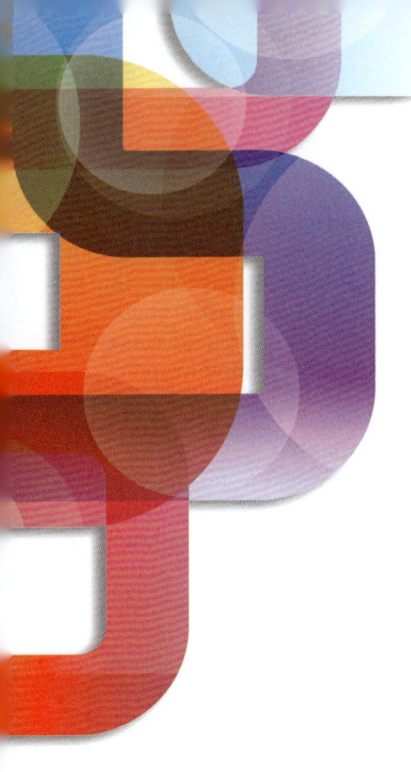

10 ASSESSING FOR VIOLENCE

Learning Objectives

1. Describe how to prepare a physically and emotionally safe environment in which to interview and assess a client who has experienced domestic violence.
2. Use the domestic violent screening tools to identify victims of violence across the lifespan.
3. Teach clients who are at risk for violence to develop a safety plan.
4. Discuss the importance of accurate documentation of physical assessment findings in clients who have experienced abuse.
5. Correctly use injury maps to document physical findings in clients.
6. Analyze data from the client interview and physical assessment of a client at risk for domestic violence or suspected to have suffered from abuse to formulate valid nursing diagnoses, collaborative problems, and/or referrals.

CASE STUDY

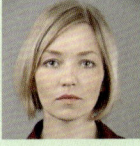

Ms. D is a 32-year-old woman who presents to the outpatient clinic with her husband and two children. She states, "My chest hurts and I cannot breathe easily." She also reports that she is "having difficulty talking." When asked about her injuries, she has poor eye contact and looks away or toward her husband. Her husband interrupts his wife frequently, preventing Ms. D from answering interview questions. The client's two children, a boy and a girl, cling to their mother.

CONCEPTUAL FOUNDATIONS

Domestic violence is defined by the U.S. Department of Justice Office on Violence against Women (FindLaw, 2016, p. 1) as "a pattern of abusive behavior in any relationship that is used by one partner to gain or maintain control over another intimate partner." Family violence in US sources tend to divide domestic violence from child abuse and elder abuse, but definitions from other countries, such as that of Australia, are broader and more readily focus on all family members. The Australian Law Reform Commission (2010) has recommended a definition for family violence: "violent or threatening behaviour, or any other form of behaviour, that coerces or controls a family member or causes that family member to be fearful." In all definitions of domestic or family violence, the abuse can be physical (e.g., slapping, hitting, kicking, punching, burning); emotional (e.g., threats of physical harm, financial harm, harm to child or pet, or suicide; harassment; insults and other verbal abuse; isolation; intimidation; mind games; throwing objects); or sexual (incest or rape).

Domestic violence or intimate partner violence (IPV) statistics (Domestic Violence Statistics, 2015) note that one in every three women worldwide has been beaten, coerced into sex, or otherwise abused at least once in her lifetime. Also noted is that "the costs of intimate partner violence in the United States alone exceed $5.8 billion per year: $4.1 billion are for direct medical and health care services, while productivity losses account for nearly $1.8 billion" (Domestic Violence Statistics, 2015). As for child abuse, Safe Horizon (2015) reports that in the United States, 1 in 10 children suffers from child maltreatment, 1 in 16 children suffers from sexual abuse, and nearly 1 in 10 children witnesses family violence. The annual cost of child abuse in the United States was estimated for 2008 to be $124 billion (Fang et al., 2012).

Theories of Family Violence

To discuss the theory of family violence, the concepts of violence and aggression need to be defined. *Violence* is "the use of physical force to harm someone, to damage property, etc." (Merriam-Webster Online, 2015). Violence tends to have a negative connotation in the context of murder, torture, or hate, but has more of a positive connotation if associated with self-defense or acts of war. American culture condemns violence in the context of murder, torture, and hate. However, some movies, television programs, and literature glorify it. *Aggression* is defined as "a forceful action or procedure (as an unprovoked attack) especially when intended to dominate or master" (Merriam-Webster Online, 2015). Aggression also has both positive and negative connotations. The positive connotation is associated with the drive for success, as in aggressive men. The negative connotation is often associated with the notion of aggressive women, which violates what is considered appropriate for gender norms in many cultures. The negative connotation is also associated with aggression against a family member when one person tries to dominate or master another.

McCue (2008) presents five theories related to domestic violence for why men batter women: (1) psychopathology theory (batterers suffer personality disorders); (2) social learning theory (violence is a learned behavior from childhood); (3) biologic theory (physiologic changes from childhood trauma, head injuries, or through heredity cause violent behavior); (4) family systems theory (violence grows through family system function, but some criticize this theory as blaming the victim); and (5) feminist theory (male/female inequity in patriarchal societies leads to violence). All of these theories help to explain domestic violence. An additional theory, Walker's Cycle of Violence (Walker, 1979; 1984) and (Devine, 2008), discuss the cyclic nature of violence. Walker explains that abuse occurs in a predictable pattern. During the beginning of a relationship, couples are rarely apart and the relationship is very intense. The abuser displays possessiveness and jealousy, and starts to separate the victim from supportive relationships. Criticism is the sign of phase 1, the tension-building phase. The abuser makes unrealistic demands. When expectations are not satisfied, criticism and/or ridicule escalate into shoving or slapping. The victims often blame themselves for failing to satisfy the unrealistic demands of the abuser. Phase 2, the acute battering stage, may be triggered by something minor but results in violence lasting up to 24 hours. The victim is rarely able to stop the abuse. Phase 3, the honeymoon phase, is described as a period of reconciliation. This phase begins after an incident of battery. The abuser is loving, promises never to abuse the victim again, and is very attentive to the victim. Then the cycle begins again.

Walker's three-stage model is also referred to as the Tension Building/Explosion Model. A more elaborate model presented by The Center for Hope and Safety organization, the Cycle of Domestic Violence Model, has seven stages (The Center for Hope and Safety, n.d.). In this model, the seven stages are: Abuse, guilt, rationalization, "normal" behavior, fantasy, planning, and set-up. In the fantasy stage, the abuser fantasizes about the abuse, then planning begins to accomplish the fantasy of abusing the victim. The abuser then sets up the victim to fail at whatever he expects, such as sending her to the grocery store, but under a time limit, at a high traffic time. The victim returns late and the next episode of abuse begins.

Culture, race, ethnicity, and the economy must be considered in the evaluation for suspected family violence. One needs to conduct a cultural assessment (using assessment guidelines) before attempting to understand a client's particular case of family violence, especially for family members of an ethnic origin different from that of the nurse. Note that health care providers are more likely to report child abuse in minority populations or in persons of lower socioeconomic levels (CME Resource, 2012), even though studies show little difference in rates of abuse in racial groups when income levels are included (National Institutes of Health, 2012).

Types of Family Violence

Types of family violence include physical abuse, psychological abuse, economic abuse, and sexual abuse. Abandonment, physical and emotional neglect, and parental substance abuse are added by CME Resources (2012) in an overview of types of abuse.

Physical Abuse

Physical abuse includes pushing, shoving, slapping, kicking, choking, punching, and burning. It may also involve holding, tying, or other methods of restraint. The victim may be left in a dangerous place without resources. The abuser may refuse to help the victim when sick, injured, or in need. Physical abuse may also involve attacking the victim with household items (lamps, radios, ashtrays, irons, etc.) or with common weapons (knives or guns).

Psychological Abuse

Psychological abuse involves the use of constant insults or criticism, blaming the victim for things that are not the victim's fault, threats to hurt children or pets, isolation from supporters (family, friends, or coworkers), deprivation, humiliation, stalking and intimidation, and manipulation of various kinds, such as threats of suicide. Psychological abuse, also known as emotional abuse, has been defined by Vancouver Coastal Health (2013) as "any act including confinement, isolation, verbal assault, humiliation, intimidation, infantilization, or any other treatment which may diminish the sense of identity, dignity, and self-worth" (para. 1). Tracy (2012) provides lists of short- and long-term effects of emotional abuse in adults (Box 10-1).

Dr. Harriet McMillan reports on a new study declaring psychological abuse of children as "acts such as belittling, denigrating, terrorizing, exploiting, emotional unresponsiveness, or corrupting a child to the point a child's well-being is at risk.... behavior that makes a child feel worthless, unloved, or unwanted," (para. 2) and that such abuse "interferes with a child's development path, has been linked with disorders of attachment, developmental and educational problems, socialization problems and disruptive behaviour" (para. 6) (Science News, 2012). This type of abuse is difficult to assess because of the lack of a clearly defined diagnosis. Legal definitions of psychological abuse differ from state to state, which results in an underestimated number of cases reported. The majority of children who suffer from psychological abuse use effective coping mechanisms and will not exhibit pathologic behaviors, but many have lingering psychological and behavioral problems and even posttraumatic stress disorder (PTSD).

Economic Abuse

Economic abuse may be evidenced by preventing the victim from getting or keeping a job, controlling money and limiting access to funds, spending the victim's money, and controlling knowledge of family finances. Economic abuse, also known as financial abuse, is the improper exploitation of another person's personal assets, properties, or funds. Examples of this type of abuse include the cashing of another person's checks without authorization or permission, forging signatures, and misusing or stealing money or possessions. Economic abuse may also occur if someone deceives another into signing a will or contract, coerces a person into signing a will or contract, or controls another person's money and demands a detailed accounting of the funds. Statistics of economic abuse are difficult to find due to underreporting by abused elders.

Sexual Abuse

Sexual abuse involves forcing the victim to perform sexual acts against her or his will, pursuing sexual activity after the victim has said no, using violence during sex, and using weapons

BOX 10-1 EFFECTS OF EMOTIONAL ABUSE ON ADULTS

SHORT-TERM EFFECTS OF EMOTIONAL ABUSE

- Surprise and confusion
- Questioning of one's own memory: "Did that really happen?"
- Anxiety or fear; hypervigilance
- Shame or guilt
- Aggression (as a defense to the abuse)
- Becoming overly passive or compliant
- Frequent crying
- Avoidance of eye contact
- Feeling powerless and defeated, as nothing you do ever seems to be right (learned helplessness)
- Feeling like you're "walking on eggshells"
- Feeling manipulated, used, and controlled
- Feeling undesirable
- Partners may also find themselves trying to do anything possible to bring the relationship back to the way it was before the abuse.

LONG-TERM EFFECTS OF EMOTIONAL ABUSE

- Depression
- Withdrawal
- Low self-esteem and self-worth
- Emotional instability
- Sleep disturbances
- Physical pain without cause
- Suicidal ideation, thoughts, or attempts
- Extreme dependence on the abuser
- Underachievement
- Inability to trust
- Feeling trapped and alone
- Substance abuse
- Stockholm syndrome is also common in long-term abuse situations. In Stockholm syndrome, the victim is so terrified of the abuser that the victim overly identifies and becomes bonded with the abuser in an attempt to stop the abuse. Victims will even defend their abuser and their emotionally abusive actions.

Modified and used with permission from Tracy, N. (2012). Effects of emotional abuse on adults. Available at http://www.healthyplace.com/abuse/emotional-psychological-abuse/effects-of-emotional-abuse-on-adults/

vaginally, orally, or anally. Sexual abuse is not limited to family members or intimate partners but can be stranger abuse such as assault and rape as well. Sexual violence may occur in any type of relationship, but most perpetrators of sexual assault are known to their victims. The Bureau of Justice Statistics (BJS) reports that 6 in 10 rape or sexual assault victims said that they were assaulted by an intimate partner, relative, friend, or acquaintance (National Institute of Justice, 2010).

Categories of Family Violence

Categories of family violence include IPV, child abuse, and elder mistreatment. Family violence affects people of all ages, sexes, religions, ethnicities, and socioeconomic levels.

Intimate Partner Violence

Intimate partner violence, as defined by the CDC (2015b) is "physical, sexual, or psychological harm by a current or former partner or spouse" (para. 1). Forms of the harm may be psychological abuse, sexual assault, progressive isolation, stalking, deprivation, intimidation, and reproductive coercion. IPV affects millions of women regardless of age, economic status, race, religion, ethnicity, sexual orientation, or educational background. Over time, IPV escalates in both severity and frequency unless intervention occurs. The National Intimate Partner and Sexual Violence Survey (NISVS) conducted by the Centers for Disease Control and Prevention (CDC, 2014) found that IPV, sexual violence, and stalking are widespread. Significant impacts related to violence were reported by 81% of the women surveyed who had experienced the violence. It was estimated that more than 1.3 million women were raped in the year prior to the NISVS and 1 million women sought medical care for injuries related to abuse, resulting in 100,000 days of hospitalization, 30,000 emergency department (ED) visits, and 40,000 primary care visits a year. Furthermore, one out of four women has been a victim of severe physical abuse by an intimate partner and one in five has been raped in her lifetime. The American Psychological Association (2015) reported that 30% of all murdered women are victims of IPV. In addition, children raised in homes with IPV are more likely to use violence as adults (Child Help, 2012). Recent studies have indicated that children experiencing violence in the home or who are exposed to violence inflicted on others have changes in their brain activity similar to veterans in combat (Sherin & Nemeroff, 2011).

When examining the problem of IPV, it is common to focus on the woman as the victim. Males also suffer from victimization. The NISVS found that 1 in 71 men have been raped in their lifetime, but that 1 out of every 7 men experience physical violence by their intimate partner (CDC, 2014). Male victims report that if they inform the police of an incident, it may not be filed and they are often ridiculed. Male victims suffer effects of trauma similar to those experienced by female victims (Douglas & Hines, 2011). When men attempt to leave their abuser, they face many of the same problems as female victims. However, they may have fewer options for assistance, as there are few if any facilities that offer shelter to male victims. Men, like women who experience any form of violence, report chronic pain, headaches, difficulty sleeping, and poor physical and mental health more than men who have not experienced violence (CDC, 2015c).

Child Abuse

The Child Abuse Prevention and Treatment Act (CAPTA) defines *child abuse* as "any recent act or failure to act on the part of a parent or caretaker which results in death, serious physical or emotional harm, sexual abuse or exploitation" or "an act or failure to act that presents an imminent risk of serious harm" (Child Abuse Prevention and Treatment Act, Public Law 104–235, §111; 42 U.S.C. 510g, 2003; and the CAPTA Reauthorization Act of 2010 [P.L. 111–320]).

The Child Welfare Information Gateway (2013b) noted that each state provides its own definition of child abuse as long as the definition is within the minimum standards set by CAPTA. Child abuse may be either by commission or by omission and is rarely an isolated incident. There are four broad categories of child abuse: neglect, emotional abuse, sexual abuse, and physical abuse. Some states add abandonment and parental substance abuse to the categories.

In 2015, the Health and Human Services Administration for Child and Families reported that for the year 2013 in the United States, 3.1 million children were referred to child protective services (p. 79) and 679,000 (p. 21) were determined to be victims of child abuse (physical, sexual, psychological abuse, or neglect), and of these, 1,520 children died. The National Conference of State Legislatures (NCSL, 2015) reports that since 2013, all 50 states have statutes that mandate reporting of child abuse and neglect. Guidelines have been developed to aid clinicians in recognizing child abuse injuries, performing comprehensive examinations, recommending tests, documenting injuries, and reporting and testifying in child abuse cases.

The long-term consequences of child abuse and neglect, according to the Child Welfare Information Gateway (2013a), include:

- Physical: chronic health conditions, and greater likelihood of suffering from cardiovascular disease, lung and liver disease, hypertension, diabetes, asthma, and obesity; impaired brain development, including difficulties with cognitive, language, and academic abilities; brain injury with head trauma; emotional conditions such as chronic fear, hypervigilance, impulsivity.
- Psychological: isolation, fear, and an inability to trust—can translate into lifelong psychological consequences, including low self-esteem, depression, and relationship difficulties; impaired psychological development during infancy; cognitive and social difficulties.
- Behavioral: adolescent issues such as grade repetition, substance abuse, delinquency, truancy, or pregnancy, and sexual risk-taking; greater likelihood of being raped in adulthood; correlation with juvenile delinquency and adult criminality; abuse of alcohol and other drugs; greater likelihood to become abusive parents.
- Societal: direct costs of child maltreatment and fatalities total $124 billion per year, but for each $1 spent in prevention, $47 are saved; indirect costs of long-term economic costs to society include costs associated with increased use of our health care system, juvenile and adult criminal activity, mental illness, substance abuse, domestic violence, employment problems, financial problems, and absenteeism from work.

Elder Mistreatment

Elder mistreatment—also known as elder abuse—includes neglect, physical abuse, sexual abuse, financial abuse, psychological abuse (including humiliation, intimidation, and threats), exploitation, abandonment, or prejudicial attitudes that decrease quality of life and are demeaning to those over the age of 65 years. The abuse may be from commission, but is frequently from omission.

The rate of violence against the elderly age 65 and older for 2003–2013, reported by the U.S. Department of Justice (Bureau of Justice Statistics [BJS], 2014), was lower than for younger groups, but significant nonetheless.

- The rates of nonfatal violent crime (3.6 per 1,000 persons) and property crime (72.3 per 1,000) against elderly persons were lower than those of younger persons.
- The ratio of the estimates of property crime to violent crime was higher for the elderly (13 to 1) than for younger persons aged 25 to 49 (3 to 1) and persons aged 50 to 64 (5 to 1).
- Elderly homicide rates declined 44%, from 3.7 homicides per 100,000 persons in 1993 to 2.1 per 100,000 in 2011.
- Persons age 65 or older experienced more incidents of identity theft (5.0%) than persons aged 16 to 24 (3.8%), but less than those aged 25 to 49 (7.9%) and 50 to 64 (7.8%).
- Among elderly violent crime victims, about 59% reported being victimized at or near their home. A smaller percentage of elderly victims (18%) suffered an injury during the incident, compared with victims aged 12 to 24 (30%) and 25 to 49 (25%).
- The elderly (56%) reported incidents of violent crime to police more often than persons aged 12 to 24 (38%). No differences were detected between the elderly and other age groups.
- About 11% of elderly victims of violent crime received assistance from victim service agencies.

As for elder abuse, including neglect and exploitation, the CDC (2015a) reports that one out of every ten people aged 60 and older who lives at home experiences abuse; and for every one case of elder abuse that is detected or reported, it is estimated that approximately 23 cases remain hidden.

Some of the consequences of elder mistreatment include both physical and psychological effects (CDC, 2015a). Physical effects include:

- injuries (e.g., bruises, lacerations, dental problems, head injuries, broken bones, pressure sores)
- persistent physical pain and soreness
- nutrition and hydration issues
- sleep disturbances
- increased susceptibility to new illnesses (including sexually transmitted diseases)
- exacerbation of pre-existing health conditions
- increased risk of premature death

Psychological effects include:

- increased risk for developing fear and anxiety reactions
- learned helplessness
- posttraumatic stress disorder

Elder abuse is often difficult to assess because of the older person's isolation from the community, immobility, fear of the perpetrator, and inability to report because of cognitive impairments. Older adults are often unwilling to report their abuser, due to mistrust of law enforcement or due to a relationship with the abuser (e.g., son or daughter) that may create feelings of guilt, burden, dependence, or fear of abandonment. They may be unsure of whom to contact to report the abuse, doubt authorities' willingness to become involved, or fear that without their caregiver they will end up in an institution. Many older adults prefer to stay in their own home even if it means suffering abuse at the hands of a caregiver.

Other Types of Violence

School Violence (Bullying and Punking)

Bullying can be defined as "unwanted aggressive behavior among school aged children that involves a real or perceived power imbalance that is either repeated or a single event," and may consist of verbal (teasing, name-calling, inappropriate sexual comments, threatening, or taunting), social (spreading rumors, leaving someone out of a group, discouraging others to not be friends with someone), physical (hitting, kicking, pinching, tripping, spitting, taking or breaking others' things, using rude hand gestures to someone), and/or cyberbullying (bullying via internet, text, or email) (Simms, Bushman, & Petersen, 2016). [1]Bullying has become quite common and a huge problem in the US school-age population, often occurring on school property but extending beyond the school, especially through cyberbullying. About 30% of students in the United States are involved in bullying on a regular basis, either as a victim, bully, or both (Bullying Statistics, 2015). Teens in sixth through tenth grade are the most likely to be involved in activities related to bullying. According to Stopbullying.gov, in 2014, the Centers for Disease Control and Department of Education released the first federal uniform definition of bullying for research and surveillance. The elements of this definition include: unwanted aggressive behavior; observed or perceived power imbalance; and repetition of behaviors or high likelihood of repetition. Four types of bullying include broad categories of physical, verbal, relational (e.g., efforts to harm the reputation or relationships of the targeted youth), and damage to property. Some levels of bullying fall into criminal categories of harassment, hazing, and assault. The relationship between bullying and suicide is complex, and the Stopbullying.gov site (2014) says that linking the two is dangerous. Many other factors play a role when suicide follows bullying.

Punking in the school aged population has been defined by Phillips (2007) as a practice of verbal and physical violence, humiliation, and shaming usually done in public by males to other males. Study findings reveal that punking terminology and behaviors are usually interchangeable with bullying terminology and behaviors.

Hate Crimes in the United States

The Federal Bureau of Investigation (FBI) report for the year 2013 noted a small decrease in hate crimes from 2012 (Federal Bureau of Investigation [FBI], 2014). There were 5,922 single bias hate crimes in 2013, falling into several categories of bias: racial, especially anti-black (48.5%); sexual orientation, especially anti-gay (20.8%); religious (17.4%); ethnicity (11.1%); disability (1.4%); gender identity (0.5%); and gender (0.3%). Six hate crimes involved multiple biases, bringing the total of hate crimes for the year 2013 in the United States to 5,928. A majority of these crimes were against individuals (e.g., intimidation, assaults, rapes, murders). About a third were property crimes, such as acts of destruction, damage to property, and vandalism. The rest were considered acts against society (drug offenses and prostitution).

Human Trafficking

Human trafficking has become a major international problem worldwide (United Nations Office on Drugs and Crime, 2014). Studies have shown 510 human trafficking flows (or pathways often extending across borders) around the world. Of the convicted traffickers, 72% are men and 28% women. The victims by age and gender are 49% women, 18% men, 21% girls, and 12% boys. Forms of exploitation include sexual exploitation, forced labor, servitude, slavery; organ removal; and other forms of exploitation. Sexual exploitation predominates, except in East Asia, South Asia, and the Pacific, where forced labor is the predominant exploitation. Often the perpetrators are nationals of the country where the trafficking begins (so traffickers and victims are from the same country), and the victims are taken to places within the country's borders or across the border to nearby countries. Trafficking operations can involve one or a few individuals or an entire organized crime organization.

According to DOsomething.org (n.d.), human trafficking is the third largest international crime industry worldwide, following illegal drugs and arms trafficking, and generates a profit of $32 billion per year. Globally, the average cost of a slave is $90. In the United States, between 14,500 and 17,500 individuals are trafficked into the country each year. The National Human Trafficking Hotline received the most calls from Texas each year, especially from the Dallas-Fort Worth area, while California has three of the FBI's highest child trafficking areas in the nation (Los Angeles, San Francisco, and San Diego).

Recognizing the Signs. Knowing the red flags and indicators of human trafficking is a key step in identifying more victims and helping them find the assistance they need. To request help or report suspected human trafficking, call the National Human Trafficking Resource Center hotline at 1-888-373-7888. Or text INFO or HELP at: BeFree (233733). The following list suggests common indicators that victims of human trafficking might exhibit:

Common Work and Living Conditions
- Is not free to leave or come and go as he/she wishes
- Is under 18 and is providing commercial sex acts
- Is in the commercial sex industry and has a pimp/manager
- Is unpaid, paid very little, or paid only through tips
- Works excessively long and/or unusual hours
- Is not allowed breaks or suffers under unusual restrictions at work
- Owes a large debt and is unable to pay it off
- Was recruited through false promises concerning the nature and conditions of his/her work
- High security measures exist in the work and/or living locations (e.g., opaque windows, boarded up windows, bars on windows, barbed wire, security cameras)

Poor Mental Health or Abnormal Behavior
- Is fearful, anxious, depressed, submissive, tense, or nervous/paranoid
- Exhibits unusually fearful or anxious behavior after law enforcement is mentioned
- Avoids eye contact

Poor Physical Health
- Lacks health care
- Appears malnourished
- Shows signs of physical and/or sexual abuse, physical restraint, confinement, or torture

Lack of Control
- Has few or no personal possessions
- Is not in control of his/her own money, no financial records or bank account
- Is not in control of his/her own identification documents (ID or passport)
- Is not allowed or able to speak for themselves (a third party may insist on being present and/or translating)

Other
- Claims of just visiting and inability to clarify where he/she is staying/address
- Lack of knowledge of whereabouts (e.g., does not know what city he/she is in)
- Loss of sense of time
- Has numerous inconsistencies in his/her story

This list is not exhaustive and represents only a selection of possible indicators. Also, the red flags in this list may not be present in all trafficking cases and are not cumulative. Learn more at www.traffickingresourcecenter.org.

War Crimes

Within the United States, there may be some victims of war crimes who have come in as immigrants or are returning from military service. This is a category that is complex and depends on the theater of war to determine what crimes may have been committed. Torture, poison gases, and other crimes against humanity are being practiced in several areas of the world today. Asking clients who appear to be suffering from PTSD about their experiences may not be helpful. Should PTSD be detected in clients, referral to an appropriate health care provider is essential.

A self-assessment test for PTSD has been provided online by the Anxiety and Depression Society of America (2015) (Box 10-2).

BOX 10-2 SCREENING FOR POSTTRAUMATIC STRESS DISORDER (PTSD)

If you suspect that you might suffer from PTSD, answer the questions below, print out the results and share them with your health care professional.

To locate a specialist who treats PTSD, visit the ADAA Find a Therapist.

Are you troubled by the following?

Yes ○	No ○	You have experienced or witnessed a life-threatening event that caused intense fear, helplessness, or horror.

Do you re-experience the event in at least one of the following ways?

Yes ○	No ○	Repeated, distressing memories, or dreams
Yes ○	No ○	Acting or feeling as if the event were happening again (flashbacks or a sense of reliving it)
Yes ○	No ○	Intense physical and/or emotional distress when you are exposed to things that remind you of the event

Do reminders of the event affect you in at least three of the following ways?

Yes ○	No ○	Avoiding thoughts, feelings, or conversations about it
Yes ○	No ○	Avoiding activities and places or people who remind you of it
Yes ○	No ○	Blanking on important parts of it
Yes ○	No ○	Losing interest in significant activities of your life
Yes ○	No ○	Feeling detached from other people
Yes ○	No ○	Feeling your range of emotions is restricted
Yes ○	No ○	Sensing that your future has shrunk (for example, you don't expect to have a career, marriage, children, or normal life span)

Are you troubled by at least two of the following?

Yes ○	No ○	Problems sleeping
Yes ○	No ○	Irritability or outbursts of anger
Yes ○	No ○	Problems concentrating
Yes ○	No ○	Feeling "on guard"
Yes ○	No ○	An exaggerated startle response

Having more than one illness at the same time can make it difficult to diagnose and treat the different conditions. Depression and substance abuse are among the conditions that occasionally complicate PTSD and other anxiety disorders.

Yes ○	No ○	Have you experienced changes in sleeping or eating habits?

More days than not, do you feel…

Yes ○	No ○	sad or depressed?
Yes ○	No ○	disinterested in life?
Yes ○	No ○	worthless or guilty?

During the last year, has the use of alcohol or drugs…

Yes ○	No ○	resulted in your failure to fulfill responsibilities with work, school, or family?
Yes ○	No ○	placed you in a dangerous situation, such as driving a car under the influence?
Yes ○	No ○	gotten you arrested?
Yes ○	No ○	continued despite causing problems for you or your loved ones?

Reference: Diagnostic and Statistical Manual of Mental Disorders, Fourth Edition. Washington, DC, American Psychiatric Association, 1994. Print this form: http://www.adaa.org/screening-posttraumatic-stress-disorder-ptsd

NURSING ASSESSMENT OF FAMILY VIOLENCE

There has been a change in recommendations for universal screening for family violence. In 2013, the Office of the Assistant Secretary for Planning and Evaluation (ASPE) of the U.S. Department of Health and Human Services (HHS) recommended universal screening for domestic and IPV by any clinician in health care settings of every female patient through age 64, as opposed to only screening certain patients because of risk factors or warning signs. Health care settings include any location where health issues are addressed, including but not limited to emergency departments, patient treatment centers, and the offices of primary care clinicians and other health care practitioners. Clinicians include doctors, nurses, nurse practitioners, physician assistants, counselors, and other health care practitioners. Screening and counseling include use of a few short, open-ended questions asked by a clinician to the patient, and they can also be facilitated by the use of forms or other assessment tools. Counseling may include provision of basic information, including on how a patient's health concerns may relate to violence, and referrals for additional assistance when patients disclose abuse.

According to Neale (2012), the U.S. Preventive Services Task Force (USPSTF) has issued a draft recommendation that all childbearing women, from 14 to 46 years of age, should be screened for IPV, even if there is no obvious sign of physical, sexual, or psychological abuse. Screening for pregnant mothers should be started at the initial prenatal visit and continued periodically and postnatally (Moyer & USPSTF, 2013). New guidelines for screening for IPV and for abuse of elderly and vulnerable adults were issued in 2013 by USPSTF which support universal screening as described above.

As mentioned before, there are four areas to assess to determine the presence of family violence: physical abuse, psychological abuse, economic abuse, and sexual abuse. With physical

---

ASSESSMENT TOOL 10-1 Hurt, Insult, Threaten, Scream (HITS)

Respond to the following four questions to assess frequency of abuse.
1. How often does your partner physically hurt you?
2. How often does your partner insult or talk down to you?
3. How often does your partner threaten you with physical harm?
4. How often does your partner scream or curse at you?

Copyright © 2003 by Kevin Sherin, MD, MPH.

---

abuse, it is important to remember that it may start at any time during a relationship. The abuse may not be part of the presenting problem for which the client is being seen but may be the cause of the presenting problem. Consistent risk factors for women at risk have not been identified. Therefore, both abused and nonabused women require routine screening by health care providers. A recommended tool for IPV is the HITS screening tool, a four-item tool to assess the frequency of IPV (Assessment Tool 10-1). The HITS tool (Hurt, Insult, Threaten, and Scream) is a self-report tool that may be asked verbally or given to the client. The tool, whether self-report or verbal, may be administered to both women and men (CDC, 2007; Sherin, 2003).

When sexual abuse is suspected, a complete physical examination is required. Disclosure of the incident may not occur for months or years after the sexual abuse event. Often sexual abuse, such as fondling, oral sex, or activity without penetration, does not involve physical injury. If sexual abuse is suspected, a trained interviewer should conduct a forensic interview. Because a major intervention for sexual abuse involves having the person talk about it, both the interview and physical examination are part of the actual nursing interventions that assist the client in recovering from the sexual abuse (Evidence-Based Practice 10-1).

10-1 EVIDENCE-BASED HEALTH PROMOTION AND DISEASE PREVENTION: INTIMATE PARTNER VIOLENCE

INTRODUCTION
According to the American Congress of Obstetricians and Gynecologists (ACOG, 2012), intimate partner violence is a significant public health problem. It affects persons from all walks of life "regardless of age, economic status, race, religion, ethnicity, sexual orientation, or educational background," and causes "lifelong consequences, including emotional trauma, lasting physical impairment, chronic health problems, and even death" (p. 1).

HEALTHY PEOPLE 2020 GOAL
Healthy People 2020 (2014) discusses all types of injury, both unintentional as well as acts of violence.
   Prevent unintentional injuries and violence, and reduce their consequences.

OBJECTIVES
Healthy People 2020 injury and violence prevention objectives deal with various types of fatal and nonfatal injuries, related hospitalizations, and emergency department visits, of any cause. Objectives related to violence prevention include homicides, firearm injuries, fatal and nonfatal physical assaults, bullying, as well as a few objectives specific to child abuse and intimate partner violence. Many of the abuse objectives are new or in development, but the list indicates the interest in reducing child and intimate partner violence:
- Reduce child maltreatment deaths.
- Reduce nonfatal child maltreatment.
- (Developmental) Reduce violence by current or former intimate partners.
- (Developmental) Reduce physical violence by current or former intimate partners.
- (Developmental) Reduce sexual violence by current or former intimate partners.
- (Developmental) Reduce psychological abuse by current or former intimate partners.
- (Developmental) Reduce stalking by current or former intimate partners.
- (Developmental) Reduce sexual violence.
- (Developmental) Reduce rape or attempted rape.
- (Developmental) Reduce abusive sexual contact other than rape or attempted rape.
- (Developmental) Reduce noncontact sexual abuse.
- Reduce nonfatal intentional self-harm injuries.
- Reduce children's exposure to violence.
- Increase the number of states (as well as District of Columbia) that link data on violent deaths from death certificates, law enforcement, and coroner and medical examiner reports to inform prevention efforts at the state and local levels.

Continued on following page

| 10-1 | **EVIDENCE-BASED HEALTH PROMOTION AND DISEASE PREVENTION: INTIMATE PARTNER VIOLENCE (Continued)** |

SCREENING

The USPSTF has drafted a new proposed recommendation for screening all women of childbearing age for intimate partner violence (Neale, 2012). This is a significant change from the 2004 guidelines (USPSTF, 2004). Devi (2012) reports on the subsequent debate that has been raised by the new guidelines. Many women's groups have welcomed the guidelines, but many worry that patients will be put into legal jeopardy in some US states where health care providers are mandated to report suspicion of domestic abuse.

ACOG (2012) recommends periodic screening for physical and psychological abuse, reproductive coercion, and progressive isolation. As described earlier in this chapter, the U.S. Preventive Services Task Force (USPSTF, 2013) has revised recommendations to include universal screening for all women by all clinicians in all health care settings.

RISK ASSESSMENT

Risk factors for intimate partner violence, according to the CDC (2015c), include:

Individual Risk Factors
- Low self-esteem
- Low income
- Low academic achievement
- Young age
- Aggressive or delinquent behavior as a youth
- Heavy alcohol and drug use
- Depression
- Anger and hostility
- Antisocial personality traits
- Borderline personality traits
- Prior history of being physically abusive
- Having few friends and being isolated from other people
- Unemployment
- Emotional dependence and insecurity
- Belief in strict gender roles (e.g., male dominance and aggression in relationships)
- Desire for power and control in relationships
- Perpetrating psychological aggression
- Being a victim of physical or psychological abuse (consistently one of the strongest predictors of perpetration)
- History of experiencing poor parenting as a child
- History of experiencing physical discipline as a child

Relationship Factors
- Marital conflict: fights, tension, and other struggles
- Marital instability: divorces or separations
- Dominance and control of the relationship by one partner over the other
- Economic stress
- Unhealthy family relationships and interactions

Community Factors
- Poverty and associated factors (e.g., overcrowding)
- Low social capital: lack of institutions, relationships, and norms that shape a community's social interactions
- Weak community sanctions against IPV (e.g., unwillingness of neighbors to intervene when they witness violence)

Societal Factors
- Traditional gender norms (e.g., women should stay at home, not enter workforce, and be submissive; men support the family and make the decisions)

CLIENT EDUCATION

ACOG (2012) Recommends the Following Protocol for Nurses Handling Victims of IPV
- Screen for IPV in a private and safe setting with the woman alone and not with her partner, friends, family, or caregiver.
- Use professional language interpreters and not someone associated with the patient.
- At the beginning of the assessment, offer a framing statement to show that screening is done universally and not because IPV is suspected. Also, inform patients of the confidentiality of the discussion and exactly what state law mandates that a physician must disclose.
- Incorporate screening for IPV into the routine medical history by integrating questions into intake forms so that all patients are screened whether or not abuse is suspected.
- Establish and maintain relationships with community resources for women affected by IPV.
- Keep printed take-home resource materials—such as safety procedures, hotline numbers, and referral information—in privately accessible areas such as restrooms and examination rooms. Posters and other educational materials displayed in the office also can be helpful.
- Ensure that staff receives training about IPV and that training is regularly offered.
- Even if abuse is not acknowledged, simply discussing IPV in a caring manner and having educational materials readily accessible may be of tremendous help. Providing all patients with educational materials is a useful strategy that normalizes the conversation, making it acceptable for them to take the information without disclosure. Futures Without Violence and the American College of Obstetricians and Gynecologists have developed patient education cards about IPV and reproductive coercion for adults and teens that are available in English and Spanish. For more information visit http://fvpfstore.stores.yahoo.net/safetycards1.html.

Preparing Yourself for the Examination

Before you can begin to effectively assess for the presence of family violence, you must first examine your feelings, beliefs, and biases regarding violence. Violence is a prevalent family and community health problem that needs to be confronted by society today. No one under any circumstance should be physically, psychologically, financially, or sexually abused. As a nurse, it is imperative that you become active in interrupting or ending cycles of violence. During your assessment, be aware of "red flags" that may indicate the presence of family violence; these red flags are often hidden from others.

 Concept Mastery Alert

The first step in preparation for an interview with a client that may concern family violence is for the nurse to examine his or her own feelings and determine if there are any beliefs or biases that may interfere with the nurse's ability to "hear" what the client is saying.

SAFETY TIP *Nurses are at risk of violence in the workplace. One of the greatest risks for violence in the workplace continues to be in caring for victims of IPV. Injured IPV victims are often accompanied to the ED by their batterer. As the batterer has already shown the ability to inflict injury, he or she should be considered dangerous. By accompanying the victim, the batterer is attempting to maintain control of the victim and prevent reports from being filed.*

Collecting Subjective Data

Interview Techniques

Creating a safe and confidential environment is essential to obtain concise and valid subjective data from any client who has experienced family violence. It is important to establish a trusting rapport and to patiently listen to a client who has experienced violence. Use simple direct questions with a relaxed and calm approach. If clients share the fact that they have experienced violence, do not ask them if they want to press charges, as this decision would require an attorney and is not part of assessing the client. For any client over the age of 3 years, ask screening questions in a secure, private setting with no one else present in the room. Do not screen if there are any safety concerns for you or the client.

Prior to screening, discuss any legal, mandatory reporting requirements or other limits to confidentiality. Screening may be done orally and in a written format or through computer-generated questions. Find a reliable and appropriate interpreter if the client is non–English-speaking (see Chapter 11 for selecting interpreters).

Remember when asking questions to allow the client to answer completely. Do not interrupt; it is important to let the client talk freely as you attentively listen. Convey a concerned and nonjudgmental attitude. Show appropriate empathy and compassion (Fig. 10-1).

History of Present Health Concern

QUESTION	RATIONALE
Review the client's past health history and physical examination records if available.	Records may include documentation of past assaults; past sexual violence; punking; unexplained injuries; unexplained symptoms of pain, nausea and vomiting, or choking feeling; repeated visits to emergency department or clinic for injuries; signs and symptoms of anxiety; use of sedatives or tranquilizers; injuries during pregnancy; history of drug or alcohol abuse; history of depression and/or suicide attempts; past history of being in a war zone, subject of human trafficking. If school aged, records of school violence, such as bullying, either face-to-face or on social media.
If partner/parent/caregiver is present at the visit, observe client's interactions with partner/parent/caregiver.	Partner/parent/caregiver criticizes client about appearance, feelings, and/or actions. Partner/parent/caregiver is not sensitive to client's needs. Partner/parent/caregiver refuses to leave client's presence. Partner/parent/caregiver attempts to speak for and answer questions for client. Client appears anxious and afraid of partner/parent/caregiver; is submissive or passive to negative comments from partner/parent/caregiver.
Interview (*Perform the rest of the subjective data collection without the partner, parent, or caregiver present.*)	
Ask all clients by saying "Because violence is common in many people's lives I ask the following questions as a routine": • Has anyone in your home ever hurt you? • Do you feel unsafe in your home? • Are you afraid of anyone in your home? • Has anyone made you do anything you didn't want to do? • Has anyone ever touched you without you saying it was OK to do so? • Are you in a relationship with someone who physically or sexually hurts you? • Has anyone ever threatened you at home, in public, at school? • Have you ever been forced into dating, marital relationships, or sexual activities? • Are you or someone you know being trafficked? Is human trafficking happening in your community? • Have you ever been a victim of a hate crime or war-related violence? • Have you ever thought or suspect that you might suffer from PTSD? If the client answers yes or reveals other indicator of PSTD, ask the client to answer the self-assessment questions in Box 10-2, Screening for PTSD.	"Yes" to any of the questions indicates abuse (Fig. 10-2).

Continued on following page

History of Present Health Concern (Continued)

QUESTION	RATIONALE
For intimate partner violence, begin the screening by telling the client that it is important to routinely screen all clients for intimate partner violence because it affects so many women and men in our society. **Ask the client to fill out or help the client fill out the Abuse Assessment Screen in** Assessment Tool 10-2. ◎ **CLINICAL TIP** Sometimes no matter how carefully you prepare the client and ask the questions she or he may not disclose abuse.	"Yes" to any of the questions strongly indicates initial disclosure of abuse. If the client answers yes, then you should do the following: • Acknowledge the abuse and the client's courage in admitting that abuse is occurring. • Use supportive statements such as "I'm sorry this is happening to you. This is not your fault. You are not responsible for his behavior. You are not alone. You don't deserve to be treated this way. Help is available to you." • Acknowledge the client's autonomy and right to self-determination. • Reiterate confidentiality of disclosure. If the client replies "no" to screening questions and is not being abused, it is important for the client to know that you are available if she or he ever experiences abuse in the future. Make statements that build trust such as: "If your situation ever changes, please call me to talk about it. I am happy to hear that you are not being abused. If that should ever change, this is a safe place to talk."
To assess suspected child abuse, use the guidelines in Box 10-3. Question the child about physical abuse, sexual abuse, emotional abuse, and neglect.	Client indicates someone has hurt him or her (physically, sexually, or emotionally). Child appears neglected.
To assess suspected elder mistreatment, start out by asking the older adult to tell you about a typical day in his or her life. Ask them to describe their daily routines. Be alert for indicators placing the older adult at a high risk for abuse or neglect. Then ask the following questions • Has anyone ever made you sign papers that you did not understand? • Are you alone often? • Has anyone refused to help you when you needed help? • Has anyone ever refused to give you or let you take your medications?	"Yes" to any of the questions indicates abuse.

Personal Health History

QUESTION	RATIONALE
Have you had prior respiratory problems, thoracic surgery, trauma?	Previous surgeries or trauma to the thorax may alter the appearance of the thorax and cause changes in respiratory sounds, which may obscure evidence of physical abuse.
Have you ever experienced being harmed by another person including your spouse, parents, or anyone else before?	Episodes of abuse are usually repetitive. Abuse often runs in families with children of abuse (either personal of familial) marrying an abusive spouse.

Family History

QUESTION	RATIONALE
Is there a history of lung disease, other lung illnesses/disorders, or smoking in your family?	Family history may make the client more prone to complications of trauma to the lung and thorax.
Is there a history of child abuse, elder abuse, or intimate partner abuse in your family?	A history of abuse often is carried over from one generation of a family to the next.

Lifestyle and Health Practices

QUESTION	RATIONALE
Do you have difficulty performing your usual daily activities? Describe any difficulties.	Injury from abuse may affect breathing, movement, sight, and hearing. The trauma of abuse may affect energy levels necessary for completing activities of daily living.
What kind of stress are you experiencing at this time? How does it affect your breathing?	IPV is associated with severe emotional stress. Shortness of breath can be a manifestation of stress. Client may need education about relaxation techniques.
Do you participate in activities outside the house?	Abusive partners often control the activities of the partner and do not allow outside friendships or significant contact with others.

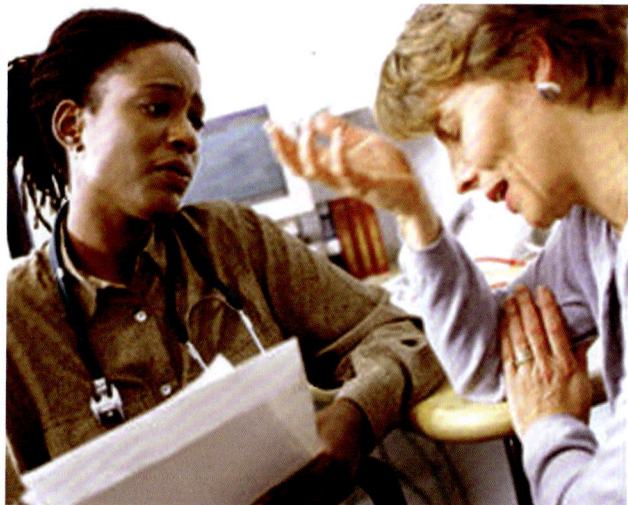

FIGURE 10-1 The nurse allows the woman to talk freely about her experience (Lippincott's Professional Development Programs, February–June 2012 releases).

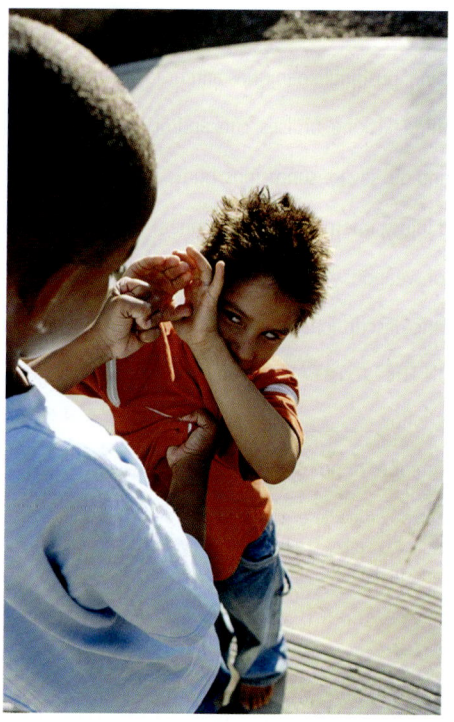

FIGURE 10-2 Child expressing fear after violence or bullying (Mohr, Psychiatric–Mental Health Nursing, Wolters Kluwer, 2012).

BOX 10-3 CONSIDERATIONS FOR INTERVIEWING CHILDREN

- It is important to establish a reassuring environment for the interview.
- Although you may be uncomfortable questioning the child about abuse, do not convey this in the interactions with the child.
- It is important that you receive any information the child may disclose to you with interest. Be calm and accepting without showing surprise or distaste.
- Do not coerce the child to answer questions by offering a reward.
- Establish the child's understanding or developmental stage by asking simple questions (name, how to spell name, age, birth date, how many eyes do you have, etc.). Then formulate questions keeping in mind child's ability to comprehend or language limitations. Use the child's comprehensive abilities and any language limitations to structure your interview/questions. Use terms for body parts or acts that the child uses.
- Questions must be direct to extract information without being leading. Children will answer questions. Studies of to whom and why children disclose abuse show that the majority disclose in answer to questions specific to direct inquiry about the person suspected of abuse or related to type of abuse (Schaeffer, Leventhal, & Asnes, 2011).
- Avoid questions that can be answered with a yes or no. Give the child as many choices during the interview as possible. Use multiple choice or open-ended questions.

The less information you supply in your questions and the more information the child gives answering the questions increases the credibility of the information gathered during the interview.

ASSESSMENT TOOL 10-2 Abuse Assessment Screen

1. **WITHIN THE LAST YEAR**, have you been hit, slapped, kicked, or otherwise physically hurt by someone?   YES   NO

   If YES, by whom? _____

   Total number of times _____

2. **SINCE YOU'VE BEEN PREGNANT**, have you been hit, slapped, kicked, or otherwise physically hurt by someone?   YES   NO

   If YES, by whom? _____

   Total number of times _____

MARK THE AREA OF INJURY ON THE BODY MAP. SCORE EACH INCIDENT ACCORDING TO THE FOLLOWING SCALE:

SCORE

1 = Threats of abuse including use of a weapon   ____

2 = Slapping, pushing: no injuries and/or lasting pain   ____

3 = Punching, kicking, bruises, cuts and/or continuing pain   ____

4 = Beating up, severe contusions, burns, broken bones   ____

5 = Head injury, internal injury, permanent injury   ____

6 = Use of weapon; wound from weapon   ____

If any of the descriptions for the higher number apply, use the higher number.

3. **WITHIN THE LAST YEAR**, has anyone forced you to have sexual activities?   YES   NO

   If YES, who? _____

   Total number of times _____

Developed by the Nursing Research Consortium on Violence and Abuse. Readers are encouraged to reproduce and use this assessment tool.
Source: McFarlane & Parker, (1994). In N. Fishwick. (1998). Assessment of women for partner abuse. *Journal of Obstetric, Gynecologic, & Neonatal Nursing, 27*, 661–670. Reproduced with permission.

CASE STUDY

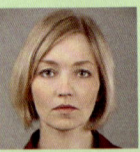

The nurse interviews Ms. D using specific probing questions. The client reports that she is experiencing chest pain due to being kicked and hit in the chest and ribs by her husband. The nurse explores Ms. D's health concerns using the COLDSPA mnemonic.

Mnemonic	Question	Data Provided
Character	Describe the sign or symptom (feeling, appearance, sound, smell, or taste if applicable).	"My chest hurts and I am having trouble breathing."
Onset	When did it begin?	"It started yesterday, but I had the same symptoms 6 months ago."
		In private, the client states, "My husband has been choking, hitting, and kicking me in the chest and stomach." She indicates this occurred "several times yesterday and many times in the past." The client indicates fear for the safety of her children and for her own life. States she was hospitalized for similar symptoms 6 months ago.
Location	Where is the pain located? Does it radiate? Does it occur anywhere else?	Well, it is hard to tell if it is from the chest, but I hurt in my stomach and back, too."

Mnemonic	Question	Data Provided
Duration	How long does the pain last? Does it recur?	"The pain lasts for a week or two after he kicks or hits me. He kicked and hit me several times yesterday and does it every so often ... maybe about every month or two."
Severity	How bad is the pain? How much does the pain bother you?	"It is bad. I can't take a deep breath. I feel like I can't talk sometimes, like now. I can't do my housework or anything for a day or two after he hits me. And I am scared he will kill me, so I try to do what I have to do, but it is hard."
Pattern	Does this chest pain occur only when your husband physically hurts you? What makes it better or worse?	"Yes, the chest pain only occurs when my husband hits or kicks me. Only then. Nothing makes it better except being left alone and putting cold on the area. But sometimes it helps to hold my arms tight to my sides with a pillow."
Associated factors/ How it **A**ffects the client	What other symptoms occur with the pain? How does the pain affect you?	When the client's husband is present, the client makes poor eye contact and looks at her husband frequently for answering questions. The children are clinging to their mother. The client is frail and thin. When answering questions without her husband present, she says she is "afraid he will kill me ... he has been saying he will kill me for the last 6 months."

After exploring the client's reports of chest pain and difficulty breathing, the nurse continues with the health history: Clara Doubtfree, a 32-year-old woman, complaining of chest pain and difficulty breathing and talking. Hygiene and dress clean and appropriate. Assisted into examination room by her husband; she is leaning on his arm. In addition to her husband, two children, 6 and 8 years old, accompany her. Denies fall or accident. Reports being hospitalized 6 months ago in another state with similar symptoms. Avoids eye contact, looks away or at husband when asked questions about injuries.

Husband interrupts client frequently, preventing her from answering interview questions. Children cling to their mother.

When interviewed alone, client states that husband has been choking her, hitting her, and kicking her in the chest and stomach several times yesterday and in the past. She states, "I know he is going to kill me; I just don't know when. I will not be able to stop him. He has been threatening to kill me for the last 6 months. Now I'm afraid he will hurt my 8-year-old, whom he choked and then locked outside in the middle of the night."

Collecting Objective Data: Physical Examination

Preparing the Client

Preparing the client for an examination after the client has experienced violence will differ for the specific circumstances. For children, make certain that the child is as comfortable as possible. Include the parent but be aware that the parent accompanying the child may be the abuser. If this is the case it may complicate the full examination, with incorrect information being provided by the parent to questions that you ask. For adults, the specific injuries involved will determine the focus of the physical examination. If possible, prepare the client for a complete physical examination. If rape is involved, arrange a consultation with, and examination by, a SANE (Sexual Assault Nurse Examiner) if at all possible, as the physical evidence obtained may be used in court (Box 10-4) (U.S. Department of Justice, Office of Victims of Crime, 2009; International Association of Forensic Nurses, 2015).

BOX 10-4 SEXUAL ASSAULT NURSE EXAMINER (SANE) PROGRAMS

When rape is suspected, you may not be adequately trained to care for the victim. Rape is a crime. Health care providers who care for rape victims have been known to inadvertently destroy the very evidence the victim needs to support a case against the rapist. In addition, providers caring for rape victims could be called to testify, taking them out of the clinical practice areas for extended times. Because of these risks and the need by the victim for support and care during this high-stress time, doctors, nurses, counsellors, and rape victim advocates recognized the need for specialized care. A program for training nurses to care for rape victims was begun in 1976; these programs have continued to spread across the United States and to other countries.

With time, the need to involve the broader community became evident. Informal support persons can serve as collaborators, or a more formally organized team is formed to respond to victims of abuse or rape. A Sexual Assault Response/Resource Team (SART) is a more formal approach. "SART team members typically include the SANE, police or sheriff, detective, prosecutor, rape crisis center advocate or counselor, and emergency department medical personnel" (U.S. Department of Justice, Office of Victims, 2009, p. 28). For details of the development and function of SANE and SART programs, refer to the Office of Victims, publication at http://www.ojp.usdoj.gov/ovc/publications/infores/sane/saneguide.pdf and the International Association of Forensic Nurses (2015).

Follow the preparations recommended for the specific physical examination needed (see chapter covering specific system affected). But be certain to make the client as comfortable as possible before and during the examination. Ask the client to remove all clothes and put on a gown allowing for full body assessment.

Equipment

Equipment needed will vary depending on the specific injuries (see chapter covering system affected). For a general examination, equipment to measure vital signs is necessary.

Physical Assessment

During examination of a client you suspect or know has been abused, it is even more essential to remember these key points:
- Provide privacy for the client.
- Keep your hands warm to promote the client's comfort during examination.
- Remain nonjudgmental regarding client's habits, lifestyle, and any revelations about abuse. At the same time, educate and inform about risks and possibilities for assistance.

General Routine Screening or Focused Specialty Assessment

The nurse performs a general survey on all clients being alert to any signs of domestic violence. If the client interview indicates the client is at risk then the nurse would proceed to further assess for IPV findings. In addition to those at risk, the Office of the Assistant Secretary for Planning and Evaluation (ASPE) of the U.S. Department of Health and Human Services (HHS) recommends universal screening for domestic and IPV by any clinician in health care settings of every female patient through age 64. Therefore, the Abuse Assessment Screen (Assessment Tool 10-2) would be used with anyone suspected to be abused in addition to every female client through age 64. The Self-Assessment: Danger Assessment (Box 10-5) would be used to determine the safety of one who is suspected to be a victim of violence. Box 10-2 would be used if the client is suspected to have PTSD.

ASSESSMENT PROCEDURE	NORMAL FINDINGS	ABNORMAL FINDINGS
Perform a General Survey		
Observe general appearance and body build.	Client appears stated age, is well developed, and appears healthy.	Abused children may appear younger than stated age due to developmental delays or malnourishment. Older clients who have been abused may appear thin and frail due to malnourishment.
Note dress and hygiene.	Client is well groomed and dressed appropriately for season and occasion.	Poor hygiene and soiled clothing may indicate neglect. Long sleeves and pants in warm weather may be an attempt to cover bruising or other injuries. Victims of sexual abuse may dress provocatively.
Assess mental status.	Client is coherent and relaxed. A child shows proper developmental level for age.	Client is anxious, depressed, suicidal, withdrawn, or has difficulty concentrating. Client has poor eye contact or soft passive speech. Client is unable to recall recent or past events. Child does not meet developmental expectations.
Evaluate vital signs.	Vital signs are within normal limits.	As with any condition of prolonged stress, hypertension may be seen in victims of abuse. Acute stress may result in elevated heart rate and respiration rate.
Inspect skin.	Skin is clean, dry, and free of lesions, bruises, or burns. People with hemophilia often have bruises and sometimes there are multiple bruises, which should not be confused with abuse. **OLDER ADULT CONSIDERATIONS** Skin fragility increases with age; bruising may occur with pressure and may mimic bruising associated with abuse. Be careful to distinguish between normal and abnormal findings.	Client has scars, bruises, burns, welts or swelling on face, breasts, arms, chest, abdomen, or genitalia, including evidence of cigarette or cigar burns; hand or finger patterns on arms, legs, or neck; or heating element patterns as though pushed against a heater or radiator.

ASSESSMENT PROCEDURE	NORMAL FINDINGS	ABNORMAL FINDINGS
	🌐 **CULTURAL CONSIDERATIONS** Mongolian spots on buttocks and back of children occur in some populations and can be confused with signs of abuse. They are normal findings. Evidence of raised red areas, either circular (from cupping) or deep scratch-like areas (coining) may be seen in some ethnic groups and are not considered abnormal. Ask the person or the parent, if on a child, about these areas to clarify their source.	
Inspect the head and neck.	Head and neck are free of injuries.	Client has hair missing in clumps, subdural hematomas, or rope marks or finger/hand strangulation marks on neck, or obvious past or present nose injuries.
Inspect the eyes.	Eyes are free of injury.	Client has bruising or swelling around eyes, unilateral ptosis of upper eyelids (due to repeated blows causing nerve damage to eyelids), or a subconjunctival hemorrhage.
Assess the ears.	Ears are clean and free of injuries.	Client has external or internal ear injuries.
Assess the abdomen.	Abdomen is free of bruises and other injuries, and is nontender.	Client has bruising in various stages of healing. Assessment reveals intra-abdominal injuries. A pregnant client has received blows to abdomen.
Assess genitalia and rectal area.	Client's genitalia and rectal areas are free of injury.	Client has irritation, tenderness, bruising, bleeding, or swelling of genitals or rectal area. Discharge, redness, or lacerations may indicate abuse in young children. Hemorrhoids are unusual in children and may be caused by sexual abuse. Extreme apprehension during this portion of the examination may indicate physical or sexual abuse.
Assess the musculoskeletal system.	Client shows full range of motion and has no evidence of injuries.	Dislocation of shoulder; old or new fractures of face, arms, or ribs; and poor range of motion of joints are indicators of abuse.
Assess the neurologic system.	Client demonstrates normal neurologic function.	Abnormal findings include tremors, hyperactive reflexes, and decreased sensations to areas of old injuries secondary to neurologic damage.
Further Assessment for Positive IPV Findings		
If screening for IPV is positive, ask the client to fill out a danger assessment questionnaire (Box 10-5). If screening for IPV is positive and the client's answers on the danger assessment questionnaire indicate a high probability for serious violence, ask the client if she has a safety plan and where she would like to go when she leaves your agency (Assessment Tool 10-3). Be sure to schedule a follow-up appointment and/or refer the client as appropriate.	Client has a safety plan.	If the client says she prefers to return home, ask her if it is safe for her to do so and have her complete Assessment Tool 10-3. Provide the client with contact information for shelters and groups. Encourage her to call with any concerns.

BOX 10-5 SELF-ASSESSMENT: DANGER ASSESSMENT

Several risk factors have been associated with increased risk of homicides (murders) of women and men in violent relationships. We cannot predict what will happen in your case, but we would like you to be aware of the danger of homicide in situations of abuse and for you to see how many of the risk factors apply to your situation.

Using the calendar, please mark the approximate dates during the past year when you were abused by your partner or ex-partner. Write on that date how bad the incident was according to the following scale:

1. Slapping, pushing; no injuries and/or lasting pain
2. Punching, kicking; bruises, cuts, and/or continuing pain
3. "Beating up"; severe contusions, burns, broken bones, miscarriage
4. Threat to use weapon; head injury, internal injury, permanent injury, miscarriage
5. Use of weapon; wounds from weapon
   (If **any** of the descriptions for the higher number apply, use the higher number.)

Mark **Yes** or **No** for each of the following. ("He" refers to your husband, partner, ex-husband, ex-partner, or whoever is currently physically hurting you.)

Yes   **No**

_____ _____ 1. Has the physical violence increased in severity or frequency over the past year?
_____ _____ 2. Does he own a gun?
_____ _____ 3. Have you left him after living together during the past year?
              3a. (If you have *never* lived with him, check here _____)
_____ _____ 4. Is he unemployed?
_____ _____ 5. Has he ever used a weapon against you or threatened you with a lethal weapon?
              5a. (If yes, was the weapon a gun? _____)
_____ _____ 6. Does he threaten to kill you?
_____ _____ 7. Has he avoided being arrested for domestic violence?
_____ _____ 8. Do you have a child that is not his?
_____ _____ 9. Has he ever forced you to have sex when you did not wish to do so?
_____ _____ 10. Does he ever try to choke you?
_____ _____ 11. Does he use illegal drugs? By drugs, I mean "uppers" or amphetamines, speed, angel dust, cocaine, "crack," street drugs, or mixtures.
_____ _____ 12. Is he an alcoholic or problem drinker?
_____ _____ 13. Does he control most or all of your daily activities? (For instance: does he tell you who you can be friends with, when you can see your family, how much money you can use, or when you can take the car? If he tries, but you do not let him, check here: _____)
_____ _____ 14. Is he violently and constantly jealous of you? (For instance, does he say, "If I can't have you, no one can.")
_____ _____ 15. Have you ever been beaten by him while you were pregnant? (If you have never been pregnant by him, check here: _____)
_____ _____ 16. Has he ever threatened or tried to commit suicide?
_____ _____ 17. Does he threaten to harm your children?
_____ _____ 18. Do you believe he is capable of killing you?
_____ _____ 19. Does he follow or spy on you, leave threatening notes or messages on answering machine, destroy your property, or call you when you don't want him to?
_____ _____ 20. Have you ever threatened or tried to commit suicide?
_____ _____ Total "Yes" Answers

Thank you. Please talk to your nurse, advocate, or counselor about what the Danger Assessment means in terms of your situation.

Campbell, J.C. (2004). Danger Assessment. Retrieved from http://www.dangerassessment.org. A danger assessment questionnaire for women in a same sex relationship and (coming soon) a danger assessment questionnaire for immigrant women, see http://www.dangerassessment.org

CASE STUDY

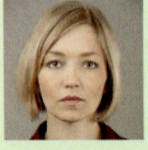

The chapter case study is now used to demonstrate a physical assessment of Ms. D for signs of IPV and thorax and lung injury. Ms. D has a large area of discoloration and swelling on the right chest wall, bruising on the right side of the abdomen and right hip, and decreased breath sounds over right lung, along with rope burn and abrasions all around the circumference of her neck. Her 8-year-old son also has abrasions around his neck. Ms. D has full range of motion but complains of pain with motion. Other than her injuries, her other body systems are intact. When questioned about what feel like old healed fractures of her right arm, the client states: "I did not come to the doctor when he broke my arm because he threatened to kill me if I went to the doctor."

Due to the nature of Ms. D answers to the interview and findings from her physical assessment, a Danger Assessment is completed (Box 10-5 for the Danger Assessment tool).

Danger Assessment: States yes for various types of physical abuse, which is increasing in severity and now has included 8-year-old son in the threats. Husband is employed but orders Ms. D to remain at home when he is not with her to take her out. Husband does not own a weapon; only uses his hands and feet to hit and kick

ASSESSMENT TOOL 10-3 Assessing a Safety Plan

Ask the client, do you:
- Have a packed bag ready? Keep it hidden but make it easy to grab quickly?
- Tell your neighbors about your abuse and ask them to call the police when they hear a disturbance?
- Have a code word to use with your kids, family, and friends? They will know to call the police and get you help?
- Know where you are going to go, if you ever have to leave?
- Remove weapons from the home?
- Have the following gathered:
  - Cash
  - Social Security cards/numbers for you and your children
  - Birth certificates for you and your children
  - Driver's license
  - Rent and utility receipts
  - Bank account numbers
  - Insurance policies and numbers
  - Marriage license
  - Jewelry
  - Important phone numbers
  - Copy of protection order

Ask children, do you:
- Know a safe place to go?
- Know who is safe to tell you are unsafe?
- Know how and when to call 911? Know how to make a collect call?

Inform children that it is their job to keep themselves safe; they should not interject themselves into adult conflict.

If the client is planning to leave:
- Remind the client this is a dangerous time that requires awareness and planning.
- Review where the client is planning to go, shelter options, and the need to be around others to curtail violence.
- Review the client's right to possessions and list of possessions to take.

---

her. Neither she nor her husband has threatened suicide. However, she has begun to think about it as a way out, except for needing to protect her children if possible. Husband has not expressed jealousy, just a need to control her every movement. Ms. D does believe he is capable of killing her or the child. Husband is a drinker and her description indicates an alcoholic.

When findings suggest that the client is in danger, ask about a safety plan, following the guidelines in Assessment Tool 10-3.

Validating and Documenting Findings

Validate any family violence data you have collected. This is necessary to verify that the data are reliable and accurate. Document your assessment data following the health care facility or agency policy.

CASE STUDY

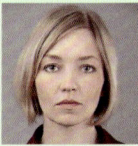

Think back to the case study. The nurse completed the following documentation of her assessment of Ms. D.

Biographic Data: CD, 32 years old, Caucasian. Married, mother of boy 8 years and girl 6 years old. Does not work outside home. Alert and oriented. Clean and neat hygiene and dress appropriate. Timid, passive interactions when husband present. Fidgeting and restless. Guarding right chest and abdomen areas.

Reason for Seeking Health care: "It hurts when I take a deep breath, and even when I try to talk. I feel like I can't get enough air in my lungs."

History of Present Health Concern: When interviewed alone without husband present, began to cry and disclosed that her husband has been choking her, hitting her, and kicking her in the chest and stomach several times today and in the past. She stated, "I know he is going to kill me; I just don't know when. I will not be able to stop him. He has been threatening to kill me for the last 6 months. Now I'm afraid he will hurt my 8-year-old, whom he choked and then locked outside in the middle of the night."

Personal Health History: Denies having had any accidents, falls, except for ongoing and present IPV. Denies any chronic chest or stomach diseases. Denies any seasonal or environmental allergies. Describes past hospitalization 6 months prior for similar symptoms of chest pain and stomach pain after being hit and kicked by husband. Acknowledges healed arm fracture for which she did not seek care. Medications include aspirin and Tylenol occasionally; two Tylenol twice today. Denies medication, food, environmental, or insect allergies.

Family History: Stated that Mr. D's father abuses his mother and her own father was very severe with her when she was a child. Denies sexual abuse, other family history of abuse. Denies history of lung problems.

Lifestyle and Health Practices: 24-hour diet recall: Breakfast—Four 8-ounce cups of coffee, 2 glazed donuts; Lunch—none today; usually a sandwich of leftovers from dinner night before. Dinner—few bites of meatloaf, mashed potatoes and gravy, cup of milk. Denies use of herbal medicines or alternative therapies to manage respiratory or other problems.

Physical Examination Findings: Large area of discoloration and swelling on the right chest wall, bruising on right side of the abdomen and right hip, decreased breath sounds over right lung, and rope burn and abrasions all around circumference of neck. Has full range of motion but complains of pain with motion. Inspection reveals no nasal flaring, shallow breathing. Skin slightly pale, but no cyanosis noted. Fingernails pale, with a 180-degree angle between the nail base and skin. Posterior thorax: Inspection reveals scapulae are symmetric and nonprotruding; ratio of anteroposterior to transverse diameter is 2:1. Upon palpation of thorax, client reports tenderness, pain over right chest wall, abdomen, and hip. Lung sounds slightly decreased on right. Chest expansion unequal with slight decrease on the right. No crepitus palpable. Diaphragmatic excursion measures 2.5 cm on the left and 1.3 cm on the right. Bronchophony, egophony, and whispered pectoriloquy nonsymmetric within normal range. Sternum is midline and straight. No sternal retractions noted. Respirations regular, shallow, and slightly tachypneic, with a respiratory rate of 20 per minute. Chest expansion equal but describes pain with deep breath. No adventitious sounds. Voice sounds same anteriorly as described posteriorly.

ANALYSIS OF DATA: DIAGNOSTIC REASONING

After collecting subjective and objective data pertaining to family violence, identify abnormal findings and client strengths. Then cluster the data to reveal any significant patterns or abnormalities. These data may be used to make clinical judgments about the status of family violence in your client's life.

Selected Nursing Diagnoses

Following is a listing of selected nursing diagnoses (health promotion, risk, or actual) that you may identify when analyzing data for assessment of family violence.

Health Promotion Diagnoses

- Readiness for Enhanced Family Relationships
- Readiness for Enhanced Family Health Management: Requests information related to safety from family violence

Risk Diagnoses

- Risk for Ineffective parent/infant/child/family Health Management related to the presence of family violence
- Risk for Violence (other directed) related to the presence of poor coping mechanisms and the misuse of alcohol and illegal drugs
- Risk for Violence (self-directed) related to ongoing history of abuse (IPV, child, elder)
- Risk for Infection (STDs and HIV) related to participation in forced sexual relationships
- Risk for Powerlessness related to control of relationships, control of children and finances by abusive significant other
- Risk for Posttrauma Syndrome related to the inability to remove self from abusive intimate relationships

Actual Diagnoses

- Dysfunctional Grieving related to loss of ideal relationship as evidenced by refusal to discuss feelings and prolonged denial
- Impaired Parenting related to choosing to remain living in the presence of an abusive marriage or intimate relationship
- Disturbed Personal Identity related to inability to function effectively outside of a victimized abusive role
- Risk for Rape-trauma Syndrome related to the forced violent penetration against the client's will secondary to the lack of a safety plan for the victim
- Risk for Rape-trauma Syndrome: silent reaction related to inability to discuss occurrences of a victim of rape
- Risk for Rape-trauma Syndrome: compound reaction related to inability to function effectively in everyday activities after being a victim of rape
- Fear of losing an ineffective abusive intimate relationship related to unrealistic expectations of self and others
- Hopelessness related to remaining in a prolonged abusive relationship and inability to seek counseling and healthy supportive relationships
- Dysfunctional Family Relationships related to family violence
- Anxiety related to inconsistency of behaviors and instability of abusive spouse or parent
- Low Self-Esteem related to lack of confidence related to presence of prolonged physical, sexual, and emotional abuse

Selected Collaborative Problems

After grouping the data, you may see various collaborative problems emerge. Remember that collaborative problems differ from nursing diagnoses in that they cannot be prevented by nursing interventions. However, these physiologic complications of medical conditions can be detected and monitored by the nurse. In addition, the nurse can use physician- and nurse-prescribed interventions to minimize the complications of these problems. The nurse may also have to refer the client in such situations for further treatment of the problem. Following is a list of collaborative problems that may be identified when assessing a victim of family violence. These problems are worded as Risk for Complications (RC), followed by the problem.

- RC: Fractures
- RC: Bruises
- RC: Concussion
- RC: Subdural hematoma
- RC: Subconjunctival hemorrhage
- RC: Intra-abdominal injury
- RC: Depression
- RC: Suicide
- RC: Death

Medical Problems

Once the data are grouped, certain signs and symptoms may become evident and may require medical diagnoses and treatment. Referral to a primary health care provider is necessary. In the case of identified abuse, both medical and abuse counseling referrals are necessary.

CASE STUDY

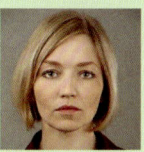

After collecting and analyzing the data for Ms. D, the nurse determines that the following conclusions are appropriate:

Nursing Diagnoses
- Acute Pain r/t physical abuse of kicking and hitting
- Risk for Other-Directed Violence related to alcoholic husband, history of past abuse by husband and father.
- Chronic Low Self-Esteem related to history of living in abusive environment as child and now as adult spouse.
- Impaired Parenting r/t abusive father and abused, fearful mother
- Risk for Suicide r/t feelings of helplessness in abusive relationship

Potential Collaborative Problems
- RC: Fracture
- RC: Hemorrhage
- RC: Intra-abdominal hemorrhages
- RC: Death

Refer to primary care providers for psychological and spiritual counseling for victims of abuse. Follow reporting guidelines for cases of abuse in your state. To view an algorithm depicting the process of diagnostic reasoning for this case, go to thePoint.

Interdisciplinary Verbal Communication of Assessment Findings Using SBAR

SITUATION: Ms. D is a 32-year-old woman who comes to outpatient clinic with her husband and two children. She states, "My chest hurts and I cannot breathe easily." She has difficulty talking. When asked questions, she has poor eye contact, looks away or toward husband, who interrupts his wife frequently. The son and daughter cling to their mother.

BACKGROUND: Mr. D's father abuses his mother and her own father was very severe with her when she was a child. Hospitalized 6 months prior for chest and stomach pain after being hit and kicked by husband. Acknowledges healed arm fracture for which she did not seek care. When interviewed alone, client states that husband has been choking her, hitting her, and kicking her in the chest and stomach several times yesterday and in the past. She states, "I know he is going to kill me; I just don't know when. I will not be able to stop him. He has been threatening to kill me for the last 6 months. Now I'm afraid he will hurt my 8-year-old, whom he choked and then locked outside in the middle of the night."

ASSESSMENT: Large area of discoloration and swelling on the right chest wall, bruising on right side of the abdomen and right hip, decreased breath sounds over right lung, and rope burn and abrasions all around circumference of neck. Has full range of motion but complains of pain with motion. Upon palpation of thorax, client reports tenderness, pain over right chest wall, abdomen, and hip. Lung sounds slightly decreased on right. Chest expansion unequal with slight decrease on the right. Eight-year old son also has neck abrasions.

DANGER ASSESSMENT: States yes for various types of physical abuse, increasing in severity and includes 8-year-old son. Husband employed but orders Ms. D to remain at home when he is not with her. Husband does not own a weapon. Neither she nor her husband has threatened suicide. However, she has begun to think about it as a way out, except for needing to protect her children. Ms. D does believe he is capable of killing her or the child. She describes her husband as an alcoholic.

RECOMMENDATION: I believe Ms. D and her children are at risk for continued abuse. They need to be referred to social services to be considered for placement in a safe environment.

Want to know more?

A wide variety of resources to enhance your learning and understanding of this book are available on thePoint. Visit thePoint to access:

- NCLEX-Style Student Review Questions
- Watch and Learn Videos
- Concepts in Action Animations
- And more!

References and Selected Readings

American College of Obstetricians & Gynecologists (ACOG). (2012). Intimate partner violence. Available at http://www.acog.org/Resources_And_Publications/Committee_Opinions/Committee_on_Health_Care_for_Underserved_Women/Intimate_Partner_Violence

American Psychological Association. (2015). Intimate partner violence: Facts and resources. Available at http://www.apa.org/topics/violence/partner.aspx

Anxiety and Depression Association of America (ADAA). (2015). Screening for posttraumatic stress disorder (PTSD). Available at http://www.adaa.org/screening-posttraumatic-stress-disorder-ptsd

Australian Law Reform Commission. (2010). Definition of family violence. Available at http://www.alrc.gov.au/publications/family-violence-and-commonwealth-laws%E2%80%94social-security-law/definition-family-violence

Bullying statistics. (2015). School bullying statistics. Available at http://www.bullyingstatistics.org/content/school-bullying-statistics.html

Bureau of Justice Statistics (BJS). (2014). Crimes against the elderly 2003–2013. Available at http://www.bjs.gov/content/pub/pdf/cae0313.pdf

Centers for Disease Control & Prevention (CDC). (2007). Intimate partner violence and sexual violence victimization assessment tools for use in healthcare settings. Available at http://www.cdc.gov/violenceprevention/pdf/ipv/ipvandsvscreening.pdf

Centers for Disease Control & Prevention (CDC). (2014). National Intimate Partner and Sexual Violence Survey (NIPSVS): Infographic. Available at http://www.cdc.gov/violenceprevention/nisvs/infographic.html

Centers for Disease Control & Prevention (CDC). (2015a). Elder abuse: Consequences. Available at http://www.cdc.gov/violenceprevention/elderabuse/consequences.html

Centers for Disease Control & Prevention (CDC). (2015b). Intimate partner violence. Available at http://www.cdc.gov/violenceprevention/intimatepartnerviolence/

Centers for Disease Control & Prevention (CDC). (2015c). Intimate partner violence: Risk and protective factors. Available at http://www.cdc.gov/violenceprevention/intimatepartnerviolence/riskprotectivefactors.html

Child Help. (2012). Child abuse statistics & facts. Available at https://www.childhelp.org/child-abuse-statistics/

Child Welfare Information Gateway. (2013a). *Long-term consequences of child abuse and neglect*. Washington, DC: U.S. Department of Health and Human Services, Children's Bureau. Available at https://www.childwelfare.gov/pubpdfs/long_term_consequences.pdf

Child Welfare Information Gateway. (2013b). *What is child abuse and neglect? Recognizing the signs and symptoms*. Washington, DC: U.S. Department of Health and Human Services, Children's Bureau. Available at https://www.childwelfare.gov/pubPDFs/whatiscan.pdf#page=2&view=How Is Child Abuse and Neglect Defined in Federal Law?

CME Resource. (2012). Child abuse in ethnic minority and immigrant communities. Available http://www.netce.com/coursecontent.php?courseid=861#chap.1

Devi, S. (2012). US guidelines for domestic violence screening spark debate. *Lancet*, 379(9815), 506. Available at http://www.thelancet.com/journals/lancet/article/PIIS0140-6736%2812%2960215-3/fulltext

Devine, J. (2008). Lenore Walker's Cycle of Violence. Available at http://ezinearticles.com/?Lenore-Walkers-Cycle-of-Violence&id=1366375

Domestic Violence Statistics. (2015). Available at http://domesticviolencestatistics.org/domestic-violence-statistics/

DOsomething.org (n.d.). 11 Facts about human trafficking. Available at https://www.dosomething.org/facts/11-facts-about-human-trafficking

Douglas, E., & Hines, D. (2011). The helpseeking experiences of men who sustain intimate partner violence: An overlooked population and implications for practice. *Journal of Family Violence*, 26(6), 473–485. Available at http://www.ncbi.nlm.nih.gov/pmc/articles/PMC3175099/

Fang, X., Brown, D., Florence, C., et al. (2012). The economic burden of child maltreatment in the United States and implications for prevention. *Child Abuse and Neglect*, 36(2). Available at http://www.sciencedirect.com/science/article/pii/S0145213411003140

Federal Bureau of Investigation (FBI). (2014). Latest hate crime statistics report released. Available at https://www.fbi.gov/news/stories/2014/december/latest-hate-crime-statistics-report-released

FindLaw. (2016). What is domestic violence? Available at http://family.findlaw.com/domestic-violence/what-is-domestic-violence.html

Healthy People 2020. (2014). Injury and violence prevention. Available at http://www.healthypeople.gov/2020/topicsobjectives2020/overview.aspx?topicid=24

International Association of Forensic Nurses (IAFN). (2015). Sexual Assault Nurse Examiners (SANE). Available at http://www.forensicnurses.org/?page=aboutsane

McCue, M. L. (2008). *Domestic violence: A reference handbook* (2nd ed.). Santa Barbara, CA: ABC-CLIO, Inc.

Merriam-Webster Online. (2015). Available at http://www.m-w.com/

Moyer, V., & USPSTF. (2013). Clinical guidelines: Screening for intimate partner violence and abuse of elderly and vulnerable adults: A U.S. Preventive Services Task Force recommendation statement. *Annals of Internal Medicine* [online]. Available at http://annals.org/article.aspx?articleid=1558517

National Conference of State Legislatures (NCSL). (2015). Mandatory reporting of child abuse and neglect 2013 introduced state legislation. Available at http://www.ncsl.org/research/human-services/redirect-mandatory-rprtg-of-child-abuse-and-neglect-2013.aspx

National Institute of Justice. (2010). Victims and perpetrators. Available at http://www.nij.gov/topics/crime/rape-sexual-violence/pages/victims-perpetrators.aspx

National Institutes of Health. (2012). Docs more likely to suspect abuse in poor kids. Available at http://www.nim.nih.gov/medlinepls/new/fullstor_121054

Neale, T. (2012). USPSTF: Screen all potential moms for abuse. Available http://www.medpagetoday.com/OBGYN/DomesticViolence/33261

Phillips, D. (2007). Punking and bullying: Strategies in middle school, high school, and beyond. *Journal of Interpersonal Violence*, 22(2), 158–178.

Safe Horizon. (2015). Child abuse facts. Available at http://www.safehorizon.org/page/child-abuse-facts-56.html

Schaeffer, P., Leventhal, J., & Asnes, A. (2011). Children's disclosures of sexual abuse: learning from direct inquiry. *Child Abuse & Neglect*, 35(5), 343–352. Available at http://www.ncbi.nlm.nih.gov/pubmed/21620161

Science News. (2012). Psychological abuse puts children at risk. Available at http://www.sciencedaily.com/releases/2012/07/120730094134.htm

Sherin, K. (2003). HITS. Available at http://www.cdc.gov/violenceprevention/pdf/ipv/ipvandsvscreening.pdf

Sherin, J., & Nemeroff, C. (2011). Post-traumatic stress disorder: The neurobiological impact of psychological trauma. *Dialogues in Clinical Neuroscience*, 13(3). Available at http://www.ncbi.nlm.nih.gov/pmc/articles/PMC3182008/

Simms, L., Bushman, S., & Petersen, S. (2016). Bullying: How to prevent it and help children who are victims. Available at http://center4research.org/violence-risky-behavior/z-other-violence/bullying-and-violence/

Stopbullying.gov. (2014). Facts about bullying. Available at http://www.stopbullying.gov/news/media/facts/

Tracy, N. (2012). Effects of emotional abuse on adults. Available at http://www.healthyplace.com/abuse/emotional-psychological-abuse/effects-of-emotional-abuse-on-adults/

The Center for Hope and Safety (n.d.). The cycle of domestic violence model. Available http://hopeandsafety.org/learn-more/the-cycle-of-domestic-violence/

United Nations Office on Drugs and Crime. (2014). Global report on trafficking in persons. Available at https://www.unodc.org/documents/data-and-analysis/glotip/GLOTIP_2014_full_report.pdf

U.S. Department of Justice, Office of Victims of Crime. (2009). Sexual Assault Nurse Examiner (SANE) development and operations guide. Available at http://www.ojp.usdoj.gov/ovc/publications/infores/sane/saneguide.pdf

U.S. Preventive Services Task Force (USPSTF). (2013). Intimate partner violence and abuse of elderly and vulnerable adults screening. Available at http://www.uspreventiveservicestaskforce.org/Page/Document/UpdateSummaryFinal/intimate-partner-violence-and-abuse-of-elderly-and-vulnerable-adults-screening

U.S. Preventive Services Task Force (USPSTF). (2004). Screening for family and intimate partner violence: Recommendation statement. Available at http://www.uspreventiveservicestaskforce.org/3rduspstf/famviolence/famviolrs.htm

Vancouver Coastal Health. (2013). About abuse & neglect: What is abuse: Psychological abuse. Available at http://www.vchreact.ca/read_psychological.htm

Walker, L. E. (1979). *The battered woman*. New York: Harper & Row.

Walker, L. E. (1984). *The battered woman syndrome*. New York: Harper & Row.

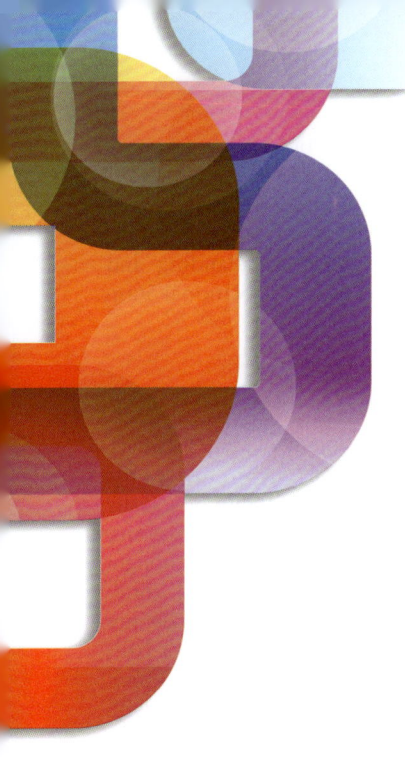

11 ASSESSING CULTURE

Learning Objectives

1. Describe culture and its basic characteristics.
2. Explain how the interaction of culture, genetics, and environmental factors affect health status.
3. Discuss how cultural competence in the role of the nurse is necessary to make accurate assessments.
4. Describe your own tendency to stereotype and be ethnocentric.
5. Be aware of your own degree of cultural competence and ways to increase it.
6. Describe the parts of a cultural assessment.
7. Interview a client modifying your questions to be culturally sensitive.
8. Complete an effective cultural assessment of a person from a different culture.
9. Recognize culture-based syndromes and the cultural groups most likely to accept them as diseases.
10. Differentiate between skills needed for a general routine cultural screening versus skills needed for a focused cultural assessment.
11. Analyze the data from the interview and assessment of a client's culture and formulate valid nursing diagnoses, collaborative problems, and/or referrals.
12. Communicate interview and assessment cultural findings through clear concise documentation and verbal reports.

CASE STUDY

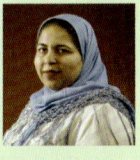

Samar Al Sayah, a 56-year-old woman who has recently emigrated from Lebanon, is diabetic. She comes to the clinic this morning seeking advice on participating in the annual Ramadan fast. She says that she has had type 2 diabetes for several years and has not tried to fast for Ramadan before, but would like to try to do so this year. She states that she has been on oral medication for elevated blood sugar for 5 years and that she has usually been in good control, but occasionally finds blood sugar fluctuations when she has bouts of diarrhea or vomiting, or when she stops exercising. She says she understands that she will have to learn much about what to do to not cause herself harm.

The month-long fast of Ramadan lasts from 29 to 30 days. This fast is one of the Pillars of Islam when people participate in spiritual reflection, prayer, charity, atone for past sins, and affirm faith in Islam. The requirements of the fast are that between dawn and sunset, Muslims abstain from all food, drink, sexual contact even with their spouses, smoking, gossip, lies, obscenity, and all sinful acts. Participation is required of all healthy, mature Muslims. However, people who are ill, traveling, and women who are menstruating or pregnant or nursing may postpone the fast until another time. Older adults or those who are too ill or weak to participate are excused from fasting, and may substitute feeding a needy person for each day they are unable to fast (if they can afford to do this).

CONCEPTUAL FOUNDATIONS

The population in the United States is made up of many cultural groups. The U.S. Census categories are as follows: White; Black or African American; American Indian or Alaska Native; Asian (including peoples from the Far East, Southeast Asia, or the Indian subcontinent); Native Hawaiian and other Pacific Islanders; and the possibility to write in other categories if identifying with more than one category (U.S. Census Bureau, 2010). The Pew Research Center (2014) has noted that the U.S. Census Bureau is considering a new category for MENA countries (those from the Middle East and North Africa), as this population group has risen from 1.19 million in 2000 to 1.80 million in 2012.

Culture affects so many aspects of life, including health-related definitions, health outcomes, and health practices. What do you believe causes illness? What do you believe is the correct way to treat minor or serious illnesses? Whom do you go to when you need to treat a minor illness, or to diagnose

181

or treat a more serious illness? What barriers do you run into when you seek care? The answers to these questions vary based on the cultural context in which you grew up or the influence of the contexts in which you have lived later in life. This has led to some confusion in the use of terminology such as disease, illness, and sickness. Albrecht et al. (2013, p. 2) noted that anthropologists have distinguished among these terms so that *disease* refers to "deviations from a biomedical norm"; *illness* refers to "the lived experience of culturally constructed categories"; and *sickness* refers to "patients' roles." All three of these terms need to be considered when talking with clients about health.

Culture affects many aspects of how people communicate, the rituals and behaviors used to express spirituality, and the main events of life, such as marriage, pregnancy, birth, death, and other celebrations. Beyond culture, there are biologic variations that affect disease susceptibility. Everyone has cultural and biologic variations. It may seem that you are the "normal" and others who are not the same are "other," or have "cultural variations," but we all vary and no one represents the norm. Based on the idea that everyone has cultural variations, and the number of variations is increasing everywhere with the large number of immigrants moving from one country to another, nurses must understand cultural variation as a basis for even minimally safe and effective care.

Why Nurses Need to Know about Culture

There are many reasons why nurses need to know about culture, including the number of cultures with which clients identify and also the growing cultural variation of health care team members (Fig. 11-1).

Why do nurses need to understand culture? Nurses interact with clients every day. A client who looks like you and comes from your community may actually hold very different beliefs about illness and health, about when and from whom to seek care, about who makes the decision about health-related issues for the family. If someone who seems so similar to you could be so different, imagine the possible differences you may encounter when you care for clients from obviously different cultural backgrounds or for immigrants to your country. In addition there has been a long history of disparity in the level of health care received by persons from certain racial groups or minorities, and the problems of ethnocentrism and stereotyping mentioned earlier. In addition, there are regulatory reasons for understanding and applying cultural knowledge, among them the National Standards for Care.

Concepts and Terms Related to Culture

Culture may be defined as a shared system of values, beliefs, and learned patterns of behavior. Purnell (2013) provides the following useful definition of culture: "the totality of socially transmitted behavioral patterns, arts, beliefs, values, customs, lifeways, and all other products of human work and thought characteristic of a population or people that guide their worldview and decision making" (p. 6). The particular culture defines *values* (learned beliefs about what is held to be good or bad) and *norms* (learned behaviors that are perceived to be appropriate or inappropriate). Culture is learned, shared, associated with adaptation to the environment, and is universal. All people have a socially transmitted culture. Our own culture forms our worldview based on the values, beliefs, and behaviors sanctioned by it. That worldview becomes, for us, reality. See Box 11-1 for more definitions related to culture and cultural assessment.

Individuals experiencing limited interaction with other cultural groups subsequently have a limited cultural worldview. The perception that one's worldview is the only acceptable truth, and that one's beliefs, values, and sanctioned behaviors are superior to all others, is called *ethnocentrism*.

Many people are aware of other cultures and their different beliefs, values, and accepted behaviors but do not recognize the considerable variation that can exist within any cultural group. Not recognizing this variation tends to lead to *stereotyping* all members of a particular culture, expecting group members to hold the same beliefs and behave in the same way. Therefore, while learning and understanding common beliefs and practices of various cultures is useful, it is imperative to view all clients as individuals and determine their views and beliefs.

Ethnicity, or a person's ethnic identity, exists when the person identifies with a "socially, culturally, and politically constructed group of individuals that holds a common set of characteristics not shared by others with whom its members come in contact" (Lipson & Dibble, 2007, p. xiv). In other words, ethnicity describes subgroups that have a common history, ancestry, or other cultural identity that may relate to geographic origin, such as Southerners, Navajos, or Mexican Americans (Fig. 11-2).

CULTURAL COMPETENCE

To provide high-quality health care, nurses must know how to assess what is normal or abnormal for all persons who seek care. This necessitates cultural competence. Cultural competence has a number of components and allows a nurse to integrate a cultural assessment into the health assessment of each client. According to Campinha-Bacote (2015), there are five constructs in the cultural competence process: cultural awareness, cultural skill, cultural knowledge, cultural encounters, and cultural desire. (For a model and description of Campinha-Bacote's "The Process of Cultural Competence in

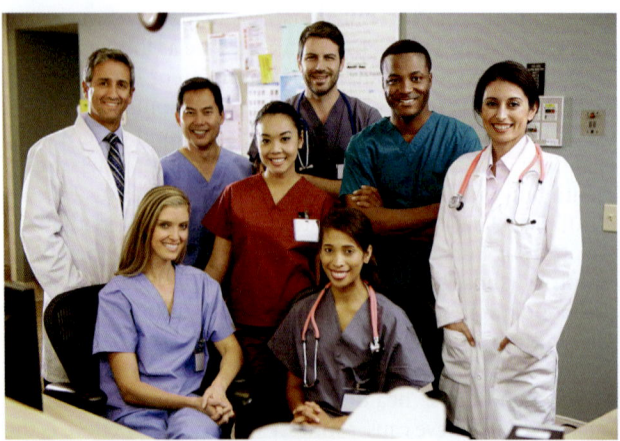

FIGURE 11-1 Example of a health care team comprised of persons from a variety of cultures.

BOX 11-1 TERMS AND DEFINITIONS RELATED TO CULTURE

Acculturation—The circumstance when a person gives up the traits of his or her culture of origin as a result of context with another culture, to variable degrees.

Assimilation—The gradual adoption and incorporation of characteristics of the prevailing culture.

Cultural diversity—The co-existence of a difference in behavior, traditions, and customs—in short, a diversity of cultures, often resulting from cross-border population flows; perhaps better referred to as "cultural pluralism" (United Nations Educational, Scientific, and Cultural Organization [UNESCO], 2016).

Cultural imposition—The intrusive application of the majority group's cultural view upon individuals and families (citing the United Nations, 1948, *Universal Declaration of Human Rights*).

Cultural relativism—The belief that the behaviors and practices of people should be judged only from the context of their cultural system.

Culture—The totality of socially transmitted behavioral patterns, arts, beliefs, values, customs, lifeways, and all other products of human work and thought characteristic of a population or people that guide their worldview and decision making

Enculturation—A natural conscious and unconscious conditioning process of learning accepted cultural norms, values, and roles in society and achieving competence in one's culture through socialization.

Ethnicity—A socially, culturally, and politically constructed group that holds in common a set of characteristics not shared by others with whom members of the group come into contact (Lipson & Dibble, 2007, p. xiv).

Ethnocentrism—The universal tendency of humans to think their ways of thinking, acting, and believing are the only right, proper, and natural ways.

Stereotyping—An oversimplified conception, opinion, or belief about some aspect of an individual or group.

Subculture—A group of people with a culture that differentiates them from the larger culture of which they are a part.

Worldview—The way individuals or groups of people look at the universe to form basic assumptions and values about their lives and the world around them; includes cosmology, relationships with nature, moral and ethical reasoning, social relationships, magicoreligious beliefs, and aesthetics.

Taken from Purnell, L. (2013). Transcultural health care: A culturally competent approach (4th ed.). Philadelphia, PA: F. A. Davis; pp. 7–11 (except where indicated by other citation).

the Delivery of Healthcare Services," visit the website at www.transculturalcare.net.)

Use the ASKED mnemonic (**a**wareness, **s**kill, **k**nowledge, **e**ncounters, and **d**esire) to examine your cultural competence (from Campinha-Bacote's website). Ask yourself how aware you are of your own biases and prejudices toward people different from you. Ask yourself if you can complete a cultural assessment being sensitive to cultural differences and sensitivities. Ask yourself how much you know about different cultures and ethnic groups, about their beliefs, customs, and biologic variations. Ask yourself what level of interest you have in interacting with people from different cultures or ethnicities. Finally, ask yourself if you really have interest in becoming culturally competent (Campinha-Bacote, 2015).

Contexts for Assessment

Culture includes contexts beyond the basic beliefs and behaviors that vary. Culture also includes family structure and function, spirituality and religion, and community, which serve as context for growth and development, health and illness, and health care delivery. Together these form the major contexts for seeing a client as an individual or from a specific group. Each individual or group is inseparable from the background contexts. The nurse must perceive the client within these contexts and be able to assess aspects of these contexts when performing a health assessment (Fig. 11-3).

Race

Race, in humans, is not a physical characteristic but a socially constructed concept that has meaning to a larger group. Anthropologists can easily show that all visible human characteristics (such as skin color; hair color and shape; eye, nose,

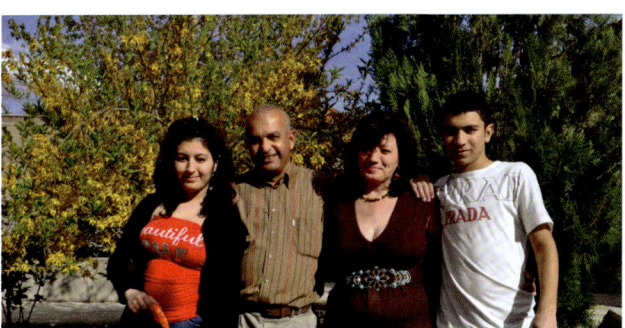

FIGURE 11-2 This Iraqi family of Armenian ethnicity is part of a subgroup of people that have a common history, ancestry, and cultural identity.

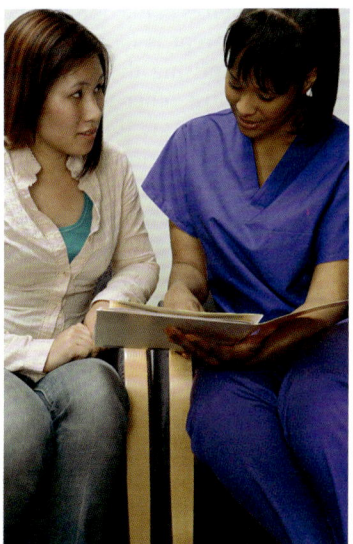

FIGURE 11-3 Cultural skill involves learning how to complete cultural assessments.

mouth shape; body shape) vary across continua of each characteristic rather than in what would be racial groupings. For instance, black skin and tightly curled black hair combines with thin lips, narrow noses, and "Caucasian-looking" faces in some of the African areas along the Nile River. And the lightly waved blond hair of northern Australian aborigines, who have dark skin and broad noses, is original to these peoples and not an admixture from intermarriage with White immigrants (author's personal experience).

The concept of race "originates from societal desire to separate people based on their looks and culture … [it is] a vague, unscientific term referring to a group of genetically related individuals who share certain physical characteristics" (Bigby, 2003). However, the genetic distinctiveness does not exist. Bigby argues that race "is reflected in American society in a way that ethnicity, culture, and class are not" (p. 2) because access to resources is often based on what are called race categories that are applied in the United States to reflect minority and skin color as opposed to genetic categories. In this case, race is more a category constructed by the society with its own meaning within that society. A prime example of this is the 15 primary "race" categories used by the U.S. Government. These categories for the 2010 U.S. Government Census (Population Reference Bureau, 2009) are: White; Black/African American/Negro; American Indian/Alaska Native; Asian Indian; Chinese; Filipino; Other Asian; Japanese; Korean; Vietnamese; Native Hawaiian; Guamanian/Chamorro; Samoan; Other Pacific Islander; and Some Other Race. In addition to race categories, the U.S. 2010 Census includes a question related to origin, "Is the person of Hispanic, Latino, or Spanish origin?" Hispanic is not considered a race because this grouping is not necessarily based on genetic variation, but on geographic origin, language spoken, or self-identity. Of course, the Census categories are not truly a reflection of genetics either, as noted above.

Minority often refers to a group that has less power or prestige within the society, but actually means a group with smaller population numbers. Because Caucasians are the majority in the United States and are expected to remain so for the next 30 or so years, all other groups would be minorities. But the term has a negative meaning in many contexts, indicating a group that does not hold the "majority" values or does not behave in "appropriate" ways; or groups whose members are considered to have less access to benefits and resources of the dominant culture.

Another important concept is *immigration*. Of the nearly 324 million people comprising the U.S. population (U.S. Census Bureau, 2016), most other than Native Americans/Alaska Natives and Hawaiians are themselves immigrants or have ancestors who came to America as immigrants (although the Native American and Alaska Native groups migrated from Asia in the far distant past). However, the category of immigrant has come to refer to those who are not native born or have not become permanent resident aliens or new citizens (naturalized). These people fall into categories based on U.S. Department of Homeland Security (2015) definitions, such as the following: nonimmigrants (those in the United States for a specific purpose with permanent residence in another country); asylees or refugees (those who have a well-founded fear of persecution should they return to their country of nationality); and illegal or undocumented aliens (the official term for those commonly referred to as illegal aliens). (The debate about this last term between the U.S. House of Representatives and the U.S. Library of Congress, which is current as of June, 2016, is described on the website ProCon.org.).

> **BOX 11-2 NATIONAL STANDARDS FOR CARE**
>
> The Office of Minority Health of the U.S. Department of Health and Human Services (USDHHS) has created standards that recommend voluntary acceptance by health care organizations of adopting standards to create systems that provide culturally and linguistically appropriate care for all persons seeking their service. Federal funds depend on adherence to the standards, thus the level of voluntary acceptance is more a mandate. Individuals who work within the health care systems are expected to follow these standards as well. "The 14 standards (known as CLAS mandates) are organized by themes: Culturally Competent Care (Standards 1 through 3), Language Access Services (Standards 4 through 7), and Organizational Supports for Cultural Competence (Standards 8 through 14). Within this framework, there are three types of standards of varying stringency: mandates, guidelines, and recommendations." (USDHHS, Office of Minority Health, 2001)

National Standards for Care

The Office of Minority Health has created standards that recommend voluntary acceptance by health care organizations of adopting standards to create systems that provide culturally and linguistically appropriate care for all persons seeking their service. Federal funds depend on adherence to the standards, thus the level of voluntary acceptance is more a mandate. Individuals who work within the health care systems are expected to follow these standards as well. "The 14 standards (known as CLAS mandates) are organized by themes: Culturally Competent Care (Standards 1 through 3), Language Access Services (Standards 4 through 7), and Organizational Supports for Cultural Competence (Standards 8 through 14). Within this framework, there are three types of standards of varying stringency: mandates, guidelines, and recommendations" (Office of Minority Health, 2001). Box 11-2 provides the standards.

> **General Routine Screening versus Focused Specialty Assessment of Culture**
>
> Every nurse–client encounter needs to include a cultural assessment, as culture affects every part of a person's health status. The degree to which cultural assessment occurs depends on the nurse's expertise and cultural experiences (Fig. 11-4). It is important to dialogue with clients to learn about their culture and cultural preferences. Next, the nurse should refer to literature to learn more about the client's culture as needed to provide culturally competent nursing care.

CULTURAL ASSESSMENT

Purposes and Scope of Assessment

The main purposes of assessing culture in a health care setting are:
- To learn about the client's beliefs and usual behaviors associated with health and illness, including beliefs about disease causes, caregiving, expected treatments (both Western

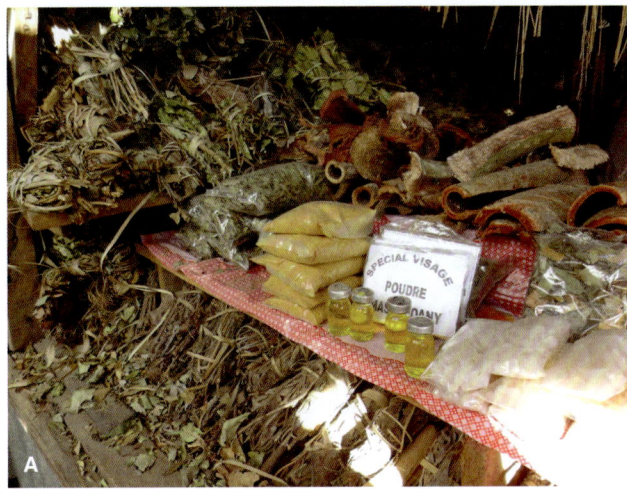

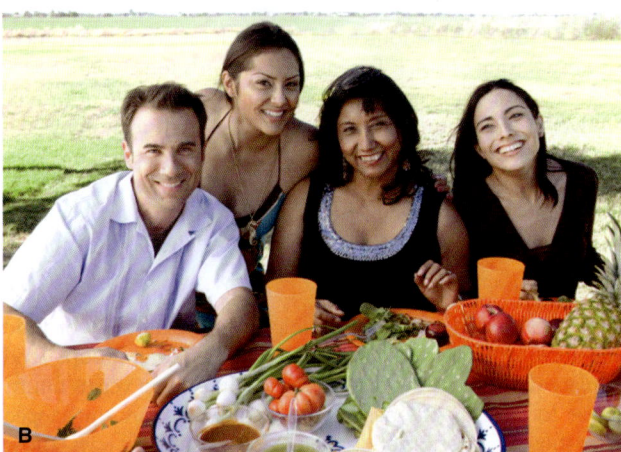

FIGURE 11-4 It is important to seek repeated encounters with people of various cultures so that awareness, knowledge, and skill continually increase. Visiting local cultural herbal medicine market (**A**), or spending times with friends of another culture (**B**) are great ways to increase awareness, knowledge, and skill.

medicine and folk practices), daily hygiene, food preferences and rituals, religious beliefs relative to health care
- To compare and contrast the client's beliefs and practices to standard Western health care
- To compare the client's beliefs and practices with those of other persons from a similar cultural background (to avoid stereotyping)
- To assess the client's health relative to diseases prevalent in the specific cultural group

does not use folk medicine or practices in her self-care for diabetes. She says that her beliefs and practices are similar to those of her friends in Beirut, where Western-style medical care is available in several hospitals and medical centers. She says that her religion, Islam, does not prevent her from pursuing the best care available.

Cultural assessment can mean adding elements of cultural assessment to the health assessment, or it can mean completing an entire cultural assessment. To know when to include cultural components—and which elements—in a health assessment, the nurse has to know how to complete an entire cultural assessment. Many of these cultural variation categories are covered in transcultural nursing and cultural anthropology texts, or can be found on the Internet. The more common cultural and biologic variations encountered in the clinical setting are described in this chapter. Knowledge of the possibilities for variation allows the nurse to select those that are most important for assessing each client.

Cultural beliefs and values to assess include:
- Value orientation (principles of what values and behaviors are considered right or wrong by a group or an individual)
- Beliefs about human nature
- Beliefs about relationship with nature
- Beliefs about purpose of life
- Beliefs about health, illness, and healing
- Beliefs about what causes disease
- Beliefs about health
- Beliefs about who serves in the role of healer or what practices bring about healing
- Beliefs about the meaning of suffering and pain

These values and beliefs can be divided into two categories: those that affect the client's approach to the health care system and provider, and those that affect the client's disease, illness, or health state. Of course there is some overlap between them. Assessing these beliefs will help the nurse to understand the client's approach to health care providers and to illness and healing. For instance, an individual who believes that diseases are punishment from God or gods may not seek help quickly or even at all. An individual who believes that evil spirits cause disease will seek out someone who can cast out evil spirits as a cure. An individual who believes that health is something that can be improved with exercise, eating the right foods, and other "healthy" behaviors will most likely seek health care for early symptoms. If a group's cultural healers play an important role, individuals belonging to that group may not accept Western-style health care without the involvement of the healer as well.

CASE STUDY

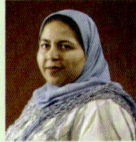

Using these categories to examine Mrs. Al Sayah's cultural beliefs and behaviors relative to health care, the nurse asks her questions or determines from her subjective assessment answers what beliefs she holds. Mrs. Al Sayah says that although she has only been in the United States for a short time, she is used to Western-style health care in Lebanon. She

CASE STUDY

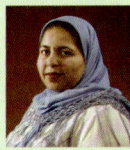

Returning to the case study of Mrs. Al Sayah, the nurse briefly asks her about her beliefs regarding the cause of her illness. Mrs. Al Sayah says that she believes it is God's will and she must accept it and do what she can to control it.

Factors Affecting Approach to Providers

The following may affect interactions between clients and their health care providers:
- Ethnicity (of both client and health care provider)
- Generational status (of both client and health care provider)
- Educational level
- Religion
- Previous health care experiences
- Occupation and income level
- Beliefs about time and space
- Communication needs/preferences

Ask clients about their cultural and ethnic backgrounds. How close to the primary culture does the person feel? To the ethnic group? To country of origin? What age was the client at immigration (if applicable)? How frequently does the client travel to and from the country of origin? If the person seeking care is from a cultural group but is well acculturated to Western values, assuming that he or she follows practices of the cultural group is stereotyping and will lead to conflict.

Generational status may be important. In some cultures, it still may be the practice that older family members have more say in health care and treatment than clients themselves, even if the client is an adult (this is especially true for females). Autonomy is assumed to be a right of all health care consumers in the United States, meaning that individuals have the right to know about diagnosis and treatment plans and to make decisions for themselves. However, autonomy is not an accepted value in many societies. In paternalistic or patriarchal societies, the father or the family is expected to be informed of diagnoses and to make decisions about treatment. In many societies, women are not decision makers. Do not assume that the client expects autonomy; clarify expectations with the client and family. Client autonomy is a legal issue in U.S. health care; thus, you will need to clearly explain this concept to the family and client. The information should be presented in such a way as to avoid a hostile response or the withdrawal of the client from Western health care. Respect is highly valued in many cultures and older age often conveys an expectation of respect. Older clients may not respect younger providers. Younger clients may fear disclosing health details to older providers. Older clients may feel uncomfortable or fail to disclose to providers of a different gender.

Education level plays an important role in health care, and it is essential to assess language proficiency. Does the client have the ability to understand spoken and written English? Can the client speak or write English? Will the individual accept an interpreter? If so, will an interpreter of a different age or gender be acceptable? For instance, some cultures do not allow a young person or a person of different gender to hear personal details.

Religious rules and norms may affect who can assess, who can treat, and what treatments are acceptable, among many other aspects of health care.

Previous experience with the primary health care system may affect provider interactions. Were past experiences positive or negative? Occupation and income level may affect ability to pay and follow prescribed care.

Ideas about time, space, and communication are especially important and necessitate specific discussion.

CASE STUDY

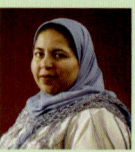

In the case study, Mrs. Al Sayah speaks as though she is well educated and has satisfactory experience with Western medical care. She speaks English well, and states that English is a second language for her, as for many in Beirut, with Arabic her first language. Due to her age and her ability to speak and comprehend English, Mrs. Al Sayah does not need translation assistance. She does state that her husband will join us in a few minutes and that all decisions about her care will have to be explained to him. He is in favor of her attempting to fast for Ramadan but is not insistent.

Communication

All communication is culturally based. Verbal communication can have many variations based on both language differences and usual tone of voice. For instance, a harsh tone of voice may be normal in some cultures and thought to be rude in others. Nonverbal communication has the most often misinterpreted variations. These variations include patterns of space, eye contact, body language and hand gestures, silence, and touch. Time is also interpreted to be a form of communication when two people from different cultures perceive time differently.

Time

Time is perceived to be measurable (Western cultures) or fluid and flowing (Eastern cultures). Different cultural groups tend to place different values on the past versus present versus future. Those focused on the past value practices that are unchanged from those of ancestors and are often resistant to new ways. Those focused on the present perceive what is happening in the present to be more important than what will occur in the future. For instance, if a person has an appointment with you but is involved in a pleasurable activity at that time, then either the appointment will be missed or the person will arrive late. Those who are future oriented place value on deferring pleasure for a later gain. They are the ones who will value the care and treatment in expectation of improvement (this reflects Western values).

Space

As noted by Davis's 1990 classic article on cultural differences in personal space, "everyone who's ever felt cramped in a crowd knows that the skin is not the body's only boundary. We each wear a zone of privacy like a hoop skirt, inviting others in or keeping them out with body language—by how closely we approach, the angle at which we face them, and speed with which we break a gaze" (p. 4). Studies show that Asians and Americans tend to keep more space between them and others when speaking. Latins, both Mediterranean and Latin American, stay closer to each other; and Middle Easterners move in the closest.

CASE STUDY

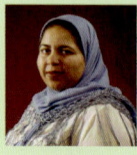

Mrs. Al Sayah sits and stands closer to the nurse than is usual in Western cultures, even more so than the many Latin clients with whom the nurse has worked.

Eye Contact and Face Positioning

Americans expect people talking to each other to maintain a fairly high level of eye contact. Those looking away and not giving "good eye contact" are thought to be rude or inattentive. But people from Eastern countries and Native Americans tend to look down to show respect to the person talking. Also, some African Americans look away when being talked to, but give a very high level of eye contact when speaking. Caucasians unfamiliar with this pattern can get the impression that the person does not care what the caregiver is saying and is aggressive when talking. However, it is just a normal cultural variation in communication pattern.

Another variation on positioning is whether persons face each other or stand with the face slightly to the side. American females (both Caucasian and Hispanic American) tend to face each other, but males, and people of some other cultures, tend to stand with the face slightly away from the other speaker.

Body Language and Hand Gestures

Two major hand gestures of note are those for indicating height and those for indicating "OK." Latins and others indicate height of an animal the way Americans indicate height of people—by putting the hand level at the indicated height. Latins indicate height for humans by bending the fingers up and putting the back of the hand at the height level. The Latin gesture is not noticed much by Americans, but the American gesture is an insult to Latins. The way Americans sign OK by making a circle with the thumb and forefinger is a definite and serious insult in many cultures around the world. Thus if any hand gesture is used, be sure to clarify if there seems to be a strange or unexpected reaction on the other person's part.

> **CASE STUDY**
>
>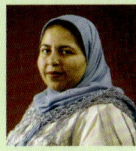
>
> Mrs. Al Sayah's body language expresses an easy manner and lack of stress in the initial interview. She uses moderate hand gestures that are appropriate to what she is saying.

Silence

There are two types of silence. One is simply remaining silent for long periods; the other is used to space talking between two people carrying on a conversation. There are three patterns of the latter. In Eastern cultures, there is a pause after each person speaks before the other does. The pause is thought to show respect and to allow for consideration of what has been said. Westerners—including English speakers in the United States—tend to interrupt this silence, leaving no pause between speakers; Americans tend to be uncomfortable with silence. In other cultures, such as Latin cultures, it is common for speakers to interrupt one another in conversation, causing overlap in speech. Within the culture, this indicates that the people are deeply engaged in the conversation, but it is perceived to be rude by other cultures.

Touch

Touch is very culturally based. How much touch is comfortable and allowable, and by whom, are all based on culture. The most modest and conservative cultures usually have religious rules about this. Touch of females by males in many of these cultures is restricted to male family members and may also be restricted among them. Even male physicians are not allowed to treat a female patient. In some religions, there are prohibitions on touching people considered to be unclean. There are prohibitions about touching parts of the body, especially the head, or touching children in some cultures because touch is a way to "give the evil eye" to another. In light of these cultural variations, a health care provider should always ask permission before touching anyone. Box 11-3 provides examples of culturally insensitive and sensitive communication.

> **CASE STUDY**
>
>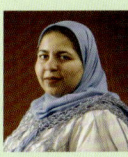
>
> In the case study, there was no difference in Mrs. Al Sayah's use of touch from that expected from Western clients. When her husband arrived, he shook hands with the nurse, which indicated that he was not a conservative Muslim. Conservative Muslim men will often cross their hands over their chests and bow instead of shaking hands to avoid touching a woman who is not a member of the immediate family.

Factors Affecting Disease, Illness, Health State

- Biomedical variations
- Nutrition/dietary habits
- Family roles and organization, patterns
- Workforce issues
- High-risk behaviors
- Pregnancy and childbirth practices
- Death rituals
- Religious and spiritual beliefs and practices
- Health care practices
- Health care practitioners
- Environment

Family content is addressed in Chapter 33, and religious and spiritual content in Chapter 12. Knowing what issues the culturally different client may have at work and what high-risk behaviors are common to the cultural group, as well as the environment from which the client comes, can give clues to current health status. Assessing health care beliefs is as important as understanding culturally based health care practices. Nutrition and biomedical variations are discussed later in this chapter. As this is an assessment text, only the most common cultural and biologic variations are covered here. More comprehensive content is available in transcultural nursing and cultural anthropology texts.

Health Care Beliefs

Cultural beliefs that affect health care involve beliefs about communication (which affect the culturally competent interview process, described previously), beliefs about the appropriate categories of persons to whom an individual goes to seek health care (Table 11-1), and beliefs about health and illness. First, a culturally competent nurse must understand the variation in beliefs about causes of illness. Then it becomes fairly easy to understand what treatments will be expected and from whom the treatments or care will be sought.

BOX 11-3 EXAMPLES OF COMMUNICATION

It is important to implement culturally sensitive communication. This box provides examples of culturally insensitive and culturally sensitive communication using a scenario between a nurse and Asami Takahashi, a young Japanese exchange student at the local university, who is being seen for a complaint of abdominal pain.

POOR COMMUNICATION

Nurse: "Good morning Asami. How are you today?"

The nurse smiles, maintains eye contact, and extends right hand to shake hands.

Asami Takahashi: "Thank you."
Nurse: "Asami, tell me why you are here today."
Asami Takahashi: "I have had a pain in my middle."
Nurse: "Whereabouts in your 'middle'?"

Asami Takahashi points to her mid to lower abdomen.

Nurse: "We call that an abdomen. So you are having pain in your abdomen. What is the pain like?"
Asami Takahashi: "It hurts."
Nurse: "Yes, I know it hurts. That is why you are here. But tell me what it feels like. Does it burn? Stab? Come and go? Stay there all the time? Does it move from where you pointed to other parts of your body?"
Asami Takahashi: "Yes, it hurts and I guess burns. Can you ask me the other questions again, please?"
Nurse: "What is the pattern of the pain? Does it stay there all the time? Does it come and go?"
Asami Takahashi: "It comes after I eat."
Nurse: "How long does it last?"
Asami Takahashi: "Sometimes it lasts a long time."
Nurse: "But how long? An hour? Two hours? All night?"
Asami Takahashi: "Sometimes an hour. Sometimes it lasts longer or comes when I haven't eaten."
Nurse: "OK. Here is a gown for you to put on. Take off your clothes, hang them on the back of the door. And put the gown on so that it ties in the back. OK? I will be back in a few minutes to take your vital signs and to examine you."

The nurse returns in 10 minutes and Asami Takahashi is not undressed.

Nurse: "Why didn't you get into the gown? I can't examine you if you keep your clothes on. Your chart says you are having abdominal pain and I have to feel your abdomen to decide what is likely going on."
Asami Takahashi: "I am uncomfortable taking my clothes off in front of strangers."
Nurse: "But how can I examine you if you don't take your clothes off? I need to take your vital signs and look you over and feel your abdomen. There are many things that could be causing your abdominal pain. I need to ask you questions and do a physical examination to see what tests you might need. Do you understand?"
Asami Takahashi: "Yes."
Nurse: "You don't sound convinced. But I thought you were a university student, so you should speak English well enough to understand. Are you afraid? Don't be. I am not here to hurt you."
Asami Takahashi: "Thank you for your time and concern, but I am feeling much better now. I think I will go back to the room and see if it has all cleared up."
Nurse: "Well, it is your choice but I advise you to stay and let me try to help you."

BETTER COMMUNICATION

Nurse: "Good morning, Ms. Takahashi. I am here to help you with your health problem."

The nurse smiles but gives only brief eye contact. She avoids touching unless Ms. Takahashi extends her hand to shake hands.

Asami Takahashi: "Thank you."
Nurse: "Can you tell me what your health problem is? Telling me what you think is the problem will help me to work with you to solve the problem."
Asami Takahashi: "I am not sure. I have this pain in my middle."
Nurse: "Can you show me?"

Asami Takahashi points to mid to lower abdominal area.

Nurse: "Can you describe the way it feels?"
Asami Takahashi: "It hurts when I eat."
Nurse: "Does it hurt right after you eat? Or does it start a few minutes later?"
Asami Takahashi: "It starts soon after I eat."
Nurse: "How long does it last?"
Asami Takahashi: "Sometimes for a long time."
Nurse: "Can you describe how long?"
Asami Takahashi: "Sometimes it lasts for more than an hour and then returns when I eat again or sometimes in between times."
Nurse: "Can you describe how it feels?"
Asami Takahashi: "It hurts."
Nurse: "If I give you some words, would you tell me if you don't understand, please? You can choose which words describe what you feel."
Asami Takahashi: "I'll try to understand."
Nurse: "Does it burn? Or feel like a knife stabbing you?"
Asami Takahashi: "If you mean, does it feel like a fire in my middle, then yes."
Nurse: "Can you tell me anything else about the feeling or when you feel it?"
Asami Takahashi: "I can tell you that it hurts."
Nurse: "To be able to tell you what may be the cause, I will need to measure your temperature, pulse, and blood pressure. And then, if you are comfortable with it, I will examine your abdomen, which means I will have to touch it to see if you feel more pain in one area than another. That way, we can see if there are blood tests or x-ray tests we need to do to make sure we are able to really find the cause, if possible. Will this be OK with you?"

Asami Takahashi remains silent for more than a minute while the nurse waits for an answer.

Asami Takahashi: "Will I have to take off my clothes?"
Nurse: "If you are uncomfortable with taking off all your clothes, then I can ask you to only rearrange them enough for me to see your abdomen."
Asami Takahashi: "Thank you. I appreciate your consideration."

The nurse proceeds with the examination, communicating with the client and asking for permission before touching her.

COMMUNICATION INTERPRETATION

Knowing some common Japanese practices helps the nurse with communication. Japanese may avoid saying "No" in order to prevent offending or embarrassing anyone—causing someone to "lose face." Many behaviors can substitute for saying no, such as ignoring the question, changing the subject, claiming that they do not understand, saying they cannot answer at this time, and stating that the question is too difficult to answer or that they have no authority to answer it.

Japanese tend to work on the assumption that too few words and silence are better than too many words. Silence is often a way of communicating. Also, the pattern of communication is for one person to talk, allow a time to process, then the other person talks, and another silence to allow the person to process. Westerners often find this pattern difficult and annoying, and unless they are aware of the pattern, assume that the person is not interested in the conversation or topic.

Japanese often do not place as much value on frankness and clarity as Westerners. Also, personal space for Japanese is much greater than for Westerners. Touch is kept to the minimum, especially from strangers. Being reserved, conservative, humble, soft spoken, and blending into the crowd are valued by Japanese. Japanese usually only nod to indicate that they are listening, and not to indicate agreement. Japanese often avoid judging information, so avoid either agreeing or disagreeing. Direct eye contact, the norm in the West, is considered rude or aggressive by the Japanese. They tend to look at areas near the face but not directly at the face.

Losing face is a very important concept in Japan; all Japanese avoid causing this or finding themselves in a situation in which they lose face. Admitting failure or error causes one to lose face. They often hesitate to admit that they do not understand something for the same reason.

Because harmony is the main desire for the Japanese, they often perceive truth to be relative. Truth depends on the circumstances and the obligations they have to others. Seeking harmony and the perception of truth being relative leads to Japanese often giving answers they think the other person wants to hear.

Japanese "give very little explanation as to what they mean and their answers are often very vague. They dislike saying no and will not tell you if they do not understand. If they disagree or do not feel they can do something, they will make a statement like 'it will be difficult.' This usually means they do not feel they can do what you requested. They often leave sentences unfinished, allowing the other person to finish it in their own mind." (Doing Business in Japan, 2004)

Based on Doing Business in Japan: Japanese communication style. (2004). Available at http://www.rikkinyman.com/training/japanese_culture/communication.htm

Causes of Illness

Western health care and medicine use the *biomedical model* as a basis for defining illness and treatments. This model is based on what science can investigate and conclude and assumes that all disease or illness has a cause and effect that can be studied. Even the usual approach of body-mind-spirit has been based on a perspective that the interaction of these components can be measured. Only recently has there been the introduction of a nonmaterialistic, nonmechanical additional perspective that allows for psychological and spiritual components in the disease process. The origin of this addition to Western medicine comes from Asian medicine beliefs.

Other beliefs about disease and illness causation, often based on Asian or indigenous populations' (such as Native Americans) beliefs, are categorized as *holistic* (or *naturalistic*) and *magicoreligious* (Fig. 11-5). In *naturalistic* belief systems, the focus is on keeping harmony or natural balance in the cosmic natural order, in which human life is only one aspect. Well-known theories associated with this belief system are the *yin/yang theory* of China (Eastern or Chinese medicine), and the *hot/cold theory* found in many other cultures that were influenced by the Greek philosopher Galen, who transmitted India-based beliefs to much of the world influenced by Greek culture. The hot/cold theory has holistic aspects, as it is based on a concept of whole person

TABLE 11-1 Cultural Variations of Traditional Healers and Practices

Culture	Traditional Healers	Preventive and Healing Practices
Asian traditions	Chinese medical practitioners, herbalists	Prevent or rebalance yin/yang, hot/cold foods and conditions, wear amulets, acupuncture, cupping, moxibustion
African traditions	Magico herbalist, Hoodoo (also known as conjurers), or other traditional healers known as "Old Lady," "granny," or lay midwife	Magical and herbal mix of herbs, roots, and rituals, talismans or amulets
Native American/Alaska Native traditions	Medicine men or shamans	Respect for nature and avoid evil spirits, use masks, herbs, sand paintings, amulets
Hispanic (Mexican, Central and South America, Spain/Portugal) traditions	Folk healers (*curandero/a, bruja/o* [witch], *yerbero/a,* partera [midwife])	Hot/cold balance for diet, herbs, amulets, prayers to God and saints and spiritual reparations for sins, avoiding "evil eye" caused by jealousy and envy
Western European traditions	Homeopathic physicians, physicians, and other health professionals	Maintain physical and emotional well-being with proper science-based modern nutrition, exercise, cleanliness, belief in and faith in God

Based on Chireau, Y. P. (2004). Natural and supernatural: African American Hoodoo narratives of sickness and healing. In C. Ember, & M. Ember (Eds.). *Encyclopedia of medical anthropology: Health & illness in the world's cultures, 2,* 3–9. New York: Springer Science + Business Media, Inc.; Galanti, G. (2015). *Caring for patients from different cultures* (5th ed.). Philadelphia, PA: University of Pennsylvania Press; Giger, J. R. (2013). *Transcultural nursing: Assessment and intervention* (6th ed.). St. Louis, MO: Mosby; Hunter-Hendrew, M. (Mama Zogbe). (1999–2006). Hoodoo: A new world name for an ancient African magical tradition. Available at http://www.mamiwata.com/hoodoo.html#hoodoois; and Purnell, L. (2013). *Transcultural health care: A culturally competent approach* (4th ed.). Philadelphia, PA: F. A. Davis.

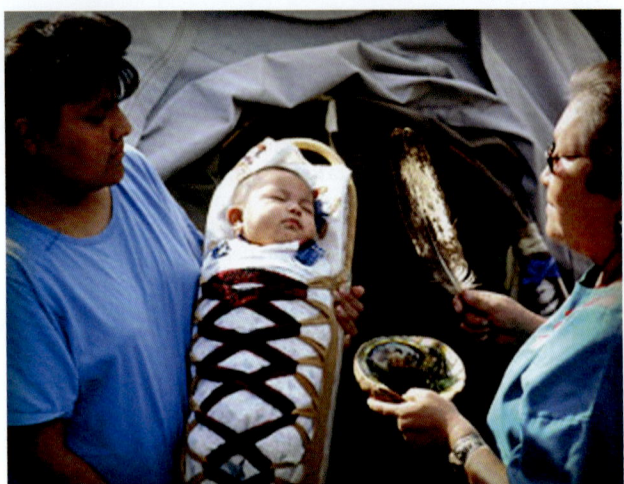

FIGURE 11-5 In the *magicoreligious* belief system, spirits and various other entities are thought to affect the status of both physical and mental health.

versus sum of the parts, and seeks a balance of all aspects of a person. There are perceived to be four "humors" of the body (blood, phlegm, black bile, and yellow bile) that work together to regulate the bodily functions. Balance is maintained by adding or subtracting substances that regulate the body's temperature, moisture, and dryness. Diet and medications are thought to have varying characteristics of hot/cold and wet/dry, and interact with diseases that are thought to be hot or cold.

In the *magicoreligious* belief system, the entire universe is seen to have supernatural forces at work, which affect all humans as well as the world in general. Spirits and various other entities are thought to affect the status of both physical and mental health.

Culture-Bound Syndromes

Culture-bound syndromes are conditions that are perceived to exist in various cultures and occur as a combination of psychiatric or psychological and physical symptoms. There is much debate over whether these syndromes are folk illnesses with behavior changes, local variations of Western psychiatric disorders, or whether they are not syndromes at all but locally accepted ways of explaining negative events in life.

Because clients perceive the syndromes to be conditions with specific symptoms, it is necessary to be familiar with them. It is important to acknowledge the client's belief that the symptoms form a disorder even if Western medicine calls it something else or does not see it as a specific disease. Table 11-2 provides a description of some of the more common culture-bound syndromes.

Many of the culture-bound syndromes are based on different beliefs about what causes disease, as described earlier. The symptoms related to the conditions are often specific to a particular culture.

Culture-Based Treatments

Culture-based treatments are often misinterpreted in Western health care settings, as they frequently produce marks on the skin that are interpreted as evidence of abuse. Assuming abuse can create a very bad nurse–client interaction and can cause the culturally different client to reject Western-style health care in the future.

Some of the more common Asian treatments are cupping, coining, and moxibustion. *Cupping*, often used to treat back pain, involves placing heated glass jars on the skin. Cooling causes suction that leaves redness and bruising. *Coining* involves rubbing ointment into the skin with a spoon or coin. It leaves bruises or red marks, but does not cause pain (Fig. 11-6). It is used for "wind illness" (a fear of being cold or of wind, which causes loss of *yang*), fever, and stress-related illnesses such as headache. *Moxibustion* is the attachment of smoldering herbs to the end of acupuncture needles or the placement of the herbs on the skin; this causes scars that look like cigarette burns. It is used to strengthen one's blood and the flow of energy, and generally to maintain good health.

The American Cancer Society (2008) has noted that in Native American culture, medicine is more about healing the person than curing a disease. There is a spiritual element at the base of their healing practices. One of the most common forms of Native American healing practices involves the use of herbal remedies. These herbal remedies include teas, tinctures, and salves. A common Native American remedy for pain uses bark from a willow tree, which contains acetylsalicylic acid, also known as aspirin (Fig. 11-7).

Other treatments are related to different beliefs about what causes disease. In many cultures an imbalance in *hot/cold* is believed to cause disease, so treatment would be to take foods, drinks, or medication of the opposite type (hot for a cold condition and cold for a hot condition). What is thought to be hot or cold has no relation to temperature. Cancer, headache, and pneumonia are described as cold, whereas diabetes mellitus, hypertension, and sore throat or infection are hot. One example of a Western versus Latino treatment belief difference is pregnancy. Pregnancy is a hot condition; iron-containing foods are also hot, thus a pregnant female should not eat iron-containing foods. In Asian societies, hot/cold is also associated with the body's energy of *yin/yang*, which must remain in balance for health. The *yin/yang* balance is maintained through diet, lifestyle, acupuncture, and herbs (Fig. 11-8).

Some standard Western treatments are unacceptable in other cultures. Counseling or psychiatric treatments are resisted by some Asians and many other cultures because psychological or psychiatric illness is considered shameful.

Death Rituals

As noted by Purnell (2013), death rituals include views on death and euthanasia along with rituals for dying, burial, and bereavement, and are unlikely to vary from the practices of the client's original ethnic group.

Practices that affect health care include such customs as ritual washing of the body, the number of family members present at the death of a family member, religious practices required during or after dying, acceptance of life- or death-prolonging treatments, beliefs about withdrawing life support, and beliefs about autopsy. Responses to death and grief vary. Some cultures expect loud wailing in grief with death (e.g., Latins, African Americans), while others expect solemn, quiet grief (e.g., Hindus). In addition, the expected duration of grief varies with culture.

Pregnancy and Childbearing

Cultural variation concerning pregnancy and childbearing practices includes "sanctioned and unsanctioned fertility

TABLE 11-2 Culture-Bound Syndromes

Syndrome	Description
Latin (American or Mediterranean)	
Ataque de nervios	Results from stressful event and build up of anger over time. Shouting, crying, trembling, verbal or physical aggression, sense of heat in chest rising to head.
Empacho	Especially in young children, soft foods believed to adhere to stomach wall. Abdominal fullness, stomach ache, diarrhea with pain, vomiting. Confirmed by rolling egg over stomach and egg appears to stick to an area.
Mal de ojo (evil eye)	Children, infants at greatest risk; women more at risk than men. Cause often thought to be stranger's touch or attention. Sudden onset of fitful sleep, crying without apparent cause, diarrhea, vomiting, and fever.
Mal puesto or *brujeria*	See rootwork entry under Africa and African Origin in Americas in this table.
Susto	Spanish word for "fright," caused by natural means (cultural stressors) or supernatural means (sorcery or witnessing supernatural phenomenon). Nervousness, anorexia, insomnia, listlessness, fatigue, muscle tics, diarrhea.
Caida de la mollera	Mexican term for fallen fontanel. Thought to be caused by midwife failing to press on the palate after delivery; falling on the head; removing the nipple from the baby's mouth inappropriately; failing to put a cap on the newborn's head. Crying, fever, vomiting, diarrhea are thought to be indications of this condition (note the similarity to dehydration).
Africa and African Origin in Americas	
Falling out or *blacking out*	Sudden collapse preceded by dizziness, spinning sensation. Eyes may remain open but unable to see. May hear and understand what is happening around them but unable to interact.
Rootwork	Belief that illnesses are supernatural in origin (witchcraft, voodoo, evil spirits, or evil person). Anxiety, gastrointestinal complaints, fear of being poisoned or killed.
Spell	Communicates with dead relatives or spirits, often with distinct personality changes (not considered pathologic in culture of origin).
High blood	Slang term for high blood pressure, but also for thick or excessive blood that rises in the body. Often believed to be caused by overly rich foods.
Low blood	Not enough or weak blood caused by diet.
Bad blood	Blood contaminated, often refers to sexually transmitted infections.
Boufeedeliriante (Haiti)	A panic disorder with sudden agitated outbursts, aggressive behavior, confusion, excitement. May have hallucinations or paranoia.
Zar (Ethiopia, Somalia, Egypt, Sudan, Iran, and other North African and Middle Eastern countries)	Spirit possession with symptoms such as dissociative episodes with laughing, shouting, hitting the head against a wall, singing, or weeping; may show apathy or withdrawal; may refuse to eat or participate in activities of daily living; may develop long-term relationship with possessing spirit. Not necessarily considered pathologic in the culture.
Native American	
Ghost sickness (Navajo)	Feelings of danger, confusion, futility, suffocation, bad dreams, fainting, dizziness, hallucinations, loss of consciousness. Possible preoccupation with death or someone who died.
Hi-Waitck (Mohave)	Unwanted separation from a loved one. Insomnia, depression, loss of appetite, and sometimes suicide.
Pibloktoq or *Arctic hysteria* (Greenland Eskimos)	An abrupt onset, extreme excitement of up to 30 minutes often followed by convulsive seizures and coma lasting up to 12 hours, with amnesia of the event. Withdrawn or mildly irritable for hours or days before attack. During the attack, may tear off clothing, break furniture, shout obscenities, eat feces, run out into snow, do other irrational or dangerous acts.
Wacinko (Oglala Sioux)	Often reaction to disappointment or interpersonal problems. Anger, withdrawal, mutism, immobility, often leads to attempted suicide.
Middle East	
Zar	Experience of spirit possession. Laughing, shouting, weeping, singing, hitting head against wall. May be apathetic, withdrawn, refuse food, unable to carry out daily tasks. May develop long-term relationship with possessing spirit (not considered pathologic in the culture).
Asian (South or East)	
Amok (Malaysia)	Occurs among males (20–45 years old) after perceived slight or insult. Aggressive outbursts, violent or homicidal, aimed at people or objects, often with ideas of persecution. Amnesia, exhaustion, finally, return to previous state.
Koro (Malaysia, Southeast Asia)	Similar to conditions in China, Thailand, and other areas. Fear that genitalia will retract into the body, possibly leading to death. Causes vary, including inappropriate sex, mass cases from belief that eating swine flu–vaccinated pork is a cause.
Latah (Malaysia)	Occurs after traumatic episode or surprise. Exaggerated startle response (usually in women). Screaming, cursing, dancing, hysterical laughter, may imitate people, hyper suggestibility.

Continued on following page

TABLE 11-2 Culture-Bound Syndromes (Continued)

Syndrome	Description
Shen kui (China) *Dhat* (India)	Similar conditions that result from the belief that semen (or "vital essence") is being lost. Anxiety, panic, sexual complaints, fatigue, weakness, loss of appetite, guilt, sexual dysfunction with no physical findings.
Taijinkyofusho (Japan)	Dread of offending or hurting others by behavior or physical condition such as body odor. Social phobia.
Illness (Asia)	Fear of wind, cold exposure causing loss of *yang* energy.
North America, Western Europe	
Anorexia nervosa	Associated with intense fear of obesity. Severely restricted food and calorie intake.
Bulimia nervosa	Associated with intense fear of obesity. Binge eating and self-induced vomiting, laxative, or diuretic use.

Modified from Andrews, M., & Boyle, J. (2016). *Transcultural concepts in nursing care* (7th ed.). Philadelphia, PA: Lippincott Williams & Wilkins; Baylor College of Medicine. (2005). Multicultural patient care: special populations: African Americans. Available at http://www.bcm.edu/mpc/special-af.html; Bigby, J. (Ed.). (2003). *Cross-cultural medicine*. Philadelphia, PA: American College of Physicians; Hall, T. M. (1996–2012). Glossary of culture bound syndromes. Available at http://www.mccajor.net/cbs_glos.html; Juckett, G. (2005). Cross-cultural medicine. *American Family Physician*, 72(11). Available at http://www.aafp.org/afp/20051201/2267.html; and O'Neill, D. (2002–2006). Culture specific diseases. Available at http://anthro.palomar.edu/medical/med_4.htm.

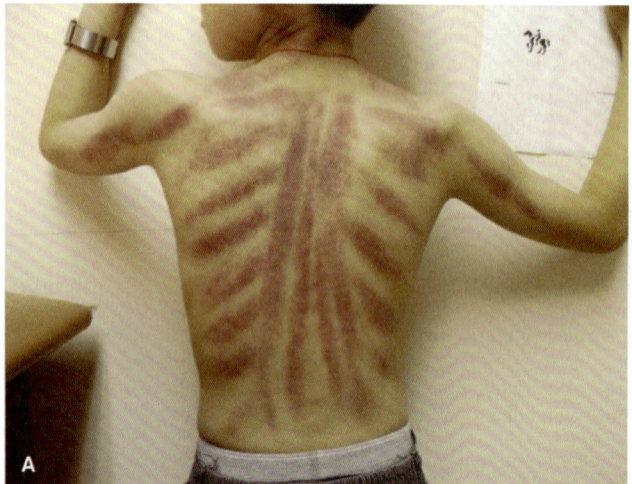
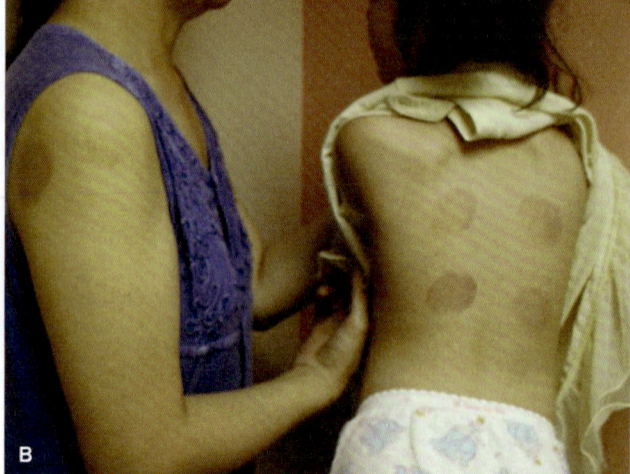

FIGURE 11-6 Two common Asian culture–based treatments that may be misinterpreted in western health care settings include coining (**A**) and cupping (**B**).

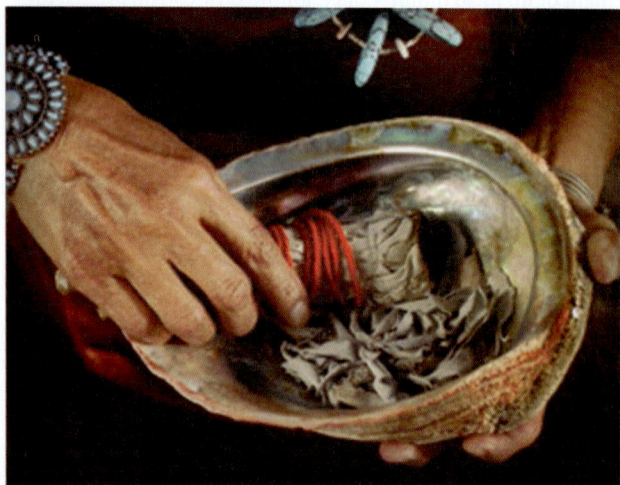

FIGURE 11-7 A common form of Native American healing practice involves the use of herbal remedies.

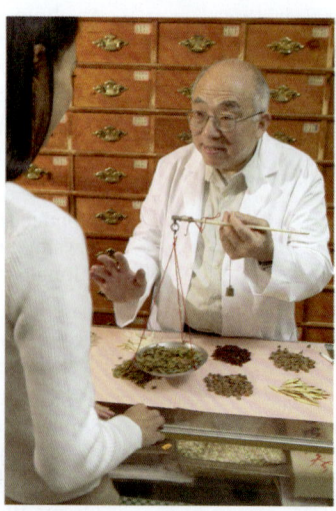

FIGURE 11-8 In Asian societies, the body's energy of *yin/yang* is balanced through diet, lifestyle, acupuncture, and herbs.

practices; views toward pregnancy; and prescriptive, restrictive, and taboo practices related to pregnancy, birthing, and the postpartum period" (Purnell, 2013, p. 32). It may be surprising to some nurses that accepted practices for getting pregnant, delivery, and childcare vary across cultures. Beliefs about conception, pregnancy, and childbearing are passed from generation to generation (an example of the transmission of culture).

Fertility control varies by culture and religion. Use of sterilization is accepted by some, rejected by others, and forcibly used in other cultures. Rituals to restrict sexuality are used in some cultures, including female circumcision (removal of the clitoris or the vulva, sewing together of the surrounding skin, leaving only a small hole for urination and menstruation). Stoning or other forms of killing women who become pregnant out of wedlock is common in some Islamic cultures.

U.S. culture has pregnancy taboos just as others do. Pregnant women are expected to avoid environments with very loud noises, avoid smoking and alcohol, avoid high caffeine and drug intake, and be cautious about taking prescription and over-the-counter medications. Other cultures have pregnancy taboos such as having the mother avoid reaching over her head to prevent the umbilical cord from going around the baby's neck, not buying baby clothes before birth (Navajo), and not permitting the father to see the mother or baby until the baby is cleaned (Belize and Panama) (Purnell, 2013).

Pain

Pain is now the fifth vital sign in U.S. health care. Assessing pain is necessary for each client (see Chapter 9). However, the experience of pain may vary by cultural conditioning. Some believe that pain is punishment for wrongdoing; others believe it is atonement for wrongdoing. The response to pain is based on cultural values. Some cultures, such as Asians, value controlling the response to pain, while others, such as Latins and Southern Europeans, value openly expressing pain. When the caregiver and the client come from different cultures, interpreting the actual level of pain being felt is difficult. It is necessary to explain the therapeutic reasons for treating pain so that a person from a stoic culture may become less reluctant to express or describe pain.

Blood Products, Transfusions, and Organ Donations

Use of blood products and blood transfusions is accepted by most religions except for Jehovah's Witnesses. Organ donation and autopsy are not accepted by certain cultural groups, including Christian Scientists, Orthodox Jews, Greeks, and some Spanish-speaking groups (because of the belief that the person will suffer in the afterlife if organs are removed or autopsy is done). African Americans (12.6% of the population) donate at a low level but make up a substantial portion of the need for donated organs (Bratton et al., 2011). Bratton et al. (2011) have listed barriers to minority donation from both deceased and living donors.

- Barriers from deceased donors:
  - Lack of awareness of transplantation
  - Religious or cultural distrust of the medical community
  - Fear of medical abandonment (if donating)
  - Fear of racism
- Barriers from living donors:
  - Unwillingness to donate
- Medical comorbid conditions
- Distrust or fear of medical community
- Loss to follow-up (not returning for follow-up appointments)
- Poor coping mechanisms
- Financial concerns
- Reluctance to ask family members and friends
- Fear of surgery
- Lack of awareness about living donor kidney transplantation

Diet and Nutrition

What we eat, how we eat it, and even when we eat are all culturally based. Dietary considerations in cultural assessment include the meaning of food to the individual, common foods eaten and rituals surrounding the eating, the distribution of food throughout a 24-hour day, religious beliefs about foods, beliefs about food and health promotion, and nutritional deficiencies associated with the ethnic group.

If possible, compare the nutrients of foods not usual in the United States with nutrition charts to understand how healthy a diet is, especially with regard to diseases such as diabetes mellitus. It is very difficult to get a client to change habitual dietary habits drastically, even with knowledge of the interaction of diet and disease. What food means to the individual can also be very important. It may serve as a comfort, as a means to stay close to ethnic roots or family. Providing food may be considered to reflect caring and love, while withdrawing food may be considered akin to torture. When meals are served can seriously affect appetite. For those who usually eat a midday meal at 2:00 or 3:00 PM, it is unappetizing to see lunch served at 11:00 AM or 12 noon, and a 5:00 or 6:00 PM dinner is considered a late lunch rather than an evening meal.

Religious beliefs affect what can and cannot be eaten, such as the prohibition of pork or pork products for Jews and Muslims and religious practices of fasting. Asking about specific diet requirements or preferences is part of cultural assessment. For dietary and nutrition practices related to religious beliefs, see Chapter 12.

CASE STUDY

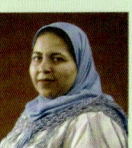
Mrs. Al Sayah is a Muslim and, therefore, will not eat pork or items that have come into contact with pork. She states that she does not drink alcohol as it is not permitted by her religion. Otherwise, she attempts to follow a diabetic diet. The normal Lebanese diet is high in fruits and vegetables, olive oil, and other foods of the Mediterranean diet. Desserts are often syrup-soaked pastries or dairy-based desserts. Mrs. Al Sayah says that she avoids Lebanese and other desserts except on occasion for holidays and celebrations.

Spirituality

Spirituality is closely associated with culture and includes religious practices, faith, and a relationship with God or a higher being and those things that bring meaning to life. See Chapter 12 for a detailed discussion of assessing spirituality.

Biologic Variations

Based on the idea that everyone is influenced by cultural variations, and the number of variations is increasing everywhere with the large number of immigrants moving from one country to another, nurses must understand cultural variation as a basis for even minimally safe and effective care. Often, biologic variations are grouped under the heading of culture; some aspects of biologic variation, in fact, affect and are affected by cultural beliefs and behaviors. Genetics and environment, and their interaction, cause humans to vary biologically. Gene variations cause obvious differences like eye color and genetic diseases, such as trisomy 21. Genes are identified increasingly as playing a role in most diseases, even if only to increase or decrease a person's susceptibility to infectious or chronic diseases. Environment has also been proved to cause disease, but modern Western thought on disease causation leans toward a mingling of genetics and environment. If, for example, a person has lungs that are genetically "hardy," then exposure to smoking may not cause lung cancer or chronic lung disease.

Physical variations (resulting from genetics or cultural behaviors) are included directly in the normal and abnormal findings in the physical assessment chapters throughout the book. Integrating the information helps the nurse to attend to the possible variations during all assessments rather than having to seek the information elsewhere if the client appears to be from a different culture.

One limitation of this approach has to be acknowledged. Because characteristics vary along a continuum with many possible points of reference, it would be cumbersome to include every possible variation as the point from which a characteristic varies. Acknowledging that this is an imperfect approach, the authors have used the U.S. population majority group as the point from which variation is assessed. As U.S. population demographics change, the baseline point will have to change in future texts.

In his model of cultural competence, Purnell (2013) includes a category called biocultural ecology. This category refers to the client's physical, biologic, and physiologic variations, such as variations in drug metabolism, disease, and health conditions. Obviously, because an assessment text cannot discuss all of the topics in biologic variation, only a sampling is included here. The variations selected for inclusion are among those most often seen or most likely to be interpreted incorrectly as normal or abnormal.

Body Surface Variation

Examples of surface variations can be seen in the following secretions: variation in apocrine and eccrine sweat secretions and the apocrine secretion of earwax. Sebaceous gland activity and secretion composition do not show significant variation.

Eccrine glands, distributed over the entire body, show no variation in number or distribution but do vary in activity based on environmental and individual adaptations (not by race; Taylor, 2006). People born in the tropics have more functioning glands than those born in other areas and those who move to the tropics later in life; persons acclimatized to hot environments have lower chloride excretion in their sweat.

Apocrine glands, opening into the hair follicles in the axilla, groin, and pubic regions; around the anus, umbilicus, and breast areola; and in the external auditory canal; vary significantly in the number of functioning glands. Asians and Native Americans have fewer functioning apocrine glands than do most Caucasians and African Americans (Preti & Leyden, 2010). The amount of sweating and body odor is directly related to the function of apocrine glands, and has a genetic base. The odor is probably related to the decomposition of lipids in the secretions. Prepubescent children, Asians, and Native Americans have no or limited underarm sweat and body odor.

Earwax, produced by the apocrine glands in the external ear, varies between dry and wet wax based on genetics. Europeans and Africans tend to have wet earwax and East Asians tend to have dry earwax (Nakano et al., 2009). The same genetic variation leads to women with dry earwax having a lower incidence of breast cancer, seen especially in East Asian women. Interestingly, the low number of Japanese women with wet earwax have been shown to have a higher risk of breast cancer than other Japanese women, apparent further evidence for the association between wet earwax and breast cancer risk (Ota et al., 2010). However, Beesley et al. (2011) found no association between a genetic variation for wet earwax and breast cancer risk in Caucasian women.

Anatomic Variation

Lower extremity venous valves vary between Caucasians and African Blacks. African Blacks have been noted to have fewer valves in the external iliac veins but many more valves lower in the leg than do Caucasians. The additional valves may account for the lower prevalence of varicose veins in African Blacks (Caggiati, 2013).

Developmental Variation

Maturity differences appear to be related to both genetics and environment. Caribbean Black, African Black, and Indian children are less likely to be experience delayed motor development than Caucasian children, but Pakistani and Bangladeshi children do not fit into this pattern (Kelly et al., 2006). African American infants and children tend to be ahead of other American groups in motor development (Martin & Fabes, 2009). However, these authors suggest that there is an interaction between biology and cultural factors that leads to this early development. Socioeconomic status has been found to have a direct relationship with fine motor skills (Ismail et al., 2016).

Biochemical Variation and Differential Disease Susceptibility

Drug metabolism differences, lactose intolerance, and malaria-related conditions—such as sickle cell disease, thalassemia, glucose-6-phosphate dehydrogenase (G6PD) deficiency, and Duffy blood group—are considered biochemical variations. The malaria-related conditions would obviously occur in populations living in or originating from mosquito-infested locales such as the Mediterranean and Africa. Lactose intolerance is another variation. Most of the world's population is lactose intolerant. The ability to digest lactose after childhood relates to a mutation that occurs mainly in those of North and Central European ancestry and in some Middle Eastern populations, with a high prevalence of lactose intolerance in South America, Africa, and the highest of all in some populations of Asia (ProCon.org, 2010, which provides results of many studies; Vesa et al., 2000).

There have been many studies on ethnic, racial, or biologic variations in drug metabolism. Purnell (2013) has provided extensive reviews of ethnic–racial group differences in drug metabolism. As Purnell noted, among other variations, Chinese are more sensitive to cardiovascular effects of some drugs and have increased absorption of antipsychotics, some narcotics, and antihypertensives. Eskimos, Native Americans, and Hispanics have increased risks for peripheral neuropathy with isoniazid. African Americans have a better response to diuretics than do Caucasians.

Many conditions can alter drug metabolism as well; for instance, smoking accelerates it, malnutrition affects it, stress affects it, and low-fat diets decrease absorption of some drugs. Cultural beliefs about taking medication affect their use. Ethnopharmacology is an entire area of study with its own society (International Society of Ethnopharmacology) and journal (Journal of Ethnopharmacology) dedicated to exchanging information about peoples' "use of plants, fungi, animals, microorganisms and minerals and their biologic and pharmacologic effects based on the principles established through international conventions" (Verpoorte, 2016, p. 1).

These brief examples of ethnic variation of diseases or susceptibility to disorders show that health status and health assessment are greatly influenced by biologic variations. Many of the chapters in this text include physical characteristics to be assessed that have normal variations or that vary in the way abnormalities are expressed. These variations are inserted into the physical assessment discussions. Also, many of the chapters include risk factor discussions addressing common illnesses associated with the content of the chapter.

Geographical and Ethnic Disease Variation

In general, chronic diseases predominate in developed countries and infectious diseases predominate in third-world countries. However, there is some genetic and ethnic variation in addition to the chronic versus infection pattern. Often the studies in developing countries and on immigrants from these countries to the United States are limited. Patterns are known, however, and are often based on body size, lifestyle, and genetics. For instance, vascular diseases tend to be higher in African Americans and populations with larger body size and lifestyle habits such as smoking. Osteoporosis is more prevalent in small-framed people such as Asians (National Institutes of Health Osteoporosis and Related Bone Diseases–National Resource Center [NIH ORBD–NRC], 2015a). Knowing that some groups will be more prone to a disease or condition can help the nurse to more carefully assess each client. Following are examples of geographic or ethnic disease variations for the physical systems.

Skin, Hair, Nails

Fair-skinned people, especially those with light eyes and freckles, are at highest risk for developing skin cancers, although all people who are exposed to high levels of intense sunlight are at risk. Because ozone depletion is a factor in skin cancer risk, people living in Australia and southern Africa are at greater risk. Worldwide, 2 to 3 million nonmelanoma and 132,000 melanoma skin cancers occur each year (WHO, 2017).

Although darker skin is not as susceptible to skin cancers, some other skin conditions occur more frequently in darker-pigmented people (Skin of color, 2006). Darker-skinned people come from many ethnic and geographic groups including African Americans, Native Americans, Asians, and Latinos or Hispanics. The conditions that are more common in darker skin are postinflammatory hyperpigmentation, vitiligo, pityriasis alba, dry or "ashy" skin, dermatosis papulosanigra (flesh moles), keloids, keloid-like acne from shaving the neck, and hair loss (in cases of tightly curled and fragile hair and use of relaxers or tight rollers).

Head and Neck

The few cultural considerations that come into play are related to dependence on poorly maintained automobiles or bicycles, lack of use of protective gear, inadequate and unsafe housing, and unsafe celebratory practices (such as shooting guns to welcome the new year). In the United States, traumatic brain injury (TBI) is especially prevalent among adolescents, young adults, and persons over 75 years of age, with males more than twice as much at risk as females. The Centers for Disease Control and Prevention (CDC, 2010) reported that falls continue to be the leading cause of TBI in the United States, causing 50% of TBIs for ages 0 to 4 years and 61% for those over 65 years. The second cause of TBI for all ages is motor vehicle accidents or traffic-related incidents. Assaults (especially firearms), head strikes, and unknown events make up the remainder of TBIs.

Eyes

Visual impairment varies across age (greater after 50), gender (more in females), and geography (more than 90% live in developing countries) (WHO, 2016b). In all but highly developed countries, cataract is the leading cause of visual disease and blindness, followed by glaucoma and age-related macular degeneration (which is the leading cause in developed countries). Other diseases include trachoma, other corneal diseases, diabetic retinopathy, and diseases of children, such as cataract, prematurity retinopathy, and vitamin A deficiency (WHO, 2016a).

Ears

The WHO (2015b) recorded that there are 360 million people across the world who have disabling hearing loss, and half of all cases are avoidable through primary prevention. Hearing loss may result from genetic causes, complications at birth, certain infectious diseases, chronic ear infections, the use of particular drugs, exposure to excessive noise and aging. As for aging, approximately one third of those over 65 years of age are affected by disabling hearing loss. There have been reports that populations with shorter, wider, and more horizontal eustachian tubes (Native Americans, Eskimos, New Zealand Maoris, one Nigerian population, and some aborigines) have higher rates of otitis media (Casselbrant et al., 1995). Shireman and Kelsey (2002) reported that African Americans have lower rates of otitis media than do Caucasians.

According to WHO (2015b), causes of hearing loss at or before birth may be from birth complications such as prematurity, reduced oxygen for the baby, or mother's infections (e.g., rubella, syphilis); use of drugs affecting the baby's hearing (more than 130 drugs including gentamicin); and severe jaundice, which can damage the baby's hearing nerve. After birth, infectious diseases, ototoxic drugs, head or ear injury, wax or foreign body blockage, excessive noise, and age can lead to hearing loss.

Mouth, Nose, Sinuses

Oral diseases are prevalent in poorer populations in developed and developing countries. They include dental caries, periodontal disease, tooth loss, oral mucosal and oropharyngeal lesions and cancers, HIV-related diseases, and trauma. Poor living conditions including diet; nutrition; hygiene; the use of alcohol, tobacco and tobacco-related products; and limited oral health care contribute to developing oral disease.

The incidence of oral cancer is different for males and females. The American Cancer Society (ACS, 2015, p. 17) reported that "an estimated 45,780 new cases of cancer of the oral cavity and pharynx (throat) are expected in 2015. Incidence rates are more than twice as high in men as in women. From 2007 to 2011, incidence rates among Whites increased in men by 1.3% per year and were stable as is in women; in contrast, among Blacks rates declined by 3.0% per year in men and by 1.4% per year in women. The increase among White men is driven by a subset of cancers in the oropharynx, including the base of the tongue and the tonsils, which are associated with human papillomavirus (HPV) infection." Although the rate of oral cancer is decreasing among African Americans, throughout the rest of the world, oral cancer is among the most prevalent cancers (WHO, 2016/2005). As in the United States, the rate is higher in males than in females and key risk factors are chewing tobacco use, smoking tobacco use, and alcohol consumption. Therefore, incidence of oral cancer is attributed to environment rather than genetics. Very high rates (five to six times higher than in the United States) are reported for South Asia, where tobacco mixed with betel nut, lime, spices, perfumes, and other substances is used for smoking and chewing (Mukherjee, 2004–2006). This practice is also used in South Asian rituals.

Sinusitis is widespread. However, the prevalence is higher in Caucasians and African Americans than in Hispanics (Sinuswars, 2012).

Thorax and Lungs

Lung cancer is directly related to smoking and to the quantity of cigarettes smoked. The highest rates for lung cancer in the United States in a study from 2013 (CDC, 2016c) are among African American men, followed by Caucasian, American Indian/Alaska Native, Asian/Pacific Islander, and Hispanic men. And among women, Caucasian women had the highest rate of developing lung cancer, followed by African American, American Indian/Alaska Native, Asian/Pacific Islander, and Hispanic women. An interesting fact is that smoking rates do not correlate with lung cancer rates when examined by ethnicity. In a 2013 study (ALA, 2016), smoking rates were highest among American Indian/Alaska Native men, followed by Caucasian and African American men, and then Hispanic men and the lowest rates were for Asian men. The same ethnic pattern for smoking rates was found in women, with lower rates for each category than for men.

The prevalence of nonmalignant lung diseases varies among different ethnic groups as well. Asthma prevalence has been found to be lowest among Asian and Hispanic adults, and highest among African American and Native American adults (Gorman & Chu, 2009). Gilkes et al. (2016) report the prevalence of chronic obstructive pulmonary disease (COPD) in the United Kingdom (where much research on COPD and ethnicity has taken place). These authors report the prevalence to be lower in Black and Asian people, with Blacks half as likely to have COPD as Caucasians when adjusting for lower smoking rates in Blacks.

Breasts and Lymphatic System

The CDC (2016a) reported a study of female breast cancer survivors and incidence and prevalence of breast cancer in the United States, noting results as follows: In 2013, Caucasian women had the highest rate of developing breast cancer, followed by African American, Hispanic, Asian/Pacific Islander, and American Indian/Alaska Native women. As for death from breast cancer, in 2013, African American women were more likely to die of breast cancer than any other group, followed by Caucasian, Hispanic, Asian/Pacific Islander, and American Indian/Alaska Native women.

There are some differences in beliefs about causes of breast cancer that vary by culture. A qualitative study by Gonzalez et al. (2015) using a focus group of Chinese, Korean, and Mexican American women found similar beliefs about cause: stress, diet, and fatalism. An interesting study done in Australia examining beliefs about causes of breast cancer compared beliefs of women without breast cancer and those with breast cancer (Thomson et al., 2014). Women without breast cancer attributed the cancer to familial and inherited factors, followed by lifestyle factors (poor diet, smoking), and environmental factors (such as food additives). Women with breast cancer attributed the cancer to mental or emotional factors (especially stress), followed by lifestyle factors and physiologic factors particularly related to hormonal history.

Heart and Neck Vessels

In the United States, heart disease causes more deaths than other conditions among all ethnic groups. However, risks vary among the groups. Heart disease and all cardiovascular diseases are higher in the southern states of the United States, known as the "Stroke Belt" (CDC, 2015a). The Harvard Health Letter (2015) described rates of hypertension, diabetes, and heart disease variations among ethnic groups, concluding that many intertwined factors likely contribute to the higher heart disease rates seen among some groups. Findings include that nearly half of all African American adults have some form of cardiovascular disease, compared with about one third of all Caucasian adults, and even after adjustment for factors related to socioeconomic differences, disparities in rates of heart disease and its risk factors persist. A possible explanation suggested by some researchers is that people who lived in equatorial Africa developed a genetic predisposition to being salt-sensitive, which means their bodies retain more sodium.

An interesting phenomenon is what has been called the "Hispanic paradox," in which those of Hispanic ethnicity have a higher prevalence of diabetes and obesity and higher death rates related to diabetes, chronic liver disease/cirrhosis, and environmental conditions conducive to disease compared with Caucasians, but have a lower overall cardiovascular disease and mortality rate by 2 years than Caucasians (CDC, 2015b).

Peripheral Vascular System

Studies of risks for chronic venous disease have remained hard to determine, according to Criqui et al. (2007). However, African American ethnicity seems to confer a protective effect. A physiologic difference in the number of lower leg veins (Africans have a higher number than do Caucasians) has been thought to account for the lower prevalence rates of varicose veins in people of African descent (1% to 2%) than in Caucasians (10% to 18%) (Caggiati, 2013).

Abdomen

Gallbladder disease and gallbladder cancer vary by ethnic group in the United States. Native Americans and Mexican Americans have higher rates of disease and cancer in this organ (ACS, 2014). Stomach cancer has an association with the prevalence of *Helicobacter pylori* (which also causes ulcers). The highest incidence of stomach cancer is in Asia, Latin America, and the Caribbean, and the lowest incidence in North America and Africa. Countries with the highest incidence are Korea,

Mongolia, and Japan (Ferlay et al., 2012; Lyons France, 2014). Ashkenazi Jews have been found to have the highest lifetime risk for developing colorectal cancer (ACS, 2016).

Cancer in general has a different pattern for Asian Americans than for those remaining in Asia. The rate of cancer is low for Asian Americans but the death rate from cancer is higher. There is a variable pattern of specific cancers across Asian groups (AANCART, 2012; ACS, 2007).

Genitalia, Anus, Rectum, Prostate

Sexually transmitted infections (chlamydia, herpes, human papilloma virus [HPV], syphilis, gonorrhea, and HIV/AIDS) vary across U.S. populations. Ethnic variation is thought to be due to rates of poverty, income inequality, unemployment, low educational attainment (CDC, 2014), use of drugs (CDC, 2016d), and other factors, but essentially to risky sexual behavior (Dariotis et al., 2011). Dariotis and colleagues reported that African American and Latino men had the consistently highest rate of sexual risk and STDs relative to their Caucasian peers, and this pattern remained even after controlling for sociodemographic variables. HIV/AIDS infection remains highest in sub-Saharan Africa, followed by Asia and the Pacific. The number of people living with HIV is highest in South Africa but other surrounding countries have high rates as well (Henry J. Kaiser Family Foundation, 2015).

The highest incidence of cervical cancer in the United States is among Hispanics and African Americans, and the lowest is among Asian/Pacific Islanders, and Native Americans/Alaska Natives, but death rates were highest among African Americans (CDC, 2016b).

In U.S. populations, incidence of prostate cancer is highest among African Americans and lowest among Native Americans/Alaska Natives, while the death rate follows the same pattern (CDC, 2016e). Forman et al. (2012) and WHO (2015a) reported worldwide prevalence of HPV and cervical cancer with the following findings: HPV infection has been identified as a definite human carcinogen for six types of cancer: cervix, penis, vulva, vagina, anus, and oropharynx (including the base of the tongue and tonsils). Cervical cancer is the third most common female malignancy and shows a strong association with level of development, rates being at least fourfold higher in countries defined within the low ranking of the Human Development Index (HDI) compared with those in the very high category; HPV varies accordingly but even in women without cervical abnormalities, HPV is most prevalent in sub-Saharan Africa, Eastern Europe, and Latin America.

Musculoskeletal System

Up to 90% of bone mass density (BMD) peaks around 18 in females and by age 20 in males (NIH ORBD–NRC, 2015b). Bone mass in women remains stable until after menopause, when it begins to decrease. Bone mass decreases in both sexes with age and some specific conditions, including lack of weight-bearing exercise. BMD is higher in men and African Americans and lowest in Asians. However, bone fracture patterns appear to be less related to bone density and size than to differences in calcium metabolism, as influenced by calcium and sodium intake, although the relative importance of calcium and sodium in calcium metabolism has not yet been determined among Asians (Walker et al., 2008).

Ethnic variation in arthritis in the United States indicates that African Americans and Caucasians have similar rates, while Hispanics have lower rates diagnosed by physicians, but higher incidence of work-related limitations and severe joint pain on diagnosis (CDC, 2005, 2011). Regarding rheumatoid arthritis, African Americans have a lower genetic predisposition (10% carry the genetic marker) compared with Caucasians (25%; The Scripps Research Institute, n.d.).

Nervous System

Cerebrovascular disease (CVD) has neurologic effects, but the cause is vascular. The same patterns of ethnic variation that occur in CVD (see Chapters 21 and 22) occur with stroke. In the United States, the states of the "stroke belt" (North Carolina, South Carolina, Georgia, Alabama, Mississippi, Louisiana, Arkansas, Tennessee; the states with highest incidence being called the "stroke buckle," which are North and South Carolina and Georgia) have greater occurrence of stroke and vascular disease, which may be due to high percentages of older adult and African American dietary factors (National Institute of Neurological Disorders and Stroke [NINDS], 2011). Children born and living in these states during childhood show greater risk for stroke in adulthood (Glymour et al., 2007).

Occurrence of dementia, including Alzheimer disease, is rising rapidly, especially in developing countries where the number of elderly is increasing (China, India, other South Asian and Pacific Island countries (Alzheimer's Disease International, 2007). Over 50% of dementia cases in Caucasians are Alzheimer's, but the rate in developing countries and in other ethnic groups has not been well studied. However, a research report from the University of Cambridge (2014) suggests that better hygiene (less exposure to bacteria, viruses, and other microorganisms) in wealthy nations may increase Alzheimer's risk.

HERITAGE ASSESSMENT VERSUS CULTURAL ASSESSMENT

Many texts include a form for a client's heritage assessment. The heritage assessment is based on the concept of acculturation and how consistent the client's lifestyle is with the cultural group from which the client originates, or the traditional habits of the client's family's culture. The country or culture of origin has cultural beliefs and practices that are common to that culture, as well as to socioeconomic, ethnic, and religious subgroups within the culture. See Rachel Spector's *Cultural Diversity in Health and Illness* (2013, Appendix D) for an example of a heritage assessment tool.

SUMMARY

To complete a culturally competent assessment, it is essential to interact with the client showing respect for the person, the family, and beliefs. Challenge yourself to learn about many of the cultural groups in your geographical area and interact with them enough to gain some understanding and appreciation for their worldviews (Fig. 11-1). Use your knowledge when meeting and assessing your clients, but be alert for behaviors, descriptions, or physical variations that need to be clarified as normal for their culture or abnormal and needing further assessment. See Box 11-4 for a complete case study of Mrs. Al Sayah, incorporating subjective data, objective data, documentation of data, and analysis of data.

BOX 11-4 CASE STUDY

Recall the case study introduced at the beginning of the chapter. The nurse uses COLDSPA to explore Mrs. Al Sayah's presenting concerns and obtains a health history.

SUBJECTIVE DATA

Mnemonic	Question	Data Provided
Character	Describe the sign or symptom.	"I don't always control my blood sugar completely."
Onset	When did it begin?	"It begins when I have bouts of vomiting or diarrhea."
Location	Where does it occur?	"No specific place."
Duration	How long does it occur?	"My blood sugar keeps fluctuating and remains out of balance until I get over the diarrhea or vomiting and get back to a regular diet and exercise program."
Severity	How bad is it? How much does it bother you?	"I have had my blood sugar go up and down between 12 and 3.8 mmol/L (180 and 68 mg/dL)."
Pattern	What makes it better or worse?	"My blood sugar is usually stable when I eat a proper diet and get regular exercise. It goes crazy with fluctuations when I have diarrhea or vomiting over several days and I take my medicine, but don't eat and drink. To stop diarrhea, I know you shouldn't eat or drink. I don't know if there is a pattern to the ups and downs of the blood sugar, but it seems to get higher when I don't eat or drink, even with the medication I usually take."
Associated factors/ How it **A**ffects the client		Only being ill and not eating, drinking, or exercising.

After exploring Mrs. Al Sayah's main concern about her occasional difficulties controlling her blood sugar during illness, the nurse continues with the past health history.

Mrs. Al Sayah denies previous treatment or hospitalization for any other condition besides type 2 diabetes. She denies any history of kidney problems, liver problems, ongoing digestive problems, or other physical system problems. The client reports occasional headache relieved with a dose of acetaminophen. Mrs. Wilson denies chest pain, palpitations, and shortness of breath.

The nurse explores Mrs. Al Sayah's family history. Her family history is significant for type 2 diabetes, coronary artery disease, and colon cancer. Her mother and sister have had type 2 diabetes. Her mother died at age 82 due to colon cancer. Her father died at age 47 due to an accident. Her maternal grandmother died at age 76 due to "unknown causes," and her maternal grandfather died at age 80 due to "heart attack." She does not know her paternal grandparents' medical history.

The nurse asks Mrs. Al Sayah to describe her typical day. She awakens at 6:00 AM, showers, dresses, and fixes her husband's breakfast before he leaves for work. She spends her day cooking and visiting friends and family, and shopping for essentials. She has a live-in housecleaner who cleans and helps with the cooking. In the evening after dinner, she often watches TV or reads. She prepares for bedtime at 10:00 PM.

Her usual 24-hour diet recall consists of: Breakfast—1 cup black coffee, 1 slice whole grain toast with peanut butter or a slice of low fat cheese, or a cup of oatmeal with fruit; lunch—a small piece of chicken with vegetables or some hummus and salad of lettuce, avocado, cucumber, tomato, lemon juice and olive oil, and a piece of fruit; dinner—a piece of meat or chicken or fish, prepared in Lebanese style with sauces that adhere to the diabetic diet, and yogurt with fruit or gelatin with fruit and a glass of milk; snacks—fruit and yogurt sometimes as a snack, and sometimes a piece of dark chocolate. Mrs. Al Sayah states that she has lost approximately 10 lb over the last 5 years since she started on her diabetic treatment and diet.

She reports rare episodes of an erratic bowel pattern: episodes of constipation alternating with diarrhea. Last bowel movement was this morning, described as "normal, soft, and brown."

Current medications include:
- Glucotrol 5 mg in morning and 5 mg in evening
- Acetaminophen: One to two 325-mg tablets every 4 hours as needed for headache/pain
- Multivitamin: 1 daily
- Correctol: 1 to 2 tablets as needed for constipation

Mrs. Al Sayah reports no known drug, food, environmental, or insect allergies.

When asked, she denies any use of recreational drugs, alcohol or tobacco products, and exposure to second-hand smoke or toxins. Her caffeine intake consists of one cup of coffee with breakfast, with a snack in the afternoon, and a cup of decaffeinated coffee with dinner.

Mrs. Al Sayah faithfully attends mosque on Fridays during Muslim holidays. She finds comfort in her faith and tries to be a good person acceptable to Allah.

Mrs. Al Sayah denies any financial or relationship problems. She says she lives near her son, who immigrated to the United States for work several years ago, and visits him and his wife and two children often. She also entertains them in her home at least once a week on the weekend.

[AT THIS POINT HER HUSBAND ARRIVES AND INTERRUPTS THE INTERVIEW.]

Mr. Al Sayah says that his wife needs to see a doctor to tell her what she should do to keep her diabetes under control while fasting during Ramadan.

The nurse explains that she will complete the interview and her physical assessment to see if she needs to see a doctor or if she, the nurse, can meet her need for the information requested.

Mr. Al Sayah expresses a perception that his wife is not having her needs met if she can only see a nurse.

The nurse calls in the doctor to explain the role of nurses in the United States and that the nurse is educated to be able to manage diets for diabetic persons who need to fast. Mr. Al Sayah seems to accept this and the assessment continues.

OBJECTIVE DATA

After asking Mrs. Al Sayah to put on a gown and then leaving the room while she does so, the nurse returns to perform a physical examination. Mrs. Al Sayah appears clean and neat, dressing and acting appropriately for her 56 years of age. She is of medium body build, weighs 134 lb. (60.1 kg), is 5 ft 4 in tall, and her muscle tone is moderate. There is even distribution of fat and firm muscle. Her skin is warm and moist, without erythema. Client is alert and cooperative, answering questions with good eye contact. Smiles and laughs appropriately. Speech is fluent, clear, and moderately paced. She speaks English, well with an accent. Thoughts are free flowing. Able to recall events earlier in day (e.g., what she had for breakfast) without difficulty.

Vital Signs: Oral temperature: 98.2°F; radial pulse: 69/min regular, bilateral and equal; respirations: 18/min regular, equal bilateral chest expansion; blood pressure: sitting position—128/72 right arm, 130/70 left arm; standing position—124/68, right arm; 125/70, left arm. She performs a blood glucose measurement with her own equipment, demonstrating good technique and a blood sugar of 126 mg/dL (7 mmol/L) 2 hours after her lunch.

DOCUMENTATION

Based on the subjective and objective data collected, the nurse documented the following assessment findings of Mrs. Al Sayah:

Biographic Data: Mrs. Al Sayah states age is 56 years, weight is 134 lb, and height is 5 ft 4 in.

Reason for Seeking Care: To find a way to safely participate in Ramadan fasting as a type 2 diabetic.

History of Present Health Concern: Mrs. Al Sayah has wanted to participate in the Ramadan fast but has been fearful of doing so since she was diagnosed 5 years ago with type 2 diabetes. She believes she has maintained blood sugar control well enough for the last year to try to modify her diet and medication regimen to allow her to fast.

Personal Health History: Other than the diabetes, Mrs. Al Sayah has been very healthy, with only occasional headaches. She says that menopause has caused her no concerns or physical effects.

Family History: Evidence of type 2 diabetes in family.

Lifestyle and Health Practices: Exercises moderately and tries to follow her diabetic diet.

Physical Examination Findings: Mrs. Al Sayah is clean and neat, dressing and acting appropriately for her 56 years of age. She is of medium body build, weighs 134 lb (60.1 kg), is 5 ft 4 in tall, and her muscle tone is moderate. There is even distribution of fat and firm muscle. Her skin is warm and moist, without erythema. Client is alert and cooperative, answering questions with good eye contact. Smiles and laughs appropriately. Speech is fluent, clear, and moderately paced. She speaks English well, with an accent. Thoughts are free flowing. Able to recall events earlier in day (e.g., what she had for breakfast) without difficulty.

Vital Signs: Oral temperature: 98.2°F; radial pulse: 69/min regular, bilateral and equal; respirations: 18/min regular, equal bilateral chest expansion; blood pressure: sitting position—128/72 right arm, 130/70 left arm; standing position—124/68, right arm; 125/70, left arm. She performs a blood glucose measurement with her own equipment, demonstrating good technique and a blood sugar of 126 mg/dL (7 mmol/L) 2 hours after her lunch.

ANALYSIS OF DATA

The nurse uses diagnostic reasoning to analyze the data collected on Mrs. Al Sayah's general status and vital signs to arrive at the following possible conclusions.

NURSING DIAGNOSES

- Readiness for Enhanced Health Management related to request for safe ways to manage diabetes when fasting for Ramadan
- Risk for Ineffective Health Maintenance related to participation in Ramadan fast
- Risk for Imbalanced Nutrition: Less or More than Body Requirements related to participation in Ramadan fast and parties after breaking the fast
- Risk for Situational Low Self-esteem related to possibility of not being able to participate fully in Ramadan fast as diabetic
- Risk for Spiritual Distress related to possibility of not being able to participate fully in Ramadan fast as diabetic

Interdisciplinary Verbal Communication of Assessment Findings Using SBAR

SITUATION: Samar Al Sayah, a 56-year-old type 2 diabetic woman who recently emigrated from Lebanon, seeks advice on participating in the 30-day Ramadan fast. (This is a time of spiritual reflection, prayer, charity, atonement for sins, and affirmation of faith in Islam. Muslims abstain from all food, drink, sexual contact, smoking, gossip, lies, obscenity, and all sinful acts between dawn and sunset.) She understands that she has much to learn to prevent complications with her diabetes.

BACKGROUND: Has had type 2 diabetes for several years and has not fasted in the past for Ramadan. Has taken oral medication for elevated blood sugar for 5 years and is usually in good control. Occasionally finds blood sugar fluctuations when she has bouts of diarrhea or vomiting, or when she stops exercising. Muslims who are ill or traveling, and women who are menstruating, pregnant, or nursing may postpone the fast until another time. She speaks English well; it is her second language with Arabic her first. Her husband is involved in all decisions about her care and is in favor of her fasting but not insistent.

ASSESSMENT: Mrs. Al Sayah, although only in the United States for a short time, is used to Western-style health care in

Beirut, Lebanon. Her religion, Islam, does not prevent her from pursuing the best care available. Believes her DM is God's will and she must accept and do what she can to manage it. Client sits and stands closer to the nurse than is usual in Western cultures. Husband shook hands with nurse, indicating he is not a conservative Muslim. She will not eat pork or items in contact with pork; does not drink alcohol as it is not permitted by her religion. Attempts to follow a diabetic diet. Eats foods of the Mediterranean diet but avoids desserts, often syrup-soaked pastries or dairy-based desserts, except on holiday occasions. Wishes to modify her diabetes diet to accommodate fasting for Ramadan, which involves fasting from food and fluids from sun up to sunset and then feasting as much as desired until the next sun up. This pattern disrupts both sleep and diet, and often exercise, as the person fasting has little energy during the day.

RECOMMENDATION: Mrs. Al Sayah is ready to learn ways she can develop a plan to safely fast and monitor her blood sugar during Ramadan. Nursing diagnosis would be: Readiness to Enhance Health Management by learning safe ways to modify diet, fluid intake, and rest/exercise during the month of Ramadan, including when to measure glucose levels and when to report findings to health care provider if necessary.

Want to know more?

A wide variety of resources to enhance your learning and understanding of this book are available on **thePoint**. Visit thePoint to access:

NCLEX-Style Student Review Questions
Watch and Learn Videos
Concept in Action Animations
And more!

References and Selected Readings

AANCART (The National Center for Reducing Asian American Cancer Health Disparities). (2012). Asian American cancer health disparities. Available at http://www.aancart.org/cancer-research/publications/asian-american-cancer-health-disparities

Albrecht, G., Fitzpatrick, R., & Scrimshaw, S. (2013). *Handbook of social studies in health and medicine: Cultural variation in the experience of health and illness.* DOI: 10.4135/9781848608412.n13

Alzheimer's Disease International. (2007). Statistics. Available at http://www.alz.co.uk/research/statistics.html.

American Cancer Society (ACS). (2008). Native American healing. Available at http://www.lung.org/stop-smoking/smoking-facts/tobacco-use-racial-and-ethnic.html

American Cancer Society (ACS). (2007). Cancer hits US Asian groups differently. Available at http://www.cancer.org/docroot/NWS/content/NWS_1_1x_Cancer_Hits_US_Asian_Groups_Differently.asp

American Cancer Society (ACS). (2014). Gallbladder cancer. Available at http://www.cancer.org/cancer/gallbladdercancer/detailedguide/gallbladder-risk-factors

American Cancer Society (ACS). (2015). Cancer facts & figures 2015. Available at http://www.oralcancerfoundation.org/facts/pdf/Us_Cancer_Facts.pdf

American Cancer Society (ACS). (2016). Colorectal cancer. Available at http://www.cancer.org/cancer/colonandrectumcancer/detailedguide/colorectal-cancer-risk-factors

American Lung Association (ALA). (2016). Tobacco use in racial and ethnic populations. Available at http://www.lung.org/stop-smoking/smoking-facts/tobacco-use-racial-and-ethnic.html

Beesley, J., Johnatty, S., Chen, X., et al. (2011). No evidence of an association between the earwax-associated polymorphism in ABCC11 and breast cancer risk in Caucasian women. *Breast Cancer Research and Treatment, 126*(1), 235–239.

Bigby, J. (Ed.). (2003). *Cross-cultural medicine.* Philadelphia, PA: American College of Physicians.

Bratton, C., Chavin, K., & Baliga, P. (2011). Racial disparities in organ donation and why. *Current Opinion in Organ Transplantation, 16*(2), 243–249.

Caggiati, A. (2013). The venous valves of the lower limbs. *Phlebotomy, 20*(2), 87–95. Available at http://www.phlebolymphology.org/wp-content/uploads/2014/09/Phlebolymphology78.pdf

Campinha-Bacote, J. (2015). The process of cultural competence in the delivery of health care services. Available at http://transculturalcare.net/the-process-of-cultural-competence-in-the-delivery-of-healthcare-services/

Casselbrant, M., Mandel, E., Kurs-Lasky, M., et al. (1995). Otitis media in a population of black American and white American infants, 0–2 years of age. *International Journal of Pediatric Otorhinolaryngology, 33,* 1–16.

Centers for Disease Control and Prevention (CDC). (2005). Racial/ethnic differences in the prevalence and impact of doctor-diagnosed arthritis—United States, 2002. *Morbidity and Mortality Weekly Report, 54*(5), 119–123. Available at http://www.cdc.gov/mmwR/preview/mmwrhtml/mm5405a3.htm.

Centers for Disease Control & Prevention (CDC). (2010). Injury prevention and control: Traumatic brain injury. Available http://www.cdc.gov/traumaticbraininjury/causes.html

Centers for Disease Control and Prevention (CDC). (2011). Prevalence of doctor-diagnosed arthritis and arthritis-attributable effects among Hispanic adults, by Hispanic subgroup — United States, 2002, 2003, 2006, and 2009. *Morbidity and Mortality Weekly Report (MMWR), 60*(6), 167–171.

Centers for Disease Control and Prevention (CDC). (2014). 2013 sexually transmitted disease surveillance: STDs in racial and ethnic minorities. Available at http://www.cdc.gov/std/stats13/minorities.htm

Centers for Disease Control and Prevention (CDC). (2015a). Stroke death rates, total population 35+. Available at http://www.cdc.gov/dhdsp/maps/national_maps/stroke_all.htm

Centers for Disease Control and Prevention (CDC). (2015b). Vital signs: Leading causes of death, prevalence of diseases and risk factors, and use of health services among Hispanics in the United States – 2009–2013. *Morbidity and Mortality Weekly Reports (MMWR), 64*(17), 469–478.

Centers for Disease Control and Prevention (CDC). (2016a). Breast cancer rates by race and ethnicity. Available at http://www.cdc.gov/cancer/breast/statistics/race.htm

Centers for Disease Control and Prevention (CDC). (2016b). Cervical cancer rates by race and ethnicity. Available at http://www.cdc.gov/cancer/cervical/statistics/race.htm

Centers for Disease Control and Prevention (CDC). (2016c). Lung cancer rates by race and ethnicity. Available at http://www.cdc.gov/cancer/lung/statistics/race.htm

Centers for Disease Control and Prevention (CDC). (2016d). Persons who use drugs. Available at http://www.cdc.gov/pwud/

Centers for Disease Control and Prevention (CDC). (2016e). Prostate cancer rates by race and ethnicity. Available at http://www.cdc.gov/cancer/prostate/statistics/race.htm

Criqui, M., Denenberg, J., Bergan, J., et al. (2007). Risk factors for chronic venous disease: the San Diego population study. *Journal of Vascular Surgery, 46*(2), 331–337.

Dariotis, J., Sifakis, F., Pleck, J., et al. (2011). Racial-ethnic disparities in sexual risk behaviors and STDs during the transition to adulthood for young men. *Perspectives on Sexual and Reproductive Health, 43*(1), 51–59.

Davis, L. (1990). Where do we stand? *Health,* 4–5.

Department of Homeland Security. (2015). Definition of terms. Available at www.dhs.gov/files/statistics/stdfdef.shtm

Ferlay, J., Soerjomataram, I., Ervik, M., et al. (2012). Cancer incidence and mortality worldwide: IARC CancerBase No. 11. [Internet]. *GLOBOCAN, 1*(1)]

Forman, D., deMartel, C., Lacey, C., et al. (2012). Global burden of human papillomavirus and related diseases. *Vaccine, 30*(Suppl 5), F12–23.

Gilkes, A., Ashworth, M., Schofield, P., et al. (2016). Does COPD risk vary by ethnicity? A retrospective cross-sectional study. *International Journal of Chronic Obstructive Pulmonary Disease, 11*(1), 739–746.

Glymour, M., Avendano, M., & Berkman, L. (2007). Is the stroke belt worn from childhood? *Stroke, 38*(9), 2415–2421. Available at http://stroke.ahajournals.org/content/38/9/2415.full

Gonzalez, P., Lim, J-W., Wang-Letzkus, M., et al. (2015). Breast cancer cause beliefs: Chinese, Korean, Mexican American breast cancer survivors. *Western Journal of Nursing Research, 37*(8), 1081–1099.

Gorman, B., & Chu, M. (2009). Racial and ethnic differences in adult asthma prevalence, problems, and medical Care. *Ethnic Health, 14*(5), 527–552.

Harvard Health Letter. (2015). Race and ethnicity: Clues to your heart disease risk. Available at http://www.health.harvard.edu/heart-health/race-and-ethnicity-clues-to-your-heart-disease-risk

Ismail, S., Sulaiman, N., & Adnan, R. (2016). The relationship between socioeconomic status and fine motor skills among six-year-old preschool children. *Proceedings of the 2nd International Colloquium on Sports Science, Exercise, Engineering and Technology 2015 (ICoSSEET 2015)* (pp. 141–148).

Kelly, Y., Sacher, A., Schoon, I., et al. (2006). Ethnic differences in achievement of milestones by 9 months of age: The Millennium Cohort study. *Developmental Medicine & Child Neurology, 48*, 825–830.

Lipson, J., & Dibble, S. (2007). *Culture & clinical care.* (6th printing). San Francisco, CA: University of California San Francisco Nursing Press.

Lyon, France: International Agency for Research on Cancer (2014). Available at http://globocan.iarc.fr

Martin, C. L., & Fabes, R. (2009). *Discovering child development* (2nd ed.). Boston, MA: Houghton Mifflin.

Mukherjee, A. (2004–2006). Cultural influences on South Asian oral health disparities. Available at http://www.umdnj.edu

Nakano, M., Miwa, N., Hirano, A., et al. (2009). A strong association of axillary osmidrosis with the wet earwax type determined by genotyping of the ABCC11 gene. *BMC Genetics,* 10–42. Available at http://www.ncbi.nlm.nih.gov/pubmed/19650936

National Institutes of Health Osteoporosis and Related Bone Diseases–National Resource Center (NIH-ORBD-NRC). (2015a). Osteoporosis and Asian American Women. Available at http://www.niams.nih.gov/health_info/bone/osteoporosis/background/asian_american_women.asp

National Institutes of Health Osteoporosis and Related Bone Diseases–National Resource Center (NIH-ORBD-NRC). (2015b). Osteoporosis: Peak bone mass in women. Available at http://www.niams.nih.gov/health_info/bone/osteoporosis/bone_mass.asp

National Institute of Neurological Disorders and Stroke (NINDS). (2011). Stroke: Hope through research. Available at http://www.ninds.nih.gov/disorders/stroke/detail_stroke.htm#170791105

Office of Minority Health. (2001). National standards on culturally and linguistically appropriate health care: Final report. Available at http://minorityhealth.hhs.gov/assets/pdf/checked/finalreport.pdf

Ota, I., Sakurai, A., Toyoda, Y., Morita, S., Sasaki, T., Chesham, T., et al. (2010). Association between breast cancer risk and the wild-type allele of human ABC transporter *ABCC11*. *Anticancer Research, 30*(12), 5189–5194.

Pew Research Center. (2014). Census bureau explores new Middle East/North Africa ethnic category. Available at http://www.pewresearch.org/fact-tank/2014/03/24/census-bureau-explores-new-middle-eastnorth-africa-ethnic-category/

Population Reference Bureau. (2009). The 2010 Census Questionnaire: Seven questions for everyone. Available http://www.prb.org/Articles/2009/questionnaire.aspx

Preti, G., & Leyden, J. (2010). Genetic influences on human body odor: From genes to the axillae. *Journal of Investigative Dermatology, 130*(2), 144–146.

ProCon.org. (2010, Feb 23). Lactose intolerance by ethnicity and region. Available at http://milk.procon.org/view.resource.php?resourceID=000661

ProCon.org. (2016, June 2). Should the term "illegal alien" be used to define persons in violation of immigration law? Available at http://immigration.procon.org/view.answers.php?questionID=000757

Purnell, L. D. (2013). *Transcultural health care: A culturally competent approach* (4th ed.). Philadelphia, PA: F. A. Davis.

Shireman, T., & Kelsey, K. (2002). Prescribing patterns and retreatment rates in patients with otitis media. *Clinical Drug Investigations, 22*(5). Available at http://www.medscape.com/viewarticle/434084_3

Sinuswars. (2012). People that may be prone to developing sinusitis. Available http://www.sinuswars.com/archive/ProneToDevelopingSinusitis.asp

Skin of Color. (2006). Available at http://aad.org [insert Skin of Color into search box].

Spector, R. (2013). *Cultural diversity in health and illness* (8th ed.). Upper Saddle River, NJ: Prentice-Hall.

Taylor, N. A. (2006). Ethnic differences in thermoregulation: Genotypic versus phenotypic heat adaptation. *Journal of Thermal Biology, 31*, 90–104.

The Henry J. Kaiser Family Foundation. (2015). The global HIV/AIDS epidemic. Available at http://kff.org/global-health-policy/fact-sheet/the-global-hivaids-epidemic/

The Scripps Research Institute. (n.d.). Philanthropy. Research advances. Arthritis. Available at http://www.scripps.edu/philanthropy/arthritis.html.

Thomson, A., Heyworth, J., Girschik, J., et al. (2014). Beliefs and perceptions about the causes of breast cancer: A case-control study. *BMC Research Notes, 7*: 558.

United Nations Educational, Scientific, and Cultural Organization (UNESCO). (2016). Cultural diversity. Available at http://www.unesco.org/new/en/social-and-human-sciences/themes/international-migration/glossary/cultural-diversity/

The United Nations. (1948). *Universal Declaration of Human Rights.*

U.S. Census Bureau. (2010). Census briefs: Overview of race and Hispanic origin: 2010. Available at http://www.census.gov/prod/cen2010/briefs/c2010br-02.pdf

U.S. Census Bureau. (2016). U.S. and world population clock. Available at http://www.census.gov/popclock/

U.S. Department of Homeland Security. (2015). Definition of terms. Available at https://www.dhs.gov/immigration-statistics/data-standards-and-definitions/definition-terms#14

University of Cambridge Research. (2014). Better hygiene in wealthy nations may increase Alzheimer's risk. Available at http://www.cam.ac.uk/research/news/better-hygiene-in-wealthy-nations-may-increase-alzheimers-risk

Verpoorte, R. (2016). Journal of Ethnopharmacology. Available at http://www.journals.elsevier.com/journal-of-ethnopharmacology

Vesa, T., Marteau, P., & Korpela, R. (2000). Lactose intolerance. *Journal of the American College of Nutrition, 19*(suppl 2), 165S–175S.

Walker, M., Novotny, R., Bilezikian, J., et al. (2008). Race and diet interactions in the acquisition, maintenance, and loss of bone. Available at http://jn.nutrition.org/content/138/6/1256S.full

World Health Organization (WHO). (2015a). Cervical cancer estimated incidence, mortality and prevalence worldwide in 2012. Available at http://globocan.iarc.fr/old/FactSheets/cancers/cervix-new.asp

World Health Organization (WHO). (2015b). Deafness and hearing loss. Available at http://www.who.int/mediacentre/factsheets/fs300/en/

World Health Organization (WHO). (2016/2005). Oral health: Global data on incidence of oral cancer (maps). Available at http://www.who.int/oral_health/publications/cancer_maps/en/

World Health Organization (WHO). (2016a). Causes of blindness and visual impairment. Available at http://www.who.int/blindness/causes/en/

World Health Organization (WHO). (2016b). Magnitude of blindness and visual impairment. Available at http://www.who.int/blindness/causes/magnitude/en/

World Health Organization (WHO). (2017). Skin cancers. Available at http://www.who.int/uv/faq/skincancer/en/index1.html

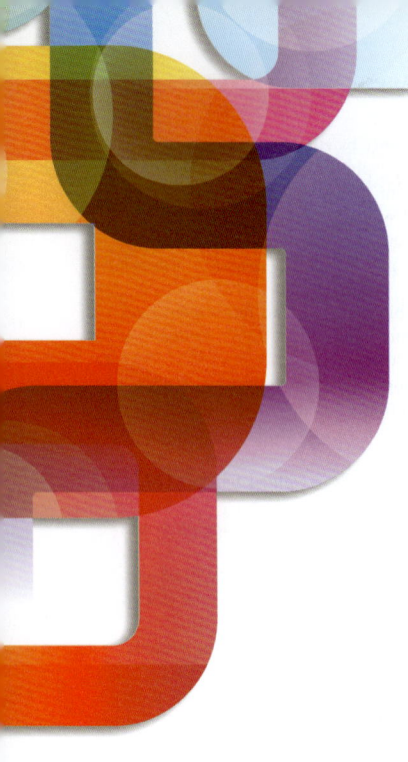

12 ASSESSING SPIRITUALITY AND RELIGIOUS PRACTICES

Learning Objectives

1. Describe the difference between religion and spirituality.
2. Review the current statistics on spiritual and religious beliefs and practices in the United States.
3. Discuss how understanding the client's spirituality assists the nurse to understand the client's decision making processes and support systems.
4. Explain why it is important for nurses to understand their own spiritual beliefs and biases.
5. Discuss risk factors associated with spiritual distress.
6. Interview a client for an accurate nursing history of his or her spirituality and religious practices.
7. Perform an objective assessment of a client's spirituality and religious practices.
8. Differentiate between skills needed for general routine screening versus skills needed for focused specialty assessment of one's spirituality and religious practices.
9. Differentiate between normal and abnormal findings of a client's spirituality and religious practices.
10. Analyze data from the interview and objective assessment of a client's spirituality and religious practices to formulate valid nursing diagnoses, collaborative problems, and/or referrals.
11. Communicate interview and assessment findings of a client's spirituality and religious practices through clear concise documentation and verbal reports.

CASE STUDY

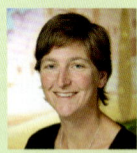 Lindsay Baird is a 40-year-old woman who lives with her two children and husband in a rural community. Mrs. Baird presents at the clinic for a routine check of her hypertension. Upon reviewing the past medical/family history, it is noted that Mrs. Baird is Catholic and believes her spirituality to be a very important part of her medical care. Entering the room, Mrs. Baird greets the nurse gracefully and continues to respond to general health questions with ease. After proceeding through relevant medical history since the last visit, a 5-lb weight gain is noted with a correlating blood pressure notably higher than the last visit. Upon questioning the recent changes in her medical condition, Mrs. Baird responds, "I just haven't felt like doing any exercise lately." Continuing to draw information out, the nurse asks particular questions related to stress levels, time restraints, and motivation. Eventually Mrs. Baird begins to tell the story of her family falling away from attending church on a regular basis and the corresponding loss of support and motivation. She states, "I used to gain such strength going to mass. It was such an encouragement. One day during the week, my friends from church and I used to walk with one another and talk about what God is doing in our lives ... now I just feel overwhelmed and busy all of the time ... and I can't talk with anyone." Mrs. Baird's case will be discussed throughout the chapter.

CONCEPTUAL FOUNDATIONS

Spirituality and religion are important factors in health and can influence health decisions and outcomes. Lifestyle practices, religious practices, dietary beliefs, and many aspects of religion and spirituality affect health. Religious practices and affiliations around the world vary, as they do within the United States due to the number of immigrants from cultures around the world in addition to the varied cultures that have coexisted within the country since its founding. To review some of the cultural variation in religious beliefs, see

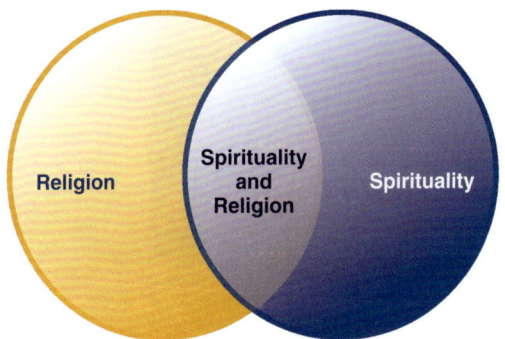

FIGURE 12-1 Interrelated yet separate concepts of religion and spirituality.

https://www.roswellpark.org/sites/default/files/node-files/page/nid940-21946-caring-across-cultures-web.pdf

Recent polls suggest a decline in religious practice and belief in God or a higher spirit in the United States. The level of religious practice in the United States has declined slightly between 2007 and 2014 (from 92% to 89%). While the percentage of adults who identify themselves as religiously affiliated declined in the same period from 83% to 77%, belief in God among those who are affiliated remained the same (97%), but belief in God among the religiously unaffiliated fell from 70% to 61% (Pew Research Center, 2015). However, this trend is not universal. The Pew Research Center (2015) reported that belief in God has been more stable among some more highly observant religious groups, such as evangelical Protestants and members of the historically black Protestant tradition—among whom nearly 90% say they are absolutely certain God exists. Eighty four percent of U.S. Muslims are certain there is a God or universal spirit, similar to 2007 (82%). Also, more than 55% of the U.S. population says they pray on a daily basis (Pew Research Center, 2016). An additional important point is that substantial portions of the unaffiliated say they believe in God or a universal spirit, and although 42% of the unaffiliated describe themselves as neither a religious nor a spiritual person, 18% say they are religious, and 37% say they are spiritual but not religious (Pew Research Center, 2012). But what is religion? What is spirituality?

Terms Related to Spirituality

It is useful to define the concepts of religion and spirituality as interconnected but separate ideas (Fig. 12-1, Box 12-1). *Religion* is defined as the rituals, practices, and experiences shared within a group that involve a search for the sacred (e.g., God, Allah, etc.). For some faiths, this idea of religion encompasses the concept of spirituality and is a natural outflow of that idea. Others may view spirituality as a separate concept, possibly disconnected from any religious institution. *Spirituality* is defined as a search for meaning and purpose in life; it seeks to understand life's ultimate questions in relation to the sacred. There has been tremendous growth in the public's conceptual understanding of spirituality during the past 20 years. Thoughts on spirituality and religion may vary immensely from one client to the next. With a growing proportion of the population identifying themselves as "spiritual but not religious," the use of the correct instrument or framework will determine the accuracy of an assessment.

The Relationship Between Spirituality, Religion, and Health

Public opinion and health care research support the importance of the relationship of religion, spirituality, and health. A very important set of concepts is involved in illness and spirituality. Wright (2005) calls suffering, beliefs, and spirituality analogous to three close cousins. Suffering, be it psychological or physical, is often associated with illness. A person's beliefs about the cause and meaning of suffering and pain affect the illness. Spiritual beliefs about the meaning of life affect the

---

BOX 12-1 FOUNDATIONAL KNOWLEDGE FOR SPIRITUAL ASSESSMENT

RELIGION

Definition: Rituals, practices, and experiences involving a search for the sacred (e.g., God, Allah, etc.)[a] that are shared within a group.

Characteristics
- Formal
- Organized
- Group oriented
- Ritualistic
- Objective, as in easily measurable (e.g., church attendance)

SPIRITUALITY

Definition: A search for meaning and purpose in life, which seeks to understand life's ultimate questions in relation to the sacred.

Characteristics
- Informal
- Nonorganized
- Self-reflective
- May involve spiritual experiences
- Subjective, as in difficult to consistently measure (e.g., daily spiritual experiences, spiritual well-being, etc.)

SPIRITUAL ASSESSMENT

Definition: Active and ongoing conversation that assesses the spiritual needs of the client.

Characteristics
- Formal or informal
- Respectful
- Nonbiased

SPIRITUAL CARE

Definition: Addressing the spiritual needs of the client as they unfold through spiritual assessment.

Characteristics
- Individualistic
- Client oriented
- Collaborative

[a]Note: God or Allah can be interchanged with universal spirit or higher power throughout this chapter as necessary to support the individual needs of the client who does not follow Christianity, Judaism, or Islam.

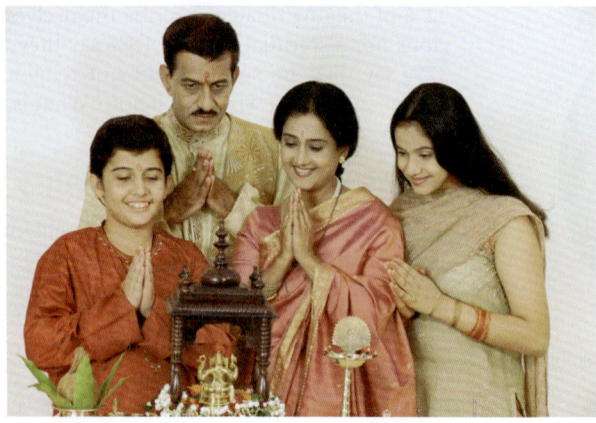
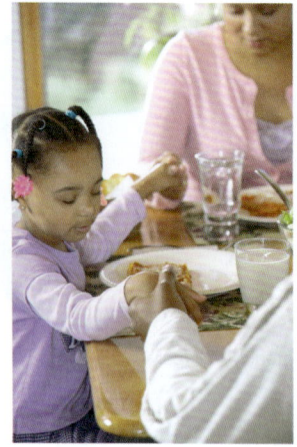
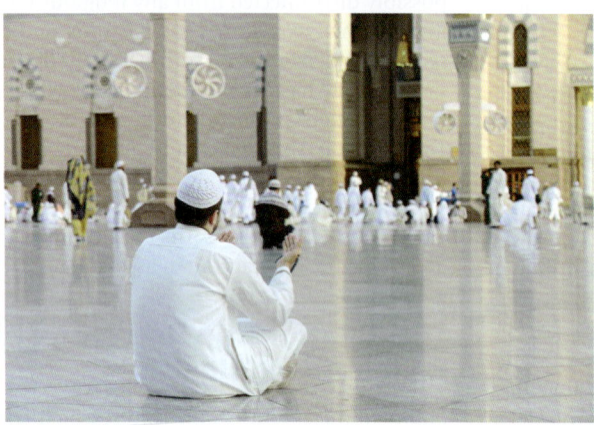

FIGURE 12-2 Prayer takes many forms.

course of illness and how a person handles suffering and pain as well. Nurses can benefit from understanding this three-part relationship when assessing a client's spiritual health.

Impact of Religion and Spirituality on Health

A large number of clients use spiritual resources during times of high stress (e.g., hospitalizations). Religion and spirituality have been shown to relate to a person's greater sense of well-being in the face of chronic disease management and ability to adhere to medical regimens. Religion and spirituality can be powerful coping mechanisms when a person faces end-of-life issues.

A substantial amount of evidence shows the positive effects of spirituality on health. Spiritual practices have the potential to encourage greater mental and physical health. A limited list of spiritual activities may include prayer (Fig. 12-2), participation in church services (Fig. 12-3), yoga (Fig. 12-4), *tai chi*

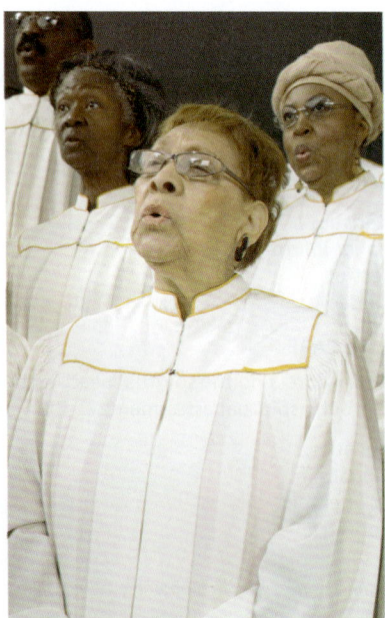
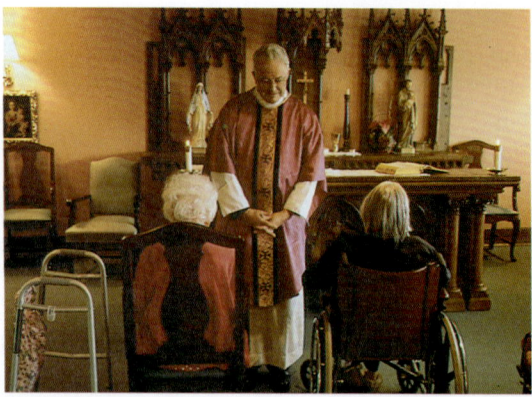

FIGURE 12-3 Many people nourish spiritually by participating in church services, such as singing in choirs and attending mass.

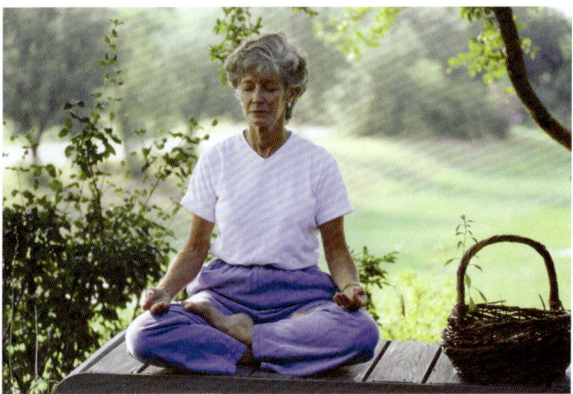

FIGURE 12-4 Yoga and meditation are practiced by many.

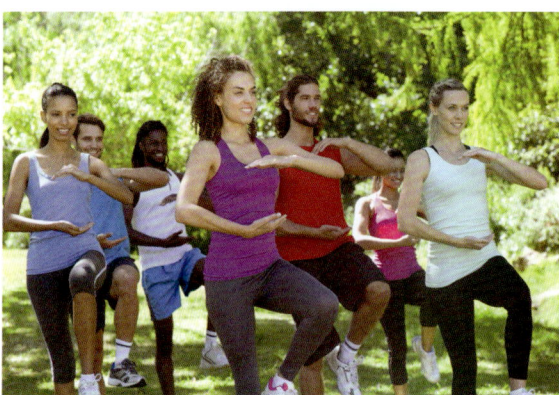

FIGURE 12-6 Fitness group doing tai chi in a park on a sunny day.

(Fig. 12-5), meditation (Fig. 12-6), dietary restrictions, pilgrimage, confessions, reflection, forgiveness, and any other activity that includes a search for meaning and purpose in life. If a client reports spiritual activities, these activities should be encouraged if found beneficial to the client's overall health.

Religious groups frequently view the body as a gift and encourage a lifestyle to mirror that belief. Avoidance of promiscuous sexual activity, shunning of alcohol and tobacco use, and following dietary guidelines each promote a healthy lifestyle. If discovered in discussion with the client, these positive health behaviors can be encouraged and supported.

Religious beliefs can express a wide variety of values and practices, including rituals (e.g., birth, death, illness) and ways of dealing with end-of-life issues that may significantly affect the religion–health relationship. Table 12-1 provides a general review of the major religions and how their beliefs affect health care decisions. A working knowledge of the ideals, beliefs, and practices of the faith followed by the majority in the nurse's community provides a useful foundation for spiritual care. When conducting any type of review of the denominations or faiths in a particular community, be aware that a client's spiritual dimension is subjective and may vary greatly among persons, even persons of the same denomination or faith. The client's spiritual experiences or spiritual history are subjective and may be the most relevant factor that guides conversation and decisions about referral or collaboration.

Particular religious views may also negatively affect health. Failure to seek timely medical care and withholding standardized medical care based on religious dogma are usually the most prominent ethical dilemmas faced by health care providers. Christian scientists frequently rely on prayer alone to heal illnesses, rarely seek mainstream medical care, and have higher rates of mortality than the general population. Jehovah's Witnesses refuse blood transfusions due to their beliefs that the body cannot be sustained by another's blood and accepting a transfusion will bar the recipient from eternal salvation. Controversy has erupted when a child of a Jehovah's Witness is in need of a blood transfusion and the parents wish to withhold a possible lifesaving therapy. The U.S. Supreme Court has generally sided against parents' withholding medical therapies for religious reasons. The hospital's ethics committee should be consulted immediately to assist in this complex decision. Members of the Faith Assembly of Indiana have a negative view of modern health care and have an especially high rate of infant mortality due to limited prenatal care. While these are only specific denominational examples of the negative impact of religion on health, there are also generalized manifestations of religion's negative effects. Religion may lead to depression or anxiety over not meeting group expectations, and certain spiritual practices or participation in complementary and alternative medical practices may delay needed medical care (Barrett et al., 2001; Koenig, 2007; Koenig et al., 2001; Williams & Sternthal, 2007).

If a nurse is presented with a situation in which religious or spiritual views have the potential to compromise adequate nursing care, the situation should be presented to a supervising staff member immediately. For complex cases, the situation may also be presented to the ethics committee of the institution or organization to assure that appropriate measures are followed. Refer to the institutional or organizational handbook for specific instructions regarding individual cases.

Incorporating Religion and Spirituality into Care

Clients have called for medical providers to address spiritual issues during client–provider interactions. Nurses generally

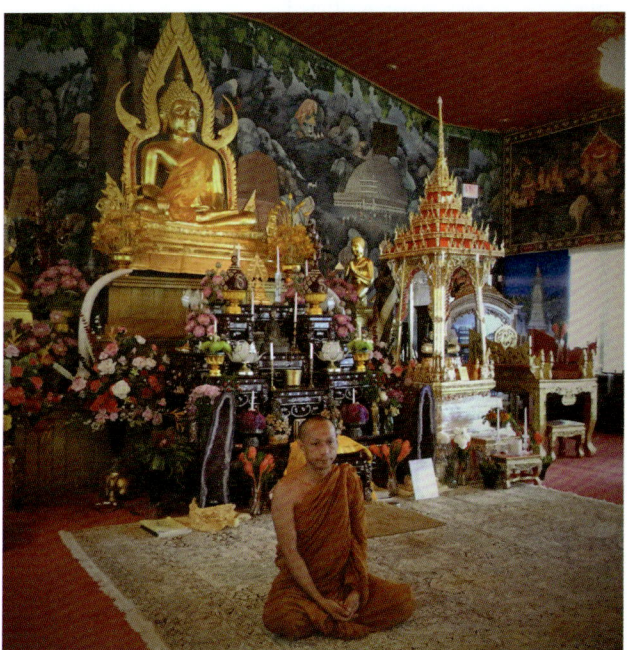

FIGURE 12-5 Formal meditation by monk in a Buddhist temple in Kissimmee, Florida.

TABLE 12-1 Major World Religions and Common Health Beliefs

	Overview	Illness	End of Life	Nutrition
Buddhism Global: ±7.1% United States: <1%	Suffering is a part of human existence, but the inward death of the self and senses leads to a state beyond suffering and existence.	Prayer and meditation are used for cleansing and healing. Terminal illness may be seen as a unique opportunity to reflect on life's ultimate meaning and the meaning of one's relation with the world. Therefore, it is important that medication does not interfere with consciousness.	Life is the opportunity to cultivate understanding, compassion, and joy for self and others. Death is associated with rebirth. Serene surroundings are important to the dignity of dying.	Many are strict vegetarians. Some holy days include fasting from dawn to dusk but considerations are allowed for the frail and elderly, for whom fasting could create problems.
Hinduism Global: ±15% United States: <1%	Nirvana (oneness with God) is the primary purpose of the religion. Many have an altar in their home for worship.	Illness is the result of past and current life actions (Karma). The right hand is seen as holy, and eating and intervention (IV) needs to be with the right hand to promote clean healing.	Death marks a passage because the soul has no beginning or end. At death the soul may be reborn as another person and one's Karma is carried forward. It is important for Karma to leave this life with as little negativity as possible to ensure a better life next birth. Holy water and basil leaves may be placed on the body; sacred threads may be tied around wrists or neck. The deceased's arms should be straightened.	Many, but not all, are vegetarians. Many holy days include fasting.
Islam Global: ±23.2% United States: ±0.6%	Mohammed is believed to be the greatest of all prophets. Worship occurs in a mosque. Prayer occurs five times a day: dawn through sunrise, noon, afternoon, sunset, and evening. Prayers are done facing east toward the sacred place in Mecca and often occur on a prayer rug with ritual washing of hands, face, and feet prior to prayer. Women are to be "modest" and are not to view men, other than their husbands, naked. The Islamic faith is presently one of the fastest growing religious groups in the United States.	Illness is often believed to be a trial sent by God, and the outcome depends on the person's attitude of pious endurance. Allah is in control of the beginning and end of life, and expressions of powerlessness are rare. To question or ask questions of health care providers is considered a sign of mistrust, thus clients and family are less likely to ask questions.	All outcomes, whether death or healing, are seen as predetermined by Allah. It is important for dying clients to face east and to die facing east. Prayer is offered but need not be done by an Imam (religious leader).	Consumption of pork or alcohol is prohibited. Other meats must meet ritual requirements and many use kosher (Jewish ritual) foods because these meet the requirements of Islamic believers as well. During the holy days of Ramadan (29 days determined by the moon), neither food nor drink is taken between sunrise and sunset, though frail, ill, and young children are exempt.
Christianity Global: ±31.5% United States: ±85%	Beliefs focus around the Old and New Testaments of the Bible and view Jesus Christ as the Savior. Prayers may be directed to one or all of the Holy Trinity (God, Holy Spirit, and Jesus Christ). Beliefs usually culturally developed vary within denominations.	Most view illness as a natural process for the body and even as a testing of faith. Others may see illness as a curse brought on by living outside the laws of God and, therefore, retribution for personal evil.	There is belief in miracles, especially through prayer. Western medicine is usually held in high regard. Memorial services rather than funerals and cremation rather than burial are more common in Christian religions than in other sects.	No special or universal food beliefs are common to Christian religions, although there may be regional or cultural beliefs.

	Overview	Illness	End of Life	Nutrition
Judaism Global: <5% United States: ±2%	Judaism includes religious beliefs and a philosophy for a code of ethics with four major groupings of Jewish beliefs: Reform, Reconstructionist, Conservative, and Orthodox. Prayer shawls are common and are often passed between generations of family. A member of the clergy is known as a Rabbi.	Restrictions related to work on holy days are removed to save a life. However, tests, signatures, and assessments for medical needs that can be scheduled to avoid holy days are appreciated.	Psalms and the last prayer of confession (vidui) are held at bedside. At death, arms are not crossed; any clothing or bandages with client's blood should be prepared for burial with the person. It is important that the whole person be buried together.	Orthodox or kosher rules involve no mixing of meat with dairy; separate cooking and eating utensils are used for food preparation and consumption. Kosher laws include special procedures for slaughter and food handling. "Keeping kosher" is predominantly an Orthodox practice. When food has passed kosher laws of preparation, a symbol (K) appears on the label. Many holy days include a fasting period.

Based on information from Alberta Health Services. (n.d.). Health care and religious beliefs. Available at http://www.albertahealthservices.ca/ps-1026227-health-care-religious-beliefs.pdf; Barrett, D., Kurlan, G., & Johnson, T. (2001). World Christian encyclopedia: A comparative survey of churches and religions in the modern world (2nd ed.). New York: Oxford; The Pew Forum on Religious & Public Life. (2010a). The global religious landscape. Available http://www.pewforum.org/global-religious-landscape-exec.aspx; The Pew Forum on Religious & Public Life. (2010b). U.S. Religious Landscape Survey: Summary of key findings. Available at http://religions.pewforum.org/reports; and World religions ranked by size. (2005). Available at www.adherents.com

have more opportunities to address spiritual concerns with clients because nurses are the primary points of contact for most clients. In fact, nursing has a long history of incorporating spirituality into client care. Florence Nightingale wrote at length about a spiritual dimension that provided an inner strength (Nightingale, 1960/1996). More recently, modern nursing theorists have used spirituality as a major determinant in the grand theories that guide nursing practice. North American Nursing Diagnosis Association (NANDA)–approved nursing diagnoses have also been formulated to assist nurses in identifying and addressing the client's spiritual dimension. These developments underlie a primary idea in nursing: clients are seen as *holistic* beings in body, mind, and spirit.

There are many ways to incorporate religion and spirituality into care. For example, providing a time of silence for the client may encourage spiritual practices such as meditation, or the nurse may gather family members or clergy to participate in a prayer ritual (Fig. 12-7). Collaboration and referral with pastoral chaplains or clergy are also extremely important when dealing with religious issues in a health care setting. Many hospitals have staff pastoral chaplains, and community resources of different faiths are usually available through the pastoral office or social work professionals. While nurses can assess and support many clients' spiritual needs, some situations are beyond the scope of nursing practice and require someone with more experience and knowledge about a particular faith. For example, a nurse from a Protestant faith faced with a Muslim client who has just been diagnosed with terminal cancer may not be able to speak to the client's end-of-life issues and may require referral to the appropriate professional.

In whatever form spirituality is incorporated into client care, the nurse should be respectful, open, and willing to discuss spiritual issues if seen as appropriate. In the process, the nurse should avoid conveying a judgmental attitude toward the client's spiritual beliefs and religious practices.

CLINICAL TIP
Plans for referral or intervention will develop out of the ongoing dialogue between the nurse and the client.

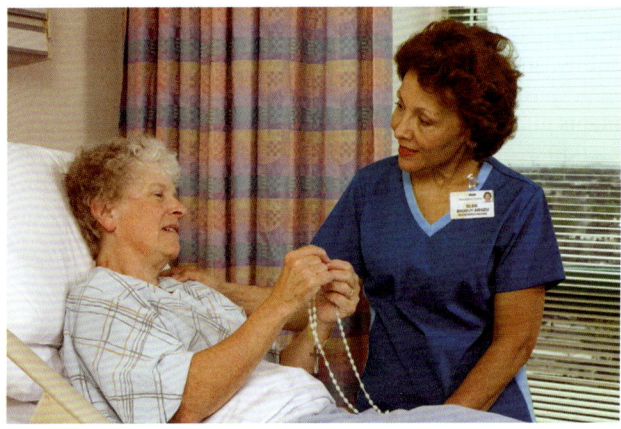

FIGURE 12-7 A nurse supports a Catholic client praying with her rosary.

Self-Understanding of Spirituality

Consistently, nurses who are more aware of their spirituality are more comfortable discussing the potential spiritual needs of the client. Introspective reflection on one's own beliefs and biases about the relationship between spirituality and health can be undertaken through journaling, meditation, or discussions with interested persons. Ask yourself:

- What are my views on the interaction between spirituality and health?
- How would I respond to someone in spiritual distress or to someone requesting an intervention relating to spirituality?
- How can I provide spiritual care?

These reflections help to provide a deeper understanding of one's spiritual dimension and build confidence for future discussions on spirituality. While many nurses view spiritual assessment and care as an important part of nursing practice, training levels vary from institution to institution. However, nurses can educate themselves to meet this vital need of the client. The nurse who understands the content of a spiritual assessment can use this knowledge also to increase self-understanding.

Concept Mastery Alert

The reason for a spiritual assessment is to better understand the client and the client's spiritual perspective related to health. The nurse must be objective during the assessment. It doesn't matter what the nurse's views are concerning the client's spiritual beliefs. Therefore the nurse would not need to share her views in open dialogue.

SPIRITUAL ASSESSMENT

Why do we complete a spiritual assessment? Spiritual care cannot be provided without a spiritual assessment. Culliford (2007) listed a few of the benefits of spiritual care to the client, which include: support for healthy grieving; support for improved self-esteem and confidence; assistance with maximization of potential in the current circumstances; support to improve relationships with self, others, and with an Absolute/God; assistance in renewing a sense of meaning and hope; enhancement of the client's sense of belonging; assistance in improving problem solving; help with enduring problems that cannot be solved and with continuing distress and disability; and help in finding renewed hope.

A spiritual assessment is similar to the many other assessments nurses perform on a daily basis. Gaining relevant information about the client's spirituality helps to identify related nursing diagnoses and needed interventions, and can improve client care. The following questions provide guidance in conducting the interview.

Approach

There is no absolute in the timing of a spiritual assessment. Some professionals recommend inclusion with the initial assessment, while others argue for a delayed assessment after the nurse–client relationship has been established. The integration of both techniques may be the most useful because the spiritual assessment should not be viewed as static but rather as an ongoing conversation between the nurse and the client. If the nurse were proceeding through an initial assessment with relevant past medical history, it would be very appropriate to include general screening questions related to clients' integration of spirituality into their personal health (e.g., Do you consider yourself to be a religious or spiritual person? If so, how is this related to your health or health care decisions?).

CLINICAL TIP
Briefly addressing a client's spirituality will establish an open dialogue, and provide a foundation for any intervention or care that may be needed in the future.

The client is the focus of the spiritual assessment. Therefore, the nurse does not have to be spiritual to take a spiritual assessment. Objectivity is a key component in a high-quality spiritual assessment. The questions in a spiritual assessment probe for beliefs that could affect client care. Divulged information is then utilized to support, encourage, or lead clients in harmonizing their personal relationship to spirituality and health. Some clients may not be connected to any religious group or have any interest in spirituality. These clients should be encouraged in whatever provides them strength in dealing with health care issues (e.g., family, friends, nature, etc.). If a client responds negatively to any aspect of the discussion of religion or spirituality, the nurse may collaborate with the hospital clergy or pastoral care department to further assess the situation and client's needs.

Techniques

Spirituality is multidimensional. It is also unique to each individual. These characteristics of spirituality can present difficulties in proper assessment. Many instruments to assess spirituality were derived within a particular faith background and may have little cross-cultural relevance. The most useful spiritual assessment techniques should begin with general introductory questions and not be specific to any religious denomination so that the nurse can avoid assumptions and ascertain the client's specific spiritual needs. Essential to taking a spiritual history or providing spiritual care to clients is maintaining an environment that fosters hope, joy, and creativity; provides a sense that the client is valued, trusted, respected, and worthy of dignity; assures confidentiality and sympathetic listening; gives assistance with making sense and finding meaning in the illness; and provides support for developing spirituality in the current circumstances (Culliford, 2007).

Nonformal

There are numerous ways to perform a spiritual assessment. Often it is helpful to have a quick reference to guide assessment. Acronyms related to the assessment of spirituality have been published (Assessment Tool 12-1: Taking a Spiritual History: SPIRIT Acronym) and can serve as excellent reminders when assessing a concept with many attributes. Techniques such as these are nonformal, yet have somewhat systematic approaches. They are nonformal in asking open-ended questions and allowing the client to disclose pertinent information. They are systematic to the extent that the client's responses guide future choices of questions, and may cover numerous practices in which the client may or may not be involved (e.g., prayer, organized religion, etc.).

> **ASSESSMENT TOOL 12-1 Taking a Spiritual History: SPIRIT Acronym**
>
> **S—Spiritual Belief System**
> Do you have a formal religious affiliation? Can you describe it?
> Do you have a spiritual life that is important to you?
> What is your clearest sense of the meaning of your life at this time?
>
> **P—Personal Spirituality**
> Describe the beliefs and practices of your religion that you personally accept.
> Describe those beliefs and practices that you do not accept or follow.
> In what ways is your spirituality/religion meaningful for you?
> How is your spirituality/religion important to you in daily life?
>
> **I—Integration with a Spiritual Community**
> Do you belong to any religious or spiritual groups or communities?
> How do you participate in this group/community? What is your role?
> What importance does this group have for you?
> In what ways is this group a source of support for you?
> What types of support and help does or could this group provide for you in dealing with health issues?
>
> **R—Ritualized Practices and Restrictions**
> What specific practices do you carry out as part of your religious and spiritual life (e.g., prayer, meditation, services, etc.)?
> What lifestyle activities or practices does your religion encourage, discourage, or forbid?
> What meaning does these practices and restrictions have for you? To what extent have you followed these guidelines?
>
> **I—Implications For Medical Care**
> Are there specific elements of medical care that your religion discourages or forbids? To what extent have you followed these guidelines?
> What aspects of your religion/spirituality would you like me to keep in mind as I care for you?
> What knowledge or understanding would strengthen our relationship as physician and patient?
> Are there barriers to our relationship based on religious or spiritual issues?
> Would you like to discuss religious or spiritual implications of health care?
>
> **T—Terminal Events Planning**
> Are there particular aspects of medical care that you wish to forgo or have withheld because of your religion/spirituality?
> Are there religious or spiritual practices or rituals that you would like to have available in the hospital or at home?
> Are there religious or spiritual practices that you wish to plan for regarding time of death, or the period following death?
> From what sources do you draw strength in order to cope with this illness?
> For what in your life do you still feel gratitude even though ill?
> When you are afraid or in pain, how do you find comfort?
> As we plan for your medical care near the end of life, in what ways will your religion and spirituality influence your decisions?

References: Maugans, T. A. (1997). The SPIRITual History. *Arch Fam Med, 5*, 11–16; Ambuel, B., & Weissman, D. E. (1999). Discussing spiritual issues and maintaining hope. In D. E. Weissman & B. Ambuel (Eds.), *Improving end-of-life care: A resource guide for physician education* (2nd ed.). Milwaukee, WI: Medical College of Wisconsin; Griffith, J. L., & Griffith, M. E. (1997). Hope in suffering/pain in health: Talking with patients about spiritual issues. Presented at The 18th Forum for the Behavioral Sciences in Family Medicine, Chicago, Illinois, October 1997.

Source: Ambuel, B. (2005). *Taking a spiritual history* (2nd ed.). Fast facts & concepts #19. Available at www.EPERC.mcw.edu/FastFactsIndex/ff_019.htm

Formal

The client's spirituality and religiosity can also be assessed with formal self-assessment instruments (Assessment Tools 12-1, 12-2, and 12-3). Other short mnemonic self-assessment tools include the HOPE Questions for Spiritual Assessment (Assessment Tool 12-4; Anadarajah & Hight, 2001) and the FICA Spiritual History Tool (Assessment Tool 12-5; Pulchalski, 1996). While many of these measures are paper-and-pencil self-response, they begin a dialogue and could be employed as important screening tools. Completion of a self-response spiritual or religious assessment instrument in conjunction with other past medical history could uncover strengths or deficiencies that may have initially gone unnoticed. For example, let's say that a client responds negatively to the question, "I find comfort in my religion or spirituality" during the initial history taking. During future conversations, the nurse could incorporate this into conversation and possibly reconnect the distressed client to an effective source of spiritual support.

Sample Format

A spiritual assessment differs substantially from a health assessment of an organ system. Spiritual well-being or distress are entirely subjective and the only objective data concern stress or depression that may accompany spiritual distress. For this reason, the format for the following spiritual assessment does not follow the same style as organ system chapters. Both normal and abnormal findings are included to provide better evidence of spiritual distress if present. The normal and abnormal findings in no way encompass all of the appropriate responses from the client. Therefore, the information in the normal and abnormal sections are only examples, as a guide.

The nurse must always approach a client's spirituality with sensitivity and acceptance (even if not in agreement with the beliefs expressed) to avoid adding further stress to the client. The following spiritual assessment does not follow any one assessment tool directly, but a tool may be incorporated into the assessment or used alone. History of present concern, related past history, family history, and lifestyle and practices are integrated into the assessment.

> **General Routine Screening versus Focused Specialty Assessment of Spirituality and Religious Practices**
>
> Nurses need to assess the client's basic religious and spiritual background. More focused questions and more advanced spiritual assessment tools are used when appropriate and time allows for this type of assessment.

ASSESSMENT TOOL 12-2 Self-Assessment: Daily Spiritual Experiences Scale

The list that follows includes items you may or may not experience. Please consider if and how often you have these experiences; try to disregard whether you feel you should or should not have them. In addition, a number of items use the word "God." If this word is not a comfortable one, please substitute another idea that calls to mind the divine or holy for you.

Scoring:
1 = Many times a day
2 = Every day
3 = Most days
4 = Some days
5 = Once in a while
6 = Never or almost never

1. I feel God's presence.	1	2	3	4	5	6
2. I experience a connection to all of life.	1	2	3	4	5	6
3. During worship or at other times when connecting with God, I feel joy that lifts me out of my daily concerns.	1	2	3	4	5	6
4. I find strength in my religion or spirituality.	1	2	3	4	5	6
5. I find comfort in my religion or spirituality.	1	2	3	4	5	6
6. I feel deep inner peace and harmony.	1	2	3	4	5	6
7. I ask for God's help in the midst of daily activities.	1	2	3	4	5	6
8. I feel guided by God in the midst of daily activities.	1	2	3	4	5	6
9. I feel God's love for me directly.	1	2	3	4	5	6
10. I feel God's love for me through others.	1	2	3	4	5	6
11. I am spiritually touched by the beauty of creation.	1	2	3	4	5	6
12. I feel thankful for my blessings.	1	2	3	4	5	6
13. I feel a selfless caring for others.	1	2	3	4	5	6
14. I accept others even when they do things I think are wrong.	1	2	3	4	5	6
15. I desire to be closer to or in union with Him.[a]	1	2	3	4		
16. In general, how close do you feel to God?[a]	1	2	3	4		

[a]For questions 15 and 16, scoring: 4 = not close at all, 3 = somewhat close, 2 = very close, 1 = as close as possible. Lower scores *represent more daily spiritual experiences*.
Adapted from: Underwood, LG, Ordinary Spiritual Experience: Qualitative Research, Interpretive Guidelines and Population Distribution for the Daily Spiritual Experience Scale. *Archive for the Psychology of Religion, 28*(1), 181–218. Do not copy without permission of the author lynn@lynnunderwood.com. Also see www.dsescale.org and Underwood, L. (2013). *Spiritual Connection in Daily Life:* 16 Little Questions that Can Make a Big Difference.

ASSESSMENT TOOL 12-3 Self-Assessment: Brief Religious Coping Questionnaire (RCOPE)

Instructions for administration: Think about how you try to understand and deal with major problems in your life. To what extent is each involved in the way you cope?

Positive Religious/Spiritual Coping Subscale
I think about how my life is part of a larger spiritual force.
1. A great deal   3. Somewhat
2. Quite a bit   4. Not at all

I work together with God as partners to get through hard times.
1. A great deal   3. Somewhat
2. Quite a bit   4. Not at all

I look to God for strength, support, and guidance in crisis.
1. A great deal   3. Somewhat
2. Quite a bit   4. Not at all

Negative Religious/Spiritual Coping Subscale
I feel that stressful situations are God's way of punishing me for my sins or lack of spirituality.
1. A great deal   3. Somewhat
2. Quite a bit   4. Not at all

I wonder if God has abandoned me.
1. A great deal   3. Somewhat
2. Quite a bit   4. Not at all

I try to make sense of the situation and decide what to do without relying on God.
1. A great deal   3. Somewhat
2. Quite a bit   4. Not at all

A more extensive form of the RCOPE exists and could be utilized for detailed analysis. Scale could be summed as a general screening tool or individual items could be identified (e.g., abandonment) and incorporated into the clinical setting.

Adapted from Pargament, K. I., Feuille, M., & Burdzy, D. (2011). The Brief RCOPE: Current psychometric status of a short measure of religious coping. *Religions,* 2, 51–76.

ASSESSMENT TOOL 12-4 HOPE Questions for Spiritual Assessment

CATEGORY	SAMPLE QUESTIONS
H: sources of hope	What are your sources of hope, strength, comfort, and peace?
	What do you hold on to during difficult times?
O: organized religion	Are you part of a religious or spiritual community?
	Does it help you? How?
P: personal spirituality and practices	Do you have personal spiritual beliefs?
	What aspects of your spirituality or spiritual practices do you find most helpful?
E: effects on medical care and end-of-life issues	Does your current situation affect your ability to do the things that usually help you spiritually? As a doctor, is there anything that I can do to help you access the resources that usually help you?
	Are there any specific practices or restrictions I should know about in providing your medical care?
	If the patient is dying: How do your beliefs affect the kind of medical care you would like me to provide over the next few days/weeks/months?

Saguil, A., & Phelps, K. (2012). The spiritual assessment. *American Family Physician, 86*(6), 546–550, Table 2, adapted with permission from Anandarajah, G., & Hight, E. Spirituality and medical practice: using the HOPE questions as a practical tool for spiritual assessment. *American Family Physician.* 2001;63(1):87.

ASSESSMENT TOOL 12-5 FICA Spiritual History Tool

The acronym FICA can help structure questions in taking a spiritual history by health care professionals.

F—Faith and Belief
"Do you consider yourself spiritual or religious?" or "Is spirituality something important to you" or "Do you have spiritual beliefs that help you cope with stress/ difficult times?" (Contextualize to reason for visit if it is not the routine history.)
If the patient responds "No," the health care provider might ask, "What gives your life meaning?" Sometimes patients respond with answers such as family, career, or nature.
(The question of meaning should also be asked even if people answer yes to spirituality.)

I—Importance
"What importance does your spirituality have in your life? Has your spirituality influenced how you take care of yourself, your health? Does your spirituality influence you in your health care decision making (e.g., advance directives, treatment, etc.)?

C—Community
"Are you part of a spiritual community? Communities such as churches, temples, and mosques, or a group of like-minded friends, family, or yoga can serve as strong support systems for some patients. Can explore further: Is this of support to you and how? Is there a group of people you really love or who are important to you?"

A—Address in Care
"How would you like me, your health care provider, to address these issues in your health care?" (With the newer models, including diagnosis of spiritual distress, **A** also refers to the Assessment and Plan of patient spiritual distress or issues within a treatment or care plan.)

© Copyright Christina M. Pulchalski, MD, 1996. Used with permission. Permission from The George Washington Institute for Spirituality and Health. FICA spiritual history tool. Available at http://www.gwumc.edu/gwish/clinical/fica.cfm

ASSESSMENT PROCEDURE	NORMAL FINDINGS	ABNORMAL FINDINGS
Explore the client's religious and spiritual background. Ask the client: Do you consider yourself to be a religious or spiritual person? If so, how is this related to your health or health care decisions? Listen to client's story and seek clarification where needed. Support client to develop trust.	Client makes reference to involvement in religious groups and/or spiritual practices that have provided comfort and social support. Describes belief that prayer reduces stress and heals disease.	Reports lost connections to religious group, while continuing to focus on the negative aspect of spirituality (e.g., suppressive religious rules). Comments and body language reveal a lack of hope with symptoms of depression. Deficiencies in the social network are identified and appear to affect the client's well-being and attitude toward recovery. Note: Not describing connections to a religious group does *not* indicate abnormal findings.
Observe nonverbal and verbal communication patterns in presence of others.	Eye contact is maintained (appropriate to cultural group) with nonverbal cues correlating with conversation.	Client displays poor eye contact. The presence of others strongly influences information client shares.

Continued on following page

ASSESSMENT PROCEDURE	NORMAL FINDINGS	ABNORMAL FINDINGS
Begin to focus questions. Use spiritual assessment tools if needed: Assessment Tools 12-1, 12-2, 12-3, 12-4, and 12-5. Begin conversation with a general dialogue about global concepts such as hope, meaning, comfort, strength, peace, love, and connection. Example: We have been discussing your support systems. What are your sources of hope, strength, comfort, and peace? What do you hold onto during difficult times? What sustains you and keeps you going? For some people, religious or spiritual beliefs act as a source of comfort and strength in dealing with life's ups and downs; is this true for you?	Reports spirituality giving a sense of peace that transcends illness or disease. Reports that meditation and exercise facilitate a sense of peace. Family frequently mentioned as source of strength and motivation. Client places a strong emphasis on spirituality as a guiding force in life.	Describes no connection to others such as God, nature, family, or peers. Shares pessimistic and fatalistic attitude toward recovery. Identifies limited coping resources with little desire to adopt new ones.
Continue to assess other dimensions of spirituality within groups. Ask about organizational (or formal) religious involvement. Reflect on previous conversations to direct questioning. (Remember that not all persons who state they are religious and/or spiritual are involved with organized religious groups or ascribe to all the religious practices of that group. Note: If there is no connection to a religious group or faith tradition, skip or modify this section and the next.) Ask the questions: Do you consider yourself part of an organized religion? How important is this to you? What aspects of your religion are helpful and not so helpful to you? Are you part of a religious or spiritual community? Does it help you? How?	Client may report regular attendance at a local mosque, church, or other religious meeting place and highlight importance of attendance as a recovery period in a very fast-paced life. States that involvement with others holding a similar worldview helps to give meaning and purpose to life.	Abnormal findings may include reporting involvement with "new religious group" in the area but being unable to provide details regarding affiliation or purpose of religious group. Client makes reference to extensive fasts and other activities that may be harmful to general health.
Ask questions about family and community support: Do you have family support for your spiritual beliefs and practices? Does your community support your spiritual beliefs and practices? Are there any stressful relationships with family, or religious or other community leaders that affect your comfort or health care?	Client relates full support for beliefs and practices (both for health care and generally) from family and religious leaders. Relates no differences with community.	Client describes disagreement among family, religious, or community members regarding choice of spiritually based health care decisions.

ASSESSMENT PROCEDURE	NORMAL FINDINGS	ABNORMAL FINDINGS
Ask transition question from organizational to personal beliefs. Ask client to specify differences or similarities in own beliefs and the beliefs of the faith or denomination with which affiliated. Ask the questions: Do you have personal spiritual beliefs independent of organized religion? What are they? Do you believe in God? What kind of relationship do you have with God? What aspects of spirituality or spiritual practices do you find most helpful to you personally (e.g., prayer, meditation, reading scripture, attending religious services, listening to music, hiking, communing with nature)?	Describes personal beliefs that coincide with denominational beliefs. Denominational beliefs do not conflict with required medical care. Reports relationship with God as healthy and positive. Desires to have time in the hospital to meditate and read scripture to gain focus and relieve stress.	Abnormal findings may include reporting very limited similarities between denomination and personal beliefs, past utilization of prayer and listening to religious music, but no current avenue for the fostering of spirituality.
Directly address beliefs that may conflict with or affect one's health care. (Assist clients with describing spiritual practices if appropriate. Attend to end-of-life issues if the condition dictates.) Ask the questions: Has being sick (or your current situation) affected your ability to do the things that usually help you spiritually? (Or affected your relationship with God?) As a nurse, is there anything I can do to help you access the resources that usually help you? Are you worried about any conflicts between your beliefs and your medical situation/care/decisions? Would it be helpful for you to speak to a clinical chaplain/community spiritual leader? Are there any specific practices or restrictions I should know about in providing your medical care? (e.g., dietary restrictions, use of blood products) *If the client is dying:* How do your beliefs affect the kind of nursing care you would like me to provide over the next few days/weeks/months?	Client views present diagnosis of cancer as "part of God's will for her life" or/and desires to continue nature walks and other spiritual practices to develop a closer relationship with God. Client makes no reference to perceived abandonment or rejection that may lead to depression. Desires to have clergy from her local church for visitation time. Client asks the nurse to contact local clergy and provides telephone number.	Client appears traumatized with cancer diagnosis and views the illness as a fault of her past lifestyle or a punishment. Refuses visits from local clergy and hospital chaplains. Declines conversation and just wants to be sent home to die.

CASE STUDY

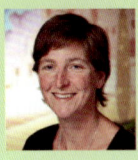

The nurse interviews Mrs. Baird, using specific probing questions. The client reports a loss of support and motivation to care about her weight gain and blood pressure elevation since her family has fallen away from regular church attendance and related loss of supportive friends she could talk to. She states, "I used to gain such strength going to our church meetings. It was such an encouragement. We used to walk with one another and talk about what God is doing in our lives ... now I just feel overwhelmed and busy all of the time ... and I can't talk with anyone." The nurse explores this health concern using the COLDSPA mnemonic.

Mnemonic	Question	Data Provided
Character	Describe the sign or symptom (feeling, appearance, sound, smell, or taste if applicable).	Loss of motivation and social support network
Onset	When did it begin?	Several months ago—the family stopped attending the church in which LB was involved.
Location	Where is it? Does it radiate? Does it occur anywhere else?	The client reports negative physical (5-lb weight gain since last routine visit for hypertension check, and blood pressure notably higher at 160/94 mmHg) and emotional consequences (feelings of isolation).
Duration	How long does it last? Does it recur?	
Severity	How bad is it? How much does it bother you?	Limited desire for exercise has resulted in weight gain, which bothers her a lot. "I have no one to share with, talk to, discuss how God is working in our lives. No one to walk with."
Pattern	What makes it better or worse?	Being with my faith family, interacting with them, walking with someone, but none of this is possible now.
Associated factors/How it **A**ffects the client	What other symptoms occur with it? How does it affect you?	She reports feeling overwhelmed and isolated.

The nurse further explores Mrs. Baird's history, asking about medical problems. The client reports mild hypertension for 3 years and states that she has no other health problems. Her current feelings are new; she has not experienced a sense of isolation, being overwhelmed, or lacking motivation in the past.

Mrs. Baird has had many years of involvement with the same church family until recently. She describes deep belief in spiritual tenets of her Catholic faith. Both her family and her husband's family follow the Catholic faith.

While attending church, Mrs. Baird walked and interacted with friends frequently. She describes beliefs about how spiritual health and physical health are related and her belief that her current physical problems are due to isolation from the faith community. She denies use of antidepressants, other medications, or recreational drugs.

During the interview, Mrs. Baird asks and answers questions appropriately and has a flat affect.

Validating and Documenting Findings

Validate the subjective and objective data collected during assessment (by asking additional questions, or comparing objective with subjective findings). Noticeably, the subjective data will be the primary source of information during a spiritual assessment, but the objective data can validate or call into question information presented to the nurse. Document both normal and abnormal findings.

CASE STUDY

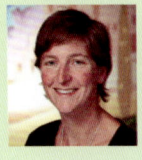

Think back to the case study of Mrs. Baird. The nurse documented the following findings.
Biographical Data: LB, 40 years old. Caucasian. Housewife with husband and two children (5 and 8 years old). Lives outside rural community.
General Survey: Awake, alert, and oriented. Asks and answers questions appropriately, with somewhat flat affect.
Reason for Seeking Care: "I just haven't felt like doing any exercise lately." Feeling overwhelmed, isolated, and lacking motivation to reduce weight and blood pressure, related to family falling away from church attendance and support.
History of Present Concern: Several months ago, the family stopped attending the church. "I used to gain such strength going to our church meetings. It was such an encouragement. We used to walk with one another and talk about what God is doing in our lives ... now I just feel overwhelmed and busy all of the time ... and I can't talk with anyone." Gained weight.

Personal Health History: Mild hypertension for 3 years. No other health problems. Denies former sense of isolation, being overwhelmed, or lacking motivation.

Family History: Both LB's family and husband's family follow the Catholic faith.

Lifestyle and Health Practices: Many years' involvement with same church family until recently. Describes deep belief in spiritual tenets of her Catholic faith.

When attending church, walked and interacted with friends frequently. Beliefs about spiritual health and physical health described and relates current physical problems to isolation from faith community. Denies use of antidepressants or other drugs.

Physical Exam Findings: A 5-lb weight gain since last visit, BP 160/94 mmHg. Flat affect.

ANALYSIS OF DATA: DIAGNOSTIC REASONING

A client's spirituality often affects his or her health. There are numerous capacities in which this occurs and frequently will go unnoticed without assessment. After collecting subjective and objective data pertaining to the client's spiritual assessment, identify abnormal findings and client strengths using diagnostic reasoning. Then, cluster the data to reveal any significant patterns or abnormalities.

The sections below provide possible conclusions that the nurse may make after assessing a client's spirituality.

Selected Nursing Diagnoses

The following is a list of selected nursing diagnoses that may be identified when analyzing data from a spiritual assessment.

Health Promotion Diagnoses
- Readiness for Enhanced Spiritual Well-being
- Readiness for Enhanced Hope

Risk Diagnoses
- Risk for Spiritual Distress
- Risk for Loneliness
- Risk for Social Isolation

Actual Diagnoses
- Spiritual Distress
- Hopelessness
- Moral Distress

Selected Collaborative Problems

After grouping the data, certain collaborative problems may become apparent. Remember that collaborative problems differ from nursing diagnoses in that they cannot be prevented or managed with independent nursing interventions. However, these physiologic complications of medical conditions can be detected and monitored by the nurse. In addition, the nurse can use physician- and nurse-prescribed interventions to minimize the complications of these problems. The nurse may also have to refer the client in such situations for further treatment of the problem. The following is a list of collaborative problems that may be identified when assessing spirituality. These problems are worded as risk for complications (RC), followed by the problem.

- RC: Depression
- RC: Hypertension
- RC: Hypoglycemia
- RC: Opportunistic infections

The RC related to spirituality is due to the psychological or physiologic responses of the body under stress. Stress induced by states such as spiritual distress will create a cascade of events within the body that produce physiologic responses and are influenced by the size and duration of the stressor as well as the client's ability to respond to that stressor.

Medical Problems

After grouping the data, it may become apparent that the client has signs and symptoms that require medical diagnosis and treatment. Referral to a primary care provider is necessary.

CASE STUDY

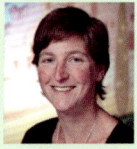

After completing the spiritual assessment, the nurse determines that the following conclusions are appropriate for Mrs. Baird.

Nursing Diagnoses
- Readiness for Enhanced Spiritual Well-Being r/t statements of desire to improve spiritual health through increasing personal interactions with others of her own faith.
- Readiness for Enhanced Hope r/t stated desire to set and achieve healthy goals for exercise and blood pressure reduction.
- Risk for Loneliness r/t separation from faith support group.
- Risk for Social Isolation r/t lack of affiliation with old or new church group.
- Spiritual Distress r/t isolation and separation from spiritual support group and church family.

Potential Collaborative Problems
- RC: Depression

To view an algorithm depicting the process for diagnostic reasoning in this case, go to thePoint.

Interdisciplinary Verbal Communication of Assessment Findings Using SBAR

SITUATION: LB, a 40-year-old woman, presents for a check of her hypertension. Reports a loss of motivation to lose weight and care about her health since her family quit attending her Catholic church several months ago. Has not felt like doing any exercise. Feels overwhelmed with no one to talk to, a lack of support, and a sense of isolation.

BACKGROUND: Lives with her two children and husband in a rural community. "Gained support and encouragement going to Catholic church meetings through group walks and talks." Has had mild hypertension for 3 years. While attending church, Mrs. Baird interacted with friends frequently.

ASSESSMENT: 5-lb weight gain. BP 160/94 mmHg. Flat affect. Describes deep belief in spiritual tenets of her Catholic faith. Describes beliefs about how spiritual health and physical health are related and belief that current physical problems are due to isolation from the faith community.

RECOMMENDATION: LB has Readiness for Enhanced Spiritual Well-Being r/t statements of desire to improve spiritual health through increasing personal interactions with others of her own faith. In addition, she has Readiness for Enhanced Hope r/t stated desire to set and achieve healthy goals for exercise and blood pressure reduction. However, she is at risk for Loneliness r/t separation from faith support group and for Social Isolation r/t lack of affiliation with old or new church group. She needs to be referred to resources in her area and may want to talk with a priest.

Want to know more?

A wide variety of resources to enhance your learning and understanding of this book are available on **thePoint**. Visit thePoint to access:

- NCLEX-Style Student Review Questions
- Watch and Learn Videos
- Concept in Action Animations
- And more!

References and Selected Readings

Anandarajah, G., & Hight, E. (2001). Spirituality and medical practice: Using the HOPE questions as a practical tool for spiritual assessment. *American Family Physician, 63*(1), 81–89.

Barrett, D., Kurlan, G., & Johnson, T. (2001). *World Christian encyclopedia: A comparative survey of churches and religions in the modern world* (2nd ed.). New York: Oxford.

Culliford, L. (2007). Taking a spiritual history. *Advances in Psychiatric Treatment, 13*, 212–219.

Koenig, H. (2007). When might religion or religious practices interfere with the health of a patient? In H. Koenig (Ed.): *Spirituality in patient care: Why, how, when, & what* (2nd ed., pp. 108–122). Philadelphia, PA: Templeton Foundation Press.

Koenig, H., McCullough, M., & Larson, D. (2001). *Handbook of religion and health*. New York: Oxford University Press.

Nightingale, F. (1960/1996). *Notes on nursing*. New York: Dover.

Pew Research Center. (2012). Religion and the unaffiliated. Available at http://www.pewforum.org/2012/10/09/nones-on-the-rise-religion/

Pew Research Center. (2015). U.S. public becoming less religious. Available at http://www.pewforum.org/2015/11/03/u-s-public-becoming-less-religious/

Pew Research Center. (2016). 5 facts about prayer. Available at http://www.pewresearch.org/fact-tank/2016/05/04/5-facts-about-prayer/

Pulchalski, C. (1996). FICA spiritual history tool. Available at https://smhs.gwu.edu/gwish/clinical/fica/spiritual-history-tool

Williams, D., & Sternthal, M. (2007). Spirituality, religion and health: Evidence and research directions. *Medical Journal of Australia, 186*(10 Suppl), S47–S50.

Wright, L. (2005). *Spirituality, suffering, and illness: Ideas for healing*. Philadelphia, PA: F. A. Davis.

13 ASSESSING NUTRITIONAL STATUS

Learning Objectives

1. Discuss the role of the essential nutrients in healthy nutrition—including carbohydrates, proteins, fats, vitamins, minerals, and water.
2. Describe various factors that affect food safety and place the client at risk for food poisoning.
3. Interview a client for an accurate nursing history of his or her nutritional status, hydration, food safety practices, and food allergies.
4. Perform a nutritional assessment—including height, body build, and other anthropometric measurements—using the correct techniques.
5. Differentiate between skills needed for routine nutritional screening versus skills needed for a comprehensive nutritional assessment.
6. Differentiate between normal and abnormal nutrition, hydration, and food safety practices.
7. Describe the findings frequently seen when assessing the older client's nutritional status.
8. Analyze the data from the nutritional interview and physical assessment to formulate valid nursing diagnoses, collaborative problems, and/or referrals.
9. Communicate interview and assessment findings of the client's nutrition, hydration, and food safety practices through clear concise documentation and verbal reports.

CASE STUDY

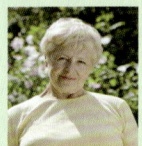

Helen Jones is a 78-year-old Caucasian woman with type 2 diabetes mellitus. When the home health nurse assesses Ms. Jones during her weekly visit, the nurse finds her weight is 138 lb, which is 7 lb less than she weighed last week. The nurse weighs Ms. Jones at the same time of day each week on her scale. Ms. Jones's case will be discussed throughout the chapter.

FOUNDATIONS

Information gathered during the nutritional assessment provides insight into the client's overall health status. Nutritional assessment identifies risk factors for obesity (excessive body fat) and for dietary deficits (malnutrition and undernutrition), and is also used to guide health promotion and disease prevention activities. Assessing hydration status is another important aspect of the nutritional assessment and an important indicator of the client's general health. Food safety is also an essential component of nutritional assessment to determine how clients store and prepare food in addition to their understanding of food contamination and allergies.

 Nutrition

Nutrition refers to the "process by which substances in food are transformed into body tissues and provide energy for the full range of physical and mental activities that make up human life" (Carpenter, 2016, p. 1). For adequate nutrition, essential nutrients—including carbohydrates, proteins, fats, vitamins, minerals, and water—must be ingested in appropriate amounts. Please refer to textbooks on nutrition and fluid and electrolyte balance for more detailed information.

Briefly, *carbohydrates* are referred to as either simple or complex, depending on their chemical structure. Simple carbohydrates, such as fruit juice, are sugar with a simple structure that raises the blood glucose level and can be converted quickly into energy. Complex carbohydrates, such as whole grains, starchy vegetables, and fiber, are composed of double or multiple sugar units and can also be used as an energy source. Carbohydrates are known as protein sparing because the body uses them for an energy source rather than breaking down proteins to fuel the body's energy needs. Additionally, carbohydrates help to burn fats more effectively and completely. Carbohydrates are stored in both the liver and muscle, where they can be converted rapidly to energy when needed. A healthy diet should consist of 45% to 65% carbohydrates with 75% of those carbohydrates being complex (Mayo Clinic, 2014b).

Fiber, both soluble and especially insoluble, helps to promote normal bowel function, reduce cholesterol levels, control blood sugar levels, and aid in weight management (Mayo Clinic, 2015a). Mayo Clinic (2015a) detailed the Institute of Medicine recommendations for adequate total fiber daily intake: For those under 50 years of age, 25 g per day for adult women and 38 g per day for men; for those over 50 years of age, 21 g for adult women and 30 g for men.

Proteins are important in a healthy diet, which is essential for normal growth and development. Proteins are made up of amino acids and are stored in muscle, skin, bone, blood, cartilage, and lymph tissue. Like carbohydrates, proteins can be broken down for energy, but protein breakdown is a less efficient form of energy production. The primary functions of protein are to provide structure to and to regulate the body's cells, tissues, and organs (specifically, to serve as antibodies, enzymes, and messengers that transmit signals that coordinate biologic processes), and to provide transport and storage of atoms and small molecules within cells and throughout the body (Genetics Home Reference, 2016).

Proteins can be obtained from plant and animal sources. Plant sources of protein include whole grains, dark green and yellow vegetables, nuts, and dried beans. Animal sources of protein include dairy products and meat, fish, poultry, and eggs. The recommended dietary allowance (RDA) for protein is 56 g per day for adult males and 46 g per day for adult females (National Academies of Science, Engineering, & Medicine [NASEM], 2016). The Dietary Reference Intake (DRI) is 0.8 g per kilogram of body weight (Gunnars, 2016).

Though controversial (see McCullogh, 2014; and discussion of guidelines controversies below), *fats* are an important part of a healthy, well-balanced diet. Fats are stored in adipose cells and are classified as triglycerides, which make up 95% of fats in foods, phospholipids, or sterols. Ingested fats are *saturated*, originating from animal sources or tropical oils and solid at room temperature; or *unsaturated*, originating from plant sources and soft or liquid at room temperature. Less desirable dietary fats are *trans fatty acids (transfats)* and, as part of the controversy, dietary cholesterol may or may not be an issue. Functions of fats include:

- Providing concentrated energy (double that of proteins and carbohydrates)
- Aiding in absorption of fat-soluble vitamins (A, D, E, and K)
- Supplying essential fatty acids for healthy skin
- Insulating skin and nerve fibers
- Protecting internal organs
- Lubricating skin to slow water loss

The RDA for fats (other than transfats, which should be avoided according to all sources) in healthy adult diets is debated. See discussion of the controversy about whether dietary fats (both saturated and unsaturated) are good or bad for us (e.g., McCullogh, 2014). Children, the elderly, and those with specific chronic illnesses require an adjusted amount of dietary fat.

Cholesterol is a fat-like substance that the liver produces. It is also found in animal food sources, such as meats, egg yolks, and dairy products. A high level of cholesterol has been thought to lead to heart attacks and strokes, but more recent studies often show this not to be true (see McCullogh, 2014). Cholesterol is important to normal bodily functions. It is necessary as a component of bile salts that aid in digestion, serves as an essential element in all cell membranes, is found in brain and nerve tissue, and is essential for the production of several hormones such as estrogen, testosterone, and cortisone.

Newer studies of the relationship of cholesterol to heart disease bring significant questions to the previous findings (e.g., McCullogh, 2014; O'Connor, 2014).

Adequate *vitamin* intake is part of a nutritionally sound diet because vitamins are required for energy to be released from carbohydrates, proteins, and fats. Additionally, they are necessary for the formation of red blood cells, hormones, and genetic material, and for a properly functioning nervous system. Vitamins are categorized as either fat- or water-soluble. Vitamins can be found across the major food groups. For instance, vitamin K, which is required for blood clotting, is found in larger amounts in green, leafy vegetables; and vitamin C is found in citrus and other fruits. Some foods are fortified with vitamins. For example, milk contains vitamin D to help with calcium metabolism. Because vitamins can be reduced or destroyed by overcooking, assessment of food preparation methods should be a part of nutritional assessment. The RDA is based on the specific vitamin, as well as age, lifestyle, and health condition.

Finally, *minerals* are essential in promoting growth and maintaining health; they can be found in all body fluids and tissues. Functions are varied and depend on the particular mineral. In general, the best sources of minerals are in unrefined and unprocessed foods, and can be found in all major food groups. They are categorized as either major or trace minerals. For example, calcium, potassium, and sodium are major minerals whereas fluoride, iron, and zinc are trace minerals. Like vitamins, the RDA depends on the specific mineral, and age, lifestyle, and health condition of the individual.

Because the body needs a consistent intake of *water*, it is one of our most basic nutritional needs. Water accounts for 50% to 75% of body weight, varying based on age and percentage of body fat. Functions of water in the body include: serving as a building block of cells, an insulator, and an internal temperature regulator; metabolizing proteins and carbohydrates; lubricating joints; insulating the brain, spinal cord, internal organs, and a fetus; and flushing toxins and waste (Mayo Clinic, 2017). On average, the daily water intake for adults living in temperate climates is 4 L for males and 2 L for females (Mayo Clinic, 2014c). Because a large number of people do not drink enough fluids, a high portion of the population is at risk for chronic mild dehydration. A thorough nutritional assessment therefore must include hydration status.

Hydration

Hydration, another important indicator of the client's general health status, may be overlooked or confused with the signs and symptoms of nutritional changes. The signs of hydration changes may also be confused with certain disease states if only one or two indicators are evaluated. For this reason, the nurse needs to look for clusters of signs and symptoms that may indicate changes in hydration status. Adequate hydration can be affected by various situations in all age groups. Some examples in adults include:

- Exposure to excessively high environmental temperatures
- Inability to access adequate fluids, especially water (e.g., clients who are unconscious, confused, or physically or mentally disabled)
- Excessive intake of alcohol or other diuretic fluids (coffee, sugar-rich and/or caffeine-rich carbonated soft drinks)
- People with impaired thirst mechanisms

- People taking diuretic medications
- Diabetic clients with severe hyperglycemia
- People with high fevers

Food Safety

Assessing how a client's food is stored and prepared is an important aspect of nutritional assessment and subsequent health. The Centers for Disease Control and Prevention ([CDC], 2015d) noted that there are more than 250 different food-borne illnesses (called also food-borne disease or poisoning). Causes are infections (bacteria, viruses, and parasites) and poisonings from contaminations with toxins or chemicals. First symptoms are usually nausea, vomiting, abdominal cramps, and diarrhea. The most common pathogens are norovirus, and bacteria *Salmonella, Clostridium perfringens*, and *Campylobacter*.

According to the CDC (2014), each year approximately 1 in 6 Americans (or 48 million) becomes ill, 128,000 are hospitalized, and 3,000 die from food-borne diseases. The CDC Surveillance Report (2015c) on widespread food outbreaks reported that in 2013, 818 food-borne disease outbreaks were reported, resulting in 13,360 illnesses, 1,062 hospitalizations, 16 deaths, and 14 food recalls.

Although these are alarming statistics, the nurse is in a unique position to assess the client's knowledge of food safety and preparation and educate clients regarding appropriate food safety measures.

Other aspects of food safety are food allergies and food intolerances. Some food allergies can be life threatening. For instance, persons with an allergy to shellfish or to peanuts can have anaphylactic reactions when exposed, often even to a small amount. Although most any food can cause an allergy in some individuals, the most likely foods to cause allergy are: peanuts, tree nuts, cow's milk, egg, wheat, soy, fish, shellfish, and sesame (Food Allergy Research & Education [FARE], 2016). Symptoms of food allergy appear from minutes to hours after ingestion.

Symptoms of a severe or anaphylactic response to a food include: obstructive swelling of the lips, tongue, and/or throat; dysphagia, cyanosis, dyspnea, hypotension, feeling faint, confused, weak, passing out; loss of consciousness; chest pain; weak or "thready" pulse; or sense of "impending doom" (FARE, 2016). There are many food allergies that have milder symptoms such as: hives (reddish, swollen, itchy areas on the skin) eczema (a persistent dry, itchy rash), redness of the skin or around the eyes, itchy mouth or ear canal, nausea or vomiting, diarrhea, stomach pain, nasal congestion or a runny nose, sneezing, slight dry cough, odd taste in mouth, or even uterine contractions. Obviously, these symptoms may be nonspecific and difficult to associate with a particular food. The nurse can ask the client about patterns of responses after eating specific foods to determine if an allergic reaction is present or has occurred in the past.

Food allergies affect about 1% of adults and 7% of children, while food intolerances are much more common, affecting about 10% of Americans (Cleveland Clinic, 2015). Where food allergy is an immune system response, food intolerance results from a digestive system irritation or when the digestive system is unable to break down or properly digest the food. Lactose intolerance, due to lack of the lactase enzyme to break down mild protein, is the most common food intolerance. Symptoms of food intolerance include: nausea, stomach pain, gas, bloating, cramps, vomiting, heartburn, diarrhea, headaches, irritability, or nervousness.

Another safety issue with food is the potential for foods and medications to have untoward interactions. There are far too many potential interactions to list, but many websites, books, and other resources are available to use for reference. All medications, whether prescribed or over the counter, should be checked online or through other sources to see if there are potential food/drug interactions. Furthermore, foods such as spices and herbs have side effects that can interfere with medications or with conditions such as coagulation. Many spices that are anti-inflammatory, such as turmeric, ginger, and cinnamon, have an anticoagulating effect (Ellis, 2013; Heidtman, 2014). Other food and supplements, such as green leafy vegetables and Coenzyme Q10, have a coagulating effect (Grey, 2013; University of Maryland Medical Center [UMMC], 2007).

NUTRITIONAL RESEARCH AND GUIDELINES

Chaos! That is the state of nutritional research conclusions in recent years. Nutritional "best practice" guidelines are in a highly controversial state due to conflicting results of research studies used to develop dietary recommendations. So which guidelines should nurses follow? Nurses need to understand the basics of nutrition and be aware of these controversial issues regarding nutritional guidelines (Cleveland Clinic, 2016; Feinman et al., 2015; Fox, 2016; Harvard Medical School, 2015; Juanola-Falgarona et al., 2014; MacClean, 2016; Mayo Clinic, 2014b; McCullogh, 2014; O'Connor, 2016; Sboros, 2015; U.S. Department of Health and Human Services [UHHS] and U.S. Department of Agriculture [USDA], 2015). Although the most current evidence will be discussed here, remember that nutritional recommendations are constantly changing. And to make matters even more confusing, a report released by the Genetics Society of America (July 13, 2016) of a study of the relationship of genetics to diet indicates that pathophysiologic responses to different dietary patterns [diets] differ according to different genetics. Although the study was done in mice, the researchers propose that the findings have implications for dietary recommendations, bringing into question various governmental and other dietary guidelines.

Table 13-1 provides the estimated calorie needs by age, gender, and physical activity. The calorie needs are the least controversial of the dietary recommendations, although some of the varied dietary recommendations suggest that calories are less important than the content of the diet.

Controversies

Low Carbohydrate/High Protein/Fat versus Low Fat Diets

Due to widespread interest in and research on nutrition, there are a number of nutritional guidelines newly developed or being developed around the world. Many of these guidelines, including the new 2015–2020 Dietary Guidelines for Americans, have been criticized by other organizations.

TABLE 13-1 Estimated Calorie Needs Per Day by Age, Gender, and Physical Activity Level[a]

Estimated amounts of calories needed to maintain calorie balance for various gender and age groups at three different levels of physical activity. The estimates are rounded to the nearest 200 calories. An individual's calorie needs may be higher or lower than these average estimates.

Gender	Age (years)	Sedentary	Moderately Active	Active
Child (female and male)	2–3	1,000–1,200[c]	1,000–1,400[c]	1,000–1,400[c]
Female[d]	4–8	1,200–1,400	1,400–1,600	1,400–1,800
	9–13	1,400–1,600	1,600–2,000	1,800–2,200
	14–18	1,800	2,000	2,400
	19–30	1,800–2,000	2,000–2,200	2,400
	31–50	1,800	2,000	2,200
	51+	1,600	1,800	2,000–2,200
Male	4–8	1,200–1,400	1,400–1,600	1,600–2,000
	9–13	1,600–2,000	1,800–2,200	2,000–2,600
	14–18	2,000–2,400	2,400–2,800	2,800–3,200
	19–30	2,400–2,600	2,600–2,800	3,000
	31–50	2,200–2,400	2,400–2,600	2,800–3,000
	51+	2,000–2,200	2,200–2,400	2,400–2,800

Physical Activity Level[b]

[a]Based on Estimated Energy Requirements (EER) equations, using reference heights (average) and reference weights (healthy) for each age/gender group. For children and adolescents, reference height and weight vary. For adults, the reference man is 5 ft 10 in tall and weighs 154 lb. The reference woman is 5 ft 4 in tall and weighs 126 lb. EER equations are from the Institute of Medicine. *Dietary reference intakes for energy, carbohydrate, fiber, fat, fatty acids, cholesterol, protein, and amino acids.* Washington, DC: The National Academies Press; 2002.
[b]Sedentary means a lifestyle that includes only the light physical activity associated with typical day-to-day life. Moderately active means a lifestyle that includes physical activity equivalent to walking about 1.5–3 miles per day at 3-4 miles per hour, in addition to the light physical activity associated with typical day-to-day life. Active means a lifestyle that includes physical activity equivalent to walking more than 3 miles per day at 3–4 miles per hour, in addition to the light physical activity associated with typical day-to-day life.
[c]The calorie ranges shown are to accommodate needs of different ages within the group. For children and adolescents, more calories are needed at older ages. For adults, fewer calories are needed at older ages.
[d]Estimates for females do not include women who are pregnant or breastfeeding.
Used with permission from Dietary Guidelines for Americans (2010), United States Department of Agriculture and Health and Human Services.

These guidelines and some of the critiques and alternatives are presented below.

The Dietary Guidelines for Americans were developed to better reflect the newer evidence for nutrition. The Executive Summary of the report lists the primary factors that are emphasized:
1. Follow a healthy eating pattern across the lifespan.
2. Focus on variety, nutrient density, and amount.
3. Limit calories from added sugars and saturated fats and reduce sodium.
4. Shift to healthier food and beverage choices.
5. Support healthy eating patterns for all.

(UHHS and USDA, 2015.) (See the full report of the 2015–2020 Dietary Guidelines for Americans. Available at http://health.gov/dietaryguidelines/2015/)

A review of these guidelines and criticisms by O'Connor (2016) summarized the guidelines as follows: Americans are urged to drastically cut back on sugar, and, for the first time, the guidelines have singled out teenage boys and men for eating too much meat, chicken, and eggs. Criticisms of the guidelines attached to the O'Connor report include a quote from an investigative journalist and Nutrition Coalition board member stating that "These dietary guidelines are virtually identical to those of the past 35 years, during which time obesity and diabetes have skyrocketed".

Fox (2016) reported that experts from the American Cancer Society Cancer Action Network and the American Institute for Cancer Research are disappointed at the guidelines' ignoring of the evidence for a strong link between cancer and diets high in red and processed meats.

However, there are many who question the relationship of eating meat or other high cholesterol foods and cholesterol in the blood. For instance, Sboros (2015) reported on studies based on the Banting diet, popularized by Dr. Tim Noakes in South Africa. Many studies are now showing that a low fat, high carbohydrate diet does little to reduce overweight and cholesterol. Total cholesterol is often shown to fall when a person follows a high fat, low carbohydrate diet.

As for the effects of a low carbohydrate diet on controlling blood glucose in diabetes mellitus, studies abound. A summary of studies was presented by Feinman et al. (2015).

Anti-Inflammatory Diet

An additional entry into the dietary guidelines is the consideration of anti-inflammatory diets. It is believed that the basis of many diseases, even beyond arthritis and autoimmune diseases, is chronic inflammation. Cancer, diabetes mellitus, heart disease, depression, Alzheimer disease, arthritis, and other diseases (Harvard Medical School, 2015), and chronic pain syndromes and fibromyalgia (Cleveland Clinic, 2016) have been linked to chronic inflammation. Eating an anti-inflammatory diet may reduce the inflammatory effects of some of these diseases.

Harvard Medical School (2015) recommended an anti-inflammatory diet that is essentially the Mediterranean diet: Include anti-inflammatory foods such as olive oil, nuts, fatty fish, leafy greens, tomatoes, and fruits. Avoid inflammatory foods and drinks such as: French fries, sodas, refined carbohydrates, lard, and processed meats.

Cleveland Clinic (2016) provides three diet basics of an anti-inflammatory diet:
1. Eat the rainbow: Consume eight to nine servings of vegetables daily, including cruciferous vegetables.
2. Restrict dairy and grains: Eat limited amounts of dairy; avoid simple carbohydrates and sugars; opt for whole grains such as barley, buckwheat, oats, quinoa, brown rice, rye, spelt, and wheat.
3. Avoid red meat: Limit red meat consumption to about twice a year. Instead eat fish and vegetarian dishes for protein. Chicken is neutral in an anti-inflammatory sense.

Other anti-inflammatory foods are herbs and spices (Maroon et al., 2010). These authors recommend natural anti-inflammatory agents for pain relief, including omega-3 EFAs in fish oil, white willow bark, curcumin (turmeric), green tea, maritime pine bark, cloves, cinnamon, Jamaican allspice, apple pie spice mixture, oregano, pumpkin pie spice, *Boswellia serrata* (frankincense), resveratrol (found in red wine, dark-skinned grapes, and other food items), cat's claw, and capsaicin (chili pepper). Other items are included in a list by the Royal Society of Chemistry (2016), including marjoram, and sage, cinnamon, ginger, allspice, and others. Care must be taken for interactions, as noted earlier. Often these spices, herbs, and supplements will have a side effect of anticoagulation that has to be considered in certain conditions or when taken concurrently with certain medications (Ellis, 2013; Heidtman, 2014).

Since chronic inflammation has been found to underlie most of the diseases that diet may affect, an anti-inflammatory diet would be the most beneficial for most people. Although the controversy about protein and fat as opposed to carbohydrates still rages, the science seems to support a diet that is low in simple carbohydrates (but does include very complex carbohydrates), high in non–red-meat sources of protein that may or may not be high in fat (saturated or not), and that includes herbs and spices if not contraindicated by condition and medication. As nurses, it is essential that we follow the discussions and the studies if we are going to be in a position to help clients recognize the need for referral for further consultation.

Low Glycemic Index Diet

The glycemic index is based on how foods affect blood glucose. The index assigns a number to carbohydrate-containing foods according to how much each food increases blood sugar. The purpose of a glycemic index diet is not to specify portion sizes or the optimal number of calories, carbohydrates, or fats for weight loss or weight maintenance, but to help a person to eat carbohydrate-containing foods that are less likely to significantly increase blood glucose (Mayo Clinic, 2014a). Because the low glycemic index diet is low in simple sugars, it is somewhat anti-inflammatory as well (Juanola-Falgarona et al., 2014).

Canada's Guideline Controversy

Canada's food guides have also been revised (for the food guides, see Government of Canada, 2015). There have been calls to further revise Canada's Food Guide as well (see MacClean, 2016). MacClean (2016) noted that the Canadian Senate Committee on Social Affairs, Science, and Technology released a report on obesity in Canada, which called obesity a crisis in the country and recommended a tax on sugar-sweetened drinks, and revision of the dietary guidelines. The major issue with the guidelines, other than format, was determined to be the lack of emphasis on restricting consumption of highly processed foods. The Senate highlights Brazil's new food guide as a shining example to follow. Brazil's guide focuses on whole foods as opposed to nutrients and food groups and has three categories: Group 1 includes all unprocessed or minimally processed foods; Group 2 includes processed items used in cooking such as flour, oils, and spices; and Group 3 includes ultra-processed foods. The Brazilian guide also advocates preparing meals from scratch and thinking of the social process of preparing food—that it is handmade and not factory made. In light of the unsettled controversies and to avoid giving nutrition advice that may be harmful, all guidelines and the *ChooseMyPlate Food Guide*, of the U.S. government and the Canadian government are omitted from this edition of the text.

> **CLINICAL TIP**
> In summary, what can the nurse take away from all the controversies? Advise clients to avoid simple sugars, transfats, processed foods, and too many calories.

Optimal Nutrition, Malnutrition, Overnutrition

Optimal Nutrition

The most beneficial nutritional status requires a balance of nutrient intake to meet daily metabolic demands. Metabolic demands vary based on developmental level, lifestyle, and other energy demands. Optimal nutrition is often thought to be a balance of calories and exercise, but metabolic demands require a variety of nutrients and not just a focus on calories.

Malnutrition

Certain diseases, disorders, or lifestyle behaviors can place clients at risk for *undernutrition* or *malnutrition* and can exacerbate or facilitate disease processes. The following is a selected list of risk factors:
- Lower socioeconomic status (SES), making nutritious foods unaffordable
- Lifestyle of long work hours and obtaining one or more meals from a fast-food chain or vending machine
- Poor food choices by children, teens, and adults, including fatty or fried meats, sugary foods, and few fruits and vegetables
- Chronic dieting, particularly with fad diets, to meet perceived societal norms for weight and appearance
- Chronic diseases (e.g., Crohn disease, cirrhosis, or cancer) that may interfere with absorption or use of nutrients
- Dental and other factors such as difficulty chewing, loss of taste sensation, depression
- Limited access to sufficient food regardless of SES such as being physically unable to shop, cook, or feed self
- Disorders whereby food is self-limited or refused (e.g., anorexia nervosa, bulimia, depression, dementia, or other psychiatric disorders)
- Illness or trauma that increases client's nutritional needs dramatically but that interferes with the ability to ingest adequate nourishment (e.g., extensive burns)

The clinical signs and symptoms of malnutrition are often confused with those of other diseases or conditions.

In addition, the signs and symptoms may not manifest until the malnutrition is profound. The nurse needs to collect as much data as possible, especially in clients who are at risk for malnutrition or show some early clinical signs. It is important to evaluate all of the information in context to avoid making judgments based on one or two isolated signs or symptoms.

Clients with cancer are a population particularly at risk for developing malnutrition. Wasting syndrome known as *cachexia* or cancerous or malignant cachexia can develop. This type of malnutrition is characterized by an abnormal metabolic rate, anorexia, muscle wasting, severe weight loss, and general decline in condition. Though this syndrome is not well understood, it is typically attributed to a combination of factors, including increased catabolism and interference with gastrointestinal function resulting from the cancer, anorexia, altered metabolism, treatment related and from psychological factors such as anxiety and depression. Nutritional assessment is the first step in providing quality care to clients with cancer.

Clients with *acquired immunodeficiency syndrome (AIDS)* are another vulnerable population that often experience malnutrition. As stated previously, early in the disease symptoms of malnourishment are subtle and often overlooked. Vitamin and mineral deficiencies and slight weight loss may be present early on. Later, as AIDS advances, symptoms of malnutrition, including fatigue, depression, diarrhea, and peripheral neuropathy, may develop (Springhouse, 2006). As with the client with cancer, malnutrition in AIDS may be multifaceted. The client's metabolic rate increases with fever, infection, and AIDS-specific cancer can all combine to increase nutritional and energy demands. Nutrient malabsorption may result from medications, diarrhea, or infections, and poor oral intake enhances the client's malnourishment. Nutritional assessment is crucial in providing the client with an appropriate nutritional intervention.

Overnutrition

Increased caloric consumption, especially of foods high in fat and sugar, with decreased energy expenditure has led to an obesity epidemic. Approximately two thirds of the adult population in the United States is *overweight* and nearly a third of this group is *obese*, a rate that has remained high and has not changed from 2003–2004 to 2010–2011, according to data from the CDC (2015a). In addition, the CDC (2015b) noted that the rate for childhood obesity has remained at approximately 17%, even though there has been a decrease in obesity in children from 2 to 5 years of age. Obesity is defined as excessive body fat in relation to lean body mass. The amount of body fat, or adipose tissue, includes both the fat distribution throughout the body as well as the size of the fat deposits. The health risks of obesity are numerous and include diabetes, heart disease, stroke, hypertension, some forms of cancers, osteoarthritis, and sleep apnea. The American Cancer Society (ACS) Guidelines on Nutrition and Physical Activity for Cancer Prevention (2016) recommend that individuals achieve and maintain a healthy weight (as lean as possible without being underweight) throughout life, be physically active, eat a healthy diet (with emphasis on plant foods (but this may be contradicted by the variable findings of the nutrition guidelines controversies), and limiting consumption of alcohol to one drink for women and two drinks for men daily (see Evidence-Based Health Promotion and Disease Prevention 13-1).

Generally, a person who is 10% over *ideal body weight* (IBW) is considered overweight, whereas one who is 20% over IBW is considered obese (see Table 13-2 for a determination of obesity based on body mass index [BMI]). However, weight alone is not a completely reliable criterion. Muscle, bone, fat, and body fluid can account for excess body weight. For example, because muscle is heavier than fat, an athlete who has increased muscle mass may be inaccurately categorized as overweight when referring to a standard weight chart. Therefore, although evaluating nutritional status by a client's weight can inform you about obvious alterations at either end of the weight–nutrition continuum, the client with subtle deviations from a healthy-appearing body may benefit from more extensive and varied examination.

Optimal Hydration

Dehydration

Dehydration can have a seriously damaging effect on body cells and the execution of body functions. Because the thirst mechanism is poorly developed in humans, dehydration can develop unnoticed in normal people under adverse conditions. Often a person may experience a sense of thirst only after dangerous excess or deficit of various serum electrolyte levels has occurred. A chronically and seriously ill client who is not receiving adequate fluids either orally or parenterally is at high risk for dehydration unless monitored carefully.

Overhydration

Overhydration in a healthy person is usually not a problem because the body is effective in maintaining a correct fluid balance. It does this by shifting fluids in and out of physiologic third spaces, such as extracellular tissues, the pleural and pericardial spaces, the tongue and the eyeball, and by excreting fluid in the urine, stool, and through respiration and perspiration. Clients at risk for overhydration or fluid retention are those with kidney, liver, and cardiac diseases in which the fluid dynamic mechanisms are impaired.

Seriously ill clients who are on humidified ventilation or who are receiving large volumes of parenteral fluids without close monitoring of their hydration status are also at risk. The health history interview provides an ideal time to teach home-care clients and their caregivers how to monitor hydration by keeping records of fluid intake and output.

HEALTH ASSESSMENT

Components of a Nutritional Assessment

Nutritional assessment is composed of nutritional screening and a comprehensive nutritional assessment that includes collection of subjective data through a health history interview; collection of objective data, including anthropometric measurements, used to evaluate the client's physical growth, development, and nutritional status; and laboratory tests. The nurse works closely with the registered dietitian (RD) through consultation and collaboration to evaluate nutritional status and identify clients needing instruction and/or nutritional support.

13-1 EVIDENCE-BASED HEALTH PROMOTION AND DISEASE PREVENTION: OBESITY

Obesity is defined as a weight more than 20% above normal body weight, and is also determined by a BMI over 30 (MedicalNewsToday, 2016).

The epidemic of obesity has become a global health challenge. Tucker (2014) reported that studies show that there has been a rise in the combined worldwide prevalence of overweight and obesity of 27.5% for adults and 47.1% for children between the years 2008 and 2013.

Approximately one third of the adult population in the United States is *obese*, according to data from the Centers for Disease Control and Prevention ([CDC] 2015a). The CDC (2015a) also reported that among U.S. adults, the obesity prevalence is highest for middle-aged people between 40 and 59 years of age, and non–Hispanic Blacks have the highest age-adjusted rates of obesity (47.8%) followed by Hispanics (42.5%), non–Hispanic Whites (32.6%), and non–Hispanic Asians (10.8%).

In addition, the CDC (2015b) reported that approximately 17% of children in the United States between 2 and 19 years of age are obese. However, a study in the *Journal of Childhood Obesity* (Asieba, 2016) reports that 33.05% of children in the United States are overweight or obese, with ethnicity playing a role in prevalence. The pattern reflects the pattern for adult obesity, with 39% of Hispanic children and 37% of non–Hispanic Black children being obese (in article's Discussion section). Educational background of the parents was found to play a role in obesity as well.

The causes for obesity are attributed to consuming too many calories, leading a sedentary lifestyle, not getting enough sleep, endocrine disruptors, lower rates of smoking (smoking suppresses appetite), medications that affect weight gain, or an obesity gene (MedicalNewsToday, 2016).

Many things influence food consumption, including access to food, knowledge and beliefs about food, beliefs about weight, societal and cultural beliefs, places where one eats, and marketing or advertising. In addition, the level of exercise in relationship to calorie intake varies with access to safe places to exercise, beliefs about weight and beauty, and level of fatigue with daily activities or health status.

HEALTHY PEOPLE 2020 GOAL

(The updated Healthy People topic of Nutrition and Weight Status contains recommendations that fall into the issues discussed in the guidelines controversy. Please note this when using the following information.)

Promote health and reduce chronic disease risk through the consumption of healthful diets and achievement and maintenance of healthy body weights.

OBJECTIVES

According to Healthy People 2020 (2016), the Nutrition and Weight Status objectives for Healthy People 2020 reflect strong science supporting the health benefits of eating a healthful diet and maintaining a healthy body weight. The objectives also emphasize that efforts to change diet and weight should address individual behaviors, as well as the policies and environments that support these behaviors in settings such as schools, worksites, health care organizations, and communities. The objectives also include promoting healthful diets and healthy weight through increasing household food security and eliminating hunger.

Only the specific objectives for weight and nutrient consumption are included here. Examples of the objectives for weight are:

- Increase the proportion of adults who are at a healthy weight.
- Reduce the proportion of adults who are obese.
- Reduce the proportion of children and adolescents who are obese by 10% (per age group category).
- Prevent inappropriate weight gain in youth and adults (in development).

Examples of Objectives for Food and Nutrient Consumption
- Increase the contribution of fruits to the diets of the population aged 2 years and older.
- Increase the variety and contribution of vegetables to the diets of the population of persons 2 years and older.
- Increase the contribution of whole grains to the diets of the population aged 2 years and older.
- Reduce consumption of calories from solid fats and added sugars in the population aged 2 years and older.
- Reduce the consumption of saturated fat and sodium in the population aged 2 years and older.
- Reduce the consumption of sodium in the population aged 2 years and older.
- Increase consumption of calcium in the population aged 2 years and older.
- Reduce iron deficiency among young children females of childbearing age, and among pregnant females.

SCREENING

The U.S. Preventive Services Task Force (USPSTF) (2012, being updated) recommends screening all adults for obesity. Clinicians should offer or refer patients with a body mass index (BMI) of 30 kg/m^2 or higher to intensive, multi-component behavioral interventions. And the USPSTF recommends that clinicians screen children aged 6 years and older for obesity and offer them or refer them to comprehensive, intensive behavioral intervention to promote improvement in weight status.

RISK ASSESSMENT

Factors Associated with Increased Risk (Mayo Clinic, 2015b)
- Genetics (affect body fat distribution and storage)
- Family lifestyle
- Inactivity
- Unhealthy diet and eating habits
- Quitting smoking
- Pregnancy
- Lack of sleep (causes changes in hormones that affect appetite)
- Certain medications (include some antidepressants, anti-seizure medications, diabetes medications, antipsychotic medications, steroids, and beta blockers)
- Social and economic issues
- Age (especially hormonal changes, less active lifestyle, lower muscle mass leading to lower metabolism)
- Medical problems: rare disease such as Prader–Willi syndrome, Cushing syndrome, polycystic ovary syndrome, among others. Some medical problems, such as arthritis, can lead to decreased activity, which may result in weight gain. A low metabolism is unlikely to cause obesity, as is having low thyroid function.

CLIENT EDUCATION

Teach Clients
- If not morbidly obese: work with health professional or dietitian to develop a diet and exercise program for weight loss.
- If morbidly obese: work with physician to develop a plan for weight loss that may include in addition to diet and exercise either medication or obesity surgery.

TABLE 13-2 Adult Body Mass Index (BMI) Chart

Body Mass Index Table

	Normal						Overweight					Obese										Extreme Obesity										
BMI	19	20	21	22	23	24	25	26	27	28	29	30	31	32	33	34	35	36	37	38	39	40	41	42	43	44	45	46	47	48	49	50	51	52	53	54
Height (inches)												Body Weight (pounds)																								
58	91	96	100	105	110	115	119	124	129	134	138	143	148	153	158	162	167	172	177	181	186	191	196	201	205	210	215	220	224	229	234	239	244	248	253	258
59	94	99	104	109	114	119	124	128	133	138	143	148	153	158	163	168	173	178	183	188	193	198	203	208	212	217	222	227	232	237	242	247	252	257	262	267
60	97	102	107	112	118	123	128	133	138	143	148	153	158	163	168	174	179	184	189	194	199	204	209	215	220	225	230	235	240	245	250	255	261	266	271	276
61	100	106	111	116	122	127	132	137	143	148	153	158	164	169	174	180	185	190	195	201	206	211	217	222	227	232	238	243	248	254	259	264	269	275	280	285
62	104	109	115	120	126	131	136	142	147	153	158	164	169	175	180	186	191	196	202	207	213	218	224	229	235	240	246	251	256	262	267	273	278	284	289	295
63	107	113	118	124	130	135	141	146	152	158	163	169	175	180	186	191	197	203	208	214	220	225	231	237	242	248	254	259	265	270	278	282	287	293	299	304
64	110	116	122	128	134	140	145	151	157	163	169	174	180	186	192	197	204	209	215	221	227	232	238	244	250	256	262	267	273	279	285	291	296	302	308	314
65	114	120	126	132	138	144	150	156	162	168	174	180	186	192	198	204	210	216	222	228	234	240	246	252	258	264	270	276	282	288	294	300	306	312	318	324
66	118	124	130	136	142	148	155	161	167	173	179	186	192	198	204	210	216	223	229	235	241	247	253	260	266	272	278	284	291	297	303	309	315	322	328	334
67	121	127	134	140	146	153	159	166	172	178	185	191	198	204	211	217	223	230	236	242	249	255	261	268	274	280	287	293	299	306	312	319	325	331	338	344
68	125	131	138	144	151	158	164	171	177	184	190	197	203	210	216	223	230	236	243	249	256	262	269	276	282	289	295	302	308	315	322	328	335	341	348	354
69	128	135	142	149	155	162	169	176	182	189	196	203	209	216	223	230	236	243	250	257	263	270	277	284	291	297	304	311	318	324	331	338	345	351	358	365
70	132	139	146	153	160	167	174	181	188	195	202	209	216	222	229	236	243	250	257	264	271	278	285	292	299	306	313	320	327	334	341	348	355	362	369	376
71	136	143	150	157	165	172	179	186	193	200	208	215	222	229	236	243	250	257	265	272	279	286	293	301	308	315	322	329	338	343	351	358	365	372	379	386
72	140	147	154	162	169	177	184	191	199	206	213	221	228	235	242	250	258	265	272	279	287	294	302	309	316	324	331	338	346	353	361	368	375	383	390	397
73	144	151	159	166	174	182	189	197	204	212	219	227	235	242	250	257	265	272	280	288	295	302	310	318	325	333	340	348	355	363	371	378	386	393	401	408
74	148	155	163	171	179	186	194	202	210	218	225	233	241	249	256	264	272	280	287	295	303	311	319	326	334	342	350	358	365	373	381	389	396	404	412	420
75	152	160	168	176	184	192	200	208	216	224	232	240	248	256	264	272	279	287	295	303	311	319	327	335	343	351	359	367	375	383	391	399	407	415	423	431
76	156	164	172	180	189	197	205	213	221	230	238	246	254	263	271	279	287	295	304	312	320	328	336	344	353	361	369	377	385	394	402	410	418	426	435	443

Adapted from Clinical Guidelines on the Identification, Evaluation, and Treatment of Overweight and Obesity in Adults: The Evidence Report. Available at http://www.nhlbi.nih.gov/guidelines/obesity/bmi_tbl.pdf

13 Assessing Nutritional Status 225

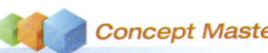 **Concept Mastery Alert**

When determining appropriate diagnoses, the nurse needs to consider all assessment data. For example, for a client who has not been eating or drinking for 24 hours and also has an elevated temperature, those assessment findings point to dehydration and the nursing diagnosis of Risk for Deficient Fluid Volume. That would be a more appropriate nursing diagnosis than the diagnosis, "Potential for Malnutrition (Deficit)," which is only related to the client's inability to tolerate food.

Nutritional Screening Tools

Using a *24-hour food recall* is an efficient and easy method of identifying a client's intake. However, this tool can only be used with a person who is able to remember all types and quantities of foods and beverages ingested in a 24-hour period. An illustration of a 24-hour food recall is provided in Assessment Tool 13-1. Additional tools used to screen a person's food habits and nutrition include:

- Sample form for a nutrition history (Assessment Tool 13-2)
- Checklist to use for nutritional screening (Assessment Tool 13-3)

ASSESSMENT TOOL 13-1 Client's 24-Hour Diet Recall

Patient's name: _____

Date taken: _____

Pregnant: ☐ ☐   Nursing: ☐ ☐
yes no   yes no

Taking nutritional supplements: ☐ ☐
yes no

Amount of money spent on food last month: _____

Check which food record: ☐ ☐
entry exit

Activity level:
☐ <30 minutes
☐ 30-60 minutes
☐ >60 minutes

| **Meal type:** | 1 = Morning
2 = Mid-morning
3 = Noon
4 = Afternoon
5 = Evening
6 = Late evening | **Serving abbreviations:** | Tablespoon
Teaspoon
Cup
Pound
Ounce
Slice | T
t
c
lb
oz
sl |

What did the patient eat and drink in the last 24 hours? (be thorough)

Describe in detail foods and beverages consumed. List one food/drink per line.	Amount eaten	Meal type

Number of lessons taught since last record:
Individual _____   Group _____   Other _____

Insert state EEO here

ASSESSMENT TOOL 13-2 Nutrition History

1. How many meals and snacks do you eat each day?
   Meals _____   Snacks _____
2. How many times a week do you eat the following meals away from home?
   Breakfast _____   Lunch _____
   Dinner _____
   What types of eating places do you frequently visit? (Check all that apply)
   Fast-food _____   Restaurant _____
   Diner/cafeteria _____   Other _____
3. On average, how many pieces of fruit or glasses of juice do you eat or drink each day?
   Fresh fruit _____   Juice (8-oz cup) _____
4. On average, how many servings of vegetables do you eat each day? _____
5. On average, how many times a week do you eat a high-fiber breakfast cereal? _____
6. How many times a week do you eat red meat (beef, lamb, veal) or pork? _____
7. How many times a week do you eat chicken or turkey? _____
8. How many times a week do you eat fish or shellfish? _____
9. How many hours of television do you watch every day? _____
   Do you usually snack while watching television?
   Yes _____ No _____
10. How many times a week do you eat desserts and sweets? _____
11. What types of beverages do you usually drink? How many servings of each do you drink a day?

    Water _____
    Juice _____
    Soda _____
    Diet soda _____
    Sports drinks _____
    Iced tea _____
    Iced tea with sugar _____

    Milk:
    Whole milk _____
    2% milk _____
    1% milk _____
    Skim milk _____

    Alcohol:
    Beer _____
    Wine _____
    Hard liquor _____

Used with permission from Hark, L. & Darwin, D. Jr. (1999). Taking a nutrition history: A practical approach for family physicians. *The American Family Physician, 59* (6), 1521–1528.

ASSESSMENT TOOL 13-3 Determine Your Nutritional Health based on the Nutritional Screening Initiative

(Developed by the American Academy of Family Physicians and the American Dietetic Association to promote the integration of nutrition screening and intervention into healthcare for older adults [Texas Department of Aging and Disability Services, 2010]). The following warning signs were identified and used to create a checklist based on these warning signs:

The Warning Signs of Poor Nutrition:
- Disease
- Eating poorly
- Tooth loss/mouth pain
- Economic hardship
- Reduced social contact
- Multiple medicines
- Involuntary weight loss/gain
- Needs assistance in self-care
- Elder years above age 80

The following checklist based on these warning signs may be used to find out if your client is at nutritional risk. Read the statements below. Circle the number in the yes column for those that apply to the client. For each yes answer, score the number in the box. Total the nutrition score.

	YES
Illness or condition that made client change the kind and/or amount of food eaten	2
Eats fewer than two meals per day	3
Eats few fruits or vegetables, or milk products	2
Has three or more drinks of beer, liquor, or wine almost every day	2
Tooth or mouth problems that make it hard to eat	2
Does not always have enough money to buy the food needed	4
Eats alone most of the time	1
Takes three or more different prescribed or over-the-counter drugs a day	1
Without wanting to, has lost or gained 10 lb in the last 6 months	2
Not physically able to shop, cook, and/or feed self	2
TOTAL	

ASSESSMENT TOOL 13-3	Determine Your Nutritional Health based on the Nutritional Screening Initiative (Continued)

Total the nutritional score.

0–2 Good. Recheck the score in 6 months.

3–5 Moderate nutritional risk. See what can be done to improve eating habits and lifestyle. Recheck score in 3 months.

6 or more High nutritional risk. Consult with physician, dietitian, or other qualified health or social service professional.

Note: Remember that warning signs suggest risk but do not represent diagnosis of any condition.
Texas Department of Aging and Disability Services. (2010). DETERMINE Your Nutritional Health Nutritional Screening Initiative (NSI). Available at https://www.dads.state.tx.us/providers/AAA/Forms/standardized/NRA.pdf. Used with permission.

For the older adult client, the *Mini Nutritional Assessment (MNA-SF)* is a valid stand-alone assessment tool that can be used to screen the nutritional status of older adults in less than 5 minutes (see Chapter 32, Assessment Tool 32-4).

Collecting Subjective Data: The Nursing Health History

The interview provides valuable information about the client's nutritional status. Nutritional assessment begins with questions regarding the client's dietary habits. Questions should solicit information about average daily intake of food and fluids, types and quantities consumed, where and when food is eaten, and any conditions or diseases that affect intake or absorption. Collection of this information can add to the evaluation of the client's risk factors as well as point to health education needs. It is important to approach the client in a respectful and nonjudgmental manner because self-esteem and body-image issues arise in part from less-than-optimal nutritional choices.

History of Present Health Concern

QUESTION	RATIONALE
Height and Weight	
What are your height and usual weight?	Answer provides a baseline for comparing client's perception with actual and current measurements. Answer also indicates client's knowledge of own health status.
Have you lost or gained weight recently? How much? Over what period of time?	Weight changes may point to changes in nutrition or hydration status, to an illness causing weight changes, or to changes in level of activity.
Diet	
Are you now or have you been on a specific diet recently? How did you decide which diet to follow?	Whether clients are following their own diet or a medically prescribed diet, the answer to the question helps to identify chronic dieters and clients with eating disorders.
How much fluid do you drink each day? How much of it is water? How many of these beverages that you consume daily contain sugar, artificial sweetener, caffeine, or alcohol?	Answers to these questions help identify clients at risk for dehydration or overhydration related to consumption of various kinds of fluids. These questions also identify those at risk for such disorders as migraine headaches related to alcohol, caffeine, or artificial-sweetener use.
Can you recall what you ate in the last 24 hours? Was this a typical 24-hour diet for you? If not what do you typically eat in a 24-hour period? How much do you drink and what types of fluids do you drink?	The client's typical daily diet indicates his or her level of nourishment, likes and dislikes, and dietary habits. A daily account of dietary and fluid intake provides insight into the client's nutrition and hydration (24-hour food recall).
Any recent changes in appetite, taste, or smell? Any recent difficulties chewing or swallowing?	Changes to taste and smell and difficulty chewing or swallowing may reduce the client's intake of food. Additionally, difficulty in swallowing can lead to serious consequences such as aspiration pneumonia.
Have you had any recent occurrences of vomiting, diarrhea, or constipation?	Each of these conditions, depending on severity, can affect nutritional and hydration status.

Continued on following page

Personal Health History

QUESTION	RATIONALE
Do you have food allergies and/or foods that you cannot eat? If so, please explain what they are and your symptoms.	Food allergies or intolerances are an immunologic response resulting in symptoms ranging from mild ones, such as rash, itching, or abdominal cramping, to very severe reactions such as life-threatening systemic anaphylaxis. Most common foods causing allergies are milk, eggs, wheat, shellfish, peanuts, and chocolate. Knowing what foods cause symptoms and how severe these symptoms are, is important in the nutritional assessment.
Do you have any chronic illnesses?	Chronic illnesses, such as digestive disorders, can negatively impact the client's nutritional status. Life-long specific diets are required to control some chronic conditions such as Crohn's, heart disease, and diabetes.
Have you experienced any recent trauma, surgery, or serious illness?	Each of these may increase the client's nutritional needs and decrease the client's ability to meet these needs.
What current medications, natural herbs, and vitamins/supplements are you taking?	Some medications or dietary supplements may decrease the client's absorption of nutrients. Other medications' therapeutic effects are affected by diet. For example, the therapeutic effects of warfarin (Coumadin) are lessened with the intake of large amounts of green, leafy vegetables.

Family History

QUESTION	RATIONALE
Are any members of your family obese?	Obesity often runs in families. In addition to genetics, families may have unhealthy eating patterns/habits that contribute to obesity.
Do any closely related family members (grandparents, parents, or siblings) have chronic illnesses such as digestive disorders, heart disease, or diabetes?	Many chronic diseases tend to be familial.

Lifestyle and Health Practices

QUESTION	RATIONALE
Do your religious beliefs or culture have dietary restrictions or requirements?	Some religions and cultures influence or dictate dietary practices.
Do you prepare your own meals? If not, who in your household typically assumes this responsibility?	Identifying who in the household prepares meals will allow the nurse to focus teaching on the correct individual.
Describe how your food is stored, cooked, and served. How is it dated and labeled?	Food storage and preparation can affect health and nutritional well-being. Food-borne illnesses are prevalent and associated with how food is handled. Overcooking can result in loss of vitamins from once vitamin-rich foods.
How often per week do you typically eat your breakfast, lunch, and dinner away from home? If you eat meals away from home, in a typical week, where do you go and which meals do you eat out?	Frequency of dining out and type of restaurant may affect the nutritional status of the client.
What types of food do you typically purchase? What is your weekly monetary budget for food purchases? Where do you typically purchase your food?	Low income may compromise the client's ability to purchase food or make healthy food choices (foods high in fat and calories, and low in nutrients are often less expensive and readily accessible).
Do you follow an exercise regimen?	Regular physical exercise is important to maintaining health and an ideal body weight.

The case study is used to demonstrate information that can be gleaned from a nursing health history.

CASE STUDY

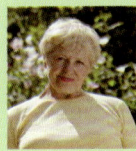

The case study introduced at the beginning of the chapter is now being used to demonstrate the mnemonic COLDSPA to interview Ms. Jones to elicit additional information. Aware that Ms. Jones has lost 7 lb since last week, the nurse interviews her using specific probing questions. The nurse explores health concerns using the COLDSPA mnemonic.

Mnemonic	Question	Data Provided
Character	Describe the sign or symptom (feeling, appearance, sound, smell, or taste if applicable). In this case, describe circumstances surrounding weight loss.	"I've lost a lot of weight since last week. I think I have a fever and the flu. I just don't feel like eating because I am so nauseous and have vomited a few times. I have to urinate frequently. My tongue is really dry as well. Since I am not eating very much, I started drinking regular (non-diet) carbonated soft drinks to keep my blood sugar up."
Onset	When did it begin?	"Haven't felt good for about 3 days. Been sick to my stomach for 3 days with a little nausea and vomiting."
Location	Where is it? Does it radiate? Does it occur anywhere else? In this case, can you describe your flu-like symptoms? Are you thirsty? Are you having problems seeing?	"I'm achy all over. I'm thirsty but my stomach is queasy so I can't drink too much at a time. No problems seeing."
Duration	How long does it last? Does it recur? In this case, how often are you nauseated? How often do you urinate?	"I'm nauseated when eating any food. I urinate every hour or two."
Severity	How bad is it? How much does it bother you? In this case, how much do you urinate at a time? How much do you vomit at a time?	"Since all of this started, I sometimes can't keep food or liquids down. I urinate larger amounts than normal and more often."
Pattern	What makes it better or worse?	"I just try not to eat so I don't get sick to my stomach. Saltine crackers do help some with the nausea."
Associated factors/How it **A**ffects the client	What other symptoms occur with it? How does it affect you?	"My clothes just hang on me now. I look sick and don't feel very well."

After discussing Ms. Jones's concern about her weight loss, increased urination, and lack of appetite, the nurse continues with the present history. Because of her type 2 diabetes mellitus, the nurse explores questions that relate to her food and fluid intake as well as her prescribed medication. The client reports that she normally has breakfast at 7:00 AM. She takes a nighttime dose of Lantus insulin 13 units (based on her weight of 145 lb). However, Ms. Jones states that she has not taken her prescribed insulin the last few days; she thought she shouldn't take it because she has not been eating much. Today she states that she has been urinating large amounts and more frequently, her mouth is dry, she is nauseated and that she feels like she has the flu. Exploring her nutritional history, Ms. Jones's 24-hour food recall consists of: Breakfast—one slice of white unbuttered toast and an 8-oz regular lemon-lime soft drink; lunch—sips of carbonated soft drink while nibbling on three to four saltine crackers to settle her stomach; dinner—4 oz of cherry gelatin, 4-oz chicken broth, one slice of dry white toast, and an 8-oz soft drink. While she has been sick, she has been using non-diet foods and drinks. Typically she often uses dietary foods and drinks with sugar substitutes.

Collecting Objective Data: Physical Examination

Physical examination includes observing body build, measuring weight and height, taking anthropometric measurements, and assessing hydration.

Preparing the Client

After the interview, ask the client to put on an examination gown. The client should be in a comfortable sitting position on the examination table (or on a bed in the home setting). Unless the client is bed-bound in the hospital, nursing home, or home-care setting, explain that he or she will need to stand and sit during the assessment, particularly during anthropometric assessments. Keep in mind that some clients may be embarrassed to be measured, especially if they are overweight or underweight.

To reassure the client, explain that the examination is necessary for evaluating overall health status. Proceed with the examination in a straightforward, nonjudgmental manner.

Equipment

- Balance beam scale with height attachment or digital scale and height measuring device.
- Metric measuring tape
- Marking pencil
- Skin fold calipers

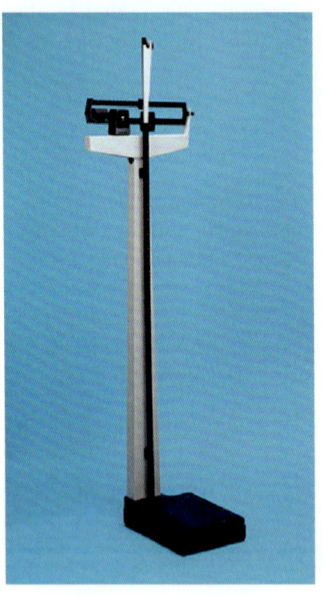

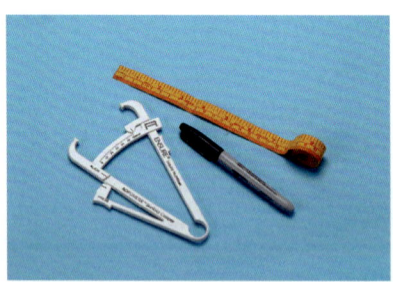

Physical Assessment

During examination of the client, remember these key points:
- Identify the equipment needed to take anthropometric measurements and the equipment's proper use.
- Explain the importance of anthropometric measurements to general health status.
- Educate the client regarding nutritional concerns and health-related risks.

General Routine Screening versus Focused Specialty Assessment of Nutritional Status

The nurse routinely assesses the client for overall appearance of body build, muscle mass, and fat distribution during the general survey when first meeting the client and on an ongoing basis for any changes. Height and weight are routinely assessed, with which the nurse can calculate the IBW and BMI. In addition, the nurse assesses the status of the client's overall hydration through measurement of intake and output and observation of skin turgor and moisture, edema, venous filling, tongue and eyeball condition, and lung sounds.

Advanced practice nurses, including nurses who have advanced experience and education in nutrition, may work as a Nutrition Nurse Advisor, Pediatric Nurse Advisor (Nutrition), Clinical Nurse Nutrition Specialist, Nurse Nutrition Practitioner, Nurse Consultant–Clinical Nutrition, or Senior Clinical Nurse Specialist. Nurses in these types of situations would measure waist circumference, determine waist-to-hip ratio, measure mid-arm circumference (MAC), measure triceps skin-fold thickness (TSF), and calculate mid-arm muscle circumference (MAMC). These same additional assessments are often made by a registered dietitian (RD). However, all nurses need to understand both how anthropometric measurements are assessed and their meaning to collaborate with other health care providers in planning effective client dietary measures.

General Routine Screening

- Observe client's general status and appearance.
- Observe body build as well as muscle mass and fat distribution.
- Measure height and weight.
- Determine IBW and percentage of IBW.
- Measure BMI.
- Observe for changes in hydration:
  - Measure I and O.
  - Assess skin turgor and moisture.
  - Check for edema.
  - Check venous filling, neck veins.
  - Check condition of tongue.
  - Check condition of eyeballs and surrounding skin.
  - Auscultate lung sounds.

Focused Specialty Assessment

- Determine waist circumference.
- Determine waist-to-hip ratio
- Measure MAC.
- Measure TSF.
- Calculate MAMC (Table 13-7).

ASSESSMENT PROCEDURE	NORMAL FINDINGS	ABNORMAL FINDINGS
General Status/Appearance		
Observe client's general status and appearance.	Alert, oriented, well developed for age, ideal weight, intact skin, normal skin tone, texture, appropriately dressed for season.	Table 13-3 provides data collected during a physical assessment that help identify nutritional disorders. Assessment Guide 13-1, compares indicators of good nutritional status with indicators of poor nutritional status.
BODY BUILD		
Observe body build as well as muscle mass and fat distribution. Note body type (Fig. 13-1).	A wide variety of body types fall within a normal range—from fat and muscle. In general, the normal body is proportional. Bilateral muscles are firm and well developed. There is equal distribution of fat with some subcutaneous fat. Body parts are intact and appear equal without obvious deformities.	A lack of subcutaneous fat with prominent bones is seen in the undernourished. Abdominal ascites is seen in starvation and liver disease. Abundant fatty tissue is noted in obesity. 🪑 **OLDER ADULT CONSIDERATIONS** Muscle tone and mass decrease with aging. There is a loss of subcutaneous fat, making bones and muscles more prominent. Fat is also redistributed with aging. Fat is lost from the face and neck and redistributed to the arms, abdomen, and hips.

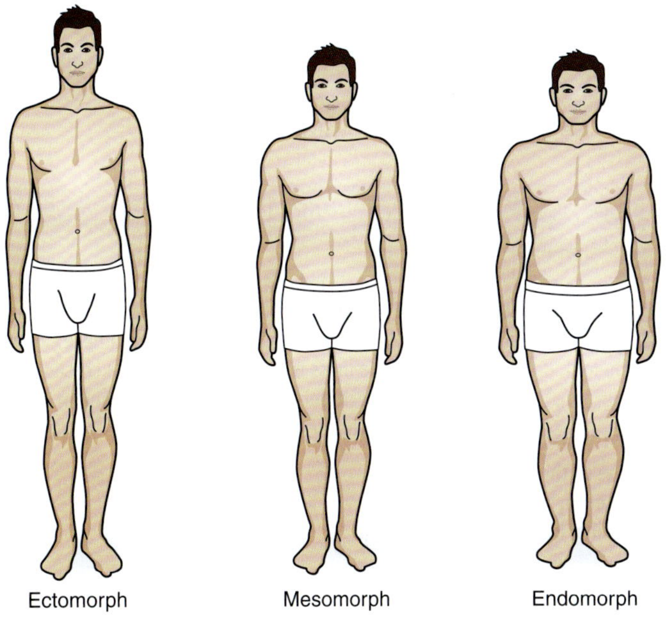

Ectomorph   Mesomorph   Endomorph

FIGURE 13-1 Body types. (Used with permission from www.bodybuilding.com.)

Anthropometric Measurements

🎯 **CLINICAL TIP**
When evaluating anthropometric data, base conclusions on a data cluster, not on individual findings. Factor in any special considerations and general health status. Although general standards are useful for making estimates, the client's overall health and well-being may be equal or more useful indicators of nutritional status.

Continued on following page

TABLE 13-3 Evaluating Nutritional Disorders

This table can help you interpret your nutritional assessment findings. Body systems are listed with signs or symptoms and implications for each.

Body System or Region	Sign or Symptom	Implications
General	• Weakness and fatigue • Weight loss	• Anemia or electrolyte imbalance • Decreased calorie intake, increased calorie use, or inadequate nutrient intake or absorption
Skin, hair, and nails	• Dry, flaky skin • Dry skin with poor turgor • Rough, scaly skin with bumps • Petechiae or ecchymoses • Sore that will not heal • Thinning, dry hair • Spoon-shaped, brittle, or ridged nails	• Vitamin A, vitamin B-complex, or linoleic acid deficiency • Dehydration • Vitamin A deficiency • Vitamin C or K deficiency • Protein, vitamin C, or zinc deficiency • Protein deficiency • Iron deficiency
Eyes	• Night blindness; corneal swelling, softening, or dryness; Bitot spots (gray triangular patches on the conjunctiva) • Red conjunctiva	• Vitamin A deficiency • Riboflavin deficiency
Throat and mouth	• Cracks at the corner of mouth • Magenta tongue • Beefy, red tongue • Soft, spongy, bleeding gums • Swollen neck (goiter)	• Riboflavin or niacin deficiency • Riboflavin deficiency • Vitamin B_{12} deficiency • Vitamin C deficiency • Iodine deficiency
Cardiovascular	• Edema • Tachycardia, hypotension	• Protein deficiency • Fluid volume deficit
Gastrointestinal	• Ascites	• Protein deficiency
Musculoskeletal	• Bone pain and bow leg • Muscle wasting	• Vitamin D or calcium deficiency • Protein, carbohydrate, and fat deficiency
Neurologic	• Altered mental status • Paresthesia	• Dehydration and thiamine or vitamin B_{12} deficiency • Vitamin B_{12}, pyridoxine, or thiamine deficiency

Springhouse. (2006). *Nutrition made incredibly easy!* (2nd ed.). Philadelphia, PA: Lippincott Williams & Wilkins.

ASSESSMENT PROCEDURE	NORMAL FINDINGS	ABNORMAL FINDINGS

Anthropometric Measurements (Continued)

Measure height. Measure the client's height by using the L-shaped measuring attachment on the balance scale. Instruct the client to stand shoeless on the balance scale platform with heels together and back straight, and to look straight ahead. Raise the attachment above the client's head. Then lower it to the top of the client's head (Fig. 13-2). Record the client's height.

CLINICAL TIP
When you do not have access to a measuring attachment on a scale, have the client stand shoeless with his back and heels against the wall. Balance a straight, level object (ruler) atop the client's head—parallel to the floor—and mark the object's position on the wall. Measure the distance between the mark and the floor.

If the client cannot stand, measure the arm span to estimate height. Have the client stretch one arm straight out sideways. Measure from the tip of one middle finger to the tip of the nose. Multiply by 2 and record the arm span height.

Height is within range for age, and ethnic and genetic heritage. Children are usually within the range of parents' height.

OLDER ADULT CONSIDERATIONS
Height begins to wane in the fifth decade of life because the intervertebral discs become thinner and spinal kyphosis increases.

Extreme shortness is seen in achondroplastic dwarfism and Turner syndrome. Extreme tallness is seen in gigantism (excessive secretion of growth hormone) and in Marfan syndrome.

13 Assessing Nutritional Status   233

ASSESSMENT PROCEDURE	NORMAL FINDINGS	ABNORMAL FINDINGS
Measure weight. Level the balance beam scale at zero before weighing the client. Do this by moving the weights on the scale to zero and adjusting the knob by turning it until the balance beam is level. Ask the client to remove shoes and heavy outer clothing and to stand on the scale. Adjust the weights to the right and left until the balance beam is level again (Fig. 13-3). Record weight (2.2 lb = 1 kg). ◎ **CLINICAL TIP** If you are weighing a client at home, you may have to use an electronic scale with an automatically adjusting true zero.	Desirable weights for men and women are listed in the BMI table (see Table 13-2). ◎ **CLINICAL TIP** Body weight may decrease with aging because of a loss of muscle or lean body tissue.	Weight does not fall within range of desirable weights for women and men. Excessive weight increases one's risks for additional health problems. See Abnormal Findings 13-1.

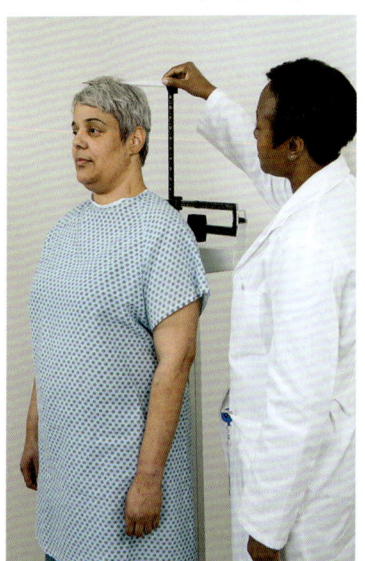

FIGURE 13-2 Measuring height.

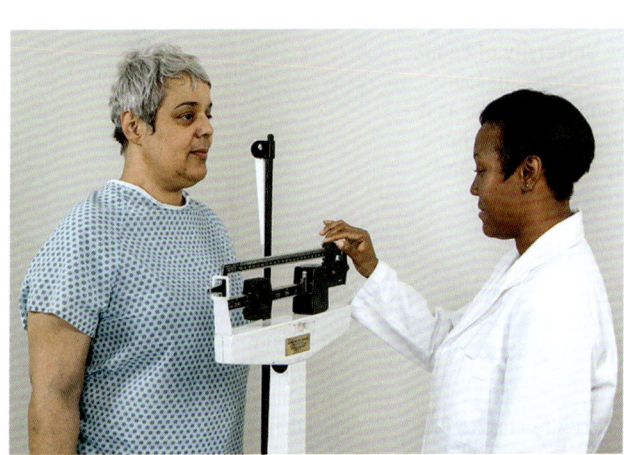

FIGURE 13-3 Measuring weight.

Determine ideal body weight (IBW) and percentage of IBW. Use this formula to calculate the client's IBW: *Female:* 100 lb for 5 ft + 5 lb for each inch over 5 ft ± 10% for small or large frame *Male:* 106 lb for 5 ft + 6 lb for each inch over 5 ft ± 10% for small or large frame. Calculate the client's percentage of IBW by the following formula: $$\frac{\text{Actual weight}}{\text{IBW}} \times 100 = \%\text{IBW}$$	Body weight is within 10% of ideal range.	A current weight that is 80% to 90% of IBW indicates a lean client and possibly mild malnutrition. Weight that is 70% to 80% indicates moderate malnutrition; less than 70% may indicate severe malnutrition, possibly from systemic disease, eating disorders, cancer therapies, and other problems. Weight exceeding 10% of the IBW range is considered overweight; weight exceeding 20% of IBW is considered obesity.
Measure body mass index (BMI). Though a number of methods are available to evaluate weight status, the most commonly used screening method is the BMI (NIDDK, 2012). BMI is calculated based on height and weight regardless of gender. It is a practical measure for estimating total body fat and is calculated as weight in kilograms and divided by the square height in meters.	BMI is between 18.5 and 24.9 (see Table 13-2).	BMI <18.5 is considered underweight. BMI between 25.0 and 29.9 is considered overweight and increases risk for health problems. A BMI of 30 or greater is considered obese and places the client at a much higher risk for type 2 diabetes, cardiovascular disease, osteoarthritis, and sleep apnea.

Continued on following page

ASSESSMENT PROCEDURE	NORMAL FINDINGS	ABNORMAL FINDINGS
Anthropometric Measurements (Continued)		
Quickly determine BMI by accessing the National Institutes of Health's website: http://nhlbisupport.com/bmi/bmicalc.htm. Alternatively, after measuring the client's height and weight, compare these findings to a standard table as seen in Table 13-2, or determine BMI using one of these formulas: $$\frac{\text{Weight in kilograms}}{\text{Height in meters}^2} = \text{BMI}$$ $$\frac{\text{Weight in pounds}}{\text{Height in inches}^2} \times 703 = \text{BMI}$$ **◎ CLINICAL TIP** The use of BMI alone is not diagnostic of a client's health status. According to Nordqvist (2013), quoting researchers from the University of Pennsylvania, BMI is an inaccurate measurement of health and body fat status, as it does not account for muscle mass, bone density, overall body composition, and racial and sex differences.		
Determine waist circumference. Waist circumference is the most common measurement used to determine the extent of abdominal visceral fat in relation to body fat. **◎ CLINICAL TIP** Adding waist circumference to BMI adds little to the predictive power of disease risk beyond using BMI alone (National Heart, Lung, and Blood Institute [NHLBI], n.d.). Yet measurements of waist circumference and waist size compared with hip size (also known as the waist-to-hip ratio) are still recommended to measure abdominal obesity (Harvard University, T. H. Chan School of Public Health, 2016). Have client stand straight with feet together and arms at sides. Place the measuring tape snugly around the waist at the umbilicus, yet not compressing the skin (Fig. 13-4). Instruct the client to relax the abdomen and take a normal breath. When the client exhales, record the waist circumference. See Table 13-4 for an interpretation of waist circumference, BMI, and associated risks.	*Females:* Less than or equal to 35 in (88 cm) *Males:* Less than or equal to 40 in (102 cm) These findings are associated with reduced disease risk. Waist circumference can be used alone as a predictor of health risk or used in conjunction with waist-to-hip ratio. See below for this technique.	*Females:* Greater than 35 in (88 cm) *Males:* Greater than 40 in (102 cm) These findings are associated with such disorders as diabetes, hypertension, hyperlipidemia, and cardiovascular disease. Table 13-4 presents some of these health risks. Excess fat deep within the abdominal cavity known as visceral fat as illustrated in Figure 13-5, is associated with higher health risks than subcutaneous fat and may be an independent predictor of health risks even when BMI falls within the normal range. This visceral belly fat releases chemicals associated with inflammation and metabolic stress, as opposed to some subcutaneous fat that releases chemicals that help balance the harmful effects of the visceral fat (Corleone, 2016). Adults with large visceral fat stores located mainly around the waist (android obesity) are more likely to develop health-related problems than if the fat is located in the hips or thighs (gynoid obesity). These problems

ASSESSMENT PROCEDURE	NORMAL FINDINGS	ABNORMAL FINDINGS

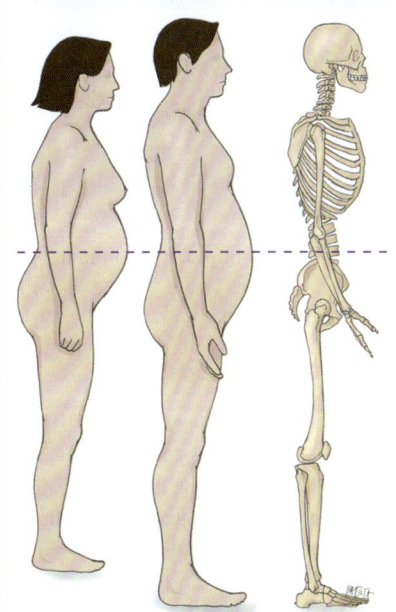

FIGURE 13-4 Positioning of measuring tape for waist circumference.

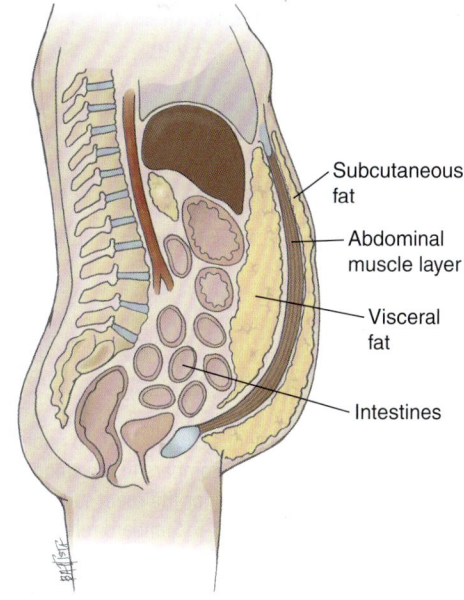

FIGURE 13-5 Visceral fat within the abdominal cavity increases health risks.

include an increased risk of type 2 diabetes, abnormal cholesterol and triglyceride levels, hypertension, and cardiovascular disease such as heart attack or stroke (see Table 13-4).

Determine waist-to-hip ratio.

After measuring the client's waist circumference, measure the hip circumference at the largest area of the buttocks. To obtain the ratio, divide the waist measurement by the hip measurement.

$$\frac{\text{Waist circumference}}{\text{Hip circumference}} = \text{Waist-to-Hip Ratio}$$

Females: Less than or equal to 0.80

Males: Less than or equal to 0.90

These findings are associated with reduced disease risk.

Using fruit as an example of this body shape concept, it is healthier to be shaped more like a pear than an apple (Fig. 13-6).

Females: Greater than 0.80

Males: Greater than 0.90

Same risk factors related to obesity as listed under waist circumference.

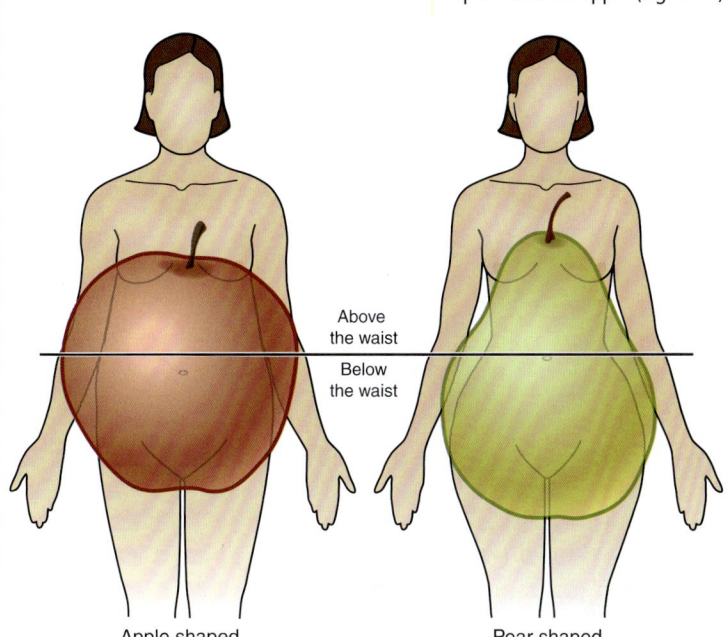

FIGURE 13-6 Waist-to-hip ratio (pear vs. apple shape).

Continued on following page

TABLE 13-4 Disease Risk for Type 2 Diabetes, Hypertension, and Cardiovascular Diseases Relative to BMI and Waist Circumference

BMI	WAIST SIZE Women: ≤35 in; Men: ≤40 in	WAIST SIZE Women: >35 in; Men: >40 in
25.0–29.9	Increased	High
30.0–34.9	High	Very high
35.0–39.9	Very high	Very high
40.0 and above	Extremely high	Extremely high

Compiled from National Heart, Lung, and Blood Institute (n.d.). Assessing your weight and health risk. Available at https://www.nhlbi.nih.gov/health/educational/lose_wt/risk.htm

ASSESSMENT PROCEDURE	NORMAL FINDINGS	ABNORMAL FINDINGS
Anthropometric Measurements (Continued)		
Measure mid-arm circumference (MAC). MAC evaluates skeletal muscle mass and fat stores. Have the client fully extend and dangle the nondominant arm freely next to the body. Locate the arm's midpoint (halfway between the top of the acromion process and the olecranon process). Mark the midpoint (Fig. 13-7A) and measure the MAC (Fig. 13-7B), holding the tape measure firmly around, but not pinching, the arm. Record the measurement in centimeters. Refer to Table 13-5 to compare with the standard reference. For example: Record both the MAC and the standard reference number. "MAC = 25 cm; 88% of standard. Standard = 28.5" (25/28.5 = 88%).	Compare the client's current MAC to prior measurements and compare to the standard MAC measurements for the client's age and sex listed in Table 13-5. Standard reference is 29.3 cm for men and 28.5 for women.	Measurements less than 90% of the standard reference are in the category of moderately malnourished. Less than 60% of the standard reference indicates severe malnourishment.

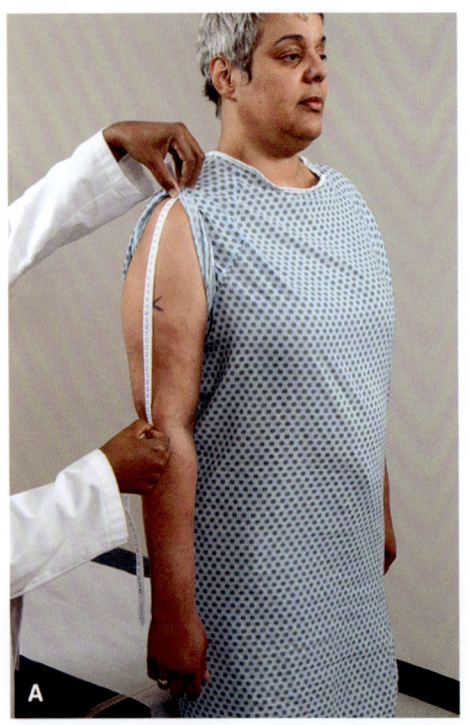
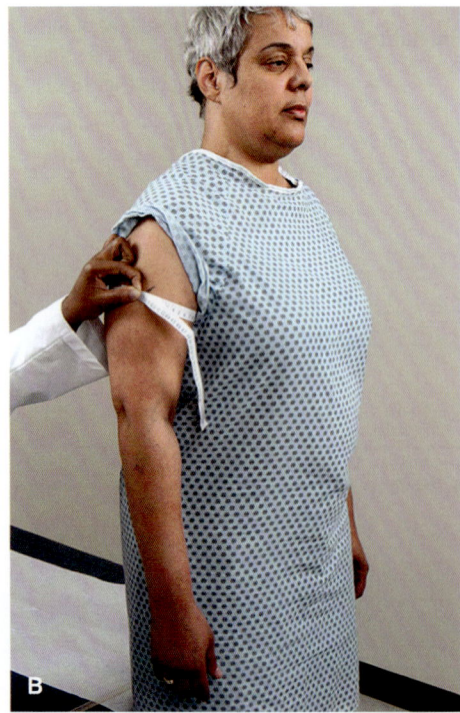

FIGURE 13-7 Measuring mid-arm circumference.

TABLE 13-5 Mid-Arm Circumference (MAC) Standard Reference

Adult MAC (cm)	Standard Reference	90% of Standard Reference—Moderately Malnourished	60% of Standard Reference—Severely Malnourished
Men	29.3	26.3	17.6
Women	28.5	25.7	17.1

ASSESSMENT PROCEDURE	NORMAL FINDINGS	ABNORMAL FINDINGS
CLINICAL TIP Though used less often, mid-arm circumference, triceps skin-fold measurements, and mid-arm muscle circumference calculations are helpful in evaluating the client's nutritional status. **Measure triceps skin-fold thickness (TSF).** Take the TSF measurement to evaluate the degree of subcutaneous fat stores. Instruct the client to stand and hang the nondominant arm freely. Grasp the skin fold and subcutaneous fat between the thumb and forefinger midway between the acromion process and the tip of the elbow. Pull the skin away from the muscle (ask client to flex arm: if you feel a contraction with this maneuver, you still have the muscle) and apply the calipers (Fig. 13-8). Repeat three times and average the three measurements. Record the measurements in millimeters. Refer to Table 13-6 to compare with the standard reference. For example: Record both the TSF and the standard reference number: "TSF = 15 mm; 91% of standard. Standard = 16.5" (15/16.5 = 91%). **CLINICAL TIP** A more accurate measurement can be obtained from the suprailiac region of the abdomen or the subscapular area.	Compare the client's current measurement to past measurements and to the standard TSF measurements for the client's gender listed in Table 13-6. Standard reference is 13.5 mm for men and 16.5 mm for women.	Measurements less than 90% of the standard reference indicate a loss of fat stores and place the client in the moderately malnourished category. Less than 60% of the standard reference indicates severe malnourishment. See Abnormal Findings 13-1 for examples of marasmus (protein/calorie malnutrition) and kwashiorkor (protein malnutrition) Measurements greater than 130% of the standard indicate obesity.

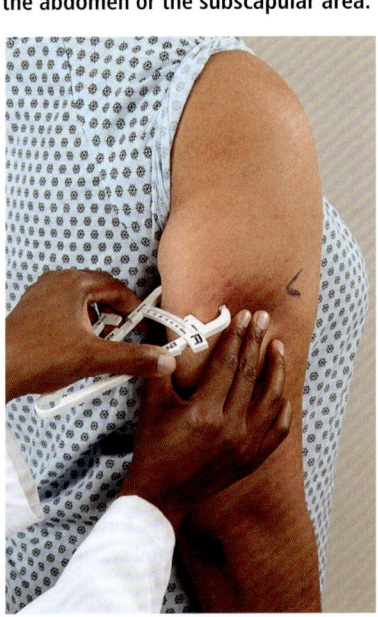

FIGURE 13-8 Measuring triceps skin-fold thickness.

Continued on following page

TABLE 13-6 Triceps Skinfold Thickness (TSF) Standard Reference

Adult TSF (mm)	Standard Reference	90% of Standard Reference—Moderately Malnourished	60% of Standard Reference—Severely Malnourished
Men	13.5	11.3	7.5
Women	16.5	14.9	9.9

ASSESSMENT PROCEDURE	NORMAL FINDINGS	ABNORMAL FINDINGS
Anthropometric Measurements (Continued)		
Calculate mid-arm muscle circumference (MAMC, Table 13-7). To determine skeletal muscle reserves or the amount of lean body mass and evaluate malnourishment in clients, calculate the MAMC. MAMC is derived from MAC and TSF by the following formula: MAMC = MAC (cm) − [0.314 × TSF (mm)] For example: Record the MAC and TSF and the standard reference number: "MAMC = 25 − [0.314 × 15] = 20.29; 87% of standard." Standard = 23.2 (20.29/23.2 = 87%).	Compare the client's current MAMC with past measurements and with the data for MAMCs for the client's age and gender listed in Table 13-7. Standard reference is 25.3 cm for men and 23.2 cm for women.	The MAMC decreases to the lower percentiles with malnutrition and in obesity if TSF is high. If the MAMC is in a lower percentile and the TSF is in a higher percentile, the client may benefit from muscle-building exercises that increase muscle mass and decrease fat. Malnutrition: • Mild—MAMC of 90% to 99% • Moderate—MAMC 60% to 90% • Severe—MAMC <60% as seen in protein-calorie malnutrition.
Assessing Hydration		
INPATIENT SETTING: INTAKE AND OUTPUT		
Measure intake and output (I&O) in inpatient settings. Measure all fluids taken in by oral and parenteral routes, through irrigation tubes, as medications in solution, and through tube feedings. Also measure all fluid output (urine, stool, drainage from tubes, perspiration). Calculate insensible loss at 800 to 1,000 mL daily, and add to total output.	I&O are closely balanced over 72 hours when insensible loss is included. 🎯 **CLINICAL TIP** Fluid is normally retained during acute stress, illness, trauma, and surgery. Expect diuresis to occur in most clients in 48 to 72 hours.	Imbalances in either direction suggest impaired organ function and fluid overload or inability to compensate for losses, resulting in dehydration.
ALL SETTINGS: FLUID-RELATED CHANGES		
Weigh clients at risk for hydration changes daily.	Weight is stable or changes less than 2 to 3 lb over 1 to 5 days.	Weight gains or losses of 6 to 10 lb in 1 week or less indicate a major fluid shift. A change of 2.2 lb (1 kg) is equal to a loss or gain of 1 L of fluid.
Take blood pressure with the client in lying, sitting, and standing positions. Palpate the radial pulse. Count the client's respirations. Take the client's temperature.	There are no orthostatic changes; blood pressure and pulse rate remain within normal range for client's activity level and status.	Blood pressure registers lower than usual and/or drops more than 20 mmHg from lying to standing position, thereby indicating fluid volume deficit, especially if the pulse rate is also elevated. Radial pulse rate +1 and thready denotes dehydration. Elevated pulse rate and blood pressure indicate overhydration.
Check skin turgor. Pinch a small fold of skin, observing elasticity, and watch how quickly the skin returns to its original position.	There is no tenting; skin returns to original position.	Tenting can indicate fluid loss but is also present in malnutrition and loss of collagen in older adults. This finding must be correlated with other hydration findings.

TABLE 13-7 Mid-Arm Muscle Circumference (MAMC) Standard Reference

Adult MAMC (cm)	Standard Reference	90% of Standard Reference—Moderately Malnourished	60% of Standard Reference—Severely Malnourished
Men	25.3	22.8	15.2
Women	23.2	20.9	13.9

ASSESSMENT PROCEDURE	NORMAL FINDINGS	ABNORMAL FINDINGS
Check for pitting edema (observable swelling of body tissues due to fluid accumulation that occurs when pressure is applied to the swollen area and indentation of the tissues occurs and or persists).	No edema is present.	Pitting edema is a sign of fluid retention, especially in cardiac and renal diseases.
Observe skin for moisture.	Skin is not excessively dry.	Abnormally dry and flaky skin. Corroborate such a finding with other findings because heredity, cholesterol levels and hormone levels determine skin moistness.
Assess venous filling. Lower the client's arm or leg and observe how long it takes to fill. Then raise the arm or leg and watch how long it takes to empty.	Veins fill in 3 to 5 seconds. Veins empty in 3 to 5 seconds.	Filling or emptying that takes more than 6 to 10 seconds suggests fluid volume deficit.
Observe neck veins with client in the supine position then with the head elevated above 45 degrees.	Neck veins are softly visible in supine position. With head elevated above 45 degrees, the neck veins flatten or are slightly visible but soft.	Flat veins in supine client may indicate dehydration. Visible firm neck veins indicate distension, possibly resulting from fluid retention and heart disease.
Inspect the tongue's condition and furrows.	Tongue is moist, plump with central sulcus, and no additional furrows.	Tongue is dry with visible papillae and several longitudinal furrows, suggesting loss of normal third-space fluid and dehydration.
Observe eye position and surrounding coloration.	Eyes are not sunken and no dark circles appear under them.	Sunken eyes—especially with deep, dark circles—indicate dehydration or malnutrition.
Auscultate lung sounds.	No crackles, friction rubs, or harsh lung sounds are auscultated.	Loud or harsh breath sounds indicate decreased pleural fluid. Friction rubs may also be heard. Crackling indicates increased fluid, as in interstitial fluid sequestration (i.e., pulmonary edema).

Laboratory Tests

Reviewing certain laboratory tests can yield valuable information about the client's nutritional status. These tests can identify undernutrition or malnutrition, especially subtle changes, before they are clinically evident. For example, a person can be obese yet undernourished because of poor food choices. In this situation, laboratory tests such as hemoglobin or protein levels may indicate anemia or other nutritional disorders. Laboratory studies such as high cholesterol and triglyceride values can indicate risk factors in undernourished, normal, overweight, and obese people because these factors can be related to inherited tendencies, lack of exercise, and unhealthful dietary habits.

When people are malnourished, the body's protein stores are affected. The proteins usually sacrificed early are those that the body considers to be less essential to survival: albumen and globulins, transport proteins, skeletal muscle proteins, blood proteins, and immunoglobulins. These can be easily evaluated by blood tests. Additional tests to evaluate general immunity (immunocompetence) consist of small-dose intradermal injections of recall antigens such as those used to test for tuberculosis, mumps, and *Candida* (yeast). Because everyone has been exposed to at least one of these, a delayed or absent reaction can indicate immunosuppression resulting from malnutrition. Table 13-8 summarizes laboratory values and other tests that can alert health care professionals to possible malnutrition. Please note that there may be slight variations in laboratory value ranges depending on the reference you use.

CASE STUDY

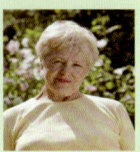

After asking Ms. Jones to put on a gown, the nurse returns to the room to perform a physical examination. The nurse observes that Ms. Jones has a well-developed body build for age with even distribution of fat and firm muscle. Height: 5 ft, 5 in (165 cm); body frame: medium; weight: 138 lb (58 kg); BMI: 22.5; IBW: 135; waist circumference 30 in; MAC: 28 cm; TSF: 16.8 mm; MAMC: 22.7 cm. Ms. Jones's blood pressure is 104/86 (usual is 150/88); her pulse is 92, and respirations are 22. Her temperature is 99.4°F. The nurse observes that Ms. Jones has soft, sunken eyeballs; her tongue is dry and furrowed; and her skin is dry, with poor skin turgor. Her blood glucose level, tested by finger-stick, is 368 mg/dL (her usual blood glucose runs high; between 200 and 250 mg/dL).

Validating and Documenting Findings

Validate the nutritional assessment data you have collected (by asking additional questions, or comparing objective with subjective findings). This is necessary to verify that the data are reliable and accurate. Documenting both normal and abnormal findings will allow for a baseline should findings change later. Following the health care facility or agency policy, document the assessment data.

CASE STUDY

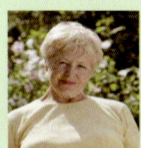

Think back to the case study of Ms. Jones. The home health care nurse completes the following documentation of her assessments.

Biologic Data: HJ, 78 years old, female Caucasian. Widow. Retired elementary school cafeteria assistant. Awake, alert, and oriented. Appropriately asks and responds to questions.

Reason for Seeking Care: "I've lost weight, I'm achy, and my stomach is queasy and sometimes I throw up. I think I have the flu."

History of Present Health Concern: Nausea with occasional vomiting that began 3 days ago. Due to feeling achy, rates her pain as a 2 on a 0–10 scale. Lost 7 lb since last week.

Personal Health History: Diagnosed with type 2 diabetes mellitus 10 years ago, treated with nighttime dose of 13 units Lantus insulin (based on weight of 145 lb) daily and a no-concentrated sweets (NCS) diet. Though in the past has declined to learn to test her blood glucose, states now she is ready to try to learn. No food or medication allergies.

Family History: Uncertain of a family history of diabetes but states her mother may have had "sugar diabetes."

Lifestyle and Health Practices: States does not exercise on a regular basis but tries to walk her dog once a day. Finds it difficult to follow a diet to control her diabetes.

Drinks four to six glasses of water daily. Avoids concentrated sugars, alcohol, and caffeinated drinks. Prior to this illness usually has a bowl of cereal with skim milk and banana for breakfast; a sandwich of low fat meat, cheese, lettuce and low fat chips for lunch. Eats moderate amount of meat, rice, and vegetables for dinner. Reports one to two snacks of fruit, vegetables, pretzels, or popcorn per day.

Physical Assessment Findings: Well-developed body build for age with even distribution of fat and firm muscle. Height: 5 ft, 5 in (165 cm); body frame: medium; weight: 138 lb (58 kg); BMI: 22.5; IBW: 135 lb; waist circumference 30 in; MAC: 28 cm; TSF: 16.8 mm; MAMC: 22.7 cm. Blood pressure is 104/86 (usual is 150/88); pulse is 92, and respirations are 22. Temperature is 99.4°F. Eyeballs are soft and sunken; dry, furrowed tongue; skin dry, with poor skin turgor. Blood glucose level, tested by finger-stick, is 368 mg/dL (her usual blood glucose runs high; between 200 and 250 mg/dL).

ANALYSIS OF DATA: DIAGNOSTIC REASONING

After collecting subjective and objective data pertaining to the nutritional and hydration status, identify abnormal findings and client strengths using diagnostic reasoning. Next, cluster the data to reveal any significant patterns or abnormalities.

Selected Nursing Diagnoses

Following is a listing of selected nursing diagnoses (health promotion risk, or actual) that you may observe when analyzing data collected for a nutritional assessment.

Health Promotion Diagnoses

- Readiness for Enhanced Health Management related to desire and request to learn more about testing blood glucose level
- Readiness for Enhanced Fluid Volume related to a desire for information pertaining to a need for increased fluids

Risk Diagnoses

- Risk for Deficient Fluid Volume related to impending dehydration secondary to nausea, vomiting, and voiding large quantities of urine
- Risk for Obesity related to increasing sedentary lifestyle and decreasing metabolic demands

Actual Diagnoses

- Disturbed Body Image related to recent weight loss
- Powerlessness related to inability to adhere to prescribed diet
- Imbalanced Nutrition: Less Than Body Requirements related to nausea, vomiting, and lack of appetite associated malignant or cancerous cachexia
- Deficient Fluid Volume related to nausea and vomiting

TABLE 13-8 Laboratory Values that Reflect Malnutrition

Laboratory Value	Normal Range	Abnormal Range	Contributing Factors
Fasting blood sugar (FBS) or blood glucose level	Adult: 65–99 mg/dL	Prediabetes: 100–135 mg/dL Critical FBS levels: <40 mg/dL or >400 mg/dL	Increased in diabetes mellitus
Hemoglobin A1c (glycosylated hemoglobin)	Nondiabetic: 4–6% Optimal diabetic control ≤7%	Correlation between % A1c and mean glucose level 6% = 126 7% = 154 8% = 183 9% = 212 10% = 240 11% = 269 12% = 298 (Group Health Foundation, 2014)	Increased in diabetes mellitus
Hemoglobin (identifies iron-carrying capacity of the blood; test helps identify anemia, malnutrition, and hydration status)	Males: 13–18 g/dL Females: 13–16 g/dL	Males: ≤13 g/dL Females: ≤11 g/dL	Increased with dehydration or polycythemia
Hematocrit (identifies volume of red blood cells/L of blood)	Males: 40—52% Females: 36–48% (Normal is usually about three times the hemoglobin level [i.e., the Hct:Hgb ratio is 1:3])	Males: ≤39% Females: ≤35%	Decreased with overhydration and blood loss, poor dietary intake of iron, protein, and certain vitamins
Serum albumin level (half-life of 14–20 days)	3.5–5.5 g/dL	Mild depletion: 2.8–3.5 Moderate depletion: 2.1–2.7 Severe depletion <2.1	Increased with dehydration. Decreased with overhydration, malnutrition, and liver disease.
Total protein level (includes globulins)	6–8 g/dL	<5.0 g/dL	Decreased in pregnancy, burns and such disorders as chronic alcoholism, cirrhosis, Crohn disease and ulcerative colitis, heart failure, malnutrition, and neoplasms. Increased with dehydration and other disorders such as some types of chronic liver disease and myeloma.
Prealbumin: Transport protein for thyroxin (T4); short half-life makes it more sensitive to changes in protein stores (half-life of 3–5 days).	15–30 mg/dL	Mild depletion: 10–15 Moderate depletion: 5–10 Severe depletion: <5	Decreased with undernutrition and malnutrition.
Transferrin: Transport protein for iron; may be more sensitive indicator of visceral protein stores than albumin because of its shorter half-life.	200–400 mg/dL	Mild depletion: 150–199 Moderate depletion: 100–149 Severe depletion: <100	Increased with pregnancy or iron deficiency. Decreased with chronic infection or cirrhosis.

Selected Collaborative Problems

After grouping the data, certain collaborative problems may become apparent. Remember that collaborative problems differ from nursing diagnoses in that they cannot be prevented by nursing interventions. However, these physiologic complications of medical conditions can be detected and monitored by the nurse. In addition, the nurse can use physician- and nurse-prescribed interventions to minimize the complications of these problems. In such situations, the nurse may also have to refer the client for further treatment. Following is a list of collaborative problems that may be identified

when obtaining a nutritional assessment. These problems are worded as Risk for Complications (or RC) followed by the problem.
- RC: Hypertension
- RC: Hyperlipidemia
- RC: Ketoacidosis
- RC: Hyperglycemia
- RC: Diabetes mellitus type 2
- RC: Morbid obesity
- RC: Bulimia; anorexia nervosa
- RC: Short bowel syndrome
- RC: Lactose intolerance
- RC: Iron deficiency anemia (any nutritional deficiency or allergy/intolerance)

Medical Problems

After you group the data, it may become apparent that the client has signs and symptoms that require medical diagnosis and treatment. Refer to a primary care provider as necessary.

CASE STUDY

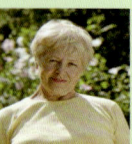

After collecting and analyzing data for Ms. Jones, the nurse determines that the following conclusions are appropriate.

Nursing Diagnoses
- Imbalanced Nutrition: Less than Body Requirements r/t queasiness, nausea, vomiting, diabetes, limited eating × 3 days
- Deficient Fluid Volume r/t nausea, vomiting, urinating large amounts of urine more frequently than normal, effects of high blood glucose on fluid balance, and inadequate fluid intake
- Readiness for Enhanced Health Management r/t statement of willingness to learn to do own blood sugar measurements at home
- Risk for Unstable Blood Glucose Level r/t deficient knowledge of and lack of adherence to diabetes management

Potential Collaborative Problems
- RC: Hypertension
- RC: Hyperlipidemia
- RC: Ketoacidosis
- RC: Hyperglycemia
- RC: Hyperosmolar nonketotic (HHNK) syndrome
- RC: Infection
- RC: Retinopathy
- RC: Diabetic neuropathy
- RC: Diabetic nephropathy

Ms. Jones needs an immediate referral to her physician to manage the acute episode of hyperglycemia, to treat her "flu," and to evaluate her diabetic treatment regimen.

To view an algorithm depicting the process of diagnostic reasoning for this case study, go to thePoint.

Interdisciplinary Verbal Communication of Assessment Findings Using SBAR

SITUATION: HJ, a 78-year-old, Caucasian widow and retired elementary school cafeteria assistant, is seeking care because of a 7-lb weight loss since last week, body aches (2 on 0–10 scale), nausea (relieved somewhat with saltine crackers) and occasional vomiting for 3 days. Urinating "large amounts every 1 to 2 hours" and has dry tongue. States "I am drinking regular (non-diet) carbonated soft drinks to keep my blood sugar up."

BACKGROUND: Diagnosed with type 2 diabetes mellitus 10 years ago, treated with daily nighttime dose of Lantus insulin 13 units (based on 145 lb) and a no-concentrated sweets (NCS) diet. Declined to learn to test her blood glucose in the past but states she now is ready to try to learn. Does not regularly exercise but walks her dog once a day. Has difficulty following a DM diet.

ASSESSMENT: Well-developed body build for age with even distribution of fat and firm muscle. Height: 5 ft, 5 in (165 cm); body frame: medium; weight: 138 lb (58 kg); BMI: 22.5; IBW: 135 lb; waist circumference 30 in; MAC: 28 cm; TSF: 16.8 mm; MAMC: 22.7 cm. Blood pressure is 104/86 (usual is 150/88); pulse is 92, and respirations are 22. Temperature is 99.4°F. Eyeballs are soft and sunken; dry, furrowed tongue; skin dry, with poor skin turgor. Blood glucose level, tested by finger-stick, is 368 mg/dL (her usual blood glucose runs high; between 200 and 250 mg/dL).

Drinks four to six glasses of water daily. Usually has a bowl of cereal with skim milk and banana for breakfast; a sandwich of low fat meat, cheese, lettuce and low fat chips for lunch. Eats moderate amount of meat, rice, and vegetables for dinner. Reports one to two snacks of fruit, vegetables, pretzels, or popcorn per day.

RECOMMENDATION: MJ has Imbalanced Nutrition: less than body requirements r/t queasiness, nausea, vomiting, diabetes, limited eating × 3 days and Deficient Fluid Volume r/t nausea, vomiting, urinating large amounts of urine more frequently than normal, effects of high blood glucose on fluid balance, and inadequate fluid intake. She is ready and willing to learn to do her own blood sugar measurements at home. She needs information on ways to adhere to her diabetes management. MJ needs to be seen by her primary care provider to manage the acute episode of hyperglycemia, to treat her "flu," and to evaluate her diabetic treatment regimen. Without management of her diabetes she will be at risk for hypertension, hyperlipidemia, ketoacidosis, hyperglycemia, HHNK syndrome, infection, retinopathy, diabetic neuropathy, and/or diabetic nephropathy.

| ABNORMAL FINDINGS | 13-1 | Malnutrition |

OBESITY
Overweight Problems

As the amount of body fat increases, especially around the abdomen, so does the risk of:

- Respiratory disease
- Obstructive sleep apnea
- Complications during surgery
- Gallbladder disease
- Stroke
- Non–insulin-dependent (type 2) diabetes
- Some forms of cancer, especially breast and colon
- Coronary heart disease
- Hypertension

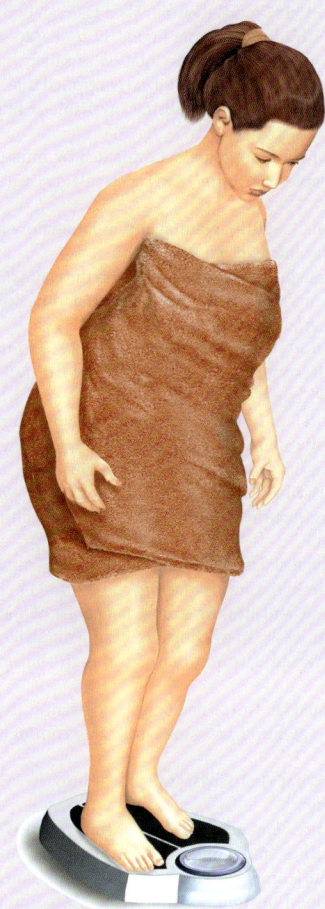

KWASHIORKOR

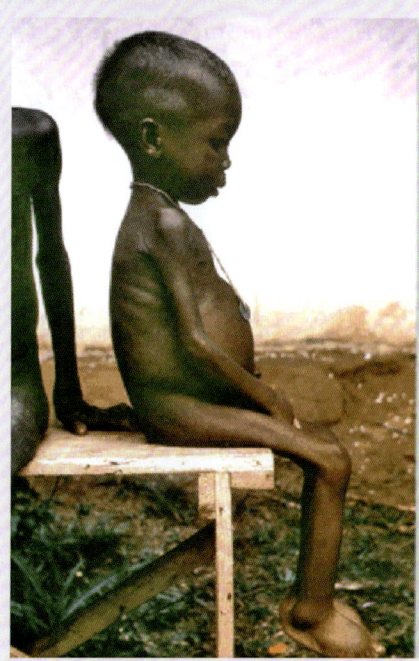

Listless child with kwashiorkor. Note the swollen belly.

MARASMUS

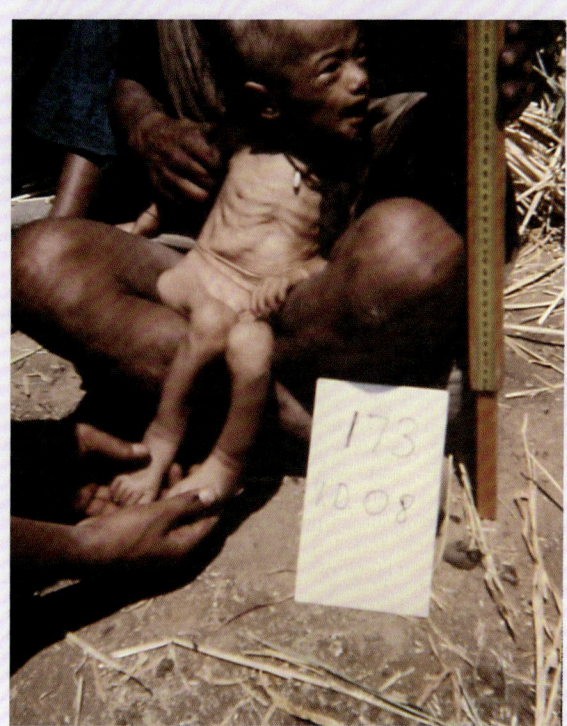

Child suffering with marasmus, which manifests with loose, folded skin and a protruding rib cage.

Illustration credits: Overweight, *from the Anatomical Chart Company. (2001). Maintaining a healthy weight. Philadelphia, PA: Lippincott Williams & Wilkins;* Kwashiorkor, *from the Centers for Disease Control and Prevention Public Health Image Library, Atlanta, Georgia;* Marasmus, *from the Centers for Disease Control and Prevention/Dr. Edward Brink.*

References and Selected Readings

American Cancer Society (ACS). (2016). Guidelines on nutrition and physical activity for cancer prevention. Available at: http://www.cancer.org/acs/groups/cid/documents/webcontent/002577-pdf.pdf

Asieba, I. O. (2016). Racial/ethnic trends in childhood obesity in the United States. *Journal of Childhood Obesity*. Available at http://childhood-obesity.imedpub.com/racialethnic-trends-in-childhood-obesity-in-the-united-states.php?aid=8597

Carpenter, K. (2016). Human nutrition. Available at http://www.britannica.com/science/human-nutrition

Centers for Disease Control and Prevention (CDC). (2014). Estimates of foodborne illness in the United States. Available at http://www.cdc.gov/foodborneburden/

Centers for Disease Control and Prevention (CDC). (2015a). Adult obesity facts. Available at http://www.cdc.gov/obesity/data/adult.html

Centers for Disease Control and Prevention (CDC). (2015b). Childhood obesity facts. Available at http://www.cdc.gov/obesity/data/childhood.html

Centers for Disease Control and Prevention (CDC). (2015c). Foodborne germs and illnesses. Available at http://www.cdc.gov/foodsafety/foodborne-germs.html

Centers for Disease Control and Prevention (CDC). (2015d). New CDC data on foodborne disease outbreaks. Available at http://www.cdc.gov/features/foodborne-diseases-data/

Cleveland Clinic. (2015). Problem foods: Is it allergy or intolerance? Available at http://my.clevelandclinic.org/health/diseases_conditions/hic_Allergy_Overview/hic_Food_Allergies/hic_Problem_Foods_Is_it_an_Allergy_or_Intolerance

Cleveland Clinic. (2016). How an anti-inflammatory diet can relieve pain as you age. Available at https://health.clevelandclinic.org/2015/11/anti-inflammatory-diet-can-relieve-pain-age/

Corleone, J. (2016). Soft belly fat vs. hard belly fat. Available at http://www.livestrong.com/article/338079-soft-belly-fat-vs-hard-belly-fat/

Ellis, M.E. (2013). Cooking up relief: Turmeric and other anti-inflammatory spices. Available at http://www.healthline.com/health/osteoarthritis/turmeric-and-anti-inflammatory-herbs#Overview1

Feinman, R., Pogozelski, W., Astrup, A., et al. (2015). Dietary carbohydrate restriction as the first approach in diabetes management: Critical review and evidence base. *Nutrition*, 31(1), 1–13. Available at http://www.nutritionjrnl.com/article/S0899–9007(14)00332–3/abstract?cc=y=

Food Allergy Research & Education (FARE). (2016). Allergens. Available at https://www.foodallergy.org/allergens

Fox, M. (2016). Who's mad about the new dietary guidelines? Cancer experts, for one. Available at http://www.nbcnews.com/health/health-news/who-s-mad-about-new-dietary-guidelines-cancer-experts-one-n492026

Genetics Home Reference. (2016). What are proteins and what do they do? Available at https://ghr.nlm.nih.gov/primer/howgeneswork/protein

Genetic Society of America. (2016, July 13). Your best diet might depend on your genetics. Available at http://www.eurekalert.org/pub_releases/2016–07/gsoa-ybd071116.php

Government of Canada. (2015). Canada's food guides. Available at http://healthycanadians.gc.ca/eating-nutrition/healthy-eating-saine-alimentation/food-guide-aliment/index-eng.php

Grey, C. (2013). Blood thinners & leafy green vegetables. Available at http://www.livestrong.com/article/541218-blood-thinners-leafy-green-vegetables/

Group Health Foundation. (2014). Why the A1c test is important. Available at http://www.ghc.org/healthAndWellness/?item=/common/healthAndWellness/conditions/diabetes/a1c.html

Gunnars, K. (2016). Protein intake—how much protein should you eat per day? Available at https://authoritynutrition.com/how-much-protein-per-day/

Harvard Medical School. (2015). Foods that fight inflammation. Available at http://www.health.harvard.edu/staying-healthy/foods-that-fight-inflammation

Harvard University, T. H. Chan School of Public Health. (2016). Waist size matters: How abdominal fat increases disease risk. Available at https://www.hsph.harvard.edu/obesity-prevention-source/obesity-definition/abdominal-obesity/

Healthy People 2020. (2016). Nutrition and weight status. Available at https://www.healthypeople.gov/2020/topics-objectives/topic/nutrition-and-weight-status

Heidtman, L. (2014). Foods to avoid when taking blood thinners. Available at http://www.livestrong.com/article/315547-foods-to-avoid-when-taking-blood-thinners/

Juanola-Falgarona, M., Salas-Salvado, J., Ibarrola-Jurado, N., et al. (2014). Effects of the glycemic index diet on weight loss, modulation of satiety, inflammation, and other metabolic risk factors: A randomized controlled trial. *American Journal of Clinical Nutrition*, 100(1), 27–35. Abstract available at http://www.ncbi.nlm.nih.gov/pubmed/24787494

MacClean, J. (2016). The Canada food guide is dominated by ultra-processed foods, says critic. Available at http://www.cantechletter.com/2016/04/canada-food-guide/

Maroon, J., Bost, J., & Maroon, A. (2010). Natural anti-inflammatory agents for pain relief. *Surgical Neurology International*, 1, 80.

Mayo Clinic. (2014a). Glycemic index diet: What's behind the claims? Available at http://www.mayoclinic.org/healthy-lifestyle/nutrition-and-healthy-eating/in-depth/glycemic-index-diet/art-20048478

Mayo Clinic. (2014b). Nutrition and healthy living. Available at http://www.mayoclinic.org/healthy-lifestyle/nutrition-and-healthy-eating/in-depth/carbohydrates/art-20045705?pg=2

Mayo Clinic. (2014c). Nutrition and healthy living: Water: How much should you drink every day? Available at http://www.mayoclinic.org/healthy-lifestyle/nutrition-and-healthy-eating/in-depth/water/art-20044256

Mayo Clinic. (2015a). Dietary fiber: Essentials for a healthy diet. Available at http://www.mayoclinic.org/healthy-lifestyle/nutrition-and-healthy-eating/in-depth/fiber/art-20043983

Mayo Clinic. (2015b). Obesity: Risk factors. Available at http://www.mayoclinic.org/diseases-conditions/obesity/basics/risk-factors/con-20014834

Mayo Clinic. (2017). Nutrition and healthy eating: Functions of water in the body. Available at http://www.mayoclinic.org/healthy-lifestyle/nutrition-and-healthy-eating/multimedia/functions-of-water-in-the-body/img-20005799

McCullogh, M. (2014). Saturated fat: Not so bad or just bad science? *Today's Dietitian*, 16(10), 32. Available at http://www.todaysdietitian.com/newarchives/111114p32.shtml

MedicalNewsToday. (2016). What is obesity? Available at http://www.medicalnewstoday.com/info/obesity

National Academies of Science, Engineering, & Medicine (NASEM). (2016). Daily reference intakes tables and application. Available at http://www.nationalacademies.org/hmd/Home/Global/News%20Announcements/DRI

National Heart, Lung, and Blood Institute (NHLBI). (n.d.). According to waist circumference. Available at http://www.nhlbi.nih.gov/health-pro/guidelines/current/obesity-guidelines/e_textbook/txgd/4142.htm

National Institute of Diabetes and Digestive and Kidney Diseases (NIDDK). (2012). Understanding adult overweight and obesity. Available at https://www.niddk.nih.gov/health-information/health-topics/weight-control/understanding/Pages/understanding-adult-overweight-and-obesity.aspx

Nordqvist, C. (2013). Why BMI is inaccurate and misleading. Available at http://www.medicalnewstoday.com/articles/265215.php

O'Connor, A. (2014). Study questions fat and heart disease link. Available at http://well.blogs.nytimes.com/2014/03/17/study-questions-fat-and-heart-disease-link/

O'Connor, A. (2016). New dietary guidelines urge less sugar for all and less protein for boys and men. Available at http://well.blogs.nytimes.com/2016/01/07/new-diet-guidelines-urge-less-sugar-for-all-and-less-meat-for-boys-and-men/?_r=1

Sboros, M. (2015). Science says Tim Noakes is right on cholesterol – and lots more. Available at http://www.biznews.com/health/2015/02/16/science-says-tim-noakes-is-right-on-cholesterol-lchf-and-a-whole-lot-else/

Springhouse. (2006). *Nutrition made incredibly easy*! (2nd ed.). Philadelphia, PA: Lippincott Williams & Wilkins.

Texas Department of Aging and Disability Services. (2010). DETERMINE your nutritional health Nutritional Screening Initiative (NSI). Available at https://www.dads.state.tx.us/providers/AAA/Forms/standardized/NRA.pdf

The Royal Society of Chemistry. (2016). The spice of life. Available at http://www.rsc.org/chemistryworld/Issues/2009/October/TheSpiceofLife.asp

Tucker, M. (2014). Obesity epidemic is global, a new study confirms. Available at http://www.medscape.com/viewarticle/825858

University of Maryland Medical Center (UMMC). (2007). Possible interactions with: Coenzyme Q10. Available at http://umm.edu/health/medical/altmed/supplement-interaction/possible-interactions-with-coenzyme-q10

U.S. Department of Health and Human Services (UHHS) and U.S. Department of Agriculture. (2015)*USDA. 2015 – 2020 Dietary Guidelines for Americans* (8th ed). (2015). Available at http://health.gov/dietaryguidelines/2015/guidelines/.

U.S. Preventive Services Task Force (USPSTF). (2010). Obesity in children and adolescents: Screening. Available at http://www.uspreventiveservicestaskforce.org/Page/Document/UpdateSummaryFinal/obesity-in-children-and-adolescents-screening

U.S. Preventive Services Task Force (USPSTF). (2012). Obesity in adults: Screening and management. Available at http://www.uspreventiveservicestaskforce.org/Page/Document/UpdateSummaryFinal/obesity-in-adults-screening-and-management

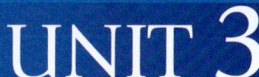

UNIT 3

Nursing Assessment of Physical Systems

14 ASSESSING SKIN, HAIR, AND NAILS

Learning Objectives

1. Review the anatomy and functions of the skin, hair, and nails.
2. Interview clients for an accurate nursing history of the skin, hair, and nails.
3. Discuss risk factors for skin cancer and methicillin-resistant Staphylococcus aureus infections.
4. Use correct techniques to perform a physical assessment of the skin, hair, and nails.
5. Teach a client to perform a self-assessment of the skin, hair, and nails.
6. Differentiate between normal and abnormal findings of the skin, hair, and nails.
7. Clearly document and verbally communicate subjective and objective data findings.
8. Recognize how assessment findings may vary in the older adult.
9. Analyze collected assessment data to formulate valid nursing diagnoses, collaborative problems, and/or referrals.

CASE STUDY

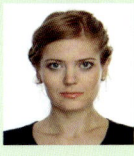

Mary Michaelson is a 29-year-old divorced woman who works as an office manager for a large, prestigious law firm. Ms. Michaelson visits the occupational health nurse at her firm. She reports she recently went to see a doctor because "my hair was falling out in chunks, and I have a red rash on my face and chest. It looks like a bad case of acne." After doing some blood work, her physician diagnosed her condition as discoid lupus erythematosus (DLE). She says she has come to see the occupational health nurse because she feels "so ugly" and she is concerned that she may lose her job because of how she looks. Ms. Michaelson's case will be discussed throughout the chapter.

STRUCTURE AND FUNCTION

The integumentary system consists of the skin, hair, and nails, which are external structures that serve a variety of specialized functions. The sebaceous and sweat glands originating within the skin also have many vital functions. Each structure's function is described separately.

Skin

The skin is the largest organ of the body. It is a physical barrier that protects the underlying tissues and organs from microorganisms, physical trauma, ultraviolet radiation (UVR), and dehydration. It plays a vital role in temperature maintenance, fluid and electrolyte balance, absorption, excretion, sensation, immunity, and vitamin D synthesis. The skin also provides individual identity to a person's appearance.

The skin is thicker on the palms of the hands and soles of the feet, and is continuous with the mucous membranes at the orifices of the body. It is composed of three layers: the epidermal, dermal, and subcutaneous tissue (Fig. 14-1A). Subcutaneous tissue, which contains varying amounts of fat, connects the skin to underlying structures.

Epidermis

The **epidermis** (Fig. 14-1B), the outer layer of skin, is composed of four distinct layers: the **stratum corneum, stratum lucidum, stratum granulosum,** and **stratum germinativum.** The outermost layer consists of dead, keratinized cells that render the skin

247

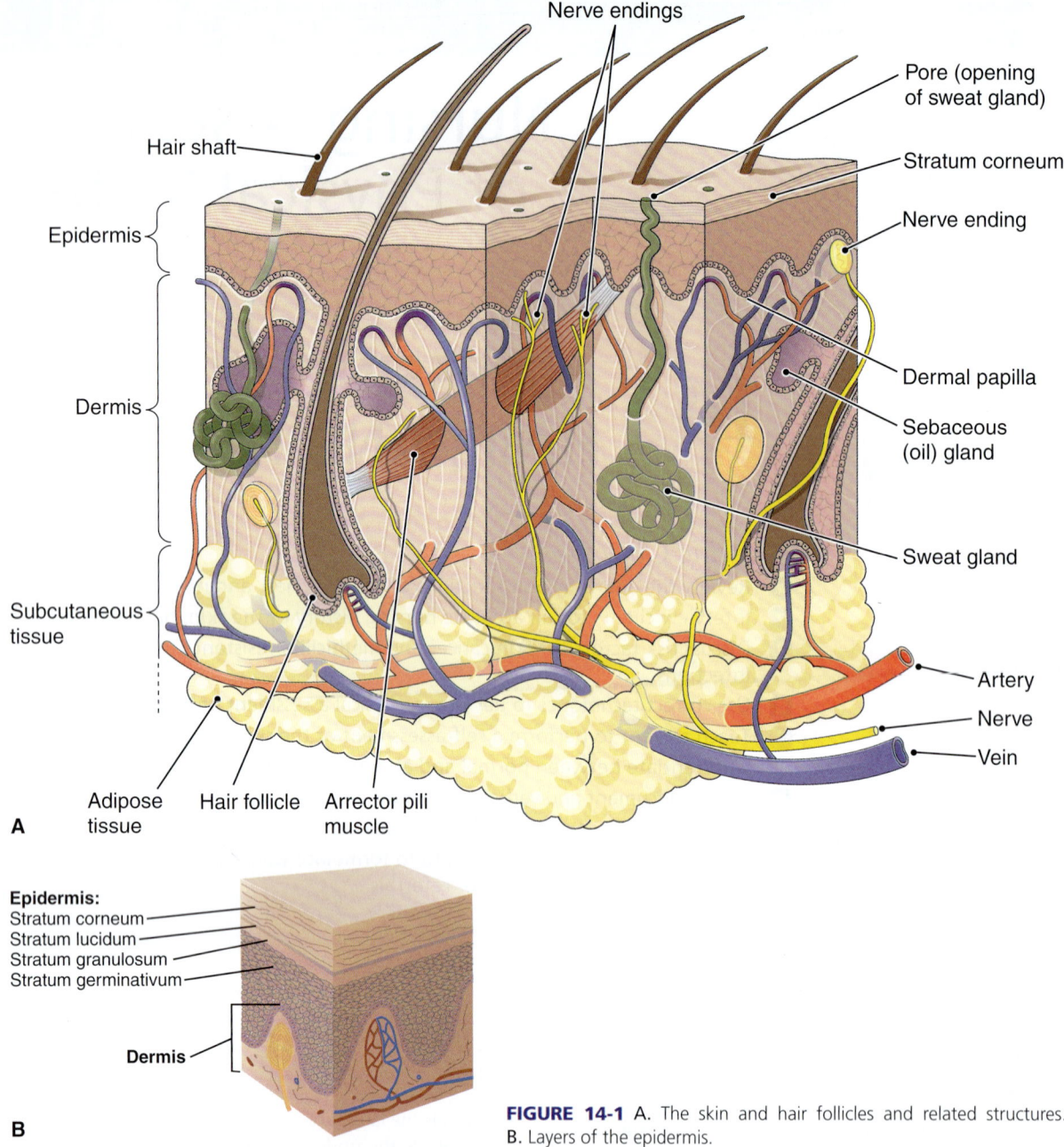

FIGURE 14-1 A. The skin and hair follicles and related structures. B. Layers of the epidermis.

waterproof. (Keratin is a scleroprotein that is insoluble in water. The epidermis, hair, nails, dental enamel, and horny tissues are composed of keratin.) The epidermal layer is almost completely replaced every 3 to 4 weeks. The innermost layer of the epidermis (stratum germinativum) is the only layer that undergoes cell division and contains melanin (brown pigment) and keratin-forming cells. The major determinant of skin color is melanin. Other significant determinants include capillary blood flow, chromophores (carotene and lycopene), and collagen.

Dermis

The inner layer of skin is the **dermis** (see Fig. 14-1B). Dermal papillae connect the dermis to the epidermis. They are visible in the hands and feet, and create the unique pattern of friction ridges commonly known as fingerprints. The dermis is a well-vascularized, connective tissue layer containing collagen, elastic fibers, nerve endings, and lymph vessels. It is also the origin of sebaceous glands, sweat glands, and hair follicles.

Sebaceous Glands

The **sebaceous glands** (see Fig. 14-1A) are attached to hair follicles and, therefore, are present over most of the body, excluding the soles and palms. They secrete an oily substance called **sebum** that waterproofs the hair and skin.

Sweat Glands

The two types of **sweat glands** (see Fig. 14-1A) are eccrine and apocrine glands. The **eccrine glands** are located over the entire skin. Their primary function is secretion of sweat and thermoregulation, which is accomplished by evaporation of sweat from the skin surface. The **apocrine glands** are associated with hair follicles in the axillae, perineum, and areolae of the breasts. Apocrine glands are small and nonfunctional until puberty, at which time they are activated and secrete a milky sweat. The interaction of sweat with skin bacteria produces a characteristic body odor. In women, apocrine secretions are linked with the menstrual cycle.

Subcutaneous Tissue

Beneath the dermis lies the **subcutaneous tissue,** a loose connective tissue containing fat cells, blood vessels, nerves, and the remaining portions of sweat glands and hair follicles (see Fig. 14-1A). The subcutaneous tissue stores fat as an energy reserve, provides insulation to conserve internal body heat, serves as a cushion to protect bones and internal organs, and contains vascular pathways for the supply of nutrients and removal of waste products to and from the skin.

Hair

Hair consists of layers of keratinized cells, found over much of the body except for the lips, nipples, soles of the feet, palms of the hands, labia minora, and penis. Hair develops within a sheath of epidermal cells called the **hair follicle.** Hair growth occurs at the base of the follicle, where cells in the hair bulb are nourished by dermal blood vessels. The hair shaft is visible above the skin; the hair root is surrounded by the hair follicle (see Fig. 14-1A). Attached to the follicle are the arrector pili muscles, which contract in response to cold or fright, decreasing skin surface area and causing the hair to stand erect (goose flesh).

There are two general types of hair: vellus and terminal. **Vellus hair (peach fuzz)** is short, pale, fine, and present over much of the body. **Terminal hair** (particularly scalp and eyebrows) is longer, generally darker, and coarser than vellus hair. Puberty initiates the growth of additional terminal hair in both sexes on the axillae, perineum, and legs. Hair color varies and is determined by the type and amount of pigment (melanin and pheomelanin) production. A reduction in production of pigment results in gray or white hair.

Vellus hair provides thermoregulation by wicking sweat away from the body. Hair on the head protects the scalp, provides insulation, and allows for self-expression. Nasal hair, auditory canal hair, eyelashes, and eyebrows filter dust and other airborne debris.

Nails

The nails, located on the distal phalanges of fingers and toes, are hard, transparent plates of keratinized epidermal cells that grow from the **cuticle** (Fig. 14-2). The **nail body** extends over the entire nail bed and has a pink tinge as a result of blood vessels underneath. The **lunula** is a crescent-shaped area

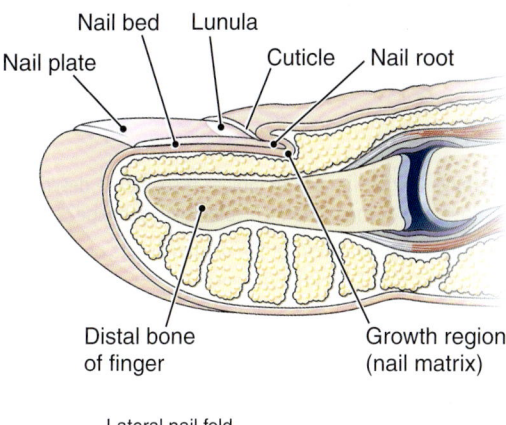
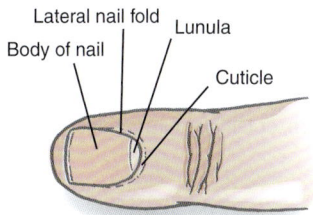

FIGURE 14-2 The nail and related structures.

located at the base of the nail. It is the visible aspect of the nail matrix. The nails protect the distal ends of the fingers and toes, enhance precise movement of the digits, and allow for an extended precision grip.

HEALTH ASSESSMENT

Collecting Subjective Data: The Nursing Health History

Diseases and disorders of the skin, hair, and nails may be local or caused by an underlying systemic condition. To perform a complete and accurate assessment it is important to collect data about current symptoms, the client's past and family history, and lifestyle and health practices. The information obtained provides clues to the client's overall level of functioning in relation to the skin, hair, and nails.

Ask questions in a straightforward manner. Keep in mind that a nonjudgmental, sensitive approach is needed if the client has abnormalities that may be associated with poor hygiene or unhealthy behaviors. Also, some skin disorders might be highly visible and potentially damaging to the person's body image and self-concept.

History of Present Health Concern	
QUESTION	**RATIONALE**
Skin	
Are you experiencing any current skin problems such as rashes, lesions, dryness, oiliness, drainage, bruising, swelling, or changes in skin color? What aggravates the problem? What relieves it?	Any of these symptoms may be related to a pathologic skin condition. Swelling, bruises, welts, or burns may indicate accidents, trauma or abuse. If these injuries cannot be explained or do not match the symptoms, or the client's explanation seems unbelievable or vague, physical abuse should be suspected. Dry, pruritic skin; stretch marks, skin tags, dark patches, and skin infections are common in obese clients (Iarocci, 2015).

Continued on following page

History of Present Health Concern (Continued)

QUESTION	RATIONALE
Skin (Continued)	
Do you have any birthmarks or moles? If so, please describe them. Have any of them changed color, size, or shape? Do you know how to check for the warning signs or characteristics (ABCDE's) of skin cancer?	Establishing normal or baseline data allows future variations to be detected. Multiple or atypical moles increase one's risk for skin cancer (American Academy of Dermatology, 2015). A change in the appearance or bleeding of any skin-lesion, especially a mole, may indicate cancer. Asymmetry, irregular borders, color variations, diameter greater than 1/4 inch or 6 mm and evolving or changing over time are characteristics of cancerous lesions (Skin Cancer Foundation, 2015a). The Skin Cancer Foundations website shows images of skin cancer (see http://www.skincancer.org/skin-cancer-information/melanoma/melanoma-warning-signs-and-images/do-you-know-your-abcdes#panel1-4).
Have you noticed any change in your ability to feel pain, pressure, light touch, or temperature variations?	Changes in sensation or temperature may indicate vascular or neurologic problems such as peripheral neuropathy related to diabetes mellitus or arterial occlusive disease. Decreased sensation may put the client at risk for developing pressure ulcers, impaired skin integrity, and skin infections.
Are you experiencing any pain, itching, tingling, or numbness?	Pruritus may be seen with dry skin, drug reactions, allergies, lice, tinea, insect bites, uremia, or obstructive jaundice. Abnormal sensations of tingling, pricking, or burning are referred to as paresthesia. Numbness or dulling of the sensations of pain, temperature, and touch to the feet may be seen in diabetic peripheral neuropathy.
Are you taking any medications (prescribed or "over the counter"), using any ointments or creams, herbal or nutritional supplements, or vitamins? If so, how long have you been taking each of these?	Some medications can cause a photosensitivity reaction if the skin is exposed to UV light. It often appears 24 hours after taking the medication and leaves after discontinuing the medication. Some clients may exhibit allergic skin reaction(s) to specific drugs, creams, or ointments.
Do you have trouble controlling body odor? Do you perceive yourself to have excessive perspiration?	Poor hygiene practices may account for body odor, and health education may be indicated. Uncontrolled body odor or excessive or insufficient perspiration (excessive perspiration: hyperhidrosis) may indicate an abnormality of the sweat glands or an endocrine problem such as hypothyroidism or hyperthyroidism. **OLDER ADULT CONSIDERATIONS** Perspiration decreases with aging because sweat gland activity decreases. **CULTURAL CONSIDERATIONS** Because of decreased sweat production, most Asians and Native Americans have mild to no body odor, whereas Caucasians and African Americans tend to have a strong body odor unless they use antiperspirant or deodorant products. Any strong body odor may indicate an abnormality (Martin et al., 2010).
Hair and Nails	
Have you had any hair loss or change in the condition of your hair? Describe.	Patchy hair loss may accompany infections, stress, hairstyles that put stress on hair roots, and some types of chemotherapy. Generalized hair loss may be seen in various systemic illnesses such as hypothyroidism and in clients receiving certain types of chemotherapy or radiation therapy. Certain medications can also contribute to hair loss. Also common with malabsorption syndromes, malnutrition, anorexia nervosa, and bulimia. Also common after gastric by-pass surgery. Hair loss is common in aging. The rate of hair growth slows and hair strands become thinner. Some hair follicles stop producing hair. A receding hairline or male pattern baldness may occur with aging. See the Norwood Scale for male pattern baldness (American Hair Loss Association, http://www.americanhairloss.org/men_hair_loss/the_norwood_scale.asp).

QUESTION	RATIONALE
Have you had any change in the condition or appearance of your nails? Describe.	Nail changes may be seen in systemic disorders such as malnutrition or with local irritation (e.g., nail biting).
	Bacterial infections cause green, black, or brown nail discoloration. Yellow, thick, crumbling nails are seen in fungal infections. Yeast infections cause a white color and separation of the nail plate from the nail bed.
	It takes 6 months to totally replace a fingernail and 12 months to totally replace a toenail.

Personal Health History

QUESTION	RATIONALE
Do you recall having severe sunburns as a child?	Severe sunburns as a child are a risk factor for skin cancer (The Skin Cancer Foundation, 2015b).
Describe any previous problems with skin, hair, or nails, including any treatment or surgery and its effectiveness.	Current problems may be a recurrence of previous ones. Visible scars may be explained by previous problems.
Have you had any recent hospitalizations or surgeries?	Hospitalization increases the client's risk for a hospital-acquired infection, such as methicillin-resistant *Staphylococcus aureus* (MRSA) (see Evidence-Based Practice 14-1).
	Major surgery or illness can cause temporary cessation of hair and nail growth.
Have you ever had any allergic skin reactions to food, medications, plants, or other environmental substances?	Various types of allergens can precipitate a variety of skin eruptions.
Have you had a recent viral or bacterial illness?	Some skin rashes or lesions may be related to viruses or bacteria.
For female clients: Are you pregnant? Are your menstrual periods regular?	Some skin and hair conditions can result from hormonal imbalance. See Chapter 29, Assessing Childbearing Women for changes to skin, hair, and nails associated with hormonal changes of pregnancy or hormonal imbalances.
Do you have a history of self-injury?	Dermatologic disorders and psychiatric conditions affect each other. Cutting or scratching the skin and skin breakouts and rashes often have an associated psychiatric condition (Greener, 2014).
	Anxiety and depression in and of themselves are not typically associated with skin issues. Self-injury, on the other hand, is classically associated with cutting, burning, or scratching and is an unhealthy way to cope with emotional pain, intense anger, and frustration. This may occur with anxiety, depression, and/or obsessive/compulsive disorder (OCD).

Family History

QUESTION	RATIONALE
Has anyone in your family had a recent illness, rash, or other skin problem or allergy? Describe.	Viruses (e.g., chickenpox, measles) can be highly contagious. Acne and atopic dermatitis tend to be familial. Some allergies may be identified from family history.
Has anyone in your family had skin cancer?	A genetic component is associated with skin cancer, especially malignant melanoma (National Cancer Institute, 2015a).
Do you have a family history of keloids?	Keloids are more common in skin of color (African, African-American, Asian descent) and in persons with a family history of keloids. Early studies indicate that keloids are more likely to form between ages 11 and 25, especially before age 18 (Tigran, 2014). Ear piercing, body piercing, and other skin wounds cause keloid formation in genetically susceptible individuals.

Continued on following page

Lifestyle and Health Practices

QUESTION	RATIONALE
Hair and Nails (Continued)	
Do you sunbathe? What is the frequency and duration of sun or tanning-booth exposure? Do you use sun block and if so what type (specify SPF)?	Excessive or unprotected exposure to ultraviolet (UV) radiation can cause premature aging of skin and increase the risk of skin cancer. Hair can also be damaged by too much sun (American Cancer Society, 2015b) (see Evidence-Based Practice 14-2).
Do you perform skin self-examination once a month?	If clients do not know how to inspect the skin, teach them how to recognize suspicious lesions early (see Box 14-1).
In your daily activities, are you regularly exposed to chemicals or irritants that may harm the skin (e.g., coal, tar, pitch, creosote, arsenic compounds, radium, alcohol, hand foam, latex, bleach, peroxide)?	Any of these substances have the potential to irritate or damage the skin, hair, or nails and increase one's risk for skin cancer (American Cancer Society, 2016).
Do you spend long periods of time sitting or lying in one position?	Older, disabled, or immobile clients who spend long periods of time in one position are at risk for impaired skin integrity (see Evidence-Based Practice 14-3).
Have you had any exposure to extreme temperatures?	Temperature extremes affect the blood supply to the skin and can damage the skin layers. Examples include frostbite and burns.
Do you have any body piercings?	Piercing needles may place clients at risk for infection.
Do you have any tattoos? ◎ **CLINICAL TIP** There are five major types of tattoos: 1. Traumatic, caused by debris embedded in skin, as after a motorcycle accident 2. Amateur, placed by nonprofessionals using India ink with a pin 3. Professional, applied by a professional or skilled tattoo artist 4. Medical, used to delineate a landmark for radiation 5. Cosmetic, used for permanent eyeliner, lipstick, hair, blush, or eyebrows	Risks involved with tattooing include infection, allergic reactions, formation of granulomas, keloid formation, swelling or burning sensations when undergoing magnetic resonance imagining (MRI) (Mayo Clinic, 2015b). Also, tattoo removal is often painful and may cause scarring. Note that tattoos have been associated with hepatitis C infection (Gardner, 2014). Clients should be informed regarding these risks.
What is your daily routine for skin, hair, and nail care? What products do you use (e.g., soaps, lotions, oils, cosmetics, self-tanning products, razor type, hair spray, shampoo, hair coloring, nail enamel)? How do you cut your nails?	Regular habits provide information on hygiene and lifestyle. 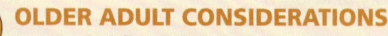 **OLDER ADULT CONSIDERATIONS** Decreased flexibility and mobility may impair the ability of some elderly clients to maintain proper hygiene practices, such as nail cutting, bathing, and hair care. The products used may also be a cause of an abnormality. Certain soaps may be drying. It is preferable to apply lotions to moist or slightly wet skin. Improper nail-cutting technique can lead to ingrown nails or infection.

QUESTION	RATIONALE
What kinds of foods do you consume in a typical day? How much fluid do you drink each day?	A balanced diet is necessary for healthy skin, hair, and nails. Adequate fluid intake is required to maintain skin elasticity.
Do you have a history of smoking and/or drinking alcohol?	A significant association between cigarette smoking, alcohol consumption, and psoriasis has been found (National Psoriasis Foundation, 2015).
Do skin problems limit any of your normal activities?	Allergens (poison oak, poison ivy) may limit certain activities such as hiking, camping, and gardening. Moreover, exposure to the sun can aggravate conditions such as scleroderma. In addition, general home maintenance (e.g., cleaning, car washing) may expose the client to certain cleaning products to which the client is sensitive or allergic.
Describe any skin disorder that prevents you from enjoying your relationships.	Skin, hair, or nail problems, especially if visible, may impair the client's ability to interact comfortably with others because of embarrassment or perceived/actual rejection by others. **CULTURAL CONSIDERATIONS** Social stigma toward some dermatologic disorders is widespread. Dermatologic diseases are found to affect quality of life in many cultures, especially of females (Ahmed et al., 2013).
How much stress do you have in your life? Describe.	Stress can cause or exacerbate skin abnormalities.

14-1 EVIDENCE-BASED HEALTH PROMOTION AND DISEASE PREVENTION: METHICILLIN-RESISTANT *STAPHYLOCOCCUS AUREUS* INFECTIONS

INTRODUCTION

Methicillin-resistant *Staphylococcus aureus* (MRSA), first noted in 1961, is a type of infection that is resistant to methicillin, as well as to many other antibiotics. MRSA can be categorized into hospital-acquired or community-acquired infections. Hospital-acquired MRSA occurs in individuals who are or have been hospitalized within the past year, receive care in a same-day surgery center or ambulatory outpatient care clinic, or are residents of long-term care facilities. MRSA hospital-acquired infections (HAIs) are associated with invasive medical devices, such as urinary catheters, as well as with surgical incisions, pneumonia, and bloodstream infections. Community-acquired MRSA occurs in individuals who have had recent medical procedures and may be otherwise healthy.

HAIs, MRSA, and other organism-based infections are a growing concern to health care professionals. Various processes to control HAIs have been put in place by US hospitals. The greatest success has been the "MRSA bundle" approach of the Veterans Administration hospitals and long-term care facilities, where MRSA infections between 2009 and 2012 fell by 69% for VA hospitals and 36% for long-term care facilities. The "MRSA bundle" includes nasal swabbing and testing for MRSA colonization in patients, contact precautions, hand hygiene, and an institutional culture of infection control for all personnel in contact with patients. The "MRSA bundle" has also been successful in detecting other pathogens and the VA's success in reducing HAIs generally is notable (Veterans Administration Health Services Research & Development, 2015).

HEALTHY PEOPLE 2020 GOAL

Prevent, reduce, and ultimately eliminate health care–associated infections (HAIs).

SCREENING

Some acute care institutions screen for MRSA, particularly in the case of ICU admissions. More institutions are using protocols for MRSA and other HAI screening since the VA "MRSA bundle" has worked so well, even though this is not a universally recommended/implemented practice.

RISK ASSESSMENT

The greatest risk factor for MRSA is impaired skin integrity.

Assess for Hospital-acquired MRSA Risk Factors
- Having an invasive medical device
- Residing in a long-term care facility
- Presence of a MRSA-positive person in the facility

Assess for Community-acquired MRSA Risk Factors
- Participating in contact sports
- Sharing personal items such as towels or razors
- Suppression of the immune system function (e.g., HIV, cancer, or chemotherapy)
- Residing in unsanitary or crowded living conditions (dormitories or military barracks)
- Working in the health care industry
- Receiving antibiotics within the past 3 to 6 months
- Young or advanced age
- Men having sex with men
- Hemodialysis

CLIENT EDUCATION

Teach Clients
- Keep wounds covered.
- Do not share personal items.
- Avoid unsanitary or unsafe nail care practices.
- If treatment has been started, do not stop until recovery is complete.
- Use Universal Precautions when touching others to avoid contact with contaminated body fluids. Wash your hands.
- Clean sports equipment between uses to avoid spread of infection.
- Wash clothes, sheets, towels, razors, and other personal items before and after use.
- Clean hands often.

14-2 EVIDENCE-BASED HEALTH PROMOTION AND DISEASE PREVENTION: SKIN CANCER

INTRODUCTION

Skin cancer is the most common of cancers. It occurs in three types: melanoma, basal cell carcinoma (BCC), and squamous cell carcinoma (SCC). BCC and SCC are nonmelanomas. Precursor lesions occur for some melanomas (benign or dysplastic nevi) and for invasive SCC (actinic keratoses or SCC in situ), but there are no precursor lesions for BCC.

BCC is the most common skin cancer in Caucasians, whereas SCC is the most common in darker skin. Asians are less susceptible to skin cancers. African Americans, Asians, and Hispanics, although less susceptible than Caucasians, are susceptible to melanoma (The Skin Cancer Foundation, 2015d). Asian Americans and African Americans tend to present with more advanced disease at diagnosis than do Caucasians. The Foundations also note that African Americans, Asians, Filipinos, Indonesians, and native Hawaiians develop melanomas on nonexposed skin with less pigmentation, such as on palms, soles, mucous membranes, and nail regions.

Nonmelanocyte skin cancers are the most common worldwide and are also increasing in populations heavily exposed to sunlight, especially in areas of ozone depletion. Malignant melanoma is the most serious skin cancer, and it is expected to account for 76,380 cases in 2016 (American Cancer Society, 2016).

HEALTHY PEOPLE 2020 GOALS

- Reduce melanoma cancer death rate.
- Increase participation in reducing exposure to harmful UV irradiation, sunburn, and use of artificial sources of UV light for tanning.
- Increase participation in protective measures that may reduce the risk of skin cancer.

SCREENING

According to the American Cancer Society (2015a), American Academy of Dermatology (2015), the National Cancer Institute (2015b), the Skin Cancer Foundation (2015a), and a number of other organizations, all people over 20 years of age should have a periodic examination of their skin by a primary care provider, and all should do routine self-examinations (see Box 14-1) for oneself or of a child. These recommendations are not supported by the U.S. Preventive Health Task Force report (U. S. Preventive Services Task Force, 2009), which provides broad reviews of studies showing insufficient evidence to support the benefits or harm of using a whole-body skin examination either by a primary care provider or self-examination for the early detection of cutaneous melanoma, BCC, or SCC in the adult general population.

RISK ASSESSMENT

Assess for the Following Risk Factors

- Sun exposure, especially intermittent pattern with sunburn; risk increases if excessive sun exposure and sunburns began in childhood. Intermittent exposure to the sun or UVR is associated with greatest risk for melanoma and for BCC, but overall amount of exposure is thought to be associated with SCC. SCC is most common on body sites with very heavy sun exposure, whereas BCC is most common on sites with moderate exposure (e.g., upper trunk or women's lower legs)
- Nonsolar sources of UVR (tanning booth, sunlamps, high-UV geographical areas). Indoor tanning has been shown to raise the risk of developing melanoma by 74% (The Skin Cancer Foundation, 2015c)
- Medical therapies such as PUVA and ionizing radiation
- Family or personal history and genetic susceptibility (especially for malignant melanoma)
- Moles, especially atypical lesions
- Pigmentation irregularities (albinism, burn scars)
- Fair skin that burns and freckles easily; light hair; light eyes
- Age; risk increases with increasing age
- Actinic keratoses
- Male gender (for nonmelanoma cancers), especially white men over 50
- Chemical exposure (arsenic, tar, coal, paraffin, some oils for nonmelanoma cancers)
- Human papillomavirus (nonmelanoma cancers)
- Xeroderma pigmentosum (rare, inherited condition)
- Long-term skin inflammation or injury (nonmelanoma)
- Alcohol intake (BCC); smoking (SCC)
- Inadequate niacin (vitamin B_3) in diet
- Bowen disease (scaly or thickened patch) (SCC)
- Depressed immune system

CLIENT EDUCATION

Teach Clients

- Reduce sun exposure; seek shade.
- Always use sunscreen (SPF 15 or higher) when sun exposure is anticipated.
- Wear long-sleeved shirts and wide-brimmed hats.
- Wear sunglasses that wrap around.
- Avoid sunburns.
- Understand the link between sun exposure and skin cancer and the accumulating effects of sun exposure on developing cancers.
- Examine the skin for suspected lesions. If there is anything unusual, seek professional advice as soon as possible.
- Ensure that diet is adequate in vitamin B_3 (M.D. Anderson Cancer Center, 2015).

NOTE: see Melanoma Risk Assessment Tool at http://www.cancer.gov/melanomarisktool/results_f.aspx?region=1&sex=2&race=1&age=62&sunburn=-1000&complexion=2&tanning=2&large_moles=-1000&small_moles_males=-1000&small_moles_females=3&freckling=2&solar_damage=-1000

BOX 14-1 SELF-ASSESSMENT: HOW TO EXAMINE YOUR OWN SKIN

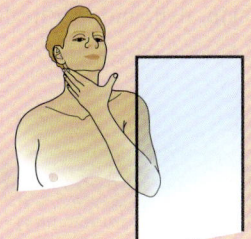
Examine head and face using one or both mirrors.
Use a blow dryer to inspect scalp.

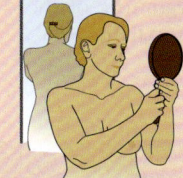
With back to the mirror, use hand mirror to inspect back of neck, shoulders, upper arms, back, buttocks, legs.

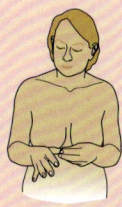
Check hands, including nails. In full-length mirror, examine elbows, arms and underarms.

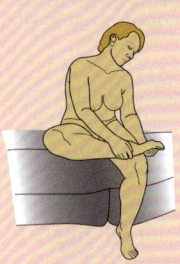
Sitting down, check legs and feet, including soles, heels, and nails.
Use hand mirror to examine genitals.

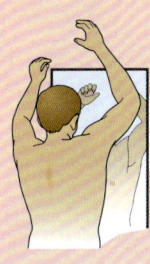
Focus on neck, chest, torso.
Women: check under breasts.

14-3 EVIDENCE-BASED HEALTH PROMOTION AND DISEASE PREVENTION: PRESSURE ULCERS

INTRODUCTION

Pressure ulcers are a major cause of morbidity and mortality. The most significant contributing factor to pressure ulcer development is unrelieved pressure, but friction and shear also can contribute or worsen the condition. Prevalence of pressure ulcers varies by bed type and clinical area, but occur more frequently in critical care, long-term care facilities, and in patients at high risk, such as those on prolonged bed rest (Berlowitz, 2014). However, a new device being developed by the U.S. Department of Veterans Affairs and General Electric may be successful at ending the problem of pressure ulcers in hospitals (U.S. Department of Veterans Affairs, 2015). Until such a device is developed, careful screening and prevention are needed.

Pressure ulcers are costly both to the client and institution in terms of pain and suffering as well as dollars. Early assessment can lead to the key element of prevention.

HEALTHY PEOPLE 2020 GOAL

Reduce the rate of pressure ulcer-related hospitalizations.

In addition to the Healthy People goal, the National Quality Measures Clearing House (2013) has the following goal for inpatients: Increase the percentage of patients with documentation in the medical record that a head-to-toe skin inspection and palpation were completed within 6 hours of admission.

SCREENING

The U.S. Preventive Services Task Force does not have recommendations for pressure ulcer screening. The Institute for Clinical Systems Improvement (2014) recommends a complete skin inspection on admission and a minimum of once every 8 to 12 hours thereafter.

RISK ASSESSMENT

The Braden Scale is often used for risk assessment (see Assessment Tool 14-1). Assess for the following risk factors:

- Prolonged pressure to body, especially bony prominences
- Decreased/absent perception or sensation
- Decreased/absent mobility
- Increased moisture
- Increased/decreased nutrition
- Friction or shearing forces
- Fragile tissues and skin due to age, vascular incompetence, diabetes mellitus, or body weight (excessive or underweight)

CLIENT EDUCATION

Teach Clients

- Bathe with mild soap or other agent; limit friction; use warm not hot water; follow set bath schedule that is individualized.
- For dry skin: Use moisturizers; avoid low humidity and cold air.
- Avoid vigorous massage; avoid massage over bony prominences.
- Complete activity as directed.
- Take nutritional supplementation, as directed.
- Use incontinence skin cleansing methods as needed: gently clean skin of all moisture, urine, feces; avoid continued moisture and dryness with protective barrier products.

For Bed- or Chair-bound Clients

- Self-reposition every 15 minutes (chair) or 2 hours (bed).
- Use repositioning schedule.
- Use pressure mattress or chair cushion.
- Use lifting devices as directed to reduce shear (trapeze bar for patient; lifts for family, if necessary).
- Use positioning with pillows or wedges to avoid bony prominence contact with surfaces and to maintain body alignment; avoid donut-type devices.
- For those who are bed bound, avoid elevating head of bed beyond 30 degrees except for brief periods.

Provide structured teaching for patient, family, and caregivers as necessary.

Recall the case study introduced at the beginning of the chapter. The nurse uses COLDSPA to explore Ms. Michaelson's presenting concerns and obtains a skin, nail, and hair health history.

CASE STUDY

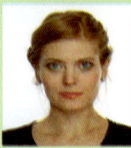

The nurse interviews Ms. Michaelson, using specific probing questions. The client reports a red rash on her face. The nurse explores this health concern using the COLDSPA mnemonic.

Mnemonic	Question	Data Provided
Character	Describe the sign or symptom (feeling, appearance, sound, smell, or taste, if applicable). In this case, describe the rash.	"Flaky red patches that look like acne."
Onset	When did it begin?	6 months ago
Location	Where is it? Does it radiate? Does it occur anywhere else?	On the face, neck, chest, above nipple line, shoulders, and upper back
Duration	How long does it last? Does it recur? How frequently does it recur?	Recurs with no pattern and each episode lasts 2 days to 2 weeks.
Severity	How bad is it? How much does it bother you?	Rates the pain as 0–1 on a 0–10 scale; rates the mental anguish as a 9–10 on a 0–10 scale.
Pattern	What makes it better or worse?	Rash worsens when exposed to sunlight while surfing. Nothing she has tried makes it better.
Associated factors/ How it **A**ffects the client	What other symptoms occur with it? How does it affect you?	Client "feels ugly." Increased level of anxiety related to the disfigurement. Reports areas of hair loss on her scalp where the rash is present.

After exploring the rash, the nurse continues with the present history. Ms. Michaelson denies birthmarks or moles. She also denies any change in ability to feel pain, pressure, light touch, or temperature changes. Ms. Michaelson has not experienced any itching, pain, tingling, or numbness. She denies issues with body odor or perspiration. Ms. Michaelson says that she does not have any tattoos but has pierced earlobes. She describes hair loss with hair "falling out in chunks." She denies any changes in appearance or condition of nails.

Next, the nurse interviews Ms. Michaelson about her past history. She was recently diagnosed with DLE. She reports one episode, 5 years ago, of a fine, raised, reddened, pruritic rash on her trunk after taking ampicillin for an ear infection. She says that the rash and pruritus resolved within 3 days after discontinuation of ampicillin and administration of antihistamines. Ms. Michaelson denies any difficulty swallowing or breathing, or edema of mouth or tongue associated with the incident. She denies any other allergies to food, medication, plants, or environmental substances. She reports a negative family history of acne, atopic dermatitis, communicable disease, skin cancer, or keloids.

Ms. Michaelson denies sunbathing, but does report tanning bed use one to two times weekly year round, and goes surfing in the summertime. She does not perform skin self-examination. She denies exposure to paint, bleach, cleaning products, weed killers, insect repellents, and petroleum. Ms. Michaelson denies long periods of immobility and exposure to extreme temperatures. The nurse asks about her routine for hygiene. She showers in AM and bathes in PM with deodorant soap. She shampoos with baby shampoo and applies conditioner each AM. Ms. Michaelson applies moisturizer to skin after each cleansing and applies antiperspirant twice daily. She shaves legs and axillae with electric razor twice weekly. Ms. Michaelson trims her toenails and fingernails and applies nail enamel weekly. She denies use of chemicals on hair to color, curl, or straighten. The nurse explores her nutritional history. Her 24-hour diet recall consists of: Breakfast—meal-replacement bar and 12 oz. of black coffee; mid-morning snack—one apple; lunch—Lean Cuisine–brand chicken and vegetables, 32 oz. diet Coke, ice cream sandwich; dinner—chicken breast, salad, baked potato with butter and sour cream, brownie; bedtime snack—one-serving bag of pretzels and 8 oz. skim milk.

She tells the nurse she feels ugly and she is concerned that she may lose her job because of how she looks.

Collecting Objective Data: Physical Examination

Physical assessment of the skin, hair, and nails provides data that may reveal local or systemic problems or alterations in a client's self-care activities. Local irritation, trauma, or disease can alter the condition of the skin, hair, or nails. Systemic problems related to impaired circulation, endocrine imbalances, allergic reactions, or respiratory disorders may also be revealed with alterations in the skin, hair, or nails. The appearance of the skin, hair, and nails also provides the nurse with data related to health maintenance and self-care activities such as hygiene, exercise, and nutrition.

A separate, comprehensive skin, hair, and nail examination, preferably at the beginning of a comprehensive physical examination, ensures that you do not inadvertently omit part of the examination. As you inspect and palpate the skin, hair, and nails, pay special attention to lesions and growths.

Preparing the Client

To prepare for the skin, hair, and nail examination, ask the client to remove all clothing and jewelry and put on an examination gown. To respect the client's modesty or desire for privacy, provide a long examination gown or robe. In addition, ask the client to remove nail enamel, artificial nails, wigs, toupees, or hairpieces as appropriate.

Have the client sit comfortably on the examination table or bed for the beginning of the examination. The client may remain in a sitting position for most of the examination. However, to assess the skin on the buttocks and dorsal surfaces of the legs properly, the client may lie on the side or abdomen.

During the skin examination, ensure privacy by exposing only the body part being examined. Make sure that the room is a comfortable temperature. If available, sunlight is best for inspecting the skin. However, a bright light that can be focused on the client works just as well. Keep the room door closed or the bed curtain drawn to provide privacy as necessary. Explain what you are going to do, and answer any questions the client may have. Wear gloves when palpating any lesions because you may be exposed to drainage.

Clients from conservative religious groups (e.g., Orthodox Jews or Muslims) may require that the nurse be the same sex as the client.

Equipment
- Examination light
- Penlight
- Mirror for client's self-examination of skin
- Magnifying glass
- Centimeter ruler
- Gloves
- Wood light
- Examination gown or drape
- Braden Scale for Predicting Pressure Sore Risk
- Pressure Ulcer Scale for Healing (PUSH) tool to measure pressure ulcer healing

Physical Assessment

When preparing to examine the skin, hair, and nails, remember these key points:
- Inspect skin color, temperature, moisture, texture.
- Check skin integrity.
- Be alert for skin lesions.

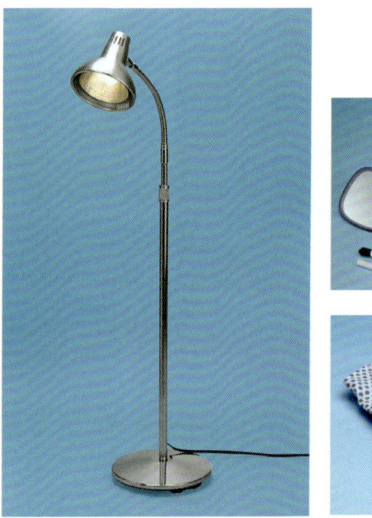
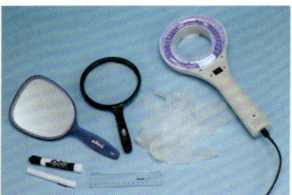
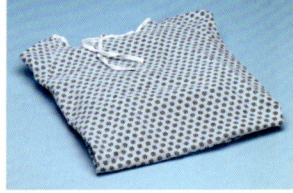

- Evaluate hair condition; loss or unusual growth.
- Note nail bed condition and capillary refill.

General Routine Screening versus Focused Specialty Assessment

The nurse completes all of the general screening for all patients as indicated in the Assessment Procedure box below. Most often the nurse does not perform a total head to toe skin, nail, and scalp examination as would a dermatologist. Yet it is essential that all nurses know how to complete a total skin examination, how to teach the client to perform a skin self-examination, and how to collaborate with other health care professionals to clearly communicate skin findings. The nurse routinely inspects exposed skin areas for temperature, turgor, and edema when caring for the client. If a lesion is noted, further assessment is completed. If the nurse suspects that a client may be at risk for developing a pressure ulcer, the Braden scale should be used to assess the patient's degree of risk. Ordinarily the nurse would not use the PUSH Scale unless a skin ulcer was identified; then the nurse would use the PUSH Scale to further assess and document the degree of skin breakdown.

The nurse also routinely inspects the patient's nails for coloration and grooming. Nail changes are often a sign of other illnesses or conditions. For example, excessive nail biting may be a sign of anxiety. The color and condition of the hair is inspected.

In certain situations, the nurse performs a more detailed examination to include scalp inspection. For example, a school nurse may inspect and palpate the scalp in situations where head lice are suspected. Or if a client reports an extremely itchy, burning scalp, the nurse would inspect and palpate the scalp.

ASSESSMENT PROCEDURE	NORMAL FINDINGS	ABNORMAL FINDINGS

Skin

INSPECTION

Inspect general skin coloration. Keep in mind that the amount of pigment in the skin accounts for the intensity of color as well as hue. Table 14-1 describes the six skin types.

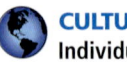 **CULTURAL CONSIDERATIONS**
Individuals with fair complexions are at an increased risk for skin cancer

Inspection reveals evenly colored skin tones without unusual or prominent discolorations.

 CULTURAL CONSIDERATIONS
Small amounts of melanin are common in pale or light skins, while large amounts of melanin are common in olive and darker skins. Carotene accounts for a yellow cast.

 OLDER ADULT CONSIDERATIONS
The older client's skin becomes pale due to decreased melanin production and decreased dermal vascularity.

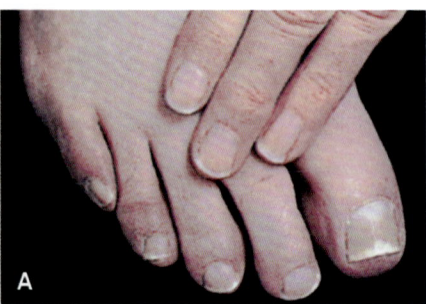
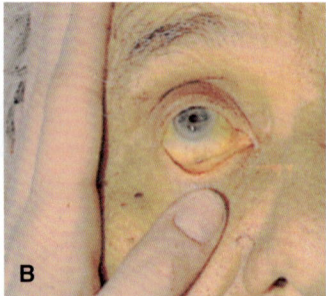
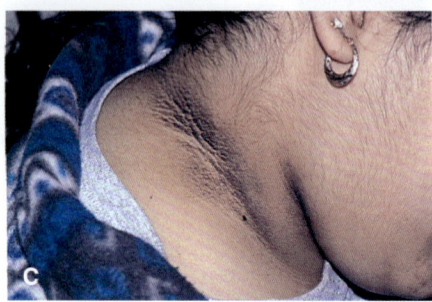

FIGURE 14-3 Abnormal findings for skin coloration: **A.** Bluish cyanotic skin associated with oxygen deficiency. **B.** Jaundice associated with hepatic dysfunction. **C.** Acanthosis nigricans (AN), a linear streak-like pattern in dark-skinned people, suggests diabetes mellitus. (Part C used with permission from Goodheart, H. P., Gonzalez, M. E. (2016). *Goodheart's photoguide of common pediatric and adult skin disorders.* (4th ed.). Philadelphia, PA: Wolters Kluwer.)

Pallor (loss of color) is seen in arterial insufficiency, decreased blood supply, and anemia. Pallid tones vary from pale to ashen without underlying pink.

Cyanosis (Fig. 14-3A) may cause white skin to appear blue-tinged, especially in the perioral, nail bed, and conjunctival areas. Dark skin may appear blue, dull, and lifeless in the same areas.

Central cyanosis results from a cardiopulmonary problem, whereas peripheral cyanosis may be a local problem resulting from vasoconstriction.

🎯 **CLINICAL TIP**
To differentiate between central and peripheral cyanosis, look for central cyanosis in the oral mucosa.

Jaundice (Fig. 14-3B) is characterized by yellow skin tones, ranging from pale to pumpkin, particularly of the sclera, oral mucosa, palms, and soles.

Acanthosis nigricans (Fig. 14-3C) is velvety darkening of skin in body folds and creases, especially the neck, groin, and axilla.

While inspecting skin coloration, note any odors emanating from the skin.

Client has slight or no odor of perspiration, depending on activity.

A strong odor of perspiration or foul odor may indicate disorder of sweat glands. Poor hygiene practices may indicate a need for client teaching or assistance with activities of daily living.

Inspect for color variations. Inspect localized parts of the body, noting any color variation (Fig. 14-4).

Common variations include suntanned areas, freckles, or white patches known as vitiligo (Box 14-2). The variations are due to different amounts of melanin in certain areas. A generalized loss of pigmentation is seen in **albinism.** Dark-skinned clients have lighter-colored palms, soles, nail beds, and lips. Freckle-like or dark streaks of pigmentation are also common in the sclera and nail beds of dark-skinned clients.

Abnormal findings include rashes, such as the reddish (in light-skinned people) or darkened (in dark-skinned people) butterfly rash (also called Malar rash) across the bridge of the nose and cheeks (Fig. 14-5), characteristic of systemic lupus erythematosus (SLE). SLE is seen in a 9:1 female-to-male ratio and is more common in black and Hispanic people (American Autoimmune Association, 2015).

ASSESSMENT PROCEDURE	NORMAL FINDINGS	ABNORMAL FINDINGS
	CULTURAL CONSIDERATIONS Pale or light-skinned clients have darker pigment around nipples, lips, and genitalia.	**CULTURAL CONSIDERATIONS** SLE prevalence is higher in Asians, Afro-Americans, Afro-Caribbeans, and Hispanics in the United States, but infrequent in blacks in Africa (Schur & Hahn, 2015). **Erythema** (skin redness and warmth) is seen in inflammation, allergic reactions, or trauma. **CLINICAL TIP** Erythema in the dark-skinned client may be difficult to see. However, the affected skin feels swollen and warmer than the surrounding skin.
Assess skin integrity. Pay special attention to pressure point areas (Fig. 14-6).	Skin is intact, and there are no reddened areas.	Skin breakdown is initially noted as a reddened area on the skin that may

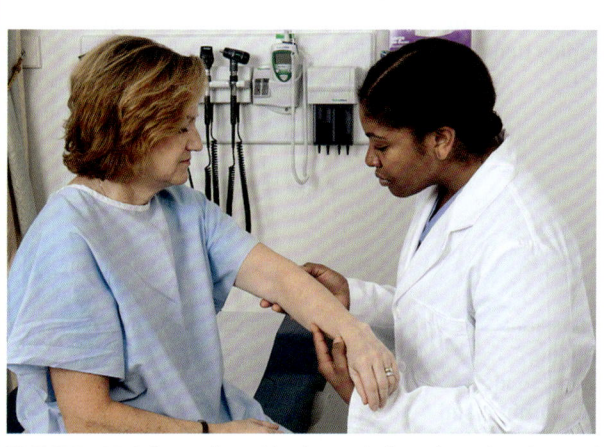

FIGURE 14-4 Inspecting skin for variations in coloration and integrity.

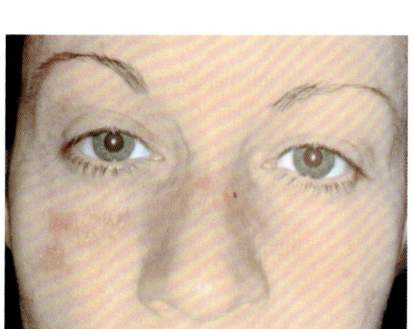

FIGURE 14-5 Characteristic butterfly rash of lupus erythematosus.

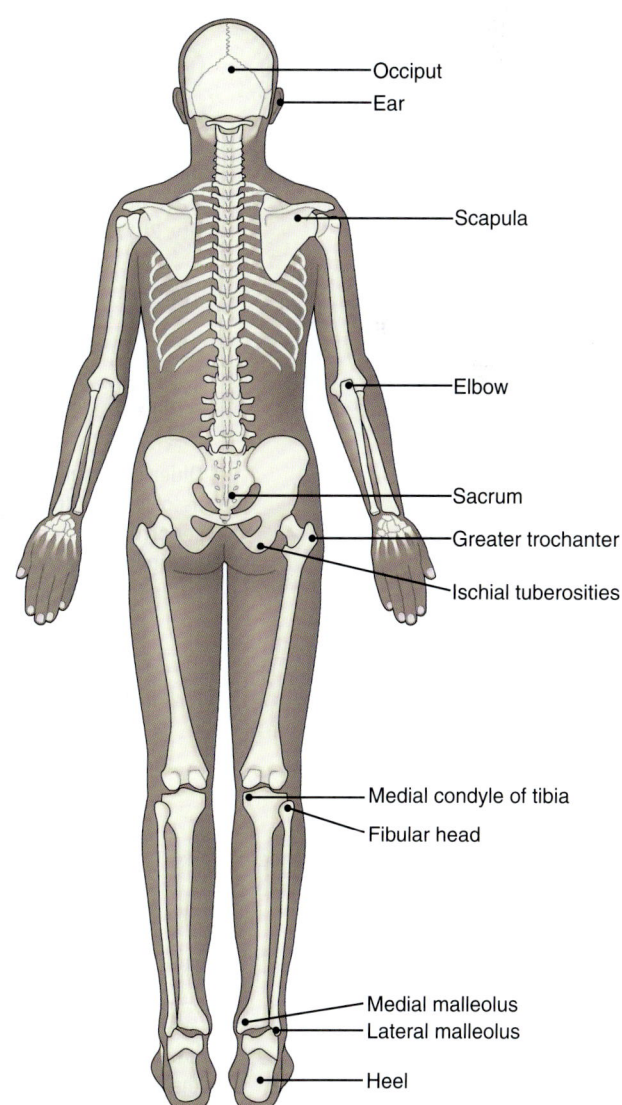

FIGURE 14-6 Common pressure ulcer sites.

Continued on following page

ASSESSMENT PROCEDURE	NORMAL FINDINGS	ABNORMAL FINDINGS
Skin (Continued)		
Use the Braden Scale (see Assessment Tool 14-1) to predict pressure sore risk. If any skin breakdown is noted, use the PUSH tool (see Assessment Tool 14-2) to document the degree of skin breakdown to provide a baseline to compare degree of healing or deterioration over time. **CLINICAL TIP** In the obese client, carefully inspect skin on the limbs, under breasts, and in the groin area where problems are frequent due to perspiration and friction.		progress to serious and painful pressure ulcers (see Abnormal Findings 14-1 for stages of pressure ulcer development). Depending on the color of the client's skin, reddened areas may not be prominent, although the skin may feel warmer in the area of breakdown than elsewhere.
Inspect for lesions. Observe the skin surface to detect abnormalities. If you observe a lesion: • Note symmetry, borders and shape, color, diameter of lesion, and change in lesion over time. • For very small lesions, use a magnifying glass to note these characteristics. • Note its location, distribution, and configuration. • Measure the lesion with a centimeter ruler.	Skin is smooth, without lesions. Stretch marks (striae), healed scars, freckles, moles, or birthmarks are common findings (see Box 14-2). Freckles or moles may be scattered over the skin in no particular pattern. **CLINICAL TIP** Scarifications may be used by some individuals who want to have a scar or keloid. These scars involve cutting or sometimes burning of the skin to leave permanent scars (Bradley University, 2017). **OLDER ADULT CONSIDERATIONS** Older clients may have skin lesions associated with aging, including seborrheic or senile keratoses, senile lentigines, cherry angiomas, purpura, and cutaneous tags and horns.	Lesions may indicate local or systemic problems. Primary lesions (see Abnormal Findings 14-2) arise from normal skin due to irritation or disease. Secondary lesions (see Abnormal Findings 14-3) arise from changes in primary lesions. Vascular lesions (see Abnormal Findings 14-4), reddish-bluish lesions, are seen with bleeding, venous pressure, aging, liver disease, or pregnancy. Cancerous lesions can be either primary or secondary lesions and are classified as squamous cell carcinoma, basal cell carcinoma, or malignant melanoma (see Abnormal Findings 14-5). See Abnormal Findings 14-5 for using the ABCDE's to detect signs of skin cancer. For abnormal lesions, distribution may be diffuse (scattered all over), localized to one area, or in sun-exposed areas. Configuration may be discrete (separate and distinct), grouped (clustered), confluent (merged), linear (in a line), annular and arciform (circular or arcing), or zosteriform (linear along a nerve route) (see Abnormal Findings 14-6).
If you suspect a fungus, shine a Wood light (an ultraviolet light filtered through a special glass) on the lesion.	Lesion does not fluoresce.	Blue-green fluorescence indicates fungal infection.
PALPATION		
Palpate skin to assess texture. Use the palmar surface of your three middle fingers to palpate skin texture.	Skin is smooth and even.	Rough, flaky, dry skin is seen in hypothyroidism. Obese clients often report dry, itchy skin.
Palpate to assess thickness.	Skin is normally thin but calluses (rough, thick sections of epidermis) are common on areas of the body that are exposed to constant pressure (e.g., the heels).	Very thin skin may be seen in clients with arterial insufficiency or in those on steroid therapy.

ASSESSMENT PROCEDURE	NORMAL FINDINGS	ABNORMAL FINDINGS
If lesions are noted when assessing skin thickness, put gloves on and palpate the lesion between the thumb and index finger for size, mobility, consistency, and tenderness (Fig. 14-7). Observe for drainage or other characteristics.	No lesions palpated.	Infected lesions may be tender to palpate. Nonmobile, fixed lesions may be cancer. (See Abnormal Findings 14-2, 14-3, and 14-4 for descriptions of lesions.)
Palpate to assess moisture. Check under skin folds and in unexposed areas. ◎ **CLINICAL TIP** Some nurses believe that using the dorsal surfaces of the hands to assess moisture leads to a more accurate result.	Skin surfaces vary from moist to dry depending on the area assessed. Recent activity or a warm environment may cause increased moisture. 🪑 **OLDER ADULT CONSIDERATIONS** The older client's skin may feel dryer than a younger client's skin because sebum production decreases with age.	Increased moisture or diaphoresis (profuse sweating) may occur in conditions such as fever or hyperthyroidism. Decreased moisture occurs with dehydration or hypothyroidism. Clammy skin is typical in shock or hypotension.
Palpate to assess temperature. Use the dorsal surfaces of your hands to palpate the skin (Fig. 14-8).	Skin is normally a warm temperature.	Cold skin may accompany shock or hypotension. Cool skin may accompany arterial disease. Very warm skin may indicate a febrile state or hyperthyroidism.

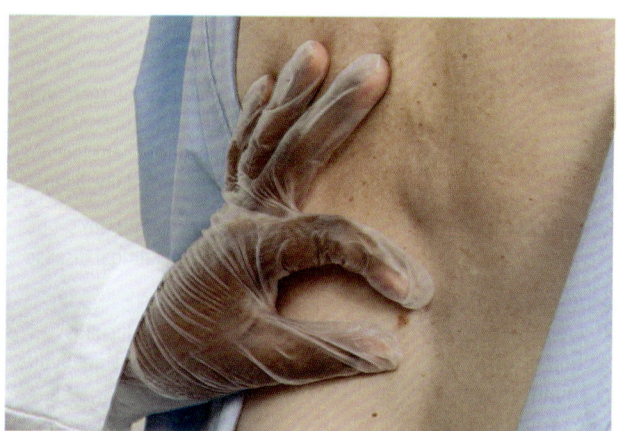

FIGURE 14-7 Palpating a lesion.

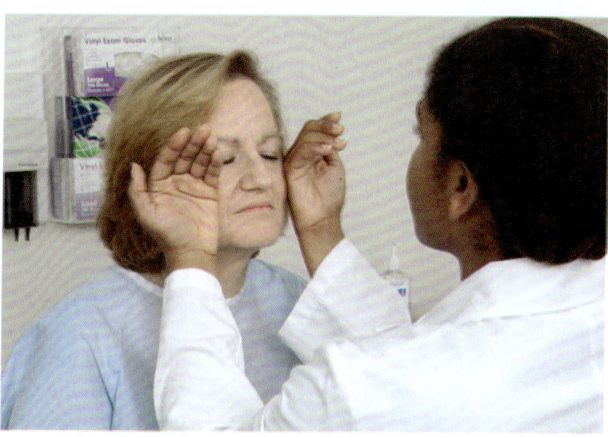

FIGURE 14-8 Assessing temperature and moisture.

Palpate to assess mobility and turgor. Ask the client to lie down. Using two fingers, gently pinch the skin over the clavicle. (Fig. 14-9).	Normally, the skin is mobile, with elasticity and returns to original shape quickly. Recoil is usually immediate.	Decreased mobility is seen with edema.

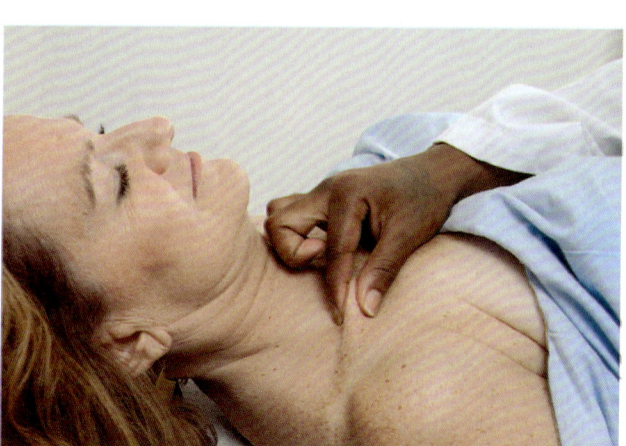

FIGURE 14-9 Palpating to assess skin turgor and mobility.

Continued on following page

ASSESSMENT PROCEDURE	NORMAL FINDINGS	ABNORMAL FINDINGS
Skin (Continued)		
Mobility refers to how easily the skin can be pinched. *Turgor* refers to the skin's elasticity and how quickly the skin returns to its original shape after being pinched.	**OLDER ADULT CONSIDERATIONS** The older client's skin loses its turgor because of a decrease in elasticity and collagen fibers. Sagging or wrinkled skin appears in the facial, breast, and scrotal areas.	Decreased turgor (a slow recoil or return of the skin to its normal state) is seen in dehydration. Recoil that occurs in less than 2 seconds suggests moderate dehydration; more than 2 seconds suggests severe dehydration; and more than 3 seconds is described as tenting.
Palpate to detect edema. Use your thumbs to press down on the skin of the feet, ankles, or pretibial area to check for edema (swelling related to accumulation of fluid in the tissue).	Skin rebounds and does not remain indented when pressure is released.	Indentations on the skin may vary from slight to great and may be in one area or all over the body. See Chapter 22, Assessing Peripheral Vascular System, for a full discussion of edema.
Scalp and Hair		
INSPECTION AND PALPATION		
Inspect the scalp and hair for general color and condition.	Natural hair color, as opposed to chemically colored hair, varies among clients from pale blond to black to gray or white. The color is determined by the amount of melanin present.	Nutritional deficiencies may cause patchy gray hair in some clients. Severe malnutrition in African American children may cause a copper-red hair color (Andrews & Boyle, 2016).
At 1-inch intervals, separate the hair from the scalp and inspect and palpate the hair and scalp for cleanliness, dryness or oiliness, parasites, and lesions (Fig. 14-10). Wear gloves if lesions are suspected or if hygiene is poor.	Scalp is clean and dry. Sparse dandruff may be visible. Hair is smooth and firm, somewhat elastic. **OLDER ADULT CONSIDERATIONS** As people age, hair feels coarser and drier. The hair is also thinner with slower growth. **CULTURAL CONSIDERATIONS** Individuals of black African descent often have very dry scalps and dry, fragile hair, which the client may condition with oil or a petroleum jelly–like product. (This kind of hair is of genetic origin and not related to thyroid disorders or nutrition. Such hair needs to be handled very gently.)	Excessive scaliness may indicate dermatitis. Raised lesions may indicate infections or tumor growth. Dull, dry hair may be seen with hypothyroidism and malnutrition. Poor hygiene may indicate a need for client teaching or assistance with activities of daily living. Pustules with hair loss in patches are seen in tinea capitis, a contagious fungal disease (ringworm, Fig. 14-11). Infections of the hair follicle (folliculitis) appear as pustules surrounded by erythema (Fig. 14-12).

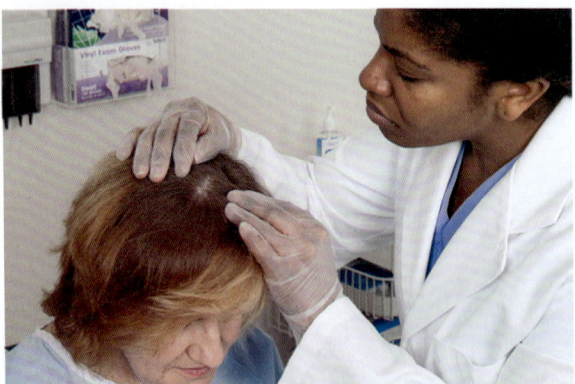

FIGURE 14-10 Inspecting the scalp and hair.

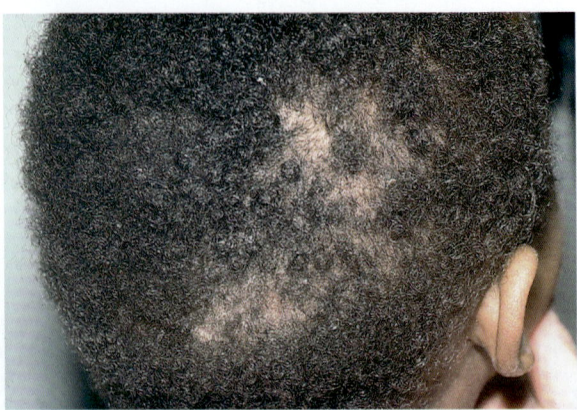

FIGURE 14-11 Tinea capitis (scalp ringworm). (Used with permission from Goodheart, H., Gonzalez, M.E. (2016). *Goodheart's photoguide to common pediatric and adult skin disorders* (4th ed.). Philadelphia, PA: Wolters Kluwer.)

14 Assessing Skin, Hair, and Nails   **263**

ASSESSMENT PROCEDURE	NORMAL FINDINGS	ABNORMAL FINDINGS

Scalp and Hair (Continued)

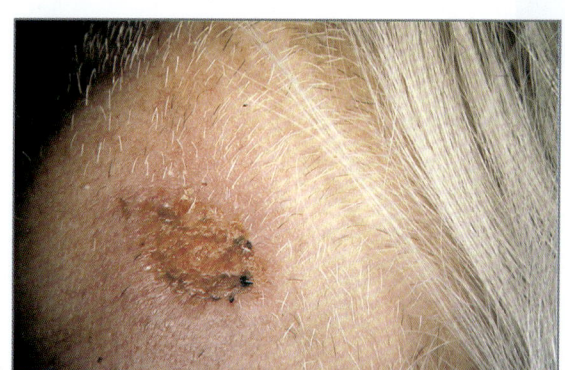 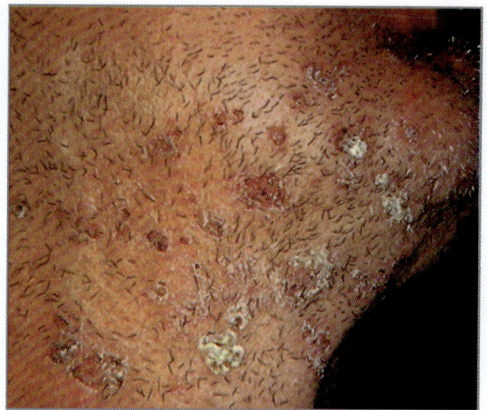

FIGURE 14-12 **A.** Folliculitis of the scalp. **B.** Folliculitis of the beard area. (Used with permission from Burroughs Wellcome Co.)

Inspect amount and distribution of scalp, body, axillae, and pubic hair. Look for unusual growth elsewhere on the body.	Varying amounts of terminal hair cover the scalp, axillae, body, and pubic areas according to normal gender distribution. Fine vellus hair covers the entire body except for the soles, palms, lips, and nipples. Normal male pattern balding is symmetric (Fig. 14-13). Individuals may shave or chemically remove axillary and genital hair. Some individuals, both male and female may also remove all body hair. **OLDER ADULT CONSIDERATIONS** Older clients have thinner hair because of a decrease in hair follicles. Pubic, axillary, and body hair also decrease with aging. Alopecia is seen, especially in men. Hair loss occurs from the periphery of the scalp and moves to the center. Older women may have terminal hair growth on the chin owing to hormonal changes.	Excessive generalized hair loss may occur with infection, nutritional deficiencies, hormonal disorders, thyroid or liver disease, drug toxicity, hepatic or renal failure. It may also result from chemotherapy or radiation therapy. Patchy hair loss (Fig. 14-14) may result from infections of the scalp, discoid or systemic lupus erythematosus, and some types of chemotherapy. Hirsutism (facial hair on females) is a characteristic of Cushing disease and polycystic ovary syndrome (PCOS) and results from an imbalance of adrenal hormones or it may be a side effect of steroids (Mayo Clinic, 2015a). 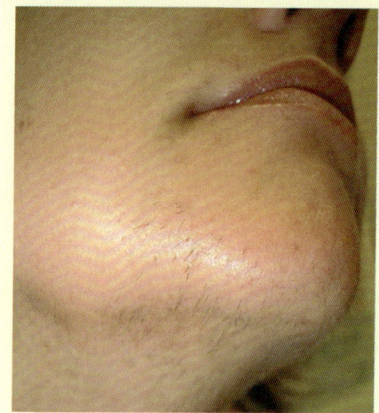

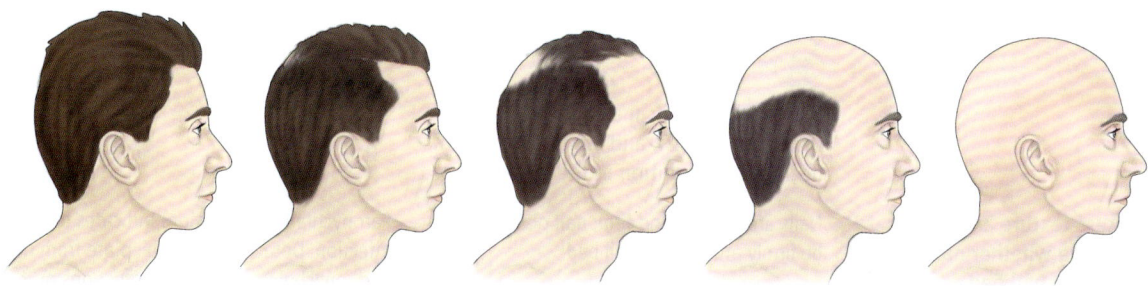

FIGURE 14-13 Male pattern balding (Used with permission from Smeltzer, S.C., et al. (2014). *Brunner & Suddarth's textbook of medical-surgical nursing* (13th ed.). Philadelphia, PA: Wolters Kluwer.)

Continued on following page

ASSESSMENT PROCEDURE	NORMAL FINDINGS	ABNORMAL FINDINGS
Scalp and Hair (Continued)		

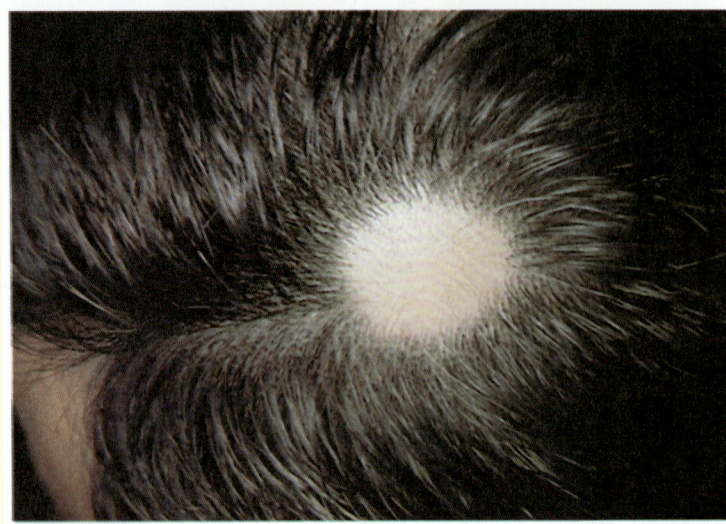

FIGURE 14-14 Patchy hair loss. (Courtesy Neutrogena Skin Care Institute.)

Nails		
INSPECTION		
Inspect nail grooming and cleanliness.	Nails are clean and manicured.	Dirty, broken, or jagged fingernails may be seen with poor hygiene. They may also result from the client's hobby or occupation.
Inspect nail color and markings.	Pink tones should be seen. Some longitudinal ridging is normal. Dark-skinned clients may have freckles or pigmented streaks in their nails.	Pale or cyanotic nails may indicate hypoxia or anemia. Splinter hemorrhages may be caused by trauma. Beau lines occur after acute illness and eventually grow out. Yellow discoloration may be seen in fungal infections or psoriasis. Nail pitting is also common in psoriasis (see Abnormal Findings 14-7).
Inspect shape of nails.	There is normally a 160-degree angle between the nail base and the skin.	Early clubbing (180-degree angle with spongy sensation) and late clubbing (greater than 180-degree angle) can occur from hypoxia. Spoon nails (concave) may be present with iron deficiency anemia (see Abnormal Findings 14-7).
PALPATION		
Palpate nail to assess texture.	Nails are hard and basically immobile. 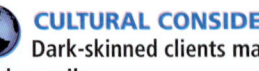 **CULTURAL CONSIDERATIONS** Dark-skinned clients may have thicker nails. **OLDER ADULT CONSIDERATIONS** Older clients' nails may appear thickened, yellow, and brittle because of decreased circulation in the extremities.	Thickened nails (especially toenails) may be caused by decreased circulation, and are also seen in onychomycosis.
Palpate to assess texture and consistency, noting whether nail plate is attached to nail bed.	Nails are smooth and firm; nail plate should be firmly attached to nail bed.	Paronychia (inflammation) indicates local infection. Detachment of nail plate from nail bed (onycholysis) is seen in infections or trauma.

ASSESSMENT PROCEDURE	NORMAL FINDINGS	ABNORMAL FINDINGS
Test capillary refill in nail beds by pressing the nail tip briefly and watching for color change (Fig. 14-15).	Pink tone returns immediately to blanched nail beds when pressure is released.	There is slow (greater than 2 seconds) capillary nail bed refill (return of pink tone) with respiratory or cardiovascular diseases that cause hypoxia.

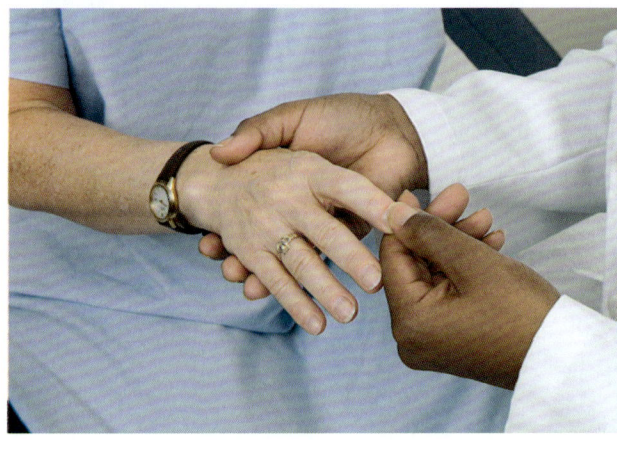

FIGURE 14-15 Testing capillary refill.

TABLE 14-1 Skin Types Classified by Their Reactions to Ultraviolet Radiation (UVR)

Type	Definition	Description
I	Always burns but never tans	Pale skin, red hair, freckles
II	Usually burns, sometimes tans	Fair skin
III	May burn, usually tans	Darker skin
IV	Rarely burns, always tans	Mediterranean
V	Moderate constitutional pigmentation	Latin American, Middle Eastern
VI	Marked constitutional pigmentation	Black

Weller, R., Hunter, H., & Mann, M. (2015). *Clinical dermatology* (5th ed.). New York: John Wiley & Sons; CDC, 2013. What are the risk factors for skin cancer. Available at http://www.cdc.gov/cancer/skin/basic_info/risk_factors.htm

BOX 14-2 COMMON VARIATIONS: SKIN VARIATIONS

Many skin assessment findings are considered normal variations in that they are not health- or life-threatening. For example, freckles are common variations in fair-skinned clients, whereas unspotted skin is considered the ideal. Scars and vitiligo, on the other hand, are not exactly normal findings because scars suggest a healed injury or surgical intervention and vitiligo may be related to a dysfunction of the immune system. However, they are common and usually insignificant. Common findings are pictured below.

Freckles—flat, small macules of pigment that appear following sun exposure.

Vitiligo depigmentation of the skin.

Striae (sometimes called stretch marks).

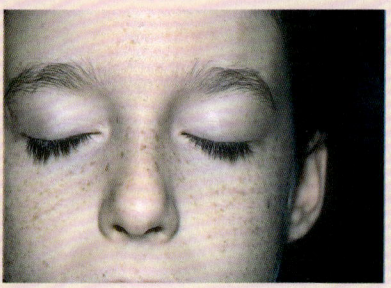
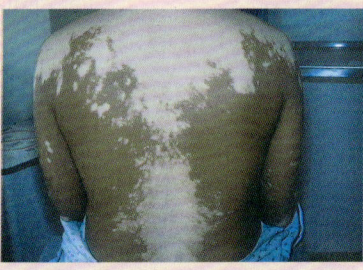
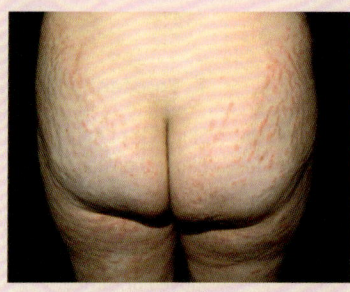

Continued on following page

BOX 14-2 COMMON VARIATIONS: SKIN VARIATIONS (Continued)

Seborrheic keratosis, a warty or crusty pigmented lesion.

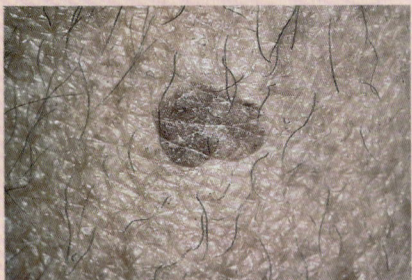

Scar.

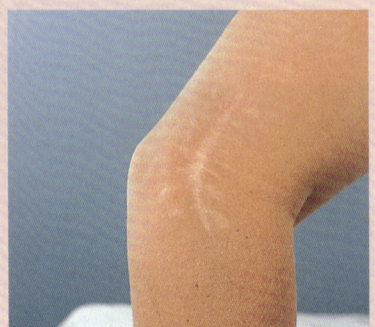

Mole (also called nevus), a flat or raised tan/brownish marking up to 6 mm wide.

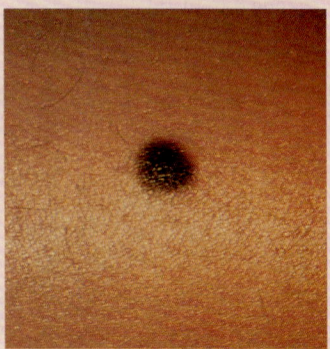

Cutaneous tag, raised papule with a depressed center.

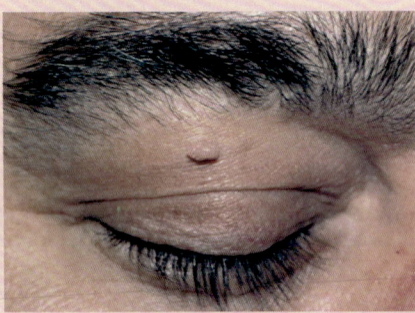

Cutaneous horn.

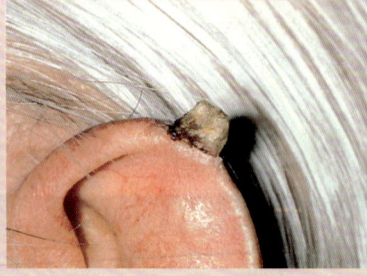

Cherry angiomas, small raised spots (1–5 mm wide) typically seen with aging.

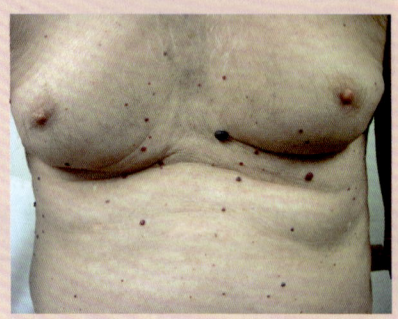

Photo credits: Used with permission from Goodheart, H., & Gonzalez, M. E. (2016). *Goodheart's photoguide to common pediatric and adult skin disorders* (4th ed.). Philadelphia, PA: Wolters Kluwer; Striae from Craft, N., Fox, L.P., Goldsmith, L.A., et al. (2010). *VisualDx: Essential Adult Dermatology*. Philadelphia, PA: Wolters Kluwer.

ASSESSMENT TOOL 14-1   Braden Scale for Predicting Pressure Sore Risk

Patient's Name _____   Evaluator's Name _____   Date of Assessment _____

SENSORY PERCEPTION	1. Completely Limited	2. Very Limited	3. Slightly Limited	4. No Impairment
Ability to respond meaningfully to pressure-related discomfort	Unresponsive (does not moan, flinch, or grasp) to painful stimuli, due to diminished level of consciousness or sedation OR limited ability to feel pain over most of body.	Responds only to painful stimuli. Cannot communicate discomfort except by moaning or restlessness OR has a sensory impairment that limits the ability to feel pain or discomfort over half of body.	Responds to verbal commands, but cannot always communicate discomfort or the need to be turned OR has some sensory impairment that limits ability to feel pain or discomfort in 1 or 2 extremities.	Responds to verbal commands. Has no sensory deficit that would limit ability to feel or voice pain or discomfort.

MOISTURE	1. Constantly Moist	2. Very Moist	3. Occasionally Moist	4. Rarely Moist
Degree to which skin is exposed to moisture	Skin is kept moist almost constantly by perspiration, urine, etc. Dampness is detected every time patient is moved or turned.	Skin is often, but not always, moist. Linen must be changed at least once per shift.	Skin is occasionally moist, requiring an extra linen change approximately once per day.	Skin is usually dry. Linen requires changing only at routine intervals.

ASSESSMENT TOOL 14-1 Braden Scale for Predicting Pressure Sore Risk (Continued)

ACTIVITY	1. Bedfast	2. Chairfast	3. Walks Occasionally	4. Walks Frequently
Degree of physical activity	Confined to bed	Ability to walk severely limited or nonexistent. Cannot bear own weight and/or must be assisted into chair or wheelchair.	Walks occasionally during day, but for very short distances, with or without assistance. Spends majority of each shift in bed or chair.	Walks outside room at least twice per day and inside room at least once every 2 hours during waking hours.

MOBILITY	1. Completely Immobile	2. Very Limited	3. Slightly Limited	4. No Limitation
Ability to change and control body position	Does not make even slight changes in body or extremity position without assistance.	Makes occasional slight changes in body or extremity position, but unable to make frequent or significant changes independently.	Makes frequent, though slight, changes in body or extremity position independently.	Makes major and frequent changes in position without assistance.

NUTRITION	1. Very Poor	2. Probably Inadequate	3. Adequate	4. Excellent
Usual food intake pattern	Never eats a complete meal. Rarely eats more than half of any food offered. Eats 2 servings or less of protein (meat or dairy products) per day. Takes fluids poorly. Does not take a liquid dietary supplement. OR Is NPO and/or maintained on clear liquids or IVs for more than 5 days.	Rarely eats a complete meal and generally eats only about half of any food offered. Protein intake includes only 3 servings of meat or dairy products per day. Occasionally will take a dietary supplement. OR Receives less than optimum amount of liquid diet or tube feeding.	Eats over half of most meals. Eats a total of 4 servings of protein (meat, dairy products) per day. Occasionally will refuse a meal, but will usually take a supplement when offered. OR Is on a tube feeding or TPN regimen that probably meets most nutritional needs.	Eats most of every meal. Never refuses a meal. Usually eats a total of 4 or more servings of meat and dairy products. Occasionally eats between meals. Does not require supplementation.

FRICTION AND SHEAR	1. Problem	2. Potential Problem	3. No Apparent Problem	
	Requires moderate to maximum assistance in moving. Complete lifting without sliding against sheets is impossible. Frequently slides down in bed or chair, requiring frequent repositioning with maximum assistance. Spasticity, contractures, or agitation leads to almost constant friction.	Moves feebly or requires minimum assistance. During a move, skin probably slides to some extent against sheets, chair, restraints, or other devices. Maintains relatively good position in chair or bed most of the time, but occasionally slides down.	Moves in bed and in chair independently and has sufficient muscle strength to lift up completely during move. Maintains good position in bed or chair.	

Total Score

Copyright: Barbara Braden and Nancy Bergstrom, 1988. Reprinted with permission. All Rights Reserved.

ASSESSMENT TOOL 14-2   PUSH Tool to Measure Pressure Ulcer Healing

PUSH Tool 3.0

Patient Name _____   Patient ID# _____

Ulcer Location _____   Date _____

Directions: Observe and measure the pressure ulcer. Categorize the ulcer with respect to surface area, exudate, and type of wound tissue. Record a subscore for each of these ulcer characteristics. Add the subscores to obtain the total score. A comparison of total scores measured over time provides an indication of the improvement or deterioration in pressure ulcer healing.

	0	1	2	3	4	5	
LENGTH × WIDTH (in cm²)	0	<0.3	0.3–0.6	0.7–1.0	1.1–2.0	2.1–3.0	Subscore
		6 3.1–4.0	7 4.1–8.0	8 8.1–12.0	9 12.1–24.0	10 >24.0	
EXUDATE AMOUNT	0 None	1 light	2 Moderate	3 Heavy			Subscore
TISSUE TYPE	0 Closed	1 Epithelial Tissue	2 Granulation Tissue	3 Slough	4 Necrotic Tissue		Subscore
							TOTAL SCORE

Length × Width: Measure the greatest length (head to toe) and the greatest width (side to side) using a centimeter ruler. Multiply these two measurements (length × width) to obtain an estimate of surface area in square centimeters (cm²). Caveat: Do not guess! Always use a centimeter ruler and always use the same method each time the ulcer is measured.

Exudate Amount: Estimate the amount of exudate (drainage) present after removal of the dressing and before applying any topical agent to the ulcer. Estimate the exudate (drainage) as none, light, moderate, or heavy.

Tissue Type: This refers to the types of tissue that are present in the wound (ulcer) bed. Score as a "4" if there is any necrotic tissue present. Score as a "3" if there is any amount of slough present and necrotic tissue is absent. Score as a "2" if the wound is clean and contains granulation tissue. A superficial wound that is re-epithelializing is scored as a "1." When the wound is closed, score as a "0."

4—Necrotic Tissue (Eschar): Black, brown, or tan tissue that adheres firmly to the wound bed or ulcer edges and may be either firmer or softer than surrounding skin.

3—Slough: Yellow or white tissue that adheres to the ulcer bed in strings or thick clumps, or is mucinous.

2—Granulation Tissue: Pink or beefy red tissue with a shiny, moist, granular appearance.

1—Epithelial Tissue: For superficial ulcers, new pink or shiny tissue (skin) that grows in from the edges or as islands on the ulcer surface.

0—Closed/Resurfaced: The wound is completely covered with epithelium (new skin).

From National Pressure Ulcer Advisory Panel. Available at www.npuap.org/PDF/push3.pdf.

The chapter case study demonstrates a physical assessment of Ms. Michaelson's skin, hair, and nails.

CASE STUDY

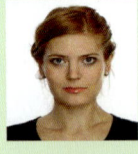

After asking Ms. Michaelson to put on a gown and then leaving the room while she does so, the nurse returns to perform a physical examination. The nurse observes that Ms. Michaelson's skin is pink and intact. There is no odor.

The nurse inspects the lesions and finds that they are circular, erythematous papules/plaques with central hypopigmentation and raised, hyperpigmented periphery with confluency covering the bridge of the nose extending to maxillary regions bilaterally, and with sparing of the paraphiltrum region. The lesions are nontender. Ms. Michaelson's skin is smooth, warm, and dry. The nurse assesses turgor and notes immediate recoil at the clavicle. There is no edema.

Ms. Michaelson's hair is dark brown, shoulder-length, clean, and shiny. The nurse inspects the hair and scalp, finding no oiliness or parasites. Ms. Michaelson's hair distribution is interrupted with five areas of alopecia, each 2 cm in diameter. The areas of alopecia exhibit circular, erythematous papules/plaques with central hypopigmentation and raised, hyperpigmented periphery. Hair has been removed from legs, axillae, and perineum.

Ms. Michaelson's nail beds are pink and her fingernails are manicured with clear enamel. The nails are hard, smooth, and immobile, forming a 160-degree angle at the base. Her cuticles are smooth, with no detachment of nail plate. Toenails are hard, smooth, immobile, clean, and trimmed. Capillary refill of toes and fingers is immediate.

Validating and Documenting Findings

Validate your normal and abnormal findings with the client, other health care workers, or your instructors. Next, document the skin, hair, and nail assessment data that you have collected on the appropriate form your school or agency uses. Document both normal and abnormal findings. Normal findings can act as a baseline for findings that may change later.

CASE STUDY

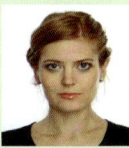

Think back to the case study. The occupational health nurse documented the following assessment findings of Ms. Michaelson's skin, hair, and nails.

Biographical Data: MM, 29 years old. Caucasian. Employed full-time as an Office Manager.

General Survey: Awake, alert, and oriented. Asks and answers questions appropriately.

Reason for Seeking Care: "My hair was falling out in chunks, and I have a red rash on my face and chest. It looks like a bad case of acne. I feel so ugly and am concerned I may lose my job because of how I look."

History of Present Health Concern: Red rash that began 6 months ago. Located on face, neck, anterior chest, above nipple line, shoulders, and upper back. Recurring, with each episode lasting from 2 days to 2 weeks. Rates the pain as 0–1 on a 0–10 scale; rates the mental anguish as a 9–10 on a 0–10 scale. Rash worsens when exposed to sunlight while surfing. Increased level of anxiety related to the disfigurement. Reports areas of hair loss on her scalp where the rash is present.

Personal Health History: Diagnosed with discoid lupus erythematosus 6 months ago. One episode, 5 years ago, of a fine, raised, reddened, pruritic rash on trunk after taking ampicillin for an ear infection. Rash and pruritus resolved within 3 days after discontinuation of ampicillin and administration of antihistamines. Denies any swallowing or breathing difficulty, edema of mouth or tongue associated with the incident. No other allergies.

Family History: Negative family history of acne, atopic dermatitis, communicable disease, skin cancer, or keloids.

Lifestyle and Health Practices: Denies sunbathing, but does use tanning bed one to two times weekly year round, and goes surfing in the summertime. Does not perform skin self-examination. Denies exposure to paint, bleach, cleaning products, weed killers, insect repellents, and petroleum; long periods of immobility; and exposure to extreme temperatures. Showers in AM and bathes in PM with deodorant soap. Shampoos with baby shampoo and applies conditioner each AM. Applies moisturizer daily after cleansing and antiperspirant twice daily. Shaves legs and axillae with electric razor twice weekly. Trims toenails and fingernails, applying nail enamel weekly. Denies use of chemicals on hair to color, curl, or straighten.

Physical Examination Findings: Skin is pink, intact, without odor. Lesions: Nontender, circular, erythematous papules/plaques with central hypopigmentation and raised, hyperpigmented periphery with confluency covering the bridge of the nose extending to maxillary regions bilaterally, with sparing of the paraphiltrum region. Skin is smooth, warm, dry. Turgor with immediate recoil at the clavicle. No edema noted. Hair is dark brown, shoulder-length, clean, shiny. Hair and scalp without oiliness or parasites. Hair distribution interrupted with five areas of alopecia, each 2 cm in diameter. Areas exhibit circular, erythematous papules/plaques with central hypopigmentation and raised, hyperpigmented periphery. Hair has been removed from legs, axillae, and perineum. Nail beds pink. Fingernails manicured with clear enamel. Nails are hard, smooth, and immobile, forming 160-degree angle at base. Cuticles smooth; no detachment of nail plate. Toenails hard, smooth, immobile, clean, and trimmed. Capillary refill of toes and fingers immediate.

ANALYSIS OF DATA: DIAGNOSTIC REASONING

After collecting subjective and objective data pertaining to the skin, hair, and nails, identify abnormal findings and client strengths using diagnostic reasoning. Then, cluster the data to reveal any significant patterns or abnormalities.

Selected Nursing Diagnoses

The following is a list of selected nursing diagnoses that may be identified when analyzing data from a skin, hair, and nail assessment.

Health Promotion Diagnoses

- Readiness for Enhanced Health Management: Skin, hair, and nail integrity related to healthy hygiene and skin care practices, avoidance of overexposure to sun.
- Readiness for Health Management: Requests information on skin reactions and effects of using a sun-tanning booth.

Risk Diagnoses

- Risk for Impaired Skin Integrity related to excessive exposure to cleaning solutions and chemicals
- Risk for Impaired Skin Integrity related to prolonged sun exposure
- Risk for Imbalanced Body Temperature related to immobility, decreased production of natural oils, and thinning skin
- Risk for Impaired Skin Integrity of toes related to thickened, dried toenails
- Risk for Imbalanced Body Temperature related to severe diaphoresis
- Risk for Infection related to scratching of rash

- Risk for Impaired Nail Integrity related to prolonged use of artificial nails
- Risk for Imbalanced Nutrition: less than body requirements related to increased vitamin and protein requirements necessary for healing of a wound
- Risk for Infection related to multiple body piercings
- Risk for Infection related to periodic skin tattooing

Actual Diagnoses

- Ineffective Health Maintenance related to lack of hygienic care of the skin, hair, and nails
- Impaired Skin Integrity related to immobility and decreased circulation
- Impaired Skin Integrity related to poor nutritional intake and bowel/bladder incontinence
- Disturbed Body Image related to scarring, rash, or other skin condition that alters skin appearance
- Disturbed Sleep Pattern related to persistent itching of the skin
- Deficient Fluid Volume related to excessive diaphoresis secondary to excessive exercise and high environmental temperatures

Selected Collaborative Problems

After grouping the data, certain collaborative problems may become apparent. Remember that collaborative problems differ from nursing diagnoses in that they cannot be prevented or managed with independent nursing interventions. However, these physiologic complications of medical conditions can be detected and monitored by the nurse. In addition, the nurse can use physician- and nurse-prescribed interventions to minimize the complications of these problems. The nurse may also have to refer the client in such situations for further treatment of the problem. The following is a list of collaborative problems that may be identified when assessing the skin, hair, and nails. These problems are worded as Risk for Complications (RC), followed by the problem.

- RC: Allergic reaction
- RC: Skin rash
- RC: Insect/animal bite
- RC: Septicemia
- RC: Hypovolemic shock
- RC: Skin infection
- RC: Skin lesion
- RC: Ischemic skin ulcers
- RC: Graft rejection
- RC: Hemorrhage
- RC: Burns

Medical Problems

After grouping the data, it may become apparent that the client has signs and symptoms that require medical diagnosis and treatment. Referral to a primary care provider is necessary.

For the chapter case study, the nurse uses diagnostic reasoning to analyze the data collected on Ms. Michaelson's skin, hair, and nails to arrive at the following possible conclusions.

CASE STUDY

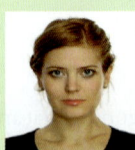

The nurse determines that the following conclusions are appropriate.

Nursing Diagnoses Include
Disturbed body image r/t changes in physical appearance
Risk for ineffective health maintenance r/t knowledge deficit of effects of sunlight on lesions
Anxiety r/t possible loss of work position secondary to perceived unattractiveness

Potential Collaborative Problems Include
RC: Skin infection/scarring
RC: Ischemic ulcers

To view an algorithm depicting the process for diagnostic reasoning in this case go to thePoint.

Interdisciplinary Verbal Communication of Assessment Findings Using SBAR

SITUATION: Mrs. Michaelson came to see me in the occupational health clinic today very concerned about feeling ugly and anxious that she will lose her job because of flaky red patches on her face, neck, chest, shoulders, and upper back, and loss of hair in patches.

BACKGROUND: She is a 29-year-old Caucasian female with a 6-month history of discoid lupus erythematosus. She is an avid surfer and reports that the lesions are exacerbated by sun exposure. She reports resolution of previous similar symptoms after taking ampicillin and antihistamines. She currently denies any current medications, constitutional symptoms, fever, allergies, pain, or change in personal hygiene products.

ASSESSMENT: The patient has multiple circular, erythematous, raised papules/plaques with central hypopigmentation and peripheral hyperpigmentation on the maxillary region, as well as five circular areas of alopecia, 2 cm in diameter, that demonstrate erythematous papules/plaques with central hypopigmentation and raised, hyperpigmented periphery.

RECOMMENDATION: Mrs. Michaelson needs to be seen for further evaluation and treatment of her rash. She may also benefit from follow-up counseling to be able to discuss her feelings of anxiety and body image disturbance.

14 Assessing Skin, Hair, and Nails   271

ABNORMAL FINDINGS 14-1   Pressure Ulcer Stage

During any skin assessment, the nurse remains watchful for signs of skin breakdown, especially in cases of limited mobility or fragile skin (e.g., in elderly or bedridden clients). Pressure ulcers, which lead to complications such as infection, are easier to prevent than to treat. Some risk factors for skin breakdown leading to pressure ulcers include poor circulation, poor hygiene, infrequent position changes, dermatitis, infection, or traumatic wounds. The stages of pressure ulcers follow.

STAGE I

Intact skin with nonblanchable redness of a localized area, usually over a bony prominence. Darkly pigmented skin may not have visible blanching; its color may differ from the surrounding area. The area may be painful, firm, soft, warmer, or cooler as compared with adjacent tissue. Stage I may be difficult to detect in individuals with dark skin tones.

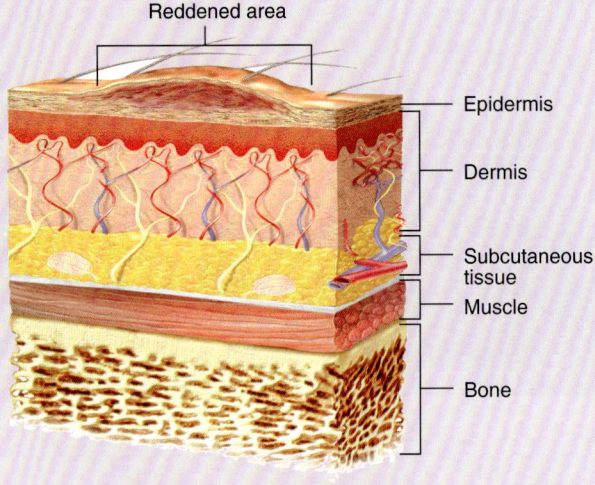
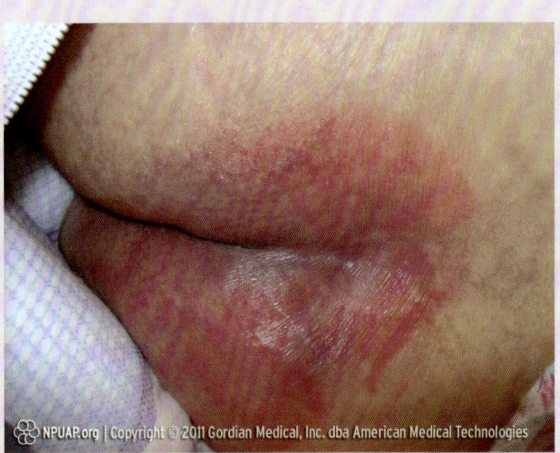

STAGE II

Partial thickness loss of dermis presenting as a shallow open ulcer with a red-pink wound bed, without slough. May also present as an intact or open/ruptured, serum-filled blister. Presents as a shiny or dry shallow ulcer without slough or bruising; bruising indicates suspected deep tissue injury. This stage should not be used to describe skin tears, tape burns, perineal dermatitis, maceration, or excoriation.

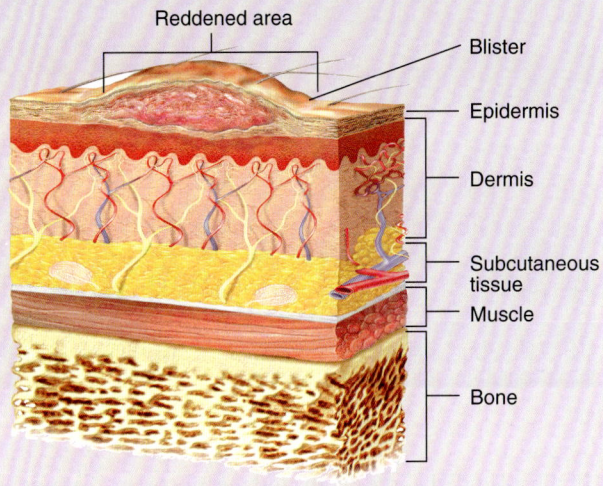
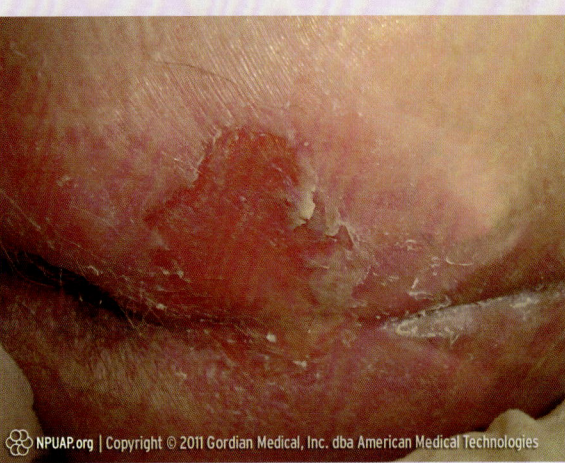

Continued on following page

ABNORMAL FINDINGS 14-1 Pressure Ulcer Stage (Continued)

STAGE III

Full-thickness tissue loss. Subcutaneous fat may be visible but bone, tendon, or muscle is not exposed. Slough may be present but does not obscure the depth of tissue loss. May include undermining and tunneling. The depth of a stage III pressure ulcer varies by anatomic location. The bridge of the nose, ear, occiput, and malleolus do not have subcutaneous tissue, and stage III ulcers can be shallow. In contrast, areas of significant adiposity can develop extremely deep stage III pressure ulcers. Bone/tendon is not visible or directly palpable.

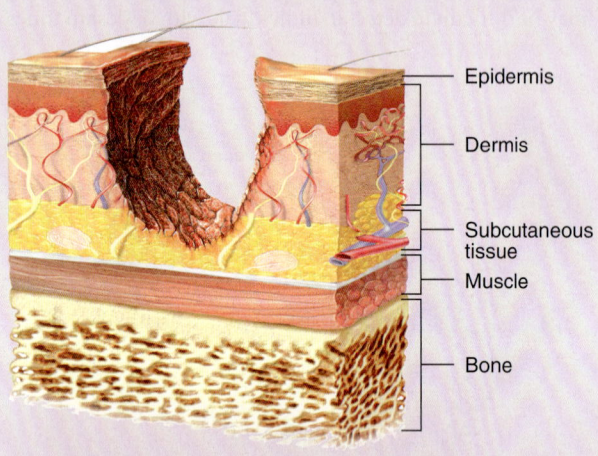

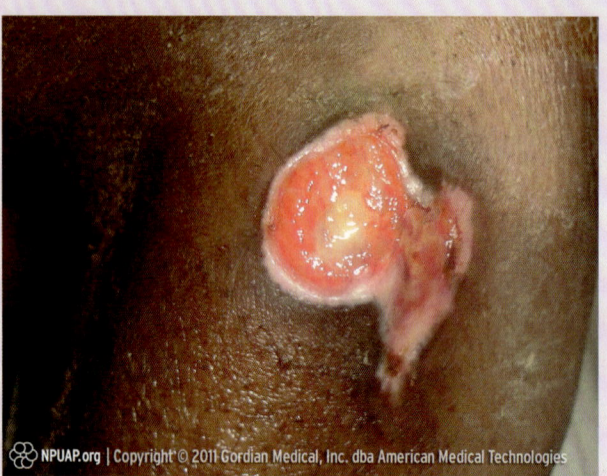

STAGE IV

Full-thickness tissue loss with exposed bone, tendon, or muscle. Slough or eschar may be present on some parts of the wound bed. Often includes undermining and tunneling. The depth of a stage IV pressure ulcer varies by anatomic location (see stage III). Stage IV ulcers can extend into muscle and/or supporting structures (e.g., fascia, tendon, or joint capsule), making osteomyelitis possible. Exposed bone/tendon is visible or directly palpable.

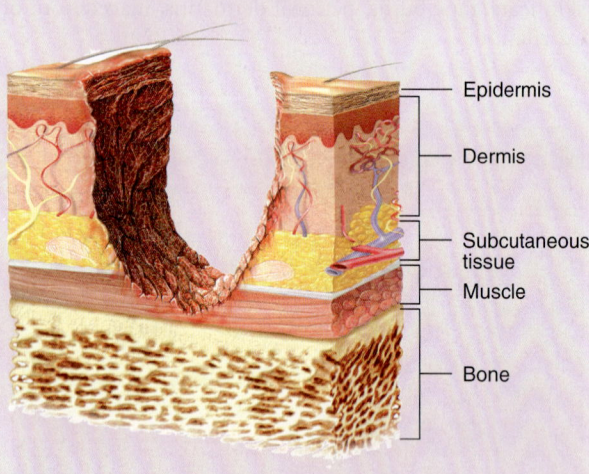

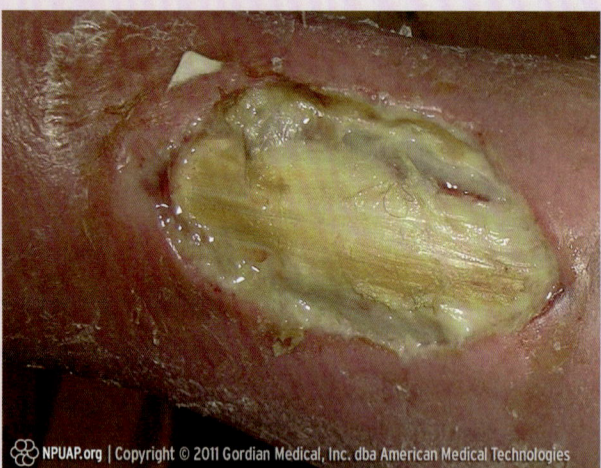

UNSTAGEABLE

Full-thickness tissue loss in which the base of the ulcer is covered by slough (yellow, tan, gray, green, or brown) and/or eschar (tan, brown, or black) in the wound bed. Until enough slough and/or eschar is removed to expose the base of the wound, the true depth, and therefore stage, cannot be determined. Stable (dry, adherent, intact without erythema or fluctuance) eschar on the heels serves as "the body's natural (biologic) cover" and should not be removed.

Photo credits: Used with permission of the National Pressure Ulcer Advisory Panel, Reston, VA.

14 Assessing Skin, Hair, and Nails **273**

ABNORMAL FINDINGS 14-2 Primary Skin Lesions

MACULE AND PATCH
Small, flat, nonpalpable skin color change (skin color may be brown, white, tan, purple, red). Macules are less than 1 cm with a circumscribed border, whereas patches are greater than 1 cm, and may have an irregular border. Examples include freckles, flat moles, petechiae, rubella (pictured below), vitiligo, port wine stains, and ecchymosis.

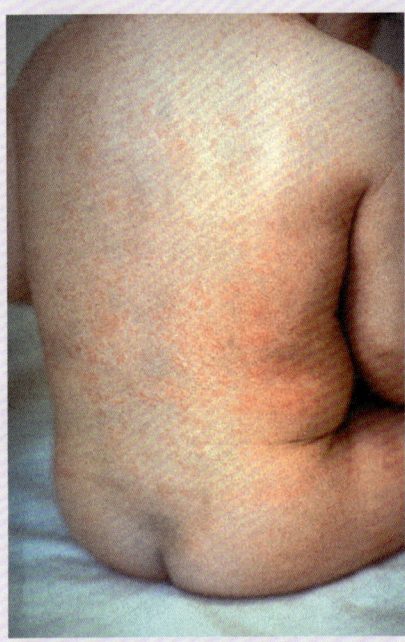
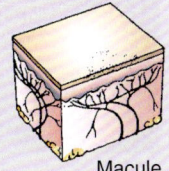
Macule

PAPULE AND PLAQUE
Elevated, palpable, solid mass. Papules have a circumscribed border and are less than 0.5 cm; plaques are greater than 0.5 cm and may be coalesced papules with a flat top. Examples of papules include elevated nevi, warts, and lichen planus. Examples of plaques include psoriasis (psoriasis vulgaris pictured below) and actinic keratosis.

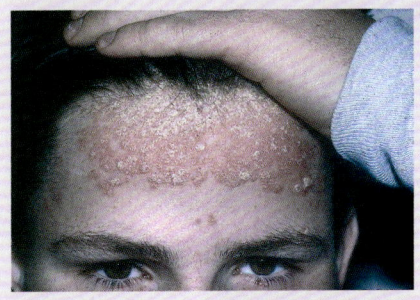
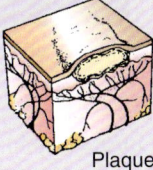
Plaque

NODULE AND TUMOR
Elevated, solid, palpable mass that extends deeper into dermis than a papule. Nodules are 0.5–2 cm and circumscribed; tumors are greater than 1–2 cm and do not always have sharp borders. Examples of nodules include keloid (pictured below), lipoma, squamous cell carcinoma, poorly absorbed injection, and dermatofibroma. Examples of tumors include larger lipoma and carcinoma.

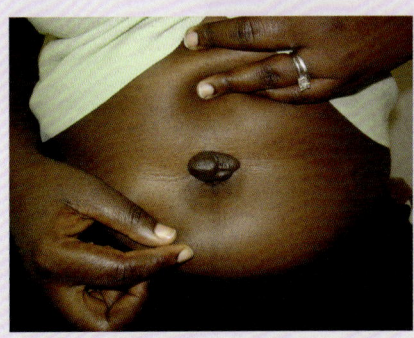
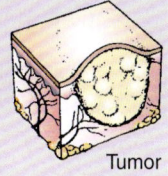
Tumor

VESICLE AND BULLA
Circumscribed elevated, palpable mass containing serous fluid. Vesicles are less than 0.5 cm; bullas are greater than 0.5 cm. Examples of vesicles include herpes simplex/zoster, varicella (chickenpox, pictured below), poison ivy, and second-degree burn. Examples of bulla include pemphigus, contact dermatitis, large burn blisters, poison ivy, and bullous impetigo.

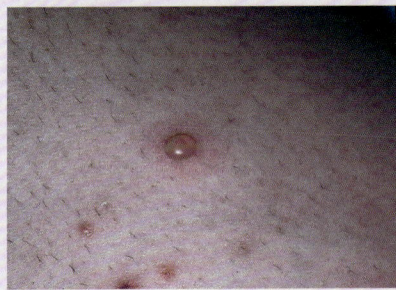
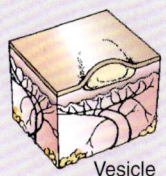
Vesicle

WHEAL
Elevated mass with transient borders that is often irregular. Size and color vary. Caused by movement of serous fluid into the dermis; it does not contain free fluid in a cavity (e.g., vesicle). Examples include urticaria (hives, pictured below) and insect bites.

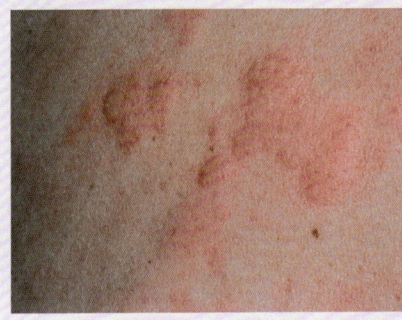
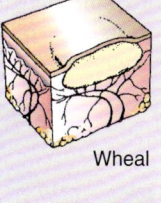
Wheal

Continued on following page

274 UNIT 3 Nursing Assessment of Physical Systems

ABNORMAL FINDINGS 14-2 Primary Skin Lesions (Continued)

PUSTULE
Pus-filled vesicle or bulla. Examples include acne (pictured below), impetigo, furuncles, and carbuncles.

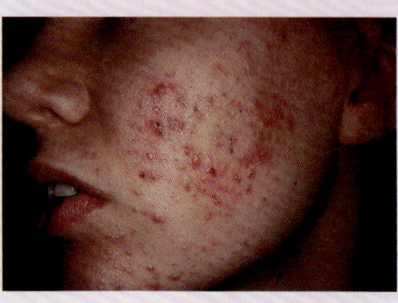
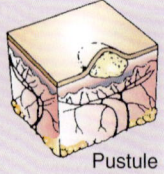
Pustule

CYST
Encapsulated fluid-filled or semisolid mass that is located in the subcutaneous tissue or dermis. Examples include sebaceous cyst and epidermoid cyst (pictured below).

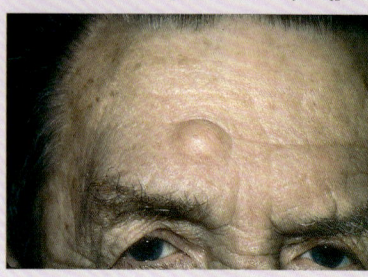
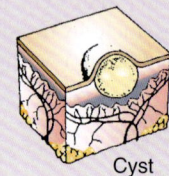
Cyst

Photo credits: Rubella and vesicle in chicken pox *used with permission from Goodheart, H. (2009). Goodheart's photoguide to common skin disorders: Diagnosis and management (3rd ed.). Philadelphia, PA: Lippincott Williams & Wilkins;* Psoriasis vulgaris, keloid, and cyst *used with permission from Goodheart, H., & Gonzalez, M.E. (2016). Goodheart's photoguide to common pediatric and adult skin disorders (4th ed.). Philadelphia, PA: Wolters Kluwer;* Urticaria and acne *used with permission from Hall, B. J., & Hall, J. C. (2010). Sauer's manual of skin diseases (10th ed.). Philadelphia, PA: Lippincott Williams & Wilkins.*

ABNORMAL FINDINGS 14-3 Secondary Skin Lesions

EROSION
Loss of superficial epidermis that does not extend to the dermis. It is a depressed, moist area. Examples include rupture vesicle, scratch mark, and aphthous ulcer (aphthous stomatitis, commonly called a canker sore, pictured below).

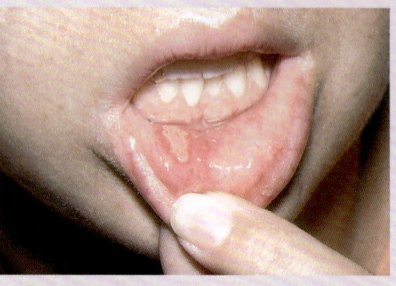
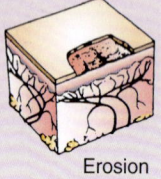
Erosion

SCAR (CICATRIX)
Skin mark left after healing of wound or lesion that represents replacement by connective tissue of the injured tissue. Young scars are red or purple, whereas mature scars (pictured below) are white or glistening. Examples include healed wound and healed surgical incision.

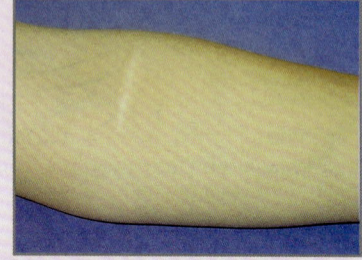
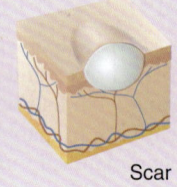
Scar

Mature healed wound.

ULCER
Skin loss extending past epidermis, with necrotic tissue loss. Bleeding and scarring are possible. Examples include stasis ulcer of venous insufficiency (stasis dermatitis with venous stasis ulcer, pictured below) and pressure ulcer.

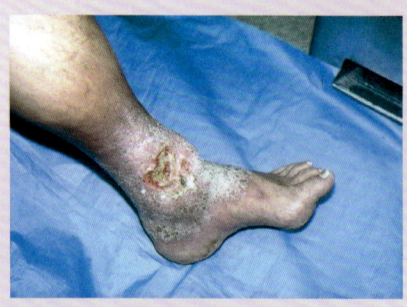
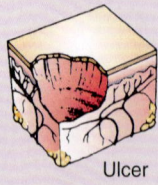
Ulcer

FISSURE
Linear crack in the skin that may extend to the dermis and may be painful. Examples include chapped lips or hands and athlete's foot. Interdigital tinea pedis with fissures and maceration is pictured below.

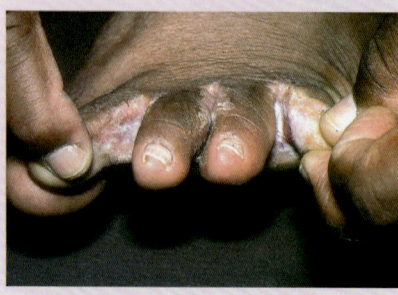
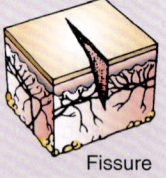
Fissure

Photo credits: Aphthous stomatitis, stasis dermatitis, and fissure *used with permission from Goodheart, H. (2009). Goodheart's photoguide to common skin disorders: Diagnosis and management (3rd ed.). Philadelphia, PA: Lippincott Williams & Wilkins.*

ABNORMAL FINDINGS 14-4 Vascular Skin Lesions

Vascular skin lesions are associated with bleeding, aging, circulatory conditions, diabetes, pregnancy, and hepatic disease, among other problems.

PETECHIA (PL. PETECHIAE)
Round red or purple macule that is 1–2 mm in size. It is secondary to blood extravasation and associated with bleeding tendencies or emboli to skin.

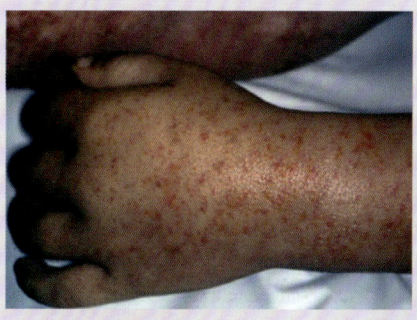
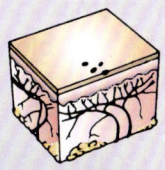
Petechiae

ECCHYMOSIS (PL. ECCHYMOSES)
Round or irregular macular lesion that is larger than petechial lesion. The color varies and changes: black, yellow, and green hues. It is secondary to blood extravasation and associated with trauma and bleeding tendencies.

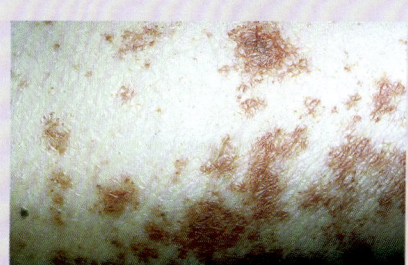
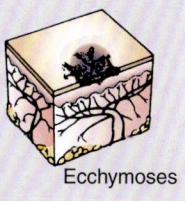
Ecchymoses

HEMATOMA
A localized collection of blood creating an elevated ecchymosis. It is associated with trauma.

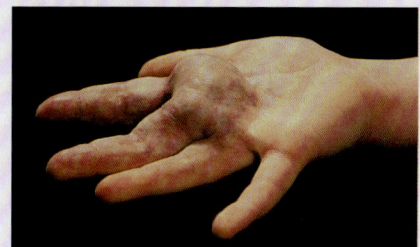
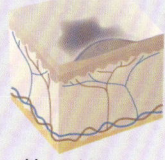
Hematoma

Hematoma. (© 1991 Patricia Barbara, RBP.)

CHERRY ANGIOMA
Papular and round, red or purple lesion found on the trunk or extremities. It may blanch with pressure. It is a normal age-related skin alteration and usually not clinically significant.

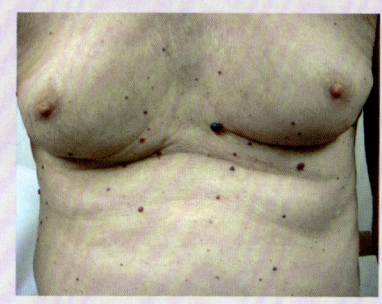
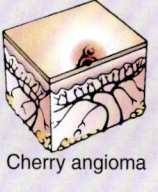
Cherry angioma

SPIDER ANGIOMA
Red arteriole lesion with a central body with radiating branches. It is usually noted on the face, neck, arms, and trunk. It is rare below the waist. Compression of the center of the arteriole completely blanches the lesion. It is associated with liver disease, pregnancy, and vitamin B deficiency.

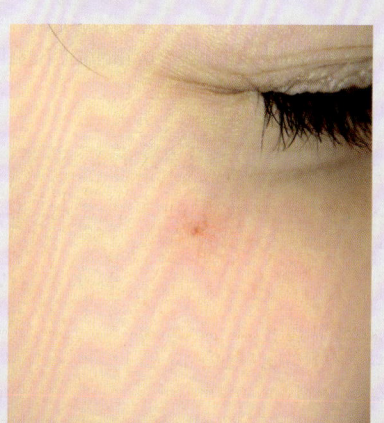
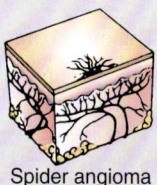
Spider angioma

TELANGIECTASIS (VENOUS STAR)
Bluish or red lesion with varying shape (spider-like or linear) found on the legs and anterior chest. It does not blanch when pressure is applied. It is secondary to superficial dilation of venous vessels and capillaries and associated with increased venous pressure states (varicosities).

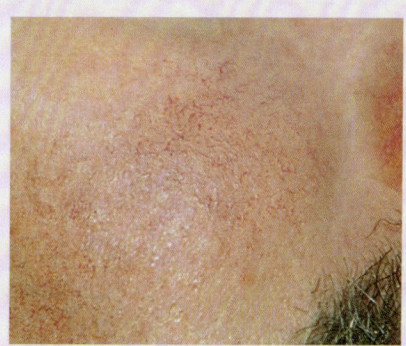
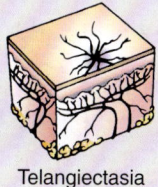
Telangiectasia

Photo credits: Cherry angioma and spider angioma used with permission from Goodheart, H., & Gonzalez, M. E. (2016). Goodheart's photoguide to common pediatric and adult skin disorders (4th ed.). Philadelphia, PA: Wolters Kluwer.

ABNORMAL FINDINGS 14-5 Skin Cancer

With the exception of malignant melanoma, most skin cancers are easily seen and easily cured, or at least controlled. Malignant melanoma can be deadly if not discovered and treated early, which is one reason why professional health assessment and skin self-assessment can be life-saving procedures.

The mnemonic ABCDE can be used to detect signs of skin cancer that indicate the need for further medical evaluation: A for asymmetrical; B for borders that are irregular (uneven or notched); C for color variations; D for diameter exceeding greater than ¼ inch or 6 mm; and E for evolution (changes over time). Danger signs of malignant melanoma include any of these factors. However, smaller areas may indicate early-stage melanomas. Other warning signs include itching, tenderness, or pain, and a change in size or bleeding of a mole. New pigmentations are also warning signs (American Cancer Society, 2015a; American Academy of Dermatology, 2015).

Asymmetry   **B**orders   **C**olor   **D**iameter, **E**levated

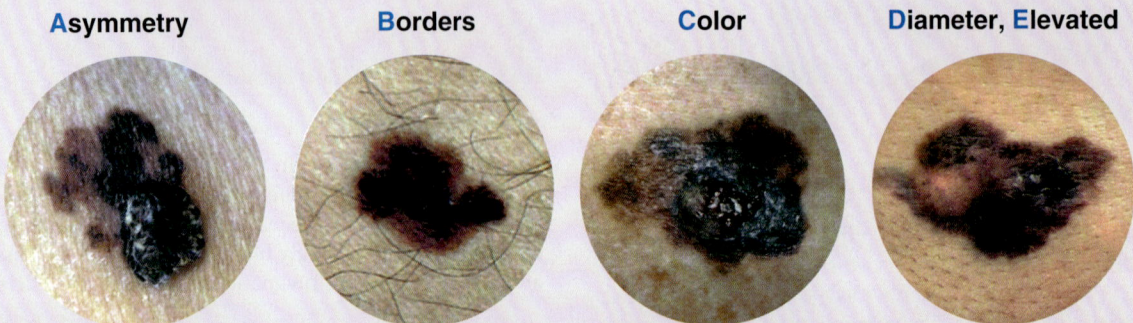

The most commonly detected skin cancers include basal cell carcinoma, squamous cell carcinoma, and melanoma.

BASAL CELL CARCINOMA

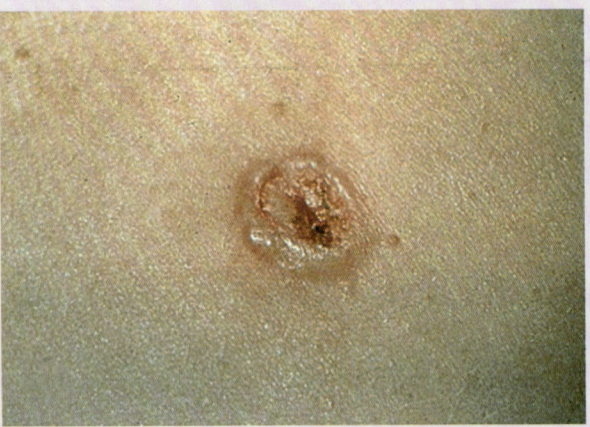

MELANOMA

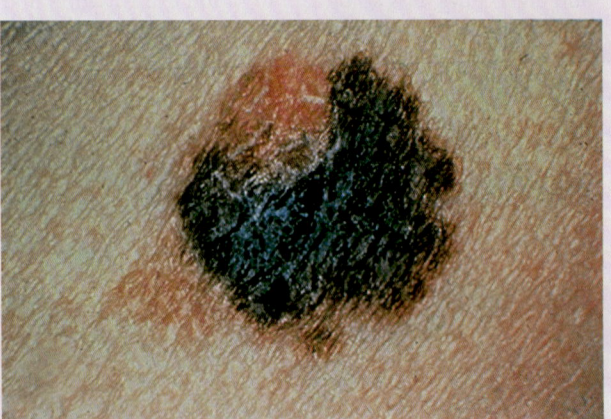

SQUAMOUS CELL CARCINOMA

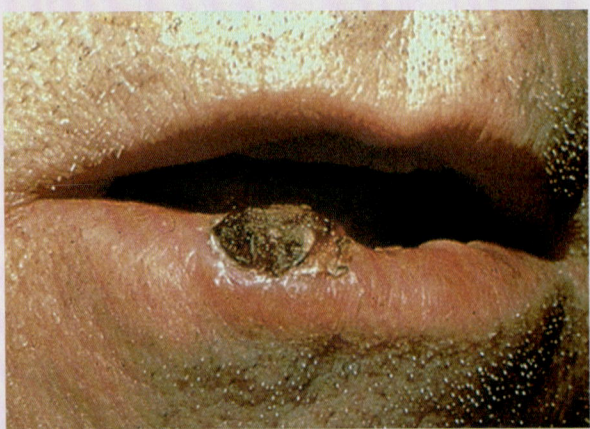

Photos courtesy of the American Cancer Society, Inc., Atlanta, GA.

14 Assessing Skin, Hair, and Nails   277

ABNORMAL FINDINGS 14-6 Configurations of Skin Lesions

Describing lesions by shape, distribution, or configuration is one way to communicate specific characteristics that can help to identify causes and treatments. Some common configurations are shown below.

Linear Configuration
Straight line, as in a scratch or streak. An example is dermatographism.

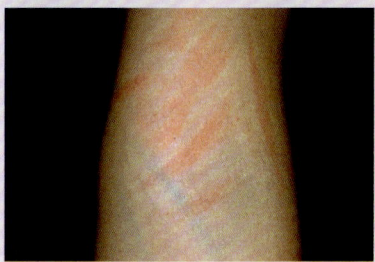

Annular Configuration
Circular lesions. An example is tinea corporis.

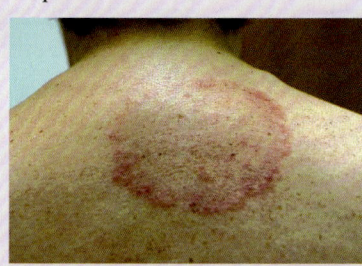

Clustered Configuration
Lesions grouped together. An example is herpes simplex.

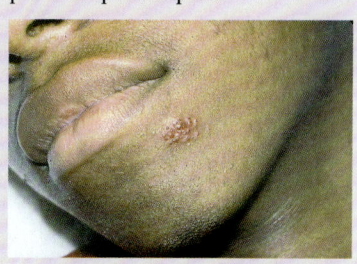

Discrete Configuration
Individual and distinct lesions. An example is multiple nevi.

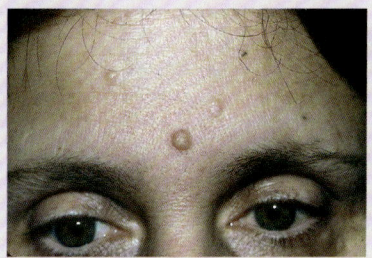

Nummular Configuration
Coin-shaped lesions. An example is nummular eczema.

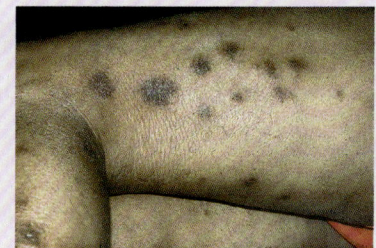

Confluent Configuration
Smaller lesions run together to form larger lesion. An example is tinea versicolor.

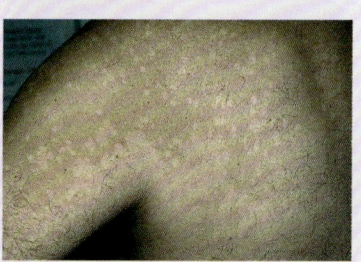

Photo credits: All photos used with permission from Goodheart, H. (2009). Goodheart's photoguide to common skin disorders: diagnosis and management (3rd ed.). Philadelphia, PA: Lippincott Williams & Wilkins.

ABNORMAL FINDINGS 14-7 Common Nail Disorders

Many clients have nails with discoloration, lines, ridges, spots, and uncommon shapes that suggest an underlying disorder. Some examples follow:

Longitudinal Ridging
Parallel ridges running lengthwise. May be seen in the elderly and some young people with no known etiology.

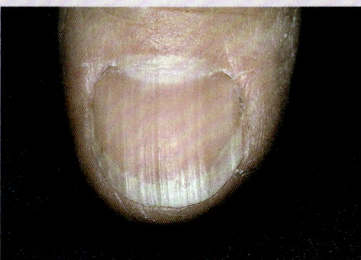

Half-and-Half Nails
Nails that are half white on the upper proximal half and pink on the distal half. May be seen in chronic renal disease.

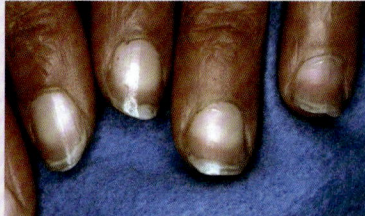

Pitting
Seen with psoriasis.

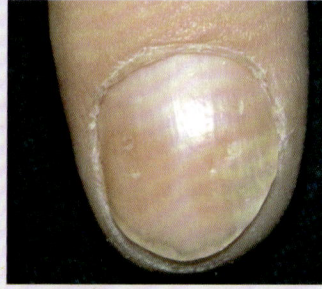

Continued on following page

ABNORMAL FINDINGS 14-7 Common Nail Disorders (Continued)

Koilonychia

Spoon-shaped nails that may be seen with trauma to cuticles or nail folds or in iron deficiency anemia, endocrine or cardiac disease.

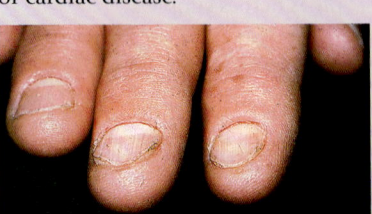

Yellow Nail Syndrome

Yellow nails grow slow and are curved. May be seen in AIDS and respiratory syndromes.

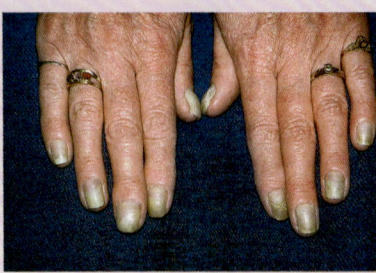

Paronychia

Local infection.

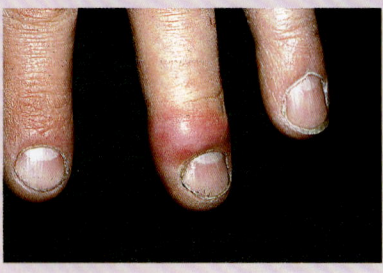

Photo credits: Half-and-half nails *used with permission from Hall, B. J., & Hall, J. C. (2010). Sauer's manual of skin diseases (10th ed.). Philadelphia, PA: Lippincott Williams & Wilkins;* All other photographs *used with permission from Goodheart, H., & Gonzalez, M. E. (2016). Goodheart's photoguide to common pediatric and adult skin disorders (4th ed.). Philadelphia, PA: Wolters Kluwer.*

Want to know more?

A wide variety of resources to enhance your learning and understanding of this book are available on **thePoint**. Visit thePoint to access:

- NCLEX-Style Student Review Questions
- Watch and Learn Videos
- Concept in Action Animations
- And more!

Unfolding Patient Stories: Kim Johnson • Part 1

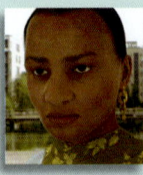

Kim Johnson is a 26-year-old police officer with paraplegia from a thoracic spinal cord injury at level 8 caused by a gunshot wound. She has started on bowel and bladder management programs. Describe the nursing assessment of the genital and rectal areas. While assessing these areas, what potential complications should the nurse consider that are associated with intermittent urinary catheterization, rectal suppositories and digital stimulation, and incontinence? (Kim Johnson's story continues in Chapter 29.)

Care for Kim and other patients in a realistic virtual environment: **vSim** *for Nursing* (http://thepoint.lww.com/vSimHealthAssessment). Practice documenting these patients' care in DocuCare (thepoint.lww.com/DocuCareEHR).

Unfolding Patient Stories: Marvin Hayes • Part 2

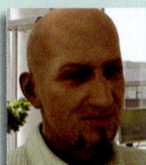

Recall from Chapter 1 Marvin Hayes, who underwent a laparoscopic abdominoperineal resection to remove a tumor in the lower rectum. A permanent sigmoid colostomy and closure of the rectum were performed. What nursing assessments are done to evaluate the status of the rectal–perineal incision? What measures can the nurse take to reduce embarrassment or anxiety and to optimize comfort when assessing the rectal–perineal area?

Care for Marvin and other patients in a realistic virtual environment: **vSim** *for Nursing* (http://thepoint.lww.com/vSimHealthAssessment). Practice documenting these patients' care in DocuCare (thepoint.lww.com/DocuCareEHR).

References and Selected Readings

Ahmed, A., Argentina, L., Butler, D., et al. (2013). Quality-of-life effects of common dermatological diseases. Available at http://www.cutis.com/fileadmin/content_pdf/san/scms_pdf/SCMS_Vol_32_No_2_QOL_Effects.pdf

American Academy of Dermatology. (2015). Moles: Who gets and types. Available at https://www.aad.org/dermatology-a-to-z/diseases-and-treatments/m—p/moles/who-gets-types

American Autoimmune Association. (2015). Autoimmune disease in women. Available at http://www.aarda.org/autoimmune-information/autoimmune-disease-in-women/

American Cancer Society. (2015a). Simple steps to reduce your skin cancer risk. Available at http://www.cancer.org/myacs/newengland/how-to-reduce-your-risk-of-skin-cancer

American Cancer Society. (2015b). What is ultraviolet (UV) radiation? Available at http://www.cancer.org/cancer/cancercauses/sunanduvexposure/skincancerprevention

andearlydetection/skin-cancer-prevention-and-early-detection-what-is-u-v-radiation

American Cancer Society. (2016). Skin cancer facts. Available at http://www.cancer.org/cancer/cancercauses/sunanduvexposure/skin-cancer-facts

Andrews, M., & Boyle, J. (2016). *Transcultural concepts in nursing care*(7th ed.). Philadelphia, PA: Wolters Kluwer.

Berlowitz, D. (2014). Incidence and prevalence of pressure ulcers. In D.R. Thomas, & G. Compton (Eds.). *Pressure ulcers in the aging population: A guide for physicians. Aging Medicine* (1). New York: Spring Science & Business Media. DOI 10.1007/978-1-62703-700-6_2

Bradley University. (2017). Body modification and body image. Available at http://www.bradley.edu/sites/bodyproject/disability/modification/

Gardner, C. (2014). Tattoos and hepatitis C: What are the risks? Available at http://www.hepmag.com/articles/tattoo_hcv_2502_25887.shtml

Greener, M. (2014). Beneath the surface: Dermatology and psychiatry. *Progress in neurology and psychiatry,* 18(1), 16–18. Available at onlinelibrary.wiley.com/doi/10.1002/pnp.316/pdf

Iarocci, T. (2015). Skin problems related to obesity. Available at www.livestrong.com/article/22070-skin-problems-related-obesity

Institute for Clinical Symptoms Improvement. (2014). Pressure ulcer prevention and treatment protocol – Revised 2012. Available at https://www.icsi.org/guidelines__more/catalog_guidelines_and_more/catalog_guidelines/catalog_patient_safetyreliability_guidelines/pressure_ulcer/

Martin, A., Saathoff, M., Kuhn, F., et al. (2010). A functional ABCC11 allele is essential in the formation of human axillary odor. *Journal of Investigative Dermatology,* 130(2), 529–540. Available at www.nature.com/jid/journal/v130/n2/abs/jid2009254a.html

Mayo Clinic. (2015a). Hair loss. Available at http://www.mayoclinic.org/diseases-conditions/hair-loss/basics/causes/con-20027666

Mayo Clinic. (2015b). Tattoos: Understanding risks and precautions. Available at http://www.mayoclinic.org/healthy-lifestyle/adult-health/in-depth/tattoos-and-piercings/art-20045067?reDate=21042015

M.D. Anderson Cancer Center. (2015). Skin cancer prevention and screening. Available at http://www.mdanderson.org/patient-and-cancer-information/cancer-information/cancer-types/skin-cancer/prevention/index.html

National Cancer Institute. (2015a). Genetics of the skin. Available at http://www.cancer.gov/cancertopics/pdq/genetics/skin/HealthProfessional/page1

National Cancer Institute. (2015b). Skin cancer screening. Available at http://www.cancer.gov/cancertopics/pdq/screening/skin/HealthProfessional/page2#_81_toc

National Psoriasis Foundation. (2015). How cigarettes and alcohol affect psoriasis. Available at http://www.psoriasis.org/advance/how-cigarettes-and-alcohol-affect-psoriasis

National Quality Measures Clearing House. (2013). Pressure ulcer prevention and treatment protocol. Available at http://www.qualitymeasures.ahrq.gov/content.aspx?id=36732

Schur, P., & Hahn, B. (2015). Epidemiology and pathogenesis of systemic lupus erythematosus. Available at http://www.uptodate.com/contents/epidemiology-and-pathogenesis-of-systemic-lupus-erythematosus

The Skin Cancer Foundation. (2015a). *Do you know your ABCDEs?* Retrieved from http://www.skincancer.org/skin-cancer-information/melanoma/melanoma-warning-signs-and-images/do-you-know-your-abcdes#panel1-4

The Skin Cancer Foundation. (2015b). Facts about sunburn and skin cancer. Available at http://www.skincancer.org/prevention/sunburn/facts-about-sunburn-and-skin-cancer

The Skin Cancer Foundation. (2015c). Indoor tanning increases melanoma risk by 74 percent. Available at http://www.skincancer.org/news/tanning/indoor-tanning-increases-melanoma-risk-by-74-percent

The Skin Cancer Foundation. (2015d). Skin cancer and skin of color. Available at http://www.skincancer.org/prevention/skin-cancer-and-skin-of-color

Tigran, M. (2014). Keloid. Available at www.keloidresearchfoundation.org/keloid.php

U.S. Department of Veterans Affairs, Office of Public & Intergovernmental Affairs. (2015). Groundbreaking device being tested by VA may put end to pressure ulcers. Available at http://www.va.gov/opa/pressrel/pressrelease.cfm?id=2686

U. S. Preventive Services Task Force. (2009). Screening for skin cancer. Available at http://www.uspreventiveservicestaskforce.org/Page/Document/UpdateSummaryFinal/skin-cancer-screening

Veterans Administration Health Services Research & Development. (2015, Feb 5). VA's MRSA reduction program features in The New York Times. Available at http://www.hsrd.research.va.gov/news/research_news/mrsa-020515.cfm

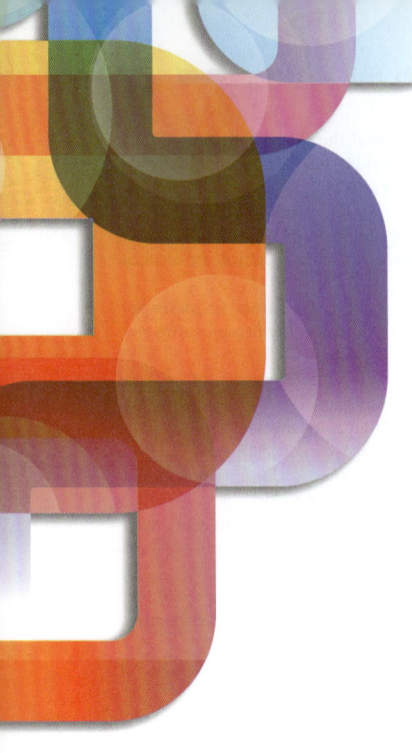

15 ASSESSING HEAD AND NECK

Learning Objectives

1. Describe the structure and function of the head and neck.
2. Discuss risk factors associated with head and neck disorders across the cultures.
3. Interview the client for an accurate nursing history of his or her head and neck.
4. Use the HEADACHE IMPACT TEST to determine how headaches affect the client's activities of daily living.
5. Use the correct technique to perform a physical assessment of the head and neck.
6. Differentiate between normal and abnormal objective and subjective findings related to the head and neck.
7. Describe subjective and objective findings frequently seen when assessing the older client's head and neck.
8. Analyze head and neck data obtained from the interview and physical assessment to formulate valid nursing diagnoses, collaborative problems, and/or referrals.

CASE STUDY

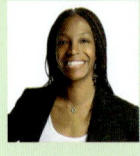

Margy Kase, a 22-year-old African American female college student, attends the annual university health screening. She has come today hoping that someone can see her because she noticed that she is fidgety and hungry all the time lately, though she thinks she has lost weight. She also noticed a swelling of the front of her neck. She denies throat pain or difficulty swallowing. She has come to the clinic today because she wants to stay healthy but has no health insurance, so she cannot see a doctor.

STRUCTURE AND FUNCTION

Head and neck assessment focuses on the cranium, face, thyroid gland, and lymph nodes contained within the head and neck. The sensory organs (eyes, ears, nose, and mouth) are discussed in separate chapters.

The Head

The framework of the head is the skull, which can be divided into two subsections: the cranium and the face (Fig. 15-1).

Cranium

The cranium houses and protects the brain and major sensory organs. It consists of eight bones:
- Frontal (1)
- Parietal (2)
- Temporal (2)
- Occipital (1)
- Ethmoid (1)
- Sphenoid (1)

In the adult client, the cranial bones are joined together by immovable sutures: the sagittal, coronal, squamosal, and lambdoid sutures.

Face

Facial bones give shape to the face. The face consists of 14 bones (see Fig. 15-1):
- Maxilla (2)
- Zygomatic (cheek) (2)
- Inferior conchae (2)
- Nasal (2)
- Lacrimal (2)
- Palatine (2)
- Vomer (1)
- Mandible (jaw) (1)

All of the facial bones are immovable except for the mandible, which has free movement (up, down, and sideways) at the temporomandibular joint (TMJ). The face also consists of many muscles that produce facial movement and expressions. The *temporal artery*, a major artery, is located between the eye and the top of the ear. Two other important structures located in the facial region are the parotid and submandibular salivary glands. The *parotid glands* are located on each side of the face, anterior and inferior to the ears and behind the mandible. The *submandibular glands* are located inferior to the mandible, underneath the base of the tongue.

The Neck

The structure of the neck is composed of muscles, ligaments, and the cervical vertebrae. Contained within the neck are the

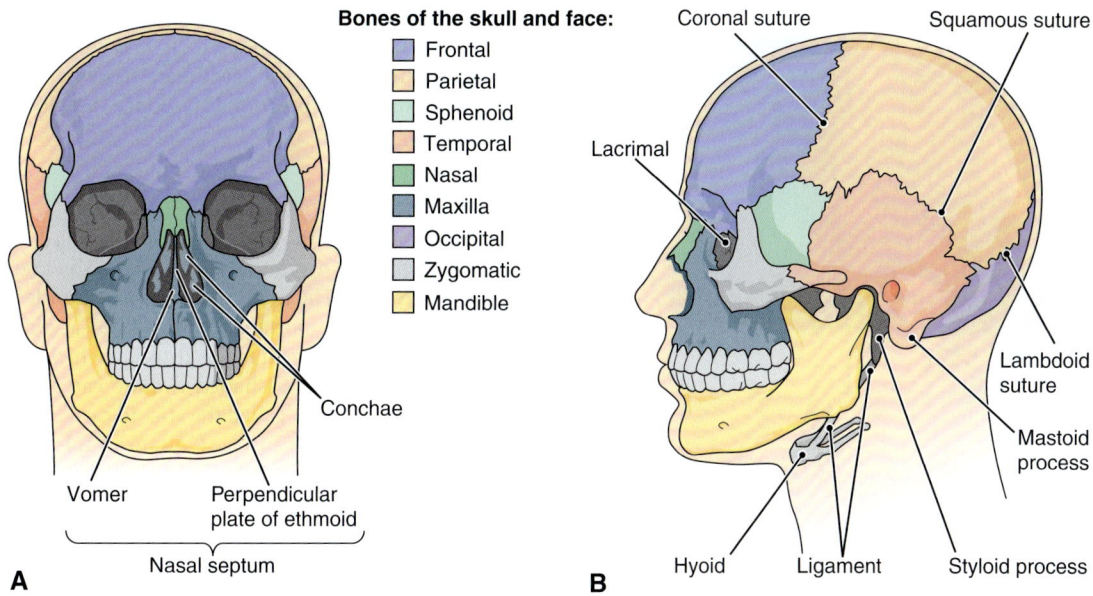

FIGURE 15-1 The skull. A. Anterior view. B. Left lateral view.

hyoid bone, several major blood vessels, the larynx, trachea, and the thyroid gland, which is in the anterior triangle of the neck (Fig. 15-2).

Muscles and Cervical Vertebrae

The sternomastoid (sternocleidomastoid) and trapezius muscles are two of the paired muscles that allow movement and provide support to the head and neck (Fig. 15-3). The *sternomastoid muscle* rotates and flexes the head, whereas the *trapezius muscle* extends the head and moves the shoulders. The *eleventh cranial nerve* is responsible for muscle movement that permits shrugging of the shoulders by the trapezius muscles and turning the head against resistance by the sternomastoid muscles. These two major muscles also form two triangles that provide important landmarks for assessment. The anterior triangle is located under the mandible, anterior to the sternomastoid muscle. The posterior triangle is located between the trapezius and sternomastoid muscles (Fig. 15-3). The cervical vertebrae (C1 through C7) are located in the posterior neck and support the cranium (Fig. 15-4). The vertebra prominens is C7, which can easily be palpated when the neck is flexed. Using C7 as a landmark will help you to locate other vertebrae.

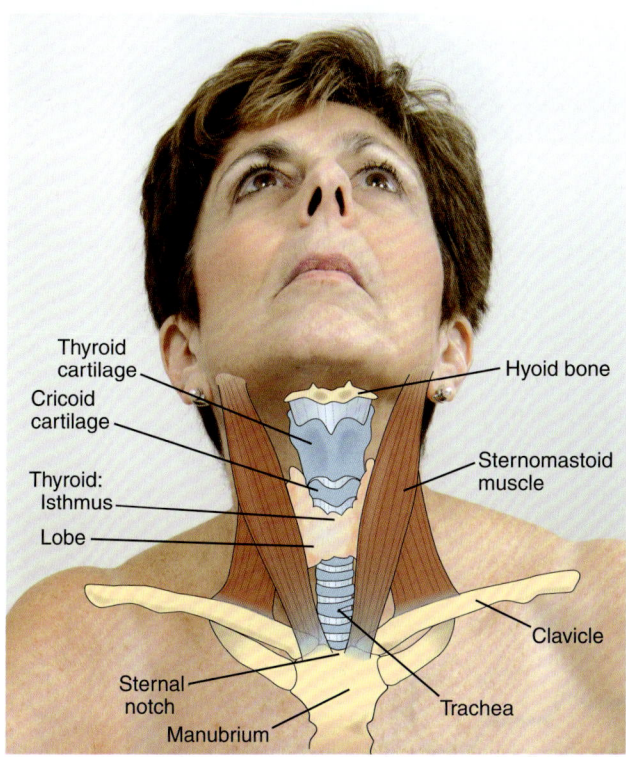

FIGURE 15-2 Structures of the neck.

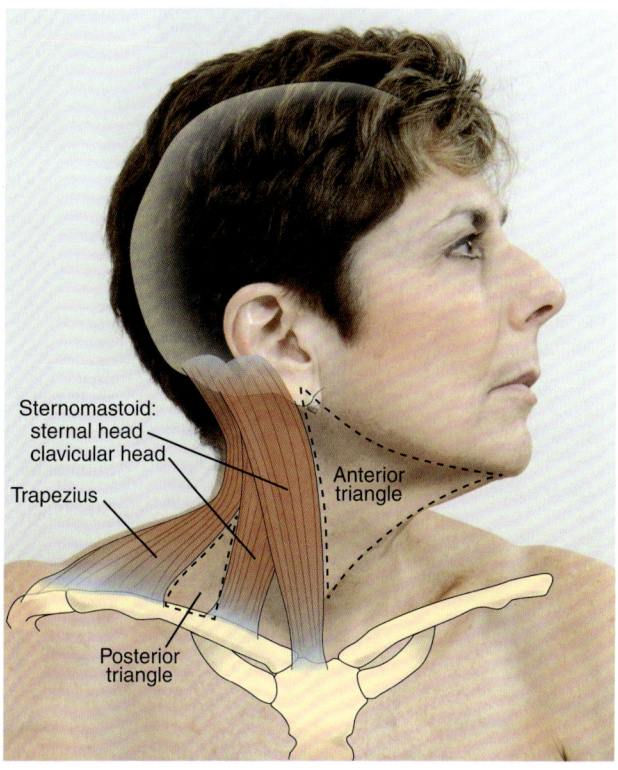

FIGURE 15-3 Neck muscles and landmarks.

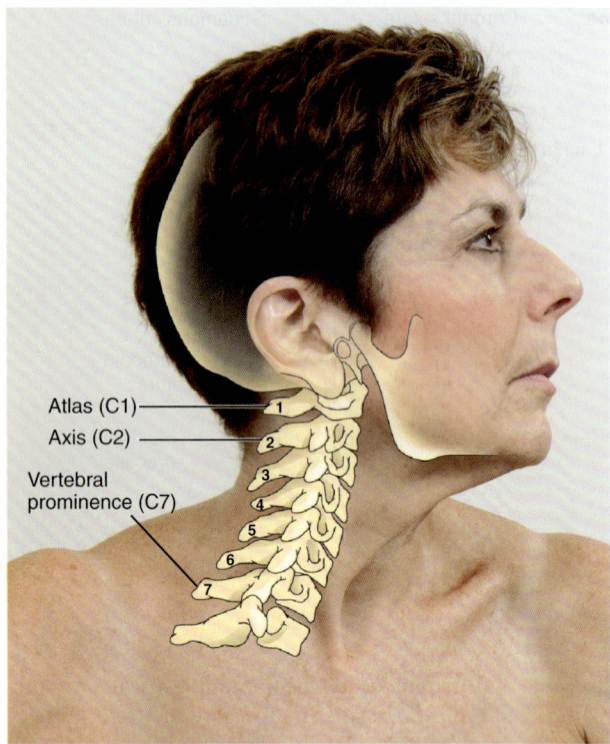

FIGURE 15-4 Cervical vertebrae.

Blood Vessels

The *internal jugular veins* and *carotid arteries* are located bilaterally, parallel and anterior to the sternomastoid muscles. The external jugular vein lies diagonally over the surface of these muscles. The purpose and assessment of these major blood vessels are discussed in Chapter 21. It is important to avoid bilaterally compressing the carotid arteries when assessing the neck, as bilateral compression can reduce the blood supply to the brain.

Thyroid Gland

The thyroid gland is the largest endocrine gland in the body. It produces thyroid hormones that increase the metabolic rate of most body cells. The thyroid gland is surrounded by several structures that are important to palpate for accurate location of the thyroid gland. The trachea, through which air enters the lungs, is composed of C-shaped hyaline cartilage rings. The first upper tracheal ring, called the cricoid cartilage, has a small notch in it. The thyroid cartilage ("Adam's apple") is larger and located just above the cricoid cartilage. The hyoid bone, which is attached to the tongue, lies above the thyroid cartilage and under the mandible (see Fig. 15-2).

The thyroid gland consists of two lateral lobes that curve posteriorly on both sides of the trachea and esophagus and are mostly covered by the sternomastoid muscles. These two thyroid lobes are connected by an isthmus that overlies the second and third tracheal rings below the cricoid cartilage. In about one third of the population, there is a third lobe that extends upward from the isthmus or from one of the two lobes.

Lymph Nodes of the Head and Neck

Several *lymph nodes* are located in the head and neck (Fig. 15-5). Lymph nodes filter lymph, a clear substance

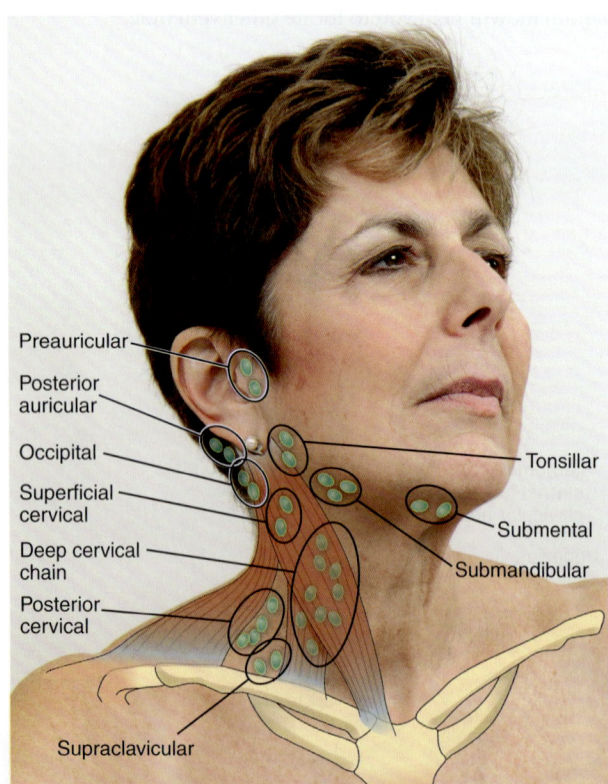
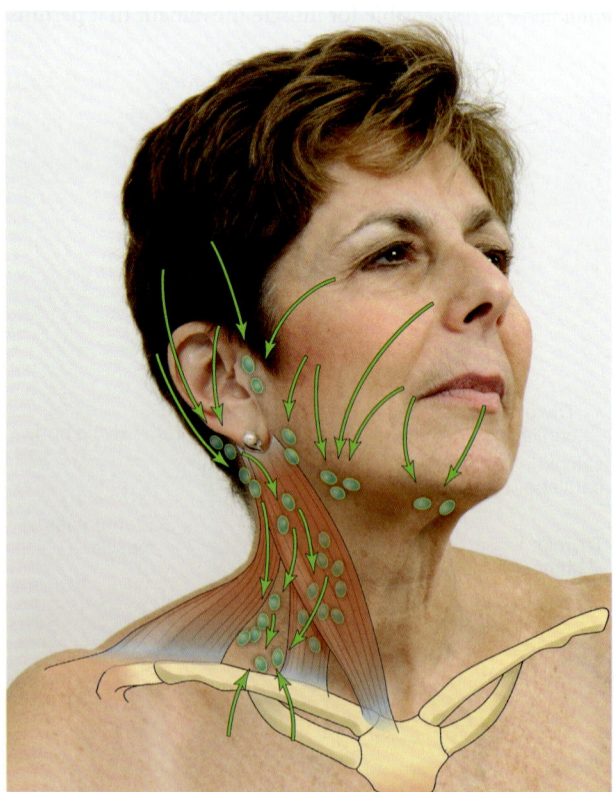

FIGURE 15-5 Lymph nodes in the neck **(left)**. Direction of lymph flow **(right)**. *Note:* Lymph nodes (*green dots*) that are covered by hair may be palpated in the scalp under the hair.

composed mostly of excess tissue fluid, after the lymphatic vessels collect it but before it returns to the vascular system. Filtering removes bacteria and tumor cells from lymph. In addition, the lymph nodes produce lymphocytes and antibodies as a defense against invasion by foreign substances. The size and shape of lymph nodes vary, but most are less than 1 cm long and are buried deep in the connective tissue. They usually appear in clusters that vary in size from 2 to 100 individual nodes.

Normally lymph nodes are either not palpable or they may feel like very small beads. If the nodes become overwhelmed by microorganisms, as happens with an infection such as mononucleosis, they swell and become painful. If cancer metastasizes to the lymph nodes, they may enlarge but not be painful. Sources vary in their reference to the names of lymph nodes. The most common head and neck lymph nodes are referred to as follows:

- Preauricular
- Postauricular
- Tonsillar
- Occipital
- Submandibular
- Submental
- Superficial cervical
- Posterior cervical
- Deep cervical
- Supraclavicular

When an enlarged lymph node is detected during assessment, the nurse needs to know from which part of the head or neck the lymph node receives drainage to assess if an abnormality (e.g., infection, disease) is in that area.

HEALTH ASSESSMENT

Collecting Subjective Data: The Nursing Health History

Abnormalities that cannot be directly observed in the physical appearance of the head and neck are often detected in the client's history. For example, a client may have no visible signs of any problems but may complain of frequent headaches. A detailed description of the type of headache and its location, intensity, and duration provides the nurse with valuable clues as to what the underlying problem might be.

In addition, because of the overlap of several body systems in this area, a thorough nursing history is needed to detect the cause of possible underlying systemic problems. For example, the client experiencing dizziness, spinning, lightheadedness, or loss of consciousness may perceive the problems as related to the head. However, these symptoms may indicate problems with the heart and neck vessels, peripheral vascular system, or neurologic system.

The history also provides an opportunity for you to evaluate activities of daily living that may affect the condition of the client's head and neck. Stress, tension, poor posture while performing work and lack of proper exercise may lead to head and neck discomfort. To prevent head and neck injuries, the nurse may inform the client of protective measures, such as wearing helmets, seat belts, and hard hats, during the history portion of the assessment.

Finally, when discussing the client's head, neck, and facial structures, recognize that the appearance of these structures often has a great influence on the client's self-image. The following questions provide guidance in conducting the interview.

History of Present Health Concern	
QUESTION	**RATIONALE**
Pain	
Do you experience neck pain? Use **COLDSPA** to further explore any neck pain. Be sure to ask about precipitating events (illness or injury), severity, and associated symptoms. **Character:** Describe how it feels. **Onset:** Did it begin after some strenuous activity, exercise, accident, or a direct injury? **Locations:** Does it radiate to the back, arms, or shoulders? **Duration:** How long does it last? Does it come and go? **Severity:** Are you able to continue your daily schedule and sleep at night? **Pattern:** Does it tend to occur more with exercise or stress? Are there any activities that relieve it or make it worse? **Associated Factors:** Do you have any limitation of movement of your head or neck or arms with this pain? Do you have any numbness or tingling with it?	Neck pain may accompany muscular problems or cervical spinal cord problems. Stress and tension may increase neck pain. Sudden head and neck pain seen with elevated temperature and neck stiffness may be a sign of meningeal inflammation. **OLDER ADULT CONSIDERATIONS** Older clients who have arthritis or osteoporosis may experience neck pain and a decreased range of motion.

Continued on following page

History of Present Health Concern (Continued)

QUESTION	RATIONALE
Pain (Continued)	
Do you experience headaches? Use **COLDSPA** to further explore the symptoms of any headache. Be sure to include assessment of severity, location, and aggravating factors.	A precise description of the symptoms can help to determine possible causes of the discomfort. Abnormal Findings 15-1 summarizes typical findings for different headaches. The most common types of headaches are related to vascular (e.g., migraine), muscle contraction (tension), traction, or inflammatory causes.
Have the client complete the Headache Impact Test at *www.bash.org.uk/wp-content/uploads/2012/07/English.pdf* and share the results with primary care provider. **Character:** Describe how the headache feels (sharp, throbbing, dull)? **Onset:** When did it first begin? Does it tend to occur with other factors (e.g., menstrual cycle, emotional or physical stress, ingestion of alcohol or certain other foods like cheese or chocolate)? **Locations:** Where does your headache begin? (Ask client to point to area in head if possible.) Does it radiate or spread to other areas? **Duration:** How long does it last? How often does it recur? Has there been any change in the duration of your headaches? Explain. **Severity:** How severe is the headache? Rate it on a scale of 1–10 (10 being most severe). Does the headache keep you from doing your usual activities of daily living? Explain. **Pattern:** What aggravates it? What makes the pain go away? What pain relievers work best for you? **Associated Factors:** Do you have other symptoms with the headache such as nausea, visual changes, dizziness, or sensitivity to noise or light?	Between 10% and 20% of women have migraine headaches provoked by hormone fluctuations and have a lifetime incidence twice as high as men (43% vs. 17%) (Sacco et al., 2012). Other vascular headaches may be caused by fever or high blood pressure ("cluster headaches"). Muscle contraction headaches may be caused by tightening of facial and neck muscles. Traction and inflammatory headaches may be warning signs of other illnesses such as stroke, sinus or gum infections, and meningitis (NINDS, 2015b). A sudden, severe headache with no known cause may be a sign of impending stroke.
Do you have any facial pain? Describe.	Trigeminal neuralgia (tic douloureux) is manifested by sharp, shooting, piercing facial pains that last from seconds to minutes. Pain occurs over the divisions of the fifth trigeminal cranial nerve (the ophthalmic, maxillary, and mandibular areas).
Other Symptoms	
Do you have any difficulty moving your head or neck?	Tension in muscles, vertebral joint dysfunction, and other disorders of the head and neck may limit mobility and affect activities of daily functioning.
Have you noticed any lumps or lesions on your head or neck that do not heal or disappear? Describe their appearance. Do you have a cough or any difficulty swallowing?	Lumps and lesions that do not heal or disappear may indicate cancer. A goiter (an enlarged thyroid gland) may appear as a large swelling at the base of the neck that the client may notice when shaving or putting on cosmetics. The client with a goiter may also have a tight feeling in the throat, a hoarse voice, cough, hoarseness, difficulty swallowing, difficulty breathing (Mayo Clinic, 2014).
Have you experienced any dizziness, lightheadedness, spinning sensation, blurred vision, or loss of consciousness? Describe.	Sudden trouble seeing or visual disturbances in one or both eyes or sudden trouble walking, dizziness, or loss of balance or coordination may be a sign of an impending stroke (National Stroke Association, 2015).
Have you noticed a change in the texture of your skin, hair, or nails? Have you noticed changes in your energy level, sleep habits, or emotional stability? Have you experienced any palpitations?	Alterations in thyroid function are manifested in many ways. Box 15-1 discusses signs and symptoms of hypo- and hyperthyroidism.

QUESTION	RATIONALE
Have you had any weakness or numbness in your face, arms, or legs or on either side of your body?	Sudden weakness or numbness in the face, arms, or legs—especially on one side of the body—may indicate an impending stroke (National Stroke Association, 2015).

Past Health History

QUESTION	RATIONALE
Describe any previous head or neck problems (trauma, injury, falls) you have had. How were they treated (surgery, medication, physical therapy)? What were the results?	Previous head and neck trauma may cause chronic pain and limitation of movement. This may affect functioning.
Have you ever undergone radiation therapy for a problem in your neck region?	Radiation therapy has been linked to the development of thyroid cancer. Radiation to the neck area may also cause esophageal strictures, leading to difficulty with swallowing. The risk of hypothyroidism increases with head and neck irradiation (Skugor, 2014).

Family History

QUESTION	RATIONALE
Do you find that you have headaches when you take any of the following medications?	Some prescription and nonprescription medicines may cause headaches as follows: • Oral contraceptives and hormone therapy for menopause • Blood-thinning medicines, such as warfarin, heparin, aspirin, and novel oral anticoagulants (NOAC) such as enoxaparin. • Caffeine (or caffeine withdrawal) • Heart and blood pressure medicines, such as nitroglycerin and antihypertensives • Medications for erectile dysfunction • Antihistamines and decongestants • Corticosteroids, such as prednisone • Ergotamine (Cafergot) therapy • Medicines to prevent organ transplant rejection • Immunosuppressants • Certain types of chemotherapy • Overuse of fat-soluble vitamins, such as vitamin A and vitamin D • Radiation therapy • Nonprescription medicines, such as acetaminophen, aspirin, or nonsteroidal anti-inflammatory drugs (NSAIDs) (especially medication overuse headache) (Auriel, Regev, & Korczyn, 2014). • Prescription pain medicines and opioids such as codeine (Kristoffersen & Lundqvist, 2014).
Is there a history of head or neck cancer in your family?	Genetic predisposition is a risk factor for head and neck cancers.
Is there a history of migraine headaches in your family?	Migraine headaches commonly have a familial association.

Lifestyle and Health Practices

QUESTION	RATIONALE
Do you smoke or chew tobacco? If yes, how much? Do you use alcohol or recreational drugs? Describe the type used and how much.	Tobacco use increases the risk of head and neck cancer. Eighty-five percent of head and neck cancers are linked to tobacco use (smoking and smokeless tobacco). Symptoms of head and neck cancer include: a lump or sore that does not heal, a sore throat that does not go away, and trouble swallowing (National Cancer Institute [NCI] at the National Institutes of Health [NIH], 2012). Alcohol use is also a risk factor for head and neck cancers (NCI, 2012). Headaches can be precipitated by the use of alcohol.

Continued on following page

Lifestyle and Health Practices (Continued)

QUESTION	RATIONALE
Do you wear a helmet when riding a horse, bicycle, motorcycle, or other open sports vehicle (e.g., four-wheeler, go-cart)? Do you wear a hard hat for hazardous occupations?	Failure to use safety precautions increases the risk for head and neck injury (see Evidence-Based Practice 15-1).
In what kinds of recreational activity do you participate? Describe the activity.	Contact or aggressive sports may increase the risk for a head or neck injury.
What is your typical posture when relaxing, during sleep, and when working?	Poor posture or body alignment can lead to or exacerbate head and neck discomfort.
Have any problems with your head or neck interfered with your relationships with others or the role you occupy at home or at work?	Head and neck pain may interfere with relationships or prevent clients from completing their usual activities of daily living.

CASE STUDY

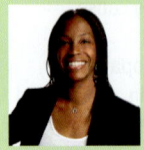

The nurse interviews Ms. Kase, using specific probing questions. The client reports that she has been fidgety, hungry all the time, but losing weight, and has a swelling in the front of her neck. The nurse explores this health concern using the COLDSPA mnemonic.

Mnemonic	Question	Client Response
Character	Describe the sign or symptom (feeling, appearance, sound, smell, or taste if applicable).	"I am hungry all the time, fidgety." Client appears thin, fidgety, and is perspiring on her forehead and upper lip in a cool examination room.
Onset	When did it begin?	"A few weeks ago. I noticed how hungry I was and then a slow weight loss, which has continued. Also, I began to notice my neck was swollen about 2 weeks ago."
Location	Where is it? Does it radiate? Does it occur anywhere else?	"The swelling is right in front and seems to cover the whole lower front of my neck." Denies neck pain or swallowing difficulty.
Duration	How long does it last? Does it recur?	"The swelling is always there now. My hunger seems to be all the time. I just can't get satisfied."
Severity	How bad is it? How much does it bother you? Rate the pain on a scale of 1–10, with 10 being the worst pain.	"I have lost about 7 pounds in the last month."
Pattern	What makes it better or worse?	"I haven't noticed anything that makes the hunger or the neck better or worse."
Associated factors/How it Affects the client	What other symptoms occur with it? How does it affect you?	"I want to stay healthy, but I don't have any health insurance and this hunger and neck swelling both worry me."

After exploring the complaint of hunger and neck swelling, the nurse continues with the health history and asks about injuries and illnesses. Ms. Kase denies any previous head or neck trauma, injury, or falls. She has not undergone radiation therapy to head or neck. She does not have a medical history of hypothyroidism/hyperthyroidism.

Ms. Kase denies any family history of head or neck cancer, or migraine headaches. Her mother had a "thyroid problem," but she does not remember what it was called or how it affected her. Her mother and father died when she was 10 years old.

Ms. Kase denies use of cigarettes, smokeless tobacco, alcohol, and recreational drugs. Ms. Kase says she is concerned that if her weight loss continues, her grades will be affected. She is also concerned about the cost of treatment since she has no health care insurance.

BOX 15-1 SIGNS AND SYMPTOMS OF ALTERED THYROID FUNCTION

HYPOTHYROIDISM

Signs and symptoms of hypothyroidism are often nonspecific and include (Skugor, 2014):
- Sleepiness
- Cold intolerance
- Weight gain
- Muscle aches
- Fatigue
- Menstrual irregularities
- Pale, dry skin
- Thin, brittle hair or nails
- Bradycardia
- Constipation
- Unintentional weight gain
- Edema (especially periorbital)
- Difficulty with concentration and memory
- Slowing of relaxation phase of tendon reflexes
- May have higher diastolic blood pressure
- Most serious form of hyperthyroidism is myxedema

HYPERTHYROIDISM (THYROTOXICOSIS)

Signs and symptoms of hypothyroidism (Skugor, 2014) include:

Symptoms
- Nervousness
- Fatigue
- Weakness
- Palpitations
- Heat intolerance
- Excessive sweating
- Dyspnea
- Diarrhea
- Insomnia
- Poor concentration
- Oligomenorrhea

Signs
- Weight loss
- Hair loss
- Tachycardia
- Proximal myopathy
- Warm, moist skin
- Hyperkinesis
- Stare, lid lag, lid retraction, and exophthalmos (with Graves disease)
- Emotional liability
- Hyperactive reflexes
- Thyroid enlargement (in most cases)

15-1 EVIDENCE-BASED HEALTH PROMOTION AND DISEASE PREVENTION: TRAUMATIC BRAIN INJURY (TBI)

INTRODUCTION

Traumatic brain injury (TBI)—which results from a bump, jolt, blow, or penetrating injury to the head—is a major public health problem (CDC, 2015a). According to the CDC, in 2010, 2.5 million TBIs occurred either as an isolated injury or along with other injuries. The CDC (2015a) says that TBI is a contributing factor in 30% of all injury-related deaths in the United States. TBI also often causes death or permanent disability.

The severity of brain injuries ranges from mild to severe, with the most common being a mild concussion. The CDC (2015b) defines mild injuries as "a brief change in mental status or consciousness," and severe injuries as "an extended period of unconsciousness or memory loss after the injury."

The largest number of TBIs are attributed to falls (40.5%). Other causes are unknown (19%); strike to head (15.5%); motor vehicle accidents (14.3%); and assaults (10.7%).

Mayo Clinic (2015) differentiates categories of sports injuries and explosive and other combat injuries. Age is a factor in TBI. Age groups most likely to have a TBI are children aged 0 to 4 years, young adults from 19 to 24 years, and adults aged 75 years and older (Mayo Clinic, 2015). The CDC reports that people over 75 years of age account for the highest rates of TBI-related hospitalizations and deaths. It is not surprising that males are more likely to sustain and/or die from a TBI than females due to more risk taking behaviors and contact sports or hazardous occupations. Falls and child abuse, such as shaken baby syndrome, account for most of the TBIs in infants and small children (CDC, 2015a).

HEALTHY PEOPLE 2020 GOAL

Healthy People 2020 (2012) includes TBI in the general topic of Injury and Violence Prevention. Elements involved in understanding injury and violence include individual behaviors, physical environment, access to services, and social environment. The specific objectives for injury and violence consider these elements.
- Prevent unintentional injury and violence, and reduce their consequences.
- Reduce fatal and nonfatal TBIs.

OBJECTIVES
- Reduce fatal and nonfatal TBIs.
- Reduce hospitalizations from nonfatal TBI.
- Reduce emergency department visits for nonfatal injuries.

SCREENING

The U.S. Preventive Services Task Force does not include screening recommendation for TBI. However, many other organizations provide screening tools for use in clinical settings to detect TBI. The USDHHS Health Resources and Services Administration (HRSA) has provided information and resources for TBI through their Traumatic Brain Injury Program, but in October, 2015, this program moved from HRSA to the Administration for Community Living (ACL). HRSA

Continued on following page

15-1 EVIDENCE-BASED HEALTH PROMOTION AND DISEASE PREVENTION: TRAUMATIC BRAIN INJURY (TBI) (Continued)

notes that there are a few questions that are found on almost all screening instruments to determine the presence of a TBI. These are:

1. Have you ever had an injury to your head or face?
2. Have you ever lost consciousness?
3. Has there been a change in your behavior?
4. Are you having difficulty concentrating, organizing your thoughts, or remembering (U.S. Department of Health and Human Services Health Resources & Services Administration, 2006)?

One short tool with instructions for use is the HELPS screening instrument (Available at: http://www2.ncdhhs.gov/dma/moneyfollows/MI-HELPS_Screening_Tool.pdf; see Instructions for use of the HELPS screening tool, original 1991 as well). There are also screening tools specific for mild concussions and for military personnel.

RISK ASSESSMENT

Risk Factors: Age-related
- Age newborn to 4 years old
- Teenagers, especially between 15 and 19 years old
- Adults over 65 years

RISK FACTORS: OTHER
- Transportation accidents involving automobiles, motorcycles, bicycles, and pedestrians
- Violence, such as firearm assaults and child abuse or self-inflicted wounds
- Falling
- Excessive alcohol ingestion
- Infants and elderly being cared for by caregivers

To assess for risk, determine the age of the individual, physical and mental health status, and lifestyle. Assess for the following factors:

Infants and Toddlers
- Environmental risks (for falls)
- Lack of parental knowledge of shaken baby syndrome
- Caregivers' risk of shaken baby syndrome

Children and Teens
- Knowledge and use of protective equipment in sports and bicycle use
- Knowledge and use of safety practices when driving

Adults and Older Adults
- Knowledge and use of safety practices when driving
- Impairment of physical or mental stability
- Potential for maltreatment or domestic violence

CLIENT EDUCATION

Teach Clients

The CDC (2015b) lists many ways to reduce the chances of a concussion or other forms of TBI, including:

- Buckling your child in the car using a child safety seat, booster seat, or seat belt (according to the child's height, weight, and age). Know the stages:
  - Birth through age 2
  - Between ages 2 and 4/until 40 lb
  - Between ages 4 and 8 or until 4' 9" tall
  - After age 8 and/or 4' 9" tall
- Wearing a seat belt every time you drive or ride in a motor vehicle
- Never driving while under the influence of alcohol or drugs
- Wearing a helmet and making sure your children wear helmets when:
  - Riding a bike, motorcycle, snowmobile, scooter, or all-terrain vehicle;
  - Playing a contact sport, such as football, ice hockey, or boxing;
  - Using in-line skates or riding a skateboard;
  - Batting and running bases in baseball or softball;
  - Riding a horse; or
  - Skiing or snowboarding.
- Making living areas safer for seniors, by:
  - Removing tripping hazards such as throw rugs and clutter in walkways;
  - Using nonslip mats in the bathtub and on shower floors;
  - Installing grab bars next to the toilet and in the tub or shower;
  - Installing handrails on both sides of stairways; and
  - Improving lighting throughout the home.
- Maintaining a regular physical activity program, if your doctor agrees, to improve lower body strength and balance.
- Making living areas safer for children, by:
  - Installing window guards to keep young children from falling out of open windows;
  - Using safety gates at the top and bottom of stairs when young children are around; and
  - Making sure the surface on your child's playground is made of shock-absorbing material, such as hardwood mulch or sand.

Collecting Objective Data: Physical Examination

Examining the head allows the nurse to evaluate the overlying protective structures (cranium and facial bones) before evaluating the underlying special senses (vision, hearing, smell, and taste) and the functioning of the neurologic system. This examination can detect head and facial shape abnormalities, asymmetry, structural changes, or tenderness. Assessment of both the head and neck assists the nurse to detect enlarged or tender lymph nodes. Thyroid enlargement, nodules, masses, or tenderness may be detected by palpating the thyroid gland. Palpation may also detect abnormalities of the neck and facial muscles. The assessment steps and findings to be described provide parameters for the examination.

Preparing the Client

Prepare the client for the head and neck examination by instructing him or her to remove any wig, hat, hair ornaments, pins, rubber bands, jewelry, and head or neck scarves.

🌐 CULTURAL CONSIDERATIONS

Take care to consider cultural norms for touch when assessing the head. Some cultures (e.g., Southeast Asian) prohibit touching the head or touching the feet before touching the head (Cotton, 2013).

Ask the client to sit in an upright position with the back and shoulders held back and straight. Explain the importance of remaining still during most of the inspection and palpation of the head and neck. However, explain the need for the client to move and bend the neck for examination of muscles and for palpation of the thyroid gland. Be aware that some clients may be anxious as you palpate the neck for lymph nodes, especially if they have a history of cancer that caused lymph node enlargement. Tell the client what you are doing and share your assessment findings.

CULTURAL CONSIDERATIONS
Keep in mind that normal facial structures and features tend to vary widely among individuals and cultures. Variations occur in the shape and size of the orbital regions, nose heights and widths, nasolabial and ear dimensions (Farkas et al., 2005; McKnight, Momoh, & Bullocks, 2009).

Equipment
- Small cup of water
- Stethoscope

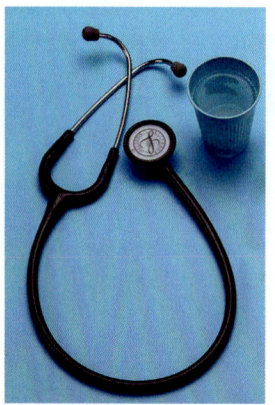

General Routine Screening or Focused/Specialty Assessment

It is difficult to separate assessment that is most useful for all nurses for general assessment as opposed to more focused and specialty area assessments. Examples of general versus focused/specialty assessments for the head and neck appear in the box below. The nurse may assess any of these; however, assessment is usually not routinely completed on a day-to day-basis for the hospitalized client with a head or neck concern for which the nurse needs additional data to report to another health care provider. In a home setting, the techniques listed below may be used to collect data to provide to primary health care providers. As can be seen, there is overlap of what a nurse in different practice settings would be required to do.

General Routine Screening
- Inspect head for size, shape, and configuration
- Palpate temporal arteries
- Palpate temporomandibular joint for swelling, tenderness, or crepitation
- Inspect neck for movement, position, symmetry, lumps, or masses
- Palpate trachea for position
- Palpate thyroid for enlargement, lumps, or masses
- Palpate for any enlarged or tender lymph nodes
- Auscultate for bruits over thyroid if enlarged

Focused Specialty Assessment
- Assess and determine type of headache client is experiencing
- Assess signs of thyroid dysfunction
- Assess signs of Bell palsy

ASSESSMENT PROCEDURE	NORMAL FINDINGS	ABNORMAL FINDINGS
Head and Face		
INSPECTION AND PALPATION		
Inspect the head. Inspect for size, shape, and configuration (Fig. 15-6).	Head size and shape vary, especially in accord with ethnicity. Usually the head is symmetric, round, erect, and in midline and appropriately related to body size (normocephalic). No lesions are visible.	An abnormally small head is called microcephaly. The skull and facial bones are larger and thicker in acromegaly (see Abnormal Findings 15-2). Acorn-shaped, enlarged skull bones are seen in Paget disease of the bone.

Continued on following page

Head and Face (Continued)

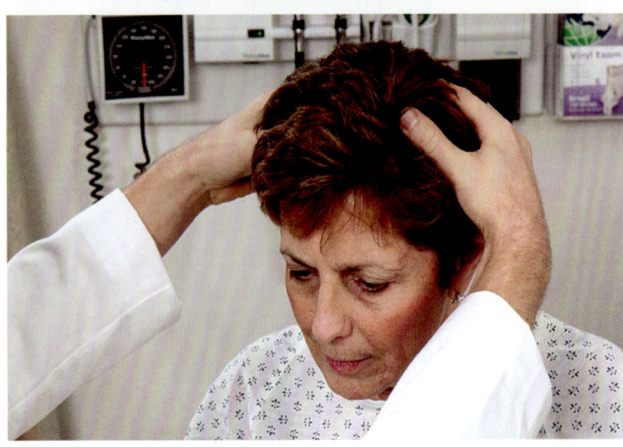

FIGURE 15-6 Inspecting the head.

ASSESSMENT PROCEDURE	NORMAL FINDINGS	ABNORMAL FINDINGS
Inspect for involuntary movement.	Head should be held still and upright.	Neurologic disorders may cause a horizontal jerking movement. An involuntary nodding movement may be seen in patients with aortic insufficiency. Head tilted to one side may indicate unilateral vision or hearing deficiency or shortening of the sternomastoid muscle.
Palpate the head. Note consistency. ◎ **CLINICAL TIP** Wear gloves to protect yourself from possible drainage.	The head is normally hard and smooth, without lesions.	Lesions or lumps on the head may indicate recent trauma or a sign of cancer.
Inspect the face. Inspect for symmetry, features, movement, expression, and skin condition. ◎ **CLINICAL TIP** The nasolabial folds and palpebral fissures are ideal places to check facial features for symmetry.	The face is symmetric with a round, oval, elongated, or square appearance. No abnormal movements noted. **OLDER ADULT CONSIDERATIONS** In older clients, facial wrinkles are prominent because subcutaneous fat decreases with age. In addition, the lower face may shrink and the mouth may be drawn inward as a result of resorption of mandibular bone, also an age-related process.	Asymmetry anterior to the earlobes occurs with parotid gland enlargement from an abscess or tumor. Unusual or asymmetric orofacial movements may be from an organic disease or neurologic problem, which should be referred for medical follow-up. Drooping, weakness, or paralysis on one side of the face may result from a stroke (cerebrovascular accident, CVA) and usually is seen with paralysis or weakness of other parts on that side of the body. Drooping, weakness, or paralysis on one side of the face may also result from a neurologic condition known as Bell palsy. A "mask-like" face marks Parkinson disease; a "sunken" face with depressed eyes and hollow cheeks is typical of cachexia (emaciation or wasting); and a pale, swollen face may result from nephrotic syndrome. See Abnormal Findings 15-2 for Bell palsy and other abnormalities of the face.

15 Assessing Head and Neck 291

ASSESSMENT PROCEDURE	NORMAL FINDINGS	ABNORMAL FINDINGS
Palpate the temporal artery, which is located between the top of the ear and the eye (Fig. 15-7).	The temporal artery is elastic and not tender. **OLDER ADULT CONSIDERATIONS** **The strength of the pulsation of the temporal artery may be decreased in the older client.**	An acute urgent condition is seen when the temporal artery is hard, thick, and tender with inflammation, as seen with temporal arteritis (inflammation of the temporal arteries that may lead to blindness).
Palpate the temporomandibular joint (TMJ). To assess the TMJ, place your index finger over the front of each ear as you ask the client to open the mouth (Fig. 15-8).	Normally there is no swelling, tenderness, or crepitation with movement. Mouth opens and closes fully (3–6 cm between upper and lower teeth). Lower jaw moves laterally 1–2 cm in each direction.	Limited range of motion, swelling, tenderness, or crepitation may indicate TMJ syndrome. 🎯 **CLINICAL TIP** When assessing TMJ syndrome, be sure to explore the client's history of headaches, if any.

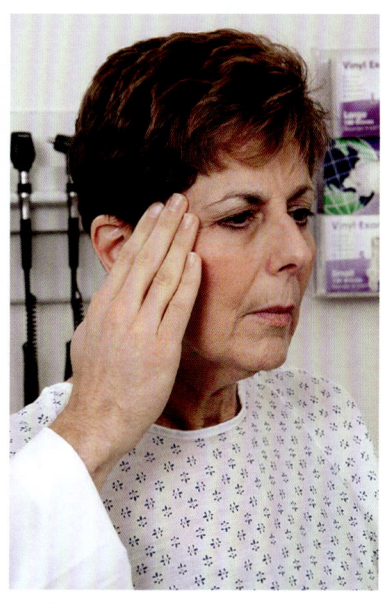

FIGURE 15-7 Palpating the temporal artery.

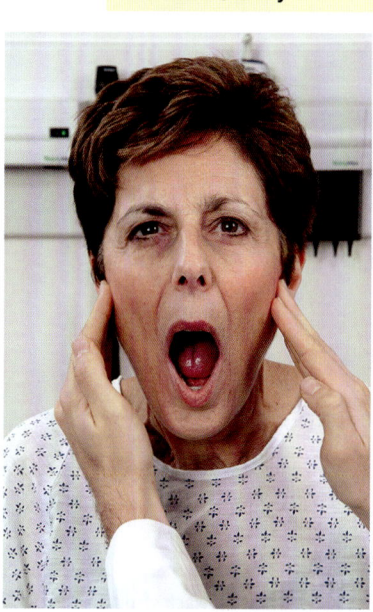

FIGURE 15-8 Palpating the temporomandibular joint (TMJ).

The Neck

INSPECTION

Inspect the neck. Observe the client's slightly extended neck for position, symmetry, and lumps or masses. Shine a light from the side of the neck across to highlight any swelling.	Neck is symmetric, with head centered and without bulging masses.	Swelling, enlarged masses—or nodules—may indicate an enlarged thyroid gland (Fig. 15-9), inflammation of lymph nodes, or a tumor.

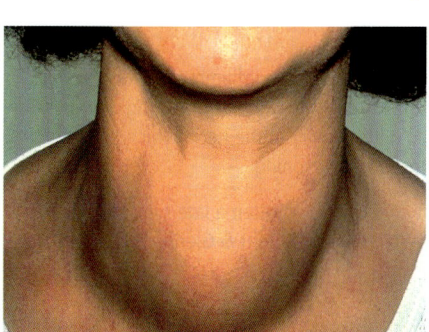

FIGURE 15-9 Diffuse enlargement of the thyroid gland.

Continued on following page

ASSESSMENT PROCEDURE	NORMAL FINDINGS	ABNORMAL FINDINGS
The Neck (Continued)		
Inspect movement of the neck structures. Ask the client to swallow a small sip of water. Observe the movement of the thyroid cartilage, thyroid gland (Fig. 15-10).	The thyroid cartilage and cricoid cartilage move upward symmetrically as the client swallows.	Asymmetric movement or generalized enlargement of the thyroid gland is considered abnormal.

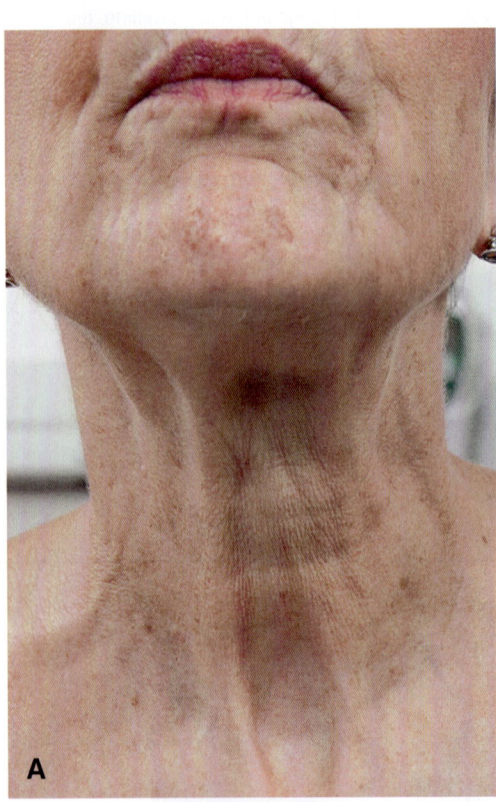 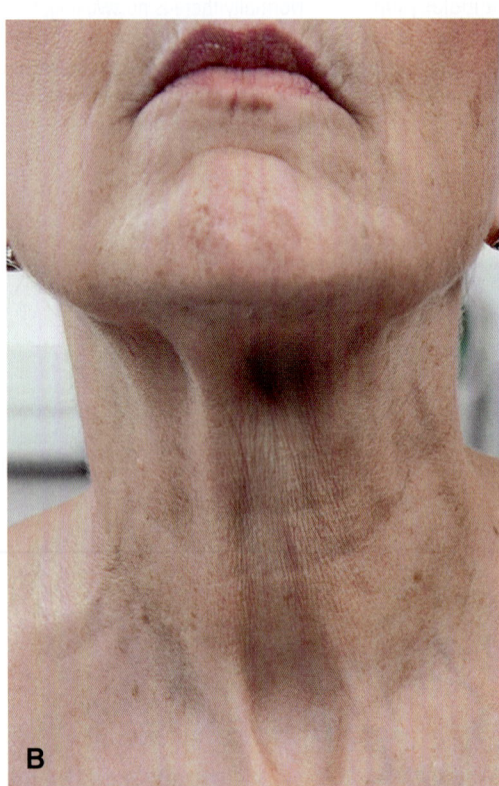

FIGURE 15-10 Neck structures move. **A.** Structures rising. **B.** Structures falling.

Inspect the cervical vertebrae. Ask the client to flex the neck (chin to chest).	C7 (vertebrae prominens) is usually visible and palpable. **OLDER ADULT CONSIDERATIONS** In older clients, cervical curvature may increase because of kyphosis of the spine. Moreover, fat may accumulate around the cervical vertebrae (especially in women). This is sometimes called a "dowager's hump."	Prominence or swellings other than the C7 vertebrae may be abnormal.
Inspect range of motion. Ask the client to turn the head to the right and to the left (chin to shoulder), touch each ear to the shoulder, touch chin to chest, and lift the chin to the ceiling.	Normally neck movement should be smooth and controlled with 45-degree flexion, 55-degree extension, 40-degree lateral abduction, and 70-degree rotation. **OLDER ADULT CONSIDERATIONS** Older clients usually have somewhat decreased flexion, extension, lateral bending, and rotation of the neck. This is usually due to arthritis.	Muscle spasms, inflammation, or cervical arthritis may cause stiffness, rigidity, and limited mobility of the neck, which may affect daily functioning. A stiff neck is often a late symptom seen in meningitis (Knight & Glennie, 2010).

ASSESSMENT PROCEDURE	NORMAL FINDINGS	ABNORMAL FINDINGS
PALPATION		
Palpate the trachea. Place your finger in the sternal notch. Feel each side of the notch and palpate the tracheal rings (Fig. 15-11). The first upper ring above the smooth tracheal rings is the cricoid cartilage.	Trachea is midline.	The trachea may be pulled to the affected side in cases of large atelectasis, fibrosis or pleural adhesions. The trachea is pushed to the unaffected side in cases of a tumor, enlarged thyroid lobe, pneumothorax, or with an aortic aneurysm.

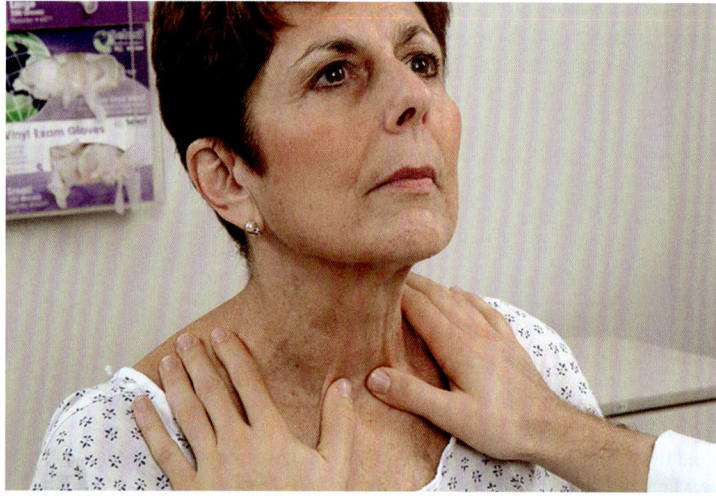

FIGURE 15-11 Palpating the trachea.

Palpate the thyroid gland. Locate key landmarks with your index finger and thumb: *Hyoid bone* (arch-shaped bone that does not articulate directly with any other bone; located high in anterior neck). *Thyroid cartilage* (under the hyoid bone; the area that widens at the top of the trachea), also known as the "Adam's apple." *Cricoid cartilage* (smaller upper tracheal ring under the thyroid cartilage). To palpate the thyroid, use a posterior approach. Stand behind the client and ask the client to lower the chin to the chest and turn the neck slightly to the right. This will relax the client's neck muscles. Then place your thumbs on the nape of the client's neck with your other fingers on either side of the trachea below the cricoid cartilage. Use your left fingers to push the trachea to the right. Then use your right fingers to feel deeply in front of the sternomastoid muscle (Fig. 15-12).	Landmarks are positioned midline. Unless the client is extremely thin with a long neck, the thyroid gland is usually not palpable. However, the isthmus may be palpated in midline. If the thyroid can be palpated, the lobes are smooth, firm, and nontender. The right lobe is often 25% larger than the left lobe. **OLDER ADULT CONSIDERATIONS** If palpable, the older client's thyroid may feel more nodular or irregular because of fibrotic changes that occur with aging; the thyroid may also be felt lower in the neck because of age-related structural changes.	Landmarks deviate from midline or are obscured because of masses or abnormal growths. In cases of diffuse enlargement, such as hyperthyroidism (see Fig. 15-9), Graves' disease, or an endemic goiter, the thyroid gland may be palpated. An enlarged, tender gland may result from thyroiditis. Multiple nodules of the thyroid may be seen in metabolic processes. However, rapid enlargement of a single nodule suggests a malignancy and must be evaluated further.

Continued on following page

ASSESSMENT PROCEDURE	NORMAL FINDINGS	ABNORMAL FINDINGS

The Neck (Continued)

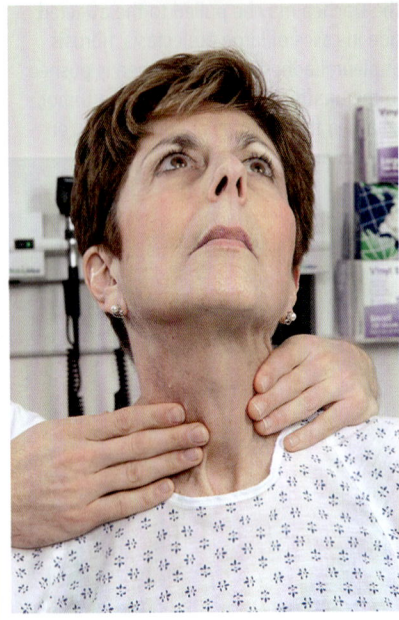

FIGURE 15-12 Palpating the thyroid.

Ask the client to swallow as you palpate the right side of the gland. Reverse the technique to palpate the left lobe of the thyroid.	Glandular thyroid tissue may be felt rising underneath your fingers. Lobes should feel smooth, rubbery, and free of nodules.	Coarse tissue or irregular consistency may indicate an inflammatory process. Nodules should be described in terms of location, size, and consistency.

AUSCULTATION

Auscultate the thyroid only if you find an enlarged thyroid gland during inspection or palpation. Place the bell of the stethoscope over the lateral lobes of the thyroid gland (Fig. 15-13). Ask the client to hold his or her breath (to obscure any tracheal breath sounds while you auscultate).	No bruits are auscultated.	A soft, blowing, swishing sound auscultated over the thyroid lobes is often heard in hyperthyroidism because of an increase in blood flow through the thyroid arteries.

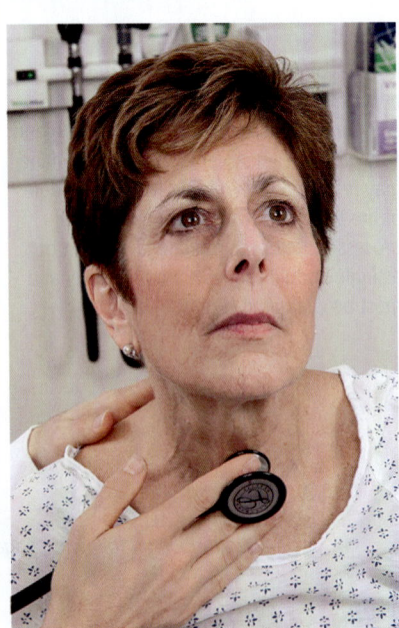

FIGURE 15-13 Auscultating for bruits over the thyroid gland.

ASSESSMENT PROCEDURE	NORMAL FINDINGS	ABNORMAL FINDINGS
Lymph Nodes of the Head and Neck		
Palpate the lymph nodes. Assessment Guide 15-1 describes general technique for palpating the lymph nodes.		Head and neck cancer includes cancers of the mouth, nose, sinuses, salivary glands, throat, and lymph nodes in the neck.
Palpate the *preauricular nodes* (in front of the ear), *postauricular nodes* (behind the ears), *occipital nodes* (at the posterior base of the skull).	There is no swelling or enlargement and no tenderness.	Enlarged nodes are abnormal.
Palpate the *tonsillar nodes* at the angle of the mandible on the anterior edge of the sternomastoid muscle (Fig. 15-14).	No swelling, no tenderness, no hardness is present.	Swelling, tenderness, hardness, immobility are abnormal.
Palpate the *submandibular nodes* located on the medial border of the mandible (Fig. 15-15).	No enlargement or tenderness is present.	Enlargement and tenderness are abnormal.
⦿ **CLINICAL TIP** Do not confuse the submandibular nodes with the lobulated submandibular gland.		

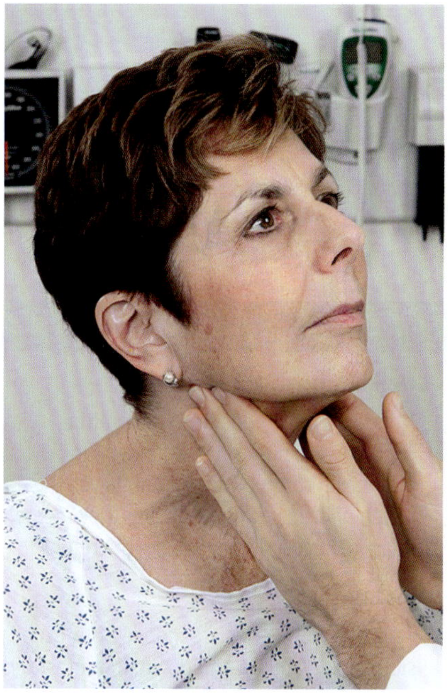

FIGURE 15-14 Palpating the tonsillar nodes.

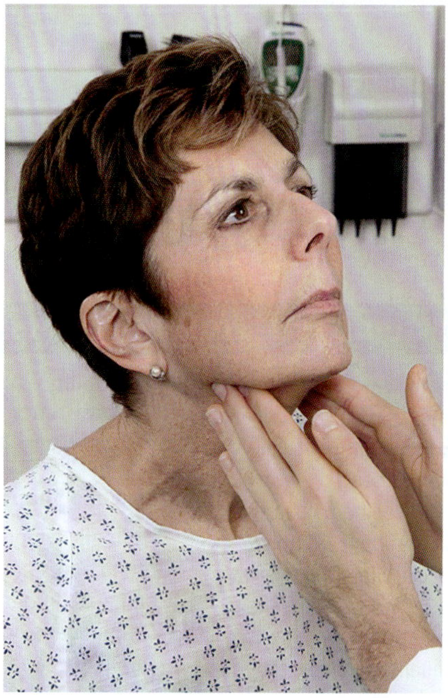

FIGURE 15-15 Palpating the submandibular nodes.

Palpate the *submental nodes*, which are a few centimeters behind the tip of the mandible.	No enlargement or tenderness is present.	Enlargement and tenderness are abnormal.
⦿ **CLINICAL TIP** It is easier to palpate these nodes using one hand.		
Palpate the *superficial cervical nodes* in the area superficial to the sternomastoid muscle.	No enlargement or tenderness is present.	Enlargement and tenderness are abnormal.
Palpate the *posterior cervical nodes* in the area posterior to the sternomastoid and anterior to the trapezius in the posterior triangle.	No enlargement or tenderness is present.	Enlargement and tenderness are abnormal.

Continued on following page

UNIT 3 Nursing Assessment of Physical Systems

ASSESSMENT PROCEDURE	NORMAL FINDINGS	ABNORMAL FINDINGS
Lymph Nodes of the Head and Neck (Continued)		
Palpate the *deep cervical chain nodes* deeply within and around the sternomastoid muscle.	No enlargement or tenderness is present.	Enlargement and tenderness are abnormal.
Palpate the *supraclavicular nodes* by hooking your fingers over the clavicles and feeling deeply between the clavicles and the sternomastoid muscles (Fig. 15-16).	No enlargement or tenderness is present.	An enlarged, hard, nontender node, particularly on the left side, may indicate a metastasis from a malignancy in the abdomen or thorax.

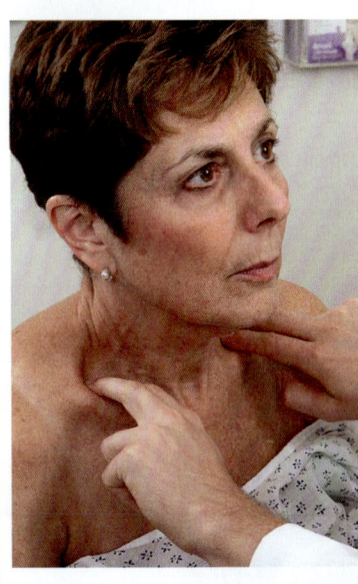

FIGURE 15-16 Palpating the supraclavicular nodes.

ASSESSMENT GUIDE 15-1 Palpating Lymph Nodes

Have the client remain seated upright. Then palpate the lymph nodes with your finger pads in a slow walking, gentle, circular motion. Ask the client to bend the head slightly toward the side being palpated to relax the muscles in that area. Compare lymph nodes that occur bilaterally. As you palpate each group of nodes, assess their size and shape, delimitation (whether they are discrete or confluent), mobility, consistency, and tenderness. Choose a particular palpation sequence. This chapter presents a sequence that proceeds in a superior to inferior order (from 1 to 10).

🎯 CLINICAL TIP
Which sequence you choose is not important. What is important is that you establish a specific sequence that does not vary from assessment to assessment. This helps to guard against skipping a group of nodes.

While palpating the lymph nodes, note the following:
- Size and shape
- Delimitation
- Mobility
- Consistency
- Tenderness and location

Size and Shape
Normally lymph nodes, which are round and smaller than 1 cm, are not palpable. In older clients especially, the lymph nodes become fibrotic, fatty, and smaller because of a loss of lymphoid elements related to aging. (This may decrease the older person's resistance to infection.)

When lymph node enlargement exceeds 1 cm, the client is said to have *lymphadenopathy*, which may be caused by acute or chronic infection, an autoimmune disorder, or metastatic disease. If one or two lymphatic groups enlarge, the client is said to have *regional lymphadenopathy*. Enlargement of three or more groups is *generalized lymphadenopathy*. Generalized lymphadenopathy that persists for more than 3 months may be a sign of human immunodeficiency virus (HIV) infection.

Delimitation
Normally lymph node delimitation (the lymph node's position or boundary) is discrete. In chronic infection, however, the lymph nodes become confluent (they merge). In acute infection, they remain discrete.

Mobility
Typical lymph nodes are mobile both from side to side and up and down. In metastatic disease, the lymph nodes enlarge and become fixed in place.

Consistency
Somewhat more fibrotic and fatty in older clients, the normal lymph node is soft, whereas the abnormal node is hard and firm. Hard, firm, unilateral nodes are seen with metastatic cancers.

Tenderness and Location
Tender, enlarged nodes suggest acute infections; normally lymph nodes are not sore or tender. Of course, you need to document the location of the lymph node being assessed.

CASE STUDY

The nurse inspects Ms. Kase's head and finds it to be symmetric, round, erect and midline (normocephalic). Ms. Kase does not display any involuntary movements. Her head is hard and smooth, without lesions. Ms. Kase's face appears symmetric and oval, with no abnormal or asymmetric orofacial movements noted. Her temporal arteries are elastic and nontender to palpation. On palpation, her temporal mandibular joints are nonedematous, nontender, and without crepitation. Her mouth opens 5 cm with lateral deviation of 2 cm both left and right.

The nurse inspects Ms. Kase's neck. It is symmetric, centered. Her thyroid gland appears to be slightly enlarged when palpated, and a bruit is detected upon auscultation. The cricoid cartilage and thyroid cartilage move upward symmetrically as she swallows, and along with the hyoid are midline. Her C7 is visible and nontender. Ms. Kase denies pain with flexion, extension, lateral movement, and rotation of cervical spine. No decreased range of motion is noted with flexion, extension, abduction, or rotation. There is no enlargement or tenderness of the preauricular, postauricular, occipital, tonsillar, submandibular, submental, superficial cervical, posterior cervical, deep cervical, or supraclavicular nodes.

The nurse takes Ms. Kase's measurements and vital signs. Her height is 5 ft 9 in, weight is 110 lb (putting her in the 5th percentile for weight for her height). Her BP is 132/82; radial pulse 96; respirations 18.

Validating and Documenting Findings

Validate the head and neck assessment data that you have collected. This is necessary to verify that the data are reliable and accurate. Document the assessment data following the health care facility or agency policy.

CASE STUDY

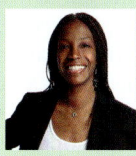

Think back to the case study. The nurse documented the following assessment findings of Ms. Kase's head and neck.
Biographical Data: MK, 22 years old. African American. Full-time college student with a part-time job as a student worker on campus.
General Survey: Awake, alert, and oriented. Makes and maintains eye contact. Asks and answers questions appropriately.
Reason for Seeking Care: "I am hungry and fidgety all the time, and my neck has started swelling."
History of Present Health Concern: "A few weeks ago. I noticed how hungry I was and then a slow weight loss, which has continued. Also, I began to notice my neck was swollen about 2 weeks ago."
Personal Health History: Denies any previous head or neck trauma, injury, or falls. Denies radiation therapy to head or neck. Denies any history of hypothyroidism/hyperthyroidism. Does not know her normal blood pressure.
Family History: Denies any family history of head or neck cancer, or migraine headaches. Mother suffered from "thyroid problems," but died when client was 10 years of age, so she does not know any details.
Lifestyle and Health Practices: Denies use of cigarettes, smokeless tobacco, drugs, or any medications except an occasional Tylenol.
Physical Examination Findings: Head is symmetric, round, erect, and midline (normocephalic). No involuntary movement noted. Head is hard and smooth, without lesions. Face is symmetric and oval, with no abnormal or asymmetric orofacial movements noted. Bilateral temporal arteries are elastic and nontender to palpation. Temporal mandibular joints are nonedematous, nontender, and without crepitation. Mouth opens 5 cm with lateral deviation of 2 cm both left and right. Neck is symmetric, centered. Her thyroid gland appears to be slightly enlarged when palpated, and a bruit is detected upon auscultation. The cricoid cartilage and thyroid cartilage move upward symmetrically as she swallows, and along with the hyoid are midline. Her C7 is visible and nontender. Ms. Kase denies pain with flexion, extension, lateral movement, and rotation of cervical spine. No decreased range of motion is noted with flexion, extension, abduction, or rotation. There is no enlargement or tenderness of the preauricular, postauricular, occipital, tonsillar, submandibular, submental, superficial cervical, posterior cervical, deep cervical, or supraclavicular nodes. Height is 5 ft 9 in, weight is 110 lb (putting her in the 5th percentile for weight for her height). BP is 132/82; radial pulse 96; respirations 18.

ANALYSIS OF DATA: DIAGNOSTIC REASONING

After collecting the assessment data, identify abnormal findings and client strengths using diagnostic reasoning. Then, cluster the data to reveal any significant patterns or abnormalities. The following sections provide possible conclusions that the nurse may make after assessing a client's head and neck.

Selected Nursing Diagnoses

The following is a list of selected nursing diagnoses that may be identified when analyzing data from a head and neck assessment.

Health Promotion Diagnoses

- Readiness for Enhanced Health Management: Requests assistance and information on how to quit smoking

Risk Diagnoses

- Risk for Injury to head and neck related to poor posture
- Risk for Injury to head and neck related to not wearing protective devices (e.g., head gear during contact sports, seat belts, eye goggles)

Actual Diagnoses

- Ineffective Health Maintenance related to refusing to wear protective gear during contact sports or seat belt while driving or riding as a passenger
- Ineffective Health Maintenance related to disregard for the effects and dangers associated with smoking and using smokeless tobacco
- Ineffective Tissue Perfusion: Cerebral related to impaired circulation to brain
- Imbalanced Nutrition: Less Than Body Requirements related to increased metabolism secondary to hyperthyroidism
- Imbalanced Nutrition: More Than Body Requirements related to decreased metabolism secondary to hypothyroidism
- Imbalanced Nutrition: Less Than Body Requirements related to difficulty swallowing, which limits consumption of food
- Activity Intolerance related to fatigue and weakness secondary to slowed metabolic rate secondary to hypothyroidism or to surgery of head, neck, or face
- Constipation related to hyperthyroidism or hypothyroidism
- Chronic pain: sinus headache related to inflammation of sinuses secondary to seasonal allergies.
- Disturbed Body Image related to head injury
- Impaired Swallowing related to mechanical obstruction of the head and neck secondary to tissue swelling, tracheostomy, or abnormal growth
- Impaired Swallowing related to lack of gag reflex, paralysis of facial muscles, or decreased cognition

Selected Collaborative Problems

After grouping the data, certain collaborative problems may become apparent. Remember that collaborative problems differ from nursing diagnoses in that they cannot be prevented by nursing interventions. However, these physiologic complications of medical conditions can be detected and monitored by the nurse. In addition, the nurse can use physician- and nurse-prescribed interventions to minimize the complications of these problems. The nurse may also have to refer the client in such situations for further treatment of the problem. Following is a list of collaborative problems that may be identified when assessing the head and neck of a client. These problems are worded as Risk for Complications (RC), followed by the problem:

- RC: Hypocalcemia
- RC: Hypercalcemia
- RC: Corneal abrasion (related to inability to close eyelids secondary to exophthalmos)
- RC: Thyroid crisis
- RC: Thyroid dysfunction
- RC: Cerebral vascular accident
- RC: Seizures
- RC: Cranial nerve impairment (fifth trigeminal, seventh facial, eleventh spinal accessory)
- RC: Increased intracranial pressure

Medical Problems

After the data are grouped, it may become apparent that the client has signs and symptoms that may require medical diagnosis and treatment. Referral to a primary care provider is necessary.

CASE STUDY

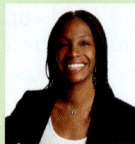

After collecting and analyzing the data for Ms. Kase, the nurse determines that the following conclusions are appropriate.

Nursing Diagnoses Include
Readiness for Enhanced Health Management r/t expressed desire to take care of health and seeking care for current symptoms.

Potential Collaborative Problems Include
Because there is no medical diagnosis, there is no collaborative problem at this time. Findings suggest CP: thyroid abnormality and referral to an appropriate health care provider is discussed with Ms. Kase.

Interdisciplinary Verbal Communication of Assessment Findings Using SBAR

SITUATION: Margy Kase, a 22-year-old African American female student came to the university health screening. She reported being fidgety and hungry all the time and thinks she has lost 7 pounds in the last week. She also noted generalized swelling of the front of her neck for 2 weeks. She denies throat pain or difficulty swallowing. Voices a need to stay healthy and is concerned how this may affect her grades. She has no health insurance and is concerned about cost.

BACKGROUND: Denies any previous head or neck trauma, injury, falls, or radiation. Has a history of hypothyroidism/hyperthyroidism. Her mother had a "thyroid problem," but she does not remember what it was called. Her parents died when she was 10 years old. Denies use of cigarettes, smokeless tobacco, alcohol, and recreational drugs.

ASSESSMENT: Neck is symmetric and centered. Thyroid gland appears to be slightly enlarged when palpated, and a bruit is detected upon auscultation. The cricoid cartilage and thyroid cartilage move upward symmetrically as she swallows, and along with the hyoid are midline. Her C7 is visible and nontender. Denies pain with flexion, extension, lateral movement, and rotation of cervical spine. No decreased range of motion is noted with flexion, extension, abduction, or rotation. There is no enlargement or tenderness of the preauricular, postauricular, occipital, tonsillar, submandibular, submental, superficial cervical, posterior cervical, deep cervical, or supraclavicular nodes. Height is 5 ft 9 in, weight is 110 lb (putting her in the 5th percentile for weight for her height). BP is 132/82; radial pulse 96; respirations 18.

RECOMMENDATION: Ms. Case fears she will not be able to make good grades related to her changes in health nor pay for health care related to lack of health insurance. She needs further evaluation of her thyroid gland and weight loss by her primary care provider.

ABNORMAL FINDINGS 15-1　Types and Characteristics of Headaches

	Sinus Headache	*Cluster Headache*	*Tension Headache*	*Migraine Headache*	*Tumor-related Headache*
Character	Deep, constant, throbbing pain; pressure-like pain in one specific area of face or head (e.g., behind eyes); face tender to the touch	Stabbing pain; may be accompanied by tearing, eyelid drooping, reddened eye, or runny nose	Dull, tight, diffuse	Accompanied by nausea, vomiting, and sensitivity to noise or light	Aching, steady; neurologic and mental symptoms as well as nausea and vomiting may develop
Onset/ Precipitating Factors	Occurs with or after a cold or acute sinusitis or acute febrile illness with purulent discharge from nose.	Has a sudden onset; may be precipitated by ingesting alcohol.	No prodromal stage; may occur with stress, anxiety, or depression.	May have prodromal stage (visual disturbances, vertigo, tinnitus, numbness or tingling of fingers or toes); may be precipitated by emotional disturbances; anxiety; or ingestion of alcohol, cheese, chocolate, or other foods and substances to which client is sensitive.	No prodromal stage; may be aggravated by coughing, sneezing, or sudden movements of the head.
Location	May occur in one area of face or along eyebrow ridge and below the cheek bone.	Localized in the eye and orbit and radiating to the facial and temporal regions.	Usually located in the frontal, temporal, or occipital region.	Located around eyes, temples, cheeks, or forehead; may affect only one side of the face.	Varies with location of tumor.

Sinus headache　　Cluster headache　　Tension headache　　Migraine headache

Continued on following page

ABNORMAL FINDINGS 15-1   Types and Characteristics of Headaches (Continued)

	Sinus Headache	Cluster Headache	Tension Headache	Migraine Headache	Tumor-related Headache
Duration	Lasts until associated condition is improved.	Typically occurs in the late evening or night.	Lasts days, months, or years.	Lasts up to 3 days.	Commonly occurs in the morning and lasts for several hours.
Severity	May be moderately severe; not debilitating.	Intense	Aching	Throbbing, severe	Variable in intensity
Pattern	Pain worse with sudden movements of the head, bending forward, lying down; in the morning (due to mucus collecting and draining all night); or with sudden temperature changes (going from warm room to cold).	Movement or walking back and forth may relieve the discomfort.	Symptomatic relief may be obtained by local heat, massage, analgesics, antidepressants, and muscle relaxants.	Rest may bring relief.	Usually subsides later in the day.
Associated factors	Associated with other symptoms of sinusitis, such as nasal drainage and congestion, fever, and foul-smelling breath. Sinus headaches may be confused with tension headaches and migraines. Hutchinson (2007) advises, "Migraines also have forehead and facial pressure over the sinuses, nasal congestion and runny nose. In the absence of fever, pus from your nose, alteration in smell or foul smelling breath you likely have a migraine headache."	Occur more in young males.	Affect women more often than men.	Occur more often in women.	

Information from Cleveland Clinic. (2015). Migraine headaches. Available at http://my.clevelandclinic.org/health/diseases_conditions/hic_Migraine_Headaches; Hutchinson, S. (2007). "Sinus headache" or migraine. Available at http://www.achenet.org/education/patients/SinusHeadacheorMigraine.asp; and University of Maryland. (2011). Sinus headache. Available at http://www.umm.edu/altmed/articles/sinus-headache-000073.htm

ABNORMAL FINDINGS 15-2 Abnormalities of the Head and Neck

During any physical examination of the head, the nurse may encounter many variations from normal as well as many abnormalities. Some of the most common abnormalities are pictured here.

ACROMEGALY

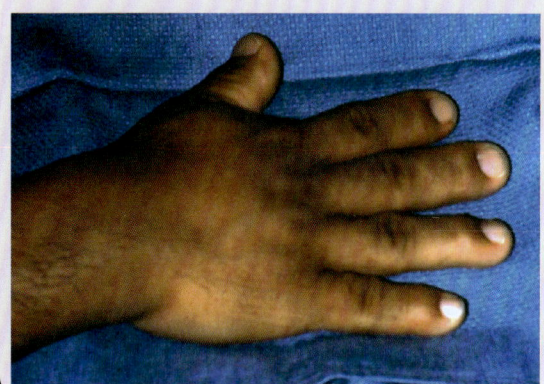

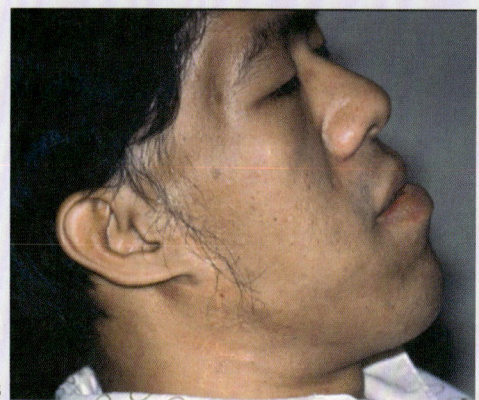

Acromegaly is characterized by enlargement of the facial features (nose, ears) and the hands and feet.

CUSHING SYNDROME

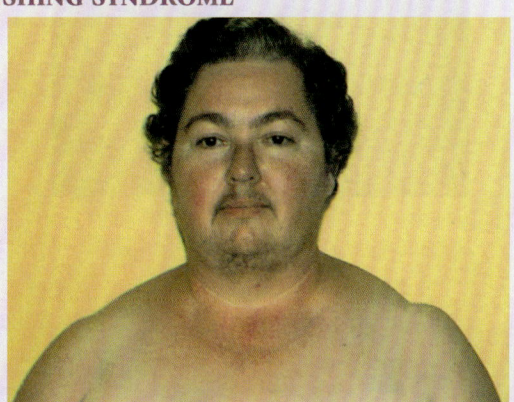

Cushing syndrome may present with a moon-shaped face with reddened cheeks and increased facial hair.

HYPERTHYROIDISM

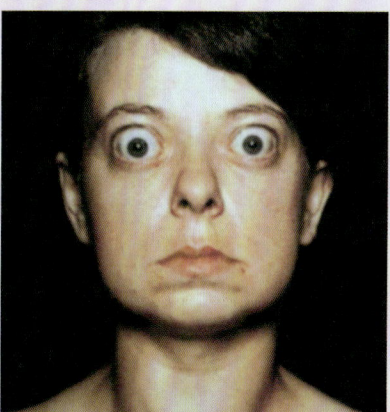

Exophthalmos is seen in hyperthyroidism.

BELL PALSY

Bell palsy usually begins suddenly and reaches a peak within 48 hours. Symptoms may include twitching, weakness, paralysis, drooping eyelid or corner of the mouth, drooling, dry eye, dry mouth, decreased ability to taste, eye tearing, and facial distortion. One-sided facial paralysis is characteristic (NINDS, 2015a).

SCLERODERMA

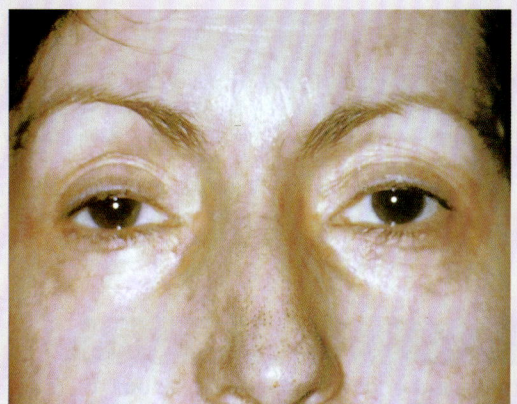

A tightened-hard face with thinning facial skin is seen in scleroderma.

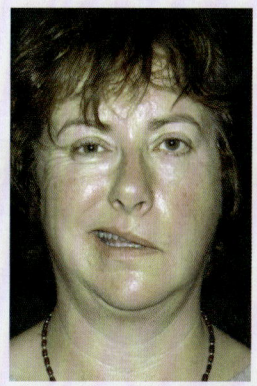

Continued on following page

ABNORMAL FINDINGS 15-2 Abnormalities of the Head and Neck (Continued)

HYPOTHYROIDISM/MYXEDEMA

Myxedema (severe hypothyroidism) is characterized by a dull, puffy face; edema around the eyes; and dry, course, and sparse hair.

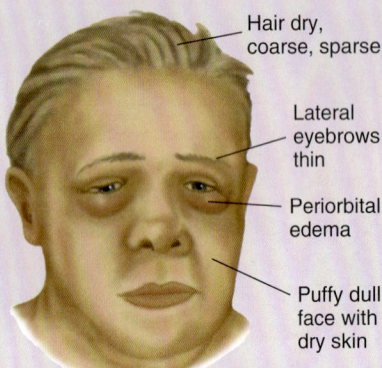

- Hair dry, coarse, sparse
- Lateral eyebrows thin
- Periorbital edema
- Puffy dull face with dry skin

PARKINSON DISEASE

Patients with Parkinson disease have a mask-like facial appearance, along with a shuffling gait, rigid muscles, and diminished reflexes.

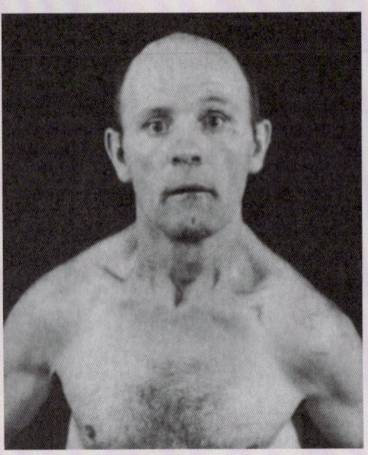

CEREBROVASCULAR ACCIDENT

Cerebrovascular accident results in neurologic damage. The symptoms depend on what part of the brain was affected.

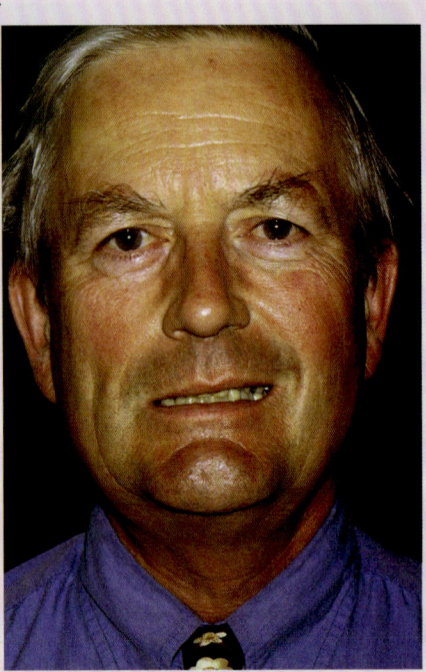

Photo credits: Acromegaly from DeLong, L., & Burkhart, N. (2012). General and Oral Pathology for the Dental Hygienist (2nd ed.). Philadelphia, PA: Wolters Kluwer Heath; Bell's palsy from Dr. P. Marazzi/Photo Researchers, Inc.; Scleroderma from Gold, D. H., & Weingeist, T. A. (2001). Color atlas of the eye in systemic disease. Baltimore, MD: Lippincott Williams & Wilkins; Hypothyroidism/myxedema from Bickley, L.S., Szilagyi, P. (2003). Bates' Guide to Physical Examination and History Taking, 8th ed. Philadelphia, PA: Lippincott Williams & Wilkins; Parkinson's disease from Jensen, S., (2014). Nursing Health Assessment: A Best Practice Approach (2nd ed.). Philadelphia, PA: Wolters Kluwer Health; Cerebrovascular accident from Dr. P. Marazzi/Photo Researchers, Inc.

Want to know more?

A wide variety of resources to enhance your learning and understanding of this book are available on **thePoint**. Visit thePoint to access:

- NCLEX-Style Student Review Questions
- Watch and Learn Videos
- Concept in Action Animations
- And more!

References and Selected Readings

Auriel, E., Regev, K., & Korczyn, A. D. (2014). Nonsteroidal anti-inflammatory drugs exposure and the central nervous system. *Handbook of Clinical Neurology*, 119, 577–584.

Centers for Disease Control & Prevention (CDC). (2015a). TBI data & statistics. Available at http://www.cdc.gov/traumaticbraininjury/data/index.html

Centers for Disease Control & Prevention (CDC). (2015b). Traumatic brain injury. Available at http://www.cdc.gov/TraumaticBrainInjury/

Cotton, G. (2013). *Say anything to anyone, anywhere*. Hoboken, NJ: John Wiley & Sons.

Farkas, L. G., Katic, M. J., Forrest, C. R., et al. (2005). International anthropometric study of facial morphology in various ethnic groups/races. *Journal of Craniofacial Surgery*, 16(4), 615–646. Available at http://www.ncbi.nlm.nih.gov/pubmed/16077306

Healthy People 2020. (2012). Injury & violence prevention: injury prevention: reduce fatal & nonfatal traumatic brain injuries. Available at http://www.healthypeople.gov/2020/topicsobjectives2020/objectiveslist.aspx?topicId=24

Hutchinson, S. (2007). "Sinus headache" or migraine. Available at http://www.achenet.org/education/patients/SinusHeadacheorMigraine.asp.

Knight, C., & Glennie, L. (2010). Early recognition of meningitis and septicaemia. Available at http://www.ncbi.nlm.nih.gov/pubmed/20397549

Kristoffersen, E., & Lundqvist, C. (2014). Medication-overuse headache: Epidemiology, diagnosis, and treatment. *Therapeutic Advances in Drug Safety*, 5(2), 87–99.

Mayo Clinic. (2014). Goiter. Available at http://www.mayoclinic.org/diseases-conditions/goiter/basics/symptoms/con-20021266

Mayo Clinic. (2015). Traumatic brain injury. Available at http://www.mayoclinic.org/diseases-conditions/traumatic-brain-injury/basics/causes/con-20029302

McKnight, A., Momoh, A., & Bullocks, J. (2009). Variations of structural components: Specific intercultural differences in facial morphology, skin type, and structures. *Seminars in Plastic Surgery*, 23(3), 163–167. Available at http://www.ncbi.nlm.nih.gov/pubmed/20676309

National Cancer Institute (NCI) at the National Institutes of Health (NIH). (2012). National Cancer Institute Fact Sheet: Head and Neck Cancers. Available at http://www.cancer.gov/cancertopics/factsheet/Sites-Types/head-and-neck

National Institute of Neurological Disorders & Stroke (NINDS). (2015a). Bell's palsy face sheet. Available at http://www.ninds.nih.gov/disorders/bells/detail_bells.htm#281243050

National Institute of Neurological Disorders & Stroke (NINDS). (2015b). Headache information page. Available at http://www.ninds.nih.gov/disorders/headache/headache.htm

National Stroke Association. (2015). Signs and symptoms of stroke. Available at http://www.stroke.org/understand-stroke/recognizing-stroke/signs-and-symptoms-stroke

Sacco, S., Ricci, S., Degan, D., et al. (2012). Migraine in women: The role of hormones and their impact on vascular diseases. *Journal of Headache Pain*, 13(3), 177–189.

Skugor, M. (2014). Hypothyroidism and hyperthyroidism. Available at http://www.clevelandclinicmeded.com/medicalpubs/diseasemanagement/endocrinology/hypothyroidism-and-hyperthyroidism/Default.htm

U.S. Department of Health and Human Services (USDHHS) Health Resources & Services Administration (HRSA). (2006). Traumatic brain injury screening: An introduction. Available at http://www.nmbiac.com/helps_screening_tool

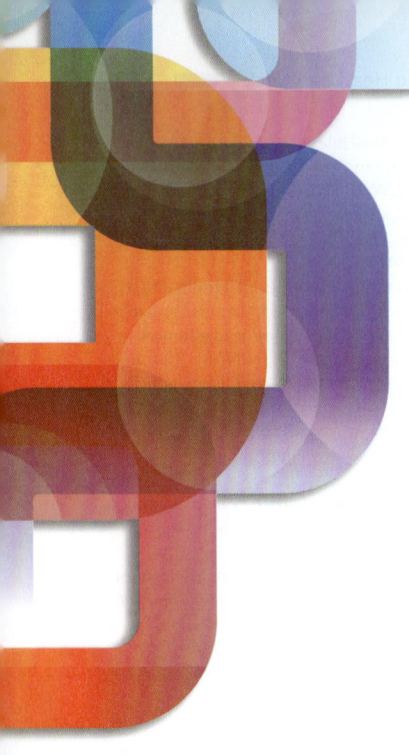

16 ASSESSING EYES

Learning Objectives

1. Describe the structures and functions of the eyes.
2. Discuss risk factors for development of cataracts and ways to reduce risk factors.
3. Interview a client for an accurate eye and vision nursing history.
4. Assess a client's distant and near visual acuity, visual fields, corneal light reflex, and eye movements.
5. Inspect the external eye structures and correctly use the ophthalmoscope to inspect internal eye structures.
6. Differentiate between normal and abnormal findings of the eye and vision.
7. Analyze interview and physical assessment data related to the eyes and vision to formulate valid nursing diagnoses, collaborative problems, and or referrals.

CASE STUDY

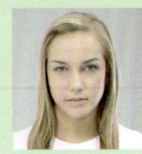

Susan Jones, a 24-year-old Caucasian woman, presents to the clinic after sustaining an injury to her right eye. She is holding her hand over her eye.

STRUCTURE AND FUNCTION

The eye transmits visual stimuli to the brain for interpretation and, in doing so, functions as the organ of vision. The eyeball is located in the eye orbit, a round, bony hollow formed by several different bones of the skull. In the orbit, a cushion of fat surrounds the eye. The bony orbit and fat cushion protect the eyeball.

To perform a thorough assessment of the eye, you need a good understanding of the external and internal structures of the eye, the visual fields and pathways, and the visual reflexes.

External Structures of the Eye

The **eyelids** (upper and lower) are two movable structures composed of skin and two types of muscle: striated and smooth. Their purpose is to protect the eye from foreign bodies and limit the amount of light entering the eye. In addition, they serve to distribute tears that lubricate the surface of the eye (Fig. 16-1). The upper eyelid is larger, more mobile, and contains *tarsal plates* made up of connective tissue. These plates contain the *meibomian glands,* which secrete an oily substance that lubricates the eyelid.

The eyelids join at two points: the *lateral (outer) canthus* and *medial (inner) canthus.* The medial canthus contains the *puncta,* two small openings that allow drainage of tears into the lacrimal system, and the *caruncle,* a small, fleshy mass that contains sebaceous glands. The white space between open eyelids is called the *palpebral fissure.* When closed, the eyelids should touch. When open, the upper lid position should be between the upper margin of the iris and the upper margin of the pupil. The lower lid should rest on the lower border of the iris. No sclera should be seen above or below the limbus (the point where the sclera meets the cornea).

Eyelashes are projections of stiff hair curving outward along the margins of the eyelids that filter dust and dirt from air entering the eye.

The *conjunctiva* is a thin, transparent, continuous membrane that is divided into two portions: a *palpebral* and a *bulbar* portion. The palpebral conjunctiva lines the inside of the eyelids, and the bulbar conjunctiva covers most of the anterior eye, merging with the cornea at the limbus. The point at which the palpebral and bulbar conjunctivae meet creates a folded recess that allows movement of the eyeball. This transparent membrane allows for inspection of underlying tissue and protects the eye from foreign bodies.

The *lacrimal apparatus* consists of glands and ducts that lubricate the eye (Fig. 16-2). The *lacrimal gland,* located in the upper outer corner of the orbital cavity just above the eye, produces tears. As the lid blinks, tears wash across the eye then drain into the *puncta,* which are visible on the upper and lower lids at the inner canthus. Tears empty into the *lacrimal canals* and are then channeled into the *nasolacrimal sac* through the *nasolacrimal duct.* They drain into the nasal meatus.

The *extraocular muscles* are the six muscles attached to the outer surface of each eyeball (Fig. 16-3). These muscles and associated nerves control six different directions of eye movement. There are four rectus muscles (superior, inferior, lateral, and medial) and two oblique muscles (superior and inferior) that are responsible for moving the eye in the direction controlled by that muscle. Each muscle coordinates with a muscle in the opposite eye. This allows for parallel movement of the eyes and thus the binocular vision characteristic of humans. Innervation for these muscles is supplied by three cranial nerves: the oculomotor (III), trochlear (IV), and abducens (VI).

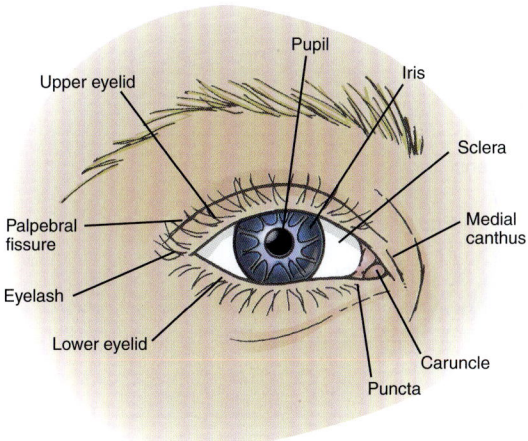

FIGURE 16-1 External structures of the eye.

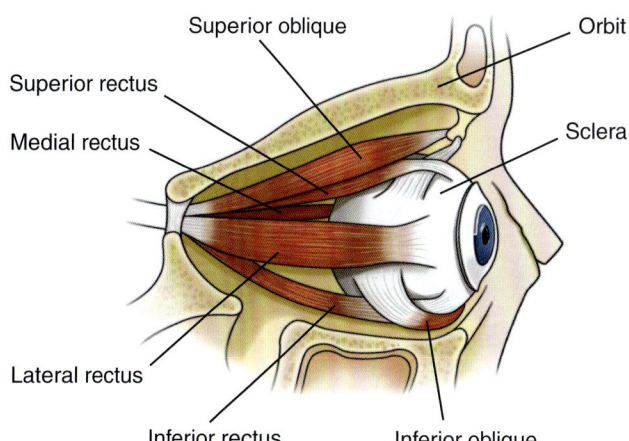

FIGURE 16-3 Extraocular muscles control the direction of eye movement.

Internal Structures of the Eye

The eyeball is composed of three separate coats or *layers* (Fig. 16-4). The external layer consists of the *sclera* and *cornea*. The sclera is a dense, protective, white covering that physically supports the internal structures of the eye. It is continuous anteriorly with the transparent cornea (the "window of the eye"). The cornea permits the entrance of light, which passes through the lens to the retina. It is well supplied with nerve endings, making it responsive to pain and touch.

> 🎯 **CLINICAL TIP**
> Because of this sensory property, contact with a wisp of cotton stimulates a blink in both eyes known as the corneal reflex. This reflex is supported by the trigeminal nerve, which carries the afferent sensation into the brain, and the facial nerve, which carries the efferent message that stimulates the blink.

The middle layer contains both an anterior portion, which includes the *iris* and the *ciliary body*, and a posterior layer, which includes the *choroid*. The ciliary body consists of muscle tissue that controls the thickness of the lens, which must be adapted to focus on objects near and far away.

The *iris* is a circular disc of muscle containing pigments that determine eye color. The central aperture of the iris is called the *pupil*. Muscles in the iris adjust to control the pupil's size, which controls the amount of light entering the eye. The muscle fibers of the iris also decrease the size of the pupil to accommodate for near vision and dilate the pupil when far vision is needed.

The *lens* is a biconvex, transparent, avascular, encapsulated structure located immediately posterior to the iris. Suspensory ligaments attached to the ciliary body support the position of the lens. The lens functions to refract (bend) light rays onto the retina. Adjustments must be made in refraction depending on the distance of the object being viewed. Refractive ability of the lens can be changed by a change in shape of the lens (which is controlled by the ciliary body). The lens bulges to focus on close objects and flattens to focus on far objects.

The *choroid layer* contains the vascularity necessary to provide nourishment to the inner aspect of the eye and prevents light from reflecting internally. Anteriorly, it is continuous with the ciliary body and the iris.

The innermost layer, the *retina*, extends only to the ciliary body anteriorly. It receives visual stimuli and sends it to the brain. The retina consists of numerous layers of nerve cells, including the cells commonly called *rods* and *cones*. These specialized nerve cells are often referred to as "photoreceptors" because they are responsive to light. The rods are highly sensitive to light, regulate black-and-white vision, and function in dim light. The cones function in bright light and are sensitive to color.

The *optic disc* is a cream-colored, circular area located on the retina toward the medial or nasal side of the eye. It is where the optic nerve enters the eyeball. The optic disc can be seen with the use of an ophthalmoscope and is normally round or oval in shape, with distinct margins. A smaller circular area that appears slightly depressed is referred to as the *physiologic cup*. This area is approximately one third the size of the entire optic disc and appears somewhat lighter/whiter than the disc borders.

The *retinal vessels* can be readily viewed with the aid of an ophthalmoscope. Four sets of *arterioles* and *venules* travel through the optic disc, bifurcate, and extend to the periphery of the fundus. Venules are dark red and grow progressively narrower as they extend out to the peripheral areas. Arterioles carry oxygenated blood and appear brighter red and narrower than the veins. The general background, or fundus (Fig. 16-5), varies in color, depending on skin color. A retinal depression known as the *fovea centralis* is located adjacent to the optic disc in the temporal section of the fundus. This area is surrounded by the *macula*, which appears darker than the rest of the fundus. The fovea centralis and macular area are highly

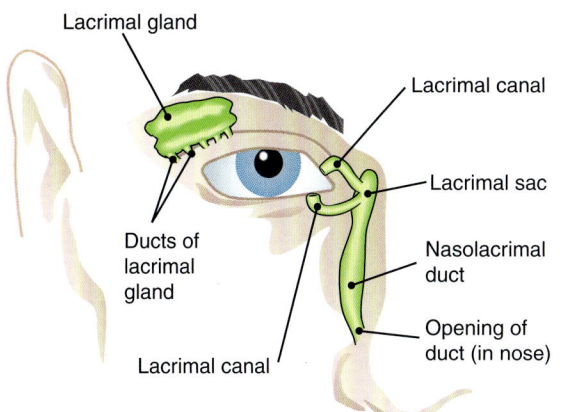

FIGURE 16-2 The lacrimal apparatus consists of tear (lacrimal) glands and ducts.

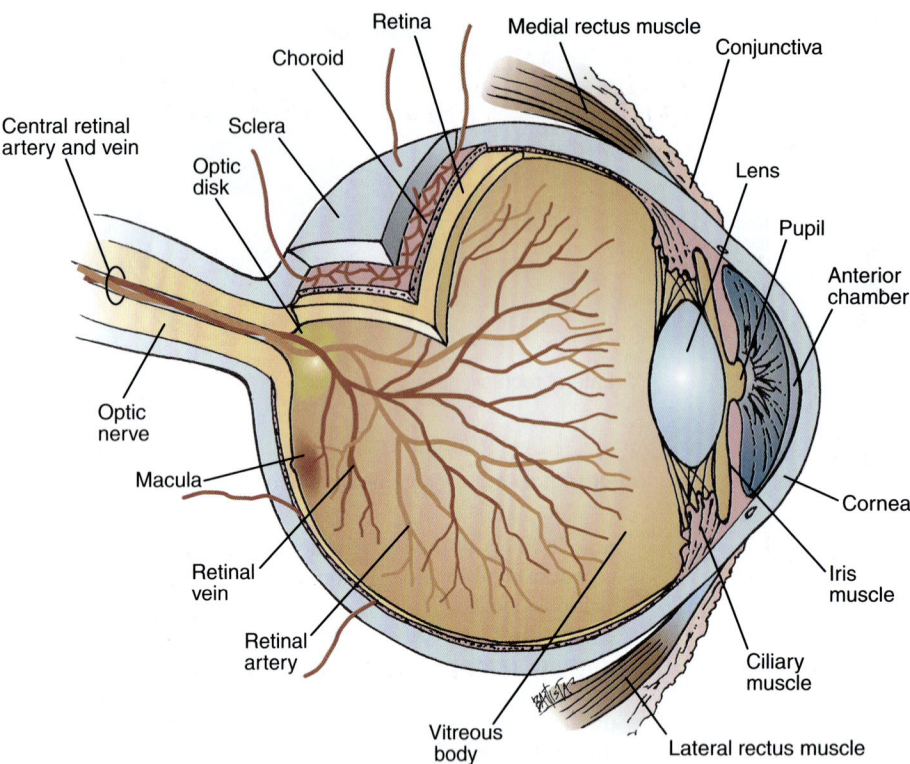

FIGURE 16-4 Anatomy of the eye.

concentrated with cones and form the area of highest visual resolution and color vision.

The eyeball contains several chambers that maintain structure, protect against injury, and transmit light rays. The *anterior chamber* is located between the cornea and iris; the *posterior chamber* is the area between the iris and the lens. These chambers are filled with *aqueous humor*, a clear liquid substance produced by the ciliary body. Aqueous humor helps to cleanse and nourish the cornea and lens as well as maintain intraocular pressure. The aqueous humor filters out of the eye from the posterior to the anterior chamber then into the *canal of Schlemm* through a filtering site called the *trabecular meshwork*. Another chamber, the *vitreous chamber*, is located in the area behind the lens to the retina. It is the largest of the chambers and is filled with a vitreous humor that is clear and gelatinous.

Vision

Visual Fields and Visual Pathways

A *visual field* refers to what a person sees with one eye. The visual field of each eye can be divided into four quadrants: upper temporal, lower temporal, upper nasal, and lower nasal (Fig. 16-6). The temporal quadrants of each visual field extend farther than the nasal quadrants. Thus, each eye sees a slightly different view but their visual fields overlap quite a bit. As a result of this, humans have binocular vision ("two-eyed" vision) in which the visual cortex fuses the two slightly different images and provides depth perception, or three-dimensional vision.

Visual perception occurs as light rays strike the retina, where they are transformed into nerve impulses, conducted to the brain through the optic nerve, and interpreted. In the eye, light must pass through transparent media (cornea, aqueous humor, lens, and vitreous body) before reaching the retina. The cornea and lens are the main eye components that refract (bend) light rays on the retina. The image projected on the retina is upside down and reversed right to left from the actual image. For example, an image from the lower temporal visual field strikes the upper temporal quadrant of the retina. At the point where the optic nerves from each eyeball cross—the *optic chiasma*—the nerve fibers from the nasal quadrant of each retina (from both temporal visual fields) cross over to the opposite side. At this point, the right optic tract contains only nerve fibers from the right side of the retina and the left optic tract contains only nerve fibers from the left side of the retina. Therefore, the left side of the brain views the right side of the world.

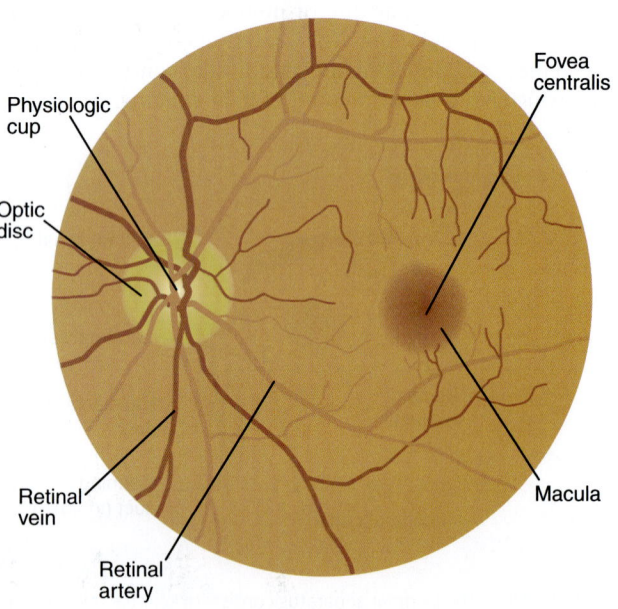

FIGURE 16-5 Normal ocular fundus.

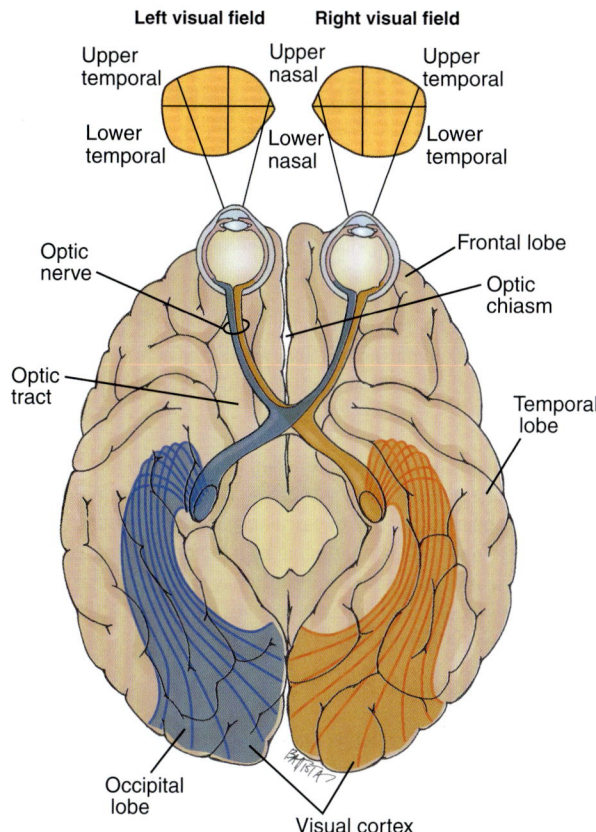

FIGURE 16-6 Visual fields and visual pathways. Each eye has a slightly different view of the same field. However, the views overlap significantly, which accounts for binocular vision.

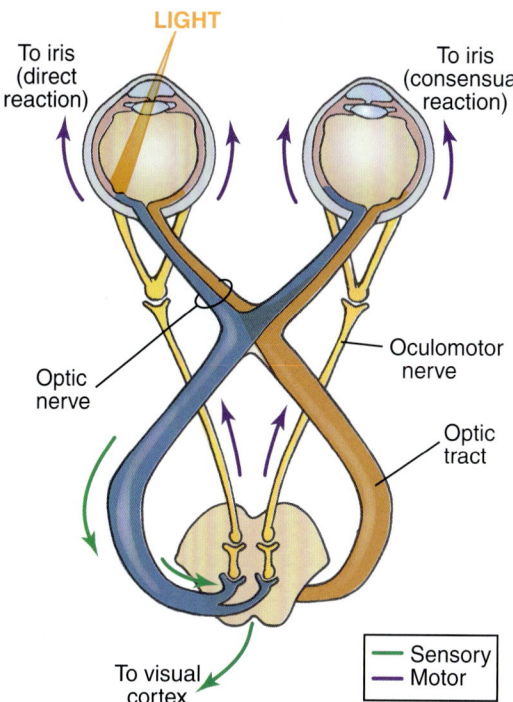

FIGURE 16-7 The pupils admit light that travels over the visual pathways. If a light focuses on only one eye, the pupil responds to ensure that the light needed for vision can enter but not so much that eye damage would result. The other pupil responds in the same manner. This phenomenon of direct pupillary response and consensual pupillary response is a reflex governed by the oculomotor nerve.

Visual Reflexes

The *pupillary light reflex* causes pupils immediately to constrict when exposed to bright light. This can be seen as a *direct reflex*, in which constriction occurs in the eye exposed to the light, or as an *indirect or consensual reflex*, in which exposure to light in one eye results in constriction of the pupil in the opposite eye (Fig. 16-7). These protective reflexes, mediated by the oculomotor nerve, prevent damage to the delicate photoreceptors by excessive light.

Accommodation is a functional reflex allowing the eyes to focus on near objects. This is accomplished through movement of the ciliary muscles, causing an increase in the curvature of the lens. This change in shape of the lens is not visible. However, convergence of the eyes and constriction of the pupils occur simultaneously and can be seen.

HEALTH ASSESSMENT

Collecting Subjective Data: The Nursing Health History

Beginning when the nurse first meets the client, assessment of vision provides important information about the client's ability to interact with the environment. Changes in vision are often gradual and go unrecognized by clients until a severe problem develops. Therefore, asking clients specific questions about their vision may help with early detection of disorders. With recent advances in medicine and surgery, early detection and intervention are increasingly important.

Visual impairments range from reduced visual acuity, which can be corrected with lenses, to total blindness. The Texas Council for Developmental Disabilities (2013) has provided a summary of definitions and conditions related to visual impairments. They define a visual impairment as any visual condition that impacts an individual's ability to successfully complete the activities of everyday life. Visual impairment may be classified as low vision, functional blindness, or total blindness. Origin of the impairment is divided into congenital (occurring in fetal development) or adventitious (occurring after having normal vision through a hereditary condition or a trauma). In the United States, legal blindness is determined to exist when an individual has a visual acuity of 20/200 or less.

There are a number of diseases that affect the eye and cause blindness. Statistics, data, and prevalence of some of these conditions can be found on the website of The National Eye Institute of NIH (https://nei.nih.gov/eyedata/pbd_tables).

First, gather data from the client about his or her current level of eye health. Also discuss any personal and family history problems that are related to the eye. Collecting data concerning environmental influences on vision as well as how any problems are influencing or affecting the client's usual activities of daily living is also important. Answers to these types of questions help to evaluate a client's risk for vision loss and, in turn, present ways that the client may modify or reduce the risk of eye problems. The following questions provide guidance in conducting the interview.

History of Present Health Concern

QUESTION	RATIONALE
Visual Problems	
Describe any recent visual difficulties or changes in your vision that you have experienced. Were they sudden or gradual?	Sudden changes in vision are associated with acute problems such as head trauma or increased intracranial pressure. Gradual changes in vision may be related to aging, diabetes, hypertension, or neurologic disorders.
Do you see spots or floaters in front of your eyes?	Spots or floaters are common among clients with myopia or in clients over age 40. In most cases, they are due to normal physiologic changes in the eye associated with aging and require no intervention.
Do you experience blind spots? Are they constant or intermittent?	A scotoma is a blind spot that is surrounded by either normal or slightly diminished peripheral vision. It may be from glaucoma. Intermittent blind spots may be associated with vascular spasms (ophthalmic migraines) or pressure on the optic nerve by a tumor or increased intracranial pressure. Consistent blind spots may indicate retinal detachment. Any report of a blind spot requires immediate attention and referral to an ophthalmologist.
Do you see halos or rings around lights?	Seeing halos around lights is associated with narrow-angle glaucoma.
Do you have trouble seeing at night?	Night blindness is associated with optic atrophy, glaucoma, and vitamin A deficiency.
Do you experience double vision (diplopia)?	Double vision (diplopia) may indicate increased intracranial pressure due to injury or a tumor.
Other Symptoms	
Do you have any eye pain or itching? Do you have pain with bright lights (photophobia)? Describe.	Burning or itching pain is usually associated with allergies or superficial irritation. Throbbing, stabbing, or deep, aching pain suggests a foreign body in the eye or changes within the eye. See procedure for assessing eye trauma and presence of foreign body at the end of the physical assessment section. Most common eye disorders are not associated with actual pain. Therefore, immediately refer reports of eye pain.
Do you have any redness or swelling in your eyes?	Redness or swelling of the eye is usually related to an inflammatory response caused by allergy, foreign body, or bacterial or viral infection.
Do you experience excessive watering or tearing of the eye? If so, is it in one eye or both eyes?	Excessive tearing (epiphora) is caused by exposure to irritants or obstruction of the lacrimal apparatus. Unilateral epiphora is often associated with foreign body or obstruction. Bilateral epiphora is often associated with exposure to irritants, such as makeup or facial cleansers, or it may be a systemic response.
Have you had any eye discharge? Describe.	Discharge other than tears from one or both eyes suggests a bacterial or viral infection.

Personal Health History

QUESTION	RATIONALE
Have you ever had problems with your eyes or vision?	A history of eye problems or changes in vision provides clues to the current health of the eye.
Have you ever had eye surgery?	Surgery may alter the appearance of the eye and the results of future examinations.

QUESTION	RATIONALE
Describe any past treatments you have received for eye problems (medication, surgery, laser treatments, corrective lenses). Were these successful? Were you satisfied?	Client may not be satisfied with past treatments for vision problems.
What types of medications do you take?	Ocular side effects of drugs are often unrecognized or overlooked. Some medications reported to have ocular side effects include alpha-1 blockers, some antiarrhythmics, anticholinergics (including antihistamines, antipsychotics, antispasmodics, cyclic antidepressants, and mydriatics), anticoagulants, antimalarials, bisphosphonates, corticosteroids, digoxin, erectile dysfunction medications, fluoroquinolones and some other antibiotics, and many other medications (Miguel et al., 2014).
When was your last eye examination?	All clients at risk for eye problems should be examined annually or as recommended by their primary care provider. A thorough eye examination is recommended for healthy clients without risk factors every 2 years, for ages 18 through 60; annually for those aged 61 and older (American Optometric Association [AOA], 2015d). However, the U.S. Preventive Services Task Force (USPSTF, 2015) asserts that the current evidence is insufficient to assess the balance of benefits and harms of screening for visual acuity for the improvement of outcomes in older adults.
Do you perform the test for macular degeneration using the Amsler chart? How do you use this chart and how often? What do you see when you use it?	To perform the Amsler test properly, clients should wear their glasses if they normally do so. They should use the bottom portion to view the chart if they wear bifocals. The Amsler chart should be posted on a wall at eye level (Fig. 16-8). Clients should stand 12–14 ft (comfortable reading distance) away from it and cover one eye. With the other eye, they should look at the center dot. Any areas of distortion, graying, blurring, or blank spots should be marked on the chart and they should notify their physician. If they have already developed a baseline with distortions that their primary care provider is aware of, then they should report any changes from their baseline to their primary care provider. Refer clients to http://www.amd.org/living-with-amd/resources-and-tools/31-amsler-grid.html to download the Amsler grid with directions to use to test for any visual changes (Macular Degeneration Partnership, 2015).
Do you have a prescription for corrective lenses (glasses or contacts)? Do you wear them regularly? If you wear contacts, how long do you wear them? How do you clean them?	Clients who do not wear the prescribed corrective lenses are susceptible to eyestrain. Improper cleaning or prolonged wearing of contact lenses can lead to infection and corneal damage.
Have you ever been tested for glaucoma? What were the results?	Tonometry is used to measure pressure within the eye. Normal eye pressures range from 10–21 mm of mercury (mm Hg). Eye pressures greater than 22 mm Hg increase one's risk for developing glaucoma. However, people with normal eye pressure may develop glaucoma (AOA, 2015b) (see Evidence-Based Practice 16-1).

Family History

QUESTION	RATIONALE
Is there a history of eye problems or vision loss in your family?	Many eye disorders have familial tendencies. Examples include glaucoma, refraction errors, allergies, and macular degeneration. Approximately 11 million people in the United States have some form of age-related macular degeneration, which is a major cause of visual impairment in the United States. It is estimated that nearly 40 million will have macular degeneration worldwide by the year 2020 (Bright Focus Foundation, 2017b). See Evidence-Based Practice 16-2.

Continued on following page

Lifestyle and Health Practices

QUESTION	RATIONALE
Are you exposed to conditions or substances in the workplace or home that may harm your eyes or vision (e.g., chemicals, fumes, smoke, dust, or flying sparks)? Do you wear safety glasses during exposure to harmful substances?	Injuries or diseases may be related to exposure in the workplace or home. These problems can be minimized or avoided altogether with hazard identification and implementation of safety measures. It is important to teach the client to use protective eyewear when engaging in recreational activities and hazardous situations (Healthy People 2020, 2015).
Do you wear sunglasses during exposure to the sun?	Exposure to ultraviolet radiation puts the client at risk for the development of cataracts (opacities of the lenses of the eyes; see Evidence-Based Practice 16-3). Consistent use of sunglasses during exposure minimizes the client's risk.
Do you have any vision loss? Has your vision loss affected your ability to care for yourself? To work?	Vision problems may interfere with the client's ability to perform usual activities of daily living. The client may be unable to read medication labels or fill insulin syringes. If the vision problem is severe, the client's ability to perform hygiene practices or prepare food may be affected. Vision problems may affect a client's ability to work if the job is one that depends on sight, such as a pilot or commercial motor vehicle operator.
What visual aids do you use to assist you with your visual loss (magnifying glasses, audiotapes, CDs, special glasses for viewing television, large-numbered phones, large-print checks, large print books)?	It is important to assist the client to access and use assistive and adaptive visual devices to improve one's activities of daily living (Healthy People 2020, 2015).
Describe your typical diet. What have you eaten in the last 24 hours? Do you take any vitamins or supplements?	The AOA (2015c) explains that research has linked nutrition to a decreased risk of age-related macular degeneration (AMD) as follows: A well-balanced diet is essential.
	Lutein and zeaxanthin (in foods or by supplements) found in green leafy vegetables, eggs, and other foods reduce the risk of chronic eye diseases, including age-related macular degeneration and cataracts. Foods rich in these nutrients include kale, spinach, collards, turnip greens, corn, green peas, broccoli, romaine lettuce, green beans, eggs, and oranges.
	Vitamin C can decrease the risk of cataracts and reduce the risk of age-related macular degeneration when taken with other essential nutrients.
	Vitamin E in its most biologically active form is a powerful antioxidant which, when taken with antioxidants beta-carotene, vitamin C, and zinc, has been found to slow progression of AMD by 25% in high-risk individuals. It is found in nuts, fortified cereals, and sweet potatoes. It is thought to protect cells of the eyes from damage caused by unstable molecules.
	Zinc is an essential trace mineral or "helper molecule." It plays a vital role in bringing vitamin A from the liver to the retina in order to produce melanin, a protective pigment in the eyes.
	Two omega-3 fatty acids have been shown to be important for proper visual development and retinal function (AOA, 2015a). Dietary deprivation of EPA and especially of DHA is related to visual impairment, retinal degradation, and even dry eye syndrome, and to the progression of advanced age-related AMD.
	Beta-carotene supplements have been known to decrease one's risk of developing cataracts and AMD. However, research shows this may increase the risk of lung cancer in people who smoke (especially those smoking more than 20 cigarettes per day), former smokers, have been exposed to asbestos, or drink one or more alcoholic beverages and also smoke. Beta-carotene from food alone does not seem to have this risk (Tanvetyanon & Bepler, 2008).
Do you smoke? How many packs and for how long?	Tobacco smoking has been found to be strongly associated with eye diseases, doubling the chance of forming cataracts and causing a three-fold risk of developing AMD (Surtenich, 2013).

Amsler's Chart to Test Your Sight

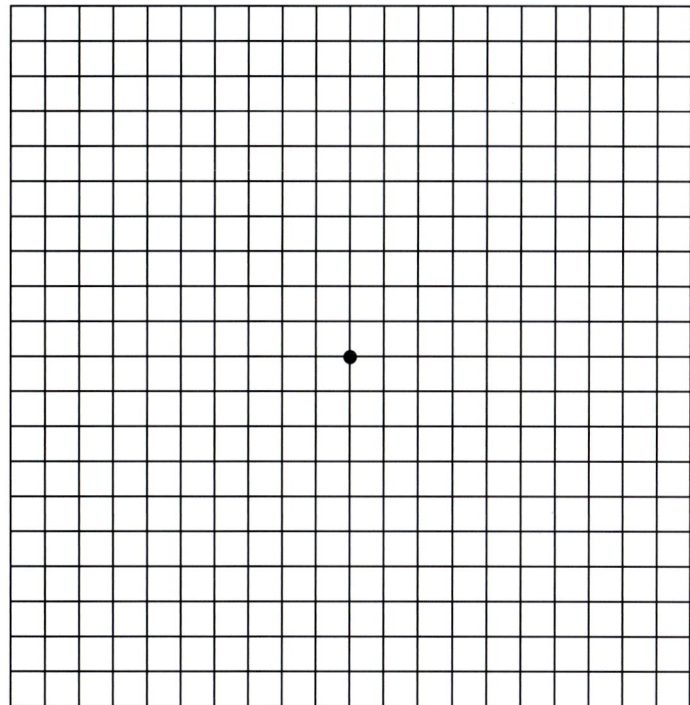

Instructions for Use

1. Tape this page at eye level where light is consistent and without glare.
2. Put on your reading glasses and cover one eye.
3. Fix your gaze on the center black dot.
4. Keeping your gaze fixed, try to see if any lines are distorted or missing.
5. Mark the defect on the chart.
6. Test each eye separately.
7. If the distortion is new or has worsened, arrange to see your ophthalmologist at once.
8. *Always* keep the Amsler's Chart the *same distance* from your eyes each time you test.

FIGURE 16-8 Amsler grid.

CASE STUDY

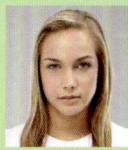

The case study introduced at the beginning of the chapter is now used to demonstrate how a nurse would use the COLDSPA mnemonic to explore Ms. Jones's presenting concerns.

Mnemonic	Question	Data Provided
Character	Describe the sign or symptom (feeling, appearance, sound, smell, or taste if applicable).	"My right eye really hurts. It feels scratchy, like there is something in my eye."
Onset	When did it begin?	"A couple of hours ago, when I accidentally poked my key in my eye."
Location	Where is it? Does it radiate? Does it occur anywhere else?	"Only my right eye."
Duration	How long does it last? Does it recur?	"It hurts constantly."
Severity	How bad is it? How much does it bother you?	Client rates pain as 4 on a scale of 0–10.
Pattern	What makes it better or worse?	"It hurts when I blink and feels better if I keep my eye shut."
Associated factors/How it **A**ffects the client	What other symptoms occur with it? How does it affect you?	"My right eye is watery and my vision is blurry, making it difficult to drive."

After investigating Susan Jones's recent eye trauma, the nurse continues with the health history. Ms. Jones reports that she has never had a problem with her eyes or vision. She states that she has never had eye surgery or any type of eye treatment. Ms. Jones reports that her father has glaucoma. She denies exposure to substances that would harm her eyes. She states that she wears sunglasses about 80% of the time when exposed to the sun. Ms. Jones reports that the only medication she takes is an occasional Tylenol for headache. Client states that her last eye examination was 2 years ago and that her vision was "perfect."

16-1 EVIDENCE-BASED HEALTH PROMOTION AND DISEASE PREVENTION: GLAUCOMA

INTRODUCTION
Glaucoma is a group of eye diseases that damage the optic nerve, often caused by abnormally high pressure (intraocular pressure) within the eye (Mayo Clinic, 2015b). There are no warning signs and its effects are so gradual that no change in vision may be noted until the condition is advanced. Vision loss caused by glaucoma is not reversible. Glaucoma is the second leading cause of blindness after cataracts. Vision loss due to glaucoma cannot be recovered, and there are no warning signs that glaucoma is developing (Mayo Clinic, 2015b). If found early, vision loss can be prevented or slowed. Referral to immediate emergency care should be made if symptoms are detected.

There are several types of glaucoma. Signs and symptoms differ for the two most common types of glaucoma—primary open-angle glaucoma (POAG) and acute angle-closure glaucoma (AACG) (Mayo Clinic, 2015b). Common signs and symptoms are:

Open-angle Glaucoma
- Patchy blind spots in your side (peripheral) or central vision, frequently in both eyes
- Tunnel vision in the advanced stages

Acute Angle-closure Glaucoma
- Severe headache
- Eye pain
- Nausea and vomiting
- Blurred vision
- Halos around lights
- Eye redness

The Glaucoma Research Foundation (2015) reports that over 3 million Americans have glaucoma, but only about half of those know that they have it. African Americans are 15 times more likely to be visually impaired by glaucoma than Caucasians. The most common form, open-angle glaucoma, accounts for 19% of all blindness among African Americans compared with 6% in Caucasians. Worldwide estimate for people with glaucoma is at least 60 million.

HEALTHY PEOPLE 2020 GOAL
Healthy People 2020 objectives (2015) related to vision focus on preserving sight and preventing blindness. The objectives are: "address screening and examinations for children and adults, early detection and timely treatment of eye diseases and conditions, injury prevention, and the use of vision rehabilitation services."

GOAL
Improve the visual health of the Nation through prevention, early detection, timely treatment, and rehabilitation.

OBJECTIVE
Reduce visual impairment due to glaucoma from a 2008 baseline of 13.9 per 1,000 population aged 45 years and over to 12.5 per 1,000.

SCREENING
The U.S. Preventive Services Task Force has found that screening is able to detect increased intraocular pressure (IOP) and early POAG in adults; however, the USPSTF finds that there is insufficient evidence to recommend for or against screening adults for glaucoma (USPSTF, 2013). This recommendation was based on the conclusion that there is insufficient evidence to know the extent that screening would reduce impaired vision or quality of life, and that treatment of increased IOP and early POAG results in some harm, including eye irritation and a risk of cataracts.

The AOA (2015b) notes that glaucoma cannot be prevented and damage or vision loss that has occurred before screening cannot be reversed. Therefore, the AOA recommends a dilated pupil eye examination for all persons at risk for glaucoma.

The American Academy of Ophthalmology (AAO, 2015a) recommends that persons younger than 40 who have no known risk factors for glaucoma should have a complete eye examination every 5 to 10 years. This includes tests that check for glaucoma. The AAO suggests more frequent routine eye examinations with increasing age.

The AAO also suggests that **people who are at risk for glaucoma** have complete eye examinations according to the schedule below:
- Ages 40 to 54, every 1 to 3 years
- Ages 55 to 64, every 1 to 2 years
- Ages 65 and older, every 6 to 12 months

For people with known risks for glaucoma (older than 40 years, African American, East Asian, high intraocular pressure, family history of glaucoma, diabetic, previous eye surgery, hypertensive, far sighted, on corticosteroids) the American Academy of Ophthalmology (Boyd, 2015) recommends following eye doctor orders for more frequent screenings.

RISK ASSESSMENT
Risk Factors for Glaucoma
Bright Focus Foundation (2017a) lists risk factors for the various types of glaucoma:

Risk Factors for Open-angle Glaucoma[a]
Strong risk factors for open-angle glaucoma include:
- High eye pressure
- Family history of glaucoma
- Age 40 and older for African Americans
- Age 60 and older for the general population, especially Mexican Americans
- Thin cornea
- Suspicious optic nerve appearance with increased cupping (size of cup, the space at the center of optic nerve, is larger than normal)

Potential risk factors for open-angle glaucoma include:
- High myopia (very severe nearsightedness)
- Diabetes
- Eye surgery or injury
- High blood pressure
- Use of corticosteroids (e.g., eye drops, pills, inhalers, and creams)

Risk Factors for Angle-closure Glaucoma
- Age 40 and older
- Family history of glaucoma
- Poor short-distance vision (farsightedness)
- Eye injury or eye surgery
- East Asian and Inuit ethnicity

Risk Factors for Normal-tension Glaucoma
- Cardiovascular disease
- Family history of glaucoma
- Low eye pressure
- Japanese ethnicity

CLIENT EDUCATION
Teach Clients
- Get regular eye examinations and treat any elevated IOP promptly.
- Wear protective eye gear if involved in activities that risk eye injury.

- Maintain optimum body weight and blood pressure to avoid diabetes, or control diabetes if present.
- Eat a varied, well-rounded, and healthy diet. The National Glaucoma Research (2011) has noted that "there is no scientific evidence suggesting that certain vitamins and minerals prevent glaucoma or delay its progress. However, carotenoids (especially lutein and zeaxanthin), antioxidants (such as vitamins C and E), vitamins A and D, zinc and omega-3 fatty acids may all contribute to better vision overall."

[a]Information from http://www.brightfocus.org/glaucoma/prevention-and-risk-factors

16-2 EVIDENCE-BASED HEALTH PROMOTION AND DISEASE PREVENTION: MACULAR DEGENERATION

INTRODUCTION

Age-related macular degeneration (AMD) is a major cause of visual impairment that affects the macula portion of the retina. AMD causes deterioration of the macula, the central area of the retina. The retina is a paper-thin tissue at the back of the eye where light-sensitive cells send visual signals to the brain. The macula processes sharp, clear, straight-ahead vision. Damage to the macula results in blind spots and blurred or distorted vision. People affected by AMD find many daily activities, such as driving and reading, increasingly difficult. According to Bright Focus Foundation (2017b), age-related macular degeneration is the leading cause of vision loss in Americans over 60 years of age. Macular degeneration currently affects 11 million Americans and the number is expected to double to 22 million by 2050.

There are two types of AMD: dry and wet. The dry form is the most common, accounting for 85% to 90% of AMD diagnoses (Bright Focus Foundation, 2017b). A person may have both dry and wet forms, which may affect one or both eyes. Also, the speed of the disease's progress may vary from slow to rapid, the dry form may advance and cause loss of vision without turning into the wet form, or the dry form in early stages or in late stages may change into the wet form of AMD. In the wet form, abnormal new blood vessels form deep in the sensory retina, which can leak or bleed and result in marked loss of central vision in one or both eyes. Each year after the onset of wet AMD in one eye, 15% of persons develop the wet form in their second eye.

HEALTHY PEOPLE 2020 GOAL

Healthy People 2020 objectives (2015) related to vision focus on preserving sight and preventing blindness. The objectives "address screening and examinations for children and adults, early detection and timely treatment of eye diseases and conditions, injury prevention, and the use of vision rehabilitation services."

GOAL

Improve the visual health of the nation through prevention, early detection, timely treatment, and rehabilitation.

OBJECTIVES

- Reduce visual impairment due to AMD by 10%.
- Increase the use of assistive and adaptive devices by people with visual impairment
- Increase the use of vision rehabilitation services by people with visual impairment

SCREENING

The U.S. Preventive Services Task Force (2009, with draft statement 2015) does not recommend screening for visual acuity in older adults due to insufficient evidence to assess the balance of benefits and harms of screening for visual acuity for the improvement of outcomes in older adults. However, the USPSTF lists the recommendations of other organizations:

- American Academy of Ophthalmology: comprehensive eye examinations every 1 to 2 years for persons 65 years or older who have no risk factors
- American Optometric Association Consensus Panel on Comprehensive Adult Eye and Vision Examination: annual eye examinations for adults 61 years or older
- American College of Obstetricians and Gynecologists: evaluation and counseling about visual acuity screening for all women 65 years or older

Visual acuity tests and the Amsler grid (Fig. 16–8) are two screening tests performed that do not require dilation of the pupils. Use of the Amsler grid is generally recommended for all individuals over 65 years.

RISK ASSESSMENT

Risk factors listed by Bright Focus Foundation (2012) include:
- Advancing age (Bright Focus Foundation, 2017b).
- Smoking (increases risk 2- to 5-fold; affects blood vessels in retina)
- Family history of AMD
- Gender (females more likely to be affected)
- Obesity (BMI >30)
- Race (Caucasians more affected than any other group)
- Light eye color
- Prolonged sun exposure (UV light directly damages retinal tissue)
- High fat, high cholesterol, high sugar/low antioxidant diet that is low in antioxidants and green leafy vegetables
- Hypertension (narrows blood vessels in retina) or blood pressure above 120/80 mm Hg
- Cardiovascular disease
- Inactivity (probably related to vascular oxygen levels)
- AMD in one eye
- Genetic predisposition (several genes associated with AMD)

CLIENT EDUCATION

Teach Clients

Bright Focus Foundation (2017b) recommends the following health habits:
- Maintain a healthy weight.
- Eat a nutritious diet that includes green leafy vegetables, yellow and orange fruit, fish, and whole grains.
- Do not smoke.
- Maintain normal blood pressure and control other medical conditions.
- Exercise regularly.
- Wear sunglasses and hats when you are outdoors.
- Get regular eye examinations, and consult your doctor if you notice vision changes.

Continued on following page

16-2 EVIDENCE-BASED HEALTH PROMOTION AND DISEASE PREVENTION: MACULAR DEGENERATION (Continued)

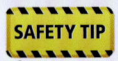 *Although beta carotene supplements have been shown to slow the progression of AMD, if you are a current or ex-smoker, you should not take these supplements because they may lead to an increased risk of lung cancer (Tanvetyanon & Bepler, 2008).*

- Two food-related research areas include:
  - Preventing AMD by eating a low glycemic index diet
  - National Eye Institute's (2003) study on the preventive effectiveness of a supplement formulation called AREDS, which "found that taking a specific high dose formula of antioxidants and zinc (500 mg of vitamin C, 400 International Units of vitamin E, 15 mg of beta-carotene, 80 mg of zinc as zinc oxide, and 2 mg of copper as cupric oxide) may delay or prevent intermediate age-related macular degeneration from progressing to the advanced stage" (see report for more details of the results).
- Have regular eye examinations as recommended by an eye doctor according to age and eye condition.
- Use the Amsler grid test at home (e.g., put it on the refrigerator door and use it daily).
- If diagnosed with AMD, vision rehabilitation and aids may be useful.
- Note: once diagnosed with AMD, there is no harm in using eyes for reading, watching TV, or other activities since eye damage will not increase.

16-3 EVIDENCE-BASED HEALTH PROMOTION AND DISEASE PREVENTION: CATARACTS

INTRODUCTION
Cataracts are the leading cause of blindness, often preventable, in the world today. More than 22 million Americans have cataracts (Gollogly et al., 2013). Furthermore, by age 80 more than half of the US population will have a cataract or will have had cataract surgery. Cataracts are a clouding of the usually clear lens of the eye, causing a person to see as though looking through a frosty or foggy window, with vision even more affected at night (Mayo Clinic, 2013a; Gollogly et al., 2013). Other symptoms include fading or yellowing of colors, sensitivity to light and glare, seeing "halos" around lights, double vision in a single eye, and frequent prescription changes in corrective lenses. Most cataracts develop slowly and are most often found in people over 65 years of age. With age, the lens becomes less flexible, thicker, and less transparent as tissues breakdown or clump together, turning the lens yellow or brown. In addition to aging, however, injury, genetics, or maternal infections (resulting in infant cataracts) may be causes. Because cataracts that impair vision are often not readily detectable, a thorough assessment is needed to determine possible preventive strategies or need for referral.

There are numerous types of cataracts. These are categorized based on location, such as center of the lens, edges of the lens, or back of the lens.

HEALTHY PEOPLE 2020 GOAL
Healthy People 2020 objectives (2015) related to vision focus on preserving sight and preventing blindness. The objectives: "address screening and examinations for children and adults, early detection and timely treatment of eye diseases and conditions, injury prevention, and the use of vision rehabilitation services."

GOAL
Improve the visual health of the nation through prevention, early detection, timely treatment, and rehabilitation. Visual impairment puts all people, especially older adults, at risk.

OBJECTIVES
- Reduce visual impairment due to cataracts (from baseline 110.0 per 1,000 population aged 65 years and over
- Increase the use of assistive and adaptive devices by people with visual impairment
- Increase the use of vision rehabilitation services by people with visual impairment

SCREENING
The American Academy of Ophthalmology (2015a) and Mayo Clinic (2013b) report that early detection and treatment of cataracts can greatly reduce the risk of partial or complete blindness and recommends that adults 65 years or more who have no symptoms have their eyes examined every 1 to 2 years. The US Preventive Services Task Force (2015) supported this screening for visual acuity in adults older than 65, as screening can lead to improved vision, function, and quality of life, even though their findings showed no direct evidence of benefits of screening. The USPSTF (2015) has issued a draft statement regarding screening for impaired visual acuity in older adults and concludes that the current evidence is still insufficient to assess the balance of benefits and harms to such screening, although there is an open period for submission of research findings to add to the final recommendation.

RISK ASSESSMENT
Mayo Clinic (2013a) lists the risk factors for cataracts as:
- Increasing age (often start developing at 30 years of age, but are most prevalent by 75 years of age)
- Diabetes
- Drinking excessive amounts of alcohol
- Excessive exposure to sunlight
- Exposure to ionizing radiation, such as that used in x-rays and cancer radiation therapy
- Family history of cataracts
- High blood pressure
- Obesity
- Previous eye injury or inflammation
- Previous eye surgery
- Prolonged use of corticosteroid medications (ingestion or applied to skin)
- Smoking

CLIENT EDUCATION
Teach Clients
- Have regular eye examinations—if generally healthy, then at least every year or two at 65 years of age. If diabetic or have other risk factors or take such medications as corticosteroids, talk with your health care provider to determine eye examination schedule.
- Wear sunglasses that block UVB rays when outdoors.
- Protect eyes if exposed to ionizing radiation sources (x-rays or radiation therapy).

- Avoid smoking or stop smoking.
- Avoid excessive alcohol intake.
- Maintain healthy weight, exercise most days, and develop a plan to lose weight if overweight.
- Eat well-rounded diet with a variety of colorful fruits and vegetables for vitamins, antioxidants, and other nutrients.
- Ask health care provider about antioxidant supplements that have been shown to prevent cataracts.
- Use eye protective equipment if necessary to prevent eye injuries.
- Seek medical care for prolonged or unusual eye inflammation or for any eye injury.

Collecting Objective Data: Physical Examination

The purpose of the eye and vision examination is to identify any changes in vision or signs of eye disorders in an effort to initiate early treatment or corrective procedures. Collected objective data should include assessment of eye function through specific vision tests, inspection of the external eye, and inspection of the internal eye using an ophthalmoscope.

For the most part, inspection and palpation of the external eye are straightforward and simple to perform. The vision tests and use of the ophthalmoscope require a great deal of skill, and thus practice, for the examiner to be capable and confident during the examination. It is a good idea for the beginning examiner to practice on friends, family, or classmates to gain experience and to become comfortable performing the examinations (see Assessment Guide 16-1).

Preparing the Client

Explain each vision test thoroughly to guarantee accurate results. For the eye examination, position the client to be seated comfortably. During examination of the internal eye with the ophthalmoscope, you will move very close to the client's face to view the retina and internal structures. Explain to the client that this may be slightly uncomfortable. To ease any client anxiety, explain in detail what you will be doing and answer any questions the client may have.

Equipment

- Snellen or E chart (see Assessment Guide 16-1)
- Hand-held Snellen card or near-vision screener
- Penlight
- Opaque cards
- Ophthalmoscope (Assessment Guide 16-2)
- Disposable gloves (wear as needed to prevent spreading infection or coming in contact with exudate)

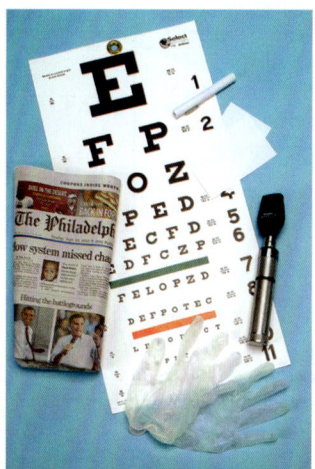

Physical Assessment

Before performing eye examination, review and recognize structures and functions of the eyes. While performing the examination, remember these key points:
- Administer vision tests competently and record the results.
- Use the ophthalmoscope correctly and confidently.
- Recognize and distinguish normal variations from abnormal findings.

General Routine Screening or Focused Specialty Assessment

Assessing the client's visual acuity and eye is always a concern to the nurse. This information may already be documented in the client's record or obtained from the client's history. However, the nurse needs to know all parts of the eye examination to be able to fully understand the status of the client's eyes and vision. In the acute care setting the nurse typically assesses the client's gross vision, peripheral vision, external eye structures, and papillary response. However, in school settings the school nurse may need to use the Snellen Chart to more accurately assess for visual loss in the child. In the home setting it may be necessary to do the additional visual and eye tests to determine the need for further assessment by the primary care provider and to detect early signs of more serious eye conditions (e.g., increased intracranial pressure). Assessment of the internal eye in intensive care settings is important to check for optic disc swelling due to intracranial swelling or in specialized settings to further assess for glaucoma. See the chart below for a general overview.

General Routine Screening

- Test distant visual acuity.
- Test near visual acuity.
- Test visual fields for gross peripheral vision.
- Inspect the eyelids and eyelashes.
- Observe the position and alignment of the eyeball in the eye socket.
- Inspect the bulbar conjunctiva and sclera.
- Inspect the lacrimal apparatus.
- Inspect the iris and pupil.
- Assess pupillary reaction to light.

Focused Specialty Assessment

- Perform corneal light reflex test.
- Perform cover test.
- Perform the cardinal fields of gaze test.
- Inspect the palpebral conjunctiva.
- Palpate the lacrimal apparatus.
- Inspect the cornea and lens.
- Assess accommodation of pupils.
- Use ophthalmoscope to inspect the optic disc, retinal vessels and background, fovea and macula, and anterior chamber.

ASSESSMENT GUIDE 16-1 Vision Charts

Snellen Chart

Used to test distant visual acuity, the Snellen chart consists of lines of different letters stacked one above the other. The letters are large at the top and decrease in size from top to bottom. The chart is placed on a wall or door at eye level in a well-lighted area. The client stands 20 ft from the chart and covers one eye with an opaque card (which prevents the client from peeking through the fingers). Then the client reads each line of letters until he or she can no longer distinguish them.

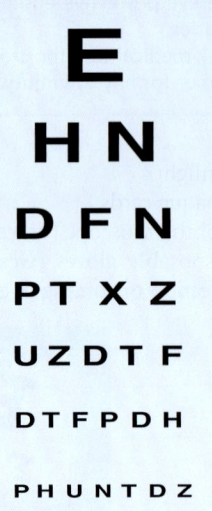

E Chart

If the client cannot read or has a handicap that prevents verbal communication, the E chart is used. The E chart is configured just like the Snellen chart but the characters on it are only Es, which face in all directions. The client is asked to indicate by pointing which way the open side of the E faces. If the client wears glasses, they should be left on, unless they are reading glasses (reading glasses blur distance vision).

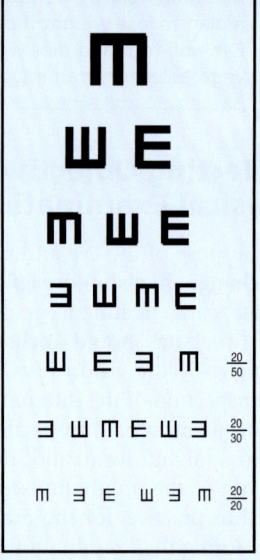

Test Results

Acuity results are recorded somewhat like blood pressure readings—in a manner that resembles a fraction (but in no way is interpreted as a fraction). A common example of an acuity test score is 20/20. The top, or first, number is always 20, indicating the distance from the client to the chart. The bottom, or second, number refers to the last full line the client could read. Usually the last line on the chart is the 20/20 line. The examiner needs to document whether the client wore glasses during the test. If any letters on a line are missed, encourage the client to continue reading until he or she cannot distinguish any letters, but record the number of letters missed by using a minus sign. If the client missed two letters on the 20/30 line, the recorded score would be 20/30 −2.

Jaeger Test

Near vision is assessed in clients over 40 years of age by holding the pocket screener (Jaeger test) or newspaper print 14 in from the eye. Clients who have decreased accommodation to view closer print will have to move the card or newspaper further away to see it.

Near Vision Test Chart
To be viewed at distance of 35 cm (14")

20/200	AbCdE35890
20/100	AbCdE35890
20/80	AbCdE35890
20/70	AbCdE35890
20/65	AbCdE357890
20/50	AbCdE357890
20/40	AbCdE357890
20/30	AbCdE357890
20/25	AbCdE357890
20/20	AbCdE357890

20/200	23 pts
20/100	14 pts
20/80	12 pts
20/70	10 pts
20/65	9 pts
20/50	8 pts
20/40	7 pts
20/30	5 pts
20/25	4 pts
20/20	3 pts

ASSESSMENT GUIDE 16-2 Ophthalmoscope

The ophthalmoscope is a hand-held instrument that allows the examiner to view the fundus of the eye by the projection of light through a prism that bends the light 90 degrees. There are several lenses arranged on a wheel that affect the focus on objects in the eye. The examiner can rotate the lenses with the index finger. Each lens is labeled with a negative or positive number, a unit of strength called a diopter. Red numbers indicate a negative diopter and are used for myopic (nearsighted) clients. Black numbers indicate a positive diopter and are used for hyperopic (farsighted) clients. The zero lens is used if neither the examiner nor the client has refractive errors.

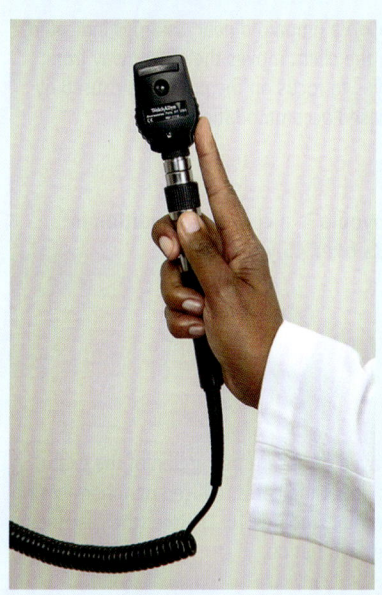

Basics of Operation

1. Turn the ophthalmoscope "on" and select the aperture with the large round beam of white light. The small round beam of white light may be used if the client has smaller pupils. There are other apertures, but they are not typically used for basic ophthalmologic screening.
2. Ask the client to remove any eyeglasses but to keep contact lenses in place. You can rotate the lenses to accommodate for any refractive errors. However, if the client has severe refractive errors, glasses should be left on. If you are wearing glasses, you should remove them, but you should keep contact lenses in place. Removing the client's and your glasses enables you to get closer to the client's eye, allowing for a more accurate inspection.
3. Ask the client to fix his or her gaze on an object that is straight ahead and slightly upward.
4. Darken the room to allow pupils to dilate. For a more thorough examination, optometrists or ophthalmologists may use mydriatic eye drops to dilate the pupils to view the posterior eye structures. However, mydriatic drops may precipitate acute angle closure glaucoma. Clients with a history of glaucoma or extreme farsightedness are at risk.
5. Hold the ophthalmoscope in your right hand with your index finger on the lens wheel and place it to your right eye (braced between the eyebrow and the nose) if you are examining the client's right eye. Use your left hand and left eye if you are examining the client's left eye. This allows you to get as close to the client's eye as possible without bumping noses with the client.

SAFETY TIP *Warn clients who receive the drops that blurring and sensitivity to sun will occur and to avoid driving for 1–2 hours following dilatation of eyes. Encourage client to wear sunglasses outside following dilatation.*

Some Do's and Don'ts

Do
- Begin about 10 to 15 in from the client at a 15-degree angle to the client's side.
- Pretend that the ophthalmoscope is an extension of your eye. Keep focused on the red reflex as you move in closer, then rotate the diopter setting to see the optic disk.

Don't
- Do not use your right eye to examine the client's left eye or your left eye to examine the client's right eye (your noses will bump).
- Do not move the ophthalmoscope around; ask the client to look into light to allow you to view the fovea and macula.
- Do not get frustrated—the ophthalmologic examination requires practice.

ASSESSMENT PROCEDURE	NORMAL FINDINGS	ABNORMAL FINDINGS
Evaluating Vision		
Test distant visual acuity. Position the client 20 ft from the Snellen or E chart (see Assessment Guide 16-1) and ask her to read each line until she cannot decipher the letters or their direction (Fig. 16-9). Document the results. 🎯 **CLINICAL TIP** If the client wears glasses, they should be left on unless they are reading glasses (reading glasses blur distance vision).	Normal distant visual acuity is 20/20 with or without corrective lenses. This means that the client can distinguish what the person with normal vision can distinguish from 20 ft away.	*Myopia* (impaired far vision) is present when the second number in the test result is larger than the first (20/40). The higher the second number, the poorer the vision. A client is considered legally blind when vision in the better eye with corrective lenses is 20/200 or less. Refer any client with vision worse than 20/30 for further evaluation. 🌐 **CULTURAL CONSIDERATIONS** Visual acuity varies by race in US populations. Japanese and Chinese Americans have the poorest corrected visual acuity (especially myopia) followed by African Americans and Hispanics. Native Americans and Caucasians have the best-corrected visual acuity. Eskimos are undergoing an epidemic of myopia (Andrews & Boyle, 2016).

Continued on following page

ASSESSMENT PROCEDURE	NORMAL FINDINGS	ABNORMAL FINDINGS

Evaluating Vision (Continued)

During the vision test, note any client behaviors (i.e., leaning forward, head tilting, or squinting) that could be unconscious attempts to see better.		**CULTURAL CONSIDERATIONS** Causes of visual impairment in the United States vary by race/ethnic groups as well: Non-Hispanic whites have lower rates of diabetic retinopathy and glaucoma, but higher rates of AMD than do African Americans and Hispanics. Hispanics have higher rates of cataracts but all three groups have a relatively high rate compared with other eye diseases. Glaucoma is much more prevalent in African Americans than in the other groups (American Academy of Ophthalmology [AAO], 2015b).
Test near visual acuity. Use this test for middle-aged clients and others who have difficulty with near vision or with reading. Give the client a hand-held vision chart (e.g., Jaeger reading card, Snellen card, or comparable chart) to hold 14 in from the eyes. Have the client cover one eye with an opaque card before reading from top (largest print) to bottom (smallest print). Repeat test for other eye (see Assessment Guide 16-1).	Normal near visual acuity is 14/14 (with or without corrective lenses). This means that the client can read what the normal eye can read from a distance of 14 in.	*Presbyopia* (impaired near vision) is indicated when the client moves the chart away from the eyes to focus on the print. It is caused by decreased accommodation. **OLDER ADULT CONSIDERATIONS** Presbyopia is a common condition in clients over 45 years of age.
CLINICAL TIP The client who wears glasses should keep them on for this test.		
Test visual fields for gross peripheral vision. To perform the confrontation test, position yourself approximately 2 ft away from the client at eye level. Have the client cover the left eye while you cover your right eye (Fig. 16-10). Look directly at each other with your uncovered eyes. Next, fully extend your left arm at midline and slowly move one finger (or a pencil) upward from below until the client sees your finger (or pencil). Test the remaining three visual fields of the client's right eye (i.e., superior, temporal, and nasal). Repeat the test for the opposite eye.	With normal peripheral vision, the client should see the examiner's finger at the same time the examiner sees it. Normal visual field degrees are approximately as follows: • Inferior: 70 degrees • Superior: 50 degrees • Temporal: 90 degrees • Nasal: 60 degrees	A delayed or absent perception of the examiner's finger indicates reduced peripheral vision (Abnormal Findings 16-1). Refer the client for further evaluation.

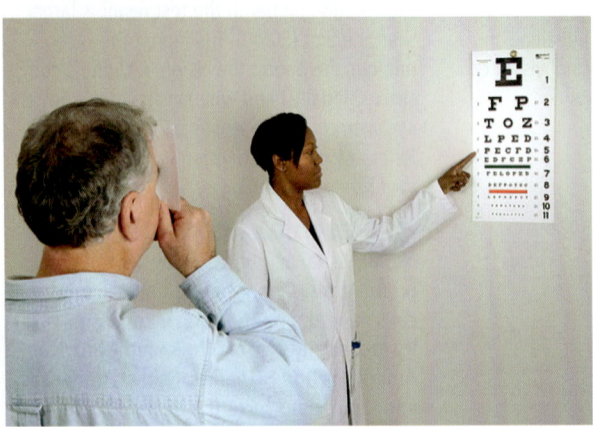

FIGURE 16-9 Testing distant visual acuity.

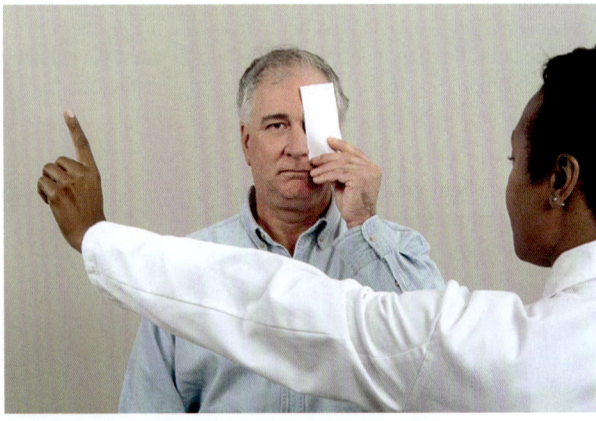

FIGURE 16-10 Performing confrontation test to assess visual fields.

16 Assessing Eyes 319

ASSESSMENT PROCEDURE	NORMAL FINDINGS	ABNORMAL FINDINGS

TESTING EXTRAOCULAR MUSCLE FUNCTION

Perform corneal light reflex test. This test assesses parallel alignment of the eyes. Hold a penlight approximately 12 in from the client's face. Shine the light toward the bridge of the nose while the client stares straight ahead. Note the light reflected on the corneas.	The reflection of light on the corneas should be in the exact same spot on each eye, which indicates parallel alignment.	Asymmetric position of the light reflex indicates deviated alignment of the eyes. This may be due to muscle weakness or paralysis (Abnormal Findings 16-2).
Perform cover test. The cover test detects deviation in alignment or strength and slight deviations in eye movement by interrupting the fusion reflex that normally keeps the eyes parallel. Ask the client to stare straight ahead and focus on a distant object. Cover one of the client's eyes with an opaque card (Fig. 16-11). As you cover the eye, observe the uncovered eye for movement. Now remove the opaque card and observe the previously covered eye for any movement. Repeat test on the opposite eye.	The uncovered eye should remain fixed straight ahead. The covered eye should remain fixed straight ahead after being uncovered.	The uncovered eye will move to establish focus when the opposite eye is covered. When the covered eye is uncovered, movement to re-establish focus occurs. Either of these findings indicates a deviation in alignment of the eyes and muscle weakness (see Abnormal Findings 16-2). *Phoria* is a term used to describe misalignment that occurs only when fusion reflex is blocked. *Strabismus* is constant malalignment of the eyes. *Tropia* is a specific type of misalignment: *esotropia* is an inward turn of the eye, and *exotropia* is an outward turn of the eye.

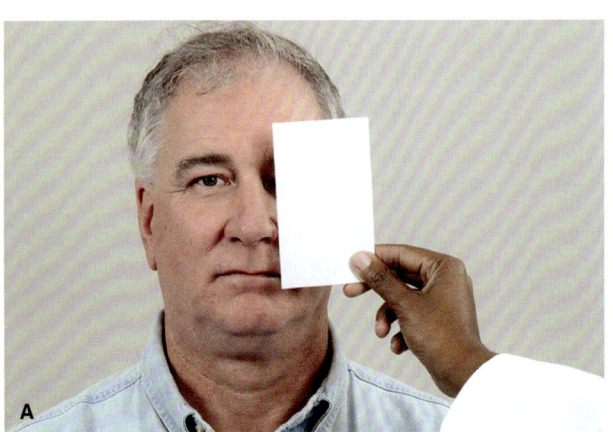 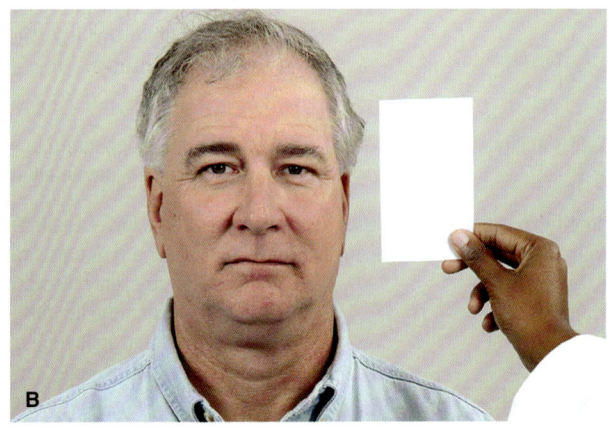

FIGURE 16-11 Performing cover test with eye covered (A) and eye uncovered (B).

Perform the cardinal fields of gaze test, which assesses eye muscle strength and cranial nerve function. Instruct the client to focus on an object you are holding (approximately 12 in from the client's face). Move the object through the six cardinal positions of gaze in a clockwise direction, and observe the client's eye movements (Fig. 16-12).	Eye movement should be smooth and symmetric throughout all six directions.	Failure of eyes to follow movement symmetrically in any or all directions indicates a weakness in one or more extraocular muscles or dysfunction of the cranial nerve that innervates the particular muscle (see Abnormal Findings 16-2). *Nystagmus*—an oscillating (shaking) movement of the eye—may be associated with an inner ear disorder, multiple sclerosis, brain lesions, or narcotics use. 🎯 **CLINICAL TIP** **A couple of oscillating movements of nystagmus at extreme lateral gaze is considered normal.**

Continued on following page

ASSESSMENT PROCEDURE	NORMAL FINDINGS	ABNORMAL FINDINGS

Evaluating Vision (Continued)

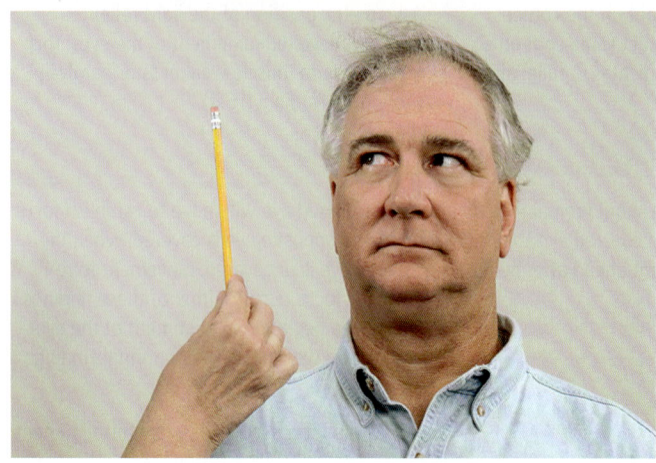

FIGURE 16-12 Performing positions test.

External Eye Structures

INSPECTION AND PALPATION

Inspect the eyelids and eyelashes. Note width and position of palpebral fissures.	The upper lid margin should be between the upper margin of the iris and the upper margin of the pupil. The lower lid margin rests on the lower border of the iris. No white sclera is seen above or below the iris. Palpebral fissures may be horizontal.	Drooping of the upper lid, called *ptosis (formal term blepharoptosis)*, may be attributed to oculomotor nerve damage, myasthenia gravis, weakened muscle or tissue, or a congenital disorder (Abnormal Findings 16-3). Retracted lid margins, which allow for viewing of the sclera when the eyes are open, suggest hyperthyroidism.
Assess ability of eyelids to close.	The upper and lower lids close easily and meet completely when closed.	Failure of lids to close completely puts client at risk for corneal damage.
Note the position of the eyelids in comparison with the eyeballs. Also note any unusual • Turnings • Color • Swelling • Lesions • Discharge	The lower eyelid is upright with no inward or outward turning. Eyelashes are evenly distributed and curve outward along the lid margins. Xanthelasma, raised yellow plaques located most often near the inner canthus, are a normal variation associated with increasing age and high lipid levels.	An inverted lower lid is a condition called an *entropion*, which may cause pain and injure the cornea as the eyelash brushes against the conjunctiva and cornea. *Ectropion*, an everted lower eyelid, results in exposure and drying of the conjunctiva. Both conditions (see Abnormal Findings 16-3) interfere with normal tear drainage. 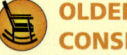 **OLDER ADULT CONSIDERATIONS** Though usually abnormal, entropion and ectropion are common in older clients.
Observe for redness, swelling, discharge, or lesions.	Skin on both eyelids is without redness, swelling, or lesions.	Redness and crusting along the lid margins suggest seborrhea or blepharitis, an infection caused by *Staphylococcus aureus*. Hordeolum (stye), a hair follicle infection, causes local redness, swelling, and pain. A chalazion, an infection of the meibomian gland (located in the eyelid), may produce extreme swelling of the lid, moderate redness, but minimal pain (see Abnormal Findings 16-3).

ASSESSMENT PROCEDURE	NORMAL FINDINGS	ABNORMAL FINDINGS
Observe the position and alignment of the eyeball in the eye socket.	Eyeballs are symmetrically aligned in sockets without protruding or sinking. **CULTURAL CONSIDERATIONS** The eyes of African Americans protrude slightly more than those of Caucasians, and those of Hispanics protrude less. Eyes of African Americans of both sexes may have eyes protruding beyond 21 mm. A difference of more than 2 mm between the two eyes is abnormal (Miller et al., 2016; Weaver et al., 2010).	Protrusion of the eyeballs accompanied by retracted eyelid margins is termed *exophthalmos* (see Abnormal Findings 16-3) and is characteristic of Graves disease (a type of hyperthyroidism). A sunken appearance of the eyes may be seen with severe dehydration or chronic wasting illnesses.
Inspect the bulbar conjunctiva and sclera. Have the client keep the head straight while looking from side to side then up toward the ceiling (Fig. 16-13). Observe clarity, color, and texture. ◎ **CLINICAL TIP** The sclera of the eye, which is normally white, is an excellent place to look for signs of jaundice or icterus.	Bulbar conjunctiva is clear, moist, and smooth. Underlying structures are clearly visible. Sclera is white. **OLDER ADULT CONSIDERATIONS** Yellowish nodules on the bulbar conjunctiva are called pinguecula. These harmless nodules are common in older clients and appear first on the medial side of the iris and then on the lateral side. **CULTURAL CONSIDERATIONS** Darker-skinned clients may have sclera with yellow or pigmented freckles.	Generalized redness of the conjunctiva suggests *conjunctivitis* (pink eye). Areas of dryness are associated with allergies or trauma. *Episcleritis* is a local, noninfectious inflammation of the sclera. The condition is usually characterized by either a nodular appearance or by redness with dilated vessels (see Abnormal Findings 16-3). Yellow sclera occurs when the client has jaundice or icterus. Bright red areas on the sclera indicate a *subconjunctival hemorrhage*. These are often caused by sneezing, coughing, or vomiting, which may break a blood vessel. This may lead to accumulation of trapped blood, which is not quickly absorbed. It is harmless and disappears in 1–2 wks (see Abnormal Findings 16-3).

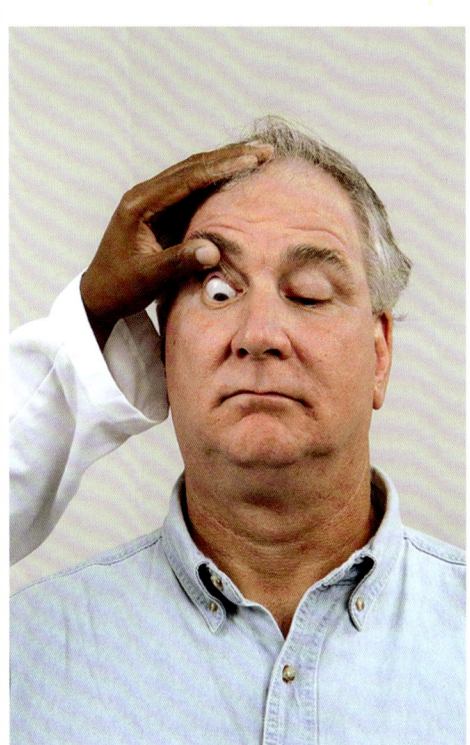

FIGURE 16-13 Inspecting the bulbar conjunctiva.

Continued on following page

ASSESSMENT PROCEDURE	NORMAL FINDINGS	ABNORMAL FINDINGS
External Eye Structures (Continued)		
Inspect the palpebral conjunctiva. 🎯 **CLINICAL TIP** This procedure is stressful and uncomfortable for the client. It is usually only done if the client complains of pain or "something in the eye."		
Put on gloves for this assessment procedure. First inspect the palpebral conjunctiva of the lower eyelid by placing your thumbs bilaterally at the level of the lower bony orbital rim and gently pulling down to expose the palpebral conjunctiva (Fig. 16-14). Avoid putting pressure on the eye. Ask the client to look up as you observe the exposed areas.	The lower and upper palpebral conjunctivae are clear and free of swelling or lesions.	Cyanosis of the lower lid suggests a heart or lung disorder.
Evert the upper eyelid. Ask the client to look down with his or her eyes slightly open. Gently grasp the client's upper eyelashes and pull the lid downward (Fig. 16-15A).	Palpebral conjunctiva is free of swelling, foreign bodies, or trauma.	A foreign body or lesion may cause irritation, burning, pain, and/or swelling of the upper eyelid.
Place a cotton-tipped applicator approximately 1 cm above the eyelid margin and push down with the applicator while still holding the eyelashes (Fig. 16-15B).		
Hold the eyelashes against the upper ridge of the bony orbit just below the eyebrow, to maintain the everted position of the eyelid. Examine the palpebral conjunctiva for swelling, foreign bodies, or trauma.		

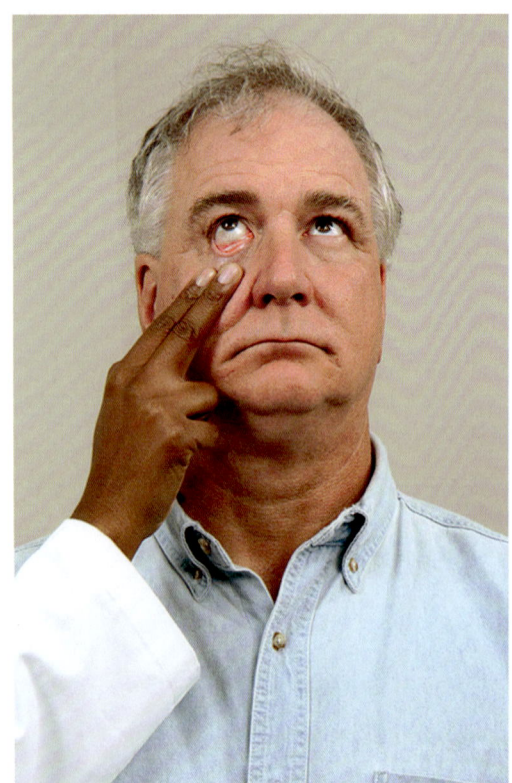

FIGURE 16-14 Inspecting palpebral conjunctiva: lower eyelid.

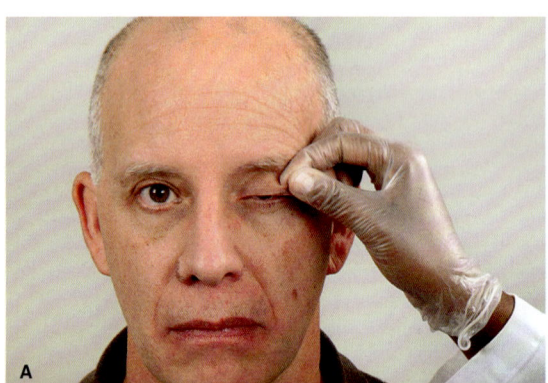

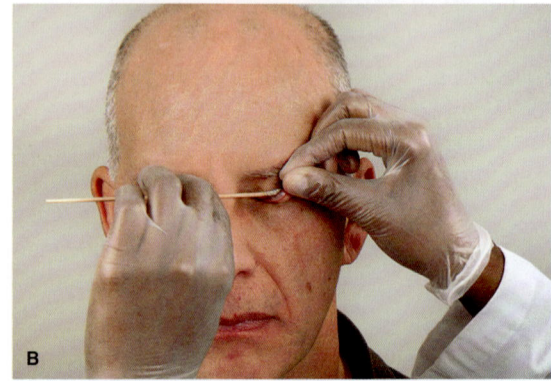

FIGURE 16-15 Everting the upper eyelid.

16 Assessing Eyes 323

ASSESSMENT PROCEDURE	NORMAL FINDINGS	ABNORMAL FINDINGS
Return the eyelid to normal by moving the lashes forward and asking the client to look up and blink. The eyelid should return to normal.		
Inspect the lacrimal apparatus. Assess the areas over the lacrimal glands (lateral aspect of upper eyelid) and the puncta (medial aspect of lower eyelid).	No swelling or redness should appear over areas of the lacrimal gland. The puncta is visible without swelling or redness and is turned slightly toward the eye.	Swelling of the lacrimal gland may be visible in the lateral aspect of the upper eyelid. This may be caused by blockage, infection, or an inflammatory condition. Redness or swelling around the puncta may indicate an infectious or inflammatory condition. Excessive tearing may indicate a nasolacrimal sac obstruction.
Palpate the lacrimal apparatus. Put on disposable gloves to palpate the nasolacrimal duct to assess for blockage. Use one finger and palpate just inside the lower orbital rim (Fig. 16-16).	No drainage should be noted from the puncta when palpating the nasolacrimal duct.	Expressed drainage from the puncta on palpation occurs with duct blockage.
Inspect the cornea and lens. Shine a light from the side of the eye for an oblique view. Look through the pupil to inspect the lens.	The cornea is transparent, with no opacities. The oblique view shows a smooth and overall moist surface; the lens is free of opacities. 🪑 **OLDER ADULT CONSIDERATIONS** **Arcus senilis, a normal condition in older clients, appears as a white arc around the limbus (Fig. 16-17). The condition has no effect on vision.**	Areas of roughness or dryness on the cornea are often associated with injury or allergic responses. Opacities of the lens are seen with cataracts (Abnormal Findings 16-4).
Inspect the iris and pupil. Inspect shape and color of iris and size and shape of pupil. Measure pupils against a gauge (Fig. 16-18) if they appear larger or smaller than normal or if they appear to be two different sizes.	The iris is typically round, flat, and evenly colored. The pupil, round with a regular border, is centered in the iris. Pupils are normally equal in size (3–5 mm). An inequality in pupil size of less than 0.5 mm occurs in 20% of clients. This condition, called *anisocoria*, is normal.	Typical abnormal findings include irregularly shaped irises, miosis, mydriasis, and anisocoria. (For a description of these abnormalities and their implications, see Abnormal Findings 16-5.) If the difference in pupil size changes throughout pupillary response tests, the inequality of size is abnormal.

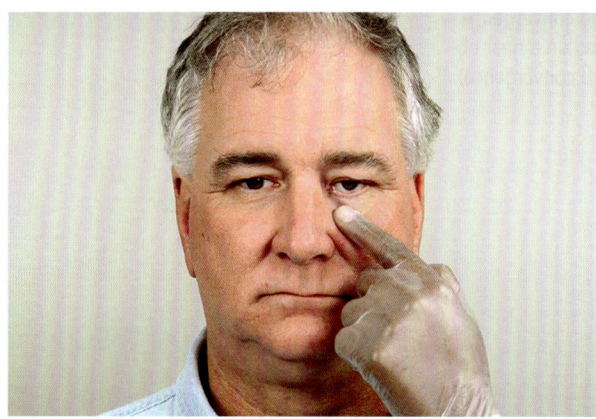

FIGURE 16-16 Palpating the lacrimal apparatus.

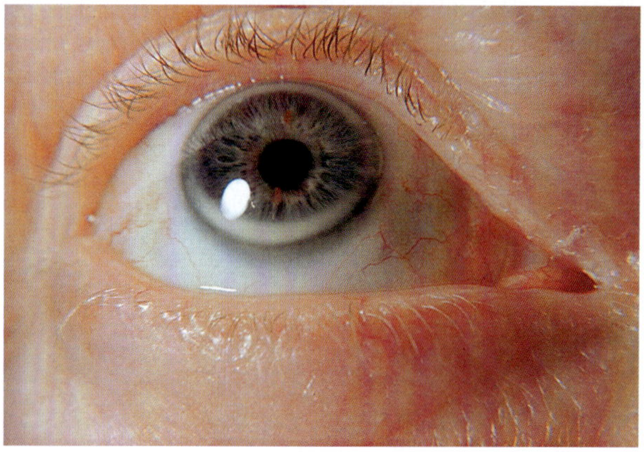

FIGURE 16-17 Arcus senilis.

Pupil Gauge (mm)

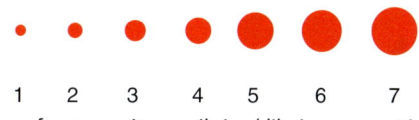

FIGURE 16-18 Pupillary gauge for measuring pupil size (dilation or constriction) in millimeters (mm).

Continued on following page

324 UNIT 3 Nursing Assessment of Physical Systems

ASSESSMENT PROCEDURE	NORMAL FINDINGS	ABNORMAL FINDINGS
External Eye Structures (Continued)		
Test pupillary reaction to light. Test for direct response by darkening the room and asking the client to focus on a distant object. To test direct pupil reaction, shine a light obliquely into one eye and observe the pupillary reaction. Shining the light obliquely into the pupil and asking the client to focus on an object in the distance ensures that pupillary constriction is a reaction to light and not a near reaction. ◎ **CLINICAL TIP** Use a pupillary gauge to measure the constricted pupil. Then, document the finding in a format similar to (but not) a fraction. The top (or first) number indicates the pupil's eye at rest, and the bottom (or second) number indicates the constricted size; for example, left eye and 3/2; right eye, 3/1. The former abbreviations O.S. (oculus sinister for left eye) and O.D. (oculus dexter, for right eye) are no longer used.	The normal direct pupillary response is constriction.	Monocular blindness can be detected when light directed to the blind eye results in no response in either pupil. When light is directed into the unaffected eye, both pupils constrict.
Assess consensual response at the same time as direct response by shining a light obliquely into one eye and observing the pupillary reaction in the opposite eye. ◎ **CLINICAL TIP** When testing for consensual response, place your hand or another barrier to light (e.g., index card) between the client's eyes to avoid an inaccurate finding.	The normal consensual pupillary response is constriction.	Pupils do not react at all to direct and consensual pupillary testing.
Test accommodation of pupils. Accommodation occurs when the client moves his or her focus of vision from a distant point to a near object, causing the pupils to constrict. Hold your finger or a pencil about 12–15 in from the client. Ask the client to focus on your finger or pencil and to remain focused on it as you move it closer in toward the eyes (Fig. 16-19).	The normal pupillary response is constriction of the pupils and convergence of the eyes when focusing on a near object (accommodation and convergence).	Pupils do not constrict; eyes do not converge.

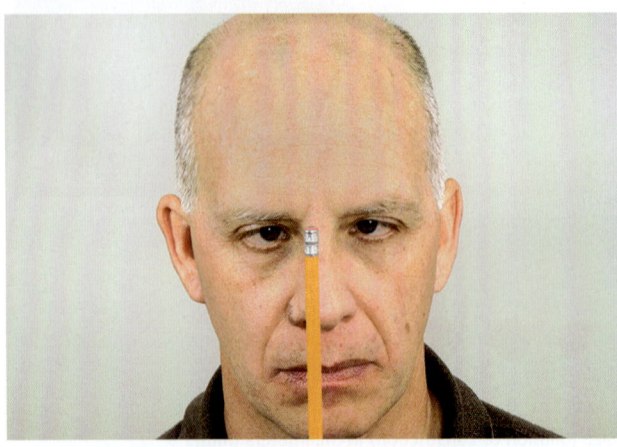

FIGURE 16-19 Testing accommodation of pupils.

16 Assessing Eyes 325

ASSESSMENT PROCEDURE	NORMAL FINDINGS	ABNORMAL FINDINGS

Internal Eye Structures

Using an ophthalmoscope (Assessment Guide 16-2), inspect the internal eye. To observe the red reflex, set the diopter at 0 and stand 10–15 in from the client's right side at a 15-degree angle. Place your free hand on the client's head, which helps limit head movement (Fig. 16-20). Shine the light beam toward the client's pupil.

> **CLINICAL TIP**
> Hold the ophthalmoscope in your right hand, to your right eye, to inspect the client's right eye. Hold the ophthalmoscope in your left hand, to your left eye, to inspect the client's left eye.

> **CLINICAL TIP**
> Visualization of the eye grounds requires much practice. Only approximately one ninth of the image of the total eye grounds will be visible to the examiner in an undilated eye.

Inspect the optic disc. Keep the light beam focused on the pupil and move closer to the client from a 15-degree angle.

You should be very close to the client's eye (about 3–5 cm), almost touching the eyelashes. Rotate the diopter setting to bring the retinal structures into sharp focus. The diopter should be 0 if neither the examiner nor the client has refractive errors. Note shape, color, size, and physiologic cup.

> **CLINICAL TIP**
> The diameter of the optic disc (DD) is used as the standard of measure for the location and size of other structures and any abnormalities or lesions within the ocular fundus. Only one-half of the optic disc is seen if the eyes are not dilated. When documenting a structure within the ocular fundus, also note the position of the structure as it relates to numbers on the clock. For example, lesion is at 2:00, 1 DD in size, 2 DD from disc.

The red reflex should be easily visible through the ophthalmoscope. The red area should appear round, with regular borders.

The optic disc should be round to oval with sharp, well-defined borders (Fig. 16-21).

The nasal edge of the optic disc may be blurred. The disc is normally creamy, yellow-orange to pink, and approximately 1.5 mm wide.

The physiologic cup, the point at which the optic nerve enters the eyeball, appears on the optic disc as slightly depressed and a lighter color than the disc. The cup occupies less than half of the disc's diameter. The disc's border may be surrounded by rings and crescents, consisting of white sclera or black retinal pigment. These normal variations are not considered in the optic disc's diameter.

 CULTURAL CONSIDERATIONS
Optic discs are larger in African Americans, which is thought to be associated with the higher rate of glaucoma in this group (Swanson, 2014).

Abnormalities of the red reflex most often result from cataracts. These usually appear as black spots against the background of the red light reflex. Two types of age-related cataracts are nuclear cataracts and peripheral cataracts (see Abnormal Findings 16-4).

Papilledema, or swelling of the optic disc, appears as a swollen disc with blurred margins, a hyperemic (blood-filled) appearance, more visible and more numerous disc vessels, and lack of visible physiologic cup. The condition may result from hypertension or increased intracranial pressure (Abnormal Findings 16-6).

The intraocular pressure associated with *glaucoma* interferes with the blood supply to optic structures and results in the following characteristics: an enlarged physiologic cup that occupies more than half of the disc's diameter, pale base of enlarged physiologic cup, and obscured or displaced retinal vessels.

Optic atrophy is evidenced by the disc being white in color and a lack of disc vessels. This condition is caused by the death of optic nerve fibers (see Abnormal Findings 16-6).

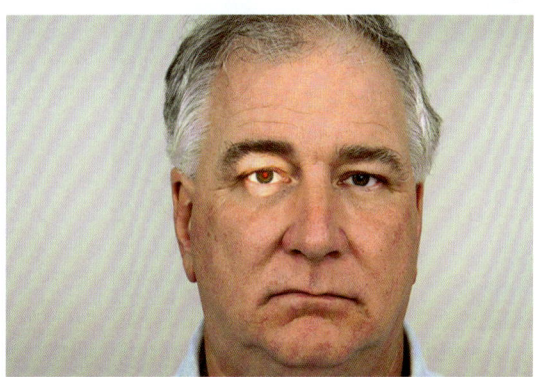
FIGURE 16-20 Inspecting the red reflex.

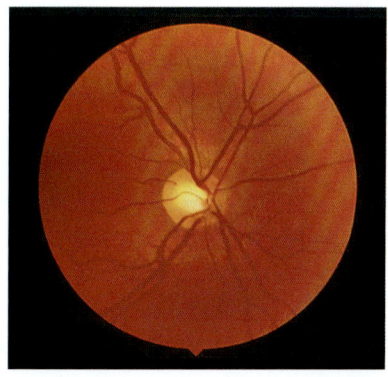
FIGURE 16-21 Normal ocular fundus (also called the optic disc).

Continued on following page

ASSESSMENT PROCEDURE	NORMAL FINDINGS	ABNORMAL FINDINGS
External Eye Structures (Continued)		
Inspect the retinal vessels. Remain in the same position as described previously. Inspect the sets of retinal vessels by following them out to the periphery of each section of the eye. Note the number of sets of arterioles and venules. Also note color and diameter of the arterioles. Observe the arteriovenous (AV) ratio.	Four sets of arterioles and venules should pass through the optic disc. Arterioles are bright red and progressively narrow as they move away from the optic disc. Arterioles have a light reflex that appears as a thin, white line in the center of the arteriole. Venules are darker red and larger than arterioles. They also progressively narrow as they move away from the optic disc. The ratio of arteriole diameter to vein diameter (AV ratio) is 2:3 or 4:5.	Changes in the blood supply to the retina may be observed in constricted arterioles, dilated veins, or absence of major vessels (Abnormal Findings 16-7). Initially hypertension may cause a widening of the arterioles' light reflex and the arterioles take on a copper color. With long-standing hypertension, arteriole walls thicken and appear opaque or silver.
Look at AV crossings.	In a normal AV crossing, the vein passing underneath the arteriole is seen right up to the column of blood on either side of the arteriole (the arteriole wall itself is normally transparent).	Arterial nicking, tapering, and banking are abnormal AV crossings caused by hypertension or arteriosclerosis (see Abnormal Findings 16-7).
Inspect retinal background. Remain in the same position described previously and search the retinal background from the disc to the macula, noting the color and the presence of any lesions.	General background appears consistent in texture. The red-orange color of the background is lighter near the optic disc.	Cotton-wool patches (soft exudates) and hard exudates from diabetes and hypertension appear as light-colored spots on the retinal background. Hemorrhages and microaneurysms appear as red spots and streaks on the retinal background (see Abnormal Findings 16-7).
Inspect fovea (sharpest area of vision) and macula. Remain in the same position described previously. Shine the light beam toward the side of the eye or ask the client to look directly into the light. Observe the fovea and the macula that surrounds it.	The macula is the darker area, one disc diameter in size, located to the temporal side of the optic disc. Within this area is a star-like light reflex called the fovea.	Excessive clumped pigment appears with detached retinas or retinal injuries. Macular degeneration may be due to hemorrhages, exudates, or cysts.
Inspect anterior chamber. Remain in the same position and rotate the lens wheel slowly to +10, +12, or higher to inspect the anterior chamber of the eye.	The anterior chamber is transparent.	*Hyphemia* occurs when injury causes red blood cells to collect in the lower half of the anterior chamber (Fig. 16-22). *Hypopyon* usually results from an inflammatory response in which white blood cells accumulate in the anterior chamber and produce cloudiness in front of the iris (Fig. 16-23).

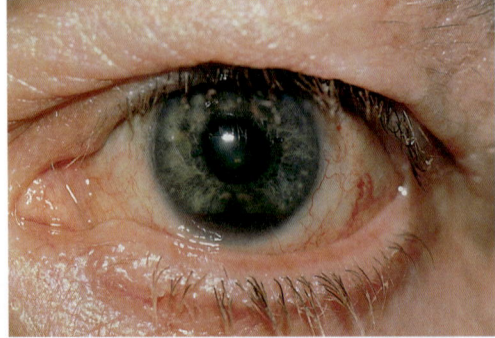

FIGURE 16-22 Hyphemia (© 1995 Science Photo Library/CMSP).

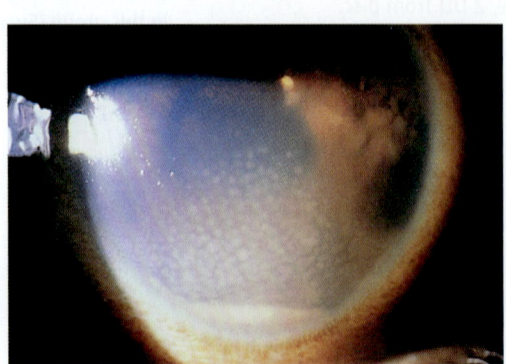

FIGURE 16-23 Hypopyon.

ASSESSMENT PROCEDURE	NORMAL FINDINGS	ABNORMAL FINDINGS
ASSESSING EYE TRAUMA		
In the event of an eye trauma in which the client is experiencing eye pain, discomfort, or feels something is in the eye, observe for: • Foreign body that remains after gentle washing • Perforated globe • Blood in eye	No foreign body is observed. The eye globe is intact with no indication of blood in eye.	Refer the client to an eye doctor immediately if a foreign body cannot be removed with gentle washing, there is perforation of globe, blood in eye, and/or client has impaired vision (Mayo Clinic, 2015a).
In the case of blunt eye trauma, observe for: • Lid swollen shut • Blood in anterior chamber • White/hazy cornea • Irregularly shaped, fixed, dilated, or constricted pupil	There is no swelling of eye, no blood in anterior chamber, cornea is clear, pupils equal and reactive to light.	Refer client to eye doctor immediately if eye is swollen, blood is observed in anterior chamber, cornea is hazy, or pupils are irregularly shaped, fixed, dilated, or constricted. See a list of common eye injuries and need for referral, especially if injury needs immediate emergency referral (Cleveland Clinic, n.d.).

CASE STUDY

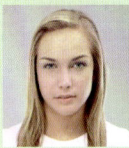

The chapter case study is now used to demonstrate the physical examination of Susan Jones's eyes.

The client's visual acuity in the left eye is 20/20. Visual acuity of the right eye is 20/30. It is noted that the client is squinting and blinking repeatedly during the examination. Peripheral vision is intact. Corneal light reflex is symmetric. Extraocular movements smooth and symmetric, with no nystagmus. Eyelids without abnormal widening or ptosis. No redness, discharge, or crusting noted on lid margins. Left eye: Bulbar conjunctiva is pink, smooth, and moist. Sclera is ivory white. Right eye: Bulbar conjunctiva is pink, smooth, and moist. Sclera is injected (vessels dilated) and tearing profusely. Inspection of right palpebral conjunctiva reveals no foreign body or edema. No swelling or redness noted over the lacrimal gland bilaterally. Puncta visible, without swelling or redness bilaterally. No drainage with nasolacrimal duct palpation bilaterally. Left cornea is transparent, smooth, and moist, without opacity. Right cornea is transparent, with an area of roughness noted; it is moist with no opacity. Irises are round, flat, and brown in color. Pupils are round, reactive to light and accommodation; 4 mm in size bilaterally. Pupils converge symmetrically. Red reflex is present bilaterally. Right eye: no internal eye structures visualized. Left eye: some internal eye vessels visualized; unable to visualize other internal eye structures. (If pupils are dilated and examiner is proficient, a normal internal eye structure examination would reveal the following: Optic discs creamy white in color, with distinct margins and vessels noted, with no crossing defects. Retinal background free of lesions and orange-red in color bilaterally. Macula 1 disc diameter in size, located temporally to the optic disc bilaterally. Anterior chambers are transparent bilaterally.)

Validating and Documenting Findings

Validate the eye assessment data that you have collected. This is necessary to verify that the data are reliable and accurate. Document the assessment data following the health care facility or agency policy.

CASE STUDY

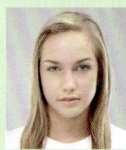

Think back to the case study. The clinic nurse documented the following subjective and objective assessment findings of Susan Jones's eye examination.

Biographic Data: SJ, 24-year-old Caucasian woman. Alert and oriented. Asks and answers questions appropriately.

Reason for Seeking Health Care: "I accidentally poked my key in my eye. My right eye really hurts. It feels scratchy, like there is something in my eye."

History of Present Health Concern: The client reports that 2 hours ago she accidentally struck her right eye with a car key. Since then, her right eye has been tearing excessively, become painful with a scratchy sensation, and vision has become blurred.

Personal Health History: Ms. Jones reports that she has never had a problem with her eyes or vision. She states that she has never had eye surgery or any type of eye treatment.

Family History: Ms. Jones reports that her father has glaucoma.

Lifestyle and Health Practices: She denies exposure to substances that would harm her eyes. She states that she wears sunglasses about 80% of the time when exposed to the sun. Ms. Jones reports that the only medication she takes is an occasional Tylenol for headache. Client states that her last eye examination was 2 years ago and that her vision was "perfect."

Physical Examination Findings: The client's visual acuity in the left eye is 20/20. Visual acuity of the right eye is 20/30. The client is squinting and blinking repeatedly during the examination. Peripheral vision is intact. Corneal light reflex is symmetric. Extraocular movements smooth and symmetric, with no nystagmus. Eyelids without abnormal widening or ptosis. No redness, discharge, or crusting noted on lid margins. Left eye: Bulbar conjunctiva is pink, smooth, and moist. Sclera is ivory white. Right eye: Bulbar conjunctiva is pink, smooth, and moist. Sclera is injected (vessels dilated) and tearing profusely. Inspection of right palpebral conjunctiva reveals no foreign body or edema. No swelling or redness noted over the lacrimal gland bilaterally. Puncta visible, without swelling or redness bilaterally. No drainage with nasolacrimal duct palpation bilaterally. Left cornea is transparent, smooth, and moist, without opacity. Right cornea is transparent, with an area of roughness noted; it is moist with no opacity. Irises are round, flat, and brown in color. Pupils are round, reactive to light and accommodation, 4 mm in size bilaterally. Pupils converge symmetrically. Red reflex is present bilaterally. Right eye: no internal eye structures visualized. Left eye: some internal eye vessels visualized; unable to visualize other internal eye structures. (If pupils are dilated and examiner is proficient, a normal internal eye structure examination would reveal the following: Optic discs creamy white in color, with distinct margins and vessels noted with no crossing defects. Retinal background free of lesions and orange-red in color bilaterally. Macula 1 disc diameter in size, located temporally to the optic disc bilaterally. Anterior chambers are transparent bilaterally.)

Interdisciplinary Verbal Communication of Assessment Findings Using SBAR

SITUATION: Susan Jones, a 24-year-old Caucasian woman, came to the clinic holding her right eye that she accidently poked with her key. She reports constant pain as a 4 on scale of 1–10 that is relieved somewhat with keeping eye shut. Reports blurry vision with watery eye.

BACKGROUND: She reports no past problems with eyes or vision, no history of eye surgery or treatment. Her father has glaucoma. She denies exposure to harmful substances. Wears sunglasses about 80% of the time when in the sun. Takes occasional Tylenol for headache, but takes no other medications. Last eye examination was 2 years ago revealing "perfect" vision.

ASSESSMENT: Visual acuity in the left eye is 20/20. Visual acuity of the right eye is 20/30. Client is squinting and blinking repeatedly during the examination. Peripheral vision is intact. Corneal light reflex is symmetric. Extraocular movements smooth and symmetric, with no nystagmus. Eyelids without abnormal widening or ptosis. No redness, discharge, or crusting noted on lid margins. No abnormalities are noted on uninjured left eye. The injured right eye conjunctiva is pink, smooth, and moist. Sclera has dilated vessels and tearing profusely. Right palpebral conjunctiva reveals no foreign body or edema. No swelling or redness noted over the lacrimal gland bilaterally. Puncta visible, without swelling or redness bilaterally. No drainage with nasolacrimal duct palpation bilaterally. Right cornea is transparent, with an area of roughness noted; it is moist with no opacity. Irises are round, flat, and brown in color. Pupils are round, reactive to light and accommodation; 4 mm in size bilaterally. Pupils converge symmetrically. Red reflex is present bilaterally. Right eye: no internal eye structures visualized. Left eye: some internal eye vessels visualized; unable to visualize other internal eye structures.

RECOMMENDATION: Client has acute right eye pain due to the car key being stuck into right eye. She needs to be further assessed by her primary health care provider because of her risk for infection and/or corneal ulceration due to trauma from foreign object.

ANALYSIS OF DATA: DIAGNOSTIC REASONING

After collecting subjective and objective data pertaining to the eyes, identify abnormal findings and client strengths. Then cluster the data to reveal any significant patterns or abnormalities. The following are some possible conclusions that the nurse may make after assessing a client's eyes.

Selected Nursing Diagnoses

The following is a list of selected nursing diagnoses that may be identified when analyzing data from eye assessment.

Health Promotion Diagnoses

- Readiness for enhanced knowledge: improved visual integrity

Risk Diagnoses

- Risk for Eye Injury related to hazardous work area or participation in high-level contact sports
- Risk for Injury related to impaired vision secondary to the aging process
- Risk for Eye Injury related to decreased tear production secondary to the aging process
- Risk for Self-Care Deficit (specify) related to vision loss

Actual Diagnoses

- Dry eye related to decreased tear production, inadequate intake of nutrients and advancing age
- Ineffective Health Maintenance related to lack of knowledge of necessity for eye examinations
- Self-Care Deficit (specify) related to poor vision
- Acute Pain related to injury from eye trauma, abrasion, or exposure to chemical irritant
- Social Isolation related to inability to interact effectively with others secondary to vision loss

Selected Collaborative Problems

After grouping the data, it may become apparent that certain collaborative problems emerge. Remember that collaborative problems differ from nursing diagnoses in that they cannot

be prevented by nursing interventions. However, these physiologic complications of medical conditions can be detected and monitored by the nurse. In addition, the nurse can use physician- and nurse-prescribed interventions to minimize the complications of these problems. The nurse may also have to refer the client in such situations for further treatment of the problem. Following is a list of collaborative problems that may be identified when assessing the eye. These problems are worded as Risk for Complications (RC), followed by the problem.
- RC: Increased intraocular pressure
- RC: Corneal ulceration or abrasion

Medical Problems

After grouping the data, it may become apparent that the client has signs and symptoms that require medical diagnosis and treatment. Referral to a primary care provider is necessary.

CASE STUDY

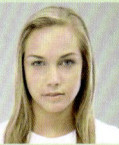

After collecting and analyzing the data for Ms. Jones, the nurse determines that the following conclusions are appropriate:

Nursing Diagnoses
- Acute Pain r/t foreign object (car key) being "stuck" into right eye.
- Risk for infection (right eye) r/t nonsterile foreign object coming into contact with eye.

Potential Collaborative Problems
- RC: Eye infection
- RC: Corneal ulceration

To view an algorithm depicting the process for diagnostic reasoning in this case, go to **thePoint**.

ABNORMAL FINDINGS 16-1 Visual Field Defects

When a client reports losing full or partial vision in one or both eyes, the nurse can usually anticipate a lesion as the cause. Some abnormal findings associated with visual field defects are illustrated here. The darker areas signify vision loss.

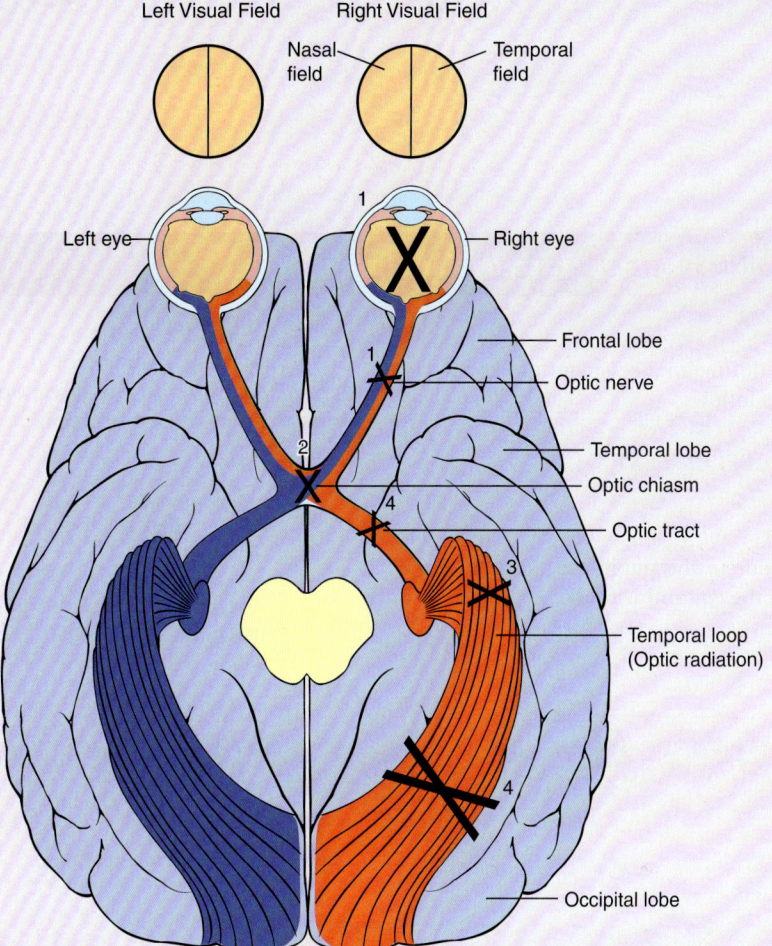

Continued on following page

ABNORMAL FINDINGS 16-1 Visual Field Defects (Continued)

Finding	Possible Source	Example (Left Eye / Right Eye)
Unilateral blindness (e.g., blind right eye)	Lesion in (right) eye or (right) optic nerve	
Bitemporal hemianopia (loss of vision in both temporal fields)	Lesion of optic chiasm	
Left superior quadrant anopia or similar loss of vision (homonymous) in quadrant of each field	Partial lesion of temporal loop (optic radiation)	
Right visual field loss—right homonymous hemianopia or similar loss of vision in half of each field	Lesion in right optic tract or lesion in temporal loop (optic radiation)	

ABNORMAL FINDINGS 16-2 Extraocular Muscle

DYSFUNCTION
Abnormalities found during an assessment of extraocular muscle function are as follows:

CORNEAL LIGHT REFLEX TEST ABNORMALITIES
Pseudostrabismus
Normal in young children, the pupils will appear at the inner canthus (due to the epicanthic fold).

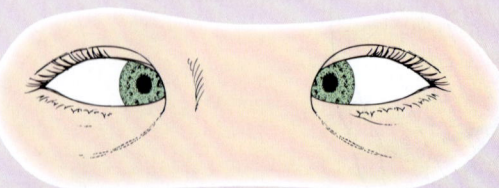

Strabismus (or Tropia)
A constant malalignment of the eye axis, strabismus is defined according to the direction toward which the eye drifts and may cause amblyopia.

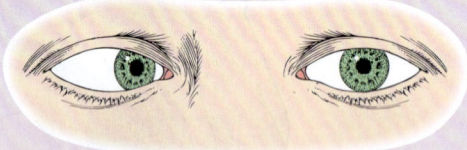
Esotropia (eye turns inward).

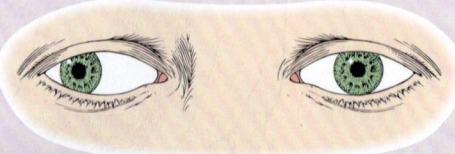
Exotropia (eye turns outward).

COVER TEST ABNORMALITIES

Phoria (Mild Weakness)

Noticeable only with the cover test, phoria is less likely to cause amblyopia than strabismus. Esophoria is an inward drift and exophoria an outward drift of the eye.

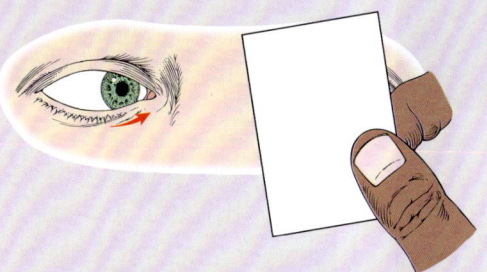

The uncovered eye is weaker; when the stronger eye is covered, the weaker eye moves to refocus.

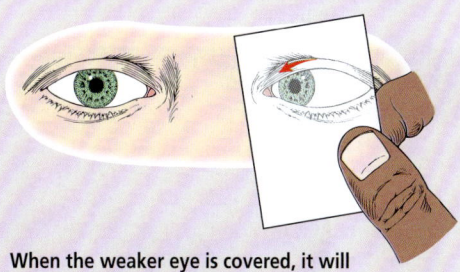

When the weaker eye is covered, it will drift to a relaxed position.

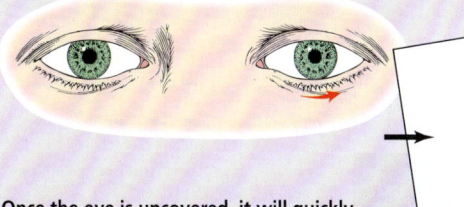

Once the eye is uncovered, it will quickly move back to reestablish fixation.

POSITIONS TEST ABNORMALITIES

Paralytic Strabismus

Noticeable with the positions test, paralytic strabismus is usually the result of weakness or paralysis of one or more extraocular muscles. The nerve affected will be on the same side as the eye affected (for instance, a right eye paralysis is related to a right-side cranial nerve). The position in which the maximum deviation appears indicates the nerve involved.

6th nerve paralysis: The eye cannot look to the outer side.

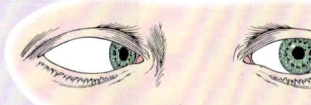

In left 6th nerve paralysis, the client tries to look to the left. The right eye moves left, but the left eye cannot move left.

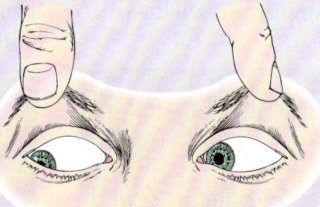

A client with left 4th nerve paralysis looks down and to the right.

4th nerve paralysis: The eye cannot look down when turned inward.

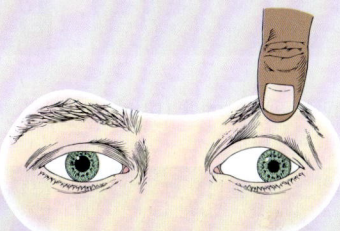

A client with left 3rd nerve paralysis looks straight ahead.

ABNORMAL FINDINGS 16-3 Abnormalities of the External Eye

Some easily recognized abnormalities that affect the external eye are as follows.

Ptosis (drooping eye)

Ectropion (outwardly turned lower lid).

Conjunctivitis (generalized inflammation of the conjunctiva).

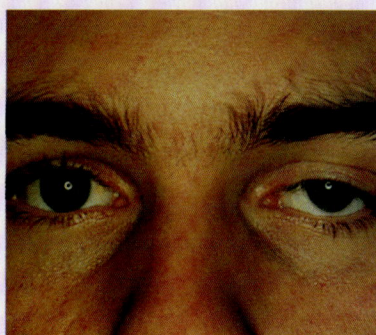
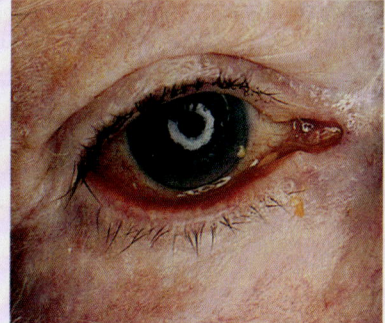
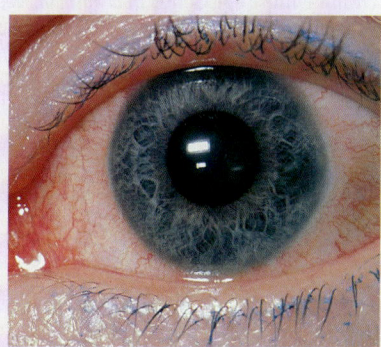

Continued on following page

| ABNORMAL FINDINGS | 16-3 | Abnormalities of the External Eye (Continued) |

Exophthalmos (protruding eyeballs and retracted eyelids)

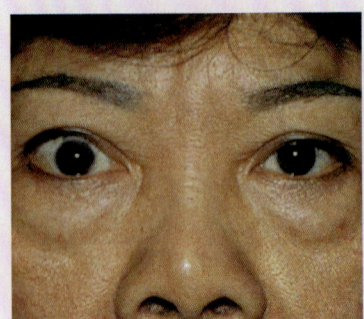

Chalazion (infected meibomian gland).

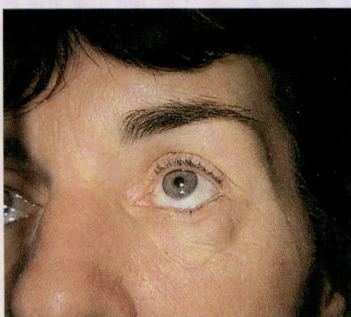

Hordeolum (stye).

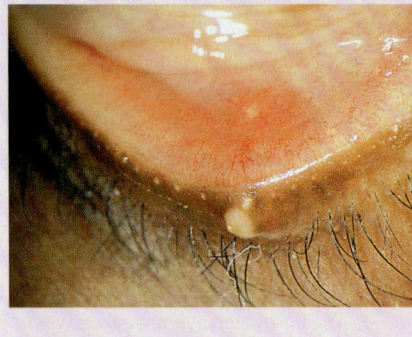

Entropion (inwardly turned lower eyelid)

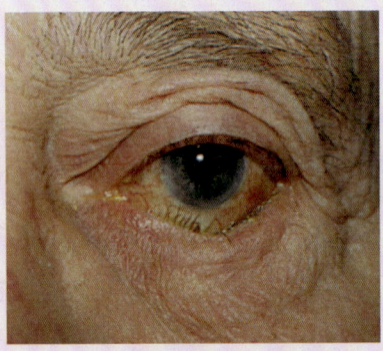

Blepharitis (staphylococcal infection of the eyelid).

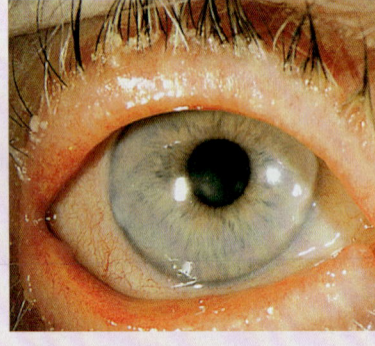

Diffuse episcleritis (inflammation of the sclera).

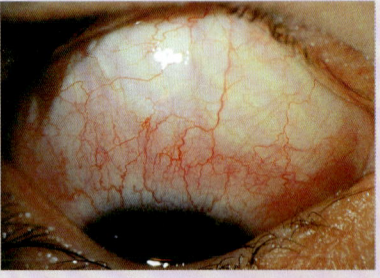

Subconjunctival hemorrhage (bright red areas of the sclera)

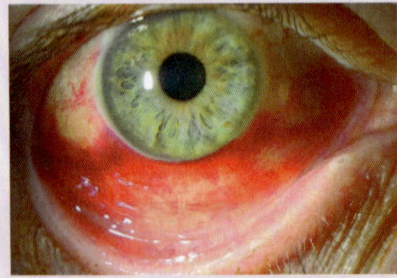

Scleral jaundice

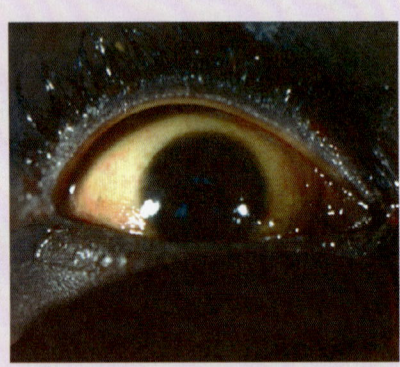

Photo credits: Diffuse episcleritis from Tasman, W., & Jaeger, E. (Eds.). (2001). The Wills Eye Hospital atlas of clinical ophthalmology (2nd ed.). Philadelphia, PA: Lippincott Williams & Wilkins; Subconjunctival hemorrhage from Rapuano, C.J., (2011). Color Atlas and Synopsis of Clinical Ophthalmology, Wills Eye Institute: Cornea (2nd ed.). Philadelphia, PA: Wolters Kluwer Health; Scleral jaundice from McConnell, T.H. (2007). The Nature of Disease Pathology for the Health Professions. Philadelphia, PA: Lippincott Williams & Wilkins.

| ABNORMAL FINDINGS | 16-4 | **Abnormalities of the Cornea and Lens** |

Representative abnormalities of the cornea are illustrated as a corneal scar and a pterygium. Lens abnormalities are represented by a nuclear cataract and a peripheral cataract. Usually, cataracts are most easily seen by the naked eye.

CORNEAL ABNORMALITIES

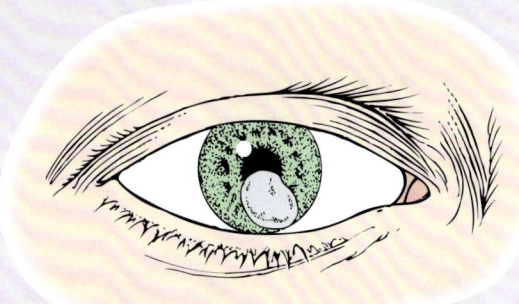

A corneal scar, which appears grayish white, usually is due to an old injury or inflammation.

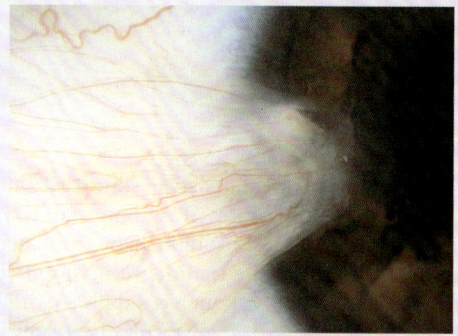

Early pterygium, a thickening of the bulbar conjunctiva that extends across the nasal side.

LENS ABNORMALITIES

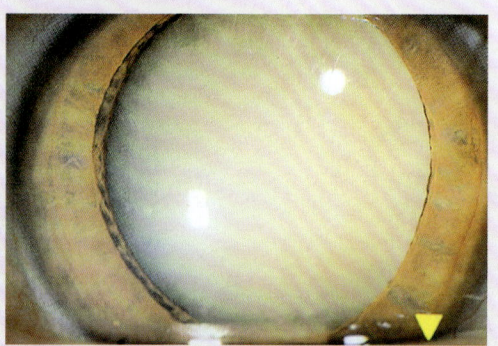

Nuclear cataracts appear gray when seen with a flashlight; they appear as a black spot against the red reflex when seen through an ophthalmoscope.

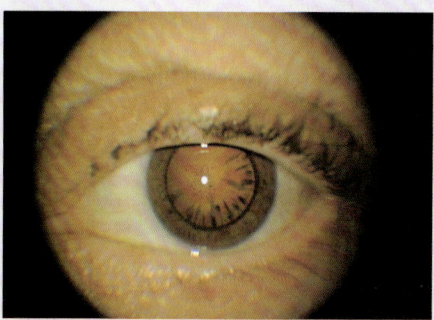

Peripheral cataracts look like gray spokes that point inward when seen with a flashlight; they look like black spokes that point inward against the red reflex when seen through an ophthalmoscope.

Photo credits: Early pterygium *and* Peripheral cataracts *from Tasman, W., & Jaeger, E. (Eds.). (2001). The Wills Eye Hospital atlas of clinical ophthalmology (2nd ed.). Philadelphia, PA: Lippincott Williams & Wilkins.*

| ABNORMAL FINDINGS | 16-5 | **Abnormalities of the Iris and Pupils** |

IRREGULARLY SHAPED IRIS

An irregularly shaped iris causes a shallow anterior chamber, which may increase the risk for narrow-angle (closed-angle) glaucoma.

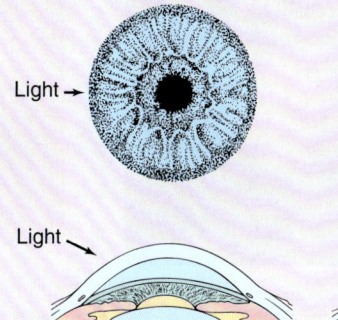
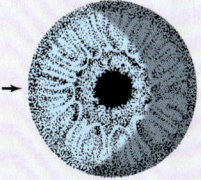
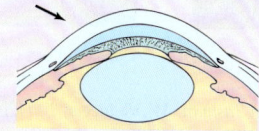

Continued on following page

| ABNORMAL FINDINGS | 16-5 | **Abnormalities of the Iris and Pupils** (Continued) |

ABNORMALITIES OF THE PUPILS

Miosis

Also known as pinpoint pupils, miosis is characterized by constricted and fixed pupils—possibly a result of narcotic drugs or brain damage.

Anisocoria

Anisocoria is pupils of unequal size. In some cases, the condition is normal; in other cases, it is abnormal. For example, if anisocoria is greater in bright light compared with dim light, the cause may be trauma, tonic pupil (caused by impaired parasympathetic nerve supply to iris), and oculomotor nerve paralysis. If anisocoria is greater in dim light compared with bright light, the cause may be Horner syndrome (caused by paralysis of the cervical sympathetic nerves and characterized by ptosis, sunken eyeball, flushing of the affected side of the face, and narrowing of the palpebral fissure).

Mydriasis

Dilated and fixed pupils, typically resulting from central nervous system injury, circulatory collapse, or deep anesthesia.

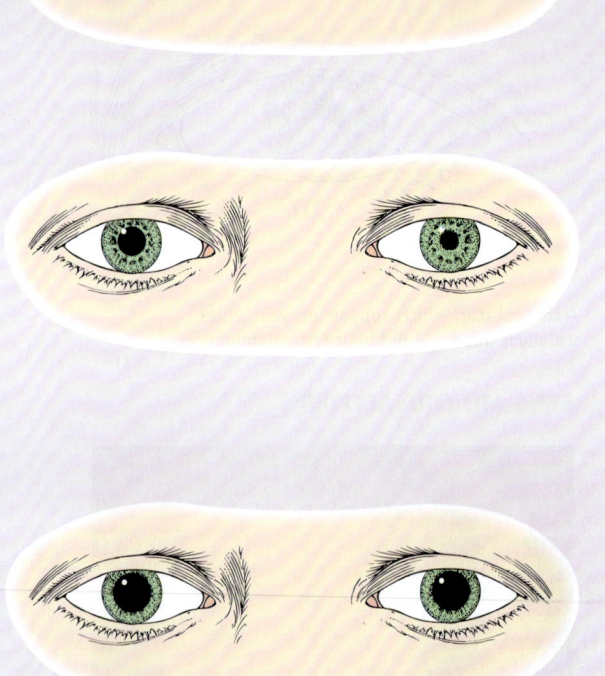

| ABNORMAL FINDINGS | 16-6 | **Abnormalities of the Optic Disc** |

Characteristic abnormal findings during an ophthalmoscopic examination include signs and symptoms of papilledema, glaucoma, and optic atrophy:

PAPILLEDEMA
- Swollen optic disc
- Blurred margins
- Hyperemic appearance from accumulation of excess blood
- Visible and numerous disc vessels
- Lack of visible physiologic cup

GLAUCOMA
- Enlarged physiologic cup occupying more than half of the disc's diameter
- Pale base of enlarged physiologic cup
- Obscured and/or displaced retinal vessels

OPTIC ATROPHY
- White optic disc
- Lack of disc vessels

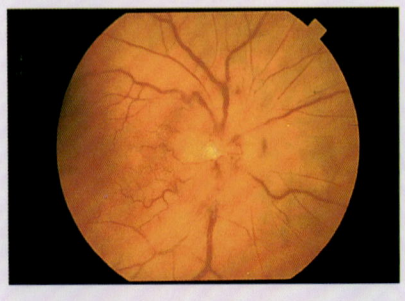
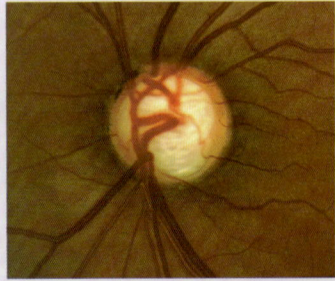
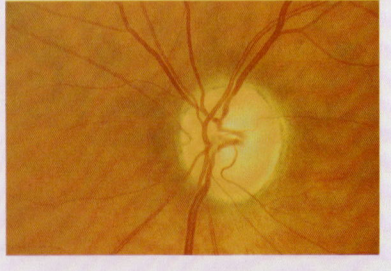

Glaucomatous cupping.

Photo credits: Glaucomatous cupping *from Tasman, W., & Jaeger, E. (Eds.). (2001). The Wills Eye Hospital atlas of clinical ophthalmology (2nd ed.). Philadelphia, PA: Lippincott Williams & Wilkins.*

ABNORMAL FINDINGS 16-7: Abnormalities of the Retinal Vessels and Background

Characteristic abnormal findings during an ophthalmoscopic examination of the retinal vessels include constricted arterioles, copper wire arterioles, silver wire arterioles, arteriovenous (AV) nicking, AV tapering, and AV banking. Signs and symptoms follow:

CONSTRICTED ARTERIOLE
- Narrowing of the arteriole
- Occurs with hypertension

COPPER WIRE ARTERIOLE
- Widening of the light reflex and a coppery color
- Occurs with hypertension

SILVER WIRE ARTERIOLE
- Opaque or silver appearance caused by thickening of arteriole wall
- Occurs with long-standing hypertension

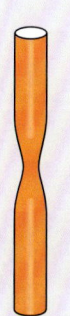
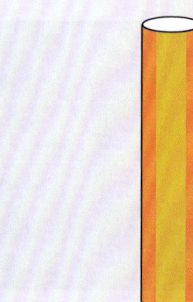
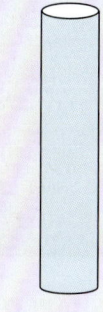

ARTERIOVENOUS NICKING
- Arteriovenous crossing abnormality characterized by vein appearing to stop short on either side of arteriole
- Caused by loss of arteriole wall transparency from hypertension

ARTERIOVENOUS TAPERING
- Arteriovenous crossing abnormality characterized by vein appearing to taper to a point on either side of the arteriole
- Caused by loss of arteriole wall transparency from hypertension

ARTERIOVENOUS BANKING
- Arteriovenous crossing abnormality characterized by twisting of the vein on the arteriole's distal side and formation of a dark, knuckle-like structure
- Caused by loss of arteriole wall transparency from hypertension

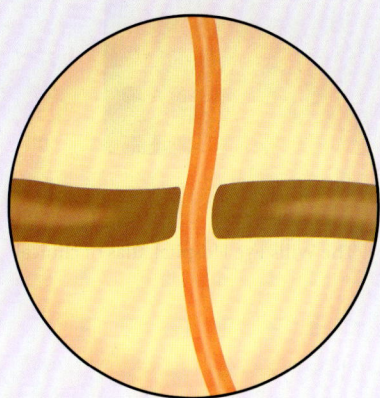
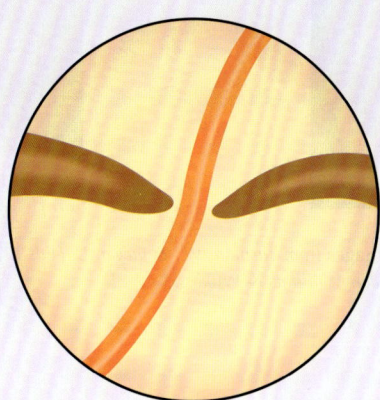
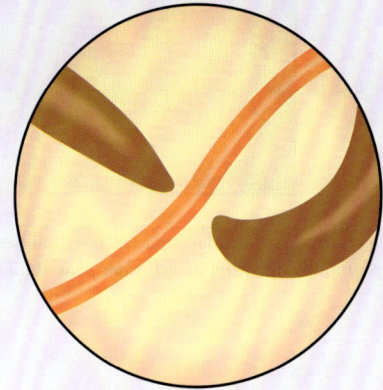

Continued on following page

| ABNORMAL FINDINGS | 16-7 | Abnormalities of the Retinal Vessels and Background (Continued) |

COTTON WOOL PATCHES

- Also known as *soft exudates*, cotton wool patches have a fluffy cotton ball appearance, with irregular edges.
- Appear as white or gray moderately sized spots on retinal background
- Caused by arteriole microinfarction
- Associated with diabetes mellitus and hypertension

HARD EXUDATE

- Solid, smooth surface and well-defined edges
- Creamy yellow-white, small, round spots typically clustered in circular, linear, or star pattern
- Associated with diabetes mellitus and hypertension

SUPERFICIAL (FLAME-SHAPED) RETINAL HEMORRHAGES

- Appear as small, flame-shaped, linear red streaks on retinal background
- Hypertension and papilledema are common causes.

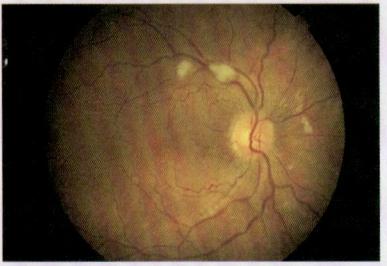 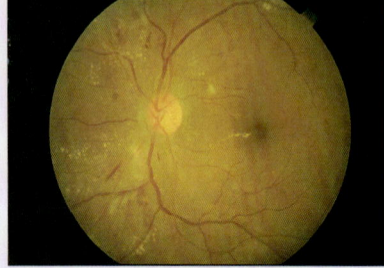 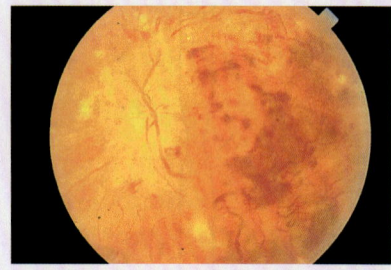

DEEP (DOT-SHAPED) RETINAL HEMORRHAGES

- Appear as small, irregular red spots with blurred edges on retinal background
- Lie deeper in retina than superficial retinal hemorrhages
- Associated with diabetes mellitus

MICROANEURYSMS

- Round, tiny red dots with smooth edges on retinal background
- Localized dilations of small vessels in retina, but vessels are too small to see
- Associated with diabetic retinopathy

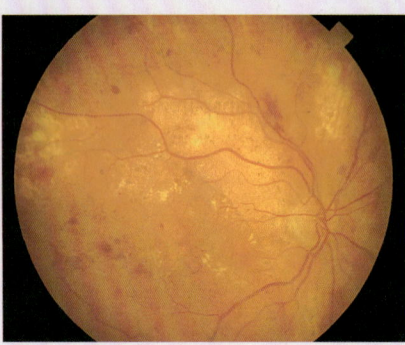 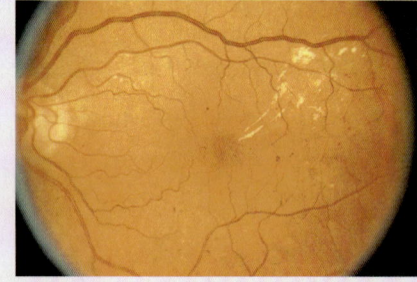

Photo credits: Hard exudate *and* Deep retinal hemorrhages *from Tasman, W., & Jaeger, E. (Eds.). (2001). The Wills Eye Hospital atlas of clinical ophthalmology (2nd ed.). Philadelphia, PA: Lippincott Williams & Wilkins.*

Want to know more?

A wide variety of resources to enhance your learning and understanding of this book are available on **the**Point. Visit thePoint to access:

| NCLEX-Style Student Review Questions | Concept in Action Animations |
| Watch and Learn Videos | And more! |

References and Selected Readings

American Academy of Ophthalmology (AAO). (2015a). Frequency of ocular examinations – 2015. Available at http://www.aao.org/clinical-statement/frequency-of-ocular-examinations–november-2009

American Academy of Ophthalmology (AAO). (2015b). US eye disease statistics. Available at http://www.aao.org/eye-disease-statistics

American Optometric Association (AOA). (2015a). Essential fatty acids: Omega-3: DHA and EPA. Available at http://www.aoa.org/patients-and-public/caring-for-your-vision/diet-and-nutrition/essential-fatty-acids?sso=y

American Optometric Association (AOA). (2015b). Glaucoma. Available at http://www.aoa.org/patients-and-public/eye-and-vision-problems/glossary-of-eye-and-vision-conditions/glaucoma?sso=y

American Optometric Association (AOA). (2015c). Nutrition and AMD. Available at http://www.aoa.org/patients-and-public/eye-and-vision-problems/glossary-of-eye-and-vision-conditions/macular-degeneration/nutrition-and-amd?sso=y

American Optometric Association (AOA). (2015d). Recommended examination frequency for the adult patient. Available at http://www.aoa.org/patients-and-public/caring-for-your-vision/comprehensive-eye-and-vision-examination/recommended-examination-frequency-for-pediatric-patients-and-adults?sso=y

Andrews, M., & Boyle, J. (2016). *Transcultural concepts in nursing care* (7th ed.). Philadelphia, PA: Lippincott Williams & Wilkins.

Boyd, K. (2015). Who is at risk for glaucoma? Available at http://www.aao.org/eye-health/diseases/glaucoma-risk

Bright Focus Foundation. (2017a). Glaucoma: Prevention and risk factors. Available at http://www.brightfocus.org/glaucoma/prevention-and-risk-factors

Bright Focus Foundation. (2017b). Macular degeneration. Available at http://www.brightfocus.org/macular/prevention-and-risk-factors

Cleveland Clinic. (n.d.). Diseases & conditions: Eye injuries. Available at https://my.clevelandclinic.org/health/diseases_conditions/eye-injury-overview

Glaucoma Research Foundation. (2015). Glaucoma facts and stats. Available at http://www.glaucoma.org/glaucoma/glaucoma-facts-and-stats.php

Gollogly, H., Hodge, D., Sauver, J., et al. (2013). Increasing incidence of cataract surgery: Population-based study. *Journal of Cataract and Refractive Surgery, 39*(9), 1383–1389. DOI: http://dx.doi.org/10.1016/j.jcrs.2013.03.027

Healthy People 2020. (2015). Vision: Objectives. Available at http://www.healthypeople.gov/2020/topics-objectives/topic/vision

Macular Degeneration Partnership. (2015). The Amsler grid. Available at http://www.amd.org/living-with-amd/resources-and-tools/31-amsler-grid.html

Mayo Clinic. (2013a). Cataracts. Available at http://www.mayoclinic.org/diseases-conditions/cataracts/basics/definition/con-20015113

Mayo Clinic. (2013b). Eye exam. Available at http://www.mayoclinic.org/tests-procedures/eye-exam/basics/definition/PRC-20014417?p=1

Mayo Clinic. (2015a). Foreign object in eye. Available at http://www.mayoclinic.org/first-aid/first-aid/basics/art-20056645

Mayo Clinic. (2015b). Glaucoma. Available at http://www.mayoclinic.org/diseases-conditions/glaucoma/basics/definition/con-20024042

Miguel, A., Henrigues, F., Acevedo, L., et al. (2014). Ophthalmic adverse reactions to systemic drugs: A systematic review. *Pharmacoepidemiology and Drug Safety, 23*(3), 221–233. DOI: 10.1002/pds.3566

Miller, N., Subramanian, P., & Patel, V. (2016). *Walsh & Hoyt's Clinical neuro-ophthalmology: The Essentials.* Vol 3. Philadelphia, PA: Wolters Kluwer, Lippincott Williams & Wilkins.

National Eye Institute. (2003). The AREDS formulation and age-related macular degeneration: Are these high levels of antioxidants and zinc right for you? Available at http://www.nei.nih.gov/amd/summary.asp

National Glaucoma Research. (2011). About glaucoma. Available at http://www.ahaf.org/glaucoma/about/

Surtenich, A. (2013). How smoking harms your vision. Available at http://www.allaboutvision.com/smoking/

Swanson, M. (2014). The changing and challenging epidemiology of glaucoma. Available at http://www.reviewofoptometry.com/content/c/49437/dnnprintmode/true/?skinsrc=%5Bl%5Dskins/ro2009/pageprint&containersrc=%5Bl%5Dcontainers/ro2009/simple

Tanvetyanon, T., & Bepler, G. (2008). Beta-carotene in multivitamins and the possible risk of lung cancer among smokers versus former smokers: A meta-analysis and evaluation of national brands. *Cancer, 113*(1), 150--157. doi: 10.1002/cncr.23527

U.S. Preventive Services Task Force (USPSTF). (2013). Glaucoma: Screening. Available at http://www.uspreventiveservicestaskforce.org/Page/Document/UpdateSummaryFinal/glaucoma-screening

U.S. Preventive Services Task Force (USPSTF). (2015). Draft recommendation statement: Impaired visual acuity in older adults: Screening. Available at http://www.uspreventiveservicestaskforce.org/Page/Document/draft-recommendation-statement161/impaired-visual-acuity-in-older-adults-screening

Weaver, A., Loftis, K., Tan, J., et al. (2010). CT based three-dimensional measurement of orbit and eye anthropometry. *Investigative Ophthalmology & Visual Science, 51*(10), 4892–4897. Available at http://www.iovs.org/content/51/10/4892.full.pdf+html

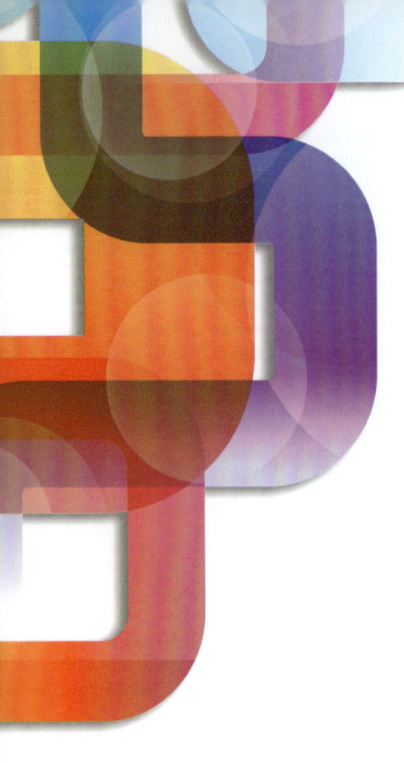

17 ASSESSING EARS

Learning Objectives

1. Describe the functions and structures of the ears.
2. Discuss the risk factors for hearing loss across cultures and ways to reduce one's risks.
3. Interview a client for an accurate nursing history of hearing and the ears.
4. Perform a physical assessment of the ears and hearing ability using the correct techniques.
5. Correctly use the otoscope to inspect the auditory canal and tympanic membrane.
6. Differentiate between normal and abnormal findings of the ear and hearing.
7. Analyze data from the ear/hearing interview and physical assessment to formulate valid nursing diagnoses, collaborative problems, and/or referrals.
8. Differentiate between general routine screening versus skills needed for focused or specialty assessment of the ear and hearing.
9. Document and verbally report accurate assessment findings of the ear and hearing.

CASE STUDY

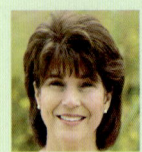

Andrea Lopez, a 47-year-old elementary school teacher, comes to the clinic reporting fever and right earache for the past 2 days. She states, "My students have been sick a lot and I think I may have caught something."

STRUCTURE AND FUNCTION

The ear is the sense organ of hearing and equilibrium. It consists of three distinct parts: the *external ear*, the *middle ear*, and the *inner ear*. The tympanic membrane separates the external ear from the middle ear. Both the external ear and the tympanic membrane can be assessed by direct inspection and by using an otoscope. The middle and inner ear cannot be directly inspected. Instead, testing hearing acuity and the conduction of sound assesses these parts of the ear. Before learning assessment techniques, it is important to understand the anatomy and physiology of the ear.

Structures of the Ear

External Ear

The external ear is composed of the following parts: the *auricle*, or *pinna*, and the *external auditory canal* (Fig. 17-1). The auricle (pinna) is the portion of the external ear visible without any tools. It is composed of a thin plate of yellow elastic cartilage covered by tight-fitting skin and is shaped with hollows, furrows, and ridges that form an irregular funnel to conduct sound waves into the external auditory canal. The external auditory canal is S shaped in the adult. The outer part of the canal curves up and back; the inner part of the canal curves down and forward. Modified sweat glands in the external ear canal secrete *cerumen*, a wax-like substance that keeps the tympanic membrane soft. Cerumen has bacteriostatic properties, and its sticky consistency serves as a defense against foreign bodies.

Middle Ear

The middle ear, or *tympanic cavity*, is a small, air-filled chamber in the temporal bone. It is separated from the external ear by the tympanic membrane (eardrum) and from the inner ear by a bony partition containing two openings, the round and oval windows. The *tympanic membrane*, or eardrum, has a translucent, pearly gray appearance and serves as a partition stretched across the inner end of the auditory canal, separating it from the middle ear. The membrane itself is concave and located at the end of the auditory canal in a tilted position such that the top of the membrane is closer to the auditory meatus than the bottom. The distinct landmarks (Fig. 17-2) of the tympanic membrane include:

- Handle and short process of the malleus—the nearest auditory ossicle that can be seen through the translucent membrane
- Umbo—the base of the malleus, also serving as a center point landmark
- Cone of light—the reflection of the otoscope light seen as a cone due to the concave nature of the membrane
- Pars flaccida—the top portion of the membrane that appears to be less taut than the bottom portion
- Pars tensa—the bottom of the membrane that appears to be taut

The middle ear contains three auditory ossicles: the *malleus*, the *incus*, and the *stapes* (Fig. 17-1). These tiny bones are responsible for transmitting sound waves from the eardrum to the inner ear through the oval window. Air pressure is

338

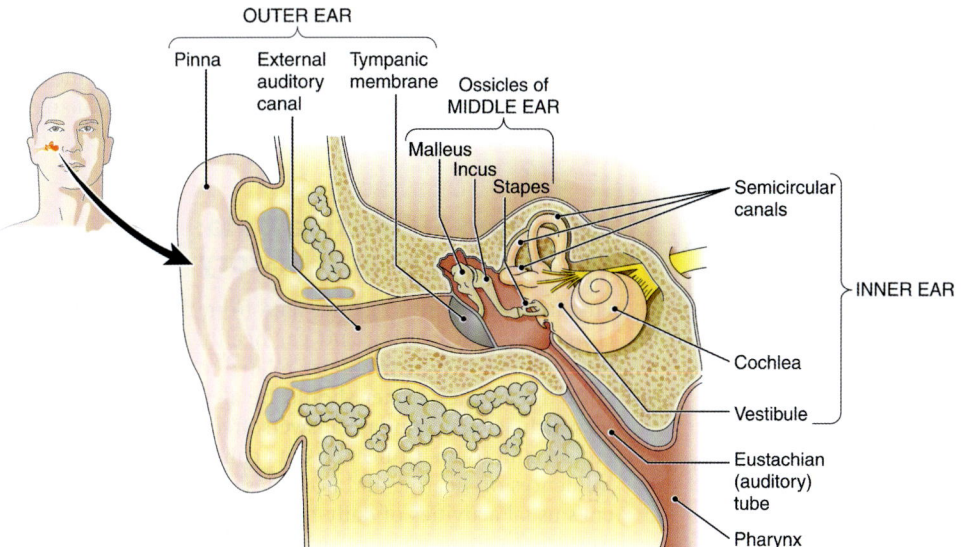

FIGURE 17-1 The ear. Structures in the outer, middle, and inner divisions are shown.

equalized on both sides of the tympanic membrane by means of the *eustachian tube*, which connects the middle ear to the nasopharynx (Fig. 17-1).

Inner Ear

The inner ear, or labyrinth, is fluid filled and made up of the bony labyrinth and an inner membranous labyrinth. The bony labyrinth has three parts: the *cochlea*, the *vestibule*, and the *semicircular canals* (Fig. 17-1). The inner cochlear duct contains the spiral organ of Corti, which is the sensory organ for hearing. *Sensory receptors*, located in the vestibule and in the membranous semicircular canals, sense position and head movements to help maintain both static and dynamic equilibrium. Nerve fibers from these areas form the *vestibular nerve*, which connects with the *cochlear nerve* to form the eighth cranial nerve (acoustic or vestibulocochlear nerve).

Hearing

Sound vibrations traveling through air are collected by and funneled through the external ear, causing the eardrum to vibrate. Sound waves are then transmitted through auditory ossicles as the vibration of the eardrum causes the malleus, the incus, and then the stapes to vibrate. As the stapes vibrates at the oval window, the sound waves are passed to the fluid in the inner ear. The movement of this fluid stimulates the hair cells of the spiral organ of Corti and initiates the nerve impulses that travel to the brain by way of the acoustic nerve.

The transmission of sound waves through the external and middle ear is referred to as *"conductive hearing,"* and the transmission of sound waves in the inner ear is referred to as "perceptive" or *"sensorineural hearing."* Therefore, a conductive hearing loss would be related to a dysfunction of the external or middle ear (e.g., impacted earwax, otitis media, foreign object, perforated eardrum, drainage in the middle ear, or otosclerosis). A sensorineural loss would be related to dysfunction of the inner ear (i.e., organ of Corti, cranial nerve VIII, or temporal lobe of brain).

In addition to the usual pathway for sound vibrations detailed previously, the bones of the skull also conduct sound waves. This bone conduction, though less efficient, serves to augment the usual pathway of sound waves through air, bone, and finally fluid (Fig. 17-3).

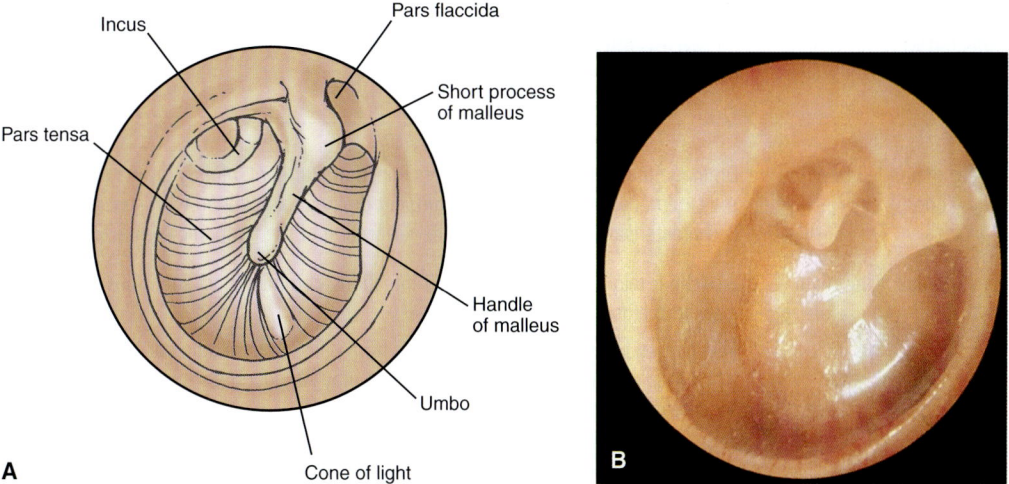

FIGURE 17-2 **A.** Right tympanic membrane. **B.** Normal otoscopic view of the right tympanic membrane. (Moore, K. L., & Agur, A. (2002). *Essential clinical anatomy* (2nd ed.). Philadelphia, PA: Lippincott Williams & Wilkins.)

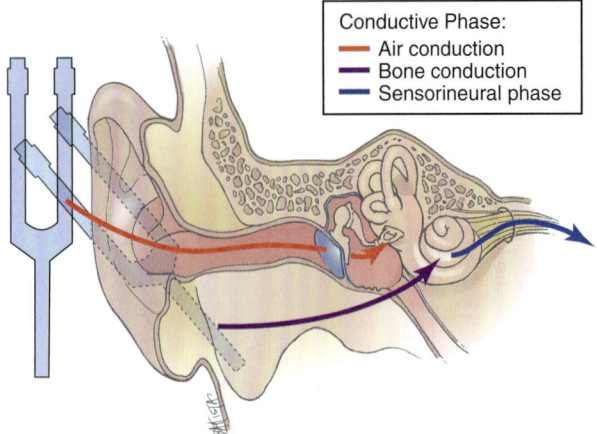

FIGURE 17-3 Pathways of hearing.

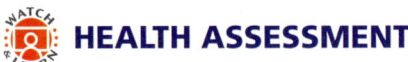

HEALTH ASSESSMENT

Beginning when the nurse first meets the client, assessment of hearing provides important information about the client's ability to interact with the environment. Changes in hearing are often gradual and go unrecognized by clients until a severe problem develops. Therefore, asking the client specific questions about hearing may help in detecting disorders at an early stage.

Collecting Subjective Data: The Nursing Health History

First it is important to gather data from the client about the current level of hearing and ear health as well as past and family health history problems related to the ear. During data collection, the examiner should be alert to signs of hearing loss such as inappropriate answers, frequent requests for repetition, and so on. Collecting data concerning environmental influences on hearing and how these problems affect the client's usual activities of daily living (ADLs) is also important. Answers to these types of questions help you to evaluate a client's risk for hearing loss and, in turn, present ways that the client may modify or lower the risk of ear and hearing problems.

History of Present Health Concern

QUESTION	RATIONALE
Changes in Hearing	
Describe any recent changes in your hearing.	A sudden decrease in ability to hear in one ear may be associated with otitis media or cerumen impaction. Sudden sensorineural hearing loss (SSHL) or sudden deafness (up to a 3-day period) may be a medical emergency and thus should be referred for immediate follow-up. Causes vary from unknown etiology to infections, trauma, toxicity, and other neurologic or circulatory disorders (National Institute on Deafness and Other Communication Disorders [NIDCD], 2015). **OLDER ADULT CONSIDERATIONS** Presbycusis, a gradual sensorineural hearing loss, is common after the age of 50 years.
Are you ever concerned that you may be losing your ability to hear well?	Have the client take the self-assessment "Ten Ways to Recognize Hearing Loss" provided by the NIDCD (2014b) (Box 17-1).
Are all sounds affected with this change or just some sounds?	Presbycusis often begins with a loss of high-frequency sounds (a woman's voice) followed later by the loss of low-frequency sounds.
Other Symptoms	
Do you have any ear drainage? Describe the amount and any odor.	Drainage (otorrhea) usually indicates infection. Purulent, bloody drainage suggests an infection of the external ear (external otitis). Purulent drainage associated with pain and a popping sensation is characteristic of otitis media with perforation of the tympanic membrane.
Do you have any ear pain? If the client answers yes, use COLDSPA to explore the symptom. **C**haracter: Describe the pain. **O**nset: When did it begin? **L**ocation: Where is it? Does it radiate? **D**uration: How long does it last?	Earache (otalgia) can occur with ear infections, cerumen blockage, sinus infections, or teeth and gum problems. Pain caused by "swimmer's ear" differs from pain felt in middle ear infections. Pain that occurs when manipulating, or wiggling, the pinna may suggest otitis externa (swimmer's ear) (Centers for Disease Control and Prevention [CDC], 2015b). Clients with ear infections may experience nausea and dizziness.

QUESTION	RATIONALE
Severity: Rate your pain on a scale of 1–10 with 10 being the most severe. Are you able to continue your usual activities? Are you able to sleep? **P**attern: Have you taken any measures to relieve it (medications, other)? Has it helped? **A**ssociated factors/How does it **A**ffect you? Do you have an accompanying sore throat, sinus infection, or problems with your teeth or gums?	
Do you experience any ringing, roaring, or crackling in your ears?	Ringing in the ears (tinnitus) may be associated with excessive earwax buildup, high blood pressure, or certain ototoxic medications (such as streptomycin, gentamicin, kanamycin, neomycin, ethacrynic acid, furosemide, indomethacin, or aspirin), loud noises, or other causes. Approximately 10% of the population experiences tinnitus reactions that vary from mild awareness to severe irritability, causing frustration, insomnia, or inability to concentrate. Some people adapt to this, while it may impair up to 5% of these people in carrying out their ADLs (Holmes & Padgham, 2011).
Do you ever feel like you are spinning or that the room is spinning? Do you ever feel dizzy or unbalanced?	Vertigo (true spinning motion) may be associated with an inner ear problem. It is termed *subjective vertigo* when clients feel that they are spinning around and *objective vertigo* when clients feel that the room is spinning around them. It is important to distinguish vertigo from dizziness. Benign paroxysmal positional vertigo (BPPV) can occur at any age, but often occurs in persons over 50 and is more common in women. Often the cause is unknown, but head injury or damage to balance organs can underlie BPPV. Crystals in the otolith organs in the ear monitor head position relative to gravity. These crystals become dislodged and create dizziness along with vertigo (sense of spinning), nausea, and vomiting. Dizziness and vertigo in rare cases are associated with serious disease. Refer to your health care provider for further assessment of unexplained dizziness that recurs or lasts for more than a week. Refer to emergency care if it is associated with new, different, or severe headache; double vision or loss of vision; hearing loss; falling or difficulty walking; or other signs of stroke (Mayo Clinic, 2015a).

Personal Health History

QUESTION	RATIONALE
Have you ever had any problems with your ears such as infections, trauma, or earaches?	A history of repeated infections can affect the tympanic membrane and hearing (Evidence-Based Health Promotion and Disease Prevention 17-1).
Describe any past treatments you have received for ear problems (medication, surgery, hearing aids). Were these successful? Were you satisfied?	Client may be dissatisfied with past treatments for ear or hearing problems. **OLDER ADULT CONSIDERATIONS** The older client may have had a bad experience with certain hearing aids and may refuse to wear one. The client may also associate a negative self-image with a hearing aid.

Family History

QUESTION	RATIONALE
Is there a history of hearing loss in your family?	Age-related hearing loss tends to run in families.

Continued on following page

Lifestyle and Health Practices

QUESTION	RATIONALE
Do you work or live in an area with frequent or continuous loud noise? How do you protect your ears from the noise?	Continuous loud noises (e.g., machinery, music, explosives) can cause a hearing loss unless the ears are protected with ear guards. Farmers were found to have a high incidence of noise-induced hearing loss, yet many do not use hearing protective devices. Clients exposed to high noise levels need to be informed of their options for using hearing protective devices (Evidence-Based Health Promotion and Disease Prevention 17-1).
Do you spend a lot of time swimming or in water? How do you protect your ears when you swim?	*Otitis externa*, often referred to as *swimmer's ear*, can occur when water stays in the ear canal for long periods of time, providing the perfect environment for germs to grow and infect the skin. Germs found in pools and at other recreational water venues are one of the most common causes of swimmer's ear. Symptoms include itchiness inside the ear, redness and swelling of the ear, pain in the ear when pressure is applied or the ear is pulled on (pain may be severe), drainage of pus (CDC, 2015b). After bathing or swimming, the external auditory canal should be dried using a hair dryer on the lowest heat setting. People who swim frequently should use a barrier to protect their ears from water. However, impermeable earplugs act as a local irritant and have been shown to predispose the ear canal to otitis externa. A tight-fitting bathing cap offers better protection (Bereznicki & Peterson, 2008). **Concept Mastery Alert** In otitis externa, the patient experiences pain when the pinna and tragus are moved. Otitis externa is also associated with submersion in water such as in swimming. This is why otitis externa is often referred to as "swimmer's ear." Tenderness behind the ear may occur with otitis media but the patient would not experience pain when wiggling the ear.
Has your hearing loss affected your ability to care for yourself? To work?	Hearing loss or ear pain may interfere with the client's ability to perform usual ADLs. Clients may not be able to drive, talk on the telephone, or operate machinery safely because of decreased hearing acuity. The ability to perform in occupations that rely heavily on hearing, such as a receptionist or telephone operator, may be affected.
Has your hearing loss affected your socializing with others?	Clients who have decreased hearing may withdraw, isolate themselves, or become depressed because of the stress of verbal communication.
When was your last hearing examination?	Annual hearing evaluations are recommended for clients who are exposed to loud noises for long periods. Knowing the date of the examination helps to determine recent changes.
Do you wear a hearing aid?	Some internal hearing aids may not be visible to the interviewer. This question will alert the nurse before doing an ear exam. Sometimes hearing aids worn are not functioning well and need to be adjusted. Clients may not be aware of this until someone indicates that they are not hearing well.
How do you care for your ears? Describe how you clean your ears.	Earwax is a natural, self-cleaning agent that should not be regularly removed unless it is causing a problem. A warm, moist washcloth should be used to clean the outside of the ears, but nothing should be inserted into the ear canal. A few drops of mineral oil, baby oil, glycerin, or commercial drops may be placed in the ear to moisten the earwax to allow it to naturally work its way out of the ear. It is important to see your primary care provider or an otolaryngologist (ear, nose, and throat [ENT] doctor) when experiencing ear discharge, fullness, ear pain, reduced hearing, or other persistent ear symptoms. The doctor may recommend ways to remove excess earwax, such as irrigation (syringing), wax-dissolving eardrops, and manual cleaning with a microscope and specialized instruments. **SAFETY TIP** *Never insert anything into your ear canal, including cotton-tipped swabs, pens, hairpins, and so on. Never use an "ear candle" to remove earwax. These are ineffective and may cause burns, obstruction of the ear canal, or perforation of the tympanic membrane. Irrigation devices should only be used by health care professionals.* (American Academy of Otolaryngology—Head and Neck Surgery [AAO-HNS], 2012.)

BOX 17-1 TEN WAYS TO RECOGNIZE HEARING LOSS

The following questions will help you determine if you need to have your hearing evaluated by a medical professional:

Do you have a problem hearing over the telephone?
Yes ☐   No ☐

Do you have trouble following the conversation when two or more people are talking at the same time?
Yes ☐   No ☐

Do people complain that you turn the TV volume up too high?
Yes ☐   No ☐

Do you have to strain to understand conversation?
Yes ☐   No ☐

Do you have trouble hearing in a noisy background?
Yes ☐   No ☐

Do you find yourself asking people to repeat themselves?
Yes ☐   No ☐

Do many people you talk to seem to mumble (or not speak clearly)?
Yes ☐   No ☐

Do you misunderstand what others are saying and respond inappropriately?
Yes ☐   No ☐

Do you have trouble understanding the speech of women and children?
Yes ☐   No ☐

Do people get annoyed because you misunderstand what they say?
Yes ☐   No ☐

If you answered "yes" to three or more of these questions, you may want to see an otolaryngologist (an ear, nose, and throat specialist) or an audiologist for a hearing evaluation.

The material on this page is for general information only and is not intended for diagnostic or treatment purposes. A doctor or other health care professional must be consulted for diagnostic information and advice regarding treatment.

Excerpt from NIH Publication No. 01-4913
For more information, contact the NIDCD Information Clearinghouse.

17-1 EVIDENCE-BASED HEALTH PROMOTION AND DISEASE PREVENTION: HEARING LOSS

INTRODUCTION

According to Healthy People 2020 (2017), at least one in six Americans has a sensory or communication disorder, and even when temporary or mild, can affect physical and mental health. Hearing affects all interpersonal communication. Personal relationships, academic and job performance, and even safety are affected when hearing is impaired, which can be frustrating or embarrassing. The National Institute on Deafness and Other Communication Disorders (NIDCD, 2014a) lists safety areas affected by hearing loss, such as difficulty following a doctor's orders, responding to warnings, and hearing doorbells or alarms. Uncorrected hearing impairment can affect childhood development as well.

The WHO (2015) defines hearing loss (sensorineural, conductive, or mixed hearing loss) as a circumstance when a person is not able to hear as well as a person with normal hearing (measured at or above 25 dB). When hearing loss reaches 40 dB, the loss is considered to be disabling. The majority of people with disabling hearing loss live in low- to middle-income countries.

The three types of hearing loss are defined by the Hearing Loss Association of America (2015) as:
- Conductive hearing loss—when hearing loss is due to problems with the ear canal, ear drum, or middle ear and its little bones (the malleus, incus, and stapes).
- Sensorineural hearing loss (SNHL)—when hearing loss is due to problems of the inner ear, also known as nerve-related hearing loss.
- Mixed hearing loss—refers to a combination of conductive and sensorineural hearing loss. This means that there may be damage in the outer or middle ear and in the inner ear (cochlea) or auditory nerve.

Causes of hearing disorders are many and include both genetic and nongenetic conditions.

Congenital hearing loss is associated with maternal rubella, syphilis, or certain other infections during pregnancy; low birth weight; birth asphyxia (a lack of oxygen at the time of birth); inappropriate use of particular drugs during pregnancy, such as aminoglycosides, cytotoxic drugs, antimalarial drugs, and diuretics; and severe jaundice in the neonatal period, which can damage the hearing nerve in a newborn infant.

Acquired causes include infectious diseases such as meningitis, measles, and mumps; chronic ear infections; collection of fluid in the ear (otitis media); use of particular drugs, such as some antibiotic and antimalarial medicines; injury to the head or ear; excessive noise, including occupational noise such as that from machinery and explosions, and recreational noise such as that from personal audio devices, concerts, nightclubs, bars, and sporting events; aging, in particular due to

Continued on following page

17-1 EVIDENCE-BASED HEALTH PROMOTION AND DISEASE PREVENTION: HEARING LOSS (Continued)

degeneration of sensory cells; wax or foreign bodies blocking the ear canal.

Hearing loss can be in one or both ears and temporary or permanent, and sudden or slow developing. Temporary hearing loss is associated with hearing loss causes such as allergies, blocked eustachian tubes, wax buildup in the ear canal, ear infections, foreign bodies in the ear canal, injuries, scarred or perforated eardrum, and reactions to certain ototoxic medications (e.g., aminoglycosides, chloroquine, quinidine).

Age-related hearing loss is called presbycusis and is caused by changes in the nerves or cells of the inner ear. Approximately one in three people between the ages of 65 and 74 has hearing loss and nearly half of those older than 75 have difficulty hearing (NIDCD, 2014a).

HEALTHY PEOPLE 2020 GOAL OVERVIEW

The Healthy People 2020 objectives (2017) relate to a broad spectrum of disorders associated with communication, including hearing, balance, smell, taste, voice, speech, and language. Specifically, these objectives concern newborn hearing screening; ear infections (otitis media); hearing and assistive device use; tinnitus; balance and dizziness; smell and taste; voice, speech, and language; and related Internet health care resource use.

GOAL

Reduce the prevalence and severity of disorders of hearing and balance; smell and taste; and voice, speech, and language.

OBJECTIVES

For newborns, the objectives include screening no later than age 1 month and follow-up audiologic examination no later than 3 months of age.

For otitis media in children and adolescents, the objective is to reduce the rate by 10%, and to reduce the proportion of adolescents who have noise-induced hearing loss.

For hearing generally, the objective is to increase the proportion of persons with hearing impairments who have ever used a hearing aid or assistive listening devices or who have cochlear implants; increase the proportion of persons who have had a hearing evaluation on schedule or who have been referred by their primary care provider for hearing evaluation and treatment; increase the use of hearing protective devices; and reduce the proportion of adults who have noise-induced hearing loss.

SCREENING

The U.S. Preventive Services Task Force (2012) report on screening guidelines for hearing loss has concluded that the current evidence is insufficient to assess the balance of benefits and harms of screening for hearing loss in asymptomatic adults aged 50 years or older (asymptomatic is emphasized in the report). As of 2015, the USPSTF has decided not to review and update recommendations for universal screening of newborns but urges primary care providers to seek other sources of recommendations for this practice (USPSTF, 2015).

OTHER SCREENING RECOMMENDATIONS

Healthy People 2020 (2017) recommends that all newborns be screened for hearing loss by no later than age 1 month, have an audiologic evaluation by age 3 months, and if necessary be enrolled in appropriate intervention services by no later than 6 months of age.

The CDC (2015a) recommends that all babies be screened for hearing before 1 month of age, and preferably before they leave the hospital, but no later than 3 months.

The American Speech-Language-Hearing Association (2015b) recommends that all infants be screened before leaving the hospital, all school-aged children be screened periodically at school, and all adults should be screened at least every decade through age 50 and at 3-year intervals thereafter.

Mayo Clinic (2015b) lists some screening methods to diagnose hearing loss. These include general screening tests (asking clients to cover one ear at a time to see how well they hear words spoken at various volumes and respond to other sounds); tuning fork tests (to differentiate types of hearing loss); and audiometer tests (completed by an audiologist). Other simple assessments easily used to identify the need for further testing include: asking the client about any decrease in their ability to hear persons' voices or television; asking if others (for instance, a spouse) have noticed a decrease in their hearing; and observing the client's behavior while completing the health assessment for evidence of diminished hearing. Chou et al. (2011) found that the "whispered voice test at 2 ft and a single question regarding perceived hearing loss were comparable with a more detailed screening questionnaire or a hand-held audiometric device for identifying at least mild (>25 dB) hearing loss."

A personal hearing questionnaire for individuals is provided by the NIDCD (2014b), called Ten Ways to Recognize Hearing Loss. This quiz is recommended for anyone. It is available on the NIDCD website.

RISK ASSESSMENT

The NIDCD (2015) describes one type of hearing loss: noise-induced hearing loss (NIHL). Long or repeated sounds at or above 85 dB can cause hearing loss. The louder the sound, the shorter amount of time is needed for hearing to be affected.

Mayo Clinic (2015c) lists:
- Aging, especially due to many years of exposure to sounds that can damage inner ear cells
- Heredity, with genetics that are related to susceptibility to ear damage
- Occupational loud noises as regular part of the working environment (e.g., farming, construction, factory work)
- Recreational noises and exposure to explosive noises (firearms and fireworks; snowmobiling, motorcycling, listening to loud music or MP3s, especially if volume is high)
- Ototoxic medications (e.g., gentamicin, some chemotherapy medications; or high-dose aspirin, some other pain relievers, antimalarial drugs, or loop diuretics can lead to tinnitus or hearing loss)
- Illnesses, especially with high fever (e.g., meningitis)

Mayo Clinic (2013); Jensen et al. (2013); and Perlstein (2015) list risks for otitis media:
- Age (between 6 months and 2 years especially, due to size and shape of eustachian tubes)
- Group childcare
- Babies fed from a bottle, especially lying down
- Seasons of fall and winter, due to exposure to colds, flu, and increased allergens
- Poor air quality, especially irritants in the air (e.g., cigarette smoke)
- Family history
- Cleft palate
- Down syndrome
- Ethnicity (Alaskan Indians and Inuits have higher incidence)
- Enlarged adenoids

CLIENT EDUCATION

Teach Clients

- Avoid sound exposure louder than a washing machine. (Your distance from the source of the sound and the length of time you are exposed to the sound are important factors in protecting your hearing. A good rule of thumb is to avoid noises that are too loud, too close, or last too long.)
- Avoid recreational risks that involve loud sounds or risks of head or ear injury.
- Avoid listening to extremely loud music for long periods of time.
- Wear hearing protectors and take breaks from the noise in loud noise environments.
- Have hearing checked periodically, especially after age 50.
- If hearing loss is detected, obtain and use devices to improve hearing.
- Immunize children against childhood diseases, including measles, meningitis, rubella, and mumps.
- Be immunized against rubella before pregnancy if a woman of child-bearing age.
- If pregnant, get screening for syphilis and other STIs, adequate antenatal and prenatal care, and diagnosis and treatment for a baby born with jaundice.
- Avoid the use of ototoxic drugs unless prescribed by a qualified health care worker and properly monitored for correct dosage.
- If you have a newborn, avoid feeding from bottle while infant is lying on back.
- Have newborn infant screened for hearing.
- Get treatment for ear infections as soon as they are noticed; follow up with health care provider after symptoms seem to be gone to make sure there is no fluid left in the ear.
- Get treatment for tonsil and adenoid infections and inflammation.
- Keep child home from day care if possible when there is an outbreak of ear infections.
- Teach child to avoid putting foreign bodies in ears.
- Avoid use of instruments to remove wax from ears due to chance of impacting it further. See professional care for wax removal.

CASE STUDY

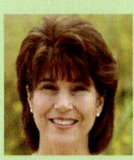

The case study introduced at the beginning of the chapter is now used to demonstrate how a nurse would use the COLDSPA mnemonic to explore Ms. Lopez's reported fever and earache.

Mnemonic	Question	Client Response
Character	Describe the sign or symptom (feeling, appearance, sound, smell, or taste if applicable).	"I have an achy pressure sensation in my right ear that pulses with every beat of my heart."
Onset	When did it begin?	"Two days ago."
Location	Where is it? Does it radiate? Does it occur anywhere else?	"Inside my right ear."
Duration	How long does it last? Does it recur?	"The pressure is constant, but the pain varies depending on when I last took ibuprofen."
Severity	How bad is it? or How much does it bother you?	"It kept me awake last night. On a scale of 1–10, I would rate the pain as 7 right now. About an hour after I take ibuprofen the pain decreases to a 3–4 out of 10."
Pattern	What makes it better or worse?	"The pain never completely goes away. Ibuprofen makes the pain tolerable. Coughing or increased activity makes the pain worse."
Associated factors/How it Affects the client	What other symptoms occur with it? How does it affect you?	"Everything sounds muffled—I can hardly hear from my right ear. I had a cold about a week ago and it went away, but now I have this earache. I really don't feel like working at school or at home. I have also been running a fever of 100°F for 2 days."

After investigating Ms. Lopez's report of fever and earache, the nurse continues with the health history. Ms. Lopez remembers a couple of ear infections as a child but has never had an ear infection as an adult. She denies any previous treatments for ear problems. She denies ear trauma. She denies a family history of hearing loss. She does not work in an area with frequent or continuous loud noises, and denies the need for hearing protection. She reports that she swims infrequently in the summer months (1–2 times per month), and denies any ear issues associated with swimming. She has never had a formal hearing evaluation and denies the use of a hearing aid. She does report the use of cotton-tipped applicators to "clean out" her ears each morning after she showers.

Collecting Objective Data: Physical Examination

The purpose of the ear and hearing examination is to evaluate the condition of the external ear, the condition and patency of the ear canal, the status of the tympanic membrane, bone and air conduction of sound vibrations, hearing acuity, and equilibrium. The external ear structures and ear canal are relatively easy to assess through inspection. Using the tuning fork to evaluate bone and air conduction is also a fairly simple procedure. However, more practice and expertise are needed to use the otoscope correctly to examine the condition of the structures of the tympanic membrane.

Preparing the Client

Make sure that the client is seated comfortably during the ear examination. This helps to promote the client's participation, which is very important in this examination. In addition, the test should be explained thoroughly to guarantee accurate results. To ease any client anxiety, explain in detail what you will be doing. Also, answer any questions the client may have. As you prepare the client for the ear examination, carefully note how the client responds to your explanations. Does the client appear to hear you well or seem to strain to catch everything you say? Does the client respond to you verbally or nonverbally or do you have to repeat what you say to get a response? This initial observation provides you with clues as to the status of the client's hearing.

Equipment
- Watch with a second hand for Romberg test
- Tuning fork (512 or 1,024 Hz)
- Otoscope

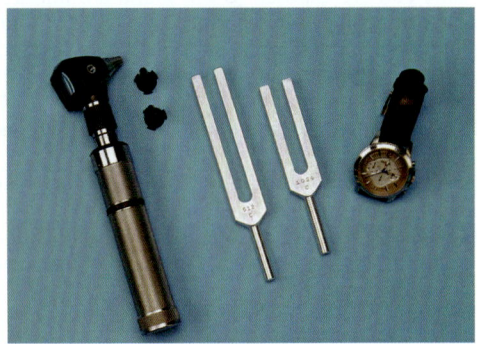

Physical Assessment

Before performing the examination, make sure to:
- Recognize the role of hearing in communication and adaptation to the environment, particularly in regard to aging.
- Know how to use the otoscope effectively when performing the ear examination (Assessment Guide 17-1).
- Understand the usefulness and significance of basic hearing tests.

ASSESSMENT GUIDE 17-1 Otoscope

The otoscope is a flashlight-type viewer used to visualize the eardrum and external ear canal. Some guidelines for using it effectively follow:

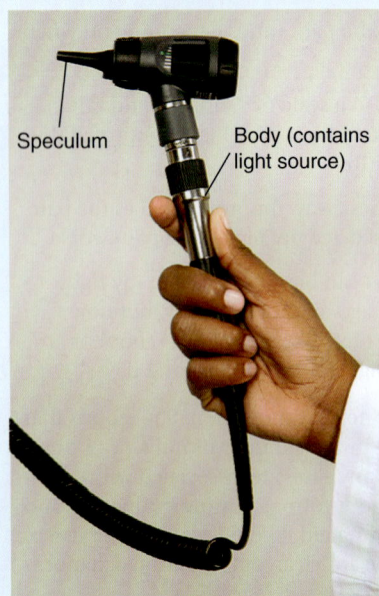

Speculum | Body (contains light source)

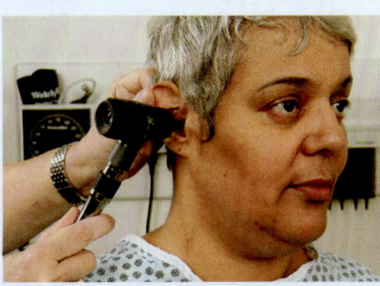

1. Ask the client to sit comfortably with the back straight and the head tilted slightly away from you toward his or her opposite shoulder.
2. Choose the largest speculum that fits comfortably into the client's ear canal (usually 5 mm in the adult) and attach it to the otoscope. Holding the instrument in your dominant hand, turn the light on the otoscope to "on."
3. Use the thumb and fingers of your opposite hand to grasp the client's auricle firmly but gently. Pull out, up, and back to straighten the external auditory canal. Do not alter this positioning at any time during the otoscopic examination.
4. Grasp the handle of the otoscope between your thumb and fingers and hold the instrument up or down.
5. Position the hand holding the otoscope against the client's head or face. This position prevents forceful insertion of the instrument and helps to steady your hand throughout the examination, which is especially helpful if the client makes any unexpected movements.
6. Insert the speculum gently down and forward into the ear canal (approximately 0.5 in). As you insert the otoscope, be careful not to touch either side of the inner portion of the canal wall. This area is bony and covered by a thin, sensitive layer of epithelium. Any pressure will cause the client pain.
7. Move your head in close to the otoscope and position your eye to look through the lens.

General Routine Screening Versus Focused Specialty Assessment for the Ear and Hearing

Assessment of hearing is always of importance to the nurse to ensure that the client is able to hear the directions and information shared by the nurse and other health care providers. If the client does not seem to hear what is being said, the nurse can perform the whisper test, followed by the Weber and Rinne tests to differentiate between a conductive and a sensorineural hearing loss. The nurse may routinely observe the external ear in any setting, such as when inspecting the skin or when attempting to take a client's temperature with a tympanic thermometer. Unless a problem was voiced by the client, the nurse would not observe the auditory canal or middle ear with an otoscope. However, the school or home nurse may be required to use the otoscope in certain situations to observe the ear canal and middle ear if the client reports ear pain or other abnormal ear sensations.

General Routine Screening
- Inspect the auricle, tragus, and lobule.
- Palpate the auricle and mastoid process.
- Perform the whisper test.

Focused Specialty Assessment
- Inspect the external auditory canal.
- Inspect the tympanic membrane (eardrum).
- Perform the Weber test if the client reports diminished or lost hearing in one ear.
- Perform the Rinne test to differentiate between conductive and sensorineural hearing loss.
- Perform the Romberg test.

ASSESSMENT PROCEDURE	NORMAL FINDINGS	ABNORMAL FINDINGS
External Ear Structures		
INSPECTION AND PALPATION		
Inspect the auricle, tragus, and lobule. Note size, shape, and position (Fig. 17-4).	Ears are equal in size bilaterally (normally 4–10 cm). The auricle aligns with the corner of each eye and within a 10-degree angle of the vertical position. Earlobes may be free, attached, or soldered (tightly attached to adjacent skin with no apparent lobe). **CULTURAL CONSIDERATIONS** Most African Americans and Caucasians have free lobes, whereas most Asians have attached or soldered lobes, although any type is possible in all cultural groups (McDonald, 2010). 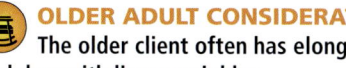 The older client often has elongated earlobes with linear wrinkles.	Ears are smaller than 4 cm or larger than 10 cm. Malaligned or low-set ears may be seen with genitourinary disorders or chromosomal defects. Microtia (see Abnormal Findings 17-1) is a congenital deformity in which the external ear and sometimes the ear canal are not fully developed. Macrotia is a congenital excessive enlargement of the external ear. Ear malformations are often related to other congenital anomalies such as face, jaw, dental, and kidney disorders (Children's National Health System, 2016).

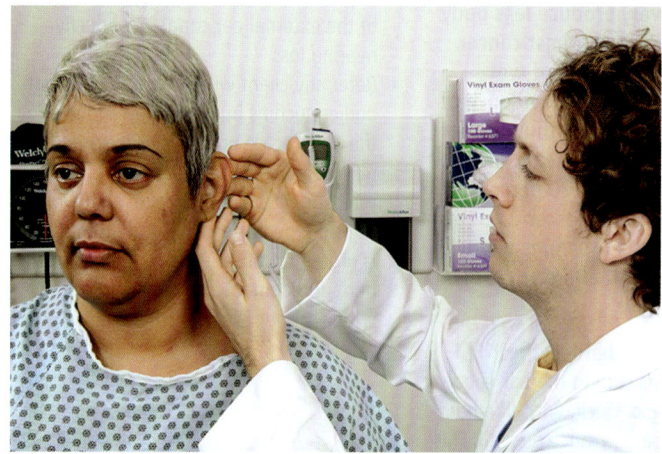

FIGURE 17-4 Inspecting the external ear.

Continued on following page

UNIT 3 Nursing Assessment of Physical Systems

ASSESSMENT PROCEDURE	NORMAL FINDINGS	ABNORMAL FINDINGS
External Ear Structures (Continued)		
Continue inspecting the auricle, tragus, and lobule. Observe for lesions, discolorations, and discharge. 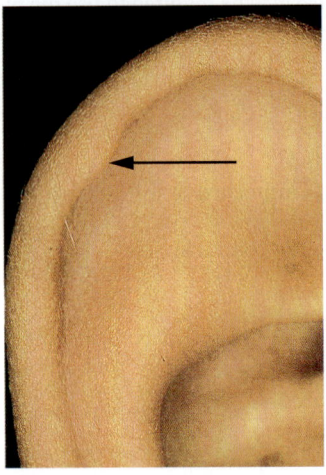 **FIGURE 17-5** Darwin's tubercle.	The skin is smooth, with no lesions, lumps, or nodules. Color is consistent with facial color. Darwin's tubercle, which is a clinically insignificant projection, may be seen on the auricle (Fig. 17-5). No discharge should be present.	Some abnormal findings suggest various disorders, including: • Enlarged preauricular and postauricular lymph nodes—infection • Tophi (nontender, hard, cream-colored nodules on the helix or antihelix, containing uric acid crystals)—gout • Blocked sebaceous glands—postauricular cysts • Ulcerated, crusted nodules that bleed—skin cancer (most often seen on the helix due to skin exposure) • Redness, swelling, scaling, or itching—otitis externa • Pale blue ear color—frostbite
Palpate the auricle and mastoid process.	Normally the auricle, tragus, and mastoid process are not tender.	A painful auricle or tragus is associated with otitis externa or a postauricular cyst. Tenderness over the mastoid process suggests mastoiditis. Tenderness behind the ear may occur with otitis media.
Internal Ear: Otoscopic Examination		
INSPECTION		
Inspect the external auditory canal. Use the otoscope (see Assessment Guide 17-1). Note any discharge along with the color and consistency of cerumen (earwax).	A small amount of odorless cerumen (earwax) is the only discharge normally present. Cerumen color may be yellow, orange, red, brown, gray, or black. Consistency may be soft, moist, dry, flaky, or even hard. 🌐 **CULTURAL CONSIDERATIONS** Earwax glands are one form of apocrine gland. Apocrine sweat glands and mammary glands are also forms of apocrine glands. Persons with lower apocrine function produce drier earwax, produce less body odor, and have lower rates of breast cancer. There seems to be an association of wet earwax and body odor, and some evidence of a relationship to breast cancer, although the relationships are not direct for breast cancer. Dry earwax occurs in about 10–20 percent of persons of western European descent, not at all in those of African descent, and is widespread in northern Asians (McDonald, 2011). **OLDER ADULT CONSIDERATIONS** In some older clients, harder, drier cerumen tends to build as cilia in the ear canal become more rigid. Coarse, thick, wire-like hair may grow at the ear canal entrance as well. This is an abnormal finding only if it impairs hearing.	Abnormal findings associated with specific disorders include: • Foul-smelling, sticky, yellow discharge—otitis externa or impacted foreign body • Bloody, purulent discharge—otitis media with ruptured tympanic membrane • Blood or watery drainage (cerebrospinal fluid)—skull trauma (refer client to physician immediately) • Impacted cerumen blocking the view of the external ear canal—conductive hearing loss • Refer any client with presence of foreign bodies such as bugs, plants, or food to the health care practitioner for prompt removal due to possible swelling and infection. If the object in the ear is a button-type battery, medical attention is urgent because leaking chemicals can burn and damage the ear canal, even within 1 hour (Cunha, 2011).

ASSESSMENT PROCEDURE	NORMAL FINDINGS	ABNORMAL FINDINGS
Observe the color and consistency of the ear canal walls and inspect the character of any nodules.	The canal walls should be pink and smooth, without nodules.	Abnormal findings in the ear canal may include: • Reddened, swollen canals—otitis externa • Exostoses (nonmalignant nodular swellings) • Polyps may block the view of the eardrum (see Abnormal Findings 17-1).
Inspect the tympanic membrane (eardrum). Note color, shape, consistency, and landmarks. 🎯 **CLINICAL TIP** The entire tympanic membrane (TM) may not be completely visible at one glance. Rotate the otoscope around to view images. The images can be "piecemealed" together to fully assess the TM. Use the largest speculum that the canal will allow. Once inserted into the ear canal, the otoscope may need to be positioned slightly anterior to see the TM.	The tympanic membrane should be pearly gray, shiny, and translucent, with no bulging or retraction. It is slightly concave, smooth, and intact. A cone-shaped reflection of the otoscope light is normally seen at 5 o'clock in the right ear and 7 o'clock in the left ear. The short process and handle of the malleus and the umbo are clearly visible (see Fig. 17-2A,B). 🪑 **OLDER ADULT CONSIDERATIONS** The older client's eardrum may appear cloudy. The landmarks may be more prominent because of atrophy of the tympanic membrane associated with the normal process of aging.	Abnormal findings in the tympanic membrane may include: • Red, bulging eardrum and distorted, diminished, or absent light reflex—acute otitis media • Yellowish, bulging membrane with bubbles behind—serous otitis media • Bluish or dark red color—blood behind the eardrum from skull trauma • White spots—scarring from infection • Perforations—trauma from infection • Prominent landmarks—eardrum retraction from negative ear pressure resulting from an obstructed eustachian tube • Obscured or absent landmarks—eardrum thickening from chronic otitis media (see Abnormal Findings 17-2).
To evaluate the mobility of the tympanic membrane, perform pneumatic otoscopy with a bulb insufflator attached by using an otoscope with bulb insufflators. Observe the position of the tympanic membrane when the bulb is inflated and again when the air is released.	The healthy membrane flutters when the bulb is inflated and returns to the resting position once the air is released.	With otitis media, the membrane does not move or flutter when the bulb is inflated.
General Observation of Hearing and Equilibrium Tests			
Box 17-2 describes hearing loss and testing.	🌎 **CULTURAL CONSIDERATIONS** Race and ethnicity have been found to be associated with hearing thresholds wherein blacks had the best hearing followed by Hispanics and whites (and darker skinned Hispanics better than lighter skinned Hispanics) even though study of skin color itself did not show significant differences (Lin et al., 2012).	More than 30% of people over age 65 have some type of hearing loss; 14% of people between 45 and 64 years of age have hearing loss. In addition, close to 8 million people between the ages of 18 and 44 have hearing loss. Adults should be screened every 10 years through age 50 and at 3-year intervals thereafter (American Speech-Language-Hearing Association [ASHA], 2015b).
Perform the whisper test (or whispered voice test) by asking the client to gently occlude the ear not being tested and rub the tragus with a finger in a circular motion. Start with testing the better hearing ear and then the poorer one. With your head 2 ft behind the client (so that the client cannot see your lips move), whisper a two-syllable word such as "popcorn" or "football." Ask the client to repeat it back to you. If the response is incorrect the first time, whisper the word one more time. Identifying three out of six whispered	Able to correctly repeat the two-syllable word as whispered.	Unable to repeat the two-syllable word after two tries indicates hearing loss and requires follow-up testing by an audiologist.

Continued on following page

ASSESSMENT PROCEDURE	NORMAL FINDINGS	ABNORMAL FINDINGS
General Observation of Hearing and Equilibrium Tests (Continued)		

words is considered passing the test. The whisper test has been studied in both pediatric and adult clients to evaluate hearing acuity and has been found to have a high sensitivity and specificity (McShefferty et al., 2013; Pirozzo et al., 2003).

Perform the Weber test if the client reports diminished or lost hearing in one ear. This test helps to evaluate the conduction of sound waves through bone to help distinguish between conductive hearing (sound waves transmitted by the external and middle ear) and sensorineural hearing (sound waves transmitted by the inner ear). Strike a tuning fork softly with the back of your hand and place it at the center of the client's head or forehead (Fig. 17-6). Centering is the important part. Ask whether the client hears the sound better in one ear or the same in both ears.

🎯 **CLINICAL TIP**
Hold the tuning fork by the handle and do not touch the tines.

Vibrations are heard equally well in both ears. No lateralization of sound to either ear.

With *conductive hearing loss,* the client reports lateralization of sound to the poor ear—that is, the client "hears" the sound in the poor ear. The good ear is distracted by background noise and conducted air, which the poor ear has trouble hearing. Thus the poor ear receives most of the sound conducted by bone vibration.

With *sensorineural hearing loss,* the client reports lateralization of sound to the good ear. This is because of limited perception of the sound due to nerve damage in the bad ear, making sound seem louder in the unaffected ear.

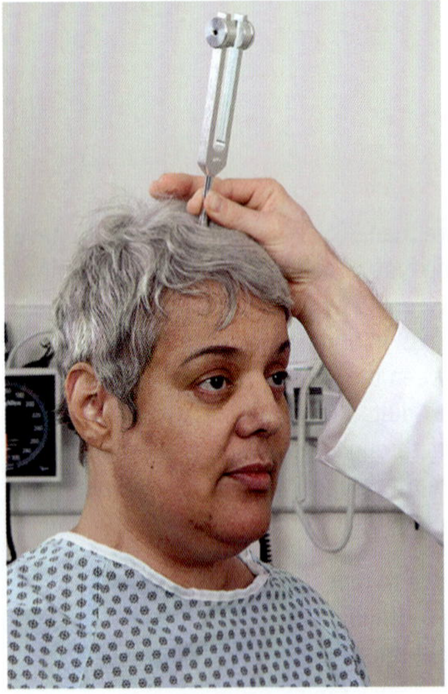

FIGURE 17-6 The Weber test assesses sound conducted via bone.

Perform the Rinne test. The Rinne test compares air and bone conduction sounds. Strike a tuning fork and place the base of the fork on the client's mastoid process (Fig. 17-7A).

Ask the client to tell you when the sound is no longer heard.

Move the prongs of the tuning fork to the front of the external auditory canal (Fig. 17-7B). Ask the client to tell you if the sound is audible after the fork is moved.

Air conduction sound is normally heard longer than bone conduction sound (AC > BC).

Although AC > BC in normal hearing, the Rinne test is used to determine the cause of the hearing loss (conduction or sensorineural) once it is determined that there is a hearing loss. If the cause is sensorineural, the finding will also be AC > BC.

With *conductive hearing loss*, bone conduction (BC) sound is heard longer than or equally as long as air conduction (AC) sound (BC ≥ AC).

ASSESSMENT PROCEDURE	NORMAL FINDINGS	ABNORMAL FINDINGS
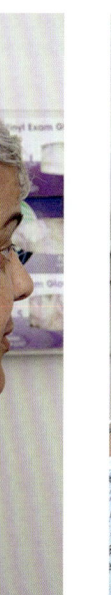 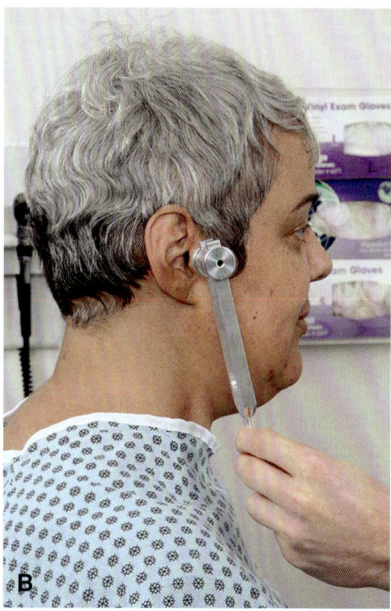 FIGURE 17-7 For the Rinne test, the tuning fork base is placed first on the mastoid process (**A**), after which the prongs are moved to the front of the external auditory canal (**B**).		Conductive hearing loss occurs when sound is not conducted through the outer ear canal to the eardrum and ossicles of the middle ear. Possible causes include fluid in middle ear, middle ear infection (otitis media), allergies (serous otitis media), eustachian tube dysfunction, perforated eardrum, benign tumors, impacted cerumen, infection in the ear canal (external otitis) or presence of a foreign body (ASHA, 2015a). If the cause is sensorineural, the finding will also be AC > BC. Sensorineural hearing loss occurs with damage to the inner ear (cochlea), or to the nerve pathways between the inner ear and brain. This is the most common type of permanent hearing loss. It decreases one's ability to hear faint sounds. Even loud speech may be muffled. Causes include ototoxic drugs, genetic hearing loss, aging, head trauma, malformation of the inner ear, and loud noise exposure (American Hearing Research Foundation, 2015).
Perform the Romberg test. This tests the client's equilibrium. Ask the client to stand with feet together, arms at sides, and eyes open, then with the eyes closed. **SAFETY TIP** *When performing this test, put your arms around the client without touching him or her to prevent falls.*	Client maintains position for 20 seconds without swaying or with minimal swaying.	Client moves feet apart to prevent falls or starts to fall from loss of balance. This may indicate a vestibular disorder.

CASE STUDY

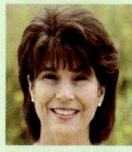

The chapter case study is now used to demonstrate the physical examination of Andrea's ears.

The client's auricle, tragus, and lobule are present and symmetric bilaterally. The auricle aligns with the lateral canthus of each eye and has a 10-degree angle of vertical position bilaterally. Earlobes are free. The skin on the ears is smooth, without lesions, lumps, or nodules; color is consistent with that of the face. Auricle, tragus, and mastoid process nontender to palpation bilaterally. Scant amount of brown cerumen lines the external auditory canals bilaterally. Bilateral canals without redness, edema, or discharge. Left tympanic membrane pearly gray, shiny, translucent, without bulging or retraction. Cone of light present at 7 o'clock. Handle of malleus and umbo visible. Right tympanic membrane red and bulging with absent light reflex. No bony landmarks visible. Whisper test: able to distinguish two-syllable words from 2 ft bilaterally. Weber test: sound lateralizes to the right ear. Rinne test: AC > BC bilaterally. Romberg test: negative.

Validating and Documenting Findings

Validate the ear assessment data that you have collected (by asking additional questions, verifying data with another health care professional, or comparing objective with subjective findings). This is necessary to verify that the data are reliable and accurate. Document the assessment data following the health care facility or agency policy.

BOX 17-2　HEARING LOSS AND TESTING

SENSORINEURAL HEARING AND HEARING LOSS

Actual hearing takes place when sound waves are channeled through the auditory canal, causing the tympanic membrane to vibrate. These vibrations are transmitted through the middle ear by the auditory ossicles to the inner ear, where they are converted into nerve impulses that travel to the brain for interpretation.

A sensorineural hearing loss results when damage is located in the inner ear. Conduction of sound waves occurs through normal pathways, but the impaired inner ear cannot make the conversion into nerve impulses. Possible causes of sensorineural hearing loss are prolonged exposure to loud noises or use of ototoxic medications.

OLDER ADULT CONSIDERATIONS
Presbycusis, a gradual sensorineural hearing loss due to degeneration of the cochlea or vestibulocochlear nerve, is common in older (over age 50) clients. The client with presbycusis has difficulty hearing consonants and whispered words; this difficulty increases over time.

CONDUCTIVE HEARING AND LOSS

Bone conduction occurs when the temporal bone vibrates with sound waves and the vibrations are picked up by the tympanic membrane and/or auditory ossicles. This type of conduction results in the perception of sound but is virtually ineffective for interpretation of sounds.

A conductive hearing loss occurs when something blocks or impairs the passage of vibrations to the inner ear. While a number of causes exist, cerumen buildup and fluid in the middle ear are the most common barriers to "vibration" transmission.

OLDER ADULT CONSIDERATIONS
Conductive hearing impairment is not uncommon in the older client due to greater incidence of cerumen buildup and/or atrophy or sclerosis of the tympanic membrane. A condition called otosclerosis often occurs with aging as the auditory ossicles develop a spongy consistency that results in conductive hearing loss.

HEARING TESTS

The tests discussed in this chapter are performed to give the examiner a basic idea of whether the client has hearing loss, what type (conduction or sensorineural) of hearing loss it might be, and whether there is a problem with equilibrium. These tests present an opportunity to educate clients about risk factors for hearing loss. These tests are not completely accurate and do not provide the examiner with an exact percentage of hearing loss. Therefore, the client should be referred to a hearing specialist for more accurate testing if a problem is suspected.

Auditory testing performed with a tuning fork is meant for screening only and should not be used for diagnostic purposes. Variations from expected findings in any tests using a tuning fork are simply an indication of the need for more elaborate testing and referral.

CASE STUDY

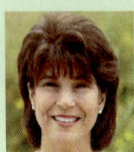

Think back to the case study. The nurse completed the following documentation of her assessment of Andrea Lopez.

Biographic Data: AL, 47-year-old, Hispanic elementary education teacher. Alert and oriented. Asks and answers questions appropriately.

Reason for Seeking Health Care: "I have an achy pressure sensation in my right ear that pulses with every beat of my heart and have had fever for 2 days."

History of Present Health Concern: Ms. Lopez reports that she developed right ear pain 2 days ago. The ear pain is described as a constant pressure sensation that varies with intensity based on last dose of ibuprofen. She reports that the pain kept her awake last evening. Has had fever of 100°F for last 2 days. Denies having been swimming. Currently rates right ear pain as 7 out of 10. Reports that ibuprofen reduces pain to 3–4 out of 10.

Personal Health History: Ms. Lopez remembers a couple of ear infections as a child but has never had an ear infection as an adult. She denies any previous treatments for ear problems. She denies ear trauma.

Family History: She denies a family history of hearing loss.

Lifestyle and Health Practices: She does not work in an area with frequent or continuous loud noises, and denies the need for hearing protection. She reports that she swims infrequently in the summer months (1–2 times per month), and denies any ear issues associated with swimming. She has never had a formal hearing evaluation and denies the use of a hearing aid. She does report the use of cotton-tipped applicators to "clean out" her ears each morning after she showers.

Physical Exam Findings: The client's auricle, tragus, and lobule are present and symmetric bilaterally. The auricle aligns with the lateral canthus of each eye and has a 10-degree angle of vertical position bilaterally. Earlobes are free. The skin on the ears is smooth, without lesions, lumps, or nodules; color is consistent with that of the face. Auricle, tragus, and mastoid process nontender to palpation bilaterally. Scant amount of brown cerumen lines the external auditory canals bilaterally. Bilateral canals without redness, edema, or discharge. Left tympanic membrane pearly gray, shiny, translucent, without bulging or retraction. Cone of light present at 7 o'clock. Handle of malleus and umbo visible. Right tympanic membrane red and bulging with absent light reflex. No bony landmarks visible. Whisper test: able to distinguish two-syllable words from 2 ft bilaterally. Weber test: sound lateralizes to the right ear. Rinne test: AC > BC bilaterally. Romberg test: negative.

ANALYSIS OF DATA: DIAGNOSTIC REASONING

After collecting subjective and objective data pertaining to the ears, identify abnormal findings and client strengths. Then cluster the data to reveal any significant patterns or abnormalities. These data will then be used to make clinical judgments (nursing diagnoses: health promotion risk, or actual) about the status of the client's ears. Following are some possible conclusions that the nurse may make after assessing a client's ears.

Selected Nursing Diagnoses

The following is a list of selected nursing diagnoses that may be identified when analyzing data from ear assessment.

Health Promotion Diagnoses

- Readiness for enhanced verbal communication related to expressed desire for hearing aid

Risk Diagnoses

- Risk for Injury related to hearing impairment
- Risk for Loneliness related to hearing loss

Actual Diagnoses

- Acute Pain related to infection of external or middle ear
- Impaired Social Interaction related to inability to interact effectively with others secondary to hearing loss
- Impaired verbal communication related to hearing loss

Selected Collaborative Problems

After grouping the data, it may become apparent that certain collaborative problems emerge. Remember that collaborative problems differ from nursing diagnoses in that nursing interventions cannot prevent them. However, these physiologic complications of medical conditions can be detected and monitored by the nurse. In addition, the nurse can use physician- and nurse-prescribed interventions to minimize the complications of these problems. The nurse may also have to refer the client in such situations for further treatment of the problem. The following is a list of collaborative problems that may be identified when assessing the ear. These problems are worded Risk for Complications (RC), followed by the problem.
- RC: Otitis media (acute, chronic, or serous)
- RC: Otitis externa
- RC: Perforated tympanic membrane

Medical Problems

If after grouping the data it becomes apparent that the client has signs and symptoms that may require medical diagnosis and treatment, referral to a primary care provider is necessary.

CASE STUDY

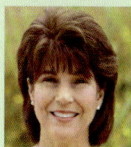

After collecting and analyzing the data for Andrea Lopez, the nurse determines that the following conclusions are appropriate:

Nursing Diagnoses
- Acute Pain r/t described pain and physical evidence of tympanic membrane inflammation
- Ineffective Health Maintenance r/t lack of knowledge about potential tympanic membrane damage from cotton-tipped applicator use in ears

Potential Collaborative Problems
- RC: Ear infection
- RC: Ruptured tympanic membrane

Refer to primary care provider to diagnose and treat her ear condition. To view an algorithm depicting the process of diagnostic reasoning for this case, go to thePoint.

Interdisciplinary Verbal Communication of Assessment Findings Using SBAR

SITUATION: AL, a 47-year-old elementary school teacher, reports "100°F fever and achy pressure sensation in right ear that pulses with each heart beat for past 2 days." Rates right ear pain as 7/10 with use of ibuprofen reducing pain to 3–4/10. Ear discomfort keeps her awake at night. Believes she may have caught something from her sick students.

BACKGROUND: Had a couple of ear infections as a child but has never as an adult. No report of other ear or hearing problems, trauma, or family history of hearing loss. No exposure to loud noises. Swims 1–2 times a month in summer without ear problems. Uses cotton-tipped applicators to "clean out" her ears daily.

ASSESSMENT: Scant amount of brown cerumen in both external auditory canals without redness, edema, or discharge. Right tympanic membrane red and bulging with absent light reflex. No bony landmarks visible. No abnormalities noted in left external auditory canal or tympanic membrane. Whisper test: able to distinguish two-syllable words from 2 ft bilaterally. Weber test: sound lateralizes to the right ear. Rinne test: AC > BC bilaterally. Romberg test: negative.

RECOMMENDATION: AL has Acute Pain related to tympanic membrane inflammation. She also has Ineffective Health Maintenance related to lack of knowledge about potential tympanic membrane damage from using cotton-tipped applicator to clean ears. Client needs to be seen by primary health care provider to diagnose and treat her ear condition (possible ear infection) and to prevent perforation of the tympanic membrane.

354 UNIT 3 Nursing Assessment of Physical Systems

ABNORMAL FINDINGS 17-1 — Abnormalities of the External Ear and Ear Canal

Many abnormalities may affect the external ear and ear canal; among them are infections and abnormal growths. Some are pictured below:

Malignant lesion.

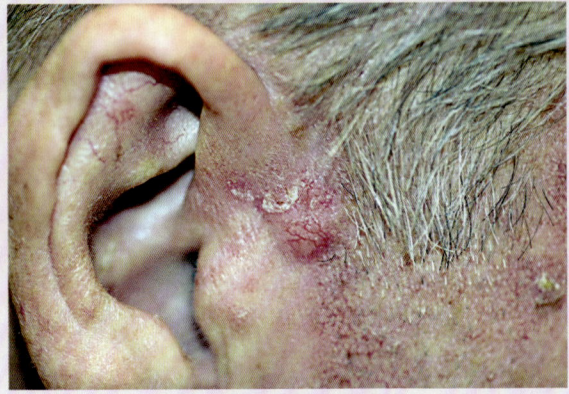

Otitis externa. (© 1992 Science Photo Library/Custom Medical Science Photography)

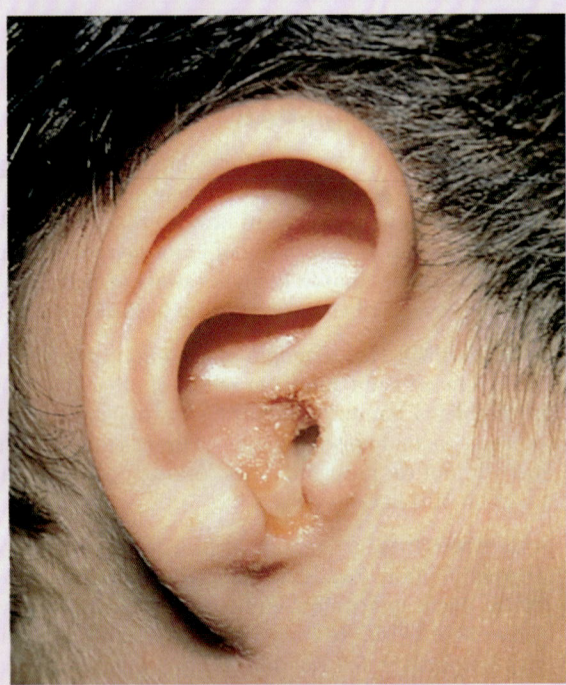

Buildup of cerumen in ear canal.

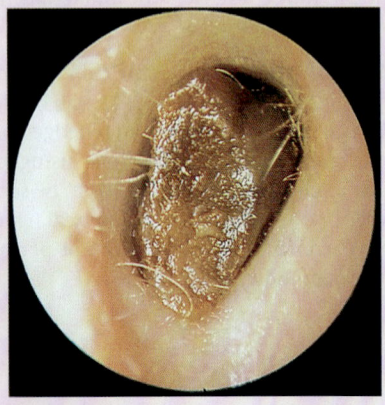

Polyp.

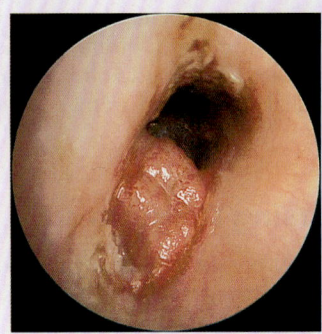

Exostosis.

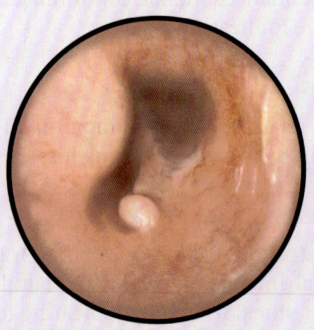

Microtia: Congenital abnormality where the external ear does not fully develop.

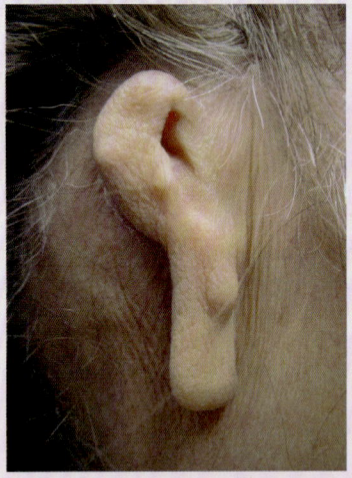

Tophi: Hard external ear nodules associated with deposits of uric acid crystals in advanced gout.

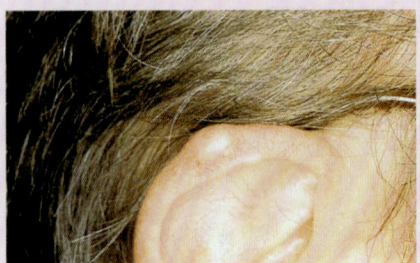

| ABNORMAL FINDINGS | 17-2 | **Abnormalities of the Tympanic Membrane** |

The thin, drum-like structure of the tympanic membrane is essential for hearing. It is also essential for promoting equilibrium and barring infection. Damage to the membrane may have grave and serious consequences.

Acute Otitis Media
Note the red, bulging membrane; decreased or absent light reflex.

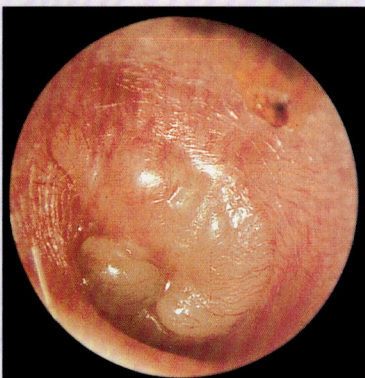

Blue/Dark Red Tympanic Membrane
Indicates blood behind eardrum due to trauma.

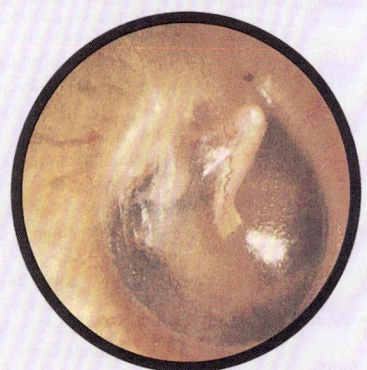

Perforated Tympanic Membrane
Perforation results from rupture caused by increased pressure, usually from untreated infection or trauma.

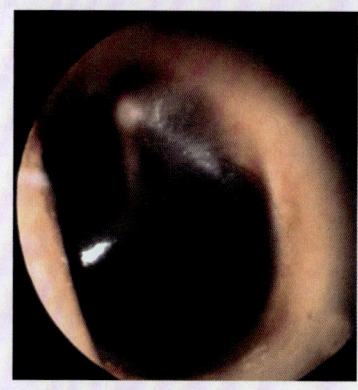

(© 1992 Science Photo Library/Custom Medical Science Photography)

Serous Otitis Media
Note the yellowish, bulging membrane with bubbles behind it.

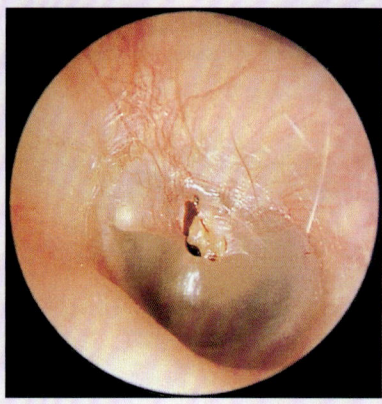

Scarred Tympanic Membrane
White spots and streaks indicate scarring from infections.

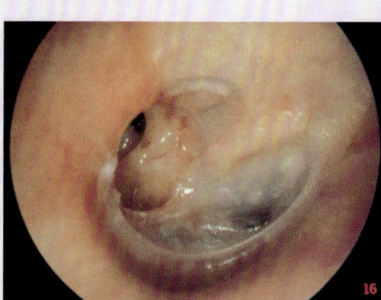

Retracted Tympanic Membrane
Prominent landmarks are caused by negative ear pressure due to obstructed eustachian tube or chronic otitis media.

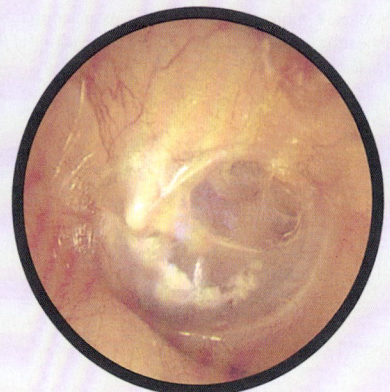

Want to know more?

A wide variety of resources to enhance your learning and understanding of this book are available on **thePoint**. Visit thePoint to access:

- NCLEX-Style Student Review Questions
- Watch and Learn Videos
- Concepts in Action Animations
- And more!

References and Selected Readings

American Academy of Otolaryngology–Head and Neck Surgery (AAO-HNS). (2012). Earwax and care. Available at http://www.entnet.org/HealthInformation/earwax.cfm

American Hearing Research Foundation. (2015). Hearing testing. Available at http://american-hearing.org/disorders/hearing-testing/

American Speech-Language-Hearing Association (ASHA). (2015a). Conductive hearing loss. Available at http://www.asha.org/public/hearing/Conductive-Hearing-Loss/

American Speech-Language-Hearing Association (ASHA). (2015b). Who should be screened for hearing loss? Available at http://www.asha.org/public/hearing/Who-Should-be-Screened/

Bereznicki, L., & Peterson, G. (2008). External ear problems. *Australian Pharmacist, 27*(10), 838–847.

Centers for Disease Control and Prevention (CDC). (2015a). Hearing loss in children. Available at http://www.cdc.gov/ncbddd/hearingloss/screening.html

Centers for Disease Control and Prevention (CDC). (2015b). "Swimmer's ear" (otitis externa). Available at http://www.cdc.gov/healthywater/swimming/rwi/illnesses/swimmers-ear.html

Children's National Health System. (2016). What is ear malformation? Available at http://childrensnational.org/choose-childrens/conditions-and-treatments/ear-nose-throat/ear-malformations

Chou, R., Dana, T., Bougatsos, C., et al. (2011). Screening for hearing loss in adults ages 50 years and older: A review of the evidence for the U.S. Preventive Services Task Force. *Annals of Internal Medicine, 154*, 347–355.

Cunha, J. (2011). Objects or insects in ear. Available at http://www.medicinenet.com/objects_or_insects_in_ear/article.htm

Healthy People 2020. (2017). Hearing and other sensory or communications disorders. Available at https://www.healthypeople.gov/2020/topics-objectives/topic/hearing-and-other-sensory-or-communication-disorders

Hearing Loss Association of American (ALAA). (2015). Hearing loss basics: Types, causes, and treatments. Available at http://www.hearingloss.org/content/types-causes-and-treatment

Holmes, S., & Padgham, N. (2011). "Ringing in the ears": Narrative review of tinnitus and its impact. *Biological Research for Nursing, 13*(1), 97–108. Available at http://www.ncbi.nlm.nih.gov/pubmed/21199815

Jensen, R., Koch, A., Homøe, P., et al. (2013).Tobacco smoke increases the risk of otitis media among Greenlandic Inuit children while exposure to organochlorines remains insignificant. Available at http://www.sciencedirect.com/science/article/pii/S0160412013000354

Lin, F., Maas, P., Chien, W., et al. (2012). Association of skin color, race/ethnicity, and hearing loss among adults in the USA. *Journal of the Association for Research in Otolaryngology, 13*(1), 109–117.

Mayo Clinic. (2013). Ear infection (middle ear): Risk factors. Available at http://www.mayoclinic.org/diseases-conditions/ear-infections/basics/risk-factors/con-20014260

Mayo Clinic. (2015a). Benign paroxysmal positional vertigo (BPPV). Available at http://www.mayoclinic.org/diseases-conditions/vertigo/basics/symptoms/con-20028216

Mayo Clinic. (2015b). Hearing loss. Available at http://www.mayoclinic.org/diseases-conditions/hearing-loss/basics/tests-diagnosis/con-20027684

Mayo Clinic. (2015c). Hearing loss: Risk factors. Available at http://www.mayoclinic.org/diseases-conditions/hearing-loss/basics/risk-factors/con-20027684

McDonald, J. (2010). Myths of human genetics. Available at http://udel.edu/~mcdonald/mythearlobe.html

McDonald, J. (2011). Earwax type. Available at http://udel.edu/~mcdonald/mythearwax.html

McShefferty, D., Whitmer, W., Swan, I., et al. (2013). The effect of experience on the sensitivity and specificity of the whispered voice test: A diagnostic accuracy study. Available at http://www.ncbi.nlm.nih.gov/pmc/articles/PMC3641455/

National Institute on Deafness and Other Communication Disorders (NIDCD). (2014a). Hearing loss and older adults. Available at http://www.nidcd.nih.gov/health/hearing/pages/older.aspx

National Institute on Deafness and Other Communication Disorders (NIDCD). (2014b). Ten ways to recognize hearing loss. Available at http://www.nidcd.nih.gov/health/hearing/pages/10ways.aspx

National Institute on Deafness and Other Communication Disorders (NIDCD). (2015). Sudden deafness. Available at http://www.nidcd.nih.gov/health/hearing/pages/sudden.aspx

Perlstein, D. (2015). Ear infections. Available at http://www.medicinenet.com/ear_infection/page3.htm

Pirozzo, S., Papinczak, T., & Glasziou, P. (2003). Whispered voice test for screening for hearing impairment in adults and children: Systematic review. *British Medical Journal, 327*(7421), 967. Available at http://www.ncbi.nlm.nih.gov/pmc/articles/PMC259166/

U.S. Preventive Services Task Force (USPSTF). (2012). Hearing loss in older adults: Screening. Available at http://www.uspreventiveservicestaskforce.org/Page/Document/UpdateSummaryFinal/hearing-loss-in-older-adults-screening

U.S. Preventive Services Task Force (USPSTF). (2015). Hearing loss in newborns: Screening. Available at http://www.uspreventiveservicestaskforce.org/BrowseRec/InactiveTopic/218

World Health Organization (WHO). (2015). Deafness and hearing loss. Available at http://www.who.int/mediacentre/factsheets/fs300/en/

18 ASSESSING MOUTH, THROAT, NOSE, AND SINUSES

Learning Objectives

1. Describe the structure and function of the mouth, throat, nose, and sinuses.
2. Discuss risk factors across cultures for oral cancer and ways to reduce one's risks.
3. Interview the client for an accurate nursing history of the mouth, throat, nose, and sinuses.
4. Use correct techniques to assess the mouth, throat, nose, and sinuses.
5. Differentiate between normal and abnormal findings of the mouth, throat, nose, and sinuses.
6. Describe cultural variations in assessment findings of the mouth, throat, nose, and sinuses.
7. Describe findings frequently seen when assessing the older client's mouth, throat, nose, and sinuses.
8. Analyze the data from the interview and physical assessment of the mouth, throat, nose, and sinuses to formulate valid nursing diagnoses, collaborative problems, and/or referrals.
9. Differentiate between general routine screening versus skills needed for focused or specialty assessment of the mouth, throat, nose, and sinuses.
10. Document and verbally report accurate assessment findings of the mouth, throat, nose, and sinuses.

CASE STUDY

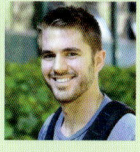

Jonathan Miller (JM), a 22-year-old college student, visits the student health service reporting severe throat pain ("like swallowing razor blades"), bad breath, neck pain and "knots" on either side of his neck, chills, fever, feeling tired all the time, and no appetite. He admitted that he had been studying "day and night" for final exams and had "only one more to go." He continued, "This is the third time I've had this problem this year. I didn't even bother coming in the first or second time. I just stayed in bed between classes and treated myself."

STRUCTURE AND FUNCTION

The mouth and throat comprise the first part of the digestive system and are responsible for receiving food (ingestion), tasting, preparing food for digestion, and aiding in speech. Cranial nerves V (trigeminal), VII (facial), IX (glossopharyngeal), and XII (hypoglossal) assist with some of these functions (the cranial nerves are discussed in Chapter 25). The nose and *paranasal sinuses* constitute the first part of the respiratory system and are responsible for receiving, filtering, warming, and moistening air to be transported to the lungs. Receptors of cranial nerve I (olfactory) are also located in the nose. These receptors are related to the sense of smell.

Mouth

The mouth—or *oral cavity*—is formed by the lips, cheeks, hard and soft palates, uvula, and the tongue and its muscles (Fig. 18-1). The mouth is the beginning of the digestive tract and serves as an airway for the respiratory tract. The upper and lower lips form the entrance to the mouth, serving as a protective gateway to the digestive and respiratory tracts. The roof of the oral cavity is formed by the anterior hard *palate* and the posterior soft palate. An extension of the soft palate is the *uvula*, which hangs in the posterior midline of the oropharynx. The cheeks form the lateral walls of the mouth, whereas the tongue and its muscles form the floor of the mouth. The *mandible* (jaw bone) provides the structural support for the floor of the mouth.

Contained within the mouth are the tongue, teeth, gums, and the openings of the salivary glands (parotid, submandibular, and sublingual). The tongue is a mass of muscle, attached to the hyoid bone and styloid process of the temporal bone. It is connected to the floor of the mouth by a fold of tissue called the frenulum. The tongue assists with moving food, swallowing, and speaking. The gums (*gingiva*) are covered by mucous membrane and normally hold 32 permanent

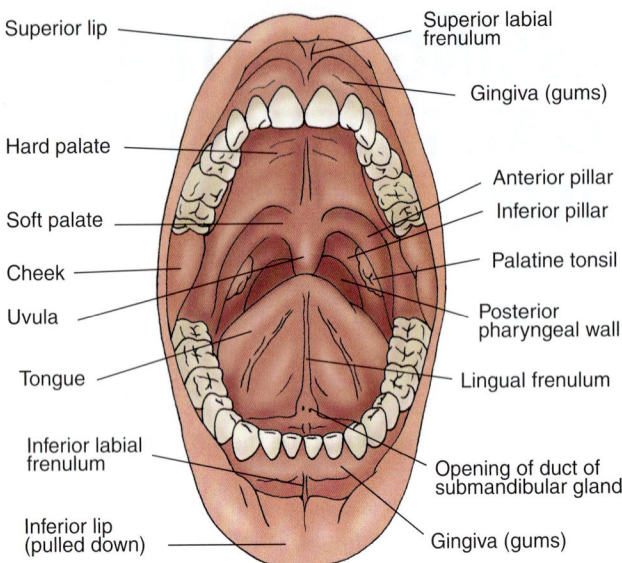

FIGURE 18-1 Structures of the mouth.

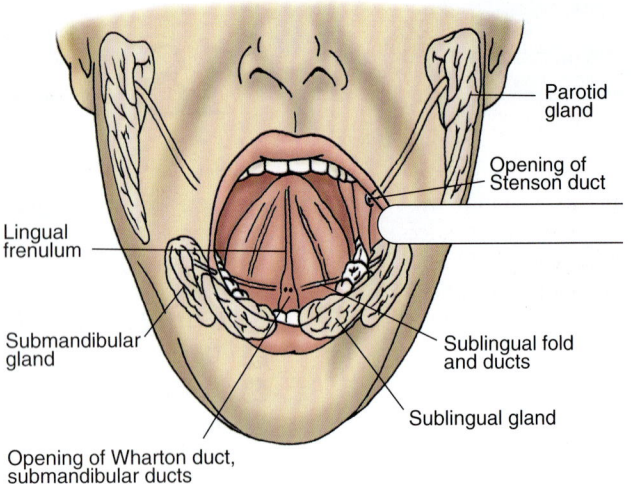

FIGURE 18-3 Salivary glands.

teeth in the adult (Fig. 18-2). The top, visible, white enameled part of each tooth is the *crown*. The portion of the tooth that is embedded in the gums is the *root*. The crown and root are connected by the region of the tooth referred to as the neck. Small bumps called papillae cover the dorsal surface of the tongue. Taste buds, scattered over the tongue's surface, carry sensory impulses to the brain. The three pairs of *salivary glands* secrete saliva (watery, serous fluid containing salts, mucus, and salivary amylase) into the mouth (Fig. 18-3). *Saliva* helps break down food and lubricates it. *Amylase* digests carbohydrates. The parotid glands, located below and in front of the ears, empty through Stensen ducts, which are located inside the cheek across from the second upper molar. The *submandibular glands*, located in the lower jaw, open under the tongue on either side of the frenulum through openings called Wharton ducts. The *sublingual glands*, located under the tongue, open through several ducts located on the floor of the mouth.

Throat

The throat (*pharynx*), located behind the mouth and nose, serves as a muscular passage for food and air. The upper part of the throat is the *nasopharynx*. Below the nasopharynx lies the *oropharynx*, and below the oropharynx lies the *laryngopharynx*. The soft palate, anterior and posterior pillars, and uvula connect behind the tongue to form arches. Masses of lymphoid tissue referred to as the *palatine tonsils* are located on both sides of the oropharynx at the end of the soft palate between the anterior and posterior pillars. The *lingual tonsils* lie at the base of the tongue. *Pharyngeal tonsils*, or adenoids, are found high in the nasopharynx. Because tonsils are masses of lymphoid tissue, they help protect against infection (Fig. 18-4).

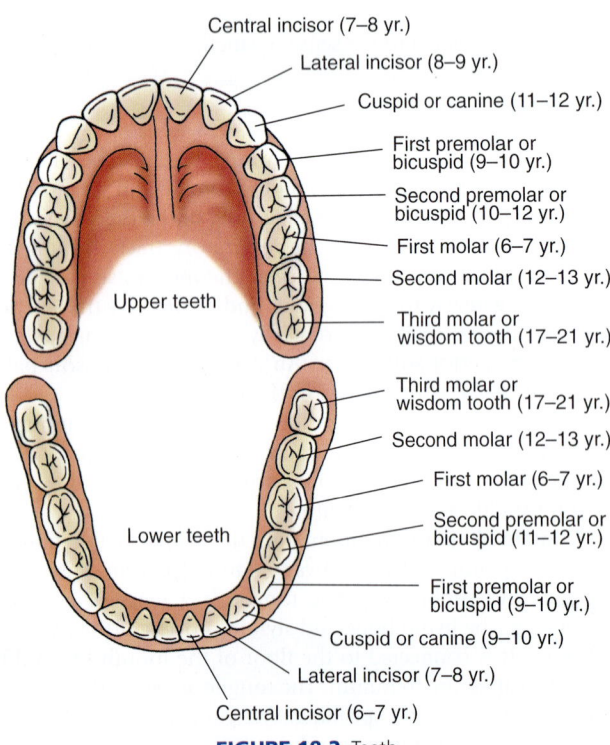

FIGURE 18-2 Teeth.

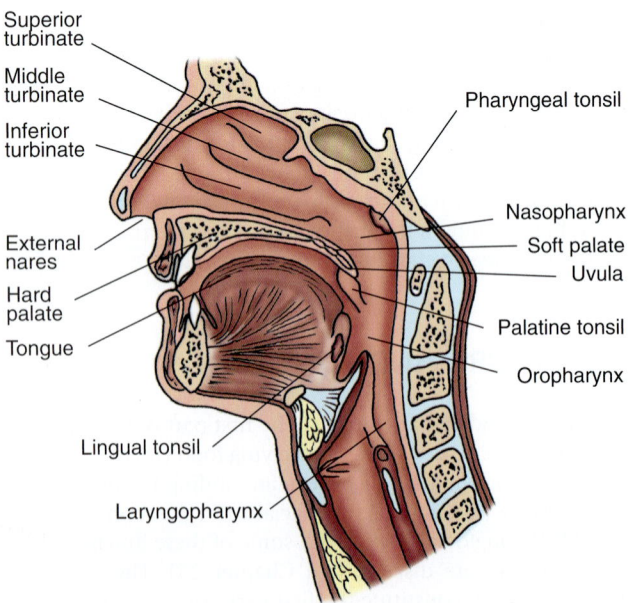

FIGURE 18-4 Nasal cavity and throat structures.

Nose

The nose consists of an external portion covered with skin and an internal nasal cavity. It is composed of bone and cartilage, and is lined with mucous membrane. The *external nose* consists of a bridge (upper portion), tip, and two oval openings called *nares*. The *nasal cavity* is located between the roof of the mouth and the cranium. It extends from the anterior nares (nostrils) to the posterior nares, which open into the nasopharynx. The nasal septum separates the cavity into two halves. The front of the nasal *septum* contains a rich supply of blood vessels and is known as Kiesselbach area. This is a common site for nasal bleeding.

The superior, middle, and inferior *turbinates* are bony lobes, sometimes called conchae, that project from the lateral walls of the nasal cavity. These three turbinates increase the surface area that is exposed to incoming air (Fig. 18-4). As the person inspires air, nasal hairs (*vibrissae*) filter large particles from the air. Ciliated mucosal cells then capture and propel debris toward the throat, where it is swallowed. The rich blood supply of the nose warms the inspired air as it is moistened by the mucous membrane. A meatus underlies each turbinate and receives drainage from the *paranasal sinuses* and the *nasolacrimal duct*. Receptors for the first cranial nerve (olfactory) are located in the upper part of the nasal cavity and septum.

Sinuses

Four pairs of *paranasal sinuses* (frontal, maxillary, ethmoidal, and sphenoidal) are located in the skull (Fig. 18-5). These air-filled cavities decrease the weight of the skull and act as resonance chambers during speech. The paranasal sinuses are also lined with ciliated mucous membrane that traps debris and propels it toward the outside. The sinuses are often a primary site of infection because they can easily become blocked. The *frontal sinuses* (above the eyes) and the *maxillary sinuses* (in the upper jaw) are accessible to examination by the nurse. The *ethmoidal* and *sphenoidal sinuses* are smaller, located deeper in the skull, and are not accessible for examination.

NURSING ASSESSMENT

Collecting Subjective Data: The Nursing Health History

Subjective data related to the mouth, throat, nose, and sinus can aid in detecting diseases and abnormalities that may affect the client's activities of daily living (ADLs). Screening for cancer of the mouth, throat, nose, and sinuses is an important area of this assessment. These cancers are highly preventable (Evidence-Based Practice 18-1). Use of tobacco and heavy alcohol consumption increases one's risk for cancer. Data collected regarding the client's risk factors may form the basis for preventive teaching.

Other problems may cause discomfort and loss of function, and can lead to serious systemic disorders. For example, malnutrition may develop in a client who cannot eat certain foods because of poorly fitting dentures, impaired dental health, or an edentulous state. A client with frequent sinus infections and headaches may have impaired concentration, which affects job or school performance.

This examination also allows the nurse to evaluate the client's health practices. For example, improper use of nasal decongestants may explain recurrent sinus congestion and infection, and improper oral hygiene practices may cause tooth decay or gum disease. The nurse should provide teaching for a client with these health practices.

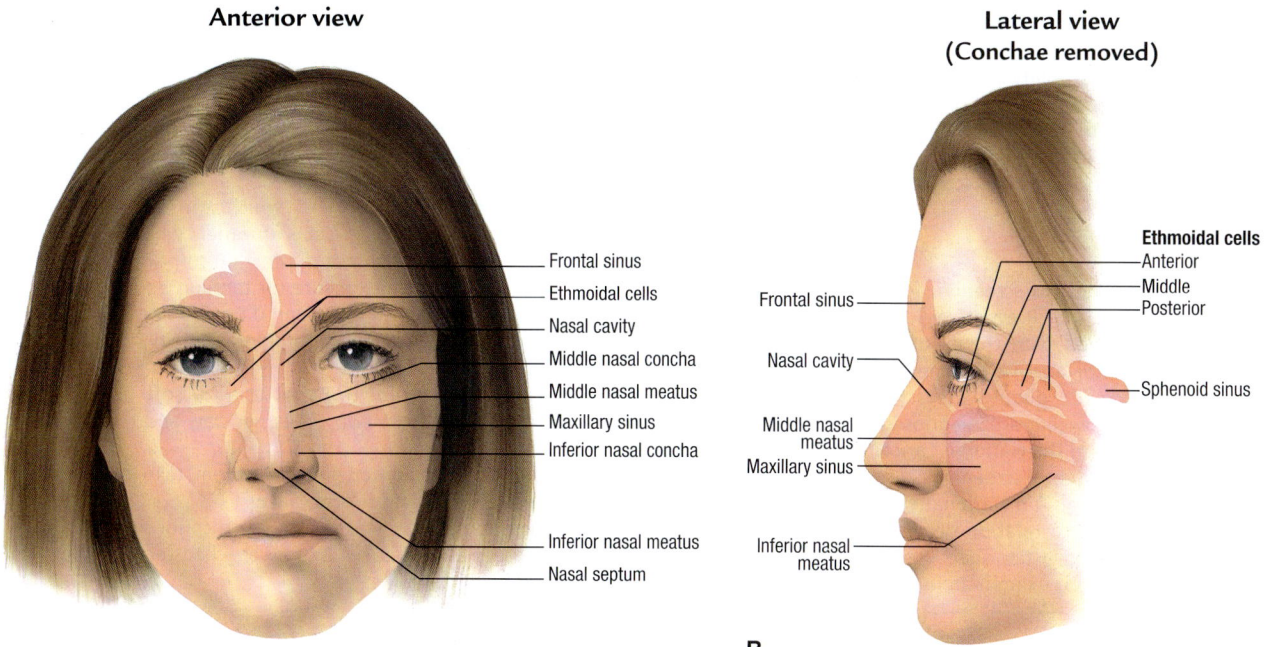

FIGURE 18-5 A. Paranasal sinuses, anterior view. **B.** Paranasal sinuses, lateral view (Asset provided by Anatomical Chart Co.).

18-1 EVIDENCE-BASED HEALTH PROMOTION AND DISEASE PREVENTION: OROPHARYNGEAL CANCER

INTRODUCTION

The fact that the oral cavity and oropharynx, along with other parts of the head and neck, contribute to the ability to chew, swallow, breathe, and talk, oropharyngeal cancer can have significant effects on well-being. American society of Clinical Oncology (ASCO, 2015) lists the following information on oropharyngeal cancer: Two of the most common types of cancer in this anatomical region are cancer of the oral cavity (mouth and tongue) and cancer of the oropharynx (the middle of the throat, from the tonsils to the tip of the larynx); more than 90% of oral and oropharyngeal cancers are squamous cell carcinoma. This year, an estimated 45,780 adults (32,670 men and 13,110 women) in the United States will be diagnosed with oral or oropharyngeal cancer and 8,650 (6,010 men and 2,640 women) will die from the diseases. Rates of oral and oropharyngeal cancer are more than twice as high in men compared with women. If diagnosed at an early stage, the 5-year survival rate is 83%. Cancer of the oral cavity ranks as the eighth most common cancer among men and is increasing, probably because of infection with the human papillomavirus (HPV).

HEALTHY PEOPLE 2020 GOAL

Healthy People 2020 (2015a) includes oral cancers within the category of oral health. Objectives are more comprehensive than simply preventing cancers.

GOAL

Prevent and control oral and craniofacial diseases, conditions, and injuries, and improve access to preventive services and dental care.

OBJECTIVES

Objectives in this topic area address a number of areas for public health improvement for adult dental health, including the need to:
- Increase awareness of the importance of oral health to overall health and well-being.
- Increase acceptance and adoption of effective preventive interventions.
- Increase accessibility and use of oral health care resources.
- Reduce disparities in access to effective preventive and dental treatment services.
- Specific to oral cancers: Increase the proportion of oral and pharyngeal cancers detected at the earliest stage by 10%.

SCREENING

The effectiveness of screening for oropharyngeal cancer is debated. The U.S. Preventive Services Task Force (USPSTF, 2015) concluded that the evidence is insufficient to recommend for or against routinely screening adults for oral cancer. However, due to the significant gains in survival when these cancers are diagnosed at an early stage, the ACS (2015a) and the National Cancer Institute (2016) recommend routine dental screenings, also including a mouth and throat screening. The National Cancer Institute (NCI, 2016) noted that the correlation between screening and mortality has not been established. Regular screening, especially at routine dental examinations, is beneficial, especially for those who are at higher risk, such as those who use tobacco, drink alcohol frequently, have had previous oral cancers, or have had heavy sun exposure. Many organizations agree with routine screening, especially in light of HPV as a cause, which makes individuals at risk somewhat hard to identify. Although dentists are often the first line of assessment, many people do not see dentists; thus, nurses can provide this assessment.

RISK ASSESSMENT

Risk factors for oropharyngeal cancer as listed by the ACS (2015b) are:
- Using tobacco products (including cigarettes, cigars, pipes, and smokeless and chewing tobacco, with pipe smoking being a significant risk factor)
- Heavy alcohol use
- Drinking alcohol and smoking together
- Being infected with a certain types of human papillomavirus (HPV)
- Being exposed to sunlight (lip cancer only)
- Being male (twice as common in men versus women)
- Age over 55
- Fair skin
- Poor oral hygiene
- Poor diet/nutrition: low in fruits and vegetables
- Chewing betel quid (betel nuts and lime wrapped in betel leaves), or chewing *gutka* (a mixture of betel quid and tobacco), both often used in South and Southeast Asia (CDC, 2016)
- Weakened immune system
- Graft-versus-host disease
- Genetic syndromes such as Fanconi anemia, dyskeratosis congenita
- Lichen planus (skin disease with an itchy rash, which can affect mouth and throat lining and is most noted in older people)
- Two controversial potential risks are use of mouthwash with high alcohol content and irritation from dentures

CLIENT EDUCATION

Teach Clients
- Avoid smoking cigarettes or using oral tobacco, or get assistance to stop if smoking or chewing currently.
- Avoid excessive alcohol use, especially if you smoke.
- Avoid chewing betel nuts.
- Avoid infection with HPV, which can be transmitted through oral sex or contact with others who are infected, or seek medical assistance if infection suspected.
- Avoid excessive sun exposure (or tanning booth exposure) to lips. Use adequate sunscreen if unable to avoid sun.
- Eat a diet rich in fruits, vegetables, vitamin A, and generally well rounded.
- Practice regular oral hygiene, using a soft tooth brush, dental floss at least two times per day, and have routine dental care.
- If you have a weakened immune system, take extra precautions to avoid risks for oral cancer.
- Avoid use of mouthwash with high alcohol content
- If wearing dentures, have them checked for good fit with no irritation to gums.

History of Present Health Concern

QUESTION	RATIONALE
Tongue and Mouth	
Do you experience tongue or mouth sores or lesions? If so, explore the symptoms using COLDSPA. **Characteristics:** Describe the size and texture of the lesions. **Onset:** When did they first occur? Do you notice these more when you are under stress or taking certain medications? Did they occur after any injury to your mouth? **Locations:** Describe exactly where these lesions are located in your mouth. **Duration:** How long have you had these lesions? Have you ever had these before and did they go away? **Severity:** Do these lesions keep you from eating, talking, or swallowing? **Palliative/relieving factors:** What aggravates these lesions or makes them go away? What over-the-counter remedies and past prescriptions have you used? **Associated Factors:** Do you have any other symptoms with these lesions such as stress, pain, bleeding? Describe.	Exploring the symptoms with COLDSPA can provide data to determine if lesions are related to medications, stress, infection, trauma, or malignancy. Lesions that last for more than 2 weeks need to be explored further and referred. Painful, recurrent ulcers in the mouth are seen with aphthous stomatitis (canker sores) and herpes simplex (cold sores). Mouth or tongue sores that do not heal; red or white patches that persist; a lump or thickening; or rough, crusty, or eroded areas are warning signs of cancer and need to be referred for further evaluation (Evidence-Based Practice 18-1).
Do you experience redness, swelling, bleeding, or pain of the gums or mouth? How long has this been happening? Do you have any toothache? Have you lost any permanent teeth?	Red, swollen gums that bleed easily occur in early gum disease (gingivitis), whereas destruction of the gums with tooth loss occurs in more advanced gum disease (periodontitis). Dental pain may occur with dental caries, abscesses, or sensitive teeth. Periodontal disease is highly correlated with cardiovascular disease. **OLDER ADULT CONSIDERATIONS** The gums recede, become ischemic, and undergo fibrotic changes as a person ages. Tooth surfaces may be worn from prolonged use. These changes make the older client more susceptible to periodontal disease and tooth loss. **CULTURAL CONSIDERATION** Periodontal disease varies in prevalence and severity by ethnic group: worldwide, blacks have a three times higher risk than whites (Marya, 2011, p. 116).
Nose and Sinuses	
Do you have pain over your sinuses (cavities around nasal passages)?	Pain, tenderness, swelling, and pressure around the eyes, cheeks, nose, or forehead are seen in acute sinusitis, which is an infection of the sinuses. In chronic sinusitis, the sinuses become inflamed and swollen, but symptoms last 12 weeks or longer even with treatment (AAAAI, 2016). See Evidence-Based Practice 18-2.
Do you experience nosebleeds? Describe the amount of bleeding you have and how often it occurs. What color is the blood?	Causes of epistaxis (nosebleeds) can be divided into local causes (e.g., trauma, mucosal irritation, septal abnormality, inflammatory diseases, tumors), systemic causes (e.g., blood dyscrasias, arteriosclerosis, hereditary hemorrhagic telangiectasia), and idiopathic causes. Local trauma is the most common cause, followed by facial trauma, foreign bodies, nasal or sinus infections, and prolonged inhalation of dry air. A large study of epistaxis found an increase in patients with allergic rhinitis, chronic sinusitis, hypertension, hematologic malignancy, coagulopathy, or hereditary hemorrhagic telangiectasia, an association with older age and colder weather (Nguyen, 2015). Refer a client who experiences frequent nosebleeds for further evaluation.

Continued on following page

History of Present Health Concern (Continued)

QUESTION	RATIONALE
Nose and Sinuses (Continued)	
Do you experience frequent clear or mucous drainage from your nose?	Thin, watery, clear nasal drainage (rhinorrhea) can indicate a chronic allergy or, in a client with a past head injury, a cerebrospinal fluid leak. Mucous drainage, especially yellow, is typical of a cold, rhinitis, or a sinus infection. The overwhelming majority of upper respiratory illnesses are viral.
Can you breathe through both of your nostrils? Do you have a stuffy nose at times during the day or night?	Inability to breathe through both nostrils may indicate sinus congestion, obstruction, or a deviated septum. Nasal congestion can interfere with daily activities or a restful sleep.
Have you experienced a change in your ability to smell or taste?	A decrease in the ability to smell may occur with lesions of the Optic nerve (I) or Facial nerve (VII), head injuries, upper respiratory tract infections, conditions affecting the nasal passages, including nasal polyps and sinusitis, and disorders associated with aging or neurologic illnesses such as Parkinson disease or Alzheimer disease. Other less common causes include cigarette smoking, radiation therapy for head and neck cancer, hormone disturbances (especially from estrogen deficiency associated with menopause), certain medications, and rarely, brain tumors (Hummel et al., 2011). Changes in perception of taste and smell also can occur from a zinc deficiency (The Taste and Smell Clinic, 2005). Olfactory dysfunction also predicts 5-year mortality in older adults, and is thus one of the strongest predictors of 5-year mortality (Pinto et al., 2014). **OLDER ADULT CONSIDERATIONS** The ability to smell and taste decreases with age. Medications can also decrease sense of smell and taste in older people. *Concept Mastery Alert* Although a decrease in the sense of both smell and taste is often seen as part of the aging process, the nurse should document any changes the client shares regarding smell and taste.
Throat	
Do you have difficulty swallowing or painful swallowing? How long have you had this?	Dysphagia (difficulty swallowing) or odynophagia (painful swallowing) may be seen with tumors of the pharynx, esophagus, or surrounding structures, narrowing of the esophagus such as in postradiation, gastroesophageal reflux disease (GERD), anxiety, poorly fitting dentures, or neuromuscular disorders. Dysphagia increases the risk for aspiration, and clients with dysphagia may require consultation with a speech therapist. Difficulty chewing, swallowing, or moving the tongue or jaws may be a late sign of oral cancer. Malocclusion may also cause difficulty chewing or swallowing.
Do you have a sore throat? How long have you had it? Describe. How long have you had it? How often do you get sore throats?	Sore throat refers to pain, itchiness, or irritation of the throat. Hoarseness may be present as well. Throat irritation and soreness are commonly seen with **viral infections** such as the flu, colds, measles, chicken pox, whooping cough, croup, or infectious mononucleosis, with bacterial infections such as streptococcus, and are often present with HIV. Additional causes include: • Allergies to pollens, molds, cat and dog dander, house dust • Irritation due to dry heat, chronic stuffy nose, pollutants, and voice straining • Reflux of stomach acids up into the back of the throat • Tumors of the throat, tongue, and larynx with pain radiating to the ear and/or difficulty swallowing • Tonsillitis A sore throat that persists without healing may signal throat cancer.
Do you experience hoarseness? For how long?	Hoarseness is associated with upper respiratory infections, allergies, hypothyroidism, overuse of the voice, smoking or inhaling other irritants, and cancer of the larynx. If hoarseness lasts 2 weeks or longer, refer the client for further evaluation.

Personal Health History

QUESTION	RATIONALE
Have you ever had any oral, nasal, or sinus surgery?	Present symptoms may be related to past problems or surgery.
Do you have a history of sinus infections? Describe your symptoms. Do you use nasal sprays? What type? How much? How often?	Some clients are more susceptible to sinus infections, which tend to recur. Overuse of nasal sprays may cause nasal irritation, nosebleeds, and rebound swelling.
Have you been diagnosed with seasonal environmental allergies (e.g., hay fever), drug allergies, food allergies, or insect allergies? Describe the timing of the allergies (e.g., spring, summer) and symptoms (e.g., sinus problems, runny nose, or watery eyes).	Pollens cause seasonal rhinitis, whereas dust may cause rhinitis year round (Evidence-Based Practice 18-2).
Do you regularly use any treatments or medications for conditions that affect the mouth, nose, or throat or to control pain in the mouth, nose, throat, or sinuses (e.g., saline spray or use of over-the-counter nasal irrigations, nasal sprays, throat spray, ibuprofen)? What are the results?	It is important to know what remedies have worked for the client in the past and what has been used that does not relieve symptoms.

Family History

QUESTION	RATIONALE
Is there a history of mouth, throat, nose, or sinus cancer in your family?	There is a genetic risk factor for mouth, throat, nose, and sinus cancers (especially those with genetic syndromes Fanconi anemia or dyskeratosis congenita) (American Cancer Society [ACS], 2015b)

Lifestyle and Health Practices

QUESTION	RATIONALE
Do you smoke or use smokeless tobacco? If so, how much? Are you interested in quitting this habit?	Cigarette, pipe, or cigar smoking and use of smokeless tobacco increase a person's risk for oral cancer. Tobacco use and heavy alcohol consumption are responsible for 74% of oral cancers (O'Neill, 2015). Cancer of the cheek is linked to chewing tobacco. Smoking a pipe is a risk factor for lip cancer. Clients who want to quit using tobacco may benefit from a referral to a smoking cessation program (Evidence-Based Practice 18-1).
Do you drink alcohol? How much and how often?	Excessive use of alcohol (more than 21 standard drinks per week) increases a person's risk for oral cancer (The Oral Cancer Foundation, 2016).

Lifestyle and Health Practices

QUESTION	RATIONALE
Do you grind your teeth?	Grinding the teeth (bruxism) may be a sign of stress or of slight malocclusion. The practice may also precipitate temporomandibular joint (TMJ) problems and pain.
Describe how you care for your teeth or dentures. How often do you brush and use dental floss? When was your last dental examination?	Brushing twice a day with a soft bristle toothbrush, flossing between teeth once a day, and oral hygiene can prevent dental caries and gum disease (American Dental Association [ADA], 2013). Regular dental checkups, as recommended by dentists, and screening can help to detect the early signs of gum disease and oral cancer, which promotes early treatment.
If the client wears braces: How do you care for your braces?	It is important that clients follow their orthodontist's prescribed routine for cleaning and caring for their teeth while wearing braces to avoid staining and cavities.
Do you avoid any specific types of foods?	Clients with braces should avoid crunchy, sticky, and chewy foods when wearing braces. These foods can damage the braces and the teeth.

Continued on following page

Lifestyle and Health Practices (Continued)

QUESTION	RATIONALE
If the client wears dentures: How do your dentures fit? **OLDER ADULT CONSIDERATIONS** Older adults and some disabled clients may have difficulty caring properly for teeth or dentures because of poor vision or impaired dexterity.	Poorly fitting dentures may lead to poor eating habits, a reluctance to speak freely, and mouth sores or leukoplakia (thick white patches of cells). Leukoplakia is a precancerous condition.
Do you brush your tongue?	Cleaning the tongue is a way to prevent halitosis (bad breath) resulting from bacteria that accumulates on the posterior tongue.
How often are you in the sun? Do you use lip sunscreen products?	Exposure to the sun is the primary risk factor associated with lip cancer.
Describe your usual dietary intake for a day.	Poor nutrition increases one's risk for oral cancers (ACS, 2015b).

18-2 EVIDENCE-BASED HEALTH PROMOTION AND DISEASE PREVENTION: SINUSITIS

INTRODUCTION

The American Academy of Allergy, Asthma & Immunology (AAAAI, 2016) describes the two types of sinusitis: acute and chronic. Acute sinusitis refers to symptoms that last less than 4 weeks, often begin with a common cold, and usually go away within 10 days. Sometimes, however, a bacterial infection develops. Chronic sinusitis (or chronic rhinosinusitis) usually lasts more than 12 weeks despite medical treatment. Sinusitis may also be caused by an infection, a fungus, a deviated nasal septum, nasal polyps, or, in rare cases, an immune system deficiency. Individuals who suffer from chronic rhinitis or asthma are at greater risk for chronic sinusitis due to prolonged inflammation of the airways.

Symptoms of Sinusitis
(AAAAI, 2016; Mayo Clinic, 2013)
- Thick yellow-green nasal discharge (which may drain into throat)
- Postnasal drip, often with a bad taste
- Cough
- Toothache
- Fever (in cases of acute sinusitis)
- Nasal obstruction or congestion, causing difficulty breathing through your nose
- Pain, tenderness, and swelling around your eyes, cheeks, nose or forehead
- Frontal headache
- Reduced sense of smell and taste

Other signs and symptoms can include:
- Ear pain
- Aching in your upper jaw and teeth
- Cough, which may be worse at night
- Sore throat
- Bad breath (halitosis)
- Fatigue or irritability

Common causes of or risk factors for chronic sinusitis include:
- Nasal polyps or tumors: These tissue growths may block the nasal passages or sinuses.
- Allergic reactions: Allergic triggers include fungal infection of the sinuses.
- Deviated nasal septum: A crooked septum—the wall between the nostrils—may restrict or block sinus passages.
- Trauma to the face: A fractured or broken facial bone may cause obstruction of the sinus passages.
- Other medical conditions: The complications of cystic fibrosis, gastroesophageal reflux disease (GERD), or HIV and other immune system–related diseases may result in nasal blockage.
- Respiratory tract infections: Infections in your respiratory tract—most commonly, colds—can inflame and thicken your sinus membranes, blocking mucus drainage and creating conditions ripe for growth of bacteria. These infections can be viral, bacterial, or fungal in nature, especially dangerous for immune-compromised persons.
- Allergies such as hay fever, chronic rhinitis, or asthma: Inflammation that occurs with allergies may block sinuses.
- Immune system cells: With certain health conditions, immune cells called eosinophils can cause sinus inflammation.

HEALTHY PEOPLE 2020 GOAL

Healthy People 2020 (2015b) has a category for respiratory diseases (asthma and COPD), but does not include sinusitis.

SCREENING

There are no recommended screening guidelines for acute or chronic sinusitis (Carson-DeWitt, 2012).

RISK ASSESSMENT

(AAAAI, 2016; Mayo Clinic, 2013)
- Nasal passage abnormality, such as a deviated nasal septum or nasal polyps
- Aspirin sensitivity that causes respiratory symptoms
- Medical condition, such as cystic fibrosis or chronic obstructive pulmonary disease (COPD)
- Immune system disorder, such as HIV/AIDS or cystic fibrosis
- Hay fever or another allergic condition, including chronic rhinitis, that affects your sinuses
- Asthma—about 1 in 5 people with chronic sinusitis have asthma
- Regular exposure to pollutants such as cigarette smoke

CLIENT EDUCATION

Teach Clients
(Harvard Medical School Patient Education Center, 2016; Mayo Clinic, 2013)
- Avoid catching colds or influenza.

- Avoid allergy triggers and indoor contamination (keep windows closed and use HEPA filter in air conditioner; in car drive with external vents closed and air conditioner on; take shower or wash hair before bed; dry clothes inside whether in dryer or on line; minimize activities with heavy exposure to pollens; avoid exposure to pollutants such as tobacco smoke, polluted air, or known sources of allergens).
- Carefully manage allergies; work to keep symptoms under control.
- Drink enough fluids to stay hydrated
- Inhale steam or rinse nose with saline solution regularly (may help to avoid symptoms)
- Use good hygiene, including frequent handwashing.
- Follow recommendations for getting an influenza vaccine.
- For frequent allergies, seek advice from your health care provider about allergy testing.
- For asthma sufferers, follow asthma protocols prescribed by your health care provider.
- Use a humidifier if home is dry (but take precautions to keep it in excellent condition to avoid growth of bacteria or other organisms).

Seek medical advice for the following conditions:
- Repeated episodes of sinusitis that do not respond to treatment
- Sinusitis symptoms last more than 7 days

Seek medical care immediately for:
- Pain or swelling around eyes
- Swollen forehead
- Severe headache
- Confusion
- Double vision or other vision changes
- Stiff neck
- Shortness of breadth

CASE STUDY

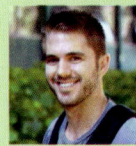

The nurse interviews Mr. Miller using specific probing questions. The client reports that he experiences severe throat pain when swallowing. He also reports bad breath, headache, neck pain, and "knots" on either side of his neck, chills, fever, no appetite, and fatigue. The nurse explores Mr. Miller's health concerns using the COLDSPA mnemonic.

Mnemonic	Question	Client Response
Character	Describe the sign or symptom (feeling, appearance, sound, smell, or taste if applicable).	"My throat feels like I am swallowing razor blades, and I have horrible smelling breath."
Onset	When did it begin?	"Last night."
Location	Where is it? Does it radiate? Does it occur anywhere else?	"My throat hurts when I swallow and my neck hurts when I turn my head. I have knots on either side of my neck."
Duration	How long does it last? Does it recur?	"The throat pain is constant. My neck only hurts when I turn my head."
Severity	How bad is it? How much does it bother you?	"I'm miserable. On a scale of 1 to 10, I would rate the throat pain at 6. When I swallow, the pain goes to 8 or 9 out of 10."
Pattern	What makes it better or worse?	"Ibuprofen helps some, but the pain never goes away completely." Upon further questioning, Jonathan reports that his throat pain decreased to 2–3 out of 10 after taking 2 ibuprofen 400 mg last night before bed.
Associated factors/How it **A**ffects the client	What other symptoms occur with it? How does it affect you?	"Headache, 101° fever, and chills. I don't have an appetite and I just want to sleep."

After exploring Jonathan's complaints of sore throat, neck pain and "knots," fever and chills, no appetite and feeling tired, the nurse continues with the health history.

He reports having had wisdom teeth removed at age 16. Denies nasal or sinus surgery. Denies any known history of sinus infections or allergies to drugs, food, environment, or insects. Denies use of nasal sprays. Reports using ibuprofen 400 mg 2 tablets every 8 hours as needed for pain. Reports two episodes of "strep throat" when in elementary school. Denies family history of mouth, throat, nose, or sinus cancer. Nutritional history reveals that he eats a lot of fast foods or whatever he can heat up out of a can. Twenty-four hour diet recall: Described a typical 24-hour diet as cereal, 1 glass of milk and 2 cups of coffee for breakfast, a medium sized hamburger, order of fries and a 16-ounce coke for lunch, and a microwaved dinner of spaghetti and meatballs with small bread. Reports drinking 2 to 6 beers on weekend nights. No known food allergies.

Denies use of smoke or smokeless tobacco or electronic cigarettes. Denies grinding teeth. Brushes teeth two times daily and sees dentist every 6 months for cleaning. Uses floss one to two times weekly. Last dental examination 3 months ago and results indicated no cavities. Uses lip sunscreen in the summer and when on annual ski vacation.

Collecting Objective Data: Physical Examination

Examination of the mouth and throat can help the nurse to detect abnormalities of the lips, gums, teeth, oral mucosa, tonsils, and uvula. This examination also allows for early detection of oral cancer. Examination of the nose and sinuses assists the nurse with detection of a deviated septum, patency of the nose and nasopharynx, and detection of sinus infection. In addition, assessment of the mouth, throat, nose, and sinuses provides the nurse with clues to the client's nutritional and respiratory status.

The mouth and nose examination can be very useful to the nurse in many situations, both in the hospital and the home. Detection of impaired oral mucous membranes or a poor dental condition may require a change in the client's diet. Additional mouth care may be needed to facilitate ingestion of food or to prevent infection of the gums (gingivitis). Detection of nasal septal deviation may help the nurse to determine which nostril to use to insert a nasogastric tube or how to suction a client. In addition, assessing for nasal obstruction may explain the reason for mouth breathing.

Assessment of the mouth, throat, nose, and sinuses usually follows the examination of the head and neck. Techniques for this examination are fairly simple to perform. However, the nurse develops proficiency in interpreting findings with continued practice.

Preparing the Client

Ask the client to assume a sitting position with the head erect. It is best if the client's head is at your eye level. Explain the specific structures you will be examining, and tell the client who wears dentures, a retainer, or rubber bands on braces that they will need to be removed for an adequate oral examination. The client wearing dentures may feel embarrassed and concerned about his or her appearance and over the possibility of breath odor on removing the dentures. A gentle, yet confident and matter-of-fact approach may help the client to feel more at ease.

Equipment

- Nonlatex gloves (wear gloves when examining any mucous membrane)
- 4 × 4-in gauze pad
- Penlight
- Short, wide-tipped speculum attached to the head of an otoscope
- Tongue depressor
- Nasal speculum

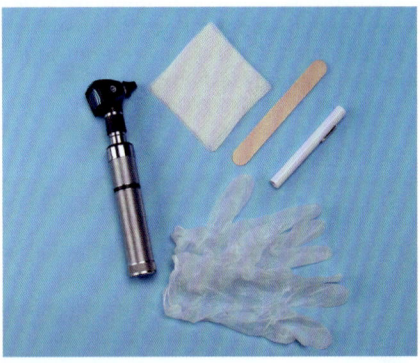

Physical Assessment

When preparing to examine the nose and mouth:
- Be able to identify and understand the relationship among the structures of the mouth and throat, nose, and sinuses.
- Know age-related changes of the oral cavity and nasal and sinus structures.
- Be aware of ethnocultural phenomena related to oral and nasal health.
- Refine examination techniques.

General Routine Screening or Focused Specialty Assessment for the Mouth, Nose, Throat, and Sinuses

The extent to which nurses perform an assessment of the mouth, nose, throat, and sinuses varies with the setting specialty area, and the situation in which they are practicing. The nurse would routinely be able to note any abnormality of the external mouth, nose, throat, and sinuses when interacting with the client on a daily basis. For instance the nurse may notice the client has an oral or tongue lesion or rhinorrhea (runny nose). While talking with the client, the nurse may notice the client has poor oral hygiene and missing teeth. This would require a more in-depth assessment of the mouth and throat. If the client voices concern about a sore throat, the nurse would inspect the internal mouth and throat. Further examination of the nose and sinuses may be needed if drainage is noted in the throat. If the nurse is providing mouth care, it is an opportunity to assess some of the client's internal mouth structures. When feeding clients, it is important to assess their swallowing abilities. When inserting a nasogastric tube, the nurse needs to assess for any nasal obstructions in addition to other assessments before inserting the tube. Inspection of the sinuses may be useful in a home or school setting when a client voices nasal stuffiness and a headache.

General Routine Screening
- Inspect the lips
- Note odor from the mouth
- Inspect the teeth, gums, and tongue, and buccal mucosa
- Inspect the external nose
- Check patency of air flow through the nostrils
- Inspect the throat

Focused Specialty Assessment
- Palpate the buccal mucosa and tongue
- Assess the ventral surface and sides of the tongue.
- Inspect for Wharton ducts and Stensen ducts
- Check the strength of the tongue.
- Check the anterior tongue's ability to taste.
- Inspect the hard (anterior) and soft (posterior) palates and uvula.
- Assess the uvula, tonsils, and posterior pharyngeal wall.
- Inspect the internal nose with an otoscope and nasal speculum
- Palpate, percuss, and transilluminate the sinuses.

ASSESSMENT PROCEDURE	NORMAL FINDINGS	ABNORMAL FINDINGS

Mouth

INSPECTION AND PALPATION

Inspect the lips. Observe lip consistency and color.	Lips are smooth and moist without lesions or swelling. 🌐 **CULTURAL CONSIDERATIONS** Pink lips are normal in light-skinned clients, as are bluish or freckled lips in some dark-skinned clients, especially those of Mediterranean descent.	Pallor around the lips (circumoral pallor) is seen in anemia and shock. Bluish (cyanotic) lips may result from cold or hypoxia. Reddish lips are seen in clients with ketoacidosis, carbon monoxide poisoning, and chronic obstructive pulmonary disease (COPD) with polycythemia. Swelling of the lips (edema) is common in local or systemic allergic or anaphylactic reactions. Additional abnormal findings are pictured in Abnormal Findings 18-1.
Inspect the teeth and gums. Ask the client to open the mouth (Fig. 18-6). Note the number of teeth, color, and condition. Note any repairs such as crowns and any cosmetics such as veneers. Ask the client to bite down as though chewing on something and note the alignment of the lower and upper jaws.	Thirty-two pearly whitish teeth with smooth surfaces and edges. Upper molars should rest directly on the lower molars and the front upper incisors should slightly override the lower incisors. Some clients normally have only 28 teeth if the four wisdom teeth do not erupt. No decayed areas; no missing teeth. Client may have appliances on the teeth (e.g., braces). Client may have evidence of repair work done on teeth (e.g., fillings, crowns, or cosmetics such as veneers). Jaws are aligned with no deviation seen with biting down.	Clients who smoke, drink large quantities of coffee or tea, or have an excessive intake of fluoride may have yellow or brownish teeth. Tooth decay (caries) may appear as brown dots or cover more extensive areas of chewing surfaces. Missing teeth can affect chewing as well as self-image. A chalky white area in the tooth surface is a cavity that will turn darker with time. Malocclusion of teeth is seen when upper or lower incisors protrude. Poor occlusion of teeth can affect chewing, wearing down of teeth, speech, and self-image. Brown or yellow stains or white spots on teeth may result from antibiotic therapy or tooth trauma.
Put on gloves and retract the client's lips (Fig. 18-7) and cheeks to check gums for color and consistency.	Color and consistency of tissues along cheeks and gums are even. **OLDER ADULT CONSIDERATIONS** In older clients, the teeth may appear longer because of age-related gingival recession, which is common. 🌐 **CULTURAL CONSIDERATIONS** A number of tooth variations occur, especially in Asian, Pacific Islanders, and Native Americans, including talon cusps on incisors and circular cusps on molars (Nimala et al., 2011).	Receding gums.

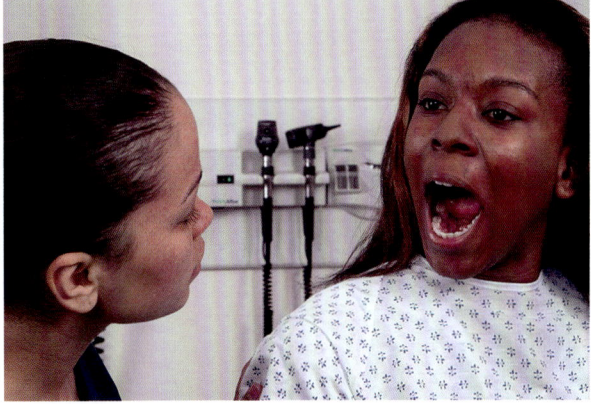

FIGURE 18-6 Inspecting the general condition of the teeth.

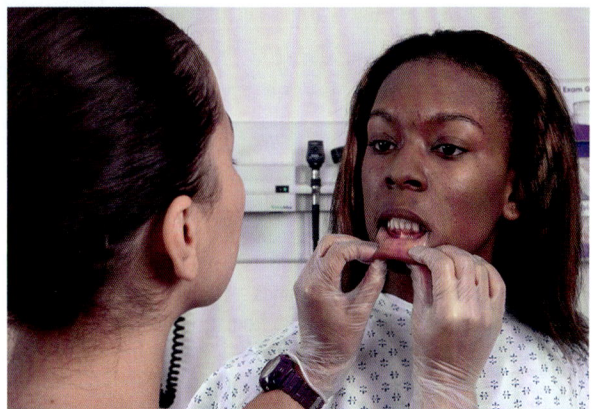

FIGURE 18-7 Lower gingiva (gums).

Continued on following page

ASSESSMENT PROCEDURE	NORMAL FINDINGS	ABNORMAL FINDINGS
Mouth (Continued)		
	Gums are pink, moist, and firm with tight margins to the tooth. No lesions or masses.	Red, swollen gums that bleed easily are seen in gingivitis, scurvy (vitamin C deficiency), and leukemia. Receding red gums with loss of teeth are seen in periodontitis. Enlarged reddened gums (hyperplasia) that may cover some of the normally exposed teeth may be seen in pregnancy, puberty, leukemia, and with use of some medications, such as phenytoin. A bluish-black or grey-white line along the gum line is seen in lead poisoning (Khalil, 2009). There is a significant link between periodontal disease and cardiovascular disease (Dhadse et al., 2010).
Inspect the buccal mucosa. Use a penlight and tongue depressor to retract the lips and cheeks to check color and consistency (Fig. 18-8).	**CULTURAL CONSIDERATIONS** The buccal mucosa should appear pink in light-skinned clients; tissue pigmentation typically increases in dark-skinned clients, which may include freckling or dark pigmentation on ventral surface of tongue and floor of mouth; hard and soft palate may also be darkly pigmented. In all clients, tissue is smooth and moist without lesions. **OLDER ADULT CONSIDERATIONS** Oral mucosa is often drier and more fragile in the older client because the epithelial lining of the salivary glands degenerates.	Leukoplakia (chalky white raised patches) may be seen in chronic irritation, heavy smoking, and alcohol use. These are precancerous lesions and should be referred to the client's primary health care provider for further assessment. Whitish, curd-like patches that scrape off over reddened mucosa and bleed easily indicate "thrush" (*Candida albicans*) infection. Koplik spots (tiny whitish spots that lie over reddened mucosa) are an early sign of the measles. Canker sores may be seen. Brown patches inside the cheeks of clients with Addison disease (chronic adrenocortical insufficiency). See Abnormal Findings 18-1.

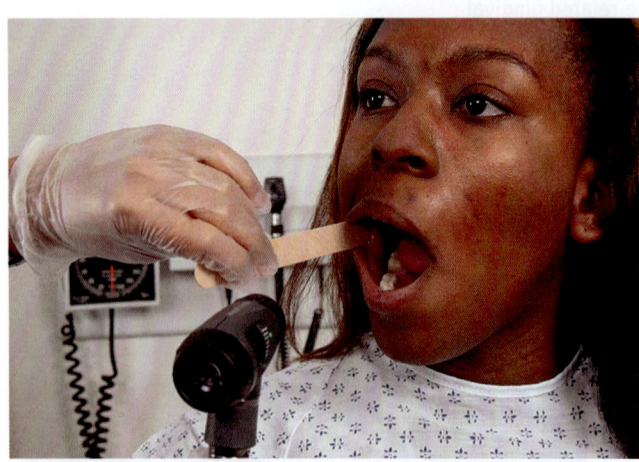

FIGURE 18-8 Inspecting the buccal mucosa.

Inspect Stensen ducts (parotid ducts), openings of the parotid salivary glands—located on the buccal mucosa across from the second upper molar.	Stensen ducts are visible with flow of saliva. No redness, swelling, pain, or moistness in area. Fordyce spots or granules, yellowish-whitish raised spots, are normal ectopic sebaceous glands.	Reddened opening of Stensen ducts is seen with mumps.

18 Assessing Mouth, Throat, Nose, and Sinuses   369

ASSESSMENT PROCEDURE	NORMAL FINDINGS	ABNORMAL FINDINGS

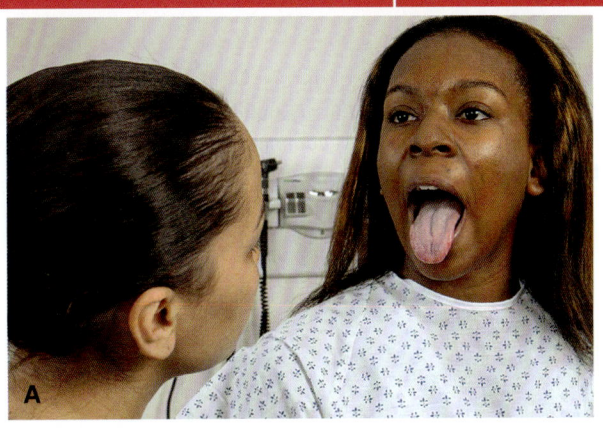 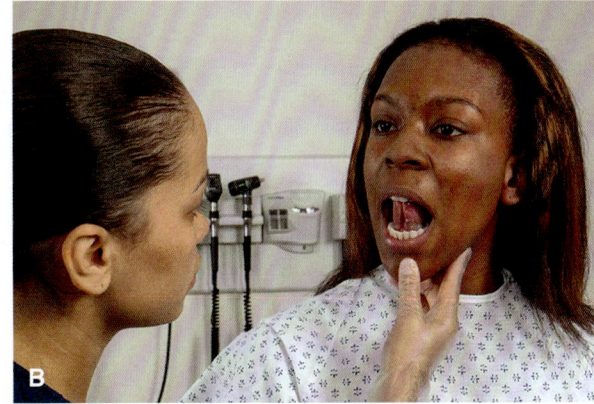

FIGURE 18-9 Inspecting the tongue. **A.** Inspecting the ventral surface of the tongue. **B.** Inspecting the dorsal surface of the tongue.

Inspect and palpate the tongue.
Ask client to stick out the tongue (Fig. 18-9A). Inspect for color, moisture, size, and texture. Observe for fasciculations (fine tremors), and check for midline protrusion.

Palpate any lesions present for induration (hardness).

Tongue should be pink, moist, a moderate size with papillae (little protuberances) present. A common variation is a fissured, topographic-map–like tongue, which is not unusual in older clients (Fig. 18-10).

No lesions are present.

Abnormalities include:

Dry; nodules, ulcers present; papillae or fissures absent; asymmetrical. Deep longitudinal fissures are seen in dehydration; *black hairy tongue* seen with conditions causing hyposalivation, heavy smoking, alcohol intake, use of antibiotics that inhibit normal bacteria leading to fungus, use of mouthwashes; also seen with bismuth intake (Pepto-Bismol) (Black hairy tongue, 2014); smooth, red, shiny tongue seen in niacin or vitamin B_{12} deficiency (see Abnormal Findings 18-1).

Raised whitish feathery areas on sides of tongue that cannot be scraped off suggest hairy leukoplakias seen in HIV infection and AIDS.

A smooth, reddish, shiny tongue without papillae is indicative of niacin or vitamin B12 deficiencies, certain anemias, and antineoplastic therapy (Stanford Medicine, 2015; Abnormal Findings 18-1). An enlarged tongue suggests hypothyroidism, acromegaly, or Down syndrome, and angioneurotic edema of anaphylaxis. A very small tongue suggests malnutrition. An atrophied tongue or fasciculations point to cranial nerve (hypoglossal, CN 12) damage.

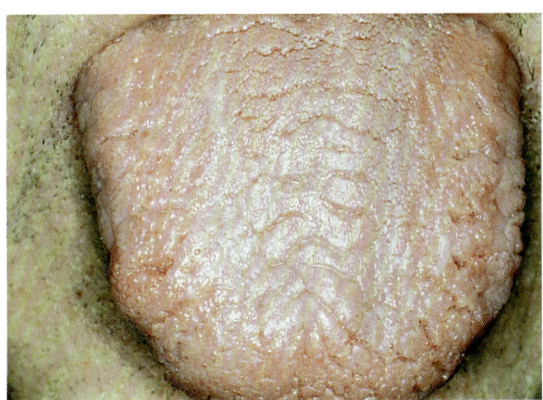

FIGURE 18-10 Fissured tongue (courtesy of Dr. Michael Bennett).

🎯 **CLINICAL TIP**
Smokers may also have a yellow-brown coating on the tongue, which is not leukoplakia.

Assess the ventral surface of the tongue. Ask the client to touch the tongue to the roof of mouth, and use a penlight to inspect the ventral surface of the tongue, frenulum, and area under the tongue (Fig. 18-9B).

The tongue's ventral surface is smooth, shiny, pink, or slightly pale, with visible veins and no lesions.

Leukoplakia, persistent lesions, ulcers, or nodules may indicate cancer and should be referred. Induration increases the likelihood of cancer.

Continued on following page

ASSESSMENT PROCEDURE	NORMAL FINDINGS	ABNORMAL FINDINGS

Mouth (Continued)

Palpate the area (Fig. 18-11) if you see lesions, if the client is over age 50, or if the client uses tobacco or alcohol. Note any induration. Check also for a short frenulum that limits tongue motion (the origin of "tongue-tied").	**OLDER ADULT CONSIDERATIONS** The older client may have varicose veins on the ventral surface of the tongue (Fig. 18-12).	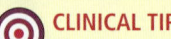 **CLINICAL TIP** The area underneath the tongue is the most common site of oral cancer.

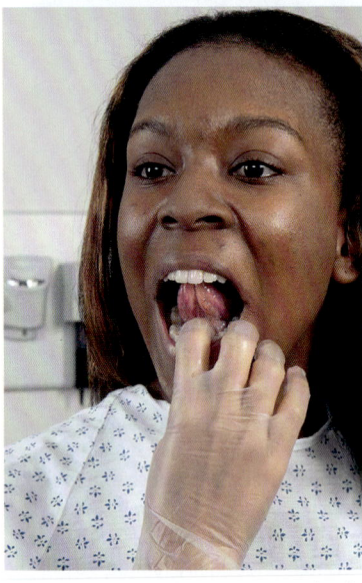

FIGURE 18-11 Palpating area under the tongue.

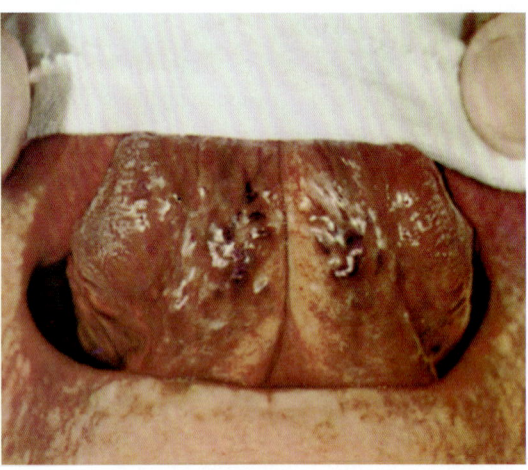

FIGURE 18-12 Varicose veins on ventral surface of the tongue.

Inspect for Wharton ducts—openings from the submandibular salivary glands—located on either side of the frenulum on the floor of the mouth. **Observe the sides of the tongue.** Use a square gauze pad to hold the client's tongue to each side (Fig. 18-13). Palpate any lesions, ulcers, or nodules for induration.	The frenulum is midline; Wharton ducts are visible, with salivary flow or moistness in the area. The client has no swelling, redness, or pain. No lesions, ulcers, or nodules are apparent.	Abnormal findings include lesions, ulcers, nodules, or hypertrophied duct openings on either side of frenulum. Canker sores may be seen on the sides of the tongue in clients receiving certain kinds of chemotherapy. Leukoplakia, persistent lesions, ulcers, or nodules may indicate cancer and should be further evaluated medically. Induration increases the likelihood of cancer (Abnormal Findings 18-1). **CLINICAL TIP** The side of the tongue is the most common site of tongue cancer.

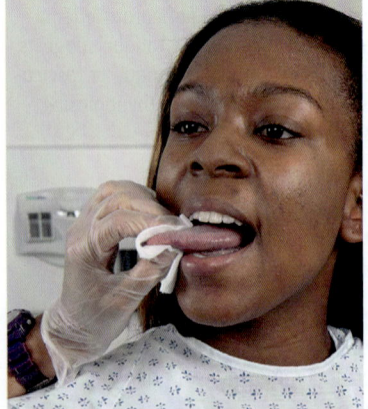

FIGURE 18-13 Inspecting the side of the tongue.

ASSESSMENT PROCEDURE	NORMAL FINDINGS	ABNORMAL FINDINGS
Check the strength of the tongue. Place your fingers on the external surface of the client's cheek. Ask the client to press the tongue's tip against the inside of the cheek to resist pressure from your fingers. Repeat on the opposite cheek.	The tongue offers strong resistance.	Decreased tongue strength may occur with a defect of the twelfth cranial nerve—hypoglossal—or with a shortened frenulum that limits motion.
Check the anterior tongue's ability to taste. Place drops of sugar and salty water on the tip and sides of tongue with a tongue depressor.	The client can distinguish between sweet and salty.	Loss of taste discrimination occurs with trauma, viral infections, sinusitis and polyposis, increasing age, neurologic illnesses such as Parkinson's or Alzheimer's; and zinc deficiency, or use of certain medication that affect smell threshold (Hummel et al., 2011).
Inspect the hard (anterior) and soft (posterior) palates and uvula. Ask the client to open the mouth wide while you use a penlight to look at the roof. Observe color and integrity.	The hard palate is pale or whitish with firm, transverse rugae (wrinkle-like folds). **CULTURAL CONSIDERATION** A bony protuberance in the midline of the hard palate, called a torus palatinus, is a normal variation. Tori, both palatinus and mandibular (also normal variation), tend to occur more in Native Americans, Eskimos, and women; in some countries, they are more prevalent in Caucasians than in Blacks (Fig. 18-14) (Smitha & Smitha, 2014). Palatine tissues are intact; the soft palate should be pinkish, movable, spongy, and smooth.	A candidal infection may appear as thick white plaques on the hard palate. Deep purple, raised, or flat lesions may indicate a Kaposi sarcoma (seen in clients with AIDS; Abnormal Findings 18-1). A yellow tint to the hard palate may indicate jaundice because bilirubin adheres to elastic tissue (collagen). An opening in the hard palate is known as a cleft palate.

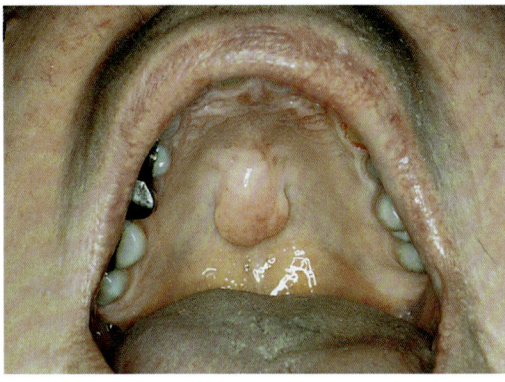

FIGURE 18-14 Torus palatinus (courtesy of Dr. Michael Bennett).

Note odor. While the mouth is wide open, note any unusual or foul odor.	No unusual or foul odor is noted.	Fruity or acetone breath is associated with diabetic ketoacidosis. An ammonia odor is often associated with kidney disease. Foul odors may indicate an oral or respiratory infection, or tooth decay. Alcohol or tobacco use may be identified by breath odor. Fecal breath odor occurs in bowel obstruction; sulfur odor (fetor hepaticus) occurs in end-stage liver disease.
Assess the uvula. Apply a tongue depressor to the tongue (halfway between the tip and back of the tongue) and shine a penlight into the client's wide-open mouth	The uvula is a fleshy, solid structure that hangs freely in the midline. No redness of or exudate from uvula or soft palate. Midline elevation of uvula and symmetric elevation of the soft palate.	Asymmetric movement or loss of movement may occur after a cerebrovascular accident (stroke). Palate fails to rise and uvula deviates to normal side with cranial nerve X (vagus) paralysis.

Continued on following page

ASSESSMENT PROCEDURE	NORMAL FINDINGS	ABNORMAL FINDINGS

Mouth (Continued)

(Fig. 18-15). Note the characteristics and positioning of the uvula. Ask the client to say "aaah" and watch for the uvula and soft palate to move.

CLINICAL TIP
Depress the tongue slightly off center to avoid eliciting the gag response.

CULTURAL CONSIDERATIONS
Native Americans and Asians may have a split (or bifid) uvula (Fig. 18-16) (Leung et al., 2014).

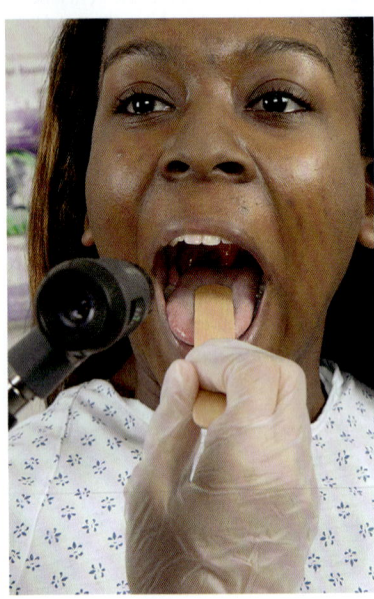

FIGURE 18-15 Inspecting the uvula.

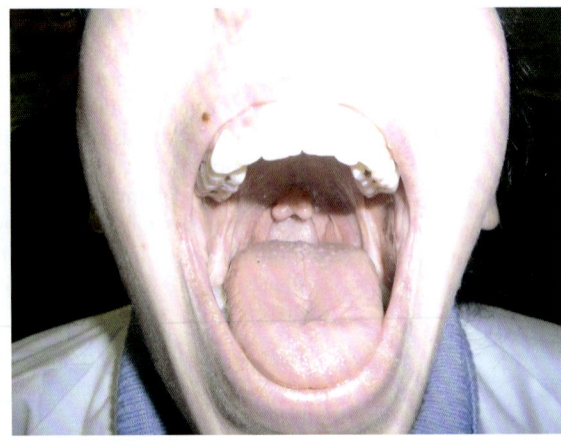

FIGURE 18-16 Bifid uvula (Courtesy of Paul S. Matz, MD).

Inspect the tonsils. Using the tongue depressor to keep the mouth open wide, inspect the tonsils for color, size, and presence of exudate or lesions. Grade the tonsils.

Tonsils may be present or absent. They are normally pink and symmetric and may be enlarged to 1+ in healthy clients (Fig. 18-17). No exudate, swelling, or lesions should be present.

Tonsils are red, enlarged (to 2+, 3+, or 4+), and covered with exudate in tonsillitis. They also may be indurated with patches of white or yellow exudate (Abnormal Findings 18-1).

Grading of tonsils in tonsillitis is depicted in Abnormal Findings 18-2.

Inspect the posterior pharyngeal wall. Keeping the tongue depressor in place, shine the penlight on the back of the throat. Observe the color of the throat, and note any exudate or lesions. Before inspecting the nose, discard gloves and perform hand hygiene.

Throat is normally pink, without exudate or lesions (Fig. 18-17).

A bright red throat with white or yellow exudate indicates pharyngitis. Yellowish mucus on throat may be seen, with postnasal sinus drainage (Abnormal Findings 18-1).

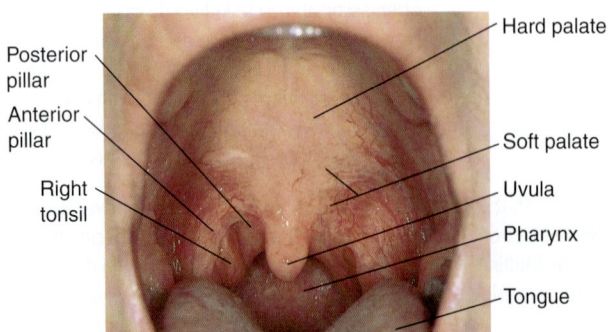

FIGURE 18-17 The normal tonsils and pharynx. (From Bickley, LS and Szilagyi, P. Bates' Guide to Physical Examination and History Taking, 8th Ed. Philadelphia: Lippincott Williams & Wilkins, 2003.)

ASSESSMENT PROCEDURE	NORMAL FINDINGS	ABNORMAL FINDINGS
Nose		
INSPECTION AND PALPATION		
Inspect and palpate the external nose. Note nasal color, shape, consistency, and tenderness.	Color is the same as the rest of the face; the nasal structure is smooth and symmetric; the client reports no tenderness.	Nasal tenderness on palpation accompanies a local infection.
Check patency of air flow through the nostrils by occluding one nostril at a time and asking client to sniff or exhale.	Client is able to sniff through each nostril while other is occluded.	Client cannot sniff through a nostril that is not occluded, nor can he or she sniff or blow air through the nostrils. This may be a sign of swelling, rhinitis, or a foreign object obstructing the nostrils. A line across the tip of the nose just above the fleshy tip is common in clients with chronic allergies.
Inspect the internal nose. To inspect the internal nose, use an otoscope with a short wide-tip attachment or you can also use a nasal speculum and penlight (Fig. 18-18). Use your nondominant hand to stabilize and gently tilt the client's head back. Insert the short wide tip of the otoscope into the client's nostril without touching the sensitive nasal septum (Fig. 18-18). Slowly direct the otoscope back and up to view the nasal mucosa, nasal septum, the inferior and middle turbinates, and the nasal passage (the narrow space between the septum and the turbinates). ⦿ **CLINICAL TIP** Position the otoscope's handle to the side to improve your view of the structures. If an otoscope is unavailable, use a penlight and hold the tip of the nose slightly up. A nasal speculum with a penlight also facilitates good visualization.	The nasal mucosa is dark pink, moist, and free of exudate. The nasal septum is intact and free of ulcers or perforations. Turbinates are dark pink (redder than oral mucosa), moist, and free of lesions. The superior turbinate will not be visible from this point of view (Fig. 18-19). A deviated septum may appear to be an overgrowth of tissue (Fig. 18-20). This is a normal finding as long as breathing is not obstructed.	Nasal mucosa is swollen and pale pink or bluish gray in clients with allergies. Nasal mucosa is red and swollen with upper respiratory infection. Exudate is common with infection and may range from large amounts of watery discharge to thick yellow-green, purulent discharge. Purulent nasal discharge is seen with acute bacterial rhinosinusitis. Bleeding (epistaxis) or crusting may be noted on the lower anterior part of the nasal septum with local irritation. Ulcers of the nasal mucosa or a perforated septum may be seen with use of cocaine, trauma, chronic infection, or chronic nose picking. Small, pale, round, firm overgrowths or masses on mucosa (polyps) are seen in clients with chronic allergies (Abnormal Findings 18-3).

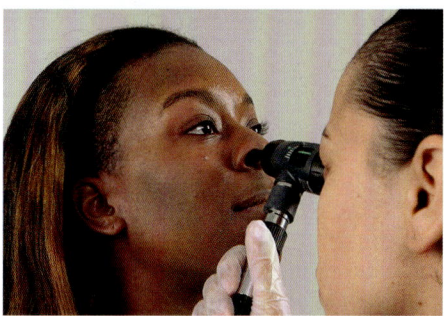

FIGURE 18-18 Inspecting the internal nose using an otoscope and wide-tipped attachment.

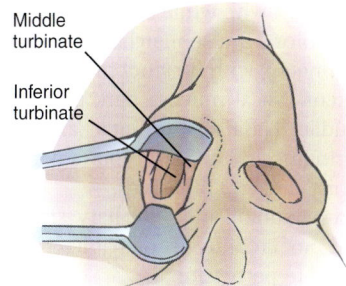

FIGURE 18-19 Normal internal nose.

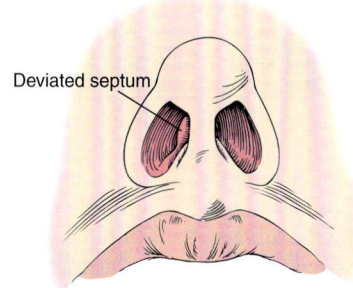

FIGURE 18-20 Deviated septum.

Continued on following page

ASSESSMENT PROCEDURE	NORMAL FINDINGS	ABNORMAL FINDINGS
Sinuses		
PALPATION		
Palpate the sinuses. When an infection is suspected, the nurse can examine the sinuses through palpation, percussion. Palpate the frontal sinuses by using your thumbs to press up on the brow on each side of nose (Fig. 18-21). Palpate the maxillary sinuses by pressing with thumbs up on the maxillary sinuses (Fig. 18-22).	Frontal and maxillary sinuses are nontender to palpation, and no crepitus is evident.	Frontal or maxillary sinuses are tender to palpation in clients with allergies or acute bacterial rhinosinusitis. If the client has a large amount of exudate, you may feel crepitus upon palpation over the maxillary sinuses. This may also be present with a viral upper respiratory infection (URI).

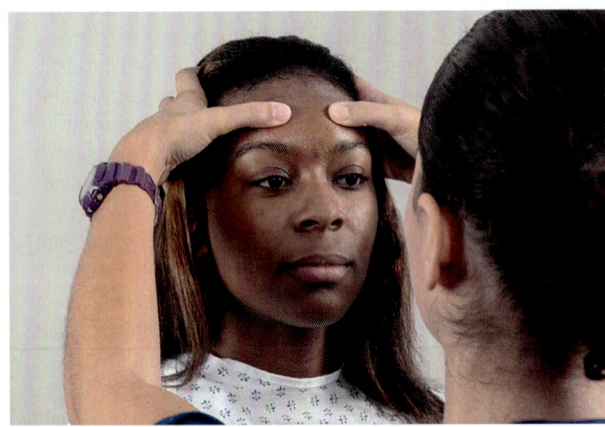

FIGURE 18-21 Palpating the frontal sinuses.

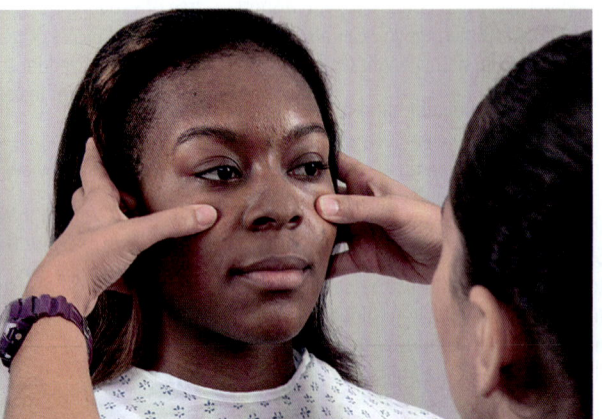

FIGURE 18-22 Palpating the maxillary sinuses.

PERCUSSION		
Percuss the sinuses. Lightly tap (percuss) over the frontal sinuses and over the maxillary sinuses for tenderness.	The sinuses are not tender on percussion.	The frontal and maxillary sinuses are tender upon percussion in clients with allergies or sinus infection.

CASE STUDY

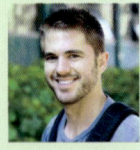

The nurse performs a physical examination of Jonathan's mouth, throat, nose, and sinuses.

Mouth: Lips are smooth, pink, and dry in appearance. Twenty-eight teeth are pearly white and smooth, with no malocclusion or obvious caries. Gums pink, moist, and firm, with tight margins to the teeth. No gum ulcerations, lesions, or masses noted. Buccal mucosa is pink. Stensen ducts are visible, with no redness or edema. "Strawberry" tongue with a white membrane and prominent red papillae noted. No tongue lesions, ulcers, or nodules noted. Frenulum is midline. Wharton ducts are visible and surrounded with moistness. Tongue strength 5/5. Able to distinguish between sweet and salty tastes. Hard palate pale pink and firm, with transverse rugae. Soft palate intact. Breath malodorous.

Throat: Uvula midline, erythemic and edematous. Uvula rises with phonation. Tonsils 3+ bilaterally and covered with patches of white exudate. Posterior pharynx erythemic with white exudates.

Nose: Color of nose matches face. Nose is smooth and symmetric, with no tenderness upon palpation. Nares patent. Nasal mucosa dark pink, moist, and free of exudate. Nasal septum intact and free of ulceration or perforations. Nasal turbinates dark pink, edematous, moist, and free of lesions.

Sinuses: Frontal and maxillary sinuses are nontender and no crepitus is palpable. No sinus tenderness noted to percussion.

Validating and Documenting Findings

Validate the mouth, throat, nose, and sinus assessment data that you have collected (by asking additional questions, verifying data with another health care professional, or comparing objective with subjective findings). This is necessary to verify that the data are reliable and accurate. Document the assessment data following the health care facility or agency policy.

> ### CASE STUDY
>
>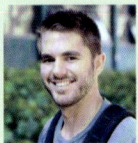
>
> Think back to the case study. The nurse completed the following documentation of her assessment of Jonathan Miller.
>
> *Biographic Data:* Jonathan Miller, 22 years old, Caucasian. Full-time student majoring in elementary education. Works part-time as a substitute teacher. Alert and oriented. Asks and answers questions appropriately.
>
> *Reason for Seeking Health Care:* "My throat feels like I am swallowing razor blades. I have horrible smelling breath, my neck hurts when I turn it and has 'knots' on either side, I have chills, and a fever and I am so tired and have no appetite."
>
> *History of Present Health Concern:* Last PM, JM developed a severe sore throat associated with fever and chills. Reports anorexia and extreme fatigue as well as foul smelling breath. States he has painful "knots" on either side of his neck and has pain when turning head. Denies nausea or vomiting. Has been taking sips of soda and water. Urinated this AM. Took two ibuprofen 400 mg at bedtime last PM.
>
> *Past Health History:* Reports having had wisdom teeth removed at age 16. Denies nasal or sinus surgery. Denies history of sinus infections or allergic rhinitis. Denies use of nasal sprays. Reports two episodes of "strep throat" when in elementary school. Denies allergies to drugs, food, environment, or insects. Medications include: ibuprofen 400 mg 2 tablets every 8 hours as needed for pain.
>
> *Family History:* Father alive and well. Mother alive and well. Sister alive and well. Paternal grandfather with hypertension. Paternal grandmother with rheumatoid arthritis. Maternal grandfather deceased at age 35 due to motor vehicle accident. Maternal grandmother with osteoarthritis, gastroesophageal reflux disease, and dementia. Denies family history of mouth, throat, nose, or sinus cancer.
>
> *Lifestyle and Health Practices:* Denies use of smoke or smokeless tobacco. Reports drinking 2 to 6 beers on weekend nights. Reports usual diet of fast and easy-to-prepare foods. Twenty-four hour diet recall only fluids, but typical 24-hour diet cereal, milk, coffee for breakfast, hamburger, fries and coke for lunch, and microwave foods for dinner. Denies grinding teeth. Brushes teeth two times daily and sees dentist every 6 months for cleaning. Uses floss occasionally. Last dental examination 3 months ago and results indicated no cavities. Uses lip sunscreen in the summer and when on annual ski vacation. Eats from drive-through fast food restaurants and whatever he can microwave from a can (soups and tamales).
>
> *Physical Examination Findings*
> *Mouth:* Lips are smooth, pink, and dry in appearance. Twenty-eight teeth are pearly white and smooth, with no malocclusion or obvious caries. Gums pink, moist, and firm, with tight margins to the teeth. No gum ulcerations, lesions, or masses noted. Buccal mucosa is pink. Stensen ducts visible, with no redness or edema. "Strawberry" tongue with a white membrane and prominent red papillae noted. No tongue lesions, ulcers, or nodules noted. Frenulum is midline. Wharton ducts visible and surrounded with moistness. Tongue strength 5/5. Able to distinguish between sweet and salty tastes. Hard palate pale pink and firm, with transverse rugae. Soft palate intact. Breath malodorous. *Throat:* Uvula midline, erythemic and edematous. Uvula rises with phonation. Tonsils 3+ bilaterally and covered with patches of white exudate. Posterior pharynx erythemic with white exudates. *Nose:* Color of nose matches face. Nose is smooth and symmetric, with no tenderness upon palpation. Nares patent. Nasal mucosa dark pink, moist, and free of exudate. Nasal septum intact and free of ulceration or perforations. Nasal turbinates dark pink, edematous, moist, and free of lesions.

ANALYSIS OF DATA: DIAGNOSTIC REASONING

After collecting subjective and objective data pertaining to the mouth, throat, nose, and sinuses, identify abnormal findings and client strengths. Then cluster the data to reveal any significant patterns or abnormalities. These data may be used to make clinical judgments about the status of the client's mouth, throat, nose, and sinuses.

Selected Nursing Diagnoses

Following is a listing of selected nursing diagnoses (health promotion, risk, or actual) that you may identify when analyzing the cue clusters.

Health Promotion Diagnoses

- Readiness for Enhanced Health Management of the teeth and gums
- Readiness for Enhanced Health Management: Requests information on how to quit smoking

Risk Diagnoses

- Risk for Aspiration related to decreased or absent gag reflex
- Risk for Imbalanced Nutrition: Less Than Body Requirements related to poorly fitting dentures or gum disease
- Risk for Infection of gums related to poor oral hygiene
- Risk for Injury to teeth and gums related to participation in active sports and lack of knowledge of protective mouth gear

Actual Diagnoses

- Ineffective Health Management related to poor oral hygiene
- Bathing/Hygiene Self-Care Deficit: Oral mouth care related to paralysis or decreased cognitive functions
- Disturbed Sensory Perception: Olfactory related to local irritation of nasal mucosa, impairment of cranial nerve I, decrease in olfactory bulb function secondary to nasal obstruction
- Impaired Oral Mucous Membranes related to poor oral hygiene or dehydration
- Impaired Swallowing related to impaired neurologic or neuromuscular function (e.g., CVA; damage to cranial nerves V, VII, IX, or X; cerebral palsy; myasthenia gravis; muscular dystrophy; cerebral palsy)
- Pain related to chronic sinusitis or inflammation of oral mucous membranes (gingivitis, periodontitis, canker sores)
- Disturbed Sensory Perception: Gustatory related to impairment of cranial nerve VII or IX, reduction of number of taste buds secondary to the aging process
- Imbalanced Nutrition: Less Than Body Requirements related to decreased appetite secondary to decreased sense of taste and smell and social isolation

Selected Collaborative Problems

After grouping the data, certain collaborative problems may become apparent. Remember that collaborative problems differ from nursing diagnoses in that they cannot be prevented by nursing intervention. However, these physiologic complications of medical conditions can be detected and monitored by the nurse. In addition, the nurse can use physician- and nurse-prescribed interventions to minimize the complications of these problems. The nurse may also have to refer the client in such situations for further treatment of the problem. Following is a list of collaborative problems that may be identified when obtaining a general impression. These problems are worded as Risk for Complications (RC) followed by the problem.

- RC: Nosebleed
- RC: Sinusitis (bacterial)
- RC: Stomatitis
- RC: Gum infection (gingivitis, periodontitis)
- RC: Oral lesions
- RC: Laryngeal edema

Medical Problems

After grouping the data, the client's signs and symptoms may clearly require medical diagnosis and treatment. Referral to a primary care provider is necessary.

CASE STUDY

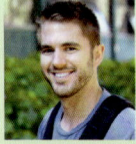

After collecting and analyzing the data for Jonathan Miller, the nurse determines that the following conclusions are appropriate:

Nursing Diagnoses
- Risk for Imbalanced Nutrition: Less Than Body Requirements r/t busy schedule with little regard to nutrition; anorexia and increased metabolic need secondary to throat pain and systemic response to possible infection.
- Acute Pain r/t possible knowledge deficit of appropriate pain-management strategies.
- Ineffective Health Management r/t inadequate knowledge of practices to promote health during periods of stress.

Potential Collaborative Problems
- RC: Streptococcal infection of throat

Refer to primary care provider to diagnose and treat his throat condition. To view an algorithm depicting the process of diagnostic reasoning for this case, go to **thePoint**.

Interdisciplinary Verbal Communication of Assessment Findings Using SBAR

SITUATION: JM, a 22-year-old male college student, reports to campus health service with severe constant throat pain ("like swallowing razor blades"), which began last night. Reports bad breath, neck pain, and "knots" on either side of his neck, chills, fever 101°F, constant fatigue, and no appetite. On scale 1–10 rates throat pain a 6 and 8–9 when swallowing. Throat pain reduced to a 2 to 3 after taking 2 ibuprofen 400 mg. Sipping soda and water. No nausea or vomiting.

BACKGROUND: Has been studying "day and night" for final exams with one more to go. This is the third time he has had these same symptoms this year but treated himself the first two times. Denies any known history of sinus infections or allergies. Tends to eat a lot of fast and canned food. Drinks 2–6 beers on weekends. Attends college full time and works part time as substitute teacher. Denies use of smoke or smokeless tobacco. Reports using ibuprofen 400 mg 2 tablets every 8 hours as needed for pain. Reports two episodes of "strep throat" when in elementary school.

ASSESSMENT: "Strawberry" tongue with a white membrane and prominent red papillae noted. Uvula midline, erythemic, edematous, and rises on phonation. Tonsils 3+ bilaterally and covered with patches of white exudates. Posterior pharynx erythemic with white exudates. Nasal mucosa dark pink, moist, and free of exudates. No sinus tenderness percussed. Breathe malodorous.

RECOMMENDATION: JM is at Risk for Imbalanced Nutrition: Less Than Body Requirements r/t busy schedule with little regard to nutrition; anorexia and increased metabolic need secondary to throat pain and systemic response to possible infection. He has Acute Pain r/t possible knowledge deficit of appropriate pain-management strategies. In addition he has Ineffective Health Management r/t inadequate knowledge of practices to promote health during periods of stress. He needs to be seen by his primary care provider to diagnose and treat his throat condition.

ABNORMAL FINDINGS 18-1 Abnormalities of the Mouth and Throat

This display depicts common abnormalities of the mouth and throat.

Herpes simplex type I (cold sores): Clear vesicles surrounded by red indurated base

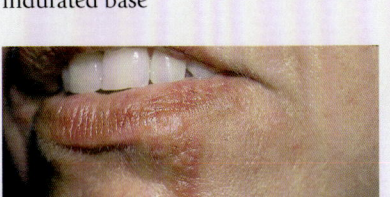

Cheilosis of lips: Scaling painful fissures at corner of lips

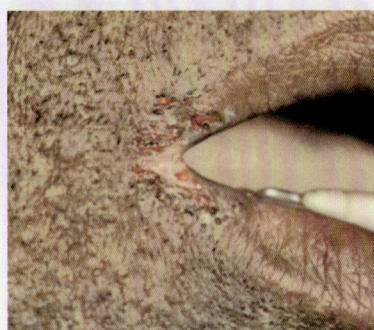

Carcinoma of lip: Round, indurated lesion becomes crusted and ulcerated with elevated border

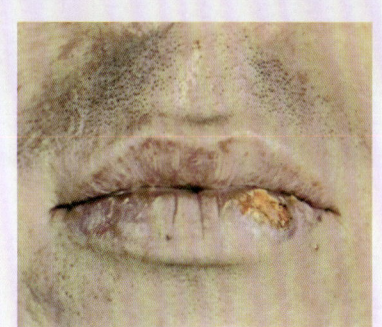

Leukoplakia (ventral surface): thick raised patch does not scrape off; seen in heavy tobacco or alcohol use

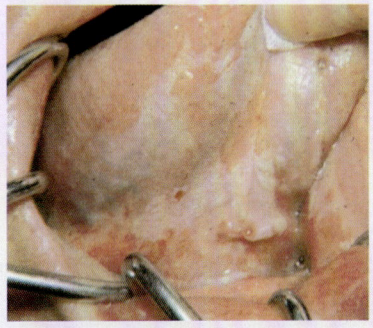

Hairy leukoplakia (lateral surface)

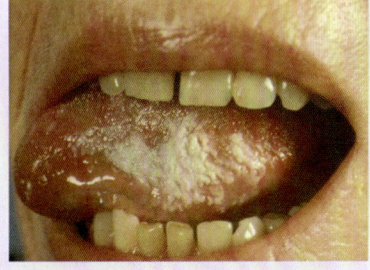

(From Goodheart, H.P. (2008). Goodheart's Photoguide to Common Skin Disorders, 3rd ed. Philadelphia: Wolters Kluwer.)

Candida albicans **infection (thrush):** Curdlike patches easily scrape off, leaving a reddened area

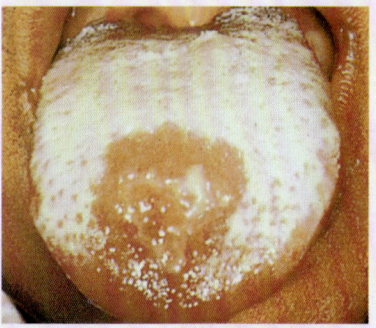

Smooth, reddish, shiny tongue without papillae due to vitamin B12 deficiency

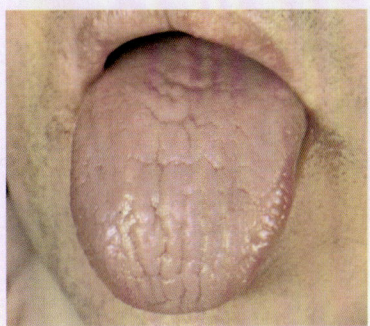

Black hairy tongue: Not hair, but elongated filiform papillae seen with use of antibiotics that inhibit normal bacteria

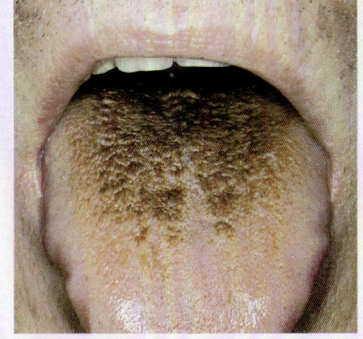

(Courtesy of Dr. Michael Bennett)

Carcinoma of tongue: Round indurated lesion becomes crusty and ulcerated with elevated border

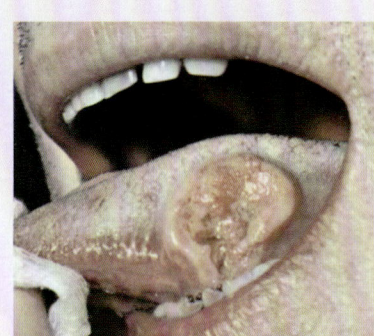

Continued on following page

378 UNIT 3 Nursing Assessment of Physical Systems

ABNORMAL FINDINGS 18-1 Abnormalities of the Mouth and Throat (Continued)

Canker sore: Painful small ulcers inside mouth; do not occur on lip surface; non-contagious

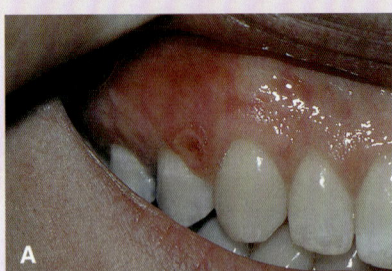
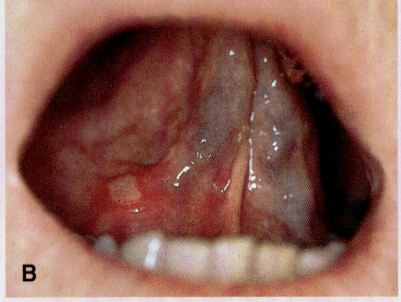
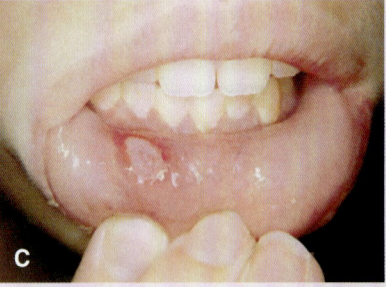

Gingivitis: Red swollen gums that easily bleed

Receding gums: Gum tissue surrounding tooth pulls back, exposing more of tooth or root of tooth

Kaposi's sarcoma lesions: Advanced lesions seen in HIV (human immunodeficiency virus)

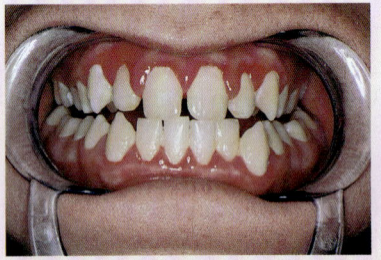
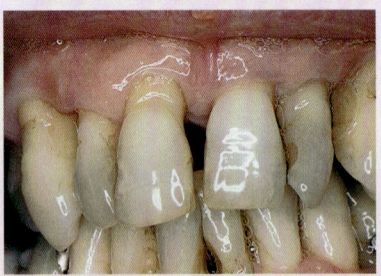
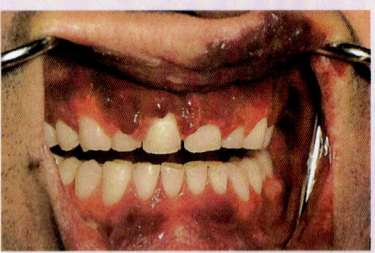

(Courtesy of Dr. Michael Bennett)

(Courtesy of Dr. Michael Bennett)

Acute tonsillitis: Acute tonsillitis secondary to infectious mononucleosis. Note the marked tonsillar enlargement with erythema and the large white-gray patches

Streptococcal pharyngitis: Characterized by an erythematous posterior pharynx (A), palatal petechiae (B), and a white strawberry tongue (C). (From Fleisher, G.R., Ludwig, W., & Baskin, M.N. (2004.) Atlas of Pediatric Emergency Medicine. Philadelphia: Lippincott Williams & Wilkins.)

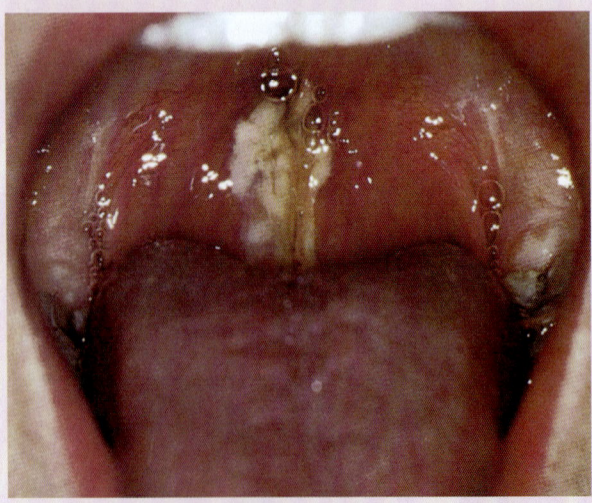
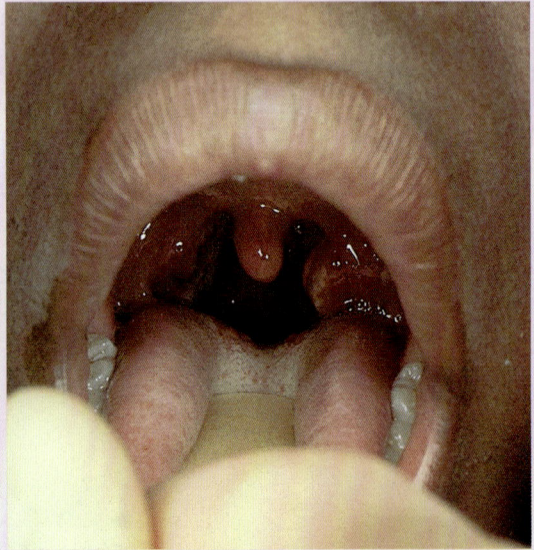

ABNORMAL FINDINGS 18-2 Tonsillitis (Detecting and Grading)

In a client who has both tonsils and a sore throat, tonsillitis can be identified and ranked with a grading scale from 1–4 as follows:

- 1+ Tonsils are visible.
- 2+ Tonsils are midway between tonsillar pillars and uvula.
- 3+ Tonsils touch the uvula.
- 4+ Tonsils touch each other.

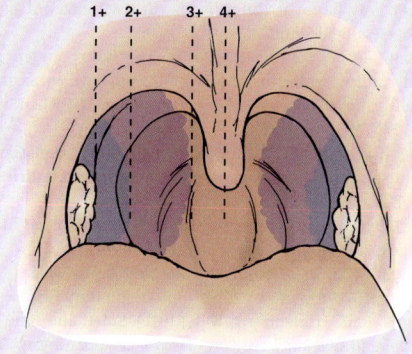

ABNORMAL FINDINGS 18-3 Common Abnormalities of the Nose

Nasal polyp

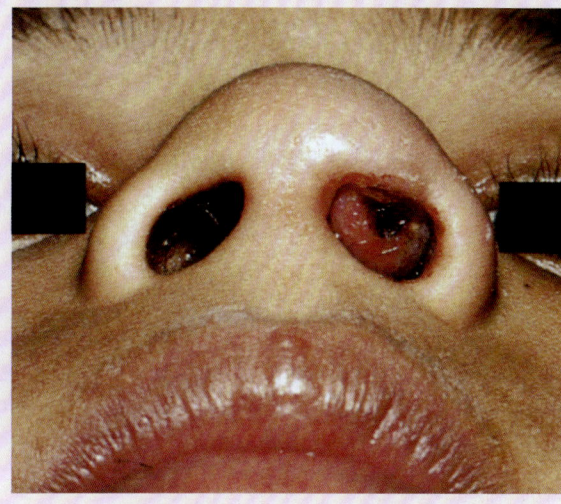

Perforated septum

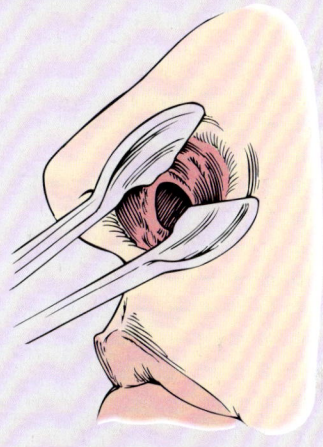

(Used with permission from Handler SD, Myer CM. Atlas of Ear, Nose and Throat Disorders in Children. Ontario, Canada: BC Decker; 1998:59.)

Want to know more?

A wide variety of resources to enhance your learning and understanding of this book are available on thePoint. Visit thePoint to access:

NCLEX-Style Student Review Questions Concepts in Action Animations
Watch and Learn Videos And more!

References and Selected Readings

American Academy of Allergy, Asthma & Immunology (AAAAI). (2016). Sinusitis. Available at http://www.aaaai.org/conditions-and-treatments/allergies/sinusitis.aspx

American Cancer Society (ACS). (2015a). Can oral cavity and pharyngeal cancers be found early? Available at http://www.cancer.org/cancer/oralcavityandoropharyngealcancer/detailedguide/oral-cavity-and-oropharyngeal-cancer-detection

American Cancer Society (ACS). (2015b). What are the risk factors for oral cavity and oropharyngeal cancers? Available at http://www.cancer.org/cancer/oralcavityandoropharyngealcancer/detailedguide/oral-cavity-and-oropharyngeal-cancer-risk-factors

American Dental Association (ADA). (2013). American Dental Association statement on regular Brushing and flossing to help prevent oral infections. Available at http://www.ada.org/en/press-room/news-releases/2013-archive/august/american-dental-association-statement-on-regular-brushing-and-flossing-to-help-prevent-oral

American Society of Clinical Oncology (ASCO). (2015). Oral and oropharyngeal cancer: Overview. Available at http://www.cancer.net/cancer-types/oral-and-oropharyngeal-cancer/overview

Black hairy tongue: Lingua villosa nigra. (2014). Available at http://www.exodontia.info/Black_Hairy_Tongue.html

Carson-DeWitt, R. (2012). Screening for sinusitis. Available at http://www.lifescript.com/health/a-z/conditions_a-z/conditionsindepth/s/sinusitis/screening.aspx

Centers for Disease Control and Prevention (CDC). (2016). Betel quid with tobacco (gutka). Available at https://www.cdc.gov/tobacco/data_statistics/fact_sheets/smokeless/betel_quid/

Dhadse, P., Gattani, D., & Mishra, R. (2010). The link between periodontal disease and cardiovascular disease: How far we have come in last two decades? *Journal of the Indian Society of Periodontology*, 14(3), 148–154. doi: 10.4103/0972-124X.75908

Harvard Medical School Patient Education Center. (2016). Chronic sinusitis (in adults). Available at http://www.patienteducationcenter.org/articles/chronic-sinusitis-in-adults/

Healthy People 2020. (2015a). Oropharyngeal cancer. Available at http://www.healthypeople.gov/2020/topics-objectives/topic/oral-health

Healthy People 2020. (2015b). Respiratory diseases. Available at http://www.healthypeople.gov/2020/topics-objectives/topic/respiratory-diseases

Hummel, T., Landis, B., & Hüttenbrink, K B. (2011). Smell and taste disorders. *GMS Current Topics in Otorhinolaryngology Head and Neck Surgery*, 10(Doc 4). doi:10.3205/cto000077

Khalil, A. (2009). Lead poisoning. *British Dental Journal*, 206, 608. doi:10.1038/sj.bdj.2009.524 Available at http://www.nature.com/bdj/journal/v206/n12/full/sj.bdj.2009.524.html

Leung, A., Wong, A., & Barankin, B. (2014). An incidental palatine finding: Benign or 'double trouble'? *Consultant for Pediatricians*, 13(2), 81–82.

Marya, C. (2011). Epidemiology of periodontal disease. In *A testbook of public health dentistry*. New Delhi, IN: Jaypee Brothers Medical Publishers.

Mayo Clinic. (2013). Chronic sinusitis. Available at http://www.mayoclinic.org/diseases-conditions/chronic-sinusitis/basics/symptoms/con-20022039

National Cancer Institute (NCI). (2016). Oral cavity and oropharyngeal cancer screening (PDQ<R>) Health professional version. Available at https://www.cancer.gov/types/head-and-neck/hp/oral-screening-pdq

Nguyen, Q. (2015). Epistaxis: Etiology. Available at http://emedicine.medscape.com/article/863220-overview#a5

Nimala, S., Challa, R., Velpula, L., et al. (2011). Unusual occurrence of accessory central cusp in the maxillary second primary molar. *Contemporary Clinical Dentistry*, 2(2), 127–130. doi:0.4103/0976–237X.83078 Available at http://www.ncbi.nlm.nih.gov/pmc/articles/PMC3180834/

O'Neill, J. (2015). Tobacco and alcohol responsible for 74% of head and neck cancers. Available at http://www.ehospice.com/ireland/ArticleView/tabid/11070/ArticleId/16134/language/en-GB/View.aspx

Pinto, J., Wroblewski, K., Kern, D., et al. (2014). Olfactory dysfunction predicts 5-year mortality in older adults. Available at http://journals.plos.org/plosone/article?id=10.1371/journal.pone.0107541

Smitha, K., & Smitha, G. (2014). Alveolar exostosis – revisited; A narrative review of the literature. *The Saudi Journal for Dental Research*, 6(1), 67–72. doi:http://dx.doi.org/10.1016/j.sjdr.2014.02.001

Stanford Medicine. (2015). The tongue in diagnosis. Available at http://stanfordmedicine25.stanford.edu/the25/tongue.html

The Oral Cancer Foundation. (2016). The alcohol connection. Available at http://www.oralcancerfoundation.org/understanding/alcohol-connection.php

The Taste and Smell Clinic. (2005). Zinc and apoptosis. Available at http://www.tasteandsmell.com/feb05.htm

U.S. Preventive Services Task Force (USPSTF). (2015). Oral cancer: Screening. Available at http://www.uspreventiveservicestaskforce.org/Page/Document/UpdateSummaryFinal/oral-cancer-screening1

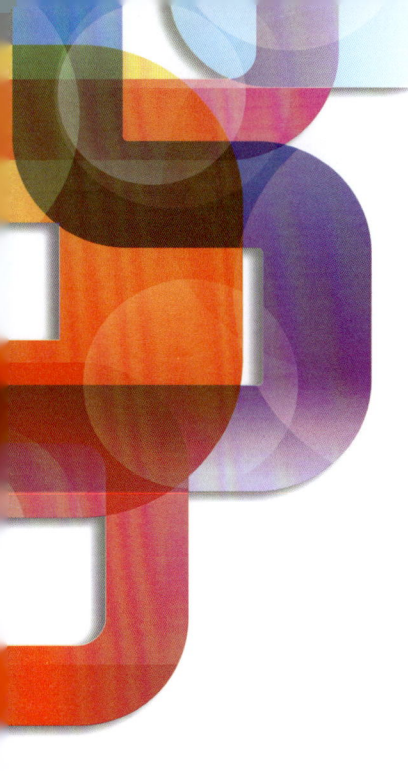

19 ASSESSING THORAX AND LUNGS

Learning Objectives

1. Describe the function and structure of the thorax and lungs.
2. Identify the thoracic landmarks in relation to the underlying thoracic structures.
3. Discuss the risk factors for lung cancer across the cultures and ways to reduce one's risks.
4. Describe the teaching opportunities to reduce risks and promote health for the thorax and lungs.
5. Interview a client for an accurate nursing history of the thorax and lungs.
6. Perform a physical assessment of the thorax and lungs using the correct techniques of inspection, auscultation, palpation, and percussion.
7. Describe the findings frequently seen when assessing the older client's thorax and lungs.
8. Analyze the data from the interview and physical assessment of the lungs and thorax to formulate valid nursing diagnoses, collaborative problems, and/or referrals.
9. Differentiate between general routine screening versus skills needed for focused or specialty assessment of the lungs and thorax.
10. Document and verbally report accurate assessment findings of the lungs and thorax.

CASE STUDY

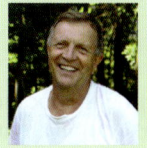

George Burney, a 67-year-old Caucasian man diagnosed by a physician with emphysema 4 years ago, reports that he has had a fever and has chest pain when he takes a deep breath or coughs. He presents to the free walk-in clinic today for an evaluation.

STRUCTURE AND FUNCTION

The term *thorax* identifies the portion of the body extending from the base of the neck superiorly to the level of the diaphragm inferiorly. The lungs, distal portion of the trachea, and the bronchi are located in the thorax and constitute the *lower respiratory system*. The outer structure of the thorax is referred to as the *thoracic cage*. The *thoracic cavity* contains the respiratory components. A thorough assessment of the lower respiratory system focuses on the external chest as well as the respiratory components in the thoracic cavity.

Thoracic Cage

The *thoracic cage* is constructed of the sternum, 12 pairs of ribs, 12 thoracic vertebrae, muscles, and cartilage. It provides support and protection for many important organs, including those of the lower respiratory system. Structures and landmarks of the anterior thoracic cage (Fig. 19-1) and the posterior thoracic cage (Fig. 19-2) are discussed in the next section.

Sternum and Clavicles

The *sternum*, or breastbone, lies in the center of the chest anteriorly and is divided into three parts: the manubrium, the body, and the xiphoid process. The manubrium connects laterally with the clavicles (collarbones) and the first two pairs of ribs. The clavicles extend from the manubrium to the acromion of the scapula.

A U-shaped indentation located on the superior border of the manubrium is an important landmark known as the *suprasternal notch*. A few centimeters below the suprasternal notch, a bony ridge can be palpated at the point where the manubrium articulates with the body of the sternum. This landmark, often referred to as the *sternal angle* (or angle of Louis), is also the location of the second pair of ribs and becomes a reference point for counting ribs and intercostal spaces.

Ribs and Thoracic Vertebrae

The 12 pairs of ribs constitute the main structure of the thoracic cage. They are numbered superiorly to inferiorly, the uppermost pair being number one. Each pair of ribs has a corresponding pair of intercostal spaces located immediately inferior to it. Anteriorly the first seven pairs articulate with the sternum by way of costal cartilages. The first pair of ribs curves up immediately under the clavicles so that only a small portion of these ribs and the first interspaces are palpable. The second ribs and intercostal spaces are easily located adjacent

381

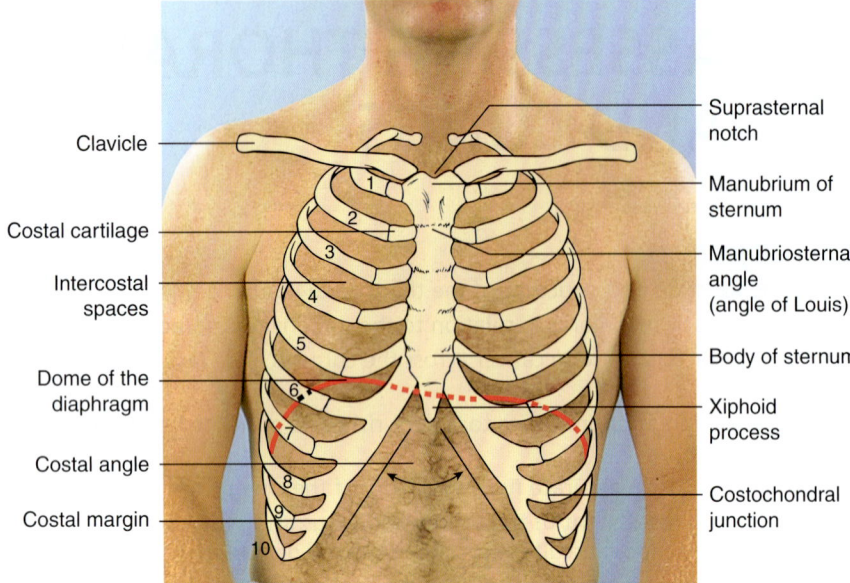

FIGURE 19-1 Anterior thoracic cage.

to the sternal angle. Ribs two through six are easy to count anteriorly because of their articulation with the sternal body.

The next four pairs of ribs (seven through ten) connect to the cartilages of the pair lying superior to them rather than to the sternum (Fig. 19-1). This configuration forms an angle between the right and left costal margins meeting at the level of the xiphoid process. This angle, commonly referred to as the *costal angle*, is an important landmark for assessment. It is normally less than 90 degrees but may be increased in instances of long-standing hyperinflation of the lungs, as in emphysema. The 11th and 12th pairs of ribs are called *"floating" ribs* because they do not connect to either the sternum or another pair of ribs anteriorly. Instead, they are attached posteriorly to the vertebra and their anterior tips are free and palpable (Fig. 19-2).

The ribs are more difficult to palpate posteriorly. Each pair of ribs articulates with its respective *thoracic vertebra*. The spinous process of the seventh cervical vertebra (C7), also called the *vertebra prominens*, can be easily felt with the client's neck flexed. The process immediately inferior to the vertebra prominens is the first thoracic vertebra, which is adjacent to the posterior aspect of the first rib.

CLINICAL TIP
When counting the spinous processes, it is helpful to know that they align with their corresponding ribs only to the fourth thoracic vertebra (T4). After this, the spinous processes angle downward from their own vertebral body and can be palpated over the vertebral body and rib below.

The lower tip of each scapula is at the level of the seventh or eighth rib when the arms are at the client's side (Fig. 19-2).

Vertical Reference Lines

By counting the ribs, an examiner can describe the location of a finding vertically. However, to describe a location around

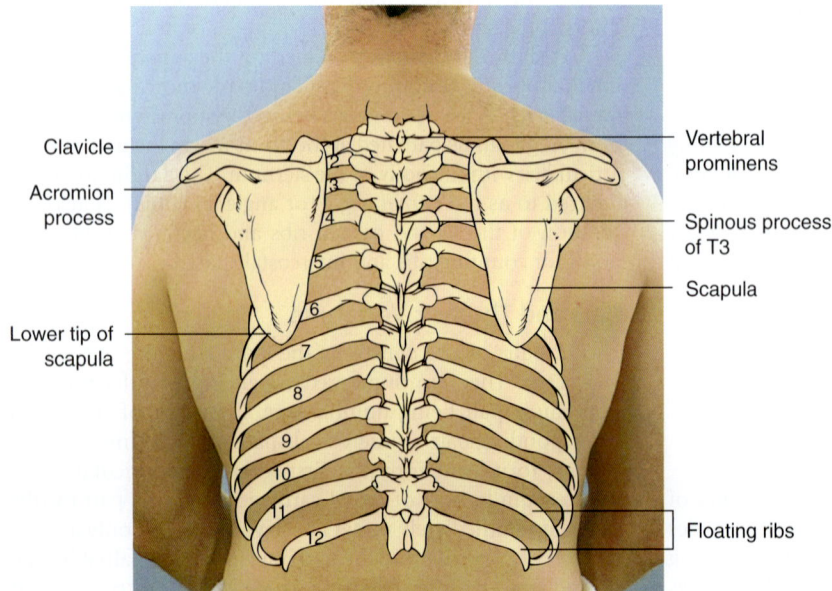

FIGURE 19-2 Posterior thoracic cage.

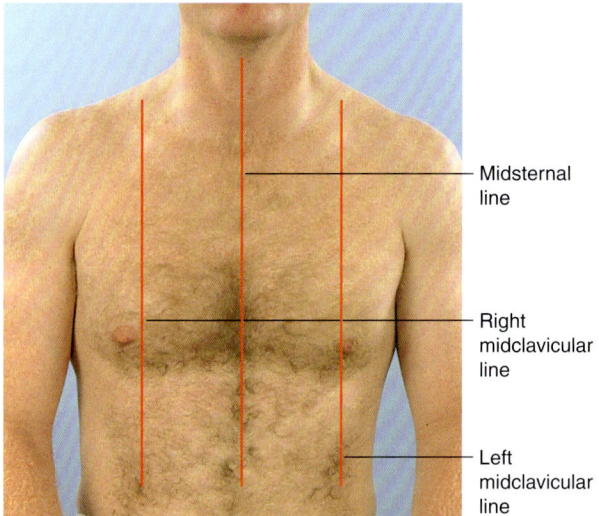

FIGURE 19-3 Anterior vertical lines (imaginary landmarks).

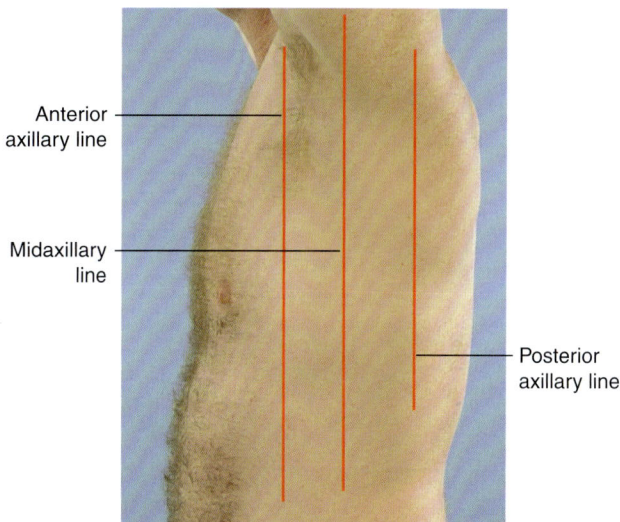

FIGURE 19-5 Lateral vertical lines (imaginary landmarks).

the circumference of the chest wall, the examiner uses imaginary lines running vertically on the chest wall. On the anterior chest, these lines are known as the *midsternal line* and the *right and left mid-clavicular lines* (Fig. 19-3).

The posterior thorax includes the *vertebral (or spinal) line* and the *right and left scapular lines*, which extend through the inferior angle of the scapulae when the arms are at the client's side (Fig. 19-4).

The lateral aspect of the thorax is divided into three parallel lines. The *mid-axillary line* runs from the apex of the axillae to the level of the 12th rib. The *anterior axillary line* extends from the anterior axillary fold along the anterolateral aspect of the thorax, whereas the *posterior axillary line* runs from the posterior axillary fold down the posterolateral aspect of the chest wall (Fig. 19-5).

Thoracic Cavity

The thoracic cavity consists of the *mediastinum* and the lungs, and is lined by the pleural membranes. The mediastinum refers to a central area in the thoracic cavity that contains the trachea, bronchi, esophagus, heart, and great vessels. The trachea and bronchi are discussed immediately following. The other structures of the mediastinum are discussed in separate chapters (Chapter 21). The lungs lie on each side of the mediastinum.

Trachea and Bronchi

The *trachea* is a flexible structure that lies anterior to the esophagus, begins at the level of the cricoid cartilage in the neck, and is approximately 10 to 12 cm long in an adult (Fig. 19-6). C-shaped rings of *hyaline cartilage* compose the trachea; they help to maintain its shape and prevent its collapse during respiration.

At the level of the sternal angle, the trachea bifurcates into the right and left main *bronchi*. Both bronchi are at an oblique position in the mediastinum and enter the lungs at the hilum. The *right main bronchus* is shorter and more vertical than the *left main bronchus*, making aspirated objects more likely to enter the right lung than the left.

The bronchi and trachea represent "dead space" in the respiratory system, where air is transported but no gas exchange takes place. They function primarily as a passageway for both inspired and expired air. In addition, the trachea and bronchi are lined with mucous membranes containing *cilia*. These hair-like projections help sweep dust, foreign bodies, and bacteria that have been trapped by the mucus toward the mouth for removal.

Inspired air travels through the trachea into the main bronchi and continues through the system. The bronchi repeatedly bifurcate into smaller passageways known as *bronchioles*. Eventually the bronchioles terminate at the alveolar ducts, and air is channeled into the alveolar sacs, which contain the *alveoli* (Fig. 19-6). Alveolar sacs contain a number of alveoli in a cluster formation (resembling grapes), creating millions of interalveolar walls that increase the surface area available for gas exchange.

Lungs

The *lungs* are two cone-shaped, elastic structures suspended within the thoracic cavity. The *apex* of each lung extends

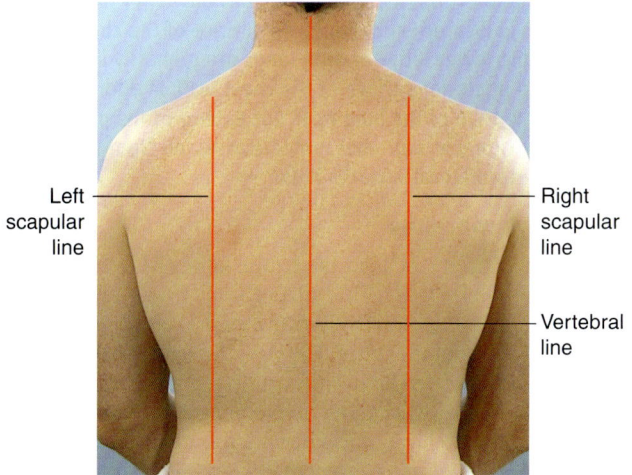

FIGURE 19-4 Posterior vertical lines (imaginary landmarks).

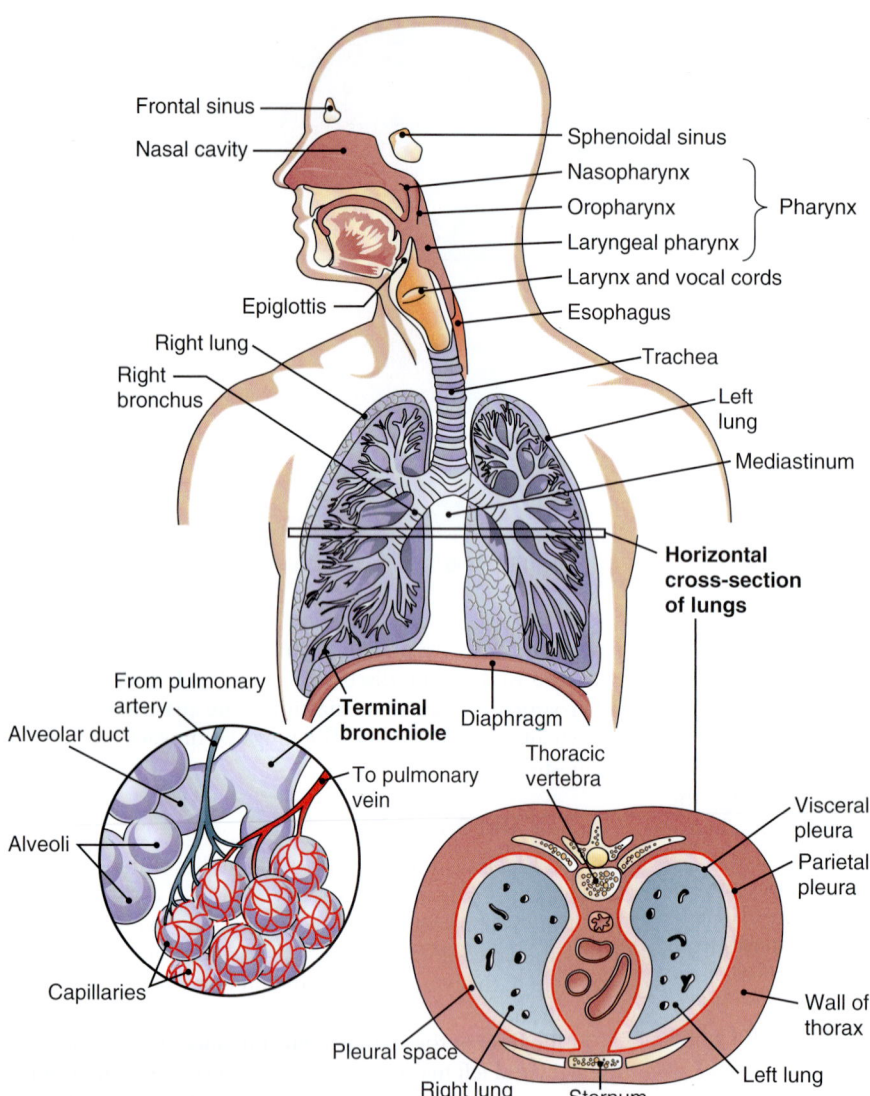

FIGURE 19-6 Major structures of the respiratory system.

slightly above the clavicle. The *base* is at the level of the *diaphragm*. At the point of the mid-clavicular line on the anterior surface of the thorax, the lung extends to approximately the sixth rib. Laterally lung tissue reaches the level of the eighth rib, and posteriorly the lung base lies at about the tenth rib (Fig. 19-7).

Although the lungs are paired, they are not completely symmetric. Both are divided into lobes by fissures. The right lung is made up of three lobes; the left lung contains only two lobes. Fissures separating the lobes run obliquely through the chest, making the lobes appear as diagonal sloping segments. Anteriorly the horizontal fissure separating the right upper lobe from the middle lobe extends from the fifth rib in the right mid-axillary line to the third intercostal space or fourth rib at the right sternal border. Posteriorly oblique fissures extend on both the right and left lungs from the level of T3 to the sixth rib at the mid-clavicular line.

In the healthy adult, during deep inspiration the lungs extend down to about the eighth intercostal space anteriorly and the twelfth intercostal space posteriorly. During expiration, the lungs rise to the fifth or sixth intercostal space anteriorly and tenth posteriorly.

CLINICAL TIP
Remember that most lung tissue in the upper lobes of both lungs is located on the anterior surface of the chest wall. Similarly, the lower lobes of both lungs are primarily located toward the posterior surface of the chest wall. In addition, the right middle lobe of the lung does not extend to the posterior side of the thoracic wall, thus must be assessed from the anterior and anterolateral surfaces alone.

Pleural Membranes

The thoracic cavity is lined by a thin, double-layered serous membrane referred to as the pleura (Fig. 19-6). The *parietal pleura* lines the chest cavity, and the *visceral pleura* covers the external surfaces of the lungs. The *pleural space* lies between the two pleural layers. In the healthy adult, the lubricating serous fluid between the layers allows movement of the visceral layer over the parietal layer during ventilation without friction. Because the pleural space is one of the physiologic third spaces

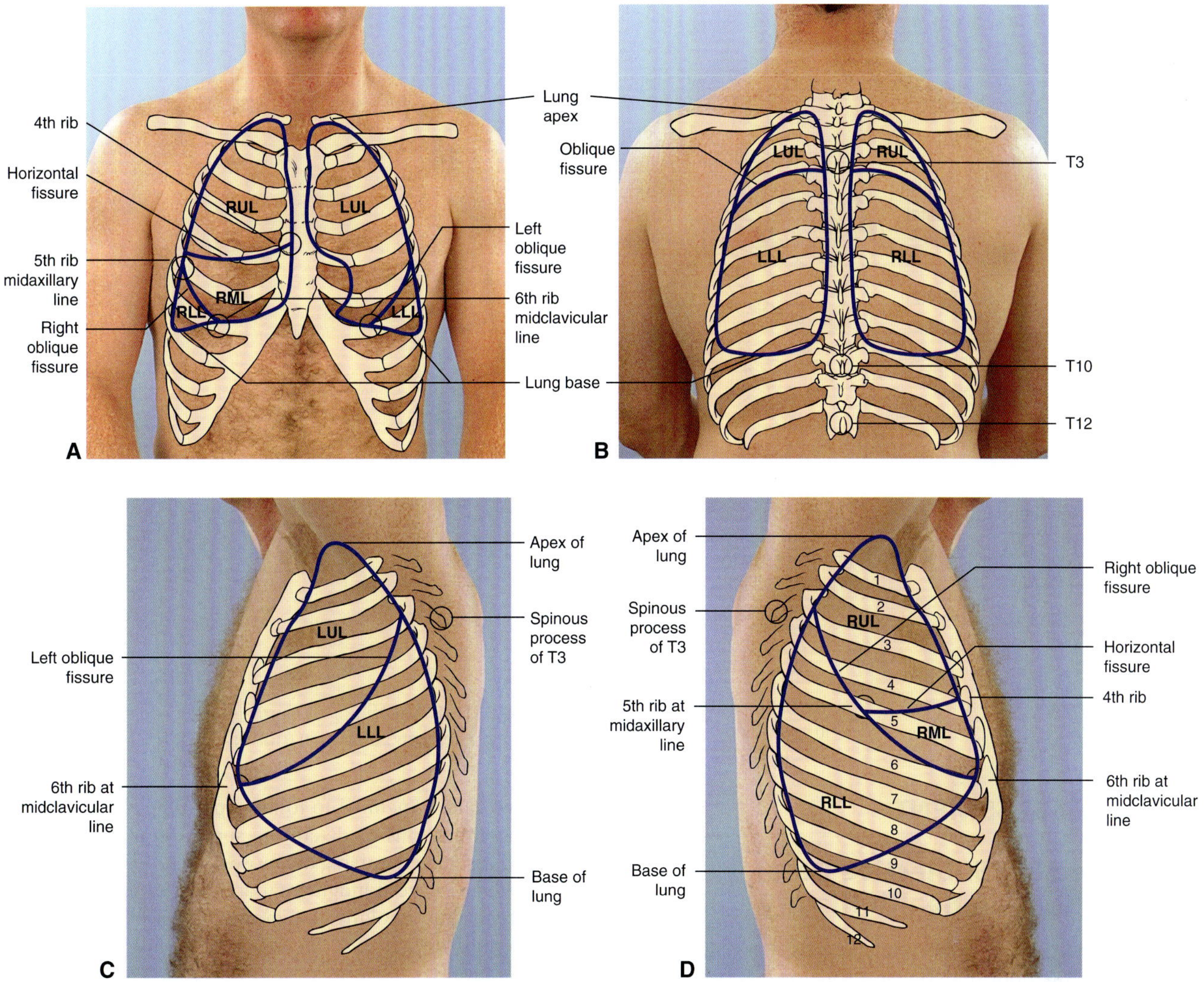

FIGURE 19-7 **A.** Anterior view of lung position. **B.** Posterior view of lung position. **C.** Lateral view of left lung position. **D.** Lateral view of right lung position.

for body fluid storage, severe dehydration will reduce the volume of pleural fluid, resulting in the increased transmission of lung sounds and a possible friction rub.

 ## Mechanics of Breathing

The purpose of respiration is to maintain an adequate oxygen level in the blood to support cellular life. By providing oxygen and eliminating carbon dioxide, respiration assists in the rapid compensation for metabolic acid–base defects. However, changes in the respiratory pattern can cause acid–base imbalances.

External respiration, or ventilation, is the mechanical act of breathing and is accomplished by expansion of the chest, both vertically and horizontally. Vertical expansion is accomplished through contraction of the diaphragm. Horizontal expansion occurs as intercostal muscles lift the sternum and elevate the ribs, resulting in an increase in anteroposterior diameter.

As a result of this enlargement of the chest cavity, a slight negative pressure is created in the lungs in relation to the atmospheric pressure, resulting in an inflow of air into the lungs. This process, called *inspiration,* is shown in Figure 19-8. *Expiration* is mostly passive in nature and occurs with relaxation of the intercostal muscles and the diaphragm. As the diaphragm relaxes, it assumes a domed shape. The resultant decrease in the size of the chest cavity creates a positive pressure, forcing air out of the lungs.

Breathing patterns change according to cellular demands—often without awareness on the part of the individual. Such involuntary control of respiration is the work of the medulla and pons, located in the brainstem. The hypothalamus and the sympathetic nervous system also play a role in involuntary control of respiration in response to emotional changes such as fear or excitement.

Hormonal regulation, changes in oxygen or carbon dioxide levels in the blood, or changes in the hydrogen ion (pH) level cause changes in breathing patterns. Under normal circumstances, the strongest stimulus to breathe is an increase of carbon dioxide in the blood (hypercapnia). A decrease in oxygen (hypoxemia) also increases respiration but is less effective than a rise in carbon dioxide levels.

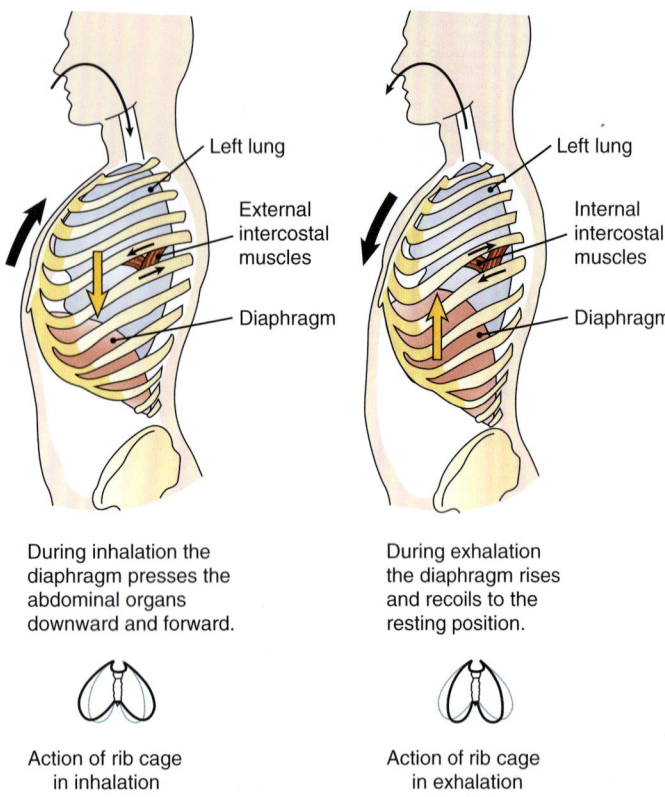

FIGURE 19-8 Mechanics of normal—not deep, not shallow—inspiration (left) and expiration (right).

HEALTH ASSESSMENT

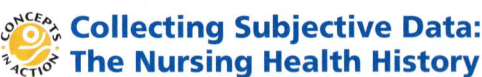 Collecting Subjective Data: The Nursing Health History

Subjective data related to thoracic and lung assessment provide many clues about underlying respiratory problems and associated nursing diagnoses as well as clues about risk for the development of lung disorders. Information regarding the client's level of functioning is also important because certain respiratory problems greatly impact a person's ability to perform activities of daily living (ADLs). When collecting subjective data, remember to follow up on the client's related signs and symptoms to determine specific respiratory problems and associated nursing diagnoses.

Be careful to avoid judgmental approaches to undesirable health practices. Smoking, for example, has become a stigmatized addiction in our society. Avoid conveying feelings of intolerance when caring for an individual with respiratory complaints who smokes. Assess smoking status for all clients at every visit. Use the 5 A's approach (Box 21-4). Based on the client's readiness for teaching, the nurse may offer information about smoking cessation methods.

History of Present Health Concern	
QUESTION	**RATIONALE**
Difficulty Breathing	
Do you ever experience difficulty breathing or a loss of breath? If the client answers yes, use COLDSPA to explore the symptom.	
Characteristics: Describe the difficulty breathing	Dyspnea (difficulty breathing) can indicate a number of health problems, including pulmonary disorders: chronic obstructive pulmonary disease (COPD), asthma, pneumonia, pneumothorax, pulmonary embolism, congestive heart failure (CHF), coronary heart disease (CHD), myocardial ischemia, and myocardial infarction (MI). Clients who have COPD may describe their dyspnea as not being able to "breathe or take a deep breath."
	Anxious clients may describe their dyspnea as feeling like they are suffocating, or they may have tingling in the lips due to a decrease in carbon dioxide level.
Onset: When did it begin?	It may occur during rest, sleep, or with mild, moderate, or extreme exertion.
	Gradual onset of dyspnea is usually indicative of lung changes such as emphysema; sudden onset is associated with viral or bacterial infections, acute asthma exacerbation, acute myocardial ischemia/infarction, pulmonary embolism (Evidence-Based Practice 19-1).

QUESTION	RATIONALE
Location: Nonapplicable	
Duration: How long did the dyspnea last?	They may have continuous coughing ("smoker's cough") with copious amounts of sputum, shortness of breath with everyday activities, and wheezing (American Lung Association [ALA] 2015c). Common symptoms of asthma are wheezing, frequent cough with or without mucous, shortness of breath, and chest tightness (ALA, 2015a).
Severity: How did it affect your ability to carry on your usual activities?	Dyspnea with exercise or strenuous activities is normal if the dyspnea subsides with resting from the activity. Dyspnea will occur with typical nonstrenuous activities (such as walking one block or climbing two stairs) of daily living in clients with lung disease or congestive heart failure.
Palliative/aggravating factors: What aggravates or relieves the dyspnea? Do any specific activities cause the difficulty in breathing? Do you have difficulty breathing when you are resting? Do you have difficulty breathing when you sleep? Do you use more than one pillow or elevate the head of the bed when you sleep? Do you snore when you sleep? Have you been told that you stop breathing at night when you snore?	**OLDER ADULT CONSIDERATIONS** Older adults may experience dyspnea with certain activities due to age-related changes of the lungs (loss of elasticity, fewer functional capillaries, and loss of lung resiliency). Dyspnea can occur with stress and anxiety.
Associated factors: Do you experience any other symptoms when you have difficulty breathing?	Associated symptoms provide clues to the underlying problem. Certain associated symptoms suggest problems in other body systems. For example, edema or angina that occurs with dyspnea may indicate a cardiovascular problem. Orthopnea (difficulty breathing when lying supine) may be associated with heart failure. Paroxysmal nocturnal dyspnea (severe dyspnea that awakens the person from sleep) also may be associated with heart failure. Changes in sleep patterns may cause the client to feel fatigued during the day. Sleep apnea (periods of breathing cessation during sleep) may be the source of snoring and gasping sounds. In general, sleep apnea diminishes the quality of sleep, which may account for fatigue or excessive tiredness, depression, irritability, loss of memory, lack of energy, and a risk for automobile and workplace accidents. Left untreated, sleep apnea can have serious and life-shortening consequences: high blood pressure, heart disease, stroke, automobile accidents caused by falling asleep at the wheel, diabetes, depression, and other ailments (American Sleep Apnea Association [ASAA], n.d.).
Chest Pain	
Do you have chest pain? Is the pain associated with a cold, fever, or deep breathing? See Chapter 21 for assessment of chest pain.	**SAFETY TIP** *Immediately assess any reports of chest pain further to determine if it is due to cardiac ischemia, which is a medical emergency requiring immediate assessment and intervention.* Pain-sensitive nerve endings are located in the parietal pleura, thoracic muscles, and tracheobronchial tree, but not in the lungs. Thus chest pain associated with a pulmonary origin may be a late sign of pulmonary disease (Evidence-Based Practice 19-2). **OLDER ADULT CONSIDERATIONS** Chest pain related to pleuritis may be absent in older clients because of age-related alterations in pain perception.
Cough	
Do you have a cough? When and how often does it occur?	Continuous coughs are usually associated with acute infections, whereas those occurring only early in the morning are often associated with chronic bronchial inflammation or smoking. Coughs late in the evening may be the result of exposure to irritants during the day. Coughs occurring at night are often related to postnasal drip or sinusitis. **OLDER ADULT CONSIDERATIONS** The ability to cough effectively may be decreased in the older client because of weaker muscles and increased rigidity of the thoracic wall.

Continued on following page

History of Present Health Concern (Continued)

QUESTION	RATIONALE
Cough (Continued)	
Do you produce any sputum when you cough? If so, what color is the sputum? How much sputum do you cough up? Has this amount increased or decreased recently? Does the sputum have an odor?	Nonproductive coughs are often associated with upper respiratory irritations and early congestive heart failure (CHF). Sputum color varies. Sputum color may have many causes, such as the following: White or mucoid sputum is often seen with common colds, viral infections, or bronchitis. Yellow or green sputum is often associated with bacterial infections. Brown or black sputum indicates blood in the sputum (hemoptysis) and is seen with more serious respiratory conditions. Rust-colored sputum is associated with tuberculosis or pneumococcal pneumonia. Pink, frothy sputum may be indicative of pulmonary edema. An increase in the amount of sputum is often seen with an increase in exposure to irritants, chronic bronchitis, and pulmonary abscess. Clients with excessive, tenacious secretions may need instruction on controlled coughing and measures to reduce viscosity of secretions.
Do you wheeze when you cough or when you are active?	Wheezing indicates narrowing of the airways due to spasm or obstruction. Wheezing is associated with CHF, asthma (reactive airway disease), or excessive secretions.
Gastrointestinal Symptoms	
Do you have any gastrointestinal symptoms such as heartburn, frequent hiccups, or chronic cough?	Studies have shown that up to 75% of clients with asthma have gastroesophageal reflux disease (GERD) or are more susceptible to GERD (Cleveland Clinic, 2017).

Personal Health History

QUESTION	RATIONALE
Have you had prior respiratory problems?	A history of respiratory disease increases the risk for a recurrence. In addition, some respiratory diseases may imitate other disorders. For example, asthma symptoms may mimic symptoms commonly associated with emphysema or heart failure.
Have you ever had any thoracic surgery, biopsy, or trauma?	Previous surgeries may alter the appearance of the thorax and cause changes in respiratory sounds. Trauma to the thorax can result in lung tissue changes.
Have you been tested for or diagnosed with allergies?	Many allergic responses are manifested with respiratory symptoms such as dyspnea, cough, or hoarseness. Clients may need education on controlling the amount of allergens in their environment.
Are you currently taking medications for breathing problems or other medications (prescription or over the counter [OTC]) that affect your breathing? Do you use any other treatments at home for your respiratory problems?	Consider all medications when determining if respiratory problems could be attributed to adverse reactions. Certain medications, for example, beta-adrenergic antagonists (beta blockers), and angiotensin-converting enzyme (ACE) inhibitors are associated with the side effect of persistent cough (Van Amburgh, 2011). These medications are contraindicated with some respiratory problems such as asthma. If the client is using oxygen or other respiratory therapy at home, it is important to evaluate knowledge of proper use and precautions as well as the client's ability to afford the therapy.
Have you ever had a chest x-ray, tuberculosis (TB) skin test, or influenza immunization? Have you had any other pulmonary studies in the past?	Information on previous chest x-rays, TB skin tests, influenza immunizations, and the like is useful for comparison with current findings, and provides insight on self-care practices and possible teaching needs.
Have you recently traveled outside of the United States?	Travel to high-risk areas such as mainland China; Hong Kong; Hanoi, Vietnam; Singapore; or Toronto, Canada may have exposed the client to severe acute respiratory syndrome (SARS).

Family History

QUESTION	RATIONALE
Is there a history of lung disease in your family?	The risk for lung cancer is thought to be partially based on genetics. A history of certain respiratory diseases (asthma, emphysema) in a family may increase the risk for development of the disease (Centers for Disease Control and Prevention [CDC], 2014a). Exposure to viral or bacterial respiratory infections in the home increases the risk for development of these conditions.

QUESTION	RATIONALE
Did any family members in your home smoke when you were growing up?	Second-hand smoke puts clients at risk for COPD (including emphysema and chronic bronchitis) or lung cancer later in life (CDC, 2016, Mayo Clinic 2015).
Is there a history of other pulmonary illnesses/disorders in the family, e.g., asthma?	Some pulmonary disorders, such as asthma, tend to run in families.

Lifestyle and Health Practices

QUESTION	RATIONALE
Describe your usual dietary intake.	Poor nutritional status (both weight loss and obesity) is frequently seen in clients with COPD and is a predictor of mortality (Divo et al., 2014).
Have you ever smoked cigarettes or other tobacco products? Do you currently smoke? At what age did you start? How much do you smoke and how much have you smoked in the past? What activities do you usually associate with smoking? Have you ever tried to quit? Have you been assessed using the 5 A's of smoking cessation (Ask, Advise, Assess, Assist, Arrange) by a health professional?	Smoking is linked to a number of respiratory conditions, including lung cancer (Evidence-Based Practice 19-2). The number of years a person has smoked and the number of cigarettes per day influence the risk for developing smoking-related respiratory problems. Information on smoking behavior and previous efforts to quit may be helpful later in identifying measures to assist with smoking cessation. Answers to the 5 A's of smoking cessation can help to determine readiness for attempting to stop smoking if currently smoking.
If the client reports a history of difficulty breathing or a history of smoking ask the client to answer the DRIVE4COPD questionnaire: https://www.copdfoundation.org/downloads/COPD_PDF_Screener.pdf	This tool will help determine the client's risk level for COPD and need for a referral.
Are you exposed to any environmental conditions that affect your breathing? Where do you work? Are you around smokers?	Exposure to certain environmental inhalants can result in an increased incidence of certain respiratory conditions. Environmental irritants commonly associated with occupations include coal dust, insecticides, paint, pollution, asbestos fibers, and the like. For example, inhaling dust contaminated with *Histoplasma capsulatum* may cause histoplasmosis, a systemic fungal disease. This disease is common throughout the world, but in the United States, it is most common in the soils of the central and eastern states, especially around the Ohio and Mississippi River valleys (CDC, 2014b). Second-hand smoke is another irritant that can seriously affect a person's respiratory health.
Do you have difficulty performing your usual daily activities? Describe any difficulties.	Respiratory problems can negatively affect a person's ability to perform the usual ADLs.
What kind of stress are you experiencing at this time? How does it affect your breathing?	Shortness of breath can be a manifestation of stress. Client may need education about relaxation techniques.
Have you used any herbal medicines or alternative therapies to manage colds or other respiratory problems?	Many people use herbal therapies, such as Echinacea, or alternative therapies, such as zinc lozenges, to decrease cold symptoms. Knowing what clients are using enables you to check for side effects or adverse interactions with prescribed medications.

19-1 EVIDENCE-BASED HEALTH PROMOTION AND DISEASE PREVENTION: COPD

INTRODUCTION

Mayo Clinic (2015) defines chronic obstructive pulmonary disease (COPD) as a chronic inflammatory lung disease that causes obstructed airflow from the lungs. Emphysema and chronic bronchitis are the two main conditions that make up COPD. Healthy People 2020 (2015b) describes COPD as a preventable and treatable disease associated with airflow limitation that is not fully reversible. This airflow limitation is usually progressive and associated with inflammatory responses of the lungs to irritants from inhaled particles and gases, usually from cigarette smoke. The inflammatory obstruction in COPD causes the airways to constrict after the air is in the lungs, making exhaling the air from the lung more difficult (American Thoracic Society, 2015).

Healthy People 2020 (2015b) notes that approximately 13.6 million adults have been diagnosed with COPD, and an approximately equal number of people have the disease but have not yet been diagnosed. COPD is a major public health problem worldwide, with high prevalence, morbidity, and mortality worldwide (Soriano & Lamprecht, 2012). However,

Continued on following page

19-1 EVIDENCE-BASED HEALTH PROMOTION AND DISEASE PREVENTION: COPD (Continued)

respiratory diseases receive little attention and funding in comparison with other major causes of global morbidity and mortality.

HEALTHY PEOPLE 2020 GOAL

- Promote respiratory health through better prevention, detection, treatment, and education efforts
  - Reduce activity limitations among adults with chronic obstructive pulmonary disease (COPD)
  - Reduce deaths from COPD among adults from 113.9 deaths per 100,000 adults aged 45 years and older (2007) to 102.6 deaths per 100,000
  - Reduce hospitalizations for COPD
  - Reduce hospital emergency department visits for COPD
  - (Developmental) Increase the proportion of adults with abnormal lung function whose underlying obstructive disease has been diagnosed (objectives being developed)

SCREENING

The U.S. Preventive Services Task Force in a revised draft recommendation statement (U.S. Preventive Services Task Force [USPSTF], 2016) recommends against screening for COPD in asymptomatic adults. However, there is a simple 5-question tool for screening clients for COPD—the COPD Population Screener (2008) provided by COPD Alliance—which can be used without invasive or costly technology. Visit https://www.copdfoundation.org/downloads/COPD_PDF_Screener.pdf.

RISK ASSESSMENT

According to Mayo Clinic (2015), the risk factors associated with developing COPD are:

- Cigarette smoke exposure (smoking cigarettes or exposure to secondhand smoke), pipe smoking, cigar smoking, marijuana smoking
- Occupational exposure to dust and chemicals
- Age of 35 to 40 years and above
- Rarely, genetics (one genetic variation)

CLIENT EDUCATION

Teach Clients
- Avoid smoking cigarettes or join a tobacco cessation program if you do smoke.
- If exposed to occupational respiratory irritants, follow all preventive measures, such as wearing masks. Seek help to modify the environment, if possible, to make it less hazardous.
  - Teach client and family about the disease, treatments, and breathing techniques, proper positioning, and energy-conserving techniques (Bauldoff, 2012):
  - Pursed lip breathing reduces respirations, improves expiratory phase, and delays small airway collapse, thereby reducing air trapping in lungs.
  - Tripod positioning (sit or stand leaning forward with the arms supported) forces diaphragm down and forward, stabilizes chest while reducing work of breathing. If shortness of breath worsens with arms raised, support arms during ADLs.
  - Energy-conserving methods: Pace activities, take frequent rests, use assistive devices, and break activities into smaller tasks to help reduce dyspnea development.

19-2 EVIDENCE-BASED HEALTH PROMOTION AND DISEASE PREVENTION: LUNG CANCER

INTRODUCTION

The ALA (2015b) reports that lung cancer is the leading cause of cancer deaths in the United States (and worldwide), and causes more deaths than breast, colorectal, and prostate cancers combined. More men and women are affected, and more blacks than whites are affected, especially black males. Age is a major factor; in 2011, 82% of those living with lung cancer were 60 years or older. Looking across states, Kentucky had the highest rate and Utah the lowest, but these rates correlate with smoking rates in these states. The 5-year survival rate for lung cancer is lower than for any other cancer.

While lung cancer is classified under cancers, Healthy People 2020 (2015a) provides a thorough set of goals and objectives for reducing tobacco use, as its use is associated with many diseases—especially lung cancer. Other Healthy People 2020 goals and objectives for cancer and respiratory diseases can be found under chapters with Evidence-Based Health Promotion and Disease Prevention conditions that relate to similar diseases.

HEALTHY PEOPLE 2020 GOALS

- Reduce lung cancer deaths from 50.6 per 100,000 population to 45.5 per 100,000.
- Reduce illness, disability, and death related to tobacco use and secondhand smoke exposure.
- Reduce cigarette smoking from 20.6% of adults to 12.0%.
- Reduce use of smokeless tobacco products (snuff, chewing tobacco) from 2.3% of adults to 0.3%.
- Reduce use of cigars by adults from 2.0% to 0.2%.
- Reduce tobacco use by adolescents in all categories of tobacco use.
- Reduce the initiation of tobacco use among children, adolescents, and young adults in all tobacco categories.
- Increase smoking cessation attempts by adult smokers from 48.3% of adult smokers who attempted to stop smoking in the past 12 months to 80.0%.
- Increase recent smoking cessation success by adult smokers from 6.0% of adult smokers who last smoked 6 months to 1 year ago to 8.0%.
- Increase smoking cessation during pregnancy.
- Increase smoking cessation attempts by adolescent smokers.

SCREENING

The USPSTF (2013) recommended annual screening for lung cancer with low-dose computed tomography (LDCT) in adults aged 55 to 80 years who have a 30 pack-year smoking history and currently smoke or have quit within the past 15 years. Screening should be discontinued once a person has not smoked for 15 years or develops a health problem that substantially limits life expectancy or the ability or willingness to have curative lung surgery. The reason for this recommendation is based on lung cancer's high mortality rate as the leading cause of cancer death in the United States and the possibility of successful treatment if nonsmall cell lung cancer is found at an early stage. The USPSTF emphasizes that lung cancer screening is not an alternative to smoking cessation.

RISK ASSESSMENT

Cigarette smoking is the primary risk factor for lung cancer. The Centers for Disease Control and Prevention (CDC, 2014a) notes that tobacco smoking accounts for 90% of lung cancer cases in the United States. Inhaling cigarette smoke offers a toxic mix of over 7,000 chemicals. Following is a list of the most important risk factors for lung cancer, in addition to age, gender, and race.
- Smoking tobacco and breathing secondhand tobacco smoke
- Exposure to asbestos, radon, arsenic, diesel exhaust, some forms of silica and chromium and other substances, in the home or at work
- Personal history of radiation exposure
- Personal or family history of lung cancer
- Diet (much research being done now, but evidence that smokers who take beta-carotene supplements are at greater risk for lung cancer)

CLIENT EDUCATION

Teach Clients
- Avoid smoking cigarettes or join a tobacco cessation program if you do smoke.
- Explain that according to a 2010 study (Parsons et al., 2010), even after early-stage diagnosis of lung cancer, stopping smoking was found to double survival rate over 5 years.
- Avoid secondhand smoke exposure.
- If you live in an older house or in an area with asbestos or radon, have home or office checked to avoid exposure.
- If work or home environment has arsenic, diesel exhaust, silica, chromium, or other environmental substances that may be irritating to the lungs, use protective gear to avoid these.
- If you do smoke, avoid taking beta-carotene supplements.
- Seek a medical assessment for respiratory symptoms such as prolonged cough or pain in the chest area.

CASE STUDY

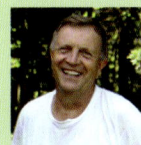

The nurse interviews Mr. Burney using specific probing questions. The client reports that he experiences chest pain when coughing and taking a deep breath. He also reports development of fever. The nurse explores Mr. Burney's health concerns using the COLDSPA mnemonic.

Mnemonic	Question	Client Response Example
Character	Describe the sign or symptom (feeling, appearance, sound, smell, or taste if applicable).	"It hurts when I cough or take a deep breath. My chest feels raw when I take a deep breath. I feel like I can't get enough air in my lungs and I'm coughing up thick, yellow phlegm."
Onset	When did it begin?	"About 6 days ago."
Location	Where is it? Does it radiate? Does it occur anywhere else?	"I have pain on the right side of my chest, but sometimes it moves to the middle of my chest."
Duration	How long does it last? Does it recur?	"Since this started, I am having a harder time breathing than I usually do. But, I only have pain in my chest with a coughing spell or when I try to take a really deep breath. I cough off and on all day and night."
Severity	How bad is it? How much does it bother you?	"I can't sleep in my bed at night because when I lie down the cough is terrible. So, I have been spending my nights in the recliner. When I am sitting, which is most of the time, my shortness of breath is not as bad. When I have to put on my clothes or eat, I can hardly catch my breath. I have been having chills off and on for a day or so."
Pattern	What makes it better or worse?	"Mucinex 600 mg every morning and Combivent 2 puffs four times a day helps me to cough up phlegm and breathe better, but I still have the pain."
Associated factors/How it **A**ffects the client	What other symptoms occur with it? How does it affect you?	"I've had a 102 temperature since yesterday. I am coughing up thick, yellow phlegm. I haven't smoked since yesterday. I usually smoke a pack a day and have for the past 51 years. I have not been able to walk in my back yard. All I do is sit around the house."

After exploring Mr. Burney's report of chest pain, cough, and fever, and long-term tobacco use, the nurse continues with the health history. Mr. Burney reports a history of shortness of breath due to emphysema first diagnosed 4 years ago and an episode of pneumonia 2 years ago. Denies having had any thoracic surgery. Mr. Burney's medication history includes: Mucinex 600 mg every AM and Combivent, 2 puffs 4 times daily. He denies medication, food, environmental, or insect allergies. Mr. Burney reports having had a chest x-ray 2 years ago that showed pneumonia and emphysema. Receives influenza vaccine annually and has had one this year. Received pneumococcal vaccine 2 years ago at age 65. Denies having had a TB skin test. Denies having had formal pulmonary function testing. Denies travel outside of the United States.

Mr. Burney's father, a smoker, suffered from emphysema and died due to lung cancer at age 67. His mother died at 74 years of age due to congestive heart failure. Mr. Burney has two younger brothers who neither smoke nor have any significant health problems. His paternal grandfather died in his 80s; the cause of death is unknown to client. His paternal grandmother died at age 85 due to "old age." Mr. Burney's maternal grandfather died at age 65 due to stomach cancer and his maternal grandmother died at age 70 due to breast cancer. Client exposed to second-hand smoke since birth. Denies any family history of asthma.

The nurse explores Mr. Burney's nutritional history. His 24-hour diet recall consists of: Breakfast—four 8-ounce cups of coffee, two glazed donuts; lunch—half of ham sandwich, 8-ounce cup of coffee; afternoon snack—chocolate chip cookies and cup of coffee; dinner—few bites of meatloaf, mashed potatoes and gravy, cup of coffee.

Mr. Burney has smoked at least one pack of cigarettes per day since he was 16 years of age (51 pack years). He has tried unsuccessfully to quit smoking a few times and states, "I like to smoke too much to quit." He reports always smoking a cigarette upon getting out of bed, after every meal, and when driving. He says that he smokes intermittently throughout the day. Denies exposure to environmental inhalants. Mr. Burney is a retired supervisor in the auto industry and worked in an office. He lives with his wife, who is a nonsmoker. He is usually able to perform ADLs with little or no difficulty. However, he reports that he has noticed having to "slow down to catch my breath" when gardening or doing yard work recently. Denies any stressors at this time. He denies use of herbal medicines or alternative therapies to manage respiratory problems.

Collecting Objective Data: Physical Examination

Examination of the thorax and lungs begins when the nurse first meets the client and observes any obvious breathing difficulties. Complete examination of the thorax and lungs consists of inspection, palpation, percussion, and auscultation of the posterior and anterior thorax to evaluate functioning of the lungs. Inspection and palpation are fairly simple skills to acquire. However, practice and experience are the best ways to become proficient with percussion and auscultation.

Preparing the Client

Have the client remove all clothing from the waist up and put on an examination gown or drape. The gown should open down the back, and is used to limit exposure. Examination of a female client's chest may create anxiety because of embarrassment related to breast exposure. Explain that exposure of the entire chest is necessary during some parts of the examination. To further ease client anxiety, explain the procedures before initiating the examination.

For the beginning of the examination, ask the client to sit in an upright position with arms relaxed at the sides. Provide explanations during the examination as you perform the various assessment techniques. Encourage the client to ask questions and to inform the examiner of any discomfort or fatigue experienced during the examination. Try to make sure that the room temperature is comfortable for the client.

Equipment

- Examination gown and drape
- Gloves
- Stethoscope
- Light source
- Mask
- Skin marker
- Metric ruler

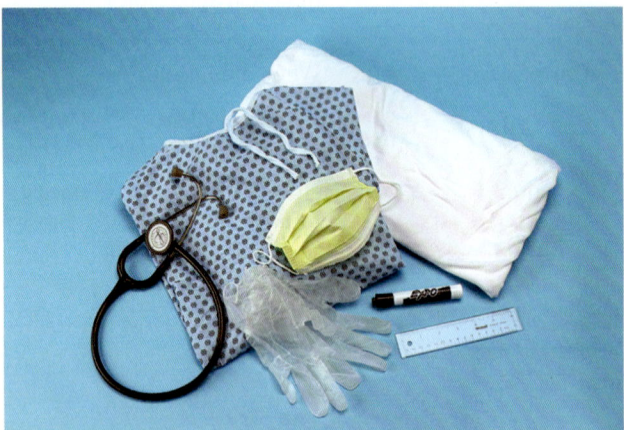

Physical Assessment

During examination of the client, remember these key points:
- Provide privacy for the client.
- Keep your hands warm to promote the client's comfort during examination.
- Remain nonjudgmental regarding the client's habits and lifestyle, particularly smoking. At the same time, educate and inform about risks, such as lung cancer and chronic obstructive pulmonary disease (COPD), related to habits.

General Routine Screening versus Focused Specialty Assessment for Lungs and Thorax

It is imperative that a nurse be able to correctly inspect, palpate, percuss, and auscultate the anterior and posterior thorax. Although inspection is more easily learned, the nurse requires additional practice and experience to become proficient at palpation, percussion, and auscultation of lung sounds. In the hospital setting the nurse auscultates lung sounds on a routine basis to determine the client's ability to adequately ventilate and to detect any complications, such as pneumonia, that would interfere with recovery. When abnormal lung sounds are detected, the nurse may proceed to palpate and percuss the thorax to further assess the problem and refer as needed. The nurse who works in an ICU or cares for clients with respiratory diseases will become more proficient with these skills and also be able to percuss for diaphragmatic excursion and auscultate voice sounds. These skills are also widely used in home health nursing, where early complications of ventilation may be detected with correct assessment of the lungs and thorax.

General Routine Screening
- Observe color of face, lips, and chest.
- Inspect color and shape of nails.
- Inspect configuration of anterior and posterior thorax.
- Observe use of accessory muscles and intercostal spaces.
- Inspect the client's positioning.
- Palpate anterior and posterior thorax for tenderness, sensation, and surface masses.
- Palpate anterior and posterior thorax for fremitus, crepitus, and surface characteristics.
- Assess anterior and posterior thorax expansion.
- Percuss for tone.
- Auscultate normal lung sounds and adventitious breath sounds.

Focused Specialty Assessment
- Percuss for diaphragmatic excursion.
- Auscultate voice sounds.

ASSESSMENT PROCEDURE	NORMAL FINDINGS	ABNORMAL FINDINGS
General		
INSPECTION		
Inspect for nasal flaring and pursed lip breathing.	Nasal flaring is not observed. Normally the diaphragm and the external intercostal muscles do most of the work of breathing. This is evidenced by outward expansion of the abdomen and lower ribs on inspiration as well as return to resting position on expiration.	Nasal flaring is seen with labored respirations (especially in small children) and is indicative of hypoxia. Pursed lip breathing may be seen in asthma, emphysema, or CHF as a physiologic response to help slow down expiration and keep alveoli open longer.
Observe color of face, lips, and chest.	The client has evenly colored skin tone, without unusual or prominent discoloration.	Ruddy to purple complexion may be seen in clients with COPD or CHF as a result of polycythemia. Cyanosis may be seen if client is cold or hypoxic. **CULTURAL CONSIDERATIONS** Cyanosis makes white skin appear blue-tinged, especially in the perioral, nailbed, and conjunctival areas. Dark skin appears blue, dull, and lifeless in the same areas.
Inspect color and shape of nails.	Pink tones should be seen in the nailbeds. There is normally a 160-degree angle between the nail base and the skin.	Pale or cyanotic nails may indicate hypoxia. Early clubbing (180-degree angle) and late clubbing (greater than a 180-degree angle) can occur from hypoxia.
Posterior Thorax		
INSPECTION		
Inspect configuration. While the client sits with arms at the sides, stand behind the client and observe the position of	Scapulae are symmetric and nonprotruding. Shoulders and scapulae are at equal horizontal positions.	Spinous processes that deviate laterally in the thoracic area may indicate scoliosis.

Continued on following page

ASSESSMENT PROCEDURE	NORMAL FINDINGS	ABNORMAL FINDINGS
Posterior Thorax (Continued)		
scapulae and the shape and configuration of the chest wall (Fig. 19-9). 🎯 **CLINICAL TIP** Some clinicians prefer to inspect the entire thorax first, followed by palpation of the anterior and posterior thorax, then percussion and auscultation of the anterior and posterior thorax.	The ratio of anteroposterior to transverse diameter is 1:2. Spinous processes appear straight, and thorax appears symmetric, with ribs sloping downward at approximately a 45-degree angle in relation to the spine. **OLDER ADULT CONSIDERATIONS** Kyphosis (an increased curve of the thoracic spine) is common in older clients (Abnormal Findings 19-1). It results from a loss of lung resiliency and a loss of skeletal muscle. It may be a normal finding. 🌐 **CULTURAL CONSIDERATIONS** Although there are definite differences in thorax size across ethnic groups, thorax size does not account for ethnic differences in lung function. Ethnic lung function differences are still being investigated (Whittaker et al., 2005).	Spinal configurations may have respiratory implications. Ribs appearing horizontal at an angle greater than 45 degrees with the spinal column are frequently the result of an increased (1 to 1) ratio between the anteroposterior and transverse diameter (barrel chest). This condition is commonly the result of emphysema due to hyperinflation of the lungs. Abnormal Findings 19-1 depicts various thoracic configurations. Trapezius, or shoulder, muscles are used to facilitate inspiration in cases of acute and chronic airway obstruction or atelectasis.
Observe use of accessory muscles. Watch as the client breathes and note use of muscles.	The client does not use accessory (trapezius/shoulder) muscles to assist breathing. The diaphragm is the major muscle at work. This is evidenced by expansion of the lower chest during inspiration.	Client leans forward and uses arms to support weight and lift chest to increase breathing capacity, referred to as the *tripod position* (Fig. 19-10). This is often seen in COPD (Evidence-Based Practice 19-1).

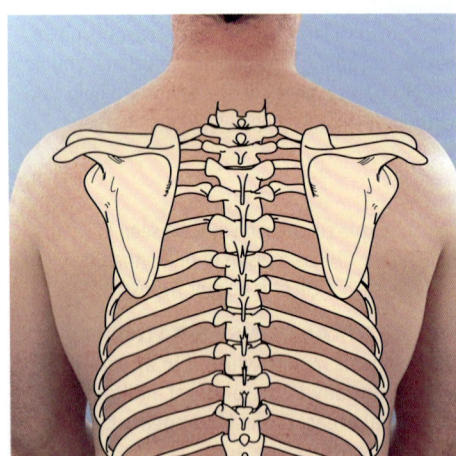

FIGURE 19-9 Observing the posterior thorax.

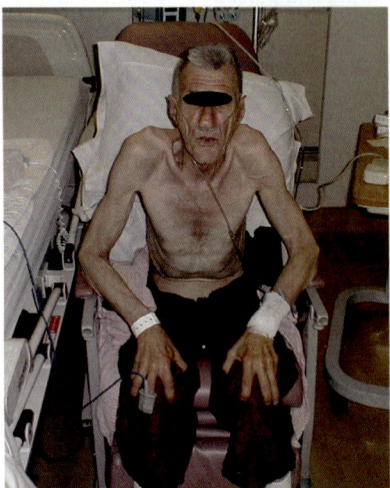

FIGURE 19-10 Tripod position seen in clients with emphysema. Leaning forward enhances use of accessory muscles to aid breathing. Loosening waistband or belt reduces abdominal constriction. There is tension in the sternocleidomastoid muscles. (Used with permission from Charles Goldberg, MD/UC San Diego. Available from http://meded.ucsd.edu/clinicalmed/lungs_tripod.jpg)

Inspect the client's positioning. Note the client's posture and ability to support weight while breathing comfortably.	Client should be sitting up and relaxed, breathing easily with arms at sides or in lap.	Tender or painful areas may indicate inflamed fibrous connective tissue. Pain over the intercostal spaces may be from inflamed pleurae. Pain over the ribs, especially at the costal chondral junctions, is a symptom of fractured ribs.

ASSESSMENT PROCEDURE	NORMAL FINDINGS	ABNORMAL FINDINGS
PALPATION		
Palpate for tenderness and sensation. Palpation may be performed with one or both hands, but the sequence of palpation is established (Fig. 19-11). Use your fingers to palpate for tenderness, warmth, pain, or other sensations. Start toward the midline at the level of the left scapula (over the apex of the left lung) and move your hand left to right, comparing findings bilaterally. Move systematically downward and out to cover the lateral portions of the lungs at the bases.	Client reports no tenderness, pain, or unusual sensations. Temperature should be equal bilaterally.	Muscle soreness from exercise or the excessive work of breathing (as in COPD) may be palpated as tenderness. Increased warmth may be related to local infection.

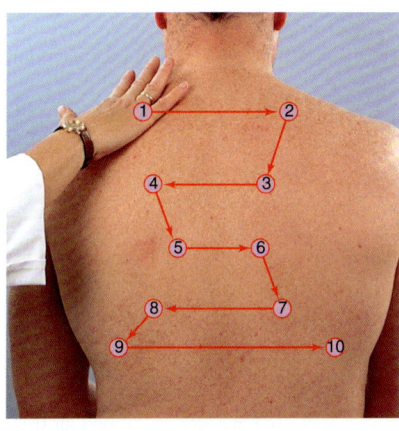

FIGURE 19-11 Sequence for palpating the posterior thorax.

Palpate for crepitus. Crepitus, also called subcutaneous emphysema, is a crackling sensation (like bones or hairs rubbing against each other) that occurs when air passes through fluid or exudate. Use your fingers and follow the sequence in Figure 19-11 when palpating.	The examiner finds no palpable crepitus.	Crepitus can be palpated if air escapes from the lung or other airways into the subcutaneous tissue, as occurs after an open thoracic injury, around a chest tube, or tracheostomy. It also may be palpated in areas of extreme congestion or consolidation. In such situations, mark margins and monitor to note any decrease or increase in the crepitant area.
Palpate surface characteristics. Put on gloves and use your fingers to palpate any lesions that you noticed during inspection. Feel for any unusual masses.	Skin and subcutaneous tissue are free of lesions and masses.	A physician or other appropriate professional should evaluate any unusual palpable mass.
Palpate for fremitus. Following the sequence described previously, use the ball or ulnar edge of one hand to assess for fremitus (vibrations of air in the bronchial tubes transmitted to the chest wall). As you move your hand to each area, ask the client to say "ninety-nine." Assess all areas for symmetry and intensity of vibration. 🎯 **CLINICAL TIP** The ball of the hand is best for assessing tactile fremitus because the area is especially sensitive to vibratory sensation.	Fremitus is symmetric and easily identified in the upper regions of the lungs. If fremitus is not palpable on either side, the client may need to speak louder. A decrease in the intensity of fremitus is normal as the examiner moves toward the base of the lungs. However, fremitus should remain symmetric for bilateral positions.	Unequal fremitus is usually the result of consolidation (which increases fremitus) or bronchial obstruction, air trapping in emphysema, pleural effusion, or pneumothorax (which all decrease fremitus). Diminished fremitus even with a loud spoken voice may indicate an obstruction of the tracheobronchial tree.
Assess chest expansion. Place your hands on the posterior chest wall with your thumbs at the level of T9 or T10	When the client takes a deep breath, the examiner's thumbs should move 5 to 10 cm apart symmetrically.	Unequal chest expansion can occur with severe atelectasis (collapse or incomplete expansion), pneumonia, chest trauma, or pneumothorax (air in the pleural space).

Continued on following page

ASSESSMENT PROCEDURE	NORMAL FINDINGS	ABNORMAL FINDINGS
Posterior Thorax (Continued)		
and pressing together a small skin fold. As the client takes a deep breath, observe the movement of your thumbs (Fig. 19-12).	**OLDER ADULT CONSIDERATIONS** Because of calcification of the costal cartilages and loss of the accessory musculature, the older client's thoracic expansion may be decreased, although it should still be symmetric.	Decreased chest excursion at the base of the lungs is characteristic of COPD. This is due to decreased diaphragmatic function.

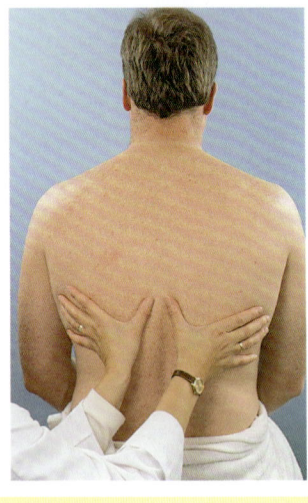

FIGURE 19-12 Starting position for assessing symmetry of chest expansion.

PERCUSSION

Percuss for tone. Start at the apices of the scapulae and percuss across the tops of both shoulders. Then percuss the intercostal spaces across and down, comparing sides. Percuss to the lateral aspects at the bases of the lungs, comparing sides. Figure 19-13 depicts the sequence for percussion.	*Resonance* is the percussion tone elicited over normal lung tissue (Fig. 19-14). Percussion elicits flat tones over the scapula.	Hyperresonance is elicited in cases of trapped air such as in emphysema or pneumothorax.

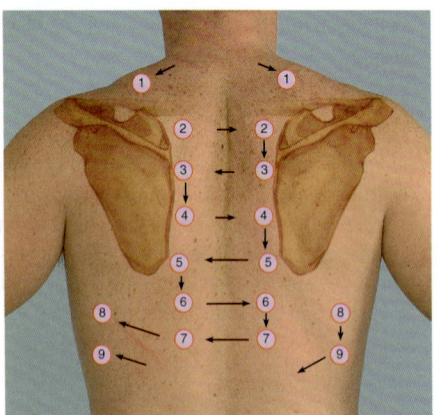

FIGURE 19-13 Percussion of the posterior thorax. With client sitting, percuss symmetrical areas of the lungs at 5 cm intervals, starting at the apex of each lung and ending at the lateral chest walls.

FIGURE 19-14 Normal percussion tones heard from the posterior thorax.

Percuss for diaphragmatic excursion. Ask the client to *exhale* forcefully and hold the breath. Beginning at the scapular line (T7), percuss the intercostal spaces of the right posterior chest wall.	Excursion should be equal bilaterally and measure 3–5 cm in adults.	Dullness is present when fluid or solid tissue replaces air in the lung or occupies the pleural space, such as in lobar pneumonia, pleural effusion, or tumor.

ASSESSMENT PROCEDURE	NORMAL FINDINGS	ABNORMAL FINDINGS
Percuss downward until the tone changes from resonance to dullness. Mark this level and allow the client to breathe. Next ask the client to *inhale* deeply and hold it. Percuss the intercostal spaces from the mark downward until resonance changes to dullness. Mark the level and allow the client to breathe. Measure the distance between the two marks (Fig. 19-15). Perform this assessment technique on both sides of the posterior thorax.	The level of the diaphragm may be higher on the right because of the position of the liver. In well-conditioned clients, excursion can measure up to 7 or 8 cm.	Diaphragmatic descent may be limited by atelectasis of the lower lobes or by emphysema, in which diaphragmatic movement and air trapping are minimal. The diaphragm remains in a low position on inspiration and expiration. Other possible causes for limited descent can be pain or abdominal changes such as extreme ascites, tumors, or pregnancy. Uneven excursion may be seen with inflammation from unilateral pneumonia, damage to the phrenic nerve, or splenomegaly.

AUSCULTATION

Auscultate for breath sounds. To best assess lung sounds, you will need to hear the sounds as directly as possible. Do not attempt to listen through clothing or a drape, which may produce additional sound or muffle lung sounds that exist. To begin, place the diaphragm of the stethoscope firmly and directly on the posterior chest wall at the apex of the lung at C7. Ask the client to breathe deeply through the mouth for each area of auscultation (each placement of the stethoscope) in the auscultation sequence so that you can best hear inspiratory and expiratory sounds. Be alert to the client's comfort and offer times for rest and normal breathing if fatigue is becoming a problem.

 OLDER ADULT CONSIDERATIONS

Deep breathing may be especially difficult for the older client, who may fatigue easily. Thus, offer rest as needed.

Auscultate from the apices of the lungs at C7 to the bases of the lungs at T10 and laterally from the axilla down to the seventh or eighth rib. Listen at each site for at least one complete respiratory cycle. Follow the auscultating sequence shown in Figure 19-17.

Three types of normal breath sounds may be auscultated—bronchial, bronchovesicular, and vesicular (Table 19-1).

◎ **CLINICAL TIP**
Breath sounds are considered normal only in the area specified. Heard elsewhere, they are considered abnormal sounds. For example, bronchial breath sounds are abnormal if heard over the peripheral lung fields.

Figure 19-16 depicts locations of normal breath sounds.

Sometimes breath sounds may be hard to hear with obese or heavily muscled clients due to increased distance to underlying lung tissue.

Diminished or absent breath sounds often indicate that little or no air is moving in or out of the lung area being auscultated. This may indicate obstruction within the lungs as a result of secretions, mucus plug, or a foreign object. It may also indicate abnormalities of the pleural space such as pleural thickening, pleural effusion, or pneumothorax. In cases of emphysema, the hyperinflated nature of the lungs, together with a loss of elasticity of lung tissue, may result in diminished inspiratory breath sounds. Increased (louder) breath sounds often occur when consolidation or compression results in a denser lung area that enhances the transmission of sound.

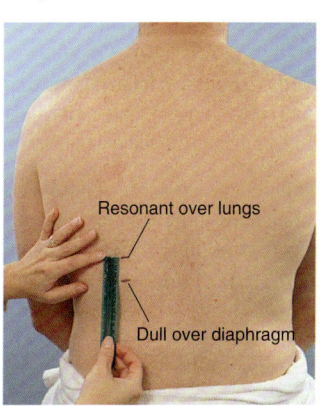

FIGURE 19-15 Measuring diaphragmatic excursion.

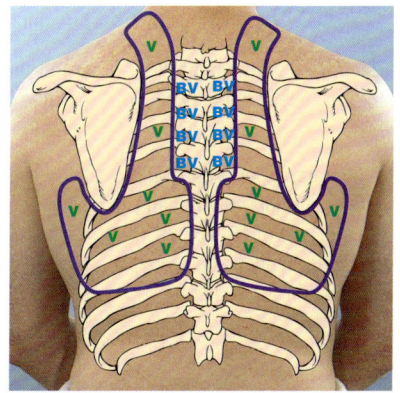

FIGURE 19-16 Location of breath sounds for the posterior thorax. V, vesicular sounds; BV, bronchovesicular sounds.

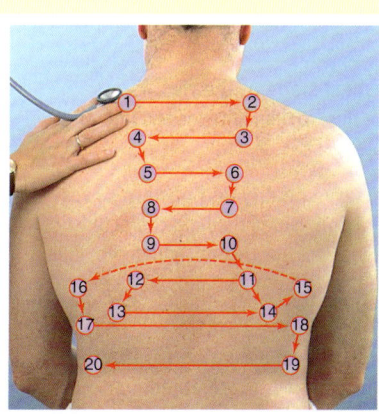

FIGURE 19-17 Sequence for auscultating the posterior thorax.

Continued on following page

ASSESSMENT PROCEDURE	NORMAL FINDINGS	ABNORMAL FINDINGS
Posterior Thorax (Continued)		
Auscultate for adventitious sounds. Adventitious sounds are sounds added or superimposed over normal breath sounds and heard during auscultation. Be careful to note the location on the chest wall where adventitious sounds are heard as well as the location of such sounds within the respiratory cycle.	No adventitious sounds, such as crackles (discrete and discontinuous sounds) or wheezes (musical and continuous), are auscultated.	Adventitious lung sounds, such as crackles (formerly called rales) and wheezes (formerly called rhonchi) are evident. See Table 19-2 for a complete description of each type of adventitious breath sound. **◎ CLINICAL TIP** If you hear an abnormal sound during auscultation, always have the client cough, then listen again and note any change. Coughing may clear the lungs.
Auscultate voice sounds.		
Bronchophony: Ask the client to repeat the phrase "ninety-nine" while you auscultate the chest wall.	Voice transmission is soft, muffled, and indistinct. The sound of the voice may be heard but the actual phrase cannot be distinguished.	The words are easily understood and louder over areas of increased density. This may indicate consolidation from pneumonia, atelectasis, or tumor.
Egophony: Ask the client to repeat the letter "E" while you listen over the chest wall.	Voice transmission will be soft and muffled but the letter "E" should be distinguishable.	Over areas of consolidation or compression, the sound is louder and sounds like "A."
Whispered pectoriloquy: Ask the client to whisper the phrase "one–two–three" while you auscultate the chest wall.	Transmission of sound is very faint and muffled. It may be inaudible.	Over areas of consolidation or compression, the sound is transmitted clearly and distinctly. In such areas, it sounds as if the client is whispering directly into the stethoscope.
Anterior Thorax		
INSPECTION		
Inspect for shape and configuration. Have the client sit with arms at the sides. Stand in front of the client and assess shape and configuration.	The anteroposterior diameter is less than the transverse diameter. The ratio of anteroposterior diameter to the transverse diameter is 1:2.	Anteroposterior equals transverse diameter, resulting in a barrel chest (Abnormal Findings 19-1). This is often seen in emphysema because of hyperinflation of the lungs.
Inspect position of the sternum. Observe the sternum from an anterior and lateral viewpoint.	Sternum is positioned at midline and straight. **◎ CLINICAL TIP** The sternum and ribs may be more prominent in the older client because of loss of subcutaneous fat.	*Pectus excavatum* is a markedly sunken sternum and adjacent cartilages (often referred to as funnel chest). It is a congenital malformation that seldom causes symptoms other than self-consciousness. *Pectus carinatum* is a forward protrusion of the sternum causing the adjacent ribs to slope backward (often referred to as pigeon chest; see Abnormal Findings 19-1 for illustrations of both conditions). Both conditions may restrict expansion of the lungs and decrease lung capacity.
Watch for sternal retractions.	Retractions not observed.	Sternal retractions are noted, with severely labored breathing.
Inspect slope of the ribs. Assess the ribs from an anterior and lateral viewpoint.	Ribs slope downward with symmetric intercostal spaces. Costal angle is within 90 degrees.	Barrel-chest configuration results in a more horizontal position of the ribs and costal angle of more than 90 degrees. This often results from long-standing emphysema.
Observe quality and pattern of respiration. Note breathing characteristics as well as rate, rhythm, and depth. Table 19-3 describes respiration patterns. **◎ CLINICAL TIP** When assessing respiratory patterns, it is more objective to describe the breathing pattern, rather than just labeling the pattern.	Respirations are relaxed, effortless, and quiet. They are of a regular rhythm and normal depth at a rate of 10–20 per minute in adults. Tachypnea and bradypnea may be normal in some clients.	Labored and noisy breathing is often seen with severe asthma or chronic bronchitis. Abnormal breathing patterns include tachypnea, bradypnea, hyperventilation, hypoventilation, Cheyne–Stokes respiration, and Biot respiration.

ASSESSMENT PROCEDURE	NORMAL FINDINGS	ABNORMAL FINDINGS
Inspect intercostal spaces. Ask the client to breathe normally and observe the intercostal spaces.	No retractions or bulging of intercostal spaces are noted.	Retraction of the intercostal spaces indicates an increased inspiratory effort. This may be the result of an obstruction of the respiratory tract or atelectasis. Bulging of the intercostal spaces indicates trapped air such as in emphysema or asthma.
Observe for use of accessory muscles. Ask the client to breathe normally and observe for use of accessory muscles.	Use of accessory muscles (sternomastoid and rectus abdominis) is not seen with normal respiratory effort. After strenuous exercise or activity, clients with normal respiratory status may use neck muscles for a short time to enhance breathing.	Neck muscles (sternomastoid, scalene, and trapezius) are used to facilitate inspiration in cases of acute or chronic airway obstruction or atelectasis. The abdominal muscles and the internal intercostal muscles are used to facilitate expiration in COPD.

PALPATION

Palpate for tenderness, sensation, and surface masses. Use your fingers to palpate for tenderness and sensation. Start with your hand positioned over the left clavicle (over the apex of the left lung) and move your hand left to right, comparing findings bilaterally. Move your hand systematically downward toward the midline at the level of the breasts and outward at the base to include the lateral aspect of the lung. The established sequence for palpating the anterior thorax (Fig. 19-18) serves as a guide for positioning your hands. 🎯 **CLINICAL TIP** Anterior and anterolateral thoracic palpation is best for assessing the right lung's middle lobe.	No tenderness or pain is palpated over the lung area with respirations.	Tenderness over thoracic muscles can result from exercising (e.g., pushups) especially in a previously sedentary client.

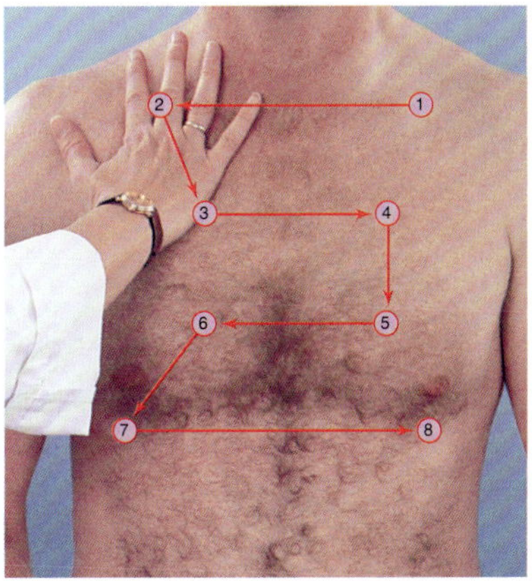

FIGURE 19-18 Sequence for palpating the anterior thorax.

Palpate for tenderness at costochondral junctions of ribs.	Palpation does not elicit tenderness.	🪑 **OLDER ADULT CONSIDERATIONS** Tenderness or pain at the costochondral junction of the ribs is seen with fractures, especially in older clients with osteoporosis.
Palpate for crepitus as you would on the posterior thorax (described previously).	No crepitus is palpated.	In areas of extreme congestion or consolidation, crepitus may be palpated, particularly in clients with lung disease.
Palpate for any surface masses or lesions.	No unusual surface masses or lesions are palpated.	Surface masses or lesions may indicate cysts or tumors.

Continued on following page

ASSESSMENT PROCEDURE	NORMAL FINDINGS	ABNORMAL FINDINGS
Anterior Thorax (Continued)		
Palpate for fremitus. Using the sequence for the anterior chest described previously, palpate for fremitus using the same technique as for the posterior thorax. 🎯 **CLINICAL TIP** When you assess for fremitus on the female client, avoid palpating the breast. Breast tissue dampens the vibrations.	Fremitus is symmetric and easily identified in the upper regions of the lungs. A decreased intensity of fremitus is expected toward the base of the lungs. However, fremitus should be symmetric bilaterally.	Diminished vibrations, even with a loud spoken voice, may indicate an obstruction of the tracheobronchial tree. Clients with emphysema may have considerably decreased fremitus as a result of air trapping.
Palpate anterior chest expansion. Place your hands on the client's anterolateral wall with your thumbs along the costal margins and pointing toward the xiphoid process (Fig. 19-19). As the client takes a deep breath, observe the movement of your thumbs.	Thumbs move outward in a symmetric fashion from the midline.	Unequal chest expansion can occur with severe atelectasis, pneumonia, chest trauma, pleural effusion, or pneumothorax. Decreased chest excursion at the bases of the lungs is seen with COPD.

PERCUSSION

Percuss for tone. Percuss the apices above the clavicles. Then percuss the intercostal spaces across and down, comparing sides (Fig. 19-20).	Resonance is the percussion tone elicited over normal lung tissue. Figure 19-21 depicts normal tones and their locations. Percussion elicits dullness over breast tissue, the heart, and the liver. Tympany is detected over the stomach, and flatness is detected over the muscles and bones. Figure 19-22 depicts locations for normal breath sounds.	Hyperresonance is elicited in cases of trapped air such as in emphysema or pneumothorax. Dullness may characterize areas of increased density such as consolidation, pleural effusion, or tumor.

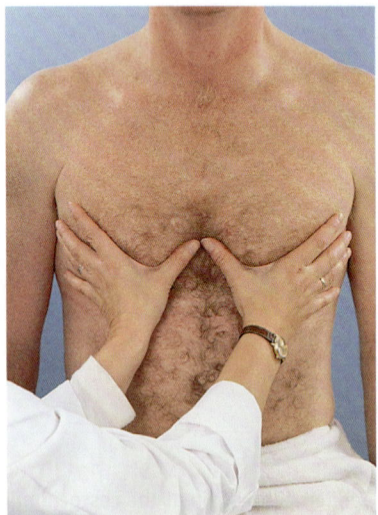

FIGURE 19-19 Palpating anterior chest expansion.

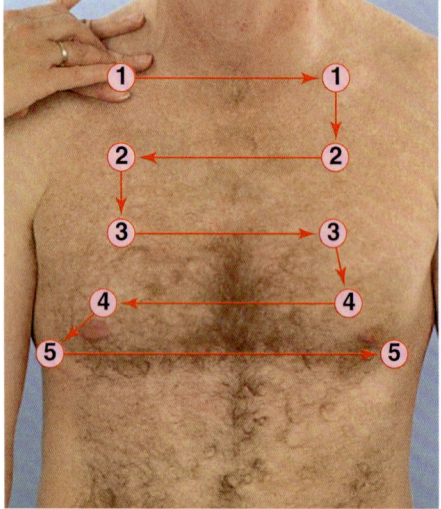

FIGURE 19-20 Sequence for percussing the anterior thorax.

AUSCULTATION

Auscultate for anterior breath sounds, adventitious sounds, and voice sounds. Place the diaphragm of the stethoscope firmly and directly on the anterior chest wall.	Refer to text in the posterior thorax section for normal voice sounds.	Refer to Table 19-2 for adventitious breath sounds.

ASSESSMENT PROCEDURE	NORMAL FINDINGS	ABNORMAL FINDINGS
Auscultate from the apices of the lungs slightly above the clavicles to the bases of the lungs at the sixth rib. Ask the client to breathe deeply through the mouth in an effort to avoid transmission of sounds that may occur with nasal breathing. Be alert to the client's comfort and offer times for rest and normal breathing if fatigue is becoming a problem, particularly for the older client. Listen at each site for at least one complete respiratory cycle. Follow the sequence for anterior auscultation shown in Figure 19-23. ◎ **CLINICAL TIP** Again, do not attempt to listen through clothing or other materials. However, if the client has a large amount of hair on the chest and/or back, listening through a thin T-shirt can decrease extraneous sounds that may be misinterpreted as crackles.		Refer to text in the posterior thorax section for abnormal voice sounds.

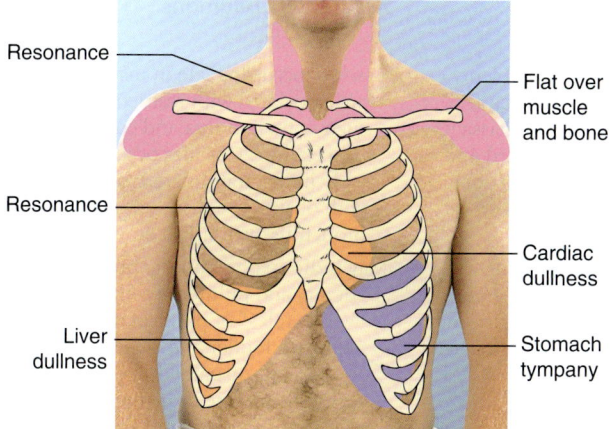

FIGURE 19-21 Normal percussion tones heard from the anterior thorax.

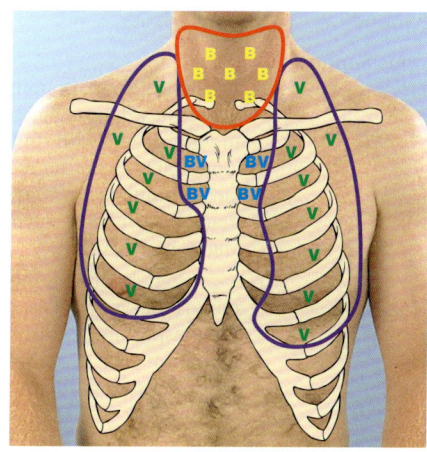

FIGURE 19-22 Location of breath sounds for the anterior thorax. B, bronchial sounds; V, vesicular sounds; BV, bronchovesicular sounds.

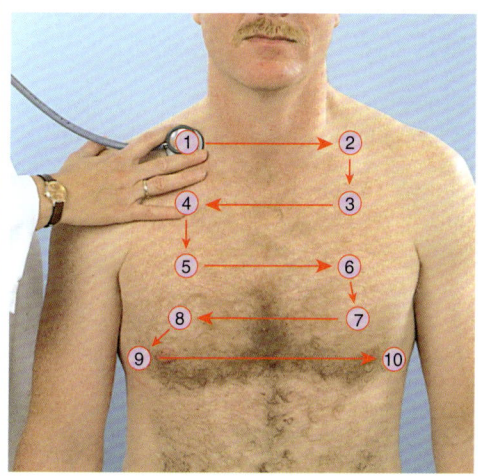

FIGURE 19-23 Sequence for auscultating the anterior thorax.

TABLE 19-1 Normal Breath Sounds

Type	Pitch	Quality	Amplitude	Duration	Location	Illustration
Bronchial	High	Harsh or hollow	Loud	Short during inspiration, long in expiration	Trachea and thorax	
Bronchovesicular	Moderate	Mixed	Moderate	Same during inspiration and expiration	Over the major bronchi—*posterior:* between the scapulae; *anterior:* around the upper sternum in the first and second intercostal spaces	
Vesicular	Low	Breezy	Soft	Long in inspiration, short in expiration	Peripheral lung fields	

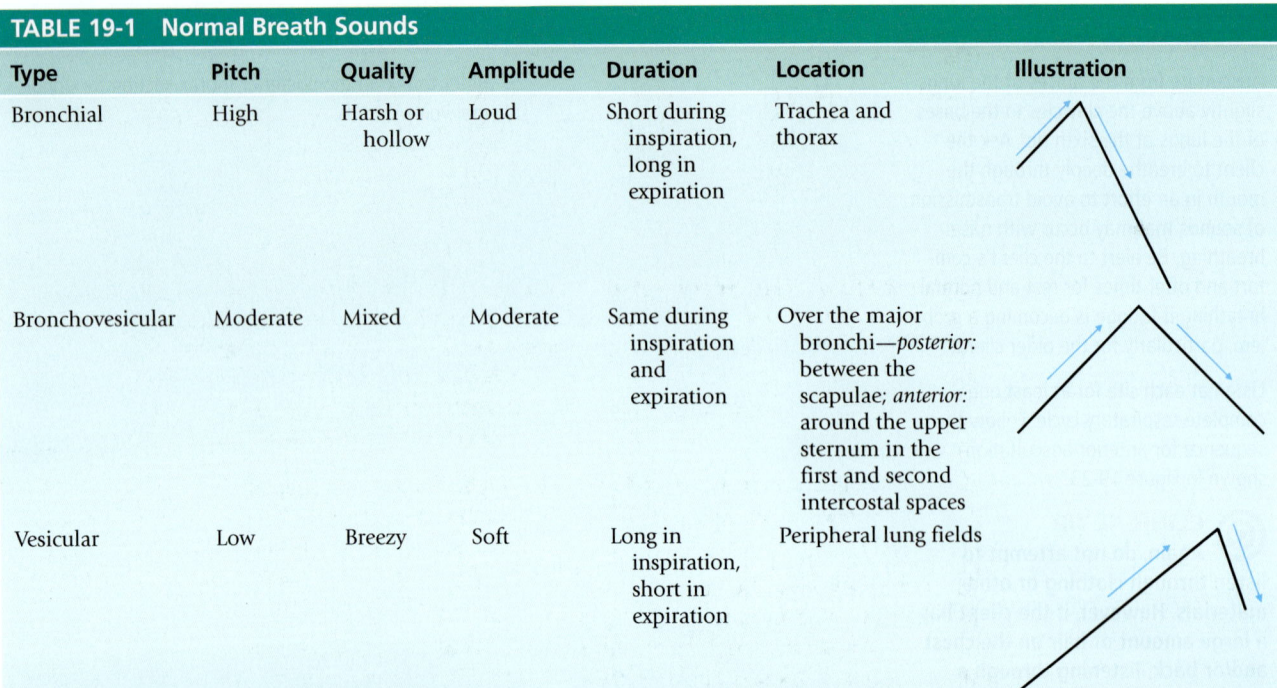

TABLE 19-2 Adventitious Breath Sounds

Abnormal Sound	Characteristics	Source	Associated Conditions
Discontinuous Sounds Crackles (fine)	High-pitched, short, popping sounds heard during inspiration and not cleared with coughing; sounds are discontinuous and can be simulated by rolling a strand of hair between your fingers near your ear.	Inhaled air suddenly opens the small, deflated air passages that are coated and sticky with exudate.	Crackles occurring late in inspiration are associated with restrictive diseases such as pneumonia and congestive heart failure. Crackles occurring early in inspiration are associated with obstructive disorders such as bronchitis, asthma, or emphysema.
Crackles (coarse)	Low-pitched, bubbling, moist sounds that may persist from early inspiration to early expiration; also described as softly separating Velcro.	Inhaled air comes into contact with secretions in the large bronchi and trachea.	May indicate pneumonia, pulmonary edema, and pulmonary fibrosis. "Velcro rales" of pulmonary fibrosis are heard louder and closer to stethoscope, usually do not change location, and are more common in clients with long-term COPD.
Continuous Sounds Pleural friction rub	Low-pitched, dry, grating sound; sound is much like crackles, only more superficial and occurring during both inspiration and expiration.	Sound is the result of rubbing of two inflamed pleural surfaces.	Pleuritis
Wheeze (sibilant)	High-pitched, musical sounds heard primarily during expiration but may also be heard on inspiration.	Air passes through constricted passages (caused by swelling, secretions, or tumor).	Sibilant wheezes are often heard in cases of acute asthma or chronic emphysema.
Wheeze (sonorous)	Low-pitched snoring or moaning sounds heard primarily during expiration but may be heard throughout the respiratory cycle. These wheezes may clear with coughing.	Same as sibilant wheeze. The pitch of the wheeze cannot be correlated to the size of the passageway that generates it.	Sonorous wheezes are often heard in cases of bronchitis or single obstructions and snoring before an episode of sleep apnea. *Stridor* is a harsh, honking wheeze with severe broncholaryngospasm, such as occurs with croup.

TABLE 19-3 Respiration Patterns

Type	Description	Pattern	Clinical Indication
Normal	12–20 breaths/min and regular		Normal breathing pattern
Tachypnea	More than 24 breaths/min and shallow		May be a normal response to fever, anxiety, or exercise Can occur with respiratory insufficiency, alkalosis, pneumonia, or pleurisy
Bradypnea	Less than 10 breaths/min and regular		May be normal in well-conditioned athletes. Can occur with medication-induced depression of the respiratory center, diabetic coma, neurologic damage
Hyperventilation	Increased rate and increased depth		Usually occurs with extreme exercise, fear, or anxiety. Causes of hyperventilation include disorders of the central nervous system, an overdose of the drug salicylate, or severe anxiety.
Kussmaul	Rapid, deep, labored		A type of hyperventilation associated with diabetic ketoacidosis
Hypoventilation	Decreased rate, decreased depth, irregular pattern		Usually associated with overdose of narcotics or anesthetics
Cheyne–Stokes respiration	Regular pattern characterized by alternating periods of deep, rapid breathing followed by periods of apnea		May result from severe congestive heart failure, drug overdose, increased intracranial pressure, or renal failure. May be noted in elderly persons during sleep, not related to any disease process
Biot respiration	Irregular pattern characterized by varying depth and rate of respirations followed by periods of apnea		May be seen with meningitis or severe brain damage
Ataxic	Significant disorganization with irregular and varying depths of respiration		A more extreme expression of Biot respirations indicating respiratory compromise
Air trapping	Increasing difficulty in getting breath out		In chronic obstructive pulmonary disease, air is trapped in the lungs during forced expiration

CASE STUDY

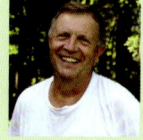

The nurse asks Mr. Burney to put on a gown, then leaves the room while he does so. The nurse returns to perform a physical examination. Inspection reveals no nasal flaring. Pursed lip breathing is noted. Client has a ruddy complexion. No cyanosis is noted. Fingernails are pale in color with a 180-degree angle between the nail base and skin.

Posterior Thorax: Inspection reveals scapulae are symmetric and nonprotruding; ratio of anteroposterior to transverse diameter is 1:1, giving a "barrel" chest appearance. Client is using accessory muscles and sitting in tripod position to facilitate breathing. Upon palpation of posterior thorax client reports no tenderness, pain, or unusual sensations. Posterior thorax skin temperature is equal bilaterally. No crepitus is palpable. Skin and subcutaneous tissue are free of lesions and masses. Fremitus is nonsymmetric, with significant decrease over right lower thorax. Chest expansion is unequal, with decrease on the right. Overall, chest expansion measures 3.5 cm. Percussion reveals hyperresonance on the left and right upper and mid-posterior thorax, with dullness over the right lower thorax. Diaphragmatic excursion measures 2.5 cm on the left and 1.3 cm on the right. Diminished vesicular breath sounds on left throughout and right upper and mid-lung, with scattered high-pitched expiratory wheezes. Breath sounds greatly diminished, with course crackles in right lower lung. Bronchophony, egophony, and whispered pectoriloquy nonsymmetric, with increased transmission and/or clarity of sounds over right lower lung.

Anterior Thorax: Inspection reveals barrel-chest configuration with anteroposterior to transverse ratio of 1:1. Sternum is midline and straight. No sternal retractions noted. Costal angle increased at 120 degrees. Respirations regular and tachypneic, with respiratory rate of 24 per minute. No tenderness or pain noted over lung area or costochondral spaces. No crepitus, masses, or lesions palpated. Fremitus diminished over right lower lung. Chest expansion is asymmetric. Hyperresonance with percussion noted with exception of dullness over right lower lung. Vesicular and bronchovesicular breath sounds diminished, with scattered expiratory wheezes described posteriorly.

Validating and Documenting Findings

If there are discrepancies between objective and subjective data or if abnormal findings are inconsistent with other data, validate your data (by asking additional questions, verifying data with another health care professional, or comparing objective with subjective findings). This is necessary to verify that the data are reliable and accurate. Document the assessment data following the health care facility or agency policy.

CASE STUDY

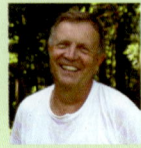

Think back to the case study. The nurse completed the following documentation of her assessment of Mr. Burney.

Biographic Data: George Burney, 67 years old, Caucasian. Retired auto manufacturing industry supervisor with high school education. Alert and oriented. Asks and answers questions appropriately.

Reason for Seeking Health Care: "It hurts when I cough or take a deep breath. My chest feels raw when I take deep breath. I feel like I can't get enough air in my lungs and I'm coughing up yellow phlegm."

History of Present Health Concern: Six days ago, Mr. Burney began to develop right-sided chest pain intermittently radiating to his mid-chest, cough with tan sputum production. Experiencing dyspnea with minimal activity and orthopnea. Has been sleeping in a recliner since onset of symptoms. Two days ago, his symptoms escalated and now has dyspnea at rest. Reports development of fever up to 102 degrees and chills in the past 24 hours. He was diagnosed with emphysema 4 years ago and continues to smoke cigarettes. Also had episode of pneumonia 2 years ago.

Past Health History: Denies having had any thoracic surgery. Denies any seasonal or environmental allergies. Reports having had a chest x-ray 2 years ago that showed pneumonia and emphysema. Receives influenza vaccine annually and has had one this year. Denies having had a TB skin test. Denies having had formal pulmonary function testing. Denies travel outside the United States.

Family History: Mr. Burney's father, a smoker, suffered from emphysema and died due to lung cancer at age 67. Mother deceased at 74 years of age due to congestive heart failure. Mr. Burney has two younger brothers who neither smoke nor have any significant health problems. His paternal grandfather died in his 80s; cause of death unknown to client. His paternal grandmother deceased at age 85 due to "old age." His maternal grandfather died at age 65 due to stomach cancer and his maternal grandmother died at age 70 due to breast cancer. Client has been exposed to secondhand smoke since birth. Denies any family history of asthma.

Lifestyle and Health Practices: Twenty-four-hour diet recall: Breakfast—Four 8-ounce cups of coffee, 2 glazed donuts; lunch—half of ham sandwich, 8-ounce cup of coffee; afternoon snack—chocolate chip cookies and cup of coffee; dinner—few bites of meatloaf, mashed potatoes and gravy, cup of coffee.

Has smoked at least one pack of cigarettes per day since the age of 16 years (51 pack years). Has tried unsuccessfully to quit smoking a few times. States, "I like to smoke too much to quit." Always smokes a cigarette upon getting out of bed, after every meal, and when driving. Smokes intermittently throughout the day. Denies exposure to environmental inhalants. Lives with his wife, who is a nonsmoker. Is usually able to perform activities of daily living with little or no difficulty. However, reports that he has noticed having to "slow down to catch my breath" when gardening or doing yard work recently. Denies any stressors at this time.

Medications include: Combivent 2 puffs four times daily. Mucinex 600 mg every morning. Denies medication, food, environmental, or insect allergies. Denies use of herbal medicines or alternative therapies to manage respiratory problems.

Physical Examination Findings: Inspection reveals no nasal flaring. Pursed lip breathing is noted. Client has a ruddy complexion. No cyanosis is noted. Fingernails are pale in color, with a 180-degree angle between the nail base and skin.

Posterior Thorax: Inspection reveals scapulae are symmetric and nonprotruding; ratio of anteroposterior to transverse diameter is 1:1, giving a "barrel" chest appearance. Client using accessory muscles and sitting in tripod position to facilitate breathing. Upon palpation of posterior thorax, client reports no tenderness, pain, or unusual sensations. Posterior thorax skin temperature is equal bilaterally. No crepitus is palpable. Skin and subcutaneous tissue are free of lesions and masses. Fremitus nonsymmetric, with significant decrease over right lower thorax. Chest expansion unequal, with decrease on the right. Overall, chest expansion measures 3.5 cm. Percussion reveals hyperresonance on the left and right upper and mid-posterior thorax, with dullness over the right lower thorax. Diaphragmatic excursion measures 2.5 cm on the left and 1.3 cm on the right. Diminished vesicular breath sounds on left throughout and right upper and mid-lung with scattered high-pitched expiratory wheezes. Breath sounds greatly diminished, with course crackles in right lower lung. Bronchophony, egophony, and whispered pectoriloquy nonsymmetric, with increased transmission and/or clarity of sounds over right lower lung.

Anterior Thorax: Inspection reveals barrel chest configuration, with anteroposterior to transverse ratio of 1:1. Sternum is midline and straight. No sternal retractions noted. Costal angle increased at 120 degrees. Respirations regular and tachypneic, with respiratory rate of 24 per minute. No tenderness or pain noted over lung area or costochondral spaces. No crepitus, masses, or lesions palpated. Fremitus diminished over right lower lung. Chest expansion asymmetric. Hyperresonance with percussion noted with exception of dullness over right lower lung. Vesicular and bronchovesicular breath sounds diminished, with scattered expiratory wheezes throughout and coarse crackles in right lower lung. Voice sounds same anteriorly as described posteriorly.

After you have collected your assessment data, you will need to use diagnostic reasoning skills to analyze it.

ANALYSIS OF DATA: DIAGNOSTIC REASONING

After collecting subjective and objective data pertaining to the thorax and lung assessment, identify abnormal findings and client strengths. Then cluster the data to reveal any significant patterns or abnormalities. These data may then be used to make clinical judgments about the status of the client's thorax and lungs.

Selected Nursing Diagnoses

Following is a listing of selected nursing diagnoses (health promotion, risk, or actual) that you may identify when analyzing the clue clusters.

Health Promotion Diagnoses

- Readiness for Enhanced Breathing Patterns
- Readiness for Enhanced Health Management: Requests information on TB skin testing, how to quit smoking, or on exercises to improve respiratory status

Risk Diagnoses

- Risk for Respiratory Infection related to exposure to environmental pollutants and lack of knowledge of precautionary measures
- Risk for Activity Intolerance related to imbalance between oxygen supply and demand
- Risk for Imbalanced Nutrition: Less Than Body Requirements related to fatigue secondary to dyspnea
- Risk for Ineffective Health Maintenance related to lack of knowledge of condition, infection transmission, and prevention of recurrence
- Risk for Impaired Oral Mucous Membranes related to mouth breathing

Actual Diagnoses

- Anxiety related to dyspnea and fear of suffocation
- Activity Intolerance related to fatigue secondary to inadequate oxygenation
- Ineffective Airway Clearance related to inability to clear thick, mucous secretions secondary to pain and fatigue
- Impaired Gas Exchange related to chronic lung tissue damage secondary to chronic smoking
- Ineffective Airway Clearance related to bronchospasm and increased pulmonary secretions
- Ineffective Breathing Pattern: Hyperventilation related to hypoxia and lack of knowledge of controlled breathing techniques
- Disturbed Sleep Pattern related to excessive coughing
- Impaired Gas Exchange related to poor muscle tone and decreased ability to remove secretions secondary to the aging process

Selected Collaborative Problems

After grouping the data, certain collaborative problems may become apparent. Remember that collaborative problems differ from nursing diagnoses in that they cannot be prevented by nursing intervention. However, these physiologic complications of medical conditions can be detected and monitored by the nurse. In addition, the nurse can use physician- and nurse-prescribed interventions to minimize the complications of these problems. The nurse may also have to refer the client in such situations for further treatment of the problem. Following is a list of collaborative problems that may be identified when obtaining a general impression. These problems are worded as Risk for Complications (RC), followed by the problem.

- RC: Atelectasis
- RC: Pneumonia
- RC: Chronic obstructive pulmonary disease
- RC: Asthma
- RC: Bronchitis
- RC: Pleural effusion
- RC: Pneumothorax
- RC: Pulmonary edema
- RC: Tuberculosis

Medical Problems

Development of RC and/or other signs and symptoms may clearly require medical treatment and referral to a primary care provider.

CASE STUDY

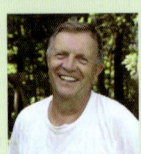

After collecting and analyzing the data for Mr. Burney, the nurse determines that the following conclusions are appropriate:

Nursing Diagnoses
- Ineffective Airway Clearance r/t knowledge deficit of energy-conserving and appropriate coughing techniques
- Ineffective Health Maintenance r/t denial of effects of cigarette smoking on current health status

Potential Collaborative Problems
- RC: Respiratory failure
- RC: Hypoxemia
- RC: Pneumonia

Refer to primary care provider for signs of COPD and potential pneumonia. To view an algorithm depicting the process of diagnostic reasoning for this case, go to **thePoint**.

Interdisciplinary Verbal Communication of Assessment Findings Using SBAR

SITUATION: GB, a 67-year-old Caucasian male, walks into free clinic reporting fever and chest pain when he takes deep breath or coughs.

BACKGROUND: Diagnosed with emphysema 4 years ago, and with pneumonia 2 years ago. Takes Mucinex 600 mg every AM and Combivent, 2 puffs four times daily. Last chest x-ray 2 years ago revealed pneumonia and emphysema. Receives influenza vaccine annually and has had one this year. Received pneumococcal vaccine at age 65. Father died from lung cancer, age 67. Mother died at age 74 with congestive heart failure. Has 51 pack years of smoking, and continues to smoke 1 pack per day. No difficulty with ADLs except to have to "slow down to catch my breath" when gardening or doing yard work recently. Pursed lip breathing and ruddy complexion present. No cyanosis. Fingernails pale with a 180-degree angle between the nail base and skin.

ASSESSMENT
Posterior Thorax: Has anteroposterior to transverse diameter of 1:1 ("barrel" chest). Uses accessory muscles and sits in tripod position. Fremitus is nonsymmetrical, with significant decrease over right lower thorax. Chest expansion unequal and decreased on right. Chest expansion 3.5 cm. Percussion hyperresonance on left and right upper and mid-posterior thorax, with dullness over right lower thorax. Diaphragmatic excursion 2.5 cm on left and 1.3 cm on right. Diminished vesicular breath sounds on left throughout and right upper and mid-lung, with scattered high-pitched expiratory wheezes. Breath sounds greatly diminished, with coarse crackles in right lower lung. Bronchophony, egophony, and whispered pectoriloquy nonsymmetric, with increased transmission and clarity of sounds over right lower lung.

Anterior Thorax: No sternal retractions noted. Costal angle increased at 120 degrees. Respirations regular and tachypneic, with respiratory rate of 24 per minute. Fremitus diminished over right lower lung. Chest expansion asymmetric. Hyperresonance percussed with exception of dullness over right lower lung. Vesicular and bronchovesicular breath sounds diminished, with scattered expiratory wheezes as described posteriorly.

RECOMMENDATION: GB has Ineffective Airway Clearance r/t knowledge deficit of energy-conserving and appropriate coughing techniques. He is at risk for complications of respiratory failure, hypoxemia, and pneumonia. He needs to be further assessed by his primary care provider for COPD and possible complications.

ABNORMAL FINDINGS 19-1 — Thoracic Deformities and Configurations

Normal chest configuration.

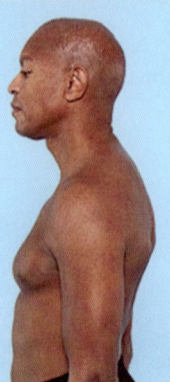

Barrel chest.

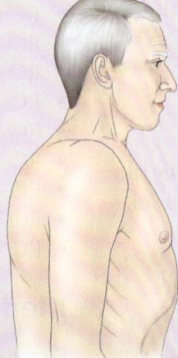

(Smeltzer, S. (2010). *Brunner & Suddarth's Textbook of Medical-Surgical Nursing* (12th ed). Philadelphia, PA: Lippincott Williams & Wilkins.)

Pectus excavatum (funnel chest).

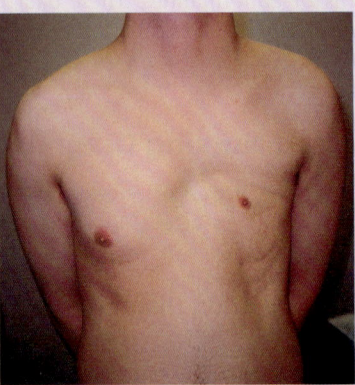

(Berg, D. & Worzala, K. (2006). *Atlas of Adult Physical Diagnosis*. Philadelphia: Lippincott Williams & Wilkins.)

Pectus carinatum (pigeon chest).

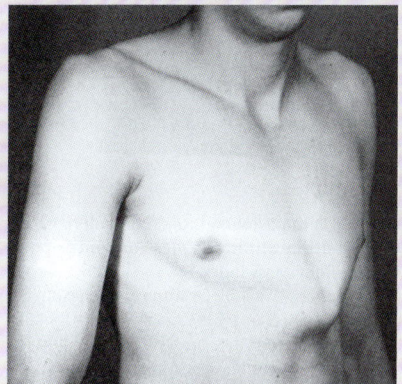

(Shamberger, R. C. Chest wall deformities. In Shields TW, ed. *General Thoracic Surgery 4th ed.* Baltimore: Lippincott Williams & Wilkins, 1994: 529–557.)

Scoliosis.

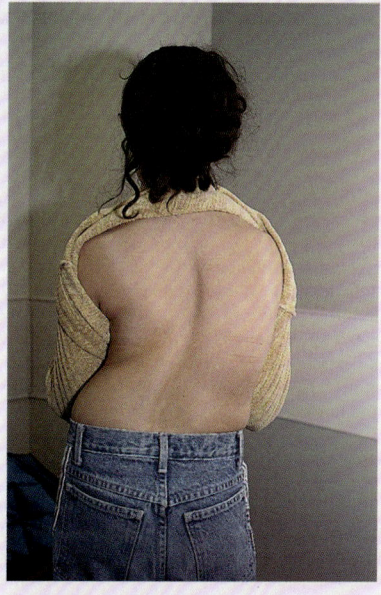

(Courtesy of George A. Datto, III, MD).

Kyphosis.

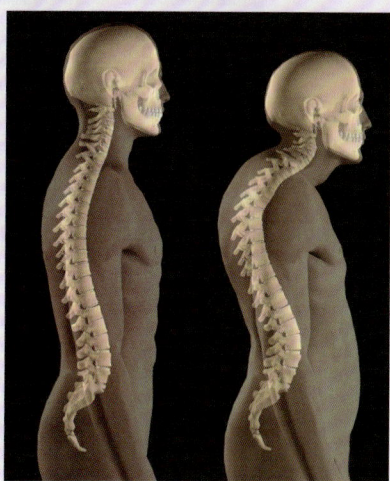

LifeART image ©2014 Lippincott Williams & Wilkins. All rights reserved.

Kyphosis, an exaggerated increased rounding of the thoracic spine, often seen with osteoporosis in older women.

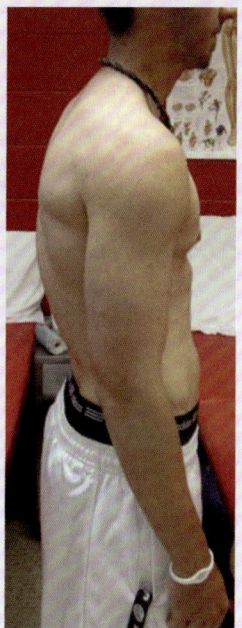

Athletes who use their arms in an overhead position, such as swimmers, often have a forward-translated head, pronounced thoracic kyphosis, lumbar lordosis, and internally rotated shoulders.

(Miniaci, A. (2013). Disorders of the Shoulder: Sports Injuries. Philadelphia: Wolters Kluwer.)

> **Concept Mastery Alert**
>
> To distinguish kyphosis from scoliosis, remember that kyphosis involves an exaggerated curvature of the thoracic vertebrae. Conversely, scoliosis involves abnormal lateral deviation of the spine. In many cases, it involves lateral deviations in cervical, thoracic, and lumbar vertebrae.

Want to know more?

A wide variety of resources to enhance your learning and understanding of this book are available on thePoint. Visit thePoint to access:

NCLEX-Style Student Review Questions
Watch and Learn Videos
Concepts in Action Animations
And more!

References and Selected Readings

American Lung Association (ALA). (2015a). Asthma: Symptoms, causes, and risk factors. Available at http://www.lung.org/lung-health-and-diseases/lung-disease-lookup/asthma/asthma-symptoms-causes-risk-factors/

American Lung Association (ALA). (2015b). Lung cancer fact sheet. Available at http://www.lung.org/lung-health-and-diseases/lung-disease-lookup/lung-cancer/learn-about-lung-cancer/lung-cancer-fact-sheet.html

American Lung Association (ALA). (2015c). Lung health and diseases. Available at http://www.lung.org/lung-health-and-diseases/

American Sleep Apnea Association (ASAA). (n.d.). Sleep apnea. Available at http://www.sleepapnea.org/learn/sleep-apnea.html

American Thoracic Society. (2015). What is chronic obstructive pulmonary disease COPD? Available at http://www.thoracic.org/copd-guidelines/for-patients/what-is-chronic-obstructive-pulmonary-disease-copd.php

Bauldoff, G. (2012). When breathing is a burden: How to help patients with COPD. Available at http://www.americannursetoday.com/when-breathing-is-a-burden-how-to-help-patients-with-copd-2/

Centers for Disease Control and Prevention (CDC). (2016). Smoking and COPD. Available at http://www.cdc.gov/tobacco/campaign/tips/diseases/copd.html

Centers for Disease Control and Prevention (CDC). (2014a). Lung cancer: Risk factors. Available at http://www.cdc.gov/cancer/lung/basic_info/risk_factors.htm

Centers for Disease Control and Prevention (CDC). (2014b). Sources of histoplasmosis. Available at http://www.cdc.gov/fungal/diseases/histoplasmosis/causes.html

Cleveland Clinic. (2017). GERD and asthma. Available at http://my.clevelandclinic.org/health/articles/gerd-and-asthma

COPD Population Screener. (2008). Available at http://copd.org/sites/default/files/COPD-Screener.pdf

Divo, M., Cabrera, C., Casanova, C., et al. (2014). Comorbidity distribution, clinical expression and survival in COPD patients with different body mass index. *Journal of the COPD Foundation*, 1(2), 229–238. doi: doi.org/10.15326/jcopdf.1.2.2014.0117. Available at http://journal.copdfoundation.org/jcopdf/id/1036/Comorbidity-Distribution-Clinical-Expression-and-Survival-in-COPD-Patients-with-Different-Body-Mass-Index

Healthy People 2020. (2015a). Cancer. Available at http://www.healthypeople.gov/2020/topics-objectives/topic/cancer

Healthy People 2020. (2015b). Respiratory diseases. Available at http://www.healthypeople.gov/2020/topics-objectives/topic/respiratory-diseases

Mayo Clinic. (2015). COPD. Available at http://www.mayoclinic.org/diseases-conditions/copd/basics/definition/con-20032017

Parsons, A., Daley, A., Begh, R., et al. (2010). Influence of smoking cessation after diagnosis of early stage lung cancer on prognosis. *British Medical Journal*, 340, b5569. doi:10.1136/bmj.b5569. Available at http://www.lungcanceralliance.org/assets/docs/get-information/Influence%20of%20smoking%20cessation%20after%20diagnosis%20of%20early%20stage%20lung%20cancer%20on%20prognosis.pdf

Soriano, J., & Lamprecht, B. (2012). Chronic obstructive pulmonary disease: A worldwide problem. *Medical Clinics of North America*, 96(4), 671–680. doi: 10.1016/j.mcna.2012.02.005. Available at http://www.ncbi.nlm.nih.gov/pubmed/22793937

U.S. Preventive Services Task Force (USPSTF). (2016). Draft recommendation statement: Chronic obstructive pulmonary disease: Screening. Available at http://www.uspreventiveservicestaskforce.org/Page/Document/draft-recommendation-statement159/chronic-obstructive-pulmonary-disease-screening

U.S. Preventive Services Task Force (USPSTF). (2013). Lung cancer screening. Available at http://www.uspreventiveservicestaskforce.org/Page/Document/RecommendationStatementFinal/lung-cancer-screening

Van Amburgh, J. (2011). Why do antihypertensives cause cough? Available at http://www.medscape.com/viewarticle/739521

Whittaker, A., Sutton, A., & Beardsmore, C. (2005). Are ethnic differences in lung function explained by chest size? *Archives of Disease in Children – Fetal and Neonatal*, 90(5), F423–F428. doi: 10.1136/adc.2004.062497. Available at http://www.ncbi.nlm.nih.gov/pmc/articles/PMC1721951/

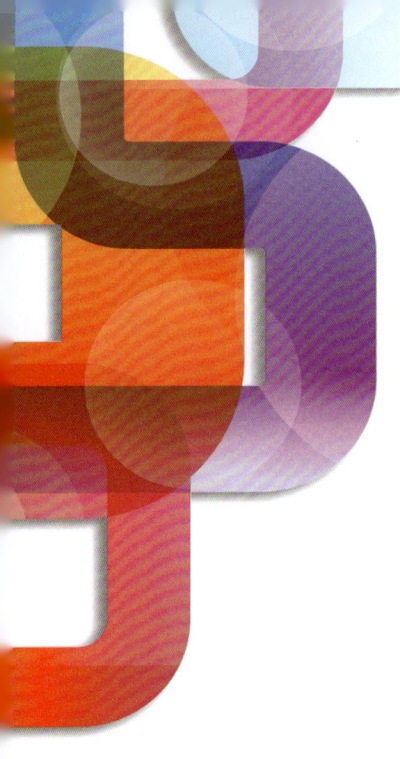

20 ASSESSING BREASTS AND LYMPHATIC SYSTEM

Learning Objectives

1. Describe the structure and the function of the breast and major axillary lymph nodes.
2. Discuss risk factors associated with breast cancer across the cultures and ways to reduce one's risks.
3. Interview a client for an accurate nursing history of the breasts and axillary lymph nodes.
4. Perform a physical assessment of the breasts and axillary lymph nodes using the correct techniques.
5. Differentiate between normal and abnormal findings of breasts and axillary lymph nodes.
6. Explain the correct method for teaching a client how to perform self breast examination.
7. Describe the findings frequently seen with assessing the older client's breasts and axillary lymph nodes.
8. Analyze the data from the interview and physical assessment of the breasts and axillary lymph nodes to formulate valid nursing diagnoses, collaborative problems, and/or referrals.
9. Differentiate between general routine screening versus skills needed for focused or specialty assessment of the breasts and axillary lymph nodes.
10. Document and verbally report accurate assessment findings of the breasts and axillary lymph nodes.

CASE STUDY

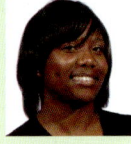

Nicole Barnes, a 31-year-old African American woman, is concerned with breast lumps and tenderness that occur each month before her menses. She comes to the office for her annual well-woman examination. Ms. Barnes's case will be discussed throughout the chapter.

STRUCTURE AND FUNCTION

The *breasts* are paired mammary glands that lie over the muscles of the anterior chest wall, anterior to the pectoralis major and serratus anterior muscles. Depending on their size and shape, the breasts extend vertically from the second to the sixth rib and horizontally from the sternum to the mid-axillary line (Fig. 20-1).

The male and female breasts are similar until puberty, when female breast tissue enlarges in response to the hormones estrogen and progesterone, which are released from the ovaries. The female breast is an accessory reproductive organ with two functions: to produce and store milk that provides nourishment for newborns and to aid in sexual stimulation. The male breasts have no functional capability.

For purposes of describing the location of assessment findings, the breasts are divided into four quadrants by drawing horizontal and vertical imaginary lines that intersect at the nipple. The upper outer quadrant, which extends into the axillary area, is referred to as the *tail of Spence*. Most breast tumors occur in this quadrant (Fig. 20-2).

Lymph nodes are present in both male and female breasts. These structures drain lymph from the breasts to filter out microorganisms and return water and protein to the blood.

External Breast Anatomy

The skin of the breasts is smooth and varies in color depending on the client's skin tones. The *nipple*, which is located in the center of the breast, contains the tiny openings of the lactiferous ducts through which milk passes. The *areola* surrounds the nipple (generally 1- to 2-cm radius) and contains elevated sebaceous glands (Montgomery glands) that secrete a protective lipid substance during lactation. Hair follicles commonly appear around the areola. Smooth muscle fibers in the areola cause the nipple to become more erectile during stimulation.

409

410   UNIT 3 Nursing Assessment of Physical Systems

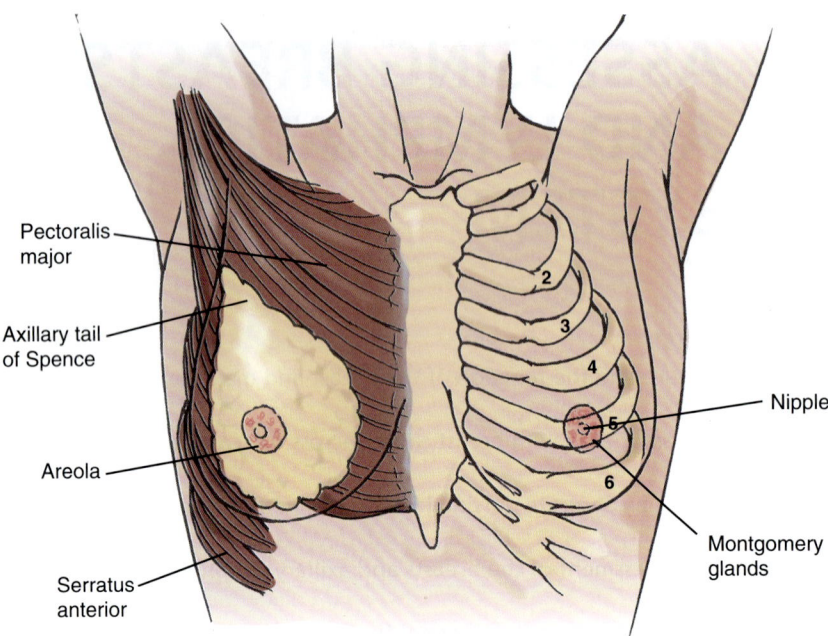

FIGURE 20-1 Anatomic breast landmarks and their position in the thorax.

The nipple and areola typically have darker pigment than the surrounding breast. Their color ranges from dark pink to dark brown, depending on the person's skin color. The amount of pigmentation increases with pregnancy, then decreases after lactation. It does not, however, entirely return to its original coloration.

During embryonic development, a milk line or ridge extends from each axilla to the groin area (Fig. 20-3). It gradually atrophies and disappears as the person grows and develops. However, in some clients, *supernumerary nipples* or other breast tissue may appear along this "milk line" (see physical examination section).

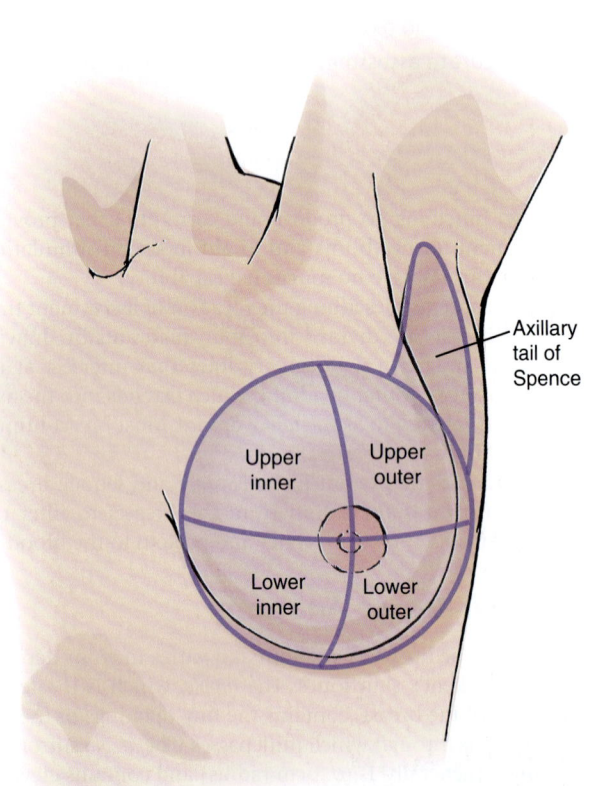

FIGURE 20-2 Breast quadrants. The upper outer quadrant is the area most targeted by breast cancer.

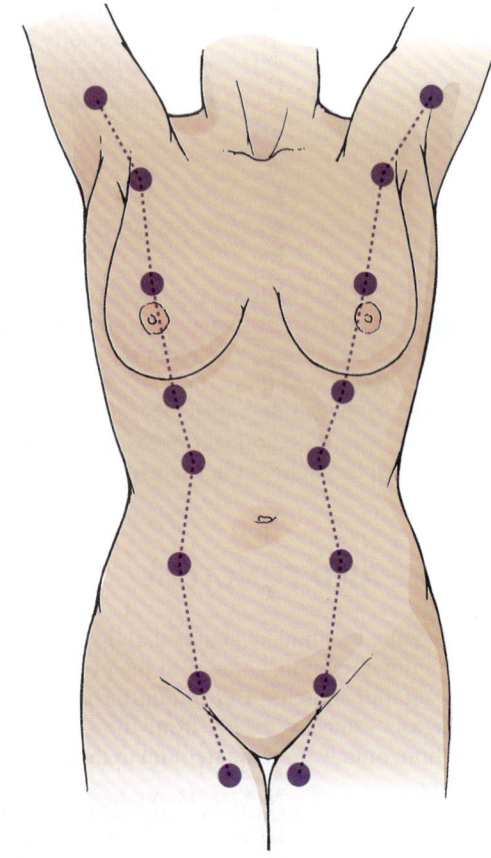

FIGURE 20-3 Supernumerary nipples along the "milk line," which extends bilaterally from the axilla to the groin.

20 Assessing Breasts and Lymphatic System   411

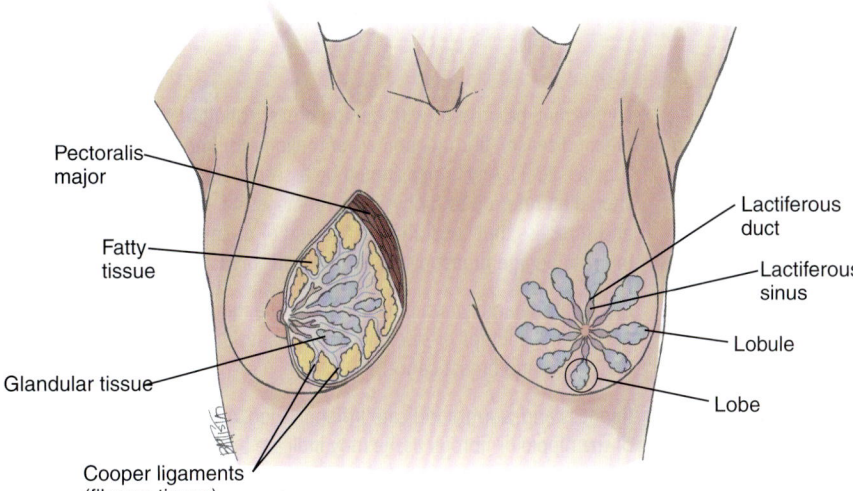

FIGURE 20-4 Internal anatomy of the breast.

Internal Breast Anatomy

Female breasts consist of three types of tissue: glandular, fibrous, and fatty (adipose) (Fig. 20-4). *Glandular tissue* constitutes the functional part of the breast, allowing for milk production. Glandular tissue is arranged in 15 to 20 lobes that radiate in a circular fashion from the nipple. Each lobe contains several lobules in which the secreting alveoli (acini cells) are embedded in grape-like clusters.

Mammary ducts from the alveoli converge into a single lactiferous duct that leaves each lobe and conveys milk to the nipple. The slight enlargement in each duct before it reaches the nipple is called the *lactiferous sinus*. The milk can be stored in the lactiferous sinus (or ampullae) until stimulated to be released from the nipple.

The *fibrous tissue* provides support for the glandular tissue largely by way of bands called Cooper ligaments (suspensory ligaments). These ligaments run from the skin through the breast and attach to the deep fascia of the muscles of the anterior chest wall.

Fatty tissue is the third component of the breast. The glandular tissue is embedded in the fatty tissue. This subcutaneous and retromammary fat provides most of the substance to the breast, determining the size and shape of the breasts. The functional capability of the breast is not related to size but rather to the glandular tissue present.

The amount of glandular, fibrous, and fatty tissue varies according to various factors including the client's age, body build, nutritional status, hormonal cycle, and whether she is pregnant or lactating.

Lymph Nodes

The major *axillary lymph nodes* consist of the anterior (pectoral), posterior (subscapular), lateral (brachial), and central (mid-axillary) nodes (Fig. 20-5). The anterior nodes drain the anterior chest wall and breasts. The posterior chest wall and part of the arms are drained by the posterior nodes.

The lateral nodes drain most of the arms, and the central nodes receive drainage from the anterior, posterior, and lateral lymph nodes. A small proportion of the lymph also flows into the infraclavicular or supraclavicular lymph nodes or deeper into nodes within the chest or abdomen.

HEALTH ASSESSMENT

This chapter covers the examination of the nonpregnant woman's breasts. Subjective and objective data related to breast changes associated with pregnancy are covered in Chapter 29.

Collecting Subjective Data: The Nursing Health History

When interviewing clients—especially females—about the breasts, keep in mind that this topic may evoke a wide spectrum of emotions from the client. Explore your own feelings regarding body image, fear of breast cancer, and the influence of the breasts on self-esteem. Western culture emphasizes the breasts for femininity and beauty as well as lactation. Fear, anxiety, or embarrassment may influence the client's ability to discuss the condition of the breasts and breast self-examination (BSE, if done) or breast self-awareness. Men with gynecomastia or cancer of the breast may be embarrassed to have what they consider a "female condition." The following questions provide guidance in conducting the interview.

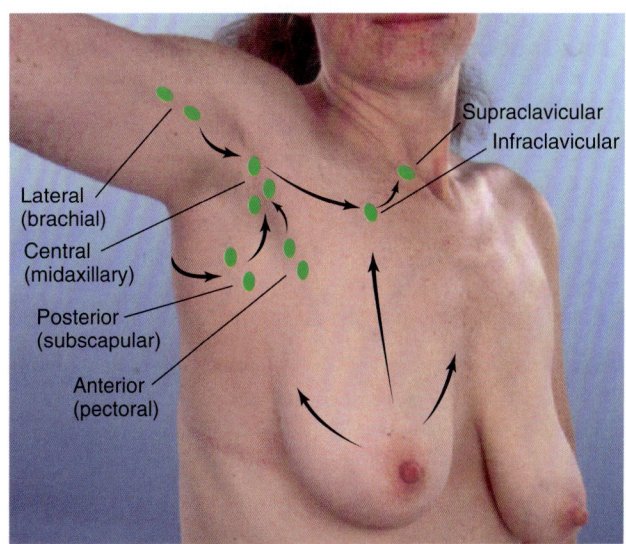

FIGURE 20-5 The lymph nodes drain impurities from the breasts (*arrows* show direction).

History of Present Health Concern

QUESTION	RATIONALE
Have you noticed any lumps or swelling in your breasts? If so, where? When did you first notice it? Has the lump grown or swelling increased? Is the lump or swelling associated with other problems? Does the lump or swelling change during your menstrual cycle?	Lumps may be present with benign breast conditions (fibrocystic breast disease), fibroadenomas, or malignant tumors (Evidence-Based Practice 20-1). Any lumps should be assessed further, and the client should be referred to a physician. Premenstrual breast lumpiness and soreness that subside after the end of the menstrual cycle may indicate benign breast disease (fibrocystic breast changes).
Have you noticed any lumps or swelling in the underarm area?	Breast tissue and lymph nodes in the axilla may become enlarged, appearing as lumps or swelling with inflammation, fibroadenomas, infections, and breast cancer.
Have you noticed any redness, warmth, or dimpling of your breasts? Any rash on the breast, nipple, or axillary area?	Redness and warmth indicate inflammation. A dimpling or retraction of the nipple or fibrous tissue may indicate breast cancer.
Have you noticed any change in the size or firmness of your breasts?	A recent increase in the size of one breast may indicate inflammation, pregnancy, lactation, or abnormal growth. **OLDER ADULT CONSIDERATIONS** The older client may notice a decrease in the size and firmness of the breasts as she ages because of a decrease in estrogen levels. Glandular tissue decreases whereas fatty tissue increases. A well-fitting supportive bra can reduce breast discomfort related to sagging breasts.
Do you experience any pain in your breasts? If yes, use **COLDSPA** to further explore the symptom. **Character:** Describe the pain (dull, aching, sharp). **Onset:** When did this first begin? **Location:** Point to the area where the pain occurs. Does it radiate to other areas? **Duration:** How long does it last? Does it recur? How often? **Severity:** Describe the pain on a scale of 1–10 (10 being the most severe). Does it limit any of your activities you perform in a day's time? **Pattern:** What do you do when you have this pain? What medications do you take to relieve the pain? **Associated Factors:** Does it occur at any specific time during your menstrual cycle? Do you have any other symptoms when you have this pain (nipple discharge, changes in color of breast, swelling)?	Pain and tenderness of the breasts are common in fibrocystic breasts, especially just before and during menstruation. This is especially true for clients taking oral contraceptives. Symptoms of fibrocystic breasts may include: • Breast pain or tenderness • Lumps or areas of thickening • Fluctuating size of breast lumps • Green or dark brown nonbloody nipple discharge • Changes in both breasts (Mayo Clinic, 2013) Breast pain can also be a late sign of breast cancer.
Do you have any discharge from the nipples? If so, describe its color, consistency, and odor, if any. When did it start? Which nipple has the discharge?	If the client reports any blood or blood-tinged discharge, she should be referred for further evaluation. Sometimes, a clear benign discharge may be manually expressed from a breast that is frequently stimulated. Certain medications (oral contraceptives, phenothiazines, steroids, digitalis, and diuretics) are also associated with a clear discharge. Further evaluation is needed if the discharge is spontaneous, unilateral, is bloody or guaiac-positive discharge; if the client is over 40 or a male; or if a mass is also palpable (Kosir, 2013).

Personal Health History

QUESTION	RATIONALE
Have you had any prior breast disease? Have you ever had breast surgery, a breast biopsy, breast implants, or breast trauma? If so, when did this occur? What was the result?	A personal history of breast cancer increases the risk for recurrence of cancer. Previous surgeries may alter the appearance of the breasts. Breast problems may occur with silicone breast implants. Trauma to the breasts from sports, accidents, or physical abuse can result in breast tissue changes.
How old were you when you began to menstruate? Have you experienced menopause?	Early menses (before age 12) or delayed menopause (after age 52) increases the risk for breast cancer.

QUESTION	RATIONALE
Have you given birth to any children? At what age did you have your first child?	The risk of breast cancer is greater for women who have never given birth or for those who had their first child after age 30.
When was the first and last day of your menstrual cycle?	This information will inform you if this is the optimal time to examine the breasts. Hormone-related swelling, breast tenderness, and generalized lumpiness are reduced right after menstruation.

Family History

QUESTION	RATIONALE
Is there a history of breast cancer in your family? Who (sister, mother, maternal grandmother)?	A history of breast cancer in one's family increases one's risk for breast cancer. Hereditary forms of breast cancer constitute only 5–10% of breast cancer cases overall (Jardines et al., 2015).

Lifestyle and Health Practices

QUESTION	RATIONALE
Are you taking any hormones, contraceptives, or antipsychotic agents?	Hormones and some antipsychotic agents can cause breast engorgement in women. Hormones and oral contraceptives also increase the risk of breast cancer. Haloperidol (Haldol), an antipsychotic drug, can cause galactorrhea (persistent milk secretion whether or not the woman is breast-feeding) and lactation. This is also a side effect of medroxyprogesterone (Depo-Provera) injections. Galactorrhea usually is medication-induced. The most common pathologic cause of galactorrhea is a pituitary tumor. Other causes include hypothalamic and pituitary stalk lesions, neurogenic stimulation, thyroid disorders, and chronic renal failure (Leung & Pacaud, 2004).
Do you live or work in an area where you have excessive exposure to radiation, benzene, or asbestos?	Exposure to these environmental hazards can increase the risk of breast cancer.
What is your typical daily diet?	A high-fat diet may increase the risk for breast cancer.
How much alcohol do you consume each day? How often do you use tobacco each day?	Alcohol intake exceeding two drinks per day and tobacco use has been associated with a higher risk for breast cancer.
How much coffee, tea, cola (or other forms of caffeine) do you consume each day?	Caffeine can aggravate a fibrocystic breast condition.
Do you engage in any type of regular exercise? If so, what type of bra do you wear when you exercise?	Breast tissue can lose its elasticity if vigorous exercise (i.e., running, aerobics) is performed without support for the breast. A well-fitting, supportive bra can also reduce discomfort in the breasts during exercise.
How important are your breasts to you in relation to a positive feeling about yourself and your physical appearance? Do you have any fears regarding breast disease?	The condition of the breasts may significantly influence how a woman feels about herself. Alterations in the breasts may threaten a woman's body image and feelings of self-worth, and men may be embarrassed to have enlarged breasts.
Do you examine your own breasts? Describe when you do this. Have you noted any changes in your breasts such as a lump, swelling, skin irritation, or dimpling, nipple pain or retraction (turning inward), redness or scaliness on nipple or breast skin, or discharge? If yes, have you reported this to your health care provider? **CLINICAL TIP** If the client has breast implants, she should check her breasts regularly, paying extra attention to how breasts look and feel. The implants have a different texture than original breast tissue. In 90% of breast cancer cases, the woman finds the breast lump herself and learning to recognize changes with the implants is one of the best ways to detect cancer if it develops (MD Anderson Cancer Center, 2016).	Breast self-examination (BSE) is discouraged by some organizations, such as the U.S. Preventive Services Task Force (USPSTF, 2009), while other organizations remain neutral. An alternative called breast self-awareness (becoming familiar with the appearance, feel, and shape of one's breasts and nipples) is supported by some. For higher risk individuals, BSE is an option for women starting in their 20s (Box 20-1). Women should report any breast changes to their health professional right away. Women should be told about the following benefits and limitations of BSE: • Research has shown that BSE plays a small role in finding breast cancer. • Some women feel very comfortable doing BSE regularly (usually monthly after their period) using the systematic approach, while other women are more comfortable looking and feeling their breasts while showering or getting dressed.

Continued on following page

Lifestyle and Health Practices (Continued)

QUESTION	RATIONALE
Press firmly inward at the edges of the breast implants to feel the ribs beneath, checking for any lumps or bumps. However, be careful not to manipulate (i.e., squeeze) the valve on the implant excessively, which may cause valve leakage and make the breast implant deflate. Any new lumps or suspicious lesions (sores) should be evaluated with a biopsy. If a biopsy is performed, care must be taken to avoid puncturing the implant.	• Some women become very stressed about "doing it right." • BSE helps the woman or man become more aware of what their breast tissue is like in order to detect any changes. • The most important goal is for the client to report any breast changes to a health care professional right away. • Women or men who choose to do BSE should have their BSE technique reviewed during their physical examination by a health professional. • It is okay for clients to choose not to do BSE or not to do it on a regular schedule. Mammogram is the screening of choice for breast cancer.
CLINICAL TIP Older clients and others who no longer menstruate and who decide to continue with BSE may find it helpful to pick a set day of the month for BSE, a date they will remember each month such as the day of the month they were born.	Some women may choose not to do BSE even if knowledgeable of the benefits and limitations. This choice needs to be accepted by the examiner (American Cancer Society [ACS], 2015a). It is important for women to know their breasts and report any breast changes promptly to their health care providers. Remember that most of the time breast changes are not cancer but it is important to detect breast cancer early for effective treatment. Women who have had a breast lumpectomy, augmentation, or breast reconstruction may also perform BSE.
Have you ever had your breasts examined by a health care provider? When was your last examination?	The ACS recommends against regular clinical breast examinations based on research findings (ACS, 2015a). However, any findings from a previous examination are useful to provide a baseline comparative assessment.
	CLINICAL TIP Although rare, men can have breast cancer, which may not be caught until the late stages, because many in society are unaware of its occurrence in men (Al-Haddad, 2010).
Have you ever had a mammogram? If so, when was your last one? **CULTURAL CONSIDERATIONS** Breast cancer is a leading cause of mortality and morbidity in Canada. Breast screening may be less than optimal in Canadian women, especially in Iranian immigrant women residing in Toronto, who were found to have little knowledge of breast cancer and screening practices. It is essential that the nurse assess the client's knowledge regarding risks and recommended screenings (Vahabi, 2011). **CULTURAL CONSIDERATIONS** Genetic variation: About 5–10% of breast cancer cases are thought to be hereditary. *BRCA1* and *BRCA2* genes are the most common cause of hereditary breast cancer. In the United States, *BRCA* mutations are found most often in Jewish women of Ashkenazi (Eastern Europe) origin (Center for Jewish Genetics, 2016). Breast cancer incidence reported by the Centers for Disease Control and Prevention (CDC, 2015) shows converging rates for Caucasians and blacks, with lower rates for Hispanics and the lowest rates for Asians. Breast cancer deaths, however, are significantly higher for blacks, with Caucasians lower and Asians and Hispanics at the lowest rates. Black women were found to have various perceptions about the risks of breast cancer related to existing knowledge, stigmatization, as well as spiritual and religious beliefs, which can decrease their engagement in breast cancer screening (Banning, 2010).	Women of age 40 and older should have a screening mammogram every year and should continue to do so for as long as they are in good health (American College of Radiology [ACR], 2015). The USPSTF (2009) recommends biennial screening mammography for women aged 50–74 years. The decision to start regular, biennial screening mammography before the age of 50 years should be an individual one and take patient context into account, including the client's values regarding specific benefits and harms. The USPSTF concludes that the current evidence is insufficient to assess the additional benefits and harms of screening mammography in women 75 years or older. The USPSTF concludes that the current evidence is insufficient to assess the additional benefits and harms of either digital mammography or magnetic resonance imaging (MRI) instead of film mammography as screening modalities for breast cancer.

20-1 EVIDENCE-BASED HEALTH PROMOTION AND DISEASE PREVENTION: BREAST CANCER

INTRODUCTION

The National Cancer Institute: Surveillance Epidemiology and End Result (SEER) Stat Fact Sheets on breast cancer (2015) report that an estimated 231,840 new breast cancer cases would be diagnosed in the United States in 2015 and estimated 2015 deaths from breast cancer would be 40,290. The lifetime risk of developing breast cancer, based on data from 2010 to 2012, is 12.3%. Death rates have been slowly falling, with the 5-year survival rate for 2005–2011 at 89.4%. The median age of diagnosis for the years 2008–2012 was 61 years. Women between the ages of 55 and 64 have the highest rate of diagnosis. Incidence of breast cancer for all races is 124.8 per 100,000 US women. Caucasian women have a higher incidence then the US national average. The NCI: SEER reports that death rates by race show a higher percentage among Black females.

Breast cancer appears in various forms, and a number of classifications are used.

Breast cancer classifications:
- Breast cancer type (see below)
- Breast cancer grade (based on cell differentiation level from Grades 1–3)
- Estrogen or progesterone receptors positive or negative
- Heu2/neu positive or negative (a growth-promoting protein instructed by the Heu2/neu gene to produce too much of the protein, which causes cancers to grow faster)
- DNA and other gene expressions

Types of breast cancer:
The ACS (2015b), Mayo Clinic (2015), and National Breast Cancer Foundation (2016) describe the majority of these types as follows:

- *Ductal carcinoma in situ (DCIS):* noninvasive and confined to the linings of the milk duct system; appears early
- *Invasive (infiltrating) ductal carcinoma (IDC):* most common type (70–80% of breast cases), which spreads beyond the ductal system
- *Medullary carcinoma:* occurs in women in their late 40s and 50s and accounts for about 3–5% of cases
- *Invasive (infiltrating) lobular carcinoma (ILC):* accounts for about 10% of all invasive cases, and usually appears as a subtle thickening, feeling of fullness, change in texture or appearance of the breast or nipple skin, rather than as a discreet lump
- *Triple negative carcinoma (TNC):* cells in the tumor are negative for progesterone, estrogen, and HER2/neu receptors; accounts for between 10% and 20% of diagnosed breast cancer cases, and is more likely to affect younger people, African Americans, Hispanics, and/or those with a BRCA1 gene mutation
- *Tubular carcinoma:* usually found in women over 50 years of age, accounts for 2% of cases, and has a 95% 10-year survival rate
- *Mucinous carcinoma (colloid):* occurs in 1–2% of breast cancers, and although the cancer cells produce mucus and are poorly defined, usually has a favorable prognosis
- *Inflammatory breast carcinoma (IBC):* very rare and very aggressive, with lymph vessels in skin blocked, making the breast appear swollen, red, and inflamed. It accounts for 1–5% of cases in the United States
- *Paget disease of the breast:* rare disease affecting the skin of the nipple and often the areola; people with Paget disease of the breast often have one or more cancerous tumors in the breast itself (National Cancer Institute, 2012).

HEALTHY PEOPLE 2020 GOALS (2014)

- Reduce the female breast cancer death rate.
- Reduce late-stage female breast cancer.
- Increase the proportion of women who receive a breast cancer screening based on the most recent guidelines.
- Increase the proportion of women who were counseled by their providers about mammograms.

Based on the 2007 female breast cancer statistics (23.0 deaths per 100,000), the Healthy People 2020 target of 10% improvement translates to 20.7 deaths per 100,000 females.

SCREENING

Screening recommendations for breast cancer vary greatly from the very conservative recommendations of the U.S. Preventive Services Task Force (USPSTF) to those of other organizations, such as ACS (2016a).

The USPSTF (2009) recommends biennial screening mammography for women aged 50–74 years. The decision to start regular biennial screening mammography before the age of 50 years should be an individual one and take client context into account, including the client's values regarding specific benefits and harms. The USPSTF concludes that the current evidence is insufficient to assess the additional benefits and harms of screening mammography in women 75 years or older. The USPSTF concludes that the current evidence is insufficient to assess the additional benefits and harms of either digital mammography or magnetic resonance imaging (MRI) instead of film mammography as screening modalities for breast cancer.

The USPSTF recommends against teaching breast self-examination (BSE). The USPSTF concludes that the current evidence is insufficient to assess the additional benefits and harms of clinical breast examination (CBE) beyond screening mammography in women 50 years or older.

A report by Berkeley Wellness (2015) reviews findings of studies and of the Canadian Task Force on Preventive Health Care, which support the conclusion that breast self-examination does "more harm than good." However, they note that the American Cancer Association takes a more neutral view, saying that women should be informed of the benefits and limitations of such examinations and choose for themselves whether to do them or not. Berkeley Wellness notes a shift to a new approach of "breast self-awareness." This approach "encourages women to be mindful of what their breasts normally look and feel like so they can inform their health care providers if they detect any changes." This approach is favored by the American College of Obstetricians and Gynecologists and the National Comprehensive Cancer Network. However, the ACOG noted that this shift in approach is not based on evidence for its efficacy.

ACR (2015), along with the Society of Breast Imaging, supports starting mammograms at age 40 and recommends that women with significant risk factors for breast cancer begin screening at least by age 30, but not before age 25.

The ACS supports offering the option of yearly mammograms at age 40–45, with annual mammograms from 45 to 54, and every 2 years for those women over 55 (ACS, 2016b). The ACS (2015b) has changed its guidelines regarding BSE and clinical breast examination. It states due to lack of evidence, regular clinical breast examinations and BSE are not recommended. However, BSE is an option for women starting in their 20s, due to the fact that research has shown that BSE plays a small role in finding breast cancer.

Because studies show that dense breast tissue is six times more likely to develop cancer, and dense tissue makes it harder to detect breast cancer on mammograms, Breastcancer.org (2016) recommends that women with dense breast tissue consult with their health care provider to determine the best screening methods.

Continued on following page

20-1 EVIDENCE-BASED HEALTH PROMOTION AND DISEASE PREVENTION: BREAST CANCER (Continued)

RISK ASSESSMENT (ACS, 2016C)

Assess for the following nonmodifiable risks:
- Gender: Females are 100 times more likely to develop breast cancer than males (estrogen and progesterone are implicated).
- Age: Risk increases with age, especially for invasive breast cancers.
- Genetics: About 5–10% of breast cancer cases are thought to be hereditary. *BRCA1* and *BRCA2* genes are the most common cause of hereditary breast cancer. In the United States, *BRCA* mutations are found most often in Jewish women of Ashkenazi (Eastern Europe) origin.
- Race/ethnicity: Caucasian women are at greater risk for diagnosis of breast cancer and Black women are at greater risk for dying of breast cancer in the United States.
- Family history (genetics and ethnicity): Even if father or brother has had breast cancer, risk is increased.
- Personal history of breast cancer (three- to fourfold risk of cancer in the same or other breast)
- Breast consistency: Denser breasts increase risk.
- Early menstruation (before 12 years of age) or later menopause (older than 55 years)
- Previous chest radiation (for therapy) before age 40
- Diethylstilbestrol exposure (1940s and 1950s), used by women to avoid miscarriage, or in daughters of mothers who took this medication

Assess for modifiable risk factors (lifestyle factors):
- Having no children or giving birth to first child after 30 years of age.
- Recent oral contraceptive use (risk declines to normal after 10 years of no use).
- Use of menopausal combined hormone replacement therapy (both estrogen and progesterone; risk is highest in first 2–3 years but long use increases risk; risk reduces to normal risk after 2–3 years without therapy). Estrogen-only therapy increases risk if used for 10 years or longer.
- No history of breast-feeding. Breast-feeding may have a protective effect due to reduced lifetime number of menstrual cycles.
- Alcohol consumption (increased risk with increased intake; especially drinking 2–5 drinks a day).
- Excess weight or obesity (due to increased fat tissue after menopause, increasing estrogen levels).
- Weight gain as adult female (studies not showing same for weight gain as child).
- Limited physical activity: increasing activity to include from 1.25 to 2.5 hours of brisk walking at least 5 days per week has been shown to decrease risk by 18% (ACS, 2016b).
- Even dim light at night while sleeping has been shown to speed the growth of human breast cancer tumors implanted into rats, and makes the tumors resistant to tamoxifen (Yardell, 2014).

Unclear associations with breast cancer (under further study):
- Night work (such as nurses on night shift)
- Exposure to secondhand smoke
- Environmental chemicals with estrogen-like properties
- Diet and vitamin intake

For an easy-to-use breast cancer risk assessment model, see the Gail model at http://www.cancer.gov/bcrisktool/

CLIENT EDUCATION

Teach Clients
- Women and men can have breast cancer; both should note any changes in breast size, shape, or tissue consistency and report to health care provider.
- Inform clients of different screening recommendations and advise them to talk with their health care provider to determine the best screening protocol for them (see screening recommendations above under Screening).

Teach About the Risk Factors for Breast Cancer
- Get intentional physical exercise for least 45–60 minutes per day for 5 or more days per week.
- Avoid alcohol intake of more than one alcoholic beverage per day (e.g., 6-oz glass of wine).
- Avoid excessive weight gain, especially as an adult and especially after menopause.
- Be aware of increased risk if client has no children or had first child after 30 years of age.
- Note breast consistency and be aware that denser breasts increase risk; women with denser breast tissue should work with their health care provider to establish a recommendation for screening patterns.
- Consider family history of breast cancer and note risk if genetic kin, including father and brothers, have had breast cancer.
- Night shift work and exposure to secondhand smoke may be linked to increased risk for breast cancer.
- Avoid even dim light source while sleeping at night (Yardell, 2014).
- Advise client to talk with health care provider after completing a formal breast cancer risk assessment such as the Gail Model.

BOX 20-1 SELF-ASSESSMENT: BREAST AWARENESS AND SELF-EXAMINATION

Although newer guidelines recommend against both BSE and clinical breast examination, especially those from the USPSTF (2009), women should be told about the benefits and limitations of breast self-examination (BSE) in their twenties. Even if they do not perform full breast self-examination, women should become familiar with the way their breasts feel and report any new breast changes to a health professional. Changes do not necessarily indicate cancer. A woman can notice changes by feeling her breasts occasionally (breast awareness), or by choosing to use the guidelines below to examine her breasts on a regular basis. Her examination technique should be reviewed periodically with a health care provider. It is best to examine breasts when they are not tender or swollen. Women with breast implants may have the surgeon identify the implant edges. Pregnant or breastfeeding women may also choose to examine their breasts regularly. It is acceptable for women to choose not to do BSE or to only occasionally perform it. If women choose not to do BSE, they still need to become familiar with the normal look and feel of their breasts, and report any changes to their health care provider immediately.

THE FIVE STEPS OF A BREAST SELF-EXAMINATION

Step 1: Look at your breasts in the mirror with your shoulders straight and your arms on your hips. Check size, shape, and color. Notice if they are evenly shaped with no distortion or swelling.

Notify your doctor if you notice:
- Dimpling, puckering, or bulging of the skin
- A nipple that has changed position or an inverted nipple (pushed inward instead of sticking out)
- Redness, soreness, rash, or swelling

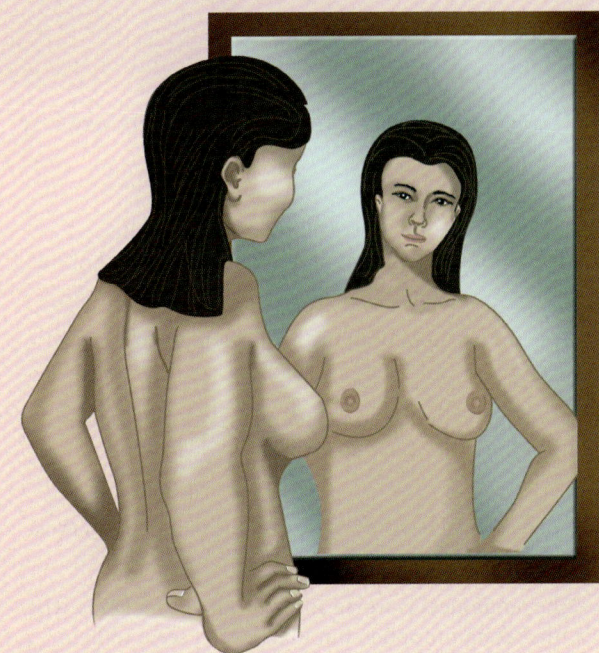

Step 2: Raise your arms and determine if you see the same changes.

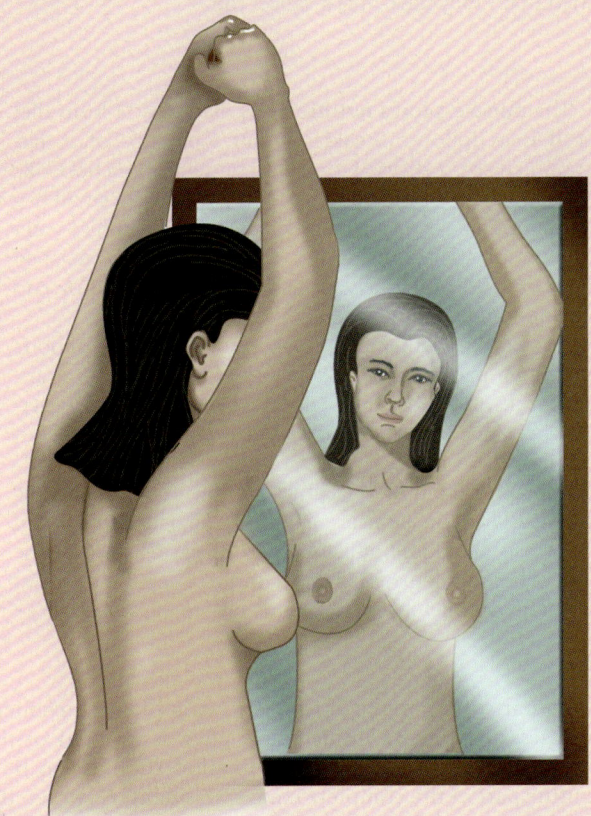

Step 3: Look for any signs of fluid coming out of one or both nipples (e.g., watery, milky, yellow fluid, or blood).

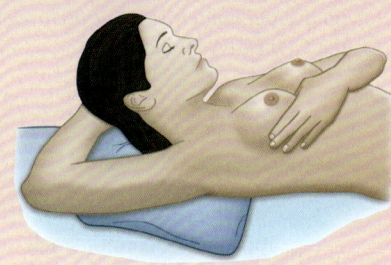

Step 4: Lie down with your right arm behind your head. Lying down spreads the breast tissue evenly over the chest wall, making it easier to feel. Use the three middle finger pads and move them in a circular motion covering the entire breast from top to bottom, side to side—from your collarbone to the top of your abdomen, and from your armpit to your cleavage.

Follow a pattern to be sure that you cover the whole breast. You can begin at the nipple, moving in larger and larger circles until you reach the outer edge of the breast.

Some women prefer to use an up-and-down approach by moving the fingers up and down vertically, in rows, as if mowing a lawn. Be sure to feel all the tissue from the front to the back of your breasts: for the skin and tissue just beneath, use light pressure; use medium pressure for tissue in the middle of your breasts; use firm pressure for the deep tissue in the back. When you have reached the deep tissue, you should be able to feel down to your ribcage.

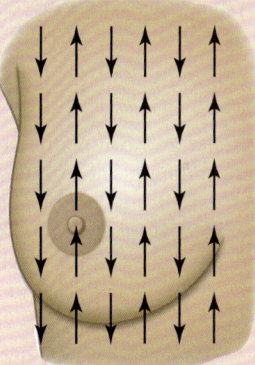

Step 5: Many women find it easiest to do this in the shower when the skin is wet and slippery. Cover the entire breast, using the same hand movements described in step 4.

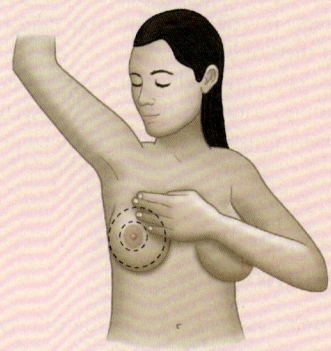

Adapted from American Cancer Society (ACS). (2016). The 5 steps of breast self-exam. Available at http://www.breastcancer.org/symptoms/testing/types/self_exam/bse_steps

CASE STUDY

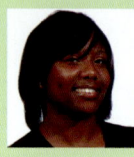

The nurse interviews Ms. Barnes, using specific probing questions. Ms. Barnes expresses concern with breast lumps and tenderness that occur each month before her menses. The nurse explores this health concern using the COLDSPA mnemonic.

Mnemonic	Question	Data Provided
Character	Describe the sign or symptom (feeling, appearance, sound, smell, or taste if applicable).	"I have lumps in both my breasts and they are very, very tender."
Onset	When did it begin?	"I have had lumpy breasts for years, but for the past 2 months, the lumps seem to be bigger and more tender."
Location	Where is it? Does it radiate? Does it occur anywhere else?	"The lumps are in both my breasts and seem to be all over."
Duration	How long does it last? Does it recur?	"I notice the lumps and tenderness 2–3 days before my period; they seem to go away 2–3 days after it starts."
Severity	How bad is it? or How much does it bother you?	"On a scale of 0–10, I would rate the pain 5–6 on those 2–3 days before my period starts."
Pattern	What makes it better or worse?	"The tenderness is worse at times but I don't know why. I tried acetaminophen but that doesn't seem to help. Ibuprofen helps a little."
Associated factors/How it Affects the client	What other symptoms occur with it? How does it affect you?	"My maternal aunt died of breast cancer and I am worried that I may have breast cancer too."

After exploring Ms. Barnes's complaint of monthly breast tenderness and lumps, the nurse continues with the health history. Ms. Barnes denies any personal history of breast cancer, breast surgeries, or breast trauma. The nurse explores her menstrual and pregnancy history, with the following findings: Menarche age 12. Gravida 3, Para 3, Aborta 0. Ms. Barnes had her first child when she was 21. Her last menstrual cycle began 2 weeks ago, with a duration of 5 days.

The nurse inquires about BSE. Ms. Barnes says that she performs BSE every month but that sometimes it is difficult to do because of bilateral breast tenderness. Her last clinical breast examination was performed 1 year ago. She has never had a mammogram. There is no history of breast cancer in sisters, mother, or maternal grandmother. Her maternal aunt died of breast cancer.

The nurse asks about medications. Ms. Barnes denies taking any hormones, contraceptives, or antipsychotic medications. She denies exposure to radiation, benzene, or asbestos.

The nurse explores nutrition. Ms. Barnes's 24-hour diet recall is as follows: Breakfast—four 6-oz cups of coffee, scrambled egg, 2 slices of toast with butter; 32-oz Diet Coke throughout the morning; lunch—ham sandwich, small bag of plain potato chips, snack cake, 6-oz cup of coffee; water throughout afternoon; dinner—fried pork chop, mashed potatoes with milk gravy, green beans, brownie, 6-oz cup of coffee, and water.

Ms. Barnes denies alcohol consumption. She reports smoking a pack of cigarettes per day for the past 10 years. She drinks approximately 50–60 oz of caffeinated beverages per day. She denies a regular exercise program, but tries to walk as much as she can.

The nurse explores Ms. Barnes's feeling about her breasts and breast health. She states that she is happy with the size of her breasts, but does not like how they have sagged since the birth of her children. Ms. Barnes is fearful of developing breast cancer because her maternal aunt died from the disease.

Collecting Objective Data: Physical Examination

The purpose of breast assessment is to identify signs of breast disease and initiate early treatment. The incidence of breast cancer in women is rising, but early detection and treatment have resulted in increased survival rates.

As part of complete assessment, it is often convenient to assess the breasts immediately after assessment of the thorax and lungs. A breast examination should also be a routine part of the complete male assessment. However, the male breast examination is not as detailed as the female breast examination. Although breast cancer in men is rare, it is often caught too late. Therefore, an awareness of the possibility and screening in men needs to be promoted (Al-Haddad, 2010). Female breast examinations are also performed by the nurse before a mammogram or by the gynecologist or nurse practitioner before a routine pelvic examination.

Keep in mind that breast palpation requires practice and skill because the consistency of the breasts varies widely from client to client. Some breasts are more difficult to palpate than others. For example, it is more difficult to palpate and inspect large, pendulous breasts to ensure adequate evaluation of all breast tissue. It may also be difficult to detect new lumps in women who have fibrocystic breast disease and who have granular, singular, or multiple mobile, tender lumps in their breasts. The following assessment steps provide parameters for the examination.

Preparing the Client

The actual hands-on physical examination of the breast may create client anxiety. The client may be embarrassed about exposing his or her breasts and may be anxious about what the assessment will reveal. Explain in detail what is happening throughout the assessment and answer any questions the client might have. In addition, provide the client with as much privacy as possible during the examination.

Prepare for the breast examination by having the client sit in an upright position. Explain that it will be necessary to expose both breasts to compare for symmetry during inspection. One breast may be draped while the other breast is palpated. Be sensitive to the fact that many women may feel embarrassed to have their breasts examined.

The breasts are first inspected in the sitting position while the client is asked to hold arms in different positions. The breasts are then palpated while the client assumes a supine position.

The final part of the examination involves teaching clients how to perform BSE and asking them to demonstrate what they have learned. If the client states that she or he already knows how to perform BSE, then ask the client to demonstrate how this is done.

Equipment

- Centimeter ruler
- Small pillow
- Gloves
- Client handout for BSE
- Slide for specimen

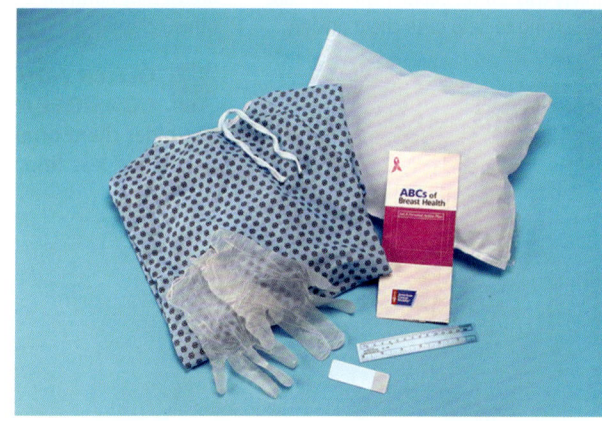

Physical Assessment

Key points for physical assessment include the following:
- Explain to the client what the steps of the examination are and the rationale for them.
- Warm your hands.
- Observe and inspect breast skin, areolas, and nipples for size, shape, rashes, dimpling, swelling, discoloration, retraction, asymmetry, and other unusual findings.
- Palpate breasts and axillary lymph nodes for swelling, lumps, masses, warmth or inflammation, tenderness, and other abnormalities.
- Remember it is important to carefully perform the breast examination on male as well as female clients.

General Routine Screening versus Focused Specialty Assessment for Breasts and Axillary Lymph Nodes

It is important that nurses know how to perform a breast examination and how to teach BSEs to clients who choose to participate. Normally, a registered nurse does not perform a complete breast examination unless working in a diagnostic breast clinic. During a head-to-toe examination, the nurse would perform a breast examination if there were concerns about a specific breast finding or if the client had breast surgery, injury, or infection. The clinicians experience and technique can affect findings. As with any examination, experience increases one's expertise with finding abnormalities. It is important to use a standard systematic method to increase one's ability to detect abnormalities. An Advanced Practice Registered Nurse (APRN) would include a complete breast examination with the client's annual examination.

General Routine Screening
- Inspect size and symmetry, color and texture.
- Inspect superficial venous pattern.
- Inspect the areolas and nipples.
- Inspect the breasts for retraction or dimpling.
- Palpate texture and elasticity.
- Palpate for tenderness and temperature.
- Ask the client who performs BSE to demonstrate how she does so, if she chooses to receive feedback on her technique and method.

Focused Specialty Assessment
- Palpate the nipples for discharge.
- Palpate the breasts for masses.
- Palpate mastectomy or lumpectomy site.
- Inspect and palpate the axillae.

ASSESSMENT PROCEDURE	NORMAL FINDINGS	ABNORMAL FINDINGS
Female Breasts		
INSPECTION		
Inspect size and symmetry. Have the client disrobe and sit with arms hanging freely (Fig. 20-6). Explain what you are observing to help ease client anxiety.	Breasts can be a variety of sizes and are somewhat round and pendulous. One breast may normally be larger than the other. **OLDER ADULT CONSIDERATIONS** The older client often has more pendulous, less firm, and saggy breasts.	A recent increase in the size of one breast may indicate inflammation or an abnormal growth.

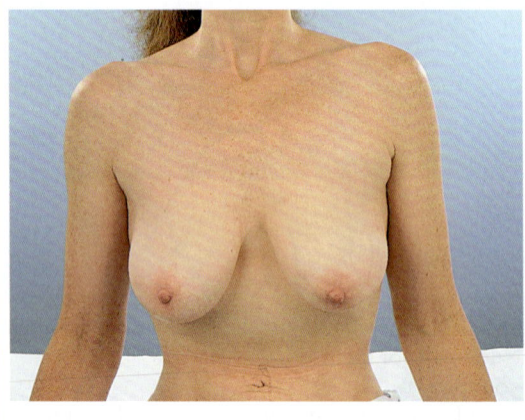

FIGURE 20-6 Client should sit with arms hanging freely at sides during assessment of breast size and symmetry.

Inspect color and texture. Be sure to note client's overall skin tone when inspecting the breast skin. Note any lesions.	Color varies depending on the client's skin tone. Texture is smooth, with no edema. Linear stretch marks may be seen during and after pregnancy or with significant weight gain or loss.	Redness is associated with breast inflammation. A pigskin-like or orange-peel (peau d'orange) appearance results from edema, which is seen in metastatic breast disease (Abnormal Findings 20-1). The edema is caused by blocked lymphatic drainage.
Inspect superficial venous pattern. Observe visibility and pattern of breast veins.	Veins radiate either horizontally and toward the axilla (transverse) or vertically with a lateral flare (longitudinal). Veins are more prominent during pregnancy. **CULTURAL CONSIDERATIONS** These two patterns are seen in varying proportions among different cultural groups. However, both patterns are normal and the transverse pattern predominates.	A prominent venous pattern may occur as a result of increased circulation due to a malignancy. An asymmetric venous pattern may be due to malignancy.
Inspect the areolas. Note the color, size, shape, and texture of the areolas of both breasts.	Areolas vary from dark pink to dark brown, depending on the client's skin tones. They are round and may vary in size. Small Montgomery tubercles are present.	Peau d'orange skin, associated with carcinoma, may be first seen in the areola. Red, scaly, crusty areas may appear in Paget disease (Abnormal Findings 20-1).
Inspect the nipples. Note the size and direction of the nipples of both breasts. Also note any dryness, lesions, bleeding, or discharge.	Nipples are nearly equal bilaterally in size and are in the same location on each breast. Nipples are usually everted, but they may be inverted or flat.	A recently retracted nipple that was previously everted suggests malignancy

ASSESSMENT PROCEDURE	NORMAL FINDINGS	ABNORMAL FINDINGS
	Supernumerary nipples (Fig. 20-7) may appear along the embryonic "milk line." No discharge should be present. ### OLDER ADULT CONSIDERATIONS **The older client may have smaller, flatter nipples that are less erectile on stimulation.**	(Abnormal Findings 20-1). Any type of spontaneous discharge should be referred for cytologic study and further evaluation.

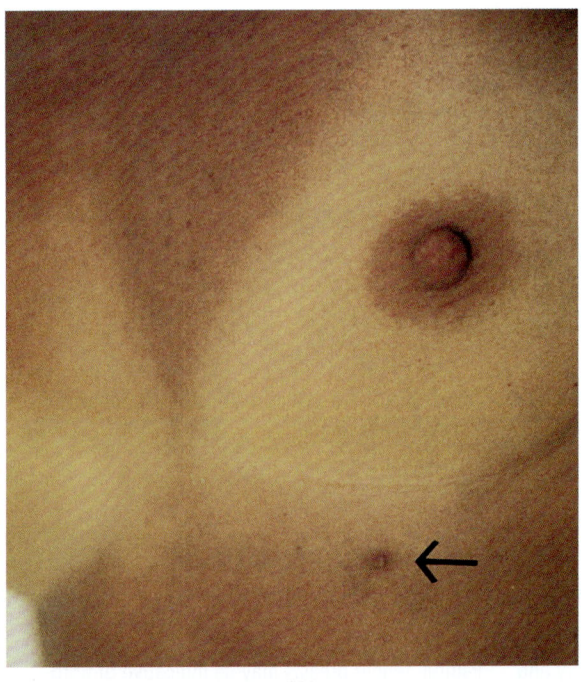

FIGURE 20-7 Supernumerary nipple (Used with permission from Logan-Young, W., & Hoffman, N.Y. (1994). Breast cancer: A practical guide to diagnosis. Rochester, NY: Mt. Hope Publishing).

Inspect for retraction and dimpling. To inspect the breasts accurately for retraction and dimpling, ask the client to remain seated while performing several different maneuvers. Ask the client to raise her arms overhead (Fig. 20-8A); then press her hands against her hips (Fig. 20-8B). Next ask her to press her hands together (Fig. 20-8C). These actions contract the pectoral muscles.	The client's breasts should rise symmetrically, with no sign of dimpling or retraction.	Dimpling or retraction (Abnormal Findings 20-1) is usually caused by a malignant tumor that has fibrous strands attached to the breast tissue and the fascia of the muscles. As the muscle contracts, it draws the breast tissue and skin with it, causing dimpling or retraction.

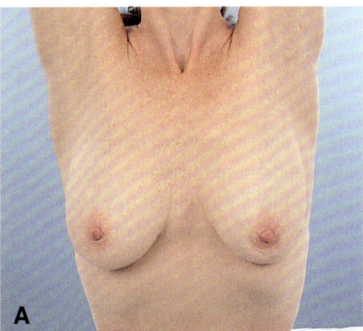 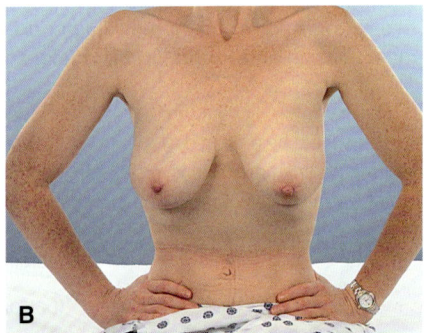 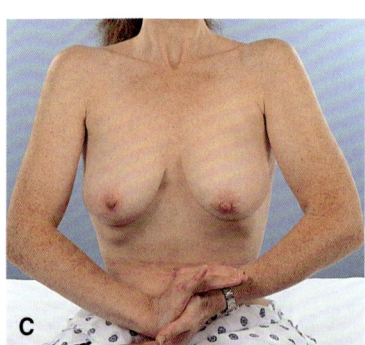

FIGURE 20-8 During assessment for retraction and dimpling, the client first (**A**) raises her arms over her head, (**B**) then lowers them and presses them against the hips, and finally (**C**) presses the hands together with the fingers of one hand pointing opposite to the fingers of the other hand.

Continued on following page

ASSESSMENT PROCEDURE	NORMAL FINDINGS	ABNORMAL FINDINGS
Female Breasts (Continued)		
Finally, ask the client to lean forward from the waist (Fig. 20-9). The nurse should support the client by the hands or forearms. This is a good position to use in women who have large, pendulous breasts.	Breasts should hang freely and symmetrically.	Restricted movement of breast or retraction of the skin or nipple indicates fibrosis and fixation of the underlying tissues. This is usually due to an underlying malignant tumor.

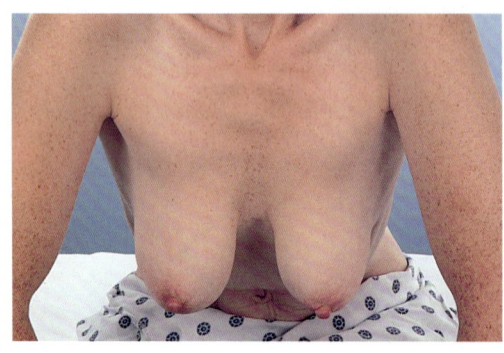

FIGURE 20-9 Forward-leaning position for breast inspection.

PALPATION		
Palpate texture and elasticity (Assessment Guide 20-1).	Palpation reveals smooth, firm, elastic tissue. 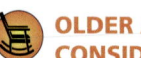 **OLDER ADULT CONSIDERATIONS** The older client's breasts may feel more granular, and the inframammary ridge may be more easily palpated as it thickens.	Thickening of the tissues may occur with an underlying malignant tumor.
Palpate for tenderness and temperature.	A generalized increase in nodularity and tenderness may be a normal finding associated with the menstrual cycle or hormonal medications. Breasts should be a normal body temperature.	Painful, tender breasts may be indicative of fibrocystic breasts, especially right before menstruation (Mayo Clinic, 2013). However, pain may also occur with a malignant tumor. Therefore, refer the client for further evaluation. Heat in the breasts of women who have not just given birth or who are not lactating indicates inflammation.

 Concept Mastery Alert

Always ask a patient who complains of lumps or swelling in the breast if the lump changes during the menstrual cycle. Women who have fibrocystic breasts will often have lumpy areas in the breast that increase in size in the two weeks prior to the menstrual period. They then decrease in size during menstruation and for the first 2 weeks after menstruation.

Palpate for masses. Note location, size in centimeters, shape, mobility, consistency, and tenderness. Also note the condition of the skin over the mass.	No masses should be palpated. However, a firm inframammary transverse ridge may normally be palpated at the lower base of the breasts.	Malignant masses or tumors are most often found in the upper outer quadrant of the breast. These masses generally are hard, immobile, and fixed to surrounding skin and soft tissue, with poorly defined or irregular margins (Barton et al.,1999). See Abnormal Findings 20-2 for masses.

ASSESSMENT PROCEDURE	NORMAL FINDINGS	ABNORMAL FINDINGS
If you detect any lump, refer the client for further evaluation. ◎ **CLINICAL TIP** More than half of women have fibrocystic breast changes at some time. The term "fibrocystic breast disease" is no longer used and is referred to as "fibrocystic breasts" or "fibrocystic breast changes" (Mayo Clinic, 2013).	Fibrocystic breast tissue that feels ropy, lumpy, or bumpy in texture is referred to as "nodular" or "glandular" breast tissue. Benign breast disease consists of bilateral, multiple, firm, regular, rubbery, mobile nodules with well-demarcated borders. Pain and fullness occurs just before menses.	**Fibroadenomas** are usually 1–5 cm, round or oval, mobile, firm, solid, elastic, nontender, single or multiple benign masses found in one or both breasts. **Milk cysts** (sacs filled with milk) and infections (mastitis), may turn into an abscess and occur if breast-feeding or recently given birth. If one's breast is bruised from an injury, there will be a blood collection that appears as a lump, which goes away in days or weeks, or the blood may have to be drained by a health care provider. **Lipomas** are a collection of fatty tissue that may also appear as a lump. **Intraductal papilloma** is a small growth inside a milk duct of the breast, often near the areola. It is harmless and occurs in women ages 35–50.
Palpate the nipples. Wear gloves to compress the nipple gently with your thumb and index finger (Fig. 20-10). Note any discharge. If spontaneous discharge occurs from the nipples, a specimen must be applied to a slide and the smear sent to the laboratory for cytologic evaluation.	The nipple may become erect and the areola may pucker in response to stimulation. A milky discharge is usually normal only during pregnancy and lactation. However, some women may normally have a clear discharge.	Common causes of nipple discharge in addition to pregnancy, include lactation, hypothyroidism, pituitary adenoma, oral contraceptives, antihypertensives, and tranquilizers (Parthasarathy & Rathnam, 2012). Nipple discharge may be bloody (possibly from a papilloma in the duct); greenish (often from a draining breast cyst); or clear (more likely associated with cancer unless from both nipples) (Johns Hopkins Medicine, n.d.).
Palpate mastectomy or lumpectomy site. If the client has had a mastectomy or lumpectomy, it is still important to perform a thorough examination. Palpate the scar and any remaining breast or axillary tissue for redness, lesions, lumps, swelling, or tenderness (Fig. 20-11).	Scar is whitish with no redness or swelling. No lesions, lumps, or tenderness noted.	Redness and inflammation of the scar area may indicate infection. Any lesions, lumps, or tenderness should be referred for further evaluation.

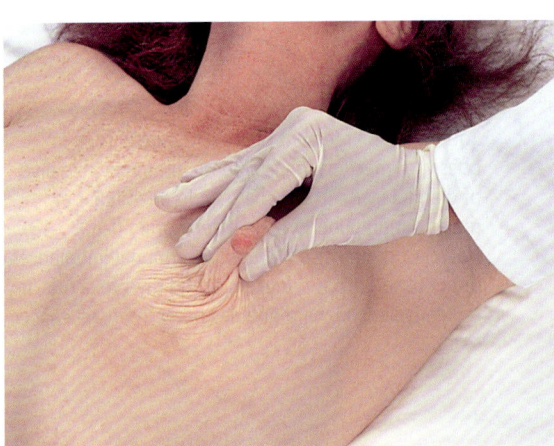

FIGURE 20-10 Palpating nipples for masses and discharge.

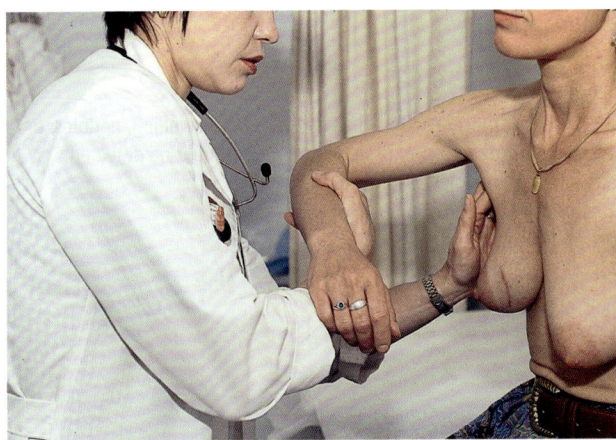

FIGURE 20-11 Palpating surgical site (© Dorothy Littell Greco 1993, Stock Boston).

Continued on following page

ASSESSMENT PROCEDURE	NORMAL FINDINGS	ABNORMAL FINDINGS
The Axillae		
INSPECTION AND PALPATION		
Inspect and palpate the axillae. Ask the client to sit up. Inspect the axillary skin for rashes or infection.	No rash or infection noted.	Redness and inflammation may be seen with infection of the sweat gland. Dark, velvety pigmentation of the axillae (acanthosis nigricans) may indicate an underlying malignancy.
Hold the client's elbow with one hand, and use the three fingerpads of your other hand to palpate firmly the axillary lymph nodes (Fig. 20-12).	No palpable nodes or one to two small (less than 1 cm), discrete, nontender, movable nodes in the central area.	Enlarged (greater than 1 cm) lymph nodes may indicate infection of the hand or arm. Large nodes that are hard and fixed to the skin may indicate an underlying malignancy.
First palpate high into the axillae, moving downward against the ribs to feel for the central nodes. Continue to move down the posterior axillae to feel for the posterior nodes. Use bimanual palpation to feel for the anterior axillary nodes. Finally palpate down the inner aspect of the upper arm.		

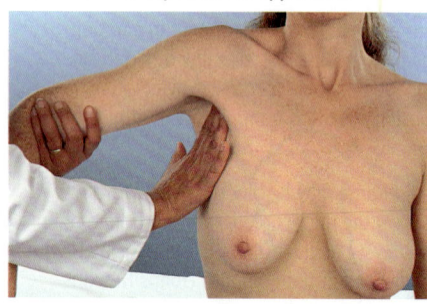

FIGURE 20-12 Palpating the axillary lymph nodes.

Breast Self-Examination		
Ask the client who performs BSE to demonstrate how she does so, if she chooses to receive feedback on her technique and method. This should be offered as an option and the client's choice accepted. This offers the nurse an opportunity to teach BSE. Give clients printed instructions (Box 20-1).	Client may request instructions on how to perform the examination or choose not to learn how to perform the examination. Either choice needs to be accepted by the examiner.	
The Male Breasts		
INSPECTION AND PALPATION		
Inspect and palpate the breasts, areolas, nipples, and axillae. Note any swelling, nodules, or ulceration. Palpate the flat disc of undeveloped breast tissue under the nipple.	No swelling, nodules, or ulceration should be detected.	Soft, fatty enlargement of breast tissue is seen in obesity. Gynecomastia, a smooth, firm, movable disc of glandular tissue, may be seen in one breast in males during puberty, usually temporary (Fig. 20-13). However, it may also be seen in hormonal imbalances, drug abuse, cirrhosis, leukemia, and thyrotoxicosis. Irregularly shaped, hard nodules occur in breast cancer.

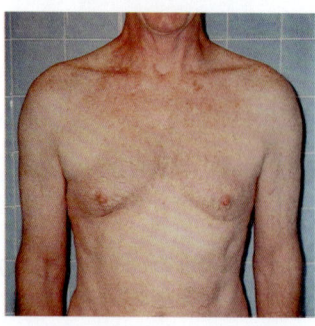

FIGURE 20-13 Gynecomastia.

20 Assessing Breasts and Lymphatic System 425

ASSESSMENT GUIDE 20-1 Palpating the Breasts

1. Ask the client to lie down and to place overhead the arm on the same side as the breast being palpated. Place a small pillow or rolled towel under the breast being palpated.
2. Use the flat pads of three fingers to palpate the client's breasts (Figure A).
3. Palpate the breasts using one of three different patterns (Figures B, C, and D). Choose one that is most comfortable for you, but be consistent and thorough with the method chosen.
4. Be sure to palpate every square inch of the breast, from the nipple and areola to the periphery of the breast tissue and up into the tail of Spence. Vary the levels of pressure as you palpate.
   Light—superficial
   Medium—mid-level tissue
   Firm—to the ribs

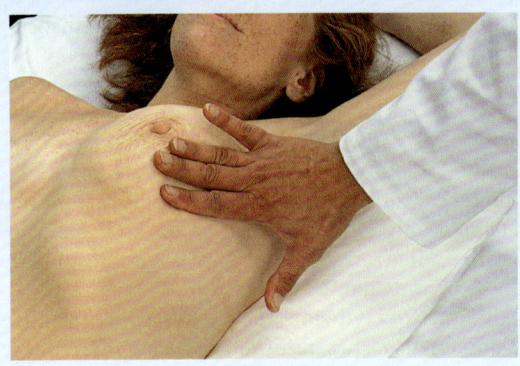

FIGURE A

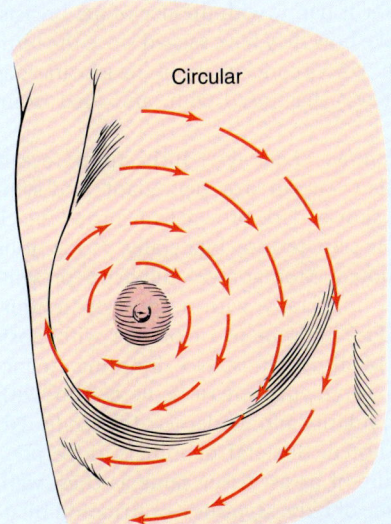

FIGURE B Circular or clockwise.

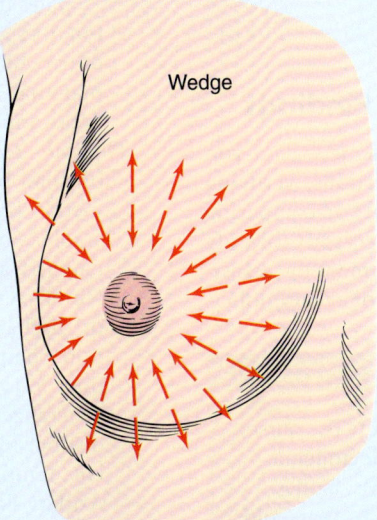

FIGURE C Wedged.

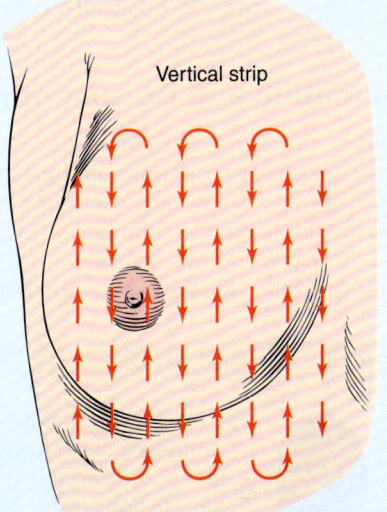

FIGURE D Vertical strip.

5. Use the bimanual technique (Figure E) if the client has large breasts. Support the breast with your nondominant hand and use your dominant hand to palpate.

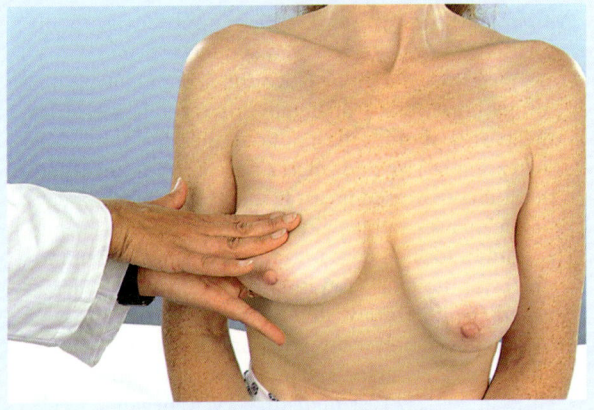

FIGURE E Bimanual palpation.

CASE STUDY

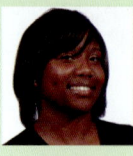

The nurse assesses Ms. Barnes. Inspection reveals bilateral breasts C cup in size, pendulant, and symmetric. Breast skin is dark brown with brown/black areola. The skin is smooth bilaterally. No venous patterns are noted. Montgomery tubercles are present. Nipples are everted bilaterally, with no dryness, lesions, or discharge. The nurse notes free movement of breasts with position changes of arms/hands. There is no dimpling, retraction, lesions, or erythema. The client's axillary skin is free of redness, rashes, or irritation bilaterally. Axillary hair has been removed bilaterally.

The nurse palpates the client's breasts. Upon palpation breast tissue is firm, with generalized nodularity and tenderness bilaterally. No distinct mass is noted. Bilateral mammary ridge is present. Temperature of breast tissue is same as chest wall. There are no palpable axillary nodes bilaterally.

Validating and Documenting Findings

Validate the breast and lymph node assessment data you have collected (by asking additional questions, verifying data with another health care professional, or comparing objective with subjective findings). This is necessary to verify that the data are reliable and accurate. Document the assessment data following the health care facility or agency policy.

CASE STUDY

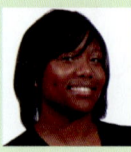

Think back to the case study. The nurse completed the following documentation of the assessment of Ms. Barnes:

Biographical Data: NB, 31 years old. African American. Employed full-time as a sales clerk. High school education. Awake, alert, and oriented. Asks and answers questions appropriately.

Reason for Seeking Care: "I have lumps in both my breasts and they are very, very tender."

History of Present Health Concern: Reports having had lumpy breast tissue bilaterally for years; however, for the past 2 months has noticed that the lumps are increasing in size and breasts have become more tender. States increased breast tenderness begins 2–3 days before menses, rating pain as 5–6 on scale of 1–10, and continues for 2–3 days into menses. Takes acetaminophen with no relief, and ibuprofen with slight relief.

Personal Health History: Reports no personal history of breast cancer, breast surgeries, or breast trauma. Menarche age 12. Gravida 3, Para 3, Aborta 0. Birth of first child at age 21. Last menstrual cycle began 2 weeks ago, with a duration of 5 days. Denies taking any hormones, contraceptives, or antipsychotic medications. Denies exposure to radiation, benzene, or asbestos. Last clinical breast examination was performed 1 year ago. Denies ever having had a mammogram.

Family History: No history of breast cancer in sisters, mother, or maternal grandmother. Maternal aunt died from breast cancer.

Lifestyle and Health Practices: Twenty-four–hour diet recall: Breakfast—four 6-oz cups of coffee, scrambled egg, 2 slices of toast with butter; 32-oz Diet Coke throughout the morning; lunch—ham sandwich, small bag of plain potato chips, snack cake, 6-oz cup of coffee; water throughout afternoon; dinner—fried pork chop, mashed potatoes with milk gravy, green beans, brownie, 6-oz cup of coffee, and water.

Denies alcohol consumption. Smokes 1 pack of cigarettes per day for the past 10 years. Drinks approximately 50–60 oz of caffeinated beverages per day. Denies a regular exercise program, but tries to walk as much as she can.

Reports performing BSEs every month but that sometimes it is difficult to do because of bilateral breast tenderness.

States that she is happy with the size of her breasts, but does not like how they have sagged since the birth of her children. Voices concern about breast cancer as maternal aunt was diagnosed with, and died from, breast cancer.

Physical Examination Findings: Inspection reveals bilateral breasts C cup in size, pendulant, and symmetric. Breast skin is dark brown with brown/black areola. Smooth skin texture bilaterally. No venous patterns are noted. Montgomery tubercles present. Nipples everted bilaterally, with no dryness, lesions, or discharge. Free movement of breasts with position changes of arms/hands. No dimpling, retraction, lesions, or erythema. Breast tissue is firm, with generalized nodularity and tenderness bilaterally. No distinct mass noted. Bilateral mammary ridge present. Temperature of breast tissue same as chest wall. Axillary skin free of redness, rashes, or irritation bilaterally. Axillary hair removed bilaterally. No palpable axillary nodes bilaterally.

ANALYSIS OF DATA: DIAGNOSTIC REASONING

After collecting subjective and objective data pertaining to the breast and lymphatic assessment, identify abnormal findings and client strengths. Then cluster the data to reveal any significant patterns or abnormalities. These data may then be used to make clinical judgments about the status of the client's breast and lymphatic health. The following sections provide possible conclusions that the nurse may make after assessing a client's breasts and axillae.

Selected Nursing Diagnoses

Following is a listing of selected nursing diagnoses (health promotion, risk, or actual) that you may identify when analyzing data collected from assessing breasts.

Health Promotion Diagnoses
- Readiness for Enhanced Knowledge: Requests information on BSE

Risk Diagnoses
- Risk for Ineffective Health Maintenance related to busy lifestyle and lack of breast self-awareness

Actual Diagnoses
- Fear of breast cancer related to increased risk factors
- Ineffective Individual Coping related to diagnosis of breast cancer
- Disturbed Body Image related to mastectomy
- Anticipatory Grieving related to anticipation of poor outcome of breast biopsy
- Ineffective Self-health Management related to lack of knowledge of BSE

Selected Collaborative Problems

After grouping the data, certain collaborative problems may become apparent. Remember that collaborative problems differ from nursing diagnoses in that they cannot be prevented or treated by nursing interventions alone. However, these physiologic complications of medical conditions can be detected and monitored by the nurse. In addition, the nurse can use physician- and nurse-prescribed interventions to minimize the complications of these problems. The nurse may also have to refer the client in such situations for further treatment of the problem. Following is a list of collaborative problems that may be identified when obtaining a general impression. These problems are worded as risk for complications (or RC), followed by the problem.
- RC: Infection (abscess)
- RC: Hematoma
- RC: Benign breast disease
- RC: Breast cancer

Medical Problems

After grouping the data, the client's signs and symptoms may clearly require medical diagnosis and treatment. Referral to a primary care provider is necessary.

CASE STUDY

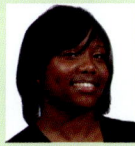

After collecting and analyzing the data for Ms. Barnes, the nurse determines that the following conclusions are appropriate.

Nursing Diagnoses
- Readiness for Enhanced Health Management r/t request for information on BSE
- Deficient knowledge r/t risk factors for benign breast disease
- Fear r/t current symptoms and family history of breast cancer

Potential Collaborative Problems
- RC: Benign breast disease
- RC: Breast cancer

Refer this client for medical evaluation, diagnosis, and possible biopsy of her breast lumps.

To view an algorithm depicting the process for diagnostic reasoning in this case, go to **thePoint**.

Interdisciplinary Verbal Communication of Assessment Findings Using SBAR

SITUATION: NB, a 31-year-old African American woman, here for annual examination, is concerned with increasing size and tenderness of bilateral breast lumps occurring monthly before menses, beginning 2–3 days before menses and continuing for 2–3 days into menses. Rates pain as 5–6 on scale of 1–10. Takes acetaminophen with no relief, and ibuprofen with slight relief.

BACKGROUND: No personal history of breast cancer, breast surgeries, or breast trauma; maternal aunt died of breast cancer. Menarche age 12. Gravida 3, Para 3, Aborta 0. Last menstrual cycle began 2 weeks ago, with a duration of 5 days. Performs BSE every month but is often difficult to do because of bilateral breast tenderness. Last clinical breast examination was 1 year ago. Never had a mammogram. Twenty-four–hour diet recall indicates high fat and caffeine intake, denies alcohol consumption. Smokes a pack of cigarettes daily for last 10 years. Drinks approximately 50–60 oz of caffeinated beverages per day. Walks for exercise when she can. Does not like how her breasts sag and is fearful of breast cancer because her maternal aunt died from it.

ASSESSMENT: Bilateral breasts C cup in size, pendulant, and symmetric. Breast skin is dark brown with brown/black areola. Smooth skin texture bilaterally. No venous patterns are noted. Montgomery tubercles present. Nipples everted bilaterally, with no dryness, lesions, or discharge. Free movement of breasts with position changes of arms/hands. No dimpling, retraction, lesions, or erythema. Breast tissue is firm, with generalized nodularity and tenderness bilaterally. No distinct mass noted. Bilateral mammary ridge present. Temperature of breast tissue same as chest wall. Axillary skin free of redness, rashes, or irritation bilaterally. Axillary hair removed bilaterally. No palpable axillary nodes bilaterally.

RECOMMENDATION: NB is ready for Enhanced Health Management r/t her request for information on BSE. She needs information provided on recommendations regarding benefits and risks of BSE as well as on risk factors associated with benign breast disease.

She needs time to voice her fears r/t current symptoms and aunt dying of breast cancer. She needs to be seen by her primary care provider for further evaluation of any diagnoses of her breast lumps.

428 UNIT 3 Nursing Assessment of Physical Systems

ABNORMAL FINDINGS 20-1 Abnormalities Noted on Inspection of the Breast

PEAU D'ORANGE
Resulting from edema, an orange peel appearance of the breast is associated with cancer.

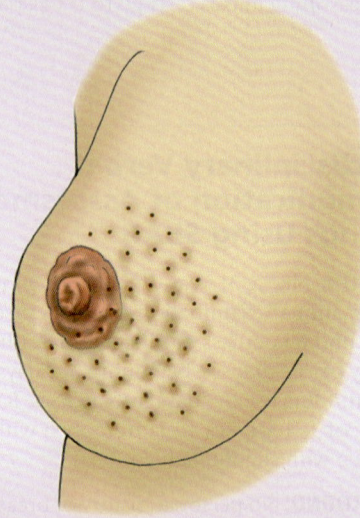

PAGET DISEASE
Redness and flaking of the nipple may be seen early in Paget disease and then disappear. However, further assessment is needed as this does not mean the disease is gone. Tingling, itching, increased sensitivity, burning, discharge, and pain in the nipple are late signs of Paget disease. It may occur in both breasts, but is rare.

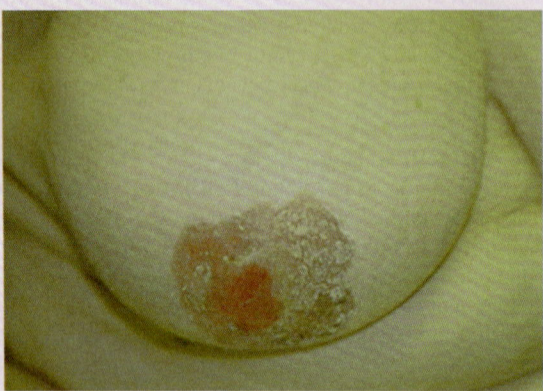

RETRACTED NIPPLE
A retracted nipple suggests malignancy.

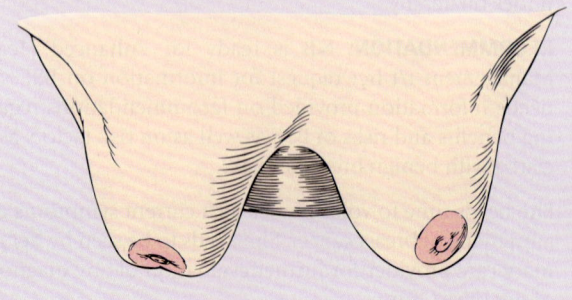

DIMPLING
Dimpling suggests malignancy. From Harris, J. R., Lippman, M.E., Morrow, M. Osborne, C.K. (2014). *Diseases of the Breast* (5th ed.). Philadelphia, PA: Lippincott Williams & Wilkins.

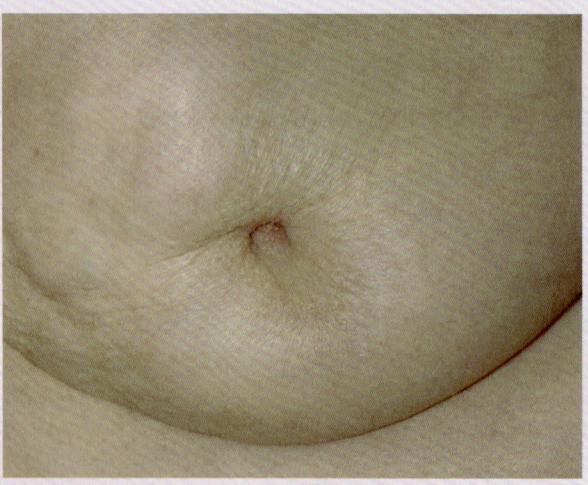

RETRACTED BREAST TISSUE
Retracted breast tissue suggests malignancy.

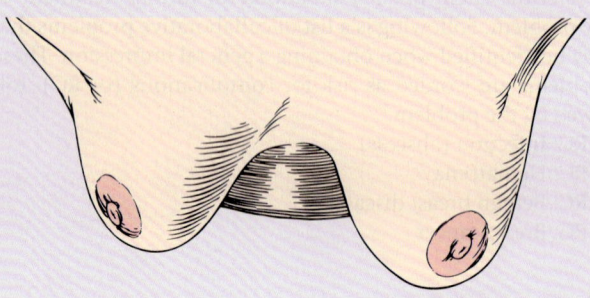

MASTITIS
Reddened, painful area on breast warm to palpation. From Hatfield, N. (2013). *Introduction Maternity and Pediatric Nursing* (3rd ed.). Philadelphia, PA: Lippincott, Williams & Wilkins.

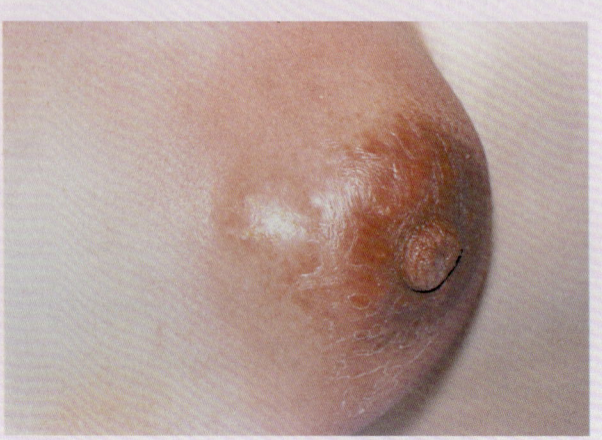

MASTECTOMY

(A) Radical mastectomy (B) Modified radical mastectomy. Berek, J.S., Hacker, N.F. *Berek and Hacker's Gynecologic Oncology* (6th ed.). Philadelphia, PA: Lippincott, Williams & Wilkins. 2014.

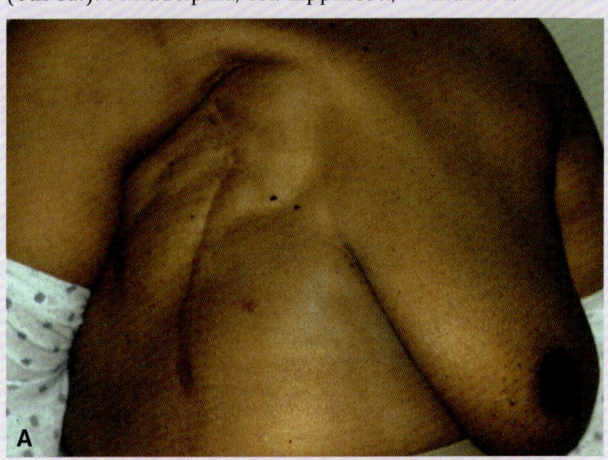
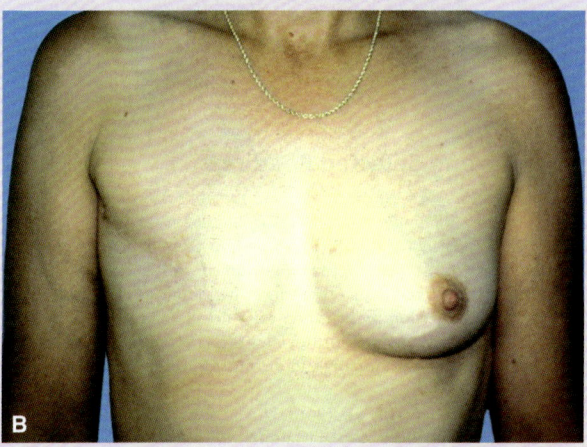

ABNORMAL FINDINGS 20-2   Abnormalities Noted on Palpation of the Breasts

Whereas some abnormalities of the breast are readily apparent, such as peau d'orange and Paget disease, some breast internal changes are detected only by palpation and mammography. The following illustrations represent breast abnormalities characteristic of tumors, fibroadenomas, and benign disease (fibrocystic breasts).

CANCEROUS TUMORS
These are irregular, firm, hard, not defined masses that may be fixed or mobile. They are not usually tender and usually occur after age 50.

FIBROADENOMAS
These lesions are lobular, ovoid, or round. They are firm, well defined, seldom tender, and usually singular and mobile. They occur more commonly between puberty and menopause.

BENIGN BREAST DISEASE
Also called fibrocystic breast disease, benign breast disease is marked by round, elastic, defined, tender, and mobile cysts. The condition is most common from age 30 to menopause, after which it decreases.

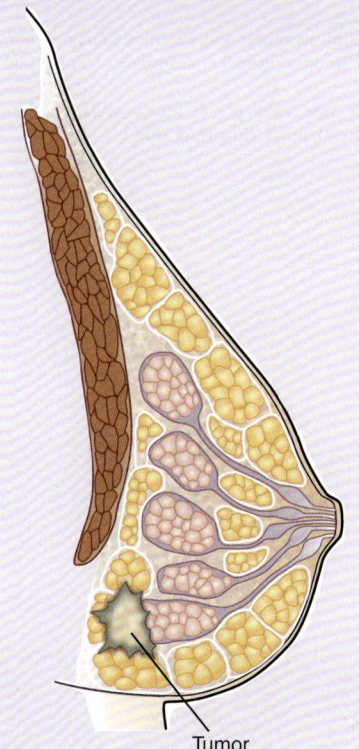

Tumor

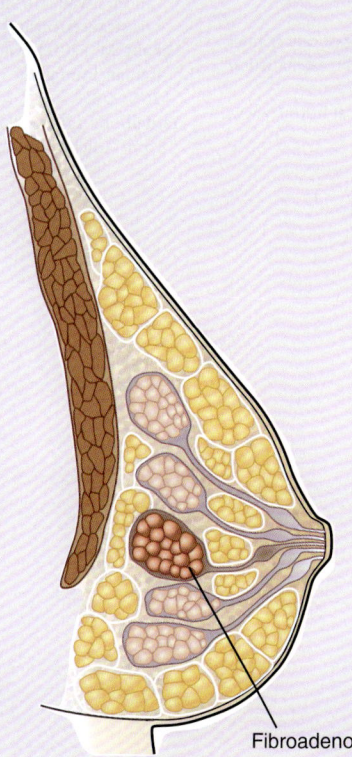

Fibroadenoma

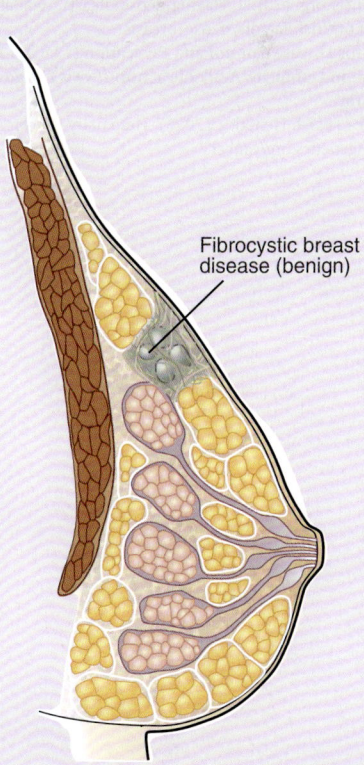

Fibrocystic breast disease (benign)

Want to know more?

A wide variety of resources to enhance your learning and understanding of this book are available on thePoint. Visit thePoint to access:

NCLEX-Style Student Review Questions
Watch and Learn Videos
Concepts in Action Animations
And more!

References and Selected Readings

Al-Haddad, M. (2010). Breast cancer in men: the importance of teaching and raising awareness. *Clinical Journal of Oncology Nursing*, 14(1), 31–32.

American Cancer Society (ACS). (2015a). American Cancer Society recommendations for early breast cancer detection in women without breast symptoms. Available at http://www.cancer.org/cancer/breastcancer/moreinformation/breastcancerearlydetection/breast-cancer-early-detection-acs-recs

American Cancer Society (ACS). (2015b). How is breast cancer classified? Available at http://www.cancer.org/cancer/breastcancer/detailedguide/breast-cancer-classifying

American Cancer Society (ACS). (2016a). American Cancer Society breast cancer screening guidelines. Available at http://www.cancer.org/cancer/news/specialcoverage/american-cancer-society-breast-cancer-screening-guidelines

American Cancer Society (ACS). (2016b). Five ways to reduce your breast cancer risk. Available at http://www.cancer.org/cancer/news/features/five-ways-to-reduce-your-breast-cancer-risk

American Cancer Society (ACS). (2016c). What are the risk factors for breast cancer? Available at http://www.cancer.org/cancer/breastcancer/detailedguide/breast-cancer-risk-factors

American College of Radiology (ACR). (2015). ACR and SBI continue to recommend regular mammography starting at age 40. Available at http://www.acr.org/About-Us/Media-Center/Press-Releases/2015-Press-Releases/20151020-ACR-SBI-Recommend-Mammography-at-Age-40

Banning, M. (2010). Black women and breast health: A review of the literature. *European Journal of Oncology Nursing*, 15(1), 16–22.

Barton, M., Harris, R., & Fletcher, S. (1999). The rational clinical examination. Does this patient have breast cancer? The screening clinical breast examination: Should it be done? How? *JAMA*, (282), 1270–1280.

Berkeley Wellness. (2015). Re-examining the breast self-exam. Available at http://www.berkeleywellness.com/self-care/preventive-care/article/re-examining-breast-self-exam

Breastcancer.org. (2016). Having dense breasts. Available at http://www.breastcancer.org/risk/factors/dense_breasts

Centers for Disease Control and Prevention (CDC). (2015). Breast cancer rates by race and ethnicity. Available at http://www.cdc.gov/cancer/breast/statistics/race.htm

Center for Jewish Genetics. (2016). Hereditary cancer. Available at https://www.jewishgenetics.org/cancer

Healthy People 2020. (2014). Cancer. Available at http://www.healthypeople.gov/node/4069/data_details#revision_history_header

Jardines, L., Goyal, S., Fisher, P., et al. (2015). Breast cancer overview: Risk factors, screening, genetic testing, and prevention. Available at http://www.cancernetwork.com/cancer-management/breast-cancer-overview-risk-factors-screening-genetic-testing-and-prevention

Johns Hopkins Medicine. (n.d.). Nipple discharge. Available at http://www.hopkinsmedicine.org/breast_center/breast_cancers_other_conditions/nipple_discharge.html

Kosir, M. (2013). Nipple discharge. Available at http://www.merckmanuals.com/professional/gynecology-and-obstetrics/breast-disorders/nipple-discharge

Leung, A., & Pacaud, D. (2004). Diagnosis and management of galactorrhea. Available at http://www.aafp.org/afp/2004/0801/p543.html

Mayo Clinic. (2013). Fibrocystic breasts. Available at http://www.mayoclinic.org/diseases-conditions/fibrocystic-breasts/basics/symptoms/con-20034681

Mayo Clinic. (2015). Invasive lobular carcinoma. Available at http://www.mayoclinic.org/diseases-conditions/invasive-lobular-carcinoma/basics/symptoms/con-20033968

MD Anderson Cancer Center. (2016). Women: Breast implants and cancer risk. Available at https://www.mdanderson.org/publications/focused-on-health/december-2014/breast-implant-cancer.html

National Breast Cancer Foundation. (2016). Types of breast cancer. Available at http://www.nationalbreastcancer.org/types-of-breast-cancer?gclid=CLWLq7WbmNICFQVZhgodpU0Law

National Cancer Institute. (2012). Paget's disease of the breast. Available at http://www.cancer.gov/cancertopics/factsheet/Sites-Types/paget-breast

National Cancer Institute: Surveillance Epidemiology and End Result (SEER). (2015). SEER stat fact sheets: Breast. Available at http://seer.cancer.gov/statfacts/html/breast.html

Parthasarathy, V., & Rathnam, U. (2012). Nipple discharge: An early sign of breast cancer. *International Journal of Preventive Medicine*, 3(11), 810–814.

U.S. Preventive Services Task Force (USPSFT). (2009). Screening for breast cancer. Available at http://www.uspreventiveservicestaskforce.org/uspstf09/breastcancer/brcanrs.htm

Vahabi, M. (2011). Knowledge of breast cancer and screening practices among Iranian immigrant women in Toronto. *Journal of Community Health*, 36(2), 265–273.

Yardell, K. (2014). Light's dark side. Available at http://www.the-scientist.com/?articles.view/articleNo/40591/title/Light-s-Dark-Side/

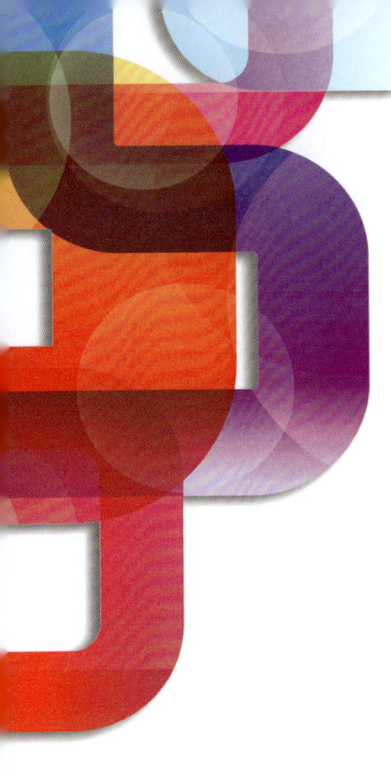

21 ASSESSING HEART AND NECK VESSELS

Learning Objectives

1. Describe the structure and function of the heart and neck vessels.
2. Discuss the risk factors for coronary heart disease (CHD) (or coronary heart disease, CAD) across cultures and ways to reduce one's risks.
3. Interview a client for an accurate nursing history of the heart and neck vessels.
4. Perform a physical assessment of the heart and neck vessels using the correct techniques of inspection, auscultation, palpation, and percussion.
5. Differentiate between normal and abnormal findings of the heart and neck vessels.
6. Describe the findings frequently seen when assessing the older client's heart and neck vessels.
7. Analyze the date from the interview and physical assessment of the heart and neck vessels to formulate valid nursing diagnoses, collaborative problems, and/or referrals.
8. Differentiate between general routine screening versus skills needed for focused or specialty assessment of the heart and neck vessels.
9. Document and verbally report accurate assessment findings of the heart and neck vessels.

CASE STUDY

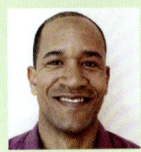

Malcolm Winchester, a 45-year-old African American man, is being admitted to the coronary care unit (CCU) with a diagnosis of chest pain and pressure. He is currently in no acute distress and wonders why he is being admitted to the CCU.

STRUCTURE AND FUNCTION

The *cardiovascular system* is highly complex, consisting of the heart and a closed system of blood vessels. To collect accurate data and correctly interpret it, the examiner must have an understanding of the structure and function of the heart, the great vessels, the electrical conduction system of the heart, the cardiac cycle, the production of heart sounds, cardiac output (CO), and the neck vessels. This information helps the examiner to differentiate between normal and abnormal findings as they relate to the cardiovascular system.

Heart and Great Vessels

The heart is a hollow, muscular, four-chambered (left and right atria, and left and right ventricles) organ located in the middle of the thoracic cavity between the lungs in the space called the *mediastinum*. It is about the size of a clenched fist and weighs approximately 255 g (9 oz) in women and 310 g (10.9 oz) in men. The heart extends vertically from the left second to the left fifth intercostal space (ICS) and horizontally from the right edge of the sternum to the left midclavicular line (MCL). The heart can be described as an inverted cone. The upper portion, near the left second ICS, is the base; the lower portion, near the left fifth ICS and the left MCL, is the apex. The anterior chest area that overlies the heart and great vessels is called the *precordium* (Fig. 21-1). The right side of the heart pumps blood to the lungs for gas exchange (pulmonary circulation); the left side of the heart pumps blood to all other parts of the body (systemic circulation).

The large veins and arteries leading directly to and away from the heart are referred to as the *great vessels*. The *superior and inferior vena cava* return blood to the right atrium from the upper and lower torso, respectively. The *pulmonary artery* exits the right ventricle, bifurcates, and carries blood to the lungs. The *pulmonary veins* (two from each lung) return oxygenated blood to the left atrium. The *aorta* transports oxygenated blood from the left ventricle to the body (Fig. 21-2).

Heart Chambers and Valves

The heart consists of four chambers, or cavities: two upper chambers, the *right and left atria*, and two lower chambers, the *right and left ventricles*. The right and left sides of the heart are separated by a partition called the *septum*. The thin-walled atria receive blood returning to the heart and pump blood into the ventricles. The thicker-walled ventricles pump blood out of the heart. The left ventricle is thicker

431

432 UNIT 3 Nursing Assessment of Physical Systems

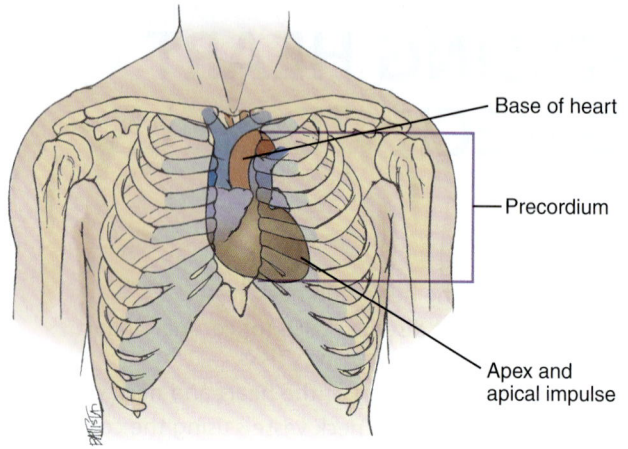

FIGURE 21-1 The heart and major blood vessels lie centrally in the chest behind the protective sternum.

than the right ventricle because the left side of the heart has a greater workload.

The entrance and exit of each ventricle are protected by one-way valves that direct the flow of blood through the heart. The *atrioventricular (AV) valves* are located at the entrance into the ventricles. There are two AV valves: the *tricuspid valve* and the *bicuspid (mitral) valve*. The tricuspid valve is composed of three cusps, or flaps, and is located between the right atrium and the right ventricle; the bicuspid (mitral) valve is composed of two cusps and is located between the left atrium and the left ventricle. Collagen fibers, called *chordae tendineae*, anchor the AV valve flaps to papillary muscles within the ventricles.

Open AV valves allow blood to flow from the atria into the ventricles. However, as the ventricles begin to contract, the AV valves snap shut, preventing the regurgitation of blood into the atria. The valves are prevented from blowing open in the reverse direction (i.e., toward the atria) by their secure anchors

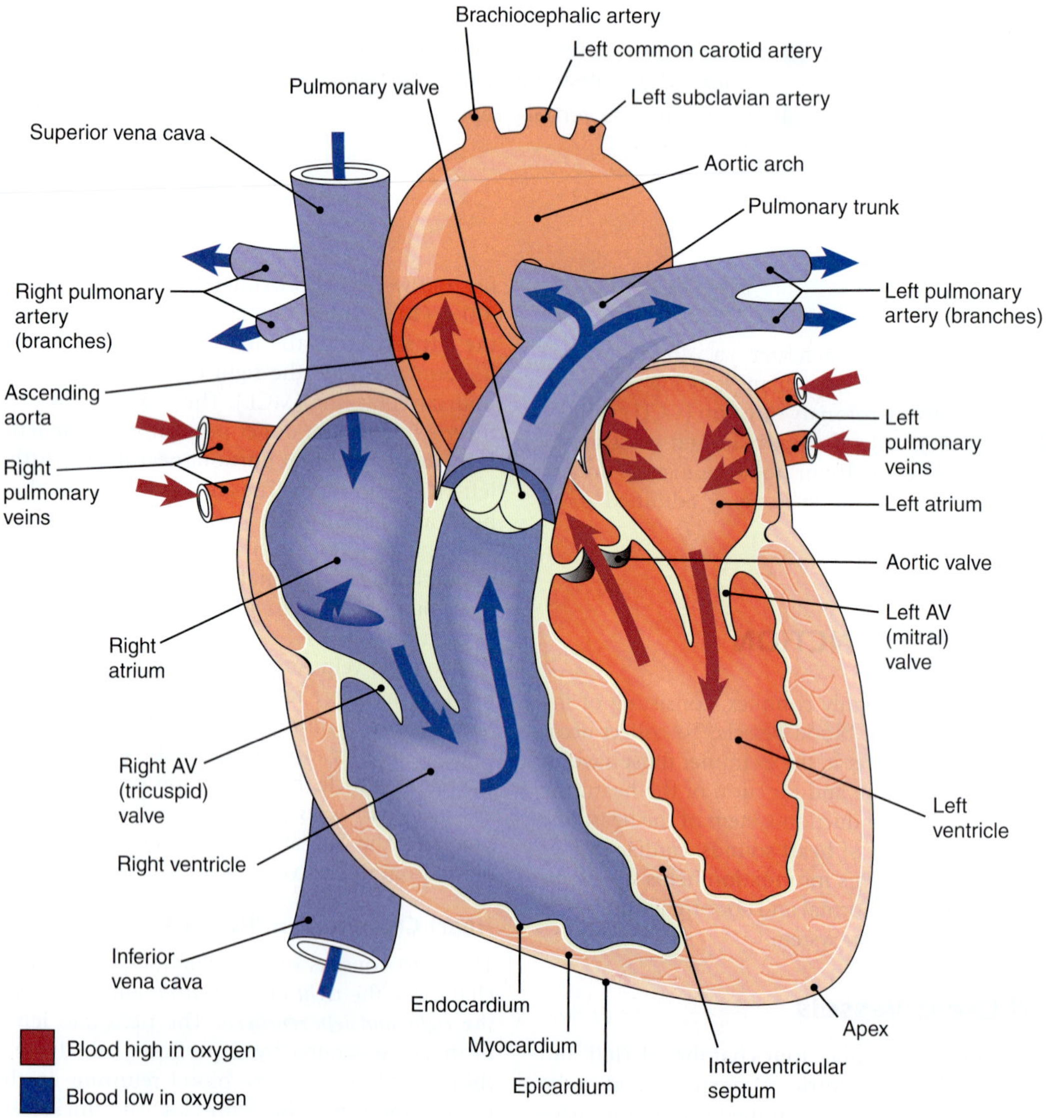

FIGURE 21-2 Heart chambers, valves, and direction of circulatory flow.

to the papillary muscles of the ventricular wall. The *semilunar valves* are located at the exit of each ventricle at the beginning of the great vessels. Each valve has three cusps that look like half-moons, hence the name "semilunar." There are two semilunar valves: the *pulmonic valve* is located at the entrance of the pulmonary artery as it exits the right ventricle and the *aortic valve* is located at the beginning of the ascending aorta as it exits the left ventricle. These valves are open during ventricular contraction and close from the pressure of blood when the ventricles relax. Blood is thus prevented from flowing backward into the relaxed ventricles (Fig. 21-2).

Heart Covering and Walls

The **pericardium** is a tough, inextensible, loose-fitting, fibroserous sac that attaches to the great vessels and surrounds the heart. A serous membrane lining, the *parietal pericardium*, secretes a small amount of pericardial fluid that allows for smooth, friction-free movement of the heart. This same type of serous membrane covers the outer surface of the heart and is known as the *epicardium*. The *myocardium* is the thickest layer of the heart, made up of contractile cardiac muscle cells. The *endocardium* is a thin layer of endothelial tissue that forms the innermost layer of the heart and is continuous with the endothelial lining of blood vessels (Fig. 21-2).

Electrical Conduction of the Heart

Cardiac muscle cells have a unique inherent ability. They can spontaneously generate an electrical impulse and conduct it through the heart. The generation and conduction of electrical impulses by specialized sections of the myocardium regulate the events associated with the filling and emptying of the cardiac chambers. The process is called the *cardiac cycle* (see description in next section).

Pathways

The *sinoatrial (SA) node* (or sinus node) is located on the posterior wall of the right atrium near the junction of the superior and inferior vena cava. The SA node, with inherent rhythmicity, generates impulses (at a rate of 60 to 100 per minute) that are conducted over both atria, causing them to contract simultaneously and send blood into the ventricles. The current, initiated by the SA node, is conducted across the atria to the **AV node** located in the lower interatrial septum (Fig. 21-3). The AV node slightly delays incoming electrical impulses from the atria and then relays the impulse to the AV bundle (bundle of His) in the upper interventricular septum. The electrical impulse then travels down the right and left bundle branches and the *Purkinje fibers* in the myocardium of both ventricles, causing them to contract almost simultaneously. Although the SA node functions as the "pacemaker of the heart," this activity shifts to other areas of the conduction system, such as the *Bundle of His* (with an inherent discharge of 40 to 60 per minute), if the SA node cannot function.

Electrical Activity

Electrical impulses, which are generated by the SA node and travel throughout the cardiac conduction circuit, can be detected on the surface of the skin. This electrical activity can be measured and recorded by *electrocardiography (ECG, also abbreviated as EKG)*, which records the depolarization and

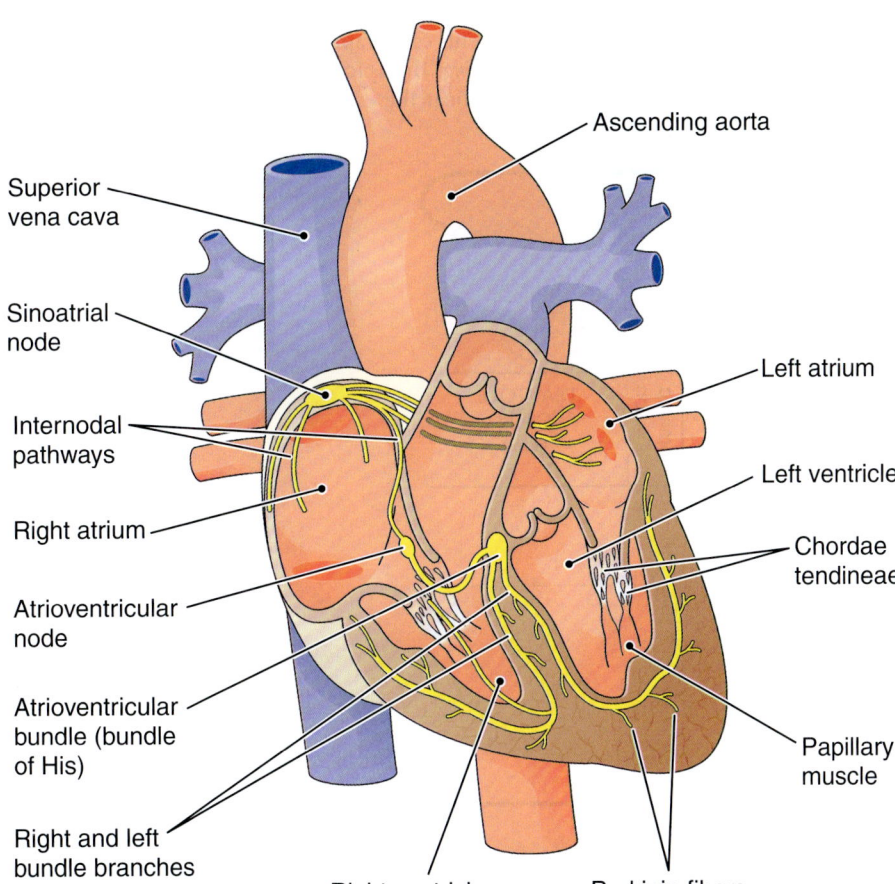

FIGURE 21-3 The electrical conduction system of the heart begins with impulses generated by the sinoatrial node (*green*) and circuited continuously over the heart.

BOX 21-1   PHASES OF THE ELECTROCARDIOGRAM

The phases of the electrocardiogram (ECG), which records depolarization and repolarization of the heart, are assigned letters: P, Q, R, S, and T.

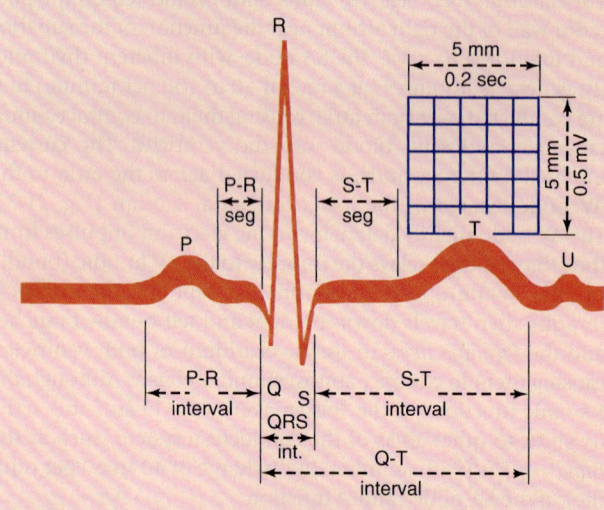

- **P wave:** Atrial depolarization; conduction of the impulse throughout the atria.
- **PR interval:** Time from the beginning of the atrial depolarization to the beginning of ventricular depolarization, that is, from the beginning of the P wave to the beginning of the QRS complex.
- **QRS complex:** Ventricular depolarization (also atrial repolarization); conduction of the impulse throughout the ventricles, which then triggers contraction of the ventricles; measured from the beginning of the Q wave to the end of the S wave.
- **ST segment:** Period between ventricular depolarization and the beginning of ventricular repolarization.
- **T wave:** Ventricular repolarization; the ventricles return to a resting state.
- **QT interval:** Total time for ventricular depolarization and repolarization, that is, from the beginning of the Q wave to the end of the T wave; the QT interval varies with HR.
- **U wave:** May or may not be present; if present, it follows the T wave and represents the final phase of ventricular repolarization.

repolarization of the cardiac muscle. The phases of the ECG are known as P, Q, R, S, and T. Box 21-1 describes the phases of the ECG.

The Cardiac Cycle

The *cardiac cycle* refers to the filling and emptying of the heart's chambers. The cardiac cycle has two phases: *diastole* (relaxation of the ventricles, known as filling) and *systole* (contraction of the ventricles, known as emptying). Diastole endures for approximately two-thirds of the cardiac cycle and systole is the remaining one-third (Fig. 21-4).

Diastole

During ventricular diastole, the AV valves are open and the ventricles are relaxed. This causes higher pressure in the atria than in the ventricles. Therefore, blood rushes through the atria into the ventricles. This early, rapid, passive filling is called *early* or *protodiastolic filling*. This is followed by a period of slow passive filling. Finally, near the end of ventricular diastole, the atria

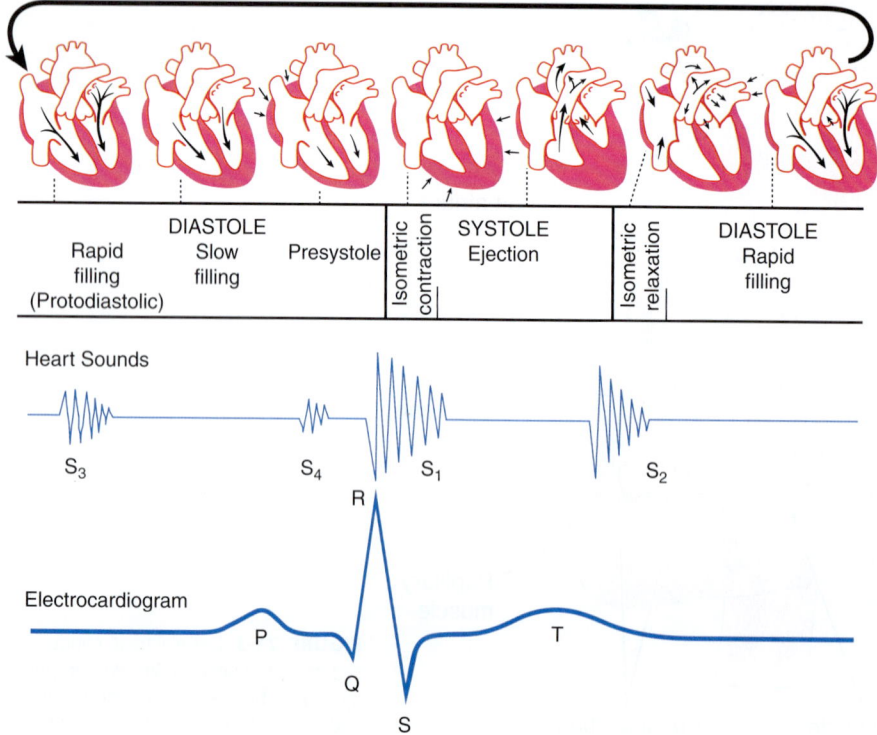

FIGURE 21-4 The cardiac cycle consists of filling and ejection. Heart sounds S_2, S_3, and S_4 are associated with diastole, while S_1 is associated with systole. The electrical activity of the heart is measured throughout diastole and systole by electrocardiography.

contract and complete the emptying of blood out of the upper chambers by propelling it into the ventricles. This final active filling phase is called *presystole, atrial systole,* or sometimes the *"atrial kick."* This action raises left ventricular pressure.

Systole

The filling phases during diastole result in a large amount of blood in the ventricles, causing the pressure in the ventricles to be higher than in the atria. This causes the AV valves (mitral and tricuspid) to shut. Closure of the AV valves produces the *first heart sound* (S_1), which is the beginning of systole. This valve closure also prevents blood from flowing backward (a process known as *regurgitation*) into the atria during ventricular contraction.

At this point in systole, all four valves are closed and the ventricles contract (isometric contraction). There is now high pressure inside the ventricles, causing the aortic valve to open on the left side of the heart and the pulmonic valve to open on the right side of the heart. Blood is ejected rapidly through these valves. With ventricular emptying, the ventricular pressure falls and the semilunar valves close. This closure produces the *second heart sound* (S_2), which signals the end of systole. After closure of the semilunar valves, the ventricles relax. Atrial pressure is now higher than the ventricular pressure, causing the AV valves to open and diastolic filling to begin again.

Heart Sounds

Heart sounds are produced by valve closure, as just described. The opening of valves is silent. Normal heart sounds, characterized as "lubdubb" (S_1 and S_2), and occasionally extra heart sounds and murmurs can be auscultated with a stethoscope over the precordium, the area of the anterior chest overlying the heart and great vessels.

Normal Heart Sounds

The first heart sound (S_1) is the result of closure of the AV valves: the mitral and tricuspid valves. As mentioned previously, S_1 correlates with the beginning of systole (see Box 21-2

BOX 21-2   UNDERSTANDING NORMAL S_1 SOUNDS AND VARIATIONS

S_1, which is the first heart sound, is produced by the AV closing. S_1 (the "lub" portion of "lubdubb") correlates with the beginning of systole.

The intensity of S_1 depends on the position of the mitral valve at the start of systole, the structure of the valve leaflets, and how quickly pressure rises in the ventricles. All of these factors influence the speed and amount of closure the valve experiences, which, in turn, determine the amount of sound produced.

🎯 **CLINICAL TIP**
Normal variations in S_1 are heard at the base and the apex of the heart. S_1 is softer at the base and louder at the apex of the heart. An S_1 may be split along the lower left sternal border, where the tricuspid component of the sound, usually too faint to be heard, can be auscultated. A split S_1 heard over the apex may be an S_4.

Accentuated S_1
An accentuated S_1 sound is louder than an S_2. This occurs when the mitral valve is wide open and closes quickly. Examples include:
- Hyperkinetic states in which blood velocity increases such as fever, anemia, and hyperthyroidism
- Mitral stenosis in which the leaflets are still mobile but increased ventricular pressure is needed to close the valve

Diminished S_1
Sometimes the S_1 sound is softer than the S_2 sound. This occurs when the mitral valve is not fully open at the time of ventricular contraction and valve closing. Examples include:
- Delayed conduction from the atria to the ventricles as in first-degree heart block, which allows the mitral valve to drift closed before ventricular contraction closes it
- Mitral insufficiency in which extreme calcification of the valve limits mobility
- Delayed or diminished ventricular contraction arising from forceful atrial contraction into a noncompliant ventricle, as in severe pulmonary or systemic hypertension

Split S_1
As named, a split S_1 occurs as a split sound. This occurs when the left and right ventricles contract at different times (asynchronous ventricular contraction). Examples include:
- Conduction delaying the cardiac impulse to one of the ventricles, as in bundle branch block
- Ventricular ectopy in which the impulse starts in one ventricle, contracting it first, and then spreading to the second ventricle

Varying S_1
This occurs when the mitral valve is in different positions when contraction occurs. Examples include:
- Rhythms in which the atria and ventricles are beating independently of each other
- Totally irregular rhythm such as atrial fibrillation

for more information about S_1 and variations of S_1). S_1 ("lub") is usually heard as one sound but may be heard as two sounds (Fig. 21-4). If heard as two sounds, the first component represents mitral valve closure (M_1) and the second component represents tricuspid closure (T_1). M_1 occurs first because of increased pressure on the left side of the heart and because of the route of myocardial depolarization. S_1 may be heard over the entire precordium but is heard best at the apex (left MCL, fifth ICS).

The second heart sound (S_2) results from closure of the semilunar valves (aortic and pulmonic) and correlates with the beginning of diastole. S_2 ("dubb") is also usually heard as one sound but may be heard as two sounds. If S_2 is heard as two sounds, the first component represents aortic valve closure (A_2) and the second component represents pulmonic valve closure (P_2). A_2 occurs first because of increased pressure on the left side of the heart and because of the route of myocardial depolarization. If S_2 is heard as two distinct sounds, it is called a *split* S_2. A splitting of S_2 may be exaggerated during inspiration and disappear during expiration. S_2 is heard best at the base of the heart. See Box 21-3 for more information about variations of S_2.

Extra Heart Sounds

S_3 and S_4 are referred to as diastolic filling sounds, or extra heart sounds, which result from ventricular vibration secondary to rapid ventricular filling. If present, S_3 can be heard early in diastole, after S_2 (Fig. 21-4). S_4 also results from ventricular vibration but, contrary to S_3, the vibration is secondary to ventricular resistance (noncompliance) during atrial contraction. If present, S_4 can be heard late in diastole, just before S_1 (Fig. 21-4). S_3 is often termed *ventricular gallop*, and S_4 is called *atrial gallop*. Extra heart sounds are described further in the Physical Assessment section of the text and in Assessment Guide 21-1.

Murmurs

Blood normally flows silently through the heart. There are conditions, however, that can create turbulent blood flow in which a swooshing or blowing sound may be auscultated over the precordium. Conditions that contribute to turbulent blood flow include (1) increased blood velocity, (2) structural valve defects, (3) valve malfunction, and (4) abnormal chamber openings (e.g., septal defect).

Cardiac Output

Cardiac output (CO) is the amount of blood pumped by the ventricles during a given period of time (usually 1 minute) and is determined by the stroke volume (SV) multiplied by the heart rate (HR): SV × HR = CO. The normal adult CO is 5 to 6 L/min.

Stroke Volume

Stroke volume (SV) is the amount of blood pumped from the heart with each contraction (SV from the left ventricle is usually 70 mL). SV is influenced by several factors:

- The degree of stretch of the heart muscle up to a critical length before contraction (preload); the greater the preload, the greater the SV. This holds true unless the heart muscle is stretched so much that it cannot contract effectively.
- The pressure against which the heart muscle has to eject blood during contraction (afterload); increased afterload results in decreased SV.
- Synergy of contraction (i.e., the uniform, synchronized contraction of the myocardium); conditions that cause an asynchronous contraction decrease SV.
- Compliance, or distensibility, of the ventricles; decreased compliance decreases SV.
- Contractility, or the force of contractions, of the myocardium under given loading conditions; increased contractility increases SV.

Although cardiac muscle has an innate pattern of contractility, cardiac activity is also mediated by the autonomic nervous system to respond to changing needs. The sympathetic impulses increase HR and, therefore, CO. The parasympathetic impulses, which travel to the heart by the vagus nerve, decrease the HR and, therefore, decrease CO.

Neck Vessels

Assessment of the cardiovascular system includes evaluation of the vessels of the neck: the *carotid artery* and the *jugular veins* (Fig. 21-5). Assessment of the pulses of these vessels reflects the integrity of the heart muscle.

BOX 21-3 VARIATIONS IN S_2

The S_2 sound depends on the closure of the aortic and pulmonic valves. Closure of the pulmonic valve is delayed by inspiration, resulting in a split S_2 sound. The components of the split sound are referred to as A_2 (aortic valve sound) and P_2 (pulmonic valve sound). If either sound is absent, no split sounds are heard. The A_2 sound is heard best over the second right ICS. P_2 is normally softer than A_2.

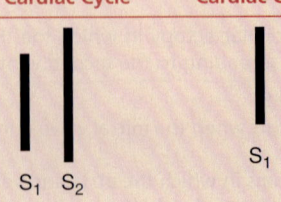

Accentuated S_2
An accentuated S_2 means that S_2 is louder than S_1. This occurs in conditions in which the aortic or pulmonic valve has a higher closing pressure. Examples include:
- Increased pressure in the aorta from exercise, excitement, or systemic hypertension (a booming S_2 is heard with systemic hypertension)
- Increased pressure in the pulmonary vasculature, which may occur with mitral stenosis or congestive heart failure
- Calcification of the semilunar valve, in which the valve is still mobile, as in pulmonic or aortic stenosis

	1st Cardiac Cycle	Beginning of Next Cardiac Cycle

Diminished S₂
A diminished S₂ means that S₂ is softer than S₁. This occurs in conditions in which the aortic or pulmonic valves have decreased mobility. Examples include:
- Decreased systemic blood pressure, which weakens the valves, as in shock
- Aortic or pulmonic stenosis, in which the valves are thickened and calcified, with decreased mobility

Normal (Physiologic) Split S₂
A normal split S₂ can be heard over the second or third left ICS. It is usually heard best during inspiration and disappears during expiration. Over the aortic area and apex, the pulmonic component of S₂ is usually too faint to be heard and S₂ is a single sound resulting from aortic valve closure. In some clients, S₂ may not become single on expiration unless the client sits up. Splitting that does not disappear during expiration is suggestive of heart disease.

Wide Split S₂
This is an increase in the usual splitting that persists throughout the entire respiratory cycle and widens on expiration. It occurs when there is delayed electrical activation of the right ventricle. An example:
- Right bundle branch block, which delays pulmonic valve closing

Fixed Split S₂
This is a wide splitting that does not vary with respiration. It occurs when there is delayed closure of one of the valves. An example:
- Atrial septal defect and right ventricular failure, which delay pulmonic valve closing

Reversed Split S₂
This is a split S₂ that appears on expiration and disappears on inspiration—also known as paradoxical split. It occurs when closure of the aortic valve is abnormally delayed, causing A₂ to follow P₂ in expiration. Normal inspiratory delay of P₂ makes the split disappear during inspiration. An example:
- Left bundle branch block

ACCENTUATED A₂
An accentuated A₂ is loud over the right, second ICS. This occurs with increased pressure, as in systemic hypertension and aortic root dilation because of the closer position of the aortic valve to the chest wall.

DIMINISHED A₂
A diminished A₂ is soft or absent over the right, second ICS. This occurs with immobility of the aortic valve in calcific aortic stenosis.

ACCENTUATED P₂
An accentuated P₂ is louder than or equal to an A₂ sound. This occurs with pulmonary hypertension, dilated pulmonary artery, and atrial septal defect. A wide split S₂, heard even at the apex, indicates an accentuated P₂.

DIMINISHED P₂
A soft or absent P₂ sound occurs with an increased anteroposterior diameter of the chest (barrel chest), which is associated with aging, pulmonic stenosis, or COPD (chronic obstructive pulmonary disease).

ASSESSMENT GUIDE 21-1   Auscultating Heart Sounds

Most nurses need many hours of practice in auscultating heart sounds to assess a client's health status and interpret findings proficiently and confidently. Practitioners may be able to recognize an abnormal heart sound but may have difficulty determining what and where it is exactly. Continued exposure and experience increase one's ability to determine the exact nature and characteristics of abnormal heart sounds. An added difficulty involves palpation, particularly of the apical impulse in clients who are obese or barrel chested. These conditions increase the distance from the apex of the heart to the precordium.

Where to Auscultate

Heart sounds can be auscultated in the traditional five areas on the precordium, which is the anterior surface of the body overlying the heart and great vessels. The traditional areas include the aortic area, the pulmonic area, Erb point, the tricuspid area, and the mitral or apical area. The four valve areas do not reflect the anatomic location of the valves. Rather, they reflect the way in which heart sounds radiate to the chest wall. Sounds always travel in the direction of blood flow. For example, sounds that originate in the tricuspid valve are usually best heard along the left lower sternal border at the fourth or fifth ICS.

Traditional Areas of Auscultation

- Aortic area: Second ICS at the right sternal border—the base of the heart
- Pulmonic area: Second or third ICS at the left sternal border—the base of the heart
- Erb point: Third ICS at the left sternal border
- Mitral (apical): Fifth ICS near the left MCL—the apex of the heart
- Tricuspid area: Fourth or fifth ICS at the left lower sternal border

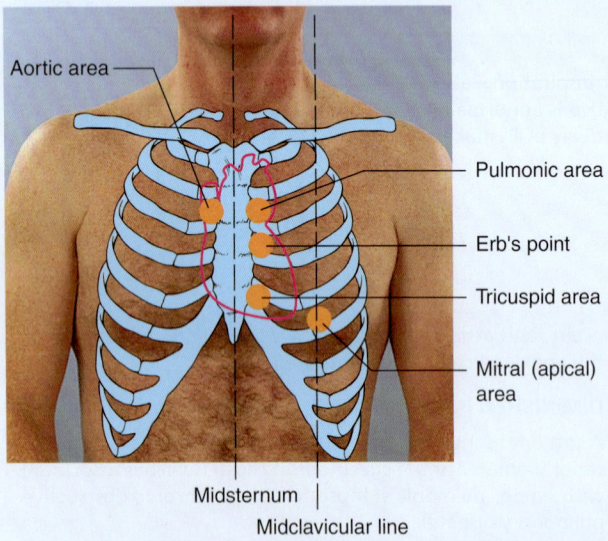

Alternative Areas of Auscultation

In reality, the areas described overlap extensively and sounds produced by the valves can be heard all over the precordium. Therefore, it is important to listen to more than just five specific points on the precordium. Keep overlap in mind and use the names of the chambers instead of Erb point, mitral, and tricuspid areas when auscultating over the precordium. "Alternative" (versus the traditional) areas of auscultation overlap and are not as discrete as the traditional areas. The alternative areas are the aortic area, pulmonic area, left atrial area, right atrial area, left ventricular area, and right ventricular area.

Cover the entire precordium. As you auscultate in all areas, concentrate on systematically moving the stethoscope from left to right across the entire heart area from the base to the apex (top to bottom) or from the apex to the base (bottom to top).

- Aortic area: Right second ICS to apex of heart
- Pulmonic area: Second and third left ICSs close to sternum but may be higher or lower
- Left atrial area: Second to fourth ICS at the left sternal border
- Right atrial area: Third to fifth ICS at the right sternal border
- Left ventricular area: Second to fifth ICSs, extending from the left sternal border to the left MCL
- Right ventricular area: Second to fifth ICSs, centered over the sternum

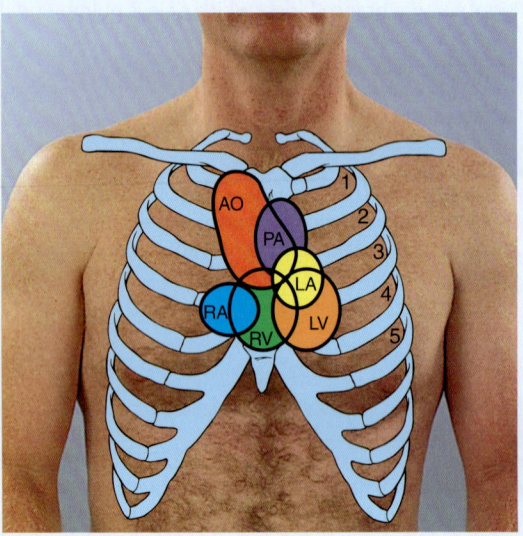

How to Auscultate

Position yourself on the client's right side. The client should be supine, with the upper trunk elevated 30 degrees. Use the diaphragm of the stethoscope to auscultate all areas of the precordium for high-pitched sounds. Use the bell of the stethoscope to detect (differentiate) low-pitched sounds or gallops. Apply the diaphragm firmly to the chest, but apply the bell lightly.

Focus on one sound at a time as you auscultate each area of the precordium. Start by listening to the heart's rate and rhythm. Then identify the first and second heart sounds, concentrate on each heart sound individually, listen for extra heart sounds, listen for murmurs, and finally listen with the client in different positions.

🎯 CLINICAL TIP
Closing your eyes reduces visual stimuli and distractions, and may enhance your ability to concentrate on auditory stimuli.

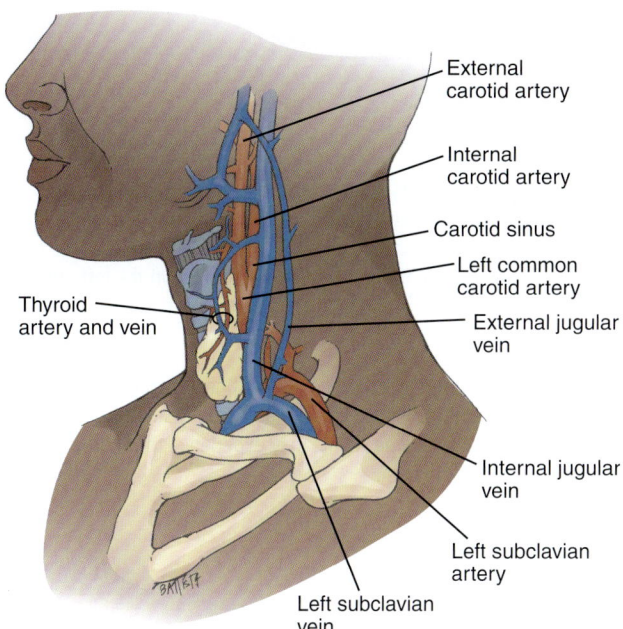

FIGURE 21-5 Major neck vessels, including the carotid arteries and jugular veins.

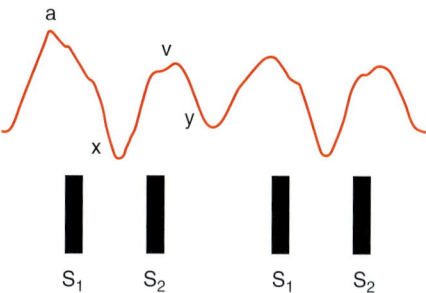

FIGURE 21-6 Jugular venous pulse wave reflects pressure levels in the heart.

Carotid Artery Pulse

The right and left common carotid arteries extend from the brachiocephalic trunk and the aortic arch, and are located in the groove between the trachea and the right and left sternocleidomastoid muscles. Slightly below the mandible, each bifurcates into an internal and external carotid artery. They supply the neck and head, including the brain, with oxygenated blood. The *carotid artery pulse* is a centrally located arterial pulse. Because it is close to the heart, the pressure wave pulsation coincides closely with ventricular systole. The carotid arterial pulse is good for assessing amplitude and contour of the pulse wave. The pulse should normally have a smooth, rapid upstroke that occurs in early systole and a more gradual downstroke.

Jugular Venous Pulse and Pressure

There are two sets of jugular veins: internal and external. The internal jugular veins lie deep and medial to the sternocleidomastoid muscle. The external jugular veins are more superficial; they lie lateral to the sternocleidomastoid muscle and above the clavicle. The jugular veins return blood to the heart from the head and neck by way of the superior vena cava.

Assessment of the *jugular venous pulse* is important for determining the hemodynamics of the right side of the heart. Observing the right internal jugular vein pulse is preferred for assessing right-sided heart hemodynamics because this vein is in direct line with the superior vena cava; however, the external jugular veins are more easily seen and provide accurate results as well (Gersh, 2016). The level of the jugular venous pressure reflects right atrial (central venous) pressure and, usually, right ventricular diastolic filling pressure. Right-sided heart failure raises pressure and volume, thus raising *jugular venous pressure*.

Decreased jugular venous pressure occurs with reduced left ventricular output or reduced blood volume. The right internal jugular vein is most directly connected to the right atrium, and provides the best assessment of pressure changes. Components of the jugular venous pulse follow:

- a wave—reflects rise in atrial pressure that occurs with atrial contraction
- x descent—reflects right atrial relaxation and descent of the atrial floor during ventricular systole
- v wave—reflects right atrial filling, increased volume, and increased atrial pressure
- y descent—reflects right atrial emptying into the right ventricle and decreased atrial pressure

NOTE: Assessment of the jugular vein pressure is often not routinely done by the nurse. The health care provider normally orders a pulmonary artery catheter when needed. However, Chiaco et al. (2016) have noted that in current medical practice, technology has come to replace low cost and effective methods of assessment such as this. This assessment by a nurse can be effective when the correct assessment technique is mastered.

Figure 21-6 illustrates the jugular venous pulse.

HEALTH ASSESSMENT

Collecting Subjective Data: The Nursing Health History

Subjective data collected about the heart and neck vessels helps the nurse to identify abnormal conditions that may affect the client's ability to perform activities of daily living (ADLs) and to fulfill his or her role and responsibilities. Data collection also provides information on the client's risk for cardiovascular disease and helps to identify areas for which health education is needed. The client may not be aware of the significant role that health promotion activities can play in preventing cardiovascular disease.

When compiling the nursing history of current complaints or symptoms, personal and family history, and lifestyle and health practices, remember to thoroughly explore signs and symptoms that the client brings to your attention either intentionally or inadvertently.

History of Present Health Concern

QUESTION	RATIONALE
Chest Pain	
Do you experience chest pain? If the client answers yes, use **COLDSPA** to explore the symptom. **C**haracter: Describe your chest pain (stabbing, burning, crushing, squeezing, or tightness). **O**nset: When did it start?	Chest pain can be cardiac, pulmonary, muscular, or gastrointestinal in origin. Angina (cardiac chest pain) is usually described as a sensation of squeezing around the heart; a steady, severe pain; and a sense of pressure. It may radiate to the left shoulder and down the left arm or to the jaw. Diaphoresis and pain worsened by activity are usually related to cardiac chest pain.
Location: Where is the pain? Does it radiate to any other area? Where? **D**uration: How long does the pain last? How often do you experience the pain? **S**everity: Rate the pain on a scale of 0 to 10, with 10 being the worst possible pain. **P**atterns: What brings on the pain (activity, stress, eating, sexual activity, weather change, extreme cold or heat, lying flat, resting)? What relieves the pain (nitroglycerin, rest)? **A**ssociated Factors: Do you have any other symptoms with this pain (shortness of breath [dyspnea], perspiration [diaphoresis], pale clammy skin, nausea, vomiting, heart beat skips or speeds up)?	Other symptoms that may occur include dyspnea, diaphoresis, pallor, nausea, palpitations, or tachycardia. Pain is usually seen in clients with angina. However, some clients may experience these other symptoms without the pain.
Tachycardia and Palpitations	
Does your heart ever beat faster? Does your heart ever skip beats, or have extra beats? When does this occur and how long does it last? What makes this better or worse?	*Tachycardia* may be seen with weak heart muscles, an attempt by the heart to increase CO. *Palpitation*s may occur with an abnormality of the heart's conduction system (arrhythmias) or during the heart's attempt to increase CO by increasing the HR. Palpitations may cause the client to feel anxious.
Other Symptoms	
Do you tire easily? Do you experience fatigue? Describe when the fatigue started. Was it sudden or gradual? Do you notice it at any particular time of day?	*Fatigue* may result from compromised CO. Fatigue related to decreased CO is worse in the evening or as the day progresses, whereas fatigue seen with depression is ongoing throughout the day.
Do you have difficulty breathing (dyspnea) or shortness of breath? When does this occur? What activities cause you to be short of breath? Do you have difficulty breathing when you are lying down? How many pillows do you use to sleep? Does the difficulty in breathing wake you up at night?	*Dyspnea* may result from congestive heart failure, pulmonary disorders, coronary artery disease, myocardial ischemia, and myocardial infarction (MI). Dyspnea may occur at rest; during sleep; or with mild, moderate, or extreme exertion. *Orthopnea* is the need to sit more upright to breathe easily due to fluid accumulation in the lungs. Waking up from dyspnea during the night (*paroxysmal nocturnal dyspnea*) is seen with heart failure due to redistribution of fluid from the ankles to the lungs when one lies down at night.
Do you cough up mucous? When does it occur? Describe the appearance.	Fluid accumulation in the lungs from heart failure can cause one to cough up white- or pink-tinged *sputum*.
Do you experience dizziness?	*Dizziness* may indicate decreased blood flow to the brain due to myocardial damage. However, there are several other causes for dizziness such as inner ear syndromes, decreased cerebral circulation, and hypotension. **SAFETY TIP** *Dizziness may put the client at risk for falls.*
Do you wake up at night with an urgent need to urinate (nocturia)? If so, how many times each night?	Increased renal perfusion during periods of rest or recumbent positions may cause *nocturia*, which occurs with heart failure.

QUESTION	RATIONALE
Do you experience swelling (edema) in your feet, ankles, or legs? When did this begin? What time of day do you have this swelling? Is it in one or both legs?	*Edema* in both lower extremities at night is seen in heart failure due to a reduction of blood flow out of the heart, causing blood returning to the heart to back up in the organs and dependent areas of the body.
Do you have frequent heartburn? When does it occur? What relieves it? How often do you experience it?	Cardiac pain may be overlooked or misinterpreted as gastrointestinal problems. Gastrointestinal pain may occur after meals and is relieved with antacids. Cardiac pain may occur anytime, is not relieved with antacids, and worsens with activity.

Personal Health History

QUESTION	RATIONALE
Have you been diagnosed with a heart defect or a murmur?	Congenital or acquired defects affect the heart's ability to pump, decreasing the oxygen supply to the tissues.
Have you ever had rheumatic fever?	Acute rheumatic fever (ARF) and rheumatic heart disease (RHD) is a significant public health concern around the world (Seckeler & Hoke, 2011). Rheumatic carditis develops after exposure to group A beta-hemolytic streptococci and results in inflammation of all layers of the heart, impairing contraction and valvular function.
Have you ever had heart surgery or cardiac balloon interventions?	Previous heart surgery may change the heart sounds heard during auscultation. Surgery and cardiac balloon interventions indicate prior cardiac compromise.
Have you ever had an electrocardiogram (ECG)? When was the last one performed? Do you know the results?	A prior ECG allows the health care team to evaluate for any changes in cardiac conduction or previous MI.
Have you ever had a blood test called a lipid profile? Based on your last test, do you know what your cholesterol levels were?	Dyslipidemia presents the greatest risk for the developing coronary artery disease. Elevated cholesterol levels have been linked to the development of atherosclerosis (American Heart Association [AHA], 2014a).
Do you take medications or use other treatments for heart disease? How often do you take them? Why do you take them?	Clients may have medications prescribed for heart disease but may not take them regularly. Clients may skip taking their diuretics because of having to urinate frequently. Beta-blockers may be omitted because of the adverse effects on sexual energy. Education about medications may be needed.
Do you monitor your own HR or blood pressure?	Self-monitoring of HR or blood pressure is recommended if the client is taking cardiotonic or antihypertensive medications. A demonstration is necessary to ensure appropriate technique.

Family History

QUESTION	RATIONALE
Is there a history of hypertension, MI, coronary heart disease (CHD), elevated cholesterol levels, or diabetes mellitus (DM) in your family?	A genetic predisposition to these risk factors increases a client's chance for developing heart disease.

Lifestyle and Health Practices

QUESTION	RATIONALE
Do you smoke? How many packs of cigarettes per day and for how many years? Are you trying to or interested in trying to quit smoking?	Cigarette smoking greatly increases the risk of heart disease (Evidence-Based Practice 21-1). If the client is trying to quit, then the 5 As of smoking cessation (Box 21-4) can be initiated, as even a brief intervention can significantly increase the rates at which patients stop smoking (ACOG, 2016).

Continued on following page

Lifestyle and Health Practices (Continued)

QUESTION	RATIONALE
What type of stress do you have in your life? How do you cope with it?	Stress has been identified as a possible risk factor for heart disease.
Describe what you usually eat in a 24-hour period.	An elevated cholesterol level increases the chance of fatty plaque formation in the coronary vessels.
How much alcohol do you consume each day/week?	Excessive intake of alcohol has been linked to hypertension. More than two drinks per day for men, or one drink per day for women, is associated with high blood pressure and other diseases (AHA, 2015a).
Do you exercise? What type of exercise and how often?	A sedentary lifestyle is a known modifiable risk factor contributing to heart disease. Aerobic exercise three times per week for 30 minutes is more beneficial than anaerobic exercise or sporadic exercise in preventing heart disease.
Describe your daily activities. How are they different from your routine 5 or 10 years ago? Does fatigue, chest pain, or shortness of breath limit your ability to perform daily activities? Describe. Are you able to care for yourself?	Heart disease may impede the ability to perform daily activities. Exertional dyspnea or fatigue may indicate heart failure. An inability to complete ADLs may necessitate a referral for home care.
Has your heart disease had any effect on your sexual activity?	Many clients with heart disease are afraid that sexual activity will precipitate chest pain. If the client can walk one block or climb two flights of stairs without experiencing symptoms, it is generally acceptable for the client to engage in sexual intercourse. Nitroglycerin can be taken before intercourse as a prophylactic for chest pain. In addition, the side-lying position for sexual intercourse may reduce the workload on the heart.
How many pillows do you use to sleep at night? Do you get up to urinate during the night? Do you feel rested in the morning?	If heart function is compromised, CO to the kidneys is reduced during episodes of activity. At rest, CO increases, as does glomerular filtration and urinary output. Orthopnea (the inability to breathe while supine) and nocturia may indicate heart failure. In addition, these two conditions may also impede the ability to get adequate rest.
How important is having a healthy heart to your ability to feel good about yourself and your appearance? What fears about heart disease do you have?	A person's feeling of self-worth may depend on the ability to perform usual daily activities and fulfill the usual roles. Of more than 1,000 adult US women surveyed, 9.7% identified heart disease as the disease they fear most (National Heart Lung and Blood Institute [NHLBI], 2012).

21-1 EVIDENCE-BASED HEALTH PROMOTION AND DISEASE PREVENTION: CORONARY HEART DISEASE

INTRODUCTION

Heart disease is a broad category used to capture a range of diseases, including diseases of blood vessels, such as coronary artery disease; heart rhythm problems (arrhythmias); heart infections; and congenital heart defects (Mayo Clinic, 2014). Furthermore, cardiovascular disease and CHD are often used interchangeably with heart disease and refers to conditions that involve narrowed or blocked blood vessels (that can lead to a heart attack, chest pain, or stroke), and those that affect heart muscles, valves, or rhythm. Heart disease is the leading cause of death in the United States (Healthy People 2020, 2014). Although the complexity of how heart disease develops is still being studied, it is well recognized that lifestyle affects the disease and healthy changes in lifestyle may reduce or reverse vascular changes leading to the disease.

HEALTHY PEOPLE 2020 GOAL

Overview
Healthy People 2020 (2014) addresses the topic of cardiovascular disease as comprised of heart disease and stroke. In this book, stroke is covered in Chapter 25.

GOAL
- Improve cardiovascular health and quality of life through prevention, detection, and treatment of risk factors for heart attack and stroke; early identification and treatment of heart attacks and strokes; and prevention of repeat cardiovascular events.

OBJECTIVES
- (Developmental) Increase overall cardiovascular health in the US population (being developed).

- Reduce CHD deaths from 129.2 per 100,000 population in 2007 to 103.4.
- Increase the proportion of adults 18 years of age and older who have had their blood pressure measured within the preceding 2 years and can state whether their blood pressure was normal or high from 90.6% in 2008 to 92.6%.
- Reduce the proportion of adults with hypertension from 26.9% to 20.9%.
- Increase the proportion of adults who have had their blood cholesterol checked within the preceding 5 years from 74.6% of adults aged 18 years and older to 82.1%.
- Reduce the proportion of adults with high total blood cholesterol levels from 15.0% in 2005–2008 to 13.5%.
- (Developmental) Increase the proportion of adults with prehypertension who meet the recommended guidelines (being developed).
- (Developmental) Increase the proportion of adults with hypertension who meet the recommended guidelines (being developed).
- Increase the proportion of adults aged 20 years and older who are aware of, and respond to, early warning symptoms and signs of a heart attack.
- (Developmental) Increase the proportion of out-of-hospital cardiac arrests in which appropriate bystander and emergency medical services were administered.
- Increase the proportion of eligible patients with heart attacks who receive timely artery-opening therapy as specified by current guidelines.
- (Developmental) Increase the proportion of adults with CHD whose low-density lipoprotein (LDL) cholesterol level is at or below recommended levels.
- Reduce hospitalizations of older adults with heart failure as the principal diagnosis.
- (Developmental and new) Increase the proportion of patients with hypertension in clinical health systems whose blood pressure is under control.

SCREENING

The U.S. Preventive Services Task Force (USPSTF, 2012) recommends against routine screening with resting ECG, exercise treadmill test (ETT), or electron-beam computerized tomography (EBCT) scanning for coronary calcium for either the presence of severe coronary artery stenosis (CAS) or the prediction of CHD events in adults at low risk for CHD events, and found insufficient evidence to recommend for or against the use of these screening techniques in adults at increased risk for CHD.

Screening for risk of heart disease includes blood tests for cholesterol level, glucose level and presence of C-reactive protein, blood pressure measurement, a health history assessing cardiovascular-related risks, and screening for peripheral artery disease.

By contrast, the AHA (2014b) notes that managing risk is the key to preventing CHD. AHA recommends that screening start at 20 years of age for blood pressure (baseline and at least every 2 years), fasting lipoprotein profile (cholesterol and triglycerides; baseline and every 4 to 6 years), and body weight (and possibly BMI); and starting at age 45, blood glucose should be measured every 3 years. Discuss smoking, diet, and physical activity with health care provider. Smoking is a major risk factor and should be avoided. If risks are elevated, then more frequent measurements are recommended.

RISK ASSESSMENT

According to AHA (2017), the risk factors for CHD are:
Factors that cannot be changed:
- Increasing age, especially over 65 years
- Gender (male)
- Heredity (including race): Parents had heart disease; African American heritage especially, but also Mexican American, Native American, native Hawaiian, and some Asian

Factors that can be modified:
- Smoking tobacco or being exposed second hand
- High blood cholesterol (total; high low-density; low high-density levels) and high triglycerides
- Hypertension
- Physical inactivity
- Obesity and overweight
- Diabetes mellitus

Factors that can contribute to heart disease:
- Stress
- Excessive alcohol consumption
- Diet and nutrition
- Diabetes mellitus

CLIENT EDUCATION

Because lifestyle has such an important effect on heart disease, it is essential to teach ways to modify the risk of developing the disease and tips on halting the progression of the disease.

Teach Clients

- Stop smoking or enroll in a smoking cessation program.
- Choose a diet that emphasizes intake of vegetables, fruits, and whole grains; includes low-fat dairy products, poultry, fish, legumes, nontropical vegetable oils, and nuts; and limits intake of sweets, sugar-sweetened beverages, and red meats (AHA, 2017).
- Reduce elevated cholesterol (through diet, activity, or per medication if prescribed).
- Lower blood pressure (through weight loss and increased activity).
- Increase physical activity; participate in at least moderate physical activity daily.
- Work to achieve or maintain a healthy weight for height.
- Manage diabetes if diagnosed.
- Limit alcohol intake to an average of one to two drinks per day for men and one drink per day for women. AHA (2015a) defines a drink as one 12 oz. beer, 4 oz. of wine, 1.5 oz. of 80-proof spirits, or 1 oz. of 100-proof spirits.
- Practice stress reducing techniques such as exercise, relaxation, meditation, yoga, recreational and diversional activities from everyday work, hobbies, and so forth.

BOX 21-4 5 A'S INTERVENTION FOR SMOKING CESSATION

Ask about current smoking status
Advise to quit and provide information on how beneficial quitting is.
Assess willingness to quit
Assist with finding resources and making a plan to quit
Arrange for follow ups to help the patient follow through and quit

Developed by the U.S. Public Health Service Supported by American College of Obstetricians and Gynecologists and the National Cancer Institute

CASE STUDY

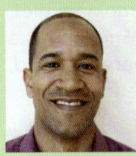

The case study introduced at the beginning of the chapter is now used to demonstrate how the nurse continues to explore Mr. Winchester, who is not in acute distress, but has the presenting symptoms of chest pain and pressure. The COLDSPA pneumonic is used as follows.

Mnemonic	Question	Data Provided
Character	Describe the sign or symptom (feeling, appearance, sound, smell, or taste if applicable).	"It feels like pressure in the middle of my chest."
Onset	When did it begin?	"The pressure-like pain started after I ate supper and sat down to watch TV. Usually I don't have any chest pain unless I'm doing something physical, like yard work."
Location	Where is it? Does it radiate? Does it occur anywhere else?	"It hurts in the middle of my chest and goes down my left arm."
Duration	How long does it last? Does it recur?	"Usually the pain only lasts a couple of minutes. But, this time it lasted a lot longer, may be 20 minutes, and that was scary. I have been having chest pain off and on for a couple of months and thought it was just indigestion."
Severity	How bad is it? or How much does it bother you?	"Right now I don't hurt, but when my wife brought me to the emergency department, I was very uncomfortable." Upon further questioning, Mr. Winchester rated his pain at the onset of this episode as 8 on a scale of 0–10. Over the past 2 months, he rated his pain as a 4–5 on a scale of 0–10. Currently, he denies any pain.
Pattern	What makes it better or worse?	"Stopping whatever I was doing made the pain go away until today."
Associated factors/How it **A**ffects the client	What other symptoms occur with it? How does it affect you?	"Before today I only had the chest pressure with the pain. Today was different. I felt light-headed, sweaty, and sick to my stomach. It was hard to take a deep breath. I hadn't been worried until today, and I have to admit that I was scared." Mr. Winchester denies having palpitations, dyspnea, nocturia, peripheral edema, or indigestion.

After investigating Malcolm Winchester's concerns about chest pain, the nurse continues with the health history.

Mr. Winchester denies heart defect, murmur, history of rheumatic fever, cardiac surgery or intervention, previous ECG, or medications for heart disease. He reports having an annual lipid profile provided by his employer. He remembers that some of the numbers were "high" but cannot recall the actual numbers. He also admits that he has been told that his blood pressure was a "little" high. However, he cannot recall any specific readings.

According to Mr. Winchester, he has a strong family history of hypertension and type 2 diabetes: Both his parents had both conditions. His mother died of a cerebral vascular accident at age 62. His father died of an acute MI at age 58. Maternal and paternal grandparents are deceased due to "heart problems."

Mr. Winchester reports that he started smoking at age 17 and quit at age 30. He smoked 2 packs per day for 13 years (26 pack years). He reports having a stressful job as a supervisor in a local factory, and relieves stress by watching television. In the past 24 hours, Mr. Winchester has eaten: Breakfast—4 cups of coffee, donut; lunch—fast-food double cheeseburger, fries, and cola; dinner—roast beef, mashed potatoes, gravy, green beans, and water; evening snack—bowl of vanilla ice cream.

Mr. Winchester has no formal exercise regimen. He reports that he exercises when he does yard work every weekend.

Mr. Winchester reports that in the past 2–3 months he has "slowed down." He wonders if may be his heart has been "acting up."

Mr. Winchester reports that there has been no change in his sexual activity. He states that he sleeps with one pillow and feels rested after sleep.

Collecting Objective Data: Physical Examination

A major purpose of this examination is to identify any sign of heart disease and initiate early referral and treatment. It is important to remember that cardiovascular disease is the number one cause of death in the United States (Healthy People 2020, 2014).

Assessment of the heart and neck vessels is an essential part of the total cardiovascular examination. It is important to remember that additional data gathered during assessment of the blood pressure, skin, nails, head, thorax and lungs, and peripheral pulses all play a part in the complete cardiovascular assessment. These additional assessment areas are covered in Chapters 8, 14, 15, 19, and 22, respectively.

This chapter encompasses inspection, palpation, and auscultation of the neck and anterior chest area (precordium). Inspection is a fairly easy skill to acquire. However, auscultation requires a lot of practice to develop expert proficiency. Novice practitioners may be able to recognize an abnormal heart sound but may have difficulty determining what and where it is exactly. Continued exposure and experience increase the practitioner's ability to determine the exact nature and characteristics of abnormal heart sounds. In addition, it may be difficult to palpate the apical impulse in clients who are obese or barrel chested: these conditions increase the distance from the apex of the heart to the precordium.

Heart and neck vessel assessment skills are useful to the nurse in all types of health care settings, including acute, clinical, and home health care.

CLINICAL TIP
When performing a total body system examination (see Chapter 28), it is often convenient to assess the heart and neck vessels immediately after assessment of the thorax and lungs.

Preparing the Client

Prepare clients for the examination by explaining that they will need to expose the anterior chest. Explain to the client that it is necessary to assume several different positions for this examination. Explain that you will need to place the client in the supine position with the head elevated to about 30 degrees during auscultation and palpation of the neck vessels and inspection, palpation, and auscultation of the precordium. Tell the client that it will be necessary to assume a left lateral position for palpation of the apical impulse if you are having trouble locating the pulse with the client in the supine position. In addition, explain to the client the necessity to assume a left lateral and sitting-up and leaning-forward position so that you can auscultate for the presence of any abnormal heart sounds. These positions may bring out an abnormal sound not detected with the client in the supine position. Make sure you explain to the client that you will be listening to the heart in a number of places and that this does not necessarily mean that anything is wrong.

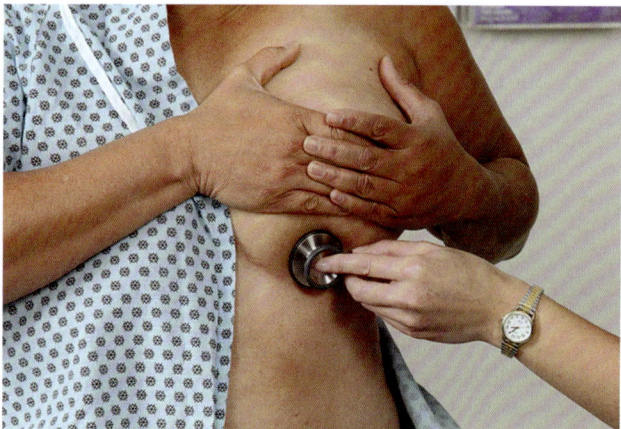

FIGURE 21-7 Asking the client to pull her breast upward and to her side facilitates auscultation of heart sounds.

CLINICAL TIP
In women with large breasts, it may be helpful to ask the client to pull her breast upward and to her side when you are auscultating for heart sounds (Fig. 21-7).

Provide the client with as much modesty as possible during the examination, describe the steps of the examination, and answer any questions the client may have. These actions will help to ease any client anxiety.

Equipment
- Stethoscope with a bell and diaphragm
- Small pillow
- Penlight or movable examination light
- Watch with second hand
- Centimeter rulers (two)

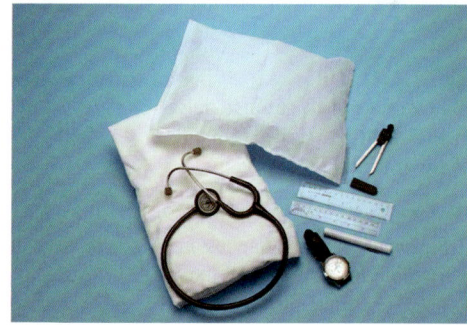

Physical Assessment

Remember these key points during examination:
- Understand the anatomy and function of the heart and major coronary vessels to identify and interpret heart sounds and electrocardiograms accurately.
- Know normal variations of the cardiovascular system in the older adult client.

General Routine Screening *versus* Focused Specialty Assessment for Heart and Neck Vessels

The nurse routinely assesses the client's heart and neck vessels through inspection and auscultation. A more detailed examination, including evaluation of jugular venous pressure and identification of the type and source of murmur and various abnormal heart sounds, would be performed by the specialized cardiovascular ICU nurse or advanced cardiovascular nurse practitioner.

General Routine Screening
- Inspect the jugular venous pulse.
- Auscultate then palpate carotid arteries.
- Inspect pulsations on anterior chest.
- Palpate the apical impulse.
- Palpate for abnormal pulsations.
- Auscultate to identify S_1 and S_2.
- Auscultate for extra heart sounds.
- Auscultate for murmurs.

Focused Specialty Assessment
- Evaluate jugular venous pressure.
- Grade and identify source of auscultated murmurs.
- Differentiate between specific split sounds, rubs, snaps, and clicks.

ASSESSMENT PROCEDURE	NORMAL FINDINGS	ABNORMAL FINDINGS
Neck Vessels		
INSPECTION		
Observe the jugular venous pulse. Inspect the jugular venous pulse by standing on the right side of the client. The client should be in a supine position with the torso elevated 30–45 degrees. Make sure the head and torso are on the same plane. Ask the client to turn the head slightly to the left. Shine a tangential light source onto the neck to increase visualization of pulsations as well as shadows. Next, inspect the suprasternal notch or the area around the clavicles for pulsations of the internal jugular veins. 🎯 **CLINICAL TIP** Be careful not to confuse pulsations of the carotid arteries with pulsations of the internal jugular veins.	The jugular venous pulse is not normally visible with the client sitting upright. This position fully distends the vein, and pulsations may or may not be discernible.	Fully distended jugular veins with the client's torso elevated more than 45 degrees indicate increased central venous pressure that may be the result of right ventricular failure, pulmonary hypertension, pulmonary emboli, or cardiac tamponade.
Evaluate jugular venous pressure (Fig. 21-8). Evaluate jugular venous pressure by watching for distention of the jugular vein. It is normal for the jugular veins to be visible when the client is supine. To evaluate jugular vein distention, position the client in a supine position with the head of the bed elevated 30, 45, 60, and 90 degrees. At each increase of the elevation, have the client's head turned slightly away from the side being evaluated. Using tangential lighting, observe for distention, protrusion, or bulging.	The jugular vein should not be distended, bulging, or protruding at 45 degrees or greater.	Distention, bulging, or protrusion at 45, 60, or 90 degrees may indicate right-sided heart failure. Document at which positions (45, 60, and/or 90 degrees) you observe distention. Clients with obstructive pulmonary disease may have elevated venous pressure only during expiration. An inspiratory increase in venous pressure, called Kussmaul sign, may occur in clients with severe constrictive pericarditis.

21 Assessing Heart and Neck Vessels   447

ASSESSMENT PROCEDURE	NORMAL FINDINGS	ABNORMAL FINDINGS
CLINICAL TIP Jugular Venous Pressure is often omitted and replaced by a medical order for pulmonary artery catheter placement. However, when performed correctly, this assessment is low cost and effective. See Chiaco et al. (2016) for a more in depth precise description of this procedure. 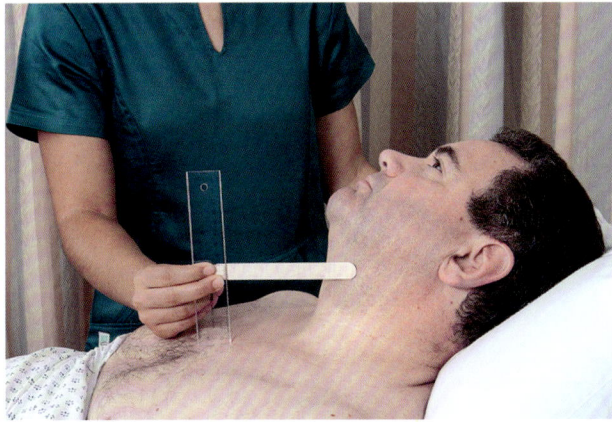 **FIGURE 21-8** Assessing jugular venous pressure.		

AUSCULTATION AND PALPATION

Auscultate the carotid arteries if the client is middle-aged or older or if you suspect cardiovascular disease. Place the bell of the stethoscope over the carotid artery and ask the client to hold his or her breath for a moment so that breath sounds do not conceal any vascular sounds (Fig. 21-9). **CLINICAL TIP** Always auscultate the carotid arteries before palpating because palpation may increase or slow the HR, changing the strength of the carotid impulse heard. 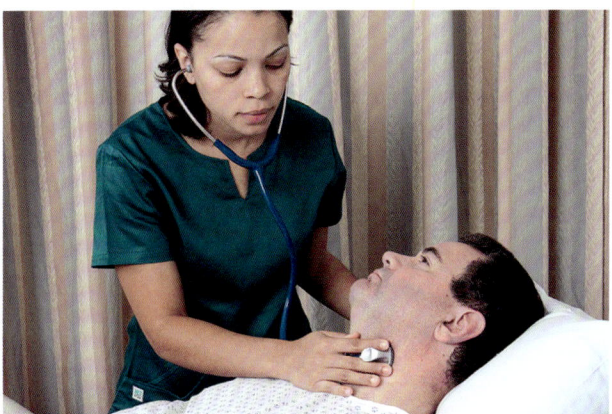 **FIGURE 21-9** Auscultating the carotid artery.	No blowing or swishing or other sounds are heard.	A bruit, a blowing or swishing sound caused by turbulent blood flow through a narrowed vessel, is indicative of occlusive arterial disease. However, if the artery is more than two-thirds occluded, a bruit may not be heard.

Continued on following page

ASSESSMENT PROCEDURE	NORMAL FINDINGS	ABNORMAL FINDINGS

Neck Vessels

Palpate the carotid arteries. Palpate each carotid artery alternately by placing the pads of the index and middle fingers medial to the sternocleidomastoid muscle on the neck (Fig. 21-10). Note amplitude and contour of the pulse, elasticity of the artery, and any thrills (which feel similar to a purring cat).

SAFETY TIP *Palpate the carotid arteries individually because bilateral palpation could result in reduced cerebral blood flow. If you detect occlusion during auscultation, palpate very lightly to avoid blocking circulation or triggering vagal stimulation and bradycardia, hypotension, or even cardiac arrest.*

 OLDER ADULT CONSIDERATIONS
Be cautious with older clients because atherosclerosis may have caused obstruction and compression may easily block circulation.

Pulses are equally strong; a 2+ or normal with no variation in strength from beat to beat. Contour is normally smooth and rapid on the upstroke and slower and less abrupt on the downstroke. The strength of the pulse is evaluated on a scale from 0 to 3 as follows:

Pulse Amplitude Scale
0 = Absent
1+ = Weak, diminished (easy to obliterate)
2+ = Normal (obliterate with moderate pressure)
3+ = Bounding (unable to obliterate or requires firm pressure)

Arteries are elastic and no thrills are noted.

Pulse inequality may indicate arterial constriction or occlusion in one carotid.

Weak pulses may indicate hypovolemia, shock, or decreased cardiac output.

A bounding, firm pulse may indicate hypervolemia or increased CO.

Variations in strength from beat to beat or with respiration are abnormal and may indicate a variety of problems (Abnormal Findings 21-1).

A delayed upstroke may indicate aortic stenosis.

Loss of elasticity may indicate arteriosclerosis. Thrills may indicate a narrowing of the artery.

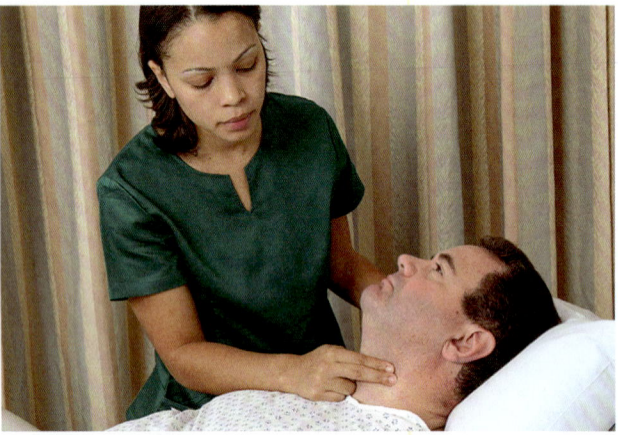

FIGURE 21-10 Palpating the carotid artery.

Heart (Precordium), Anterior Chest

INSPECTION

Inspect for any pulsations on anterior chest over heart. With the client in supine position with the head of the bed elevated between 30 and 45 degrees, stand on the client's right side and look for the apical impulse and any abnormal pulsations.

CLINICAL TIP
The apical impulse was originally called the point of maximal impulse (PMI). However, this term is no longer used because a maximal impulse may occur in other areas of the precordium as a result of abnormal conditions.

The apical impulse may or may not be visible. If apparent, it would be in the mitral area (left MCL, fourth or fifth ICS). The apical impulse is a result of the left ventricle moving outward during systole.

Pulsations, which may also be called heaves or lifts, other than the apical pulsation are considered abnormal and should be evaluated. A heave or lift may occur as the result of an enlarged ventricle from an overload of work. Abnormal Findings 21-2 describes abnormal ventricular impulses.

ASSESSMENT PROCEDURE	NORMAL FINDINGS	ABNORMAL FINDINGS
PALPATION		
Palpate the apical impulse. Remain on the client's right side and ask the client to remain supine. Use one or two finger pads to palpate the apical impulse in the mitral area (fourth or fifth ICS at the MCL) (Fig. 21-11A). You may ask the client to roll to the left side to better feel the impulse using your finger pads (Fig. 21-11B). ◎ **CLINICAL TIP** If this apical pulsation cannot be palpated, have the client assume a left lateral position. This displaces the heart toward the left chest wall and relocates the apical impulse farther to the left.	The apical impulse is palpated in the mitral area and may be the size of a nickel (1–2 cm). Amplitude is usually small—like a gentle tap. The duration is brief, lasting through the first two-thirds of systole and often less. In obese clients or clients with large breasts, the apical impulse may not be palpable. **OLDER ADULT CONSIDERATIONS** In older clients, the apical impulse may be difficult to palpate because of increased anteroposterior chest diameter.	The apical impulse may be impossible to palpate in clients with pulmonary emphysema. If the apical impulse is larger than 1–2 cm, displaced, more forceful, or of longer duration, suspect cardiac enlargement.

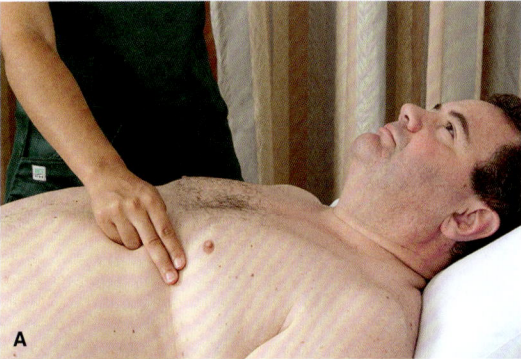
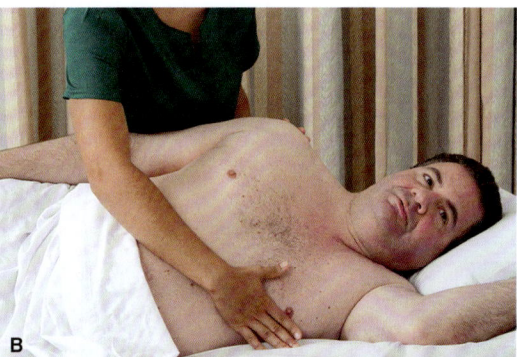

FIGURE 21-11 Locate the apical impulse with the finger pads (**A**); then palpate the apical impulse with the palmar surface (**B**).

Palpate for abnormal pulsations. Use your palmar surfaces to palpate the apex, left sternal border, and base.	No pulsations or vibrations are palpated in the areas of the apex, left sternal border, or base.	A thrill or a pulsation is usually associated with a grade IV or higher murmur.
AUSCULTATION		
Auscultate HR and rhythm. Follow the guidelines given in Assessment Guide 21-1. Place the diaphragm of the stethoscope at the apex and listen closely to the rate and rhythm of the apical impulse.	Rate should be 60–100 beats/min, with regular rhythm. A regularly irregular rhythm, such as sinus arrhythmia when the HR increases with inspiration and decreases with expiration, may be normal in young adults. Resting pulse rate (RPR) varies by age, gender, and ethnic/racial factors (Ostchega et al., 2011). Adult female RPRs are a few beats faster than male RPRs. 🌐 **CULTURAL CONSIDERATIONS** • African Americans have higher HDL levels, but paradoxically they have significantly higher rates (nearly double) of cardiovascular than white Americans (Curry, 2013). • African Americans have the world's highest rates of hypertension, which predisposes to stroke, and CHD (AHA, 2015b). • Hypertension in African Americans has a higher incidence, earlier onset, and higher mortality than in Caucasian Americans (Lackland, 2014).	Bradycardia (less than 60 beats/min) or tachycardia (more than 100 beats/min) may result in decreased CO. Refer clients with irregular rhythms (i.e., premature atrial contraction or premature ventricular contractions, atrial fibrillation, atrial flutter with varying blocks) for further evaluation. These types of irregular patterns may predispose the client to decreased CO, heart failure, or emboli (Abnormal Findings 21-3).

Continued on following page

ASSESSMENT PROCEDURE	NORMAL FINDINGS	ABNORMAL FINDINGS
Heart (Precordium), Anterior Chest (Continued)		
If you detect an irregular rhythm, auscultate for a pulse rate deficit. This is done by palpating the radial pulse while you auscultate the apical pulse. Count for a full minute.	The radial and apical pulse rates should be identical.	A pulse deficit (difference between the apical and peripheral/radial pulses) may indicate atrial fibrillation, atrial flutter, premature ventricular contractions, and varying degrees of heart block.
Auscultate to identify S_1 and S_2. Auscultate the first heart sound (S_1 or "lub") and the second heart sound (S_2 or "dubb"). Remember these two sounds make up the cardiac cycle of systole and diastole. S_1 starts systole, and S_2 starts diastole. The space, or systolic pause, between S_1 and S_2 is of short duration (thus S_1 and S_2 occur very close together); the space, or diastolic pause, between S_2 and the start of another S_1 is of longer duration. ◎ **CLINICAL TIP** If you are experiencing difficulty differentiating S_1 from S_2, palpate the carotid pulse: the harsh sound that you hear from the carotid pulse is S_1 (Fig. 21-12).	S_1 corresponds with each carotid pulsation and is loudest at the apex of the heart. S_2 immediately follows after S_1 and is loudest at the base of the heart.	See Boxes 21-2 and 21-3.

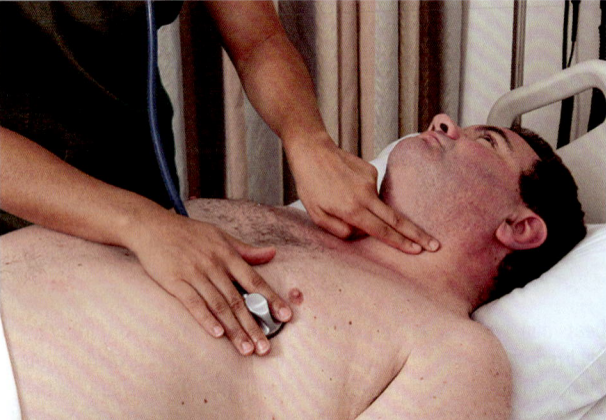

FIGURE 21-12 Palpating the carotid pulse while auscultating S_1.

Listen to S_1. Use the diaphragm of the stethoscope to best hear S_1.	A distinct sound is heard in each area but loudest at the apex. May become softer with inspiration. A split S_1 may be heard normally in young adults at the left lateral sternal border.	Accentuated, diminished, varying, or split S_1 are all abnormal findings (Box 21-2).
Listen to S_2. Use the diaphragm of the stethoscope. Ask the client to breathe regularly (Fig. 21-13). ◎ **CLINICAL TIP** Do not ask the client to hold his or her breath. Breath holding will cause any normal or abnormal split to subside.	Distinct sound is heard in each area but is loudest at the base. A split S_2 (into two distinct sounds of its components—A_2 and P_2) is normal and termed *physiologic splitting*. It is usually heard late in inspiration at the second or third left interspaces (Box 21-3).	Any split S_2 heard in expiration is abnormal. The abnormal split can be one of three types: wide, fixed, or reversed.

21 Assessing Heart and Neck Vessels 451

ASSESSMENT PROCEDURE	NORMAL FINDINGS	ABNORMAL FINDINGS
Auscultate for extra heart sounds. Use the diaphragm first, then the bell (Fig. 21-14) to auscultate over the entire heart area. Note the characteristics (e.g., location, timing) of any extra sound heard. Auscultate during the systolic pause (space heard between S_1 and S_2). Auscultate during the diastolic pause (space heard between end of S_2 and the next S_1). ◎ **CLINICAL TIP** While auscultating, keep in mind that development of a pathologic S_3 may be the earliest sign of heart failure.	Normally no sounds are heard. A physiologic S_3 heart sound is a benign finding commonly heard at the beginning of the diastolic pause in children, adolescents, and young adults. It is rare after age 40. The physiologic S_3 usually subsides upon standing or sitting up. A physiologic S_4 heart sound may be heard near the end of diastole in well-conditioned athletes and in adults older than age 40 or 50 with no evidence of heart disease, especially after exercise.	Ejection sounds or clicks (e.g., a mid-systolic click associated with mitral valve prolapse). A friction rub may also be heard during the systolic pause. Abnormal Findings 21-4 provides a full description of the extra heart sounds (normal and abnormal) of systole and diastole. A pathologic S_3 (ventricular gallop) may be heard with ischemic heart disease, hyperkinetic states (e.g., anemia), or restrictive myocardial disease. A pathologic S_4 (atrial gallop) toward the left side of the precordium may be heard with coronary artery disease, hypertensive heart disease, cardiomyopathy, and aortic stenosis. A pathologic S_4 toward the right side of the precordium may be heard with pulmonary hypertension and pulmonic stenosis. S_3 and S_4 pathologic sounds together create a quadruple rhythm, which is called a *summation gallop.* Opening snaps (OSs) occur early in diastole and indicate mitral valve stenosis. A friction rub may also be heard during the diastolic pause (Abnormal Findings 21-4).

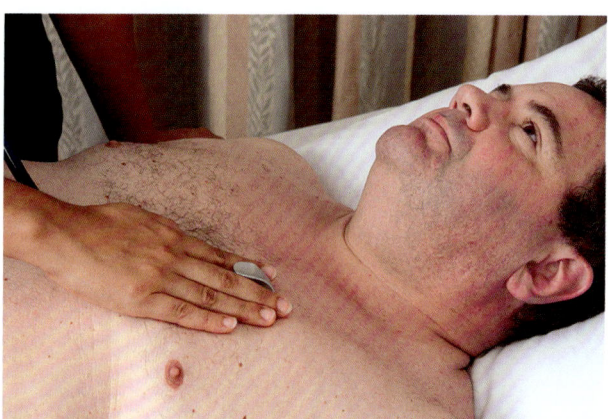

FIGURE 21-13 Auscultating S_2.

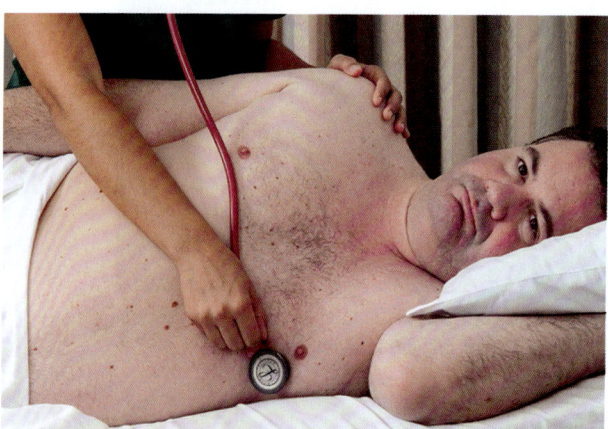

FIGURE 21-14 Listening to heart sounds with the bell of the stethoscope.

Auscultate for murmurs. A murmur is a swishing sound caused by turbulent blood flow through the heart valves or great vessels. Auscultate for murmurs across the entire heart area. Use the diaphragm and the bell of the stethoscope in all areas of auscultation because murmurs have a variety of pitches. Also auscultate with the client in different positions as described in the next section because some murmurs occur or subside according to the client's position.	Normally no murmurs are heard. However, innocent and physiologic midsystolic murmurs may be present in a healthy heart.	Pathologic midsystolic, pansystolic, and diastolic murmurs. Abnormal Findings 21-5 describes pathologic murmurs.

Continued on following page

UNIT 3 Nursing Assessment of Physical Systems

Heart (Precordium), Anterior Chest (Continued)

ASSESSMENT PROCEDURE	NORMAL FINDINGS	ABNORMAL FINDINGS
Auscultate with the client assuming other positions. Ask the client to assume a left lateral position. Use the bell of the stethoscope and listen at the apex of the heart.	S_1 and S_2 heart sounds are normally present.	An S_3 or S_4 heart sound or a murmur of mitral stenosis that was not detected with the client in the supine position may be revealed when the client assumes the left lateral position.
Ask the client to sit up, lean forward, and exhale. Use the diaphragm of the stethoscope and listen over the apex and along the left sternal border (Fig. 21-15).	S_1 and S_2 heart sounds are normally present.	Murmur of aortic regurgitation may be detected when the client assumes this position.

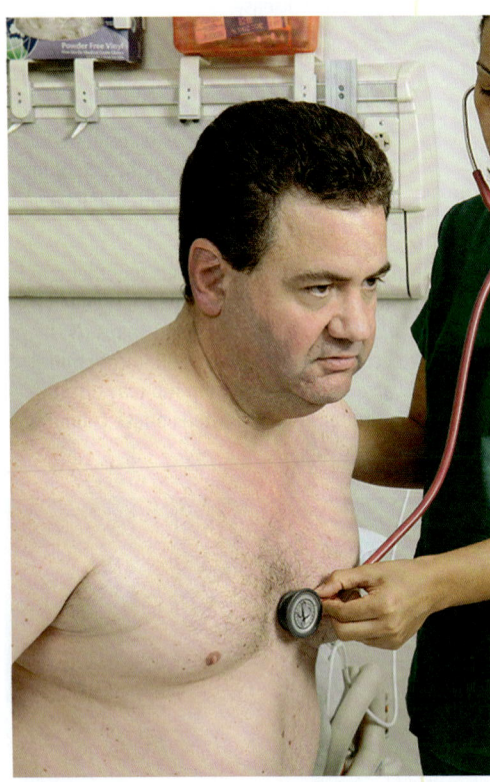

FIGURE 21-15 Auscultating at left sternal border with client sitting up, leaning forward, and exhaling.

CASE STUDY

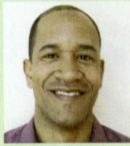

The chapter case study is now used to demonstrate the documentation of a physical assessment of Malcolm Winchester's heart and neck vessels.

No visible jugular venous pulsations or distention at 45 degrees. No carotid bruits to auscultation. Carotid pulses are 2+ bilaterally. No visible apical impulse, heaves, or lifts over the precordium. The apical impulse is palpable at the fifth ICS, MCL, and is 1.5 cm in diameter. S1 (loudest at the apex) and S2 (loudest at the base) present, with no S3 or S4. HR is regular at 72 beats per minute. No murmurs, rubs, or gallops are appreciated.

Validating and Documenting Findings

Validate the heart and neck vessel assessment data that you have collected (by asking additional questions, verifying data with another health care professional, or comparing objective with subjective findings). This is necessary to verify that the data are reliable and accurate. Document the assessment data following the health care facility or agency policy.

CASE STUDY

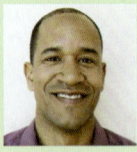

Think back to the case study. The CCU nurse documented the following subjective and objective assessment findings of Malcolm Winchester's heart and neck vessels examination.

Biographic Data: MW, 45-year-old African American male. Alert and oriented. Asks and answers questions appropriately.

Reason for Seeking Health Care: "Pressure-like pain in the middle of my chest."

History of Present Health Concern: The client presented to the emergency department with complaints of chest pressure-like pain at rest associated with left arm discomfort, nausea, and diaphoresis. He reports that the pain was in the center of his chest and lasted for 20 minutes. MW also reports that he has been having episodes of chest pain and pressure lasting 2–3 minutes and alleviated with rest for the past 2–3 months. He denies having palpitations, dyspnea, nocturia, peripheral edema, or indigestion. Mr. Winchester rated his pain at the onset of this episode as 8 on a scale of 0–10. Over the past 2 months, he rated his pain as a 4–5 on a scale of 0–10. Currently, he denies any pain.

Personal Health History: Mr. Winchester denies heart defect, murmur, history of rheumatic fever, cardiac surgery or intervention, previous ECG, or medications for heart disease. He reports having an annual lipid profile provided by his employer. He remembers that some of the numbers were "high," but cannot recall the actual numbers. He admits that he has been told that his blood pressure was a "little" high. However, he cannot recall any specific readings.

Family Health History: According to Mr. Winchester, he has a strong family history of hypertension and type 2 diabetes. Both his parents had hypertension and type 2 diabetes. His mother died of a cerebral vascular accident at age 62. His father died at age 58 of an acute MI. Maternal and paternal grandparents are deceased due to "heart problems."

Lifestyle and Health Practices: Mr. Winchester reports that he started smoking at age 17 and quit at age 30. He smoked 2 packs per day for 13 years (26 pack years). He reports having a stressful job as a supervisor in a local factory, and relieves stress by watching television. In the past 24 hours, Mr. Winchester has eaten: Breakfast—4 cups of coffee, donut; lunch—fast-food double cheeseburger, fries, and cola; dinner—roast beef, mashed potatoes, gravy, green beans, and water; evening snack—bowl of vanilla ice cream. Mr. Winchester has no formal exercise regimen. However, he reports that he exercises when he does yard work every weekend.

Mr. Winchester reports that in the past 2–3 months he has "slowed down." He wonders if maybe his heart has been "acting up."

Mr. Winchester reports that there has been no change in sexual activity. He states that he sleeps with one pillow and feels rested after sleep.

Physical Examination Findings: There are no visible jugular venous pulsations or distention at 45 degrees. There are no carotid bruits to auscultation. Carotid pulses are 2+ bilaterally. There is no visible apical impulse, heaves or lifts over precordium. The apical impulse is palpable at the fifth ICS, MCL, and is 1.5 cm in diameter. S_1 (loudest at the apex) and S_2 (loudest at the base) present, with no S_3 or S_4. HR is regular at 72 beats per minute. There are no murmurs, rubs, or gallops appreciated.

ANALYSIS OF DATA: DIAGNOSTIC REASONING

After collecting subjective and objective data pertaining to the heart and neck vessels, identify abnormal findings and client strengths. Then cluster the data to reveal any significant patterns or abnormalities. These data may be used to make clinical judgments about the status of the client's heart and neck vessels.

Selected Nursing Diagnoses

The following is a listing of selected nursing diagnoses that you may identify when analyzing data for this part of the assessment.

Health Promotion Diagnoses

- Readiness for Enhanced Health Management: Desired information on exercise and low-fat diet

Risk Diagnoses

- Risk for Sexual Dysfunction related to misinformation or lack of knowledge regarding sexual activity and heart disease
- Risk for Ineffective Denial related to smoking and obesity

Actual Diagnoses

- Fatigue related to decreased CO
- Activity Intolerance related to compromised oxygen transport secondary to heart failure
- Acute Pain: Cardiac related to an inequality between oxygen supply and demand
- Anxiety
- Impaired tissue integrity: Cardiac related to impaired circulation

Selective Collaborative Problems

After grouping the data, you may see various collaborative problems emerge. Remember that collaborative problems differ from nursing diagnoses in that they cannot be prevented by nursing interventions. However, these physiologic complications of medical conditions can be detected and monitored by the nurse. In addition, the nurse can use physician- and nurse-prescribed interventions to minimize the complications of these problems. The nurse may also have to refer the client in such situations for further treatment of the problem. Following is a list of collaborative problems that may be identified when assessing the heart and neck vessels. These problems

are worded as Risk for Complications (RC) followed by the problem.
- RC: Decreased cardiac output
- RC: Dysrhythmias
- RC: Hypertension
- RC: Congestive heart failure
- RC: Angina
- RC: Cerebrovascular accident
- RC: Cerebral hemorrhage
- RC: Renal failure

Medical Problems

Once the data are grouped, certain signs and symptoms may become evident and may require medical diagnosis and treatment. Referral to a primary care provider is necessary.

CASE STUDY

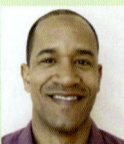

After collecting and analyzing data for Mr. Winchester, the nurse determines that the following conclusions are appropriate:

Nursing Diagnoses
- Acute Pain r/t suspected myocardial O_2 deficit
- Ineffective Health maintenance r/t unknown etiology (suspected combination of lack of knowledge and lack of perceived benefits of healthy lifestyle)

Potential Collaborative Problems
- RC: Cerebrovascular accident
- RC: Myocardial infarction
- RC: Retinal hemorrhage
- RC: Heart failure
- RC: Renal failure

To view an algorithm depicting the process of diagnostic reasoning for this case study go to thePoint.

Interdisciplinary Verbal Communication of Assessment Findings Using SBAR

SITUATION: MW, a 45-year-old African American man, is admitted to the CCU from the ER with pressure-like pain (8 on a scale of 0–10) in middle of chest lasting 20 minutes, left arm discomfort, nausea, and diaphoresis. Currently, he denies any pain.

HISTORY OF PRESENT HEALTH CONCERN: Has been having chest pain (4–5 on a scale of 0–10) and pressure lasting 2–3 minutes that was alleviated with rest over past 2–3 months. Recalls annual lipid profile and blood pressure reported to him to be "high." Mother died of CVA at age 62. Father died of an acute MI at age 58. Maternal and paternal grandparents are deceased due to "heart problems." Also has strong family history of diabetes. Smoked 2 packs per day for 13 years (26 pack years). Had stressful job as a supervisor in local factory; relieves stress by watching television. In the past 24 hours, Mr. Winchester has eaten a very high caloric and high fat breakfast, lunch, and dinner. No formal exercise regimen except for yard work every weekend. Reports slowing down in last 2–3 months.

ASSESSMENT: No visible jugular venous pulsations or distention. No carotid bruits auscultated. Carotid pulses 2+ bilaterally. No visible apical impulse, heaves, or lifts over the precordium. The apical impulse palpable at the fifth ICS, MCL, and is 1.5 cm in diameter. S1 (loudest at the apex) and S2 (loudest at the base) present, with no S3 or S4. HR is regular at 72 beats per minute. No murmurs, rubs, or gallops noted.

RECOMMENDATION: MW has Acute Pain r/t suspected myocardial O_2 deficit and Ineffective Health maintenance r/t unknown etiology (suspected combination of lack of knowledge and lack of perceived benefits of healthy lifestyle). He is at risk for Potential Complications of a cerebrovascular accident, MI, and/or heart failure. He needs to be followed up for further assessment by his primary care provider.

ABNORMAL FINDINGS 21-1 Abnormal Arterial Pulse and Pressure Waves

A normal pulse, represented in the figure, has a smooth, rounded wave with a notch on the descending slope. The pulse should feel strong and regular. The notch is not palpable. The pulse pressure (the difference between the systolic and diastolic pressure) is 30–40 mmHg. Pulse pressure may be measured in waveforms, which are produced when a pulmonary artery catheter is used to evaluate arterial pressure.

The arterial pressure waveform consists of five parts: Anacrotic limb, systolic peak, dicrotic limb, dicrotic notch, and end diastole. The initial upstroke, or anacrotic limb, occurs as blood is rapidly ejected from the ventricle through the open aortic valve into the aorta. The anacrotic limb ends at the systolic peak, the waveform's highest point. Arterial pressure falls as the blood continues into the peripheral vessels and the waveform turns downward, forming the dicrotic limb. When the pressure in the ventricle is less than the pressure in the aortic root, the aortic valve closes and a small notch (dicrotic notch) appears on the waveform. The closing of the aortic notch is the beginning of diastole. The pressure continues to fall in the aortic root until it reaches its lowest point, seen on the waveform as the diastolic peak.

Changes in circulation and heart rhythm affect the pulse and its waveform. Following are some of the variations you may find.

SMALL, WEAK PULSE

Characteristics

- Diminished pulse pressure
- Weak and small on palpation
- Slow upstroke
- Prolonged systolic peak

Causes

- Conditions causing a decreased SV
  - Heart failure
  - Hypovolemia
  - Severe aortic stenosis
- Conditions causing increased peripheral resistance
  - Hypothermia
  - Severe congestive heart failure

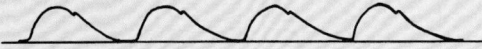

LARGE, BOUNDING PULSE

Characteristics

- Increased pulse pressure
- Strong and bounding on palpation
- Rapid rise and fall with a brief systolic peak

Causes

- Conditions that cause an increased SV or decreased peripheral resistance
  - Fever
  - Anemia
  - Hyperthyroidism
  - Aortic regurgitation
  - Patent ductus arteriosus
- Conditions resulting in increased SV due to decreased HR
  - Bradycardia
  - Complete heart block
- Conditions resulting in decreased compliance of the aortic walls
  - Aging
  - Atherosclerosis

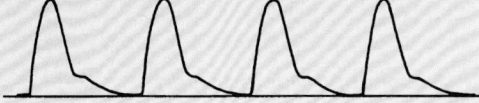

BISFERIENS PULSE

Characteristics

- Double systolic peak

Causes

- Pure aortic regurgitation
- Combined aortic stenosis and regurgitation
- Hypertrophic cardiomyopathy

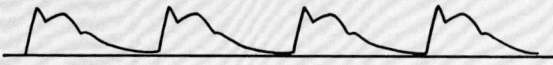

PULSUS ALTERNANS

Characteristics

- Regular rhythm
- Changes in amplitude (or strength) from beat to beat (you may need a sphygmomanometer to detect the difference)

Cause

- Left ventricular failure (usually accompanied by an S_3 sound on the left)

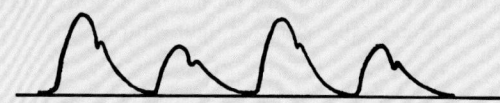

BIGEMINAL PULSE

Characteristics

- Regular, irregular rhythm (one normal beat followed by a premature contraction)
- Alternates in amplitude (one strong pulse followed by a quick, weaker one)

Cause

- Premature ventricular contractions

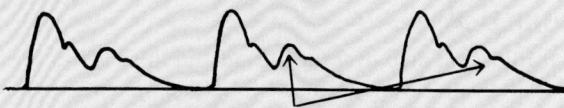

PARADOXICAL PULSE

Characteristics

- Palpable decrease in pulse amplitude on quiet inspiration
- Pulse becomes stronger with expiration
- You may need a sphygmomanometer to detect the change (the systolic pressure will decrease by more than 10 mmHg during inspiration)

Causes

- Pericardial tamponade
- Constrictive pericarditis
- Obstructive lung disease

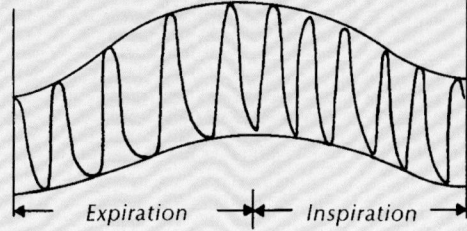

ABNORMAL FINDINGS 21-2 | Ventricular Impulses

Assessment of the chest may reveal abnormalities or variations of the ventricular impulse, signs of hypertension, hypertrophy, volume overload, and pressure overload. Some of the abnormalities or variations include the following:

LIFT

A diffuse lifting left during systole at the left lower sternal border, a lift or heave is associated with right ventricular hypertrophy caused by pulmonic valve disease, pulmonic hypertension, and chronic lung disease. You may also see retraction at the apex, from the posterior rotation of the left ventricle caused by the oversized right ventricle.

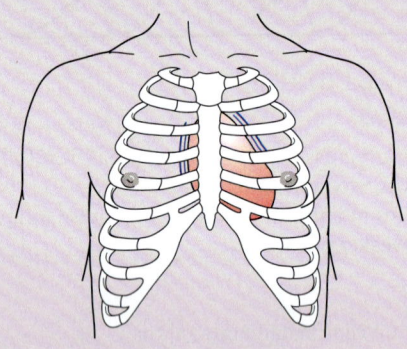

THRILL

A thrill is palpated over the second and third ICS; a thrill may indicate severe aortic stenosis and systemic hypertension. A thrill palpated over the second and third left ICSs may indicate pulmonic stenosis and pulmonic hypertension.

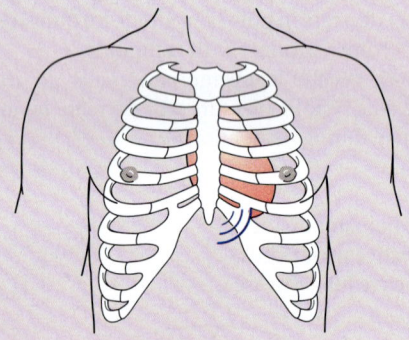

ACCENTUATED APICAL IMPULSE

A sign of pressure overload, the accentuated apical impulse has increased force and duration but is not usually displaced in left ventricular hypertrophy without dilatation associated with aortic stenosis or systemic hypertension.

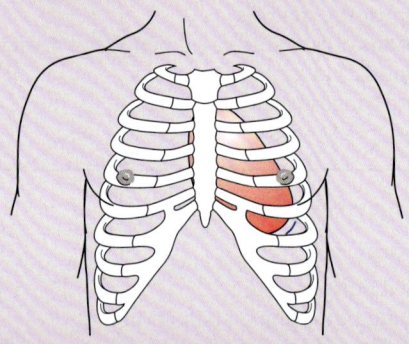

LATERALLY DISPLACED APICAL IMPULSE

A sign of volume overload, an apical impulse displaced laterally and found over a wider area is the result of ventricular hypertrophy and dilatation associated with mitral regurgitation, aortic regurgitation, or left-to-right shunts.

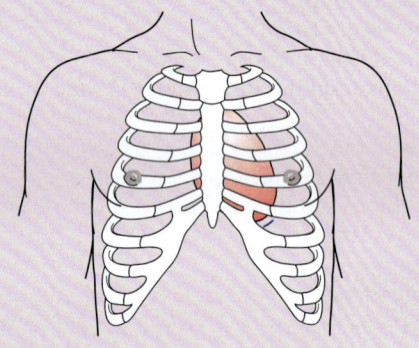

 Concept Mastery Alert

A client with ventricular hypertrophy has an apical impulse that is displaced and found over a large area. Bounding pulses are found in clients with aortic regurgitation or heart block.

ABNORMAL FINDINGS 21-3 Abnormal Heart Rhythms

Changes in the heart rhythm alter the sounds heard on auscultation.

PREMATURE ATRIAL OR JUNCTIONAL CONTRACTIONS

These beats occur earlier than the next expected beat and are followed by a pause. The rhythm resumes with the next beat.

Auscultation Tip: The early beat has an S_1 of different intensity and a diminished S_2. S_1 and S_2 are otherwise similar to normal beats.

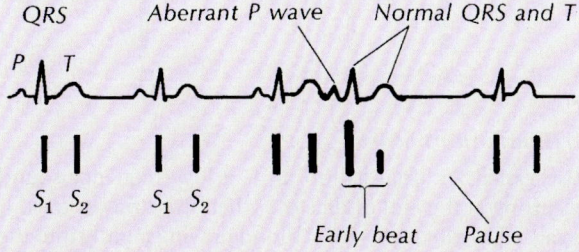

PREMATURE VENTRICULAR CONTRACTIONS

These beats occur earlier than the next expected beat and are followed by a pulse. The rhythm resumes with the next beat.

Auscultation Tip: The early beat has an S_1 of different intensity and a diminished S_2. Both sounds are usually split.

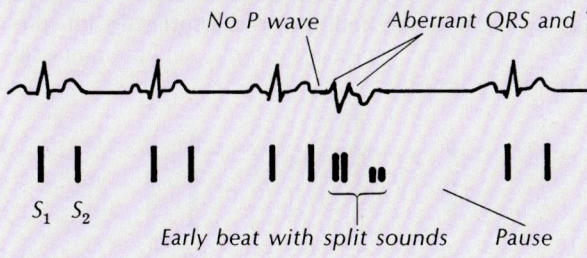

SINUS ARRHYTHMIA

With this dysrhythmia, the HR speeds up and slows down in a cycle, usually becoming faster with inhalation and slower with expiration.

Auscultation Tip: S_1 and S_2 sounds are usually normal. The S_1 may vary with the HR.

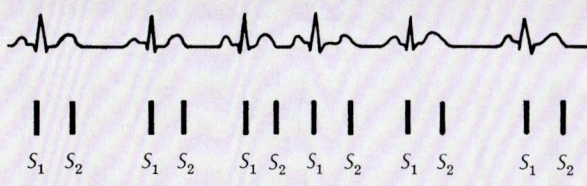

ATRIAL FIBRILLATION AND ATRIAL FLUTTER WITH VARYING VENTRICULAR RESPONSE

With this dysrhythmia, ventricular contraction occurs irregularly. At times, short runs of the irregular rhythm may appear regularly.

Auscultation Tip: S_1 varies in intensity.

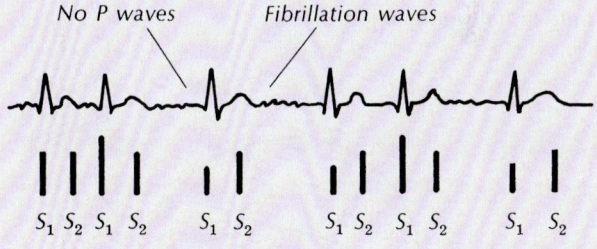

ABNORMAL FINDINGS 21-4 Extra Heart Sounds

Additional heart sounds can be classified by their timing in the cardiac cycle. The presence of the sound during systole or diastole helps in its identification. Some sounds extend into both systole and diastole.

EXTRA HEART SOUNDS DURING SYSTOLE—CLICKS

High-frequency sounds heard just after S_1 (ejection clicks) are produced by a functioning, but diseased, valve. Clicks can occur in early or mid-to-late systole and are best heard through the diaphragm of the stethoscope.

Aortic Ejection Click

Heard during early systole at the second right ICS and apex, the aortic ejection click occurs with the opening of the aortic valve and does not change with respiration.

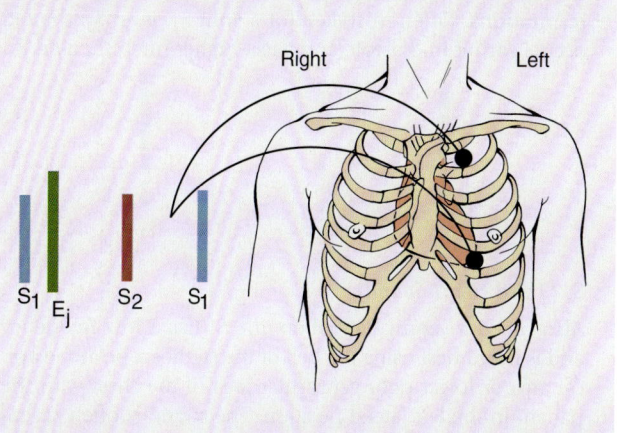

Continued on following page

458   UNIT 3   Nursing Assessment of Physical Systems

ABNORMAL FINDINGS   21-4   **Extra Heart Sounds** (Continued)

Pulmonic Ejection Click
Best heard at the second left ICS during early systole, the pulmonic ejection click often becomes softer with inspiration.

"Ken-tuc-ky." S_3 is the result of vibrations caused by the blood hitting the ventricular wall during rapid ventricular filling.

The S_3 can be a normal finding in young children, people with a high CO, and in the third trimester of pregnancy. It is rarely normal in people older than age 40 years and is usually associated with decreased myocardial contractility, myocardial failure, congestive heart failure, and volume overload of the ventricle from valvular disease.

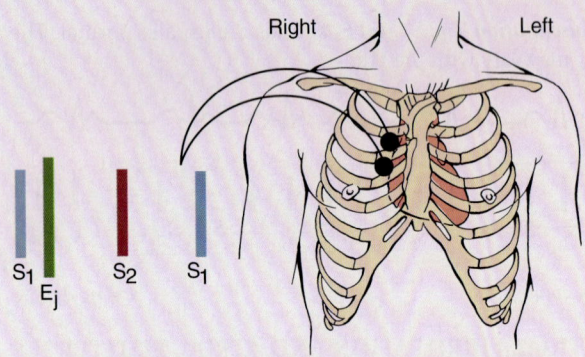

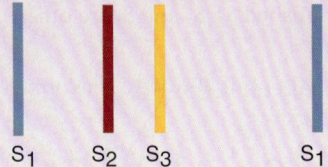

Midsystolic Click
Heard in middle or late systole, a midsystolic click can be heard over the mitral or apical area and is the result of mitral valve leaflet prolapse during left ventricular emptying. A late systolic murmur typically follows, indicating mild mitral regurgitation.

S_4 *(Fourth Heart Sound)*
Also called an atrial gallop, S_4 is a low-frequency sound occurring at the end of diastole when the atria contract. It is caused by vibrations from blood flowing rapidly into the ventricles after atrial contraction. S_4 has the rhythm of the word "Ten-nes-see" and may increase during inspiration. It is best heard with the bell of the stethoscope over the apical area with the patient in a supine or left lateral position, and is never heard in the absence of atrial contraction.

The S_4 can be a normal sound in trained athletes and some older patients, especially after exercise. However, it is usually an abnormal finding and is associated with coronary artery disease, hypertension, aortic and pulmonic stenosis, and acute MI.

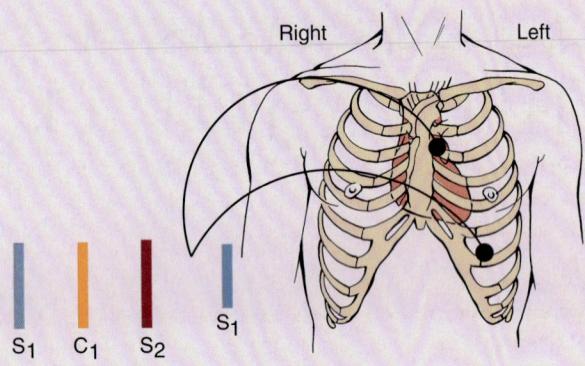

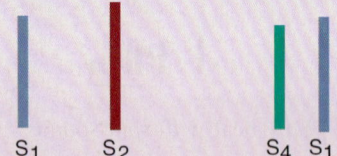

EXTRA HEART SOUNDS DURING DIASTOLE

Opening Snap
Occurring in early diastole, an opening snap (OS) is heard with the opening of a stenotic or stiff mitral valve. Heard throughout the whole precordium, it does not vary with respirations. Often mistaken for a split S_2 or an S_3, the OS occurs earlier in diastole and has a higher pitch than an S_3.

Summation Gallop
The simultaneous occurrence of S_3 and S_4 is called a summation gallop. It is brought about by rapid HRs in which diastolic filling time is shortened, moving S_3 and S_4 closer together, resulting in one prolonged sound. Summation gallop is associated with severe congestive heart disease.

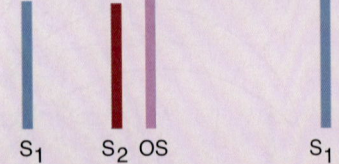

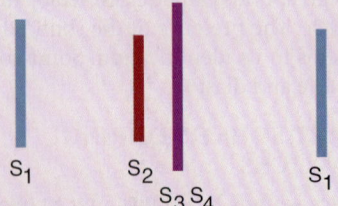

S_3 *(Third Heart Sound)*
Also called a ventricular gallop, the S_3 has a low frequency and is heard best using the bell of the stethoscope at the apical area or lower right ventricular area of the chest with the patient in the left lateral position. The sound is often accentuated during inspiration and has the rhythm of the word

EXTRA HEART SOUNDS IN BOTH SYSTOLE AND DIASTOLE

Pericardial Friction Rub
Usually heard best in the third ICS to the left of the sternum, a pericardial friction rub is caused by inflammation of the pericardial sac. A high-pitched, scratchy, scraping sound, the rub may increase with exhalation and when the

patient leans forward. For best results, use the diaphragm of the stethoscope and have the patient sit up, lean forward, exhale, and hold his or her breath.

The pericardial friction rub can have up to three components: atrial systole, ventricular systole, and ventricular diastole. These components are associated with cardiac movement. The first two components are usually present. If only one component is present, the rub may be confused with a murmur. Friction rubs are commonly heard during the first week after an MI. If a significant pericardial effusion is present, S_1 and S_2 sounds will be distant.

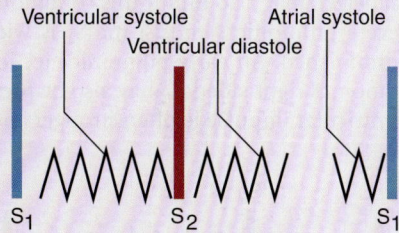

Patent Ductus Arteriosus

Patent ductus arteriosus (PDA) is a congenital anomaly that leaves an open channel between the aorta and pulmonary artery. Found over the second left ICS, the murmur of PDA may radiate to the left clavicle. It is classified as a continuous murmur because it extends through systole and into part of diastole. It has a medium pitch and a harsh, machinery-like sound. The murmur is loudest in late systole, obscures S_2, fades in diastole, and often has a silent interval in late diastole.

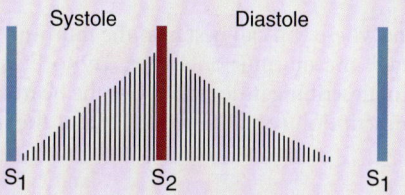

Venous Hum

Common in children, a venous hum is a benign sound caused by turbulence of blood in the jugular veins. It is heard above the medial third of the clavicles, especially on the right, and may radiate to the first and second ICSs. A low-pitched sound, it is often described as a humming or roaring continuous murmur without a silent interval, and is loudest in diastole. A venous hum can be obliterated by putting pressure on the jugular veins.

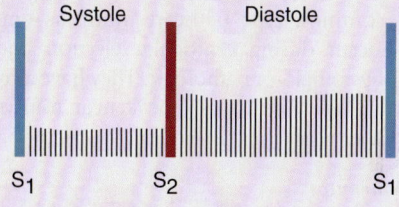

ABNORMAL FINDINGS 21-5 Heart Murmurs

Heart murmurs are typically characterized by turbulent blood flow, which creates a swooshing or blowing sound over the precordium. When listening to the heart, be alert for this turbulence and keep the characteristics of heart murmurs in mind.

CHARACTERISTICS

Heart murmurs are assessed according to various characteristics, which include timing, intensity, pitch, quality, shape or pattern, location, transmission, and ventilation and position.

Timing

A murmur can occur during systole or diastole. In addition to determining when it occurs, it is important to determine where it occurs: a systolic murmur can be present in a healthy heart whereas a diastolic murmur always indicates heart disease. Systolic murmurs can be divided into three categories: midsystolic, pansystolic, and late systolic. Diastolic murmurs can be divided into three categories: early diastolic, mid-diastolic, and late diastolic.

Intensity

Six grades describe the intensity of a murmur.
Grade 1: Very faint, heard only after the listener has "tuned in"; may not be heard in all positions
Grade 2: Quiet, but heard immediately on placing the stethoscope on the chest
Grade 3: Moderately loud
Grade 4: Loud

Grade 5: Very loud, may be heard with a stethoscope partly off the chest
Grade 6: May be heard with the stethoscope entirely off the chest

Pitch

Murmurs can assume a high, medium, or low pitch.

Quality

The sound murmurs make has been described as blowing, rushing, roaring, rumbling, harsh, or musical.

Shape or Pattern

The shape of a murmur is determined by its intensity from beginning to end. There are four different categories of shape: crescendo (growing louder), decrescendo (growing softer), crescendo–decrescendo (growing louder and then growing softer), and plateau (staying the same throughout).

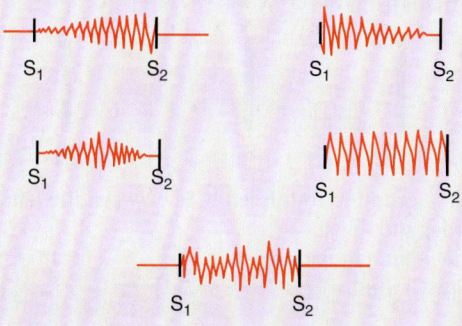

Continued on following page

ABNORMAL FINDINGS 21-5 Heart Murmurs (Continued)

Location

Determine where you can best hear the murmur; this is the point where the murmur originates. Try to be as exact as possible in describing its location. Use the heart landmarks in your description (e.g., the second ICS at the left sternal border).

Transmission

The murmur may be felt in areas other than the point of origin. If you determine where the murmur transmits, you can determine the direction of blood flow and the intensity of the murmur.

Ventilation and Position

Determine if the murmur is affected by inspiration, expiration, or a change in body position.

MIDSYSTOLIC MURMURS

The most common type of heart murmurs—midsystolic murmurs—occur during ventricular ejection and can be innocent, physiologic, or pathologic. They have a crescendo–decrescendo shape and usually peak near midsystole and stop before S_2.

Innocent Murmur

Not associated with any physical abnormality, innocent murmurs occur when the ejection of blood into the aorta is turbulent. Very common in children and young adults, they may also be heard in older people with no evidence of cardiovascular disease. A patient may have an innocent murmur and another kind of murmur.

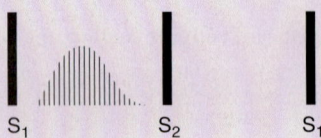

Location: Second to fourth left ICSs between the left sternal border and the apex
Radiation: Little radiation
Intensity: Grade 1 to 2
Pitch: Medium
Quality: Variable
Position: Usually disappears when the patient sits

Physiologic Murmur

Caused by a temporary increase in blood flow, a physiologic murmur can occur with anemia, pregnancy, fever, and hyperthyroidism.

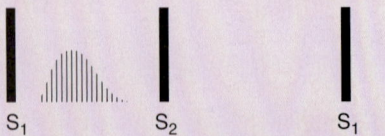

Location: Second to fourth left ICSs between the left sternal border and the apex
Radiation: Little radiation
Intensity: Grade 1 to 2
Pitch: Medium
Quality: Harsh

Murmur of Pulmonic Stenosis

A pathologic murmur, the murmur of pulmonic stenosis occurs from impeded flow across the pulmonic valve and increased right ventricular afterload. Often occurring as a congenital anomaly, the murmur is commonly found in children. Pathologic changes in flow across the valve, as in atrial septal defect, may also mimic this condition.

With severe pulmonic stenosis, the S_2 is widely split and P_2 is diminished. An early pulmonic ejection sound is also common. A right-sided S_4 may also be present, and the right ventricular impulse is often stronger and may be prolonged.

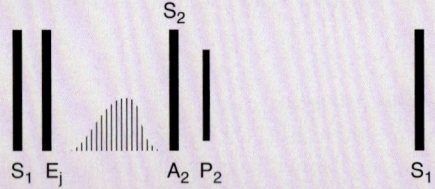

Location: Second and third ICSs
Radiation: Toward the left shoulder and neck
Intensity: Soft to loud (may be associated with a thrill if loud)
Pitch: Medium
Quality: Harsh
Position: Loudest during inspiration

Murmur of Aortic Stenosis

The murmur of aortic stenosis occurs when stenosis of the aortic valve impedes blood flow across the valve and increases left ventricular afterload. Aortic stenosis may result from a congenital anomaly, rheumatic disease, or a degenerative process. Conditions that may mimic this murmur include aortic sclerosis, a bicuspid aortic valve, a dilated aorta, or any condition that mimics the flow across the valve, such as aortic regurgitation.

If valvular disease is severe, A_2 may be delayed, resulting in an unsplit S_2 or a paradoxical split S_2. An S_4 may occur as a result of decreased left ventricular compliance. An aortic ejection sound, if present, suggests a congenital cause.

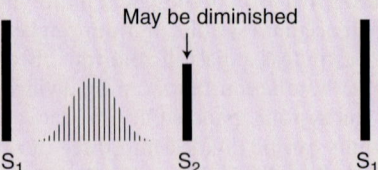

Location: Right second ICS
Radiation: May radiate to the neck and down the left sternal border to the apex
Intensity: Usually loud, with a thrill
Pitch: Medium
Quality: Harsh, may be musical at the apex
Position: Heard best with the patient sitting and leaning forward, loudest during expiration

Murmur of Hypertrophic Cardiomyopathy

Caused by unusually rapid ejection of blood from the left ventricle during systole, the murmur of cardiac hypertrophy results from massive hypertrophy of the ventricular muscle. There may be a coexisting obstruction to blood flow. If there is an accompanying distortion of the mitral valve, mitral regurgitation may result. The patient may also have an S_3 and an S_4. There may be a sustained apical impulse with two palpable components.

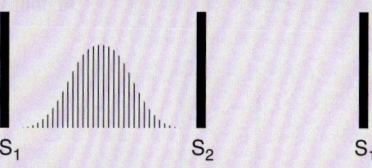

Location: Third and fourth left ICS, decreases with squatting, increases with straining down
Intensity: Variable
Pitch: Medium
Quality: Harsh

PANSYSTOLIC MURMURS

Occurring when blood flows from a chamber with high pressure to a chamber of low pressure through an orifice that should be closed, pansystolic murmurs are pathologic. Also called *holosystolic murmur*, these murmurs begin with S_1 and continue through systole to S_2.

Murmur of Mitral Regurgitation

Occurring when the mitral valve fails to close fully in systole, the murmur of mitral regurgitation is the result of blood flowing from the left ventricle back into the left atrium. Volume overload occurs in the left ventricle, causing dilatation and hypertrophy.

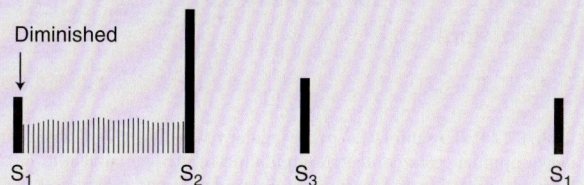

The S_1 sound is often decreased, and the apical impulse is stronger and may be prolonged. Left ventricular volume overload should be suspected if an apical S_3 is heard.
Location: Apex
Radiation: To the left axilla, less often to the left sternal border
Intensity: Soft to loud, an apical thrill is associated with loud murmurs
Pitch: Medium to high
Quality: Blowing
Position: Heard best with patient in the left lateral decubitus position; does not become louder with inspiration

Murmur of Tricuspid Regurgitation

Blood flowing from the right ventricle back into the right atrium over a tricuspid valve that is not fully closed causes the murmur of tricuspid regurgitation. Right ventricular failure with dilatation is the most common cause and usually results from pulmonary hypertension or left ventricular failure.

With this murmur, the right ventricular impulse is stronger and may be prolonged. There may be an S_3 along the lower left sternal border, and the jugular venous pressure is often elevated, with visible *v* waves.

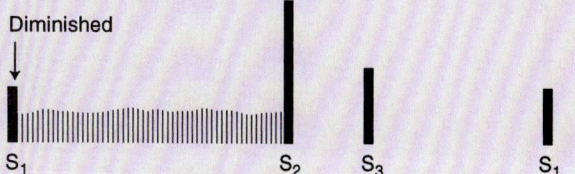

Location: Lower left sternal border
Radiation: To the right of the sternum, to the xiphoid area, and sometimes to the MCL; there is no radiation to the axilla
Intensity: Variable
Pitch: Medium to high
Quality: Blowing
Position: May increase slightly with inspiration

Ventricular Septal Defect

A congenital abnormality in which blood flows from the left ventricle into the right ventricle through a hole in the septum, a ventricular septal defect causes a loud murmur that obscures the A_2 sound. Other findings vary depending on the severity of the defect and any associated lesions.

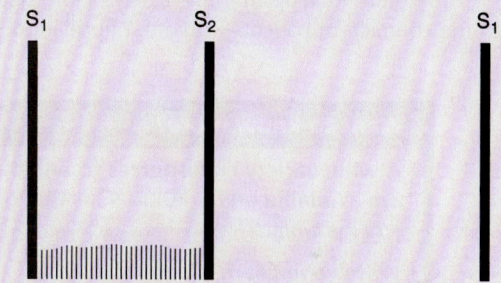

Location: Third, fourth, and fifth left ICS
Radiation: Often wide
Intensity: Very loud, with a thrill
Pitch: High
Quality: Harsh
Position: Increases with exercise

DIASTOLIC MURMURS

Usually indicative of heart disease, diastolic murmurs occur in two types. Early decrescendo diastolic murmurs indicate flow through an incompetent semilunar valve, commonly the aortic valve. Rumbling diastolic murmurs in mid- or late diastole indicate valve stenosis, usually of the mitral valve.

Murmur of Aortic Regurgitation

Occurring when the leaflets of the aortic valve fail to close completely, the murmur of aortic regurgitation is the result of blood flowing from the aorta back into the left ventricle. This results in left ventricular volume overload. An ejection sound also may be present. Severe regurgitation should be suspected if an S_3 or S_4 is also present. The apical impulse becomes displaced downward and laterally, with a widened

Continued on following page

ABNORMAL FINDINGS 21-5 Heart Murmurs (Continued)

diameter and increased duration. As the pulse pressure increases, the arterial pulses are often large and bounding.

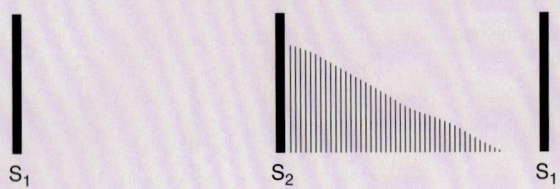

Location: Second to fourth left ICS
Radiation: May radiate to the apex or left sternal border
Intensity: Grade 1 to 3
Pitch: High
Quality: Blowing, sometime mistaken for breath sounds
Position: Heard best with the patient sitting, leaning forward. Have the patient exhale and then hold his or her breath.

Murmur of Mitral Stenosis

The murmur of mitral stenosis is the result of blood flow across a diseased mitral valve. Thickened, stiff, distorted leaflets are usually the result of rheumatic fever. The murmur is loud during mid-diastole as the ventricle fills rapidly, grows quiet, and becomes loud again immediately before systole, as the atria contract. In patients with atrial fibrillation, the second half of the murmur is absent because of the lack of atrial contraction.

The patient also has a loud S_1, which may be palpable at the apex. There is often an OS after S_2. P_2 becomes loud and the right ventricular impulse becomes palpable if pulmonary hypertension develops.

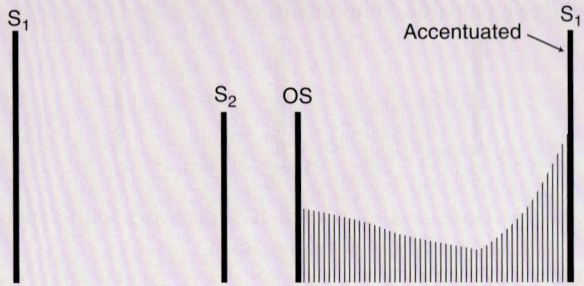

Location: Apex
Radiation: Little or none
Intensity: Grade 1 to 4
Pitch: Low
Quality: Rumbling
Position: Best heard with the bell exactly on the apex and the patient turned to a left lateral position. Mild exercise and listening during exhalation also make the murmur easier to hear.

Want to know more?

A wide variety of resources to enhance your learning and understanding of this book are available on **thePoint**. Visit thePoint to access:

NCLEX-Style Student Review Questions   Concepts in Action Animations
Watch and Learn Videos   And more!

References and Selected Readings

American Congress of Obstetricians and Gynecologists (ACOG). (2016). Tobacco and nicotine cessation toolkit. Available at https://www.acog.org/About-ACOG/ACOG-Departments/Toolkits-for-Health-Care-Providers/Tobacco-and-Nicotine-Cessation-Toolkit

American Heart Association (AHA). (2017). The American Heart Association's diet and lifestyle recommendations. Available at https://www.heart.org/HEARTORG/HealthyLiving/HealthyEating/Nutrition/The-American-Heart-Associations-Diet-and-Lifestyle-Recommendations_UCM_305855_Article.jsp

American Heart Association (AHA). (2015a). Alcohol and heart health. Available at http://www.heart.org/HEARTORG/GettingHealthy/NutritionCenter/HealthyEating/Alcohol-and-Heart-Health_UCM_305173_Article.jsp#.VowWzxV96M8

American Heart Association (AHA). (2015b). African-Americans and heart disease, stroke. Available at http://www.heart.org/HEARTORG/Conditions/More/MyHeartandStrokeNews/African-Americans-and-Heart-Disease-Stroke_UCM_444863_Article.jsp#.V_u9heB96M8

American Heart Association (AHA). (2014a). Atherosclerosis. Available at http://www.heart.org/HEARTORG/Conditions/Cholesterol/WhyCholesterolMatters/Atherosclerosis_UCM_305564_Article.jsp#.VowZ6xV96M8

American Heart Association (AHA). (2014b). Heart-health screenings. Available at http://www.heart.org/HEARTORG/Conditions/Heart-Health-Screenings_UCM_428687_Article.jsp#.VowQPRV96M8

Chiaco, J., Parikh, N., & Fergusson, D. (2016). The jugular venous pressure revisited. *Cleveland Clinic Journal of Medicine, 80*(10), 638–644. DOI:10.3949/ccjm.80a.13039

Gersh, B. (2016). Examination of the jugular venous pulse. Available at http://www.uptodate.com/contents/examination-of-the-jugular-venous-pulse

Curry, A. (2013). Can exercise improve African Americans' cholesterol? Available at http://www.diabetesforecast.org/2013/feb/can-exercise-improve-african-americans-cholesterol.html?referrer=https://www.google.com/

Healthy People 2020. (2014). Heart disease and stroke. Available at http://www.healthypeople.gov/2020/topics-objectives/topic/heart-disease-and-stroke

Lackland, D. (2014). Racial differences in hypertension: Implications for high blood pressure management. *American Journal of Medical Science, 348*(2), 135–138. DOI: 10.1097/MAJ.0000000000000308

Mayo Clinic. (2014). Heart disease. Available at http://www.mayoclinic.org/diseases-conditions/heart-disease/basics/definition/con-20034056

National Heart Lung and Blood Institute (NHLBI). (2012). Women's fear of heart disease has almost doubled in three years, but breast cancer remains most feared disease. Available at www.nhlbi.nih.gov/educational/hearttruth/about/fear-doubled.htm

Ostchega, Y., Porter, K., Hughes, J., et al. (2011). Resting pulse rate reference data for children, adolescents, and adults: United States, 1999–2008. National Health Statistics Reports, No. 41. Available at http://www.cdc.gov/nchs/data/nhsr/nhsr041.pdf

Seckeler, M. D., & Hoke, T. R. (2011). The worldwide epidemiology of acute rheumatic fever and rheumatic heart disease. *Clinical Epidemiology, 3*, 67–84.

U.S. Preventive Services Task Force (USPSTF). (2012). Screening for coronary heart disease. Available at http://www.uspreventiveservicestaskforce.org/Page/Document/RecommendationStatementFinal/coronary-heart-disease-screening-with-electrocardiography

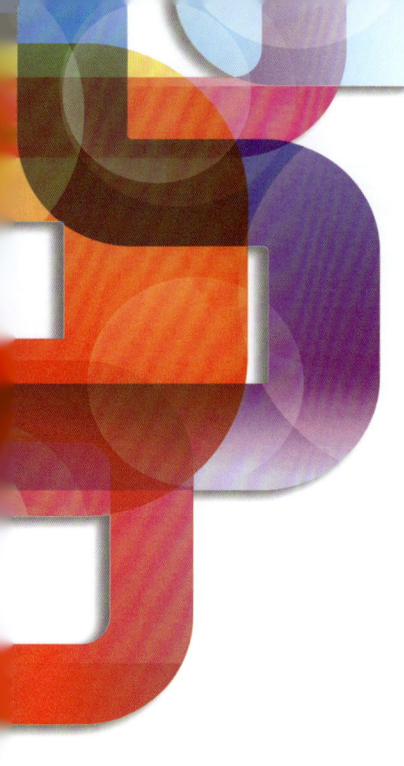

22 ASSESSING PERIPHERAL VASCULAR SYSTEM

Learning Objectives

1. Describe the structure and the function of the blood vessels, including capillaries and lymphatic circulation.
2. Discuss risk factors associated with peripheral vascular disease across the cultures and ways to reduce one's risks.
3. Interview a client for an accurate nursing history of the peripheral vascular system.
4. Perform a physical assessment of the peripheral vascular system using the correct techniques.
5. Differentiate between normal and abnormal findings of the peripheral vascular system.
6. Explain the correct method for teaching a client how to perform breast self-examination.
7. Describe the findings frequently seen with assessing the older client's peripheral vascular system.
8. Analyze the data from the interview and physical assessment of the peripheral vascular system to formulate valid nursing diagnoses, collaborative problems, and/or referrals.
9. Differentiate between general routine screening versus skills needed for focused or specialty assessment of the peripheral vascular system.
10. Document and verbally report accurate assessment findings of the peripheral vascular system.

CASE STUDY

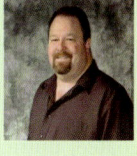

Henry Lee is a 46-year-old man who is relatively healthy, but obese (weight: 250 lb; height: 5 ft, 9 in). He comes to the clinic to see the nurse practitioner with the following statement: "I must have pulled something in my right leg. I was walking when I felt some soreness in my lower right leg, and now there is some swelling. It really hurts to walk." He states that he is a self-employed developer of computer software programs. Mr. Lee's case will be discussed throughout the chapter.

STRUCTURE AND FUNCTION

To perform a thorough peripheral vascular assessment, the nurse needs to understand the structure and function of the arteries and veins of the arms and legs, the lymphatic system, and the capillaries. Equally important is an understanding of fluid exchange. The information provided in this chapter can help you compile subjective and objective data related to the peripheral vascular system and differentiate normal vascular findings from normal variations and abnormalities.

Arteries

Arteries are the blood vessels that carry oxygenated, nutrient-rich blood from the heart to the capillaries. The arterial network is a high-pressure system. Blood is propelled under pressure from the left ventricle of the heart. Because of this high pressure, arterial walls must be thick and strong; the arterial walls also contain elastic fibers so that they can stretch. Figure 22-1 illustrates the layers and the relative thickness of arterial walls. Each heartbeat forces blood through the arterial vessels under high pressure, creating a surge. This surge of blood is the *arterial pulse*. The pulse can be felt only by lightly compressing a superficial artery against an underlying bone. Many arteries are located in protected areas, far from the surface of the skin. Therefore, the arteries discussed in this chapter include only major arteries of the arms and legs—the *peripheral arteries*—that are accessible to examination. The other major arteries accessible to examination—temporal, carotid, and aorta—are discussed in Chapters 15, 21, and 23, respectively.

463

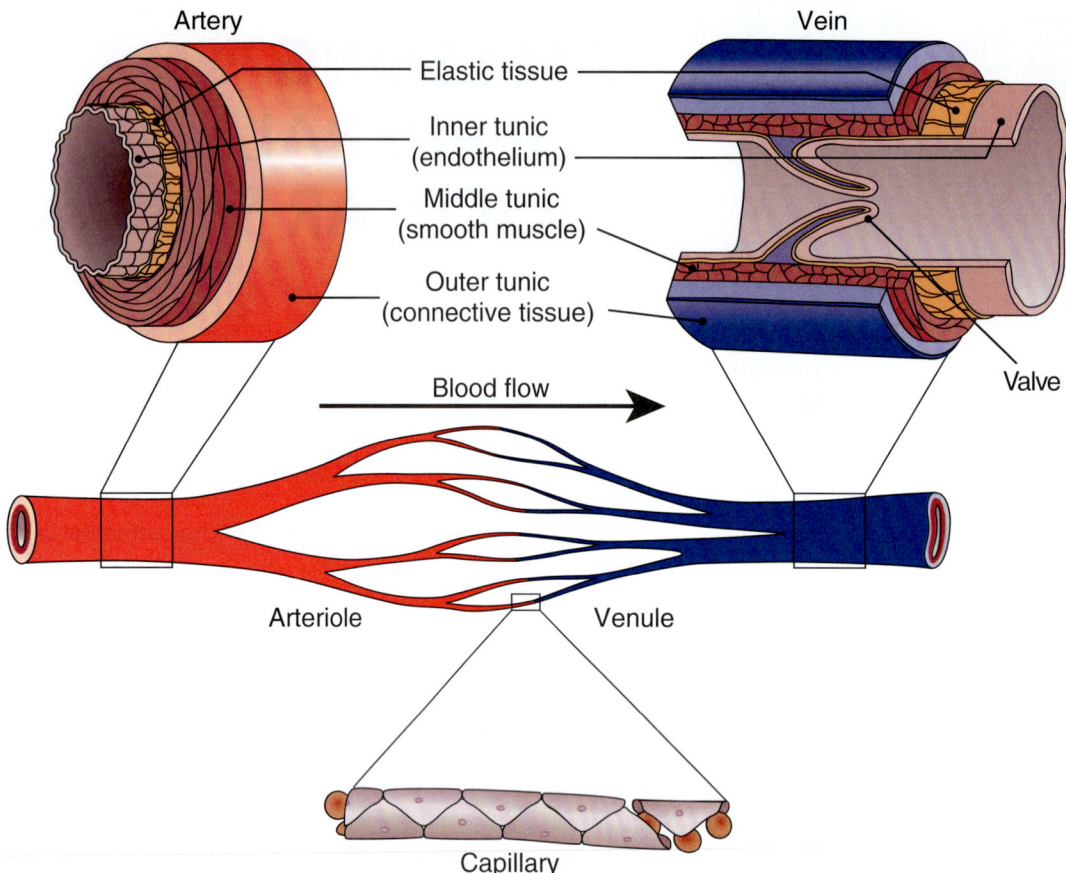

FIGURE 22-1 Blood vessel walls. Arterial walls are constructed to accommodate the high pulsing pressure of blood transported by the pumping heart, whereas venous walls are designed with valves that promote the return of blood and prevent backflow.

Major Arteries of the Arm

The *brachial artery* is the major artery that supplies the arm. The brachial pulse can be palpated medial to the biceps tendon in and above the bend of the elbow. The brachial artery divides near the elbow to become the *radial artery* (extending down the thumb side of the arm) and the *ulnar artery* (extending down the little-finger side of the arm). Both of these arteries provide blood to the hand. The *radial pulse* can be palpated on the lateral aspect of the wrist. The *ulnar pulse*, located on the medial aspect of the wrist, is a deeper pulse and may not be easily palpated. The radial and ulnar arteries join to form two arches just below their pulse sites. The superficial and deep *palmar arches* provide extra protection against arterial occlusion to the hands and fingers (Fig. 22-2).

Major Arteries of the Leg

The *femoral artery* is the major supplier of blood to the legs. Its pulse can be palpated just under the inguinal ligament. This artery travels down the front of the thigh then crosses to the back of the thigh, where it is termed the popliteal artery. The *popliteal pulse* can be palpated behind the knee. The *popliteal artery* divides below the knee into anterior and posterior branches. The anterior branch descends down the top of the foot, where it becomes the *dorsalis pedis artery*. Its pulse can be palpated on the great-toe side of the top of the foot. The posterior branch is called the *posterior tibial artery*. The posterior tibial pulse can be palpated behind the medial malleolus of the ankle. The dorsalis pedis artery and posterior tibial artery form the *dorsal arch*, which, like the superficial and deep palmar arches of the hands, provides the feet and toes with extra protection from arterial occlusion (see Fig. 22-2). For a discussion of pulse strength measurement, see Box 22-2.

Veins

Veins are the blood vessels that carry deoxygenated, nutrient-depleted, waste-laden blood from the tissues back to the heart. The veins of the arms, upper trunk, head, and neck carry blood to the superior vena cava, where it passes into the right atrium. Blood from the lower trunk and legs drains upward into the inferior vena cava. The veins contain nearly 70% of the body's blood volume. Because blood in the veins is carried under much lower pressure than in the arteries, the vein walls are much thinner (see Fig. 22-1). In addition, veins are larger in diameter than arteries and can expand if blood volume increases. This helps to reduce the workload on the heart.

This chapter focuses on those veins that are most susceptible to dysfunction: the three types of veins in the legs. Two other major veins that are important to assess—the internal and external jugular veins—are discussed in Chapter 21.

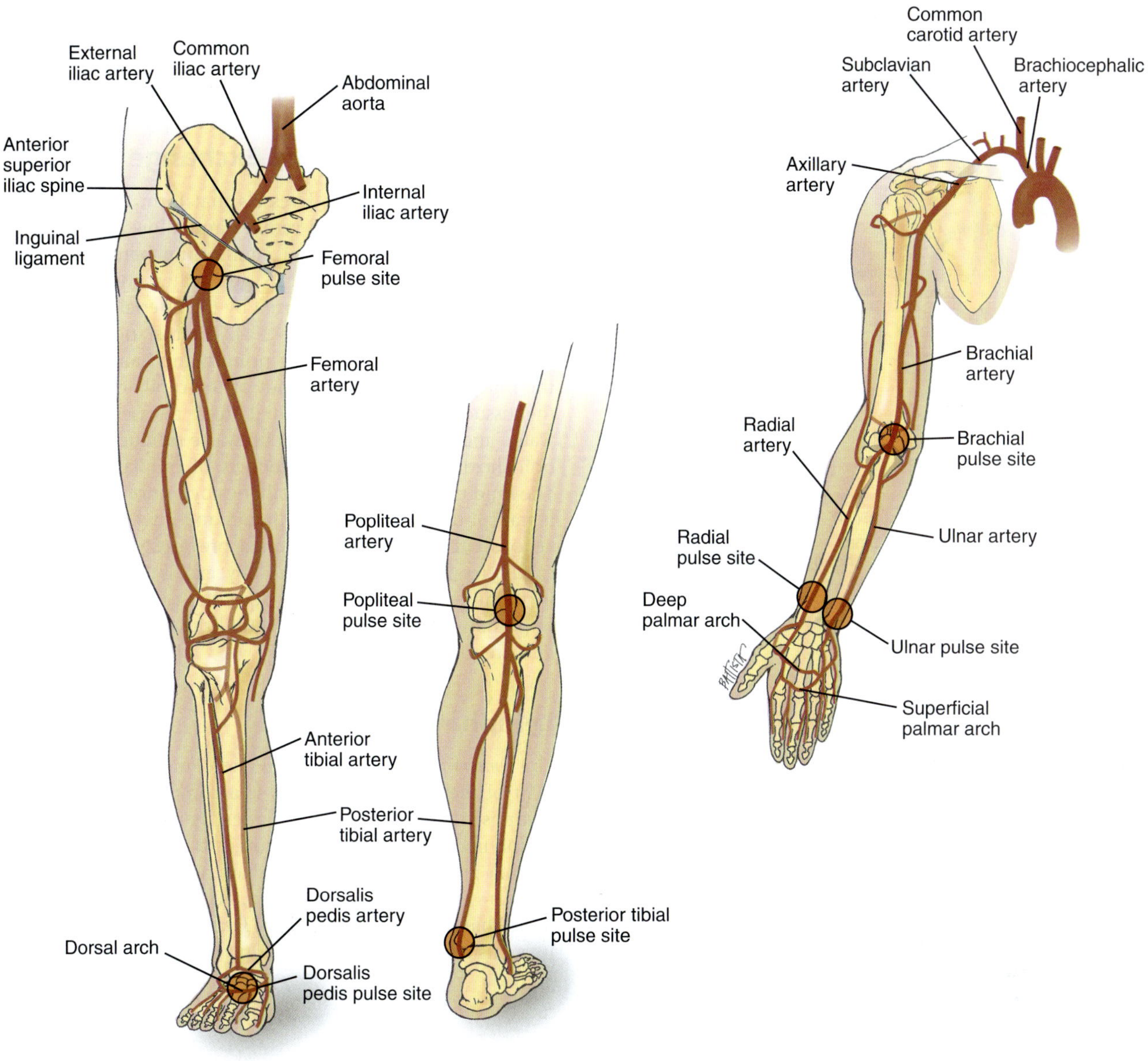

FIGURE 22-2 Major arteries of the arms and legs.

There are three types of veins: *deep veins, superficial veins,* and *perforator (or communicator) veins.* The two deep veins in the leg are the *femoral vein* in the upper thigh and the *popliteal vein* located behind the knee. These veins account for about 90% of venous return from the lower extremities. The superficial veins are the great and small *saphenous veins.* The great saphenous vein is the longest of all veins and extends from the medial dorsal aspect of the foot, crosses over the medial malleolus, and continues across the thigh to the medial aspect of the groin, where it joins the femoral vein. The small saphenous vein begins at the lateral dorsal aspect of the foot, travels up behind the lateral malleolus on the back of the leg, and joins the popliteal vein. The perforator veins connect the superficial veins with the deep veins (Fig. 22-3).

Veins differ from arteries in that there is no force that propels forward blood flow; the venous system is a low-pressure system. This fact is of special concern in the veins of the leg. Blood from the legs and lower trunk must flow upward with no help from the pumping action of the heart. Three mechanisms of venous function help to propel blood back to the heart. The first mechanism has to do with the structure of the veins. Deep, superficial, and perforator veins all contain one-way valves. These valves permit blood to pass through them on the way to the heart and prevent blood from returning through them in the opposite direction. The second mechanism is muscular contraction. Skeletal muscles contract with movement and, in effect, squeeze blood toward the heart through the one-way valves. The third mechanism is the creation of a pressure gradient through the act of breathing. Inspiration decreases intrathoracic pressure while increasing abdominal pressure, thus producing a pressure gradient.

If there is a problem with any of these mechanisms, venous return is impeded and *venous stasis* results. Risk factors for venous stasis include long periods of standing still, sitting, or lying down. Lack of muscular activity causes blood to pool in

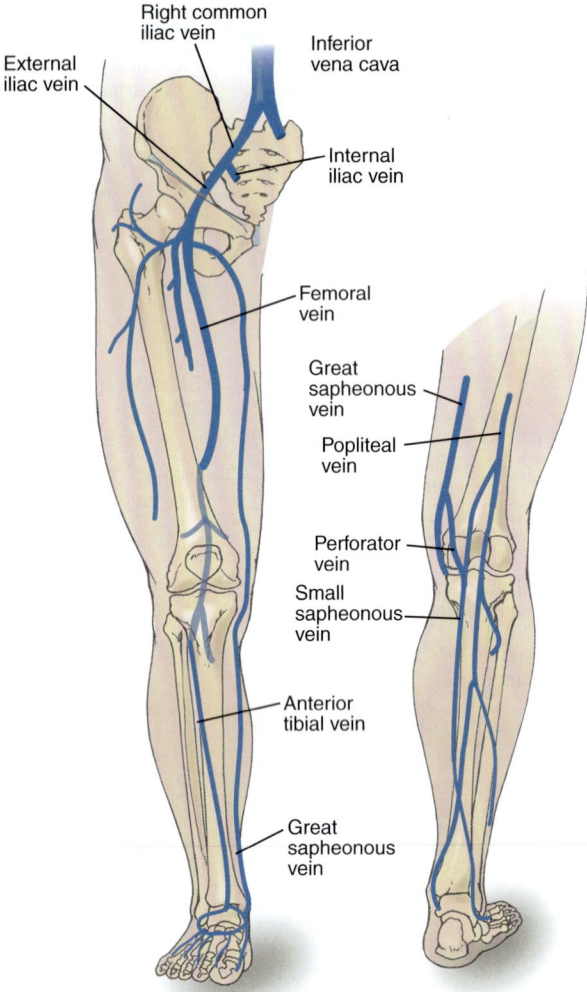

FIGURE 22-3 Major veins of the legs.

the legs, which, in turn, increases pressure in the veins. Other causes of venous stasis include varicose (tortuous and dilated) veins, which increase venous pressure. Damage to the vein wall can also contribute to venous stasis.

Capillaries and Fluid Exchange

Capillaries are small blood vessels that form the connection between the arterioles and venules and allow the circulatory system to maintain the vital equilibrium between the vascular and interstitial spaces. Oxygen, water, and nutrients in the interstitial fluid are delivered by the arterial vessels to the microscopic capillaries (Fig. 22-4). Hydrostatic force, generated by blood pressure, is the primary mechanism by which the interstitial fluid diffuses out of the capillaries and enters the tissue space. The interstitial fluid releases the oxygen, water, and nutrients and picks up waste products such as carbon dioxide and other by-products of cellular metabolism. The fluid then reenters the capillaries by osmotic pressure and is transported away from the tissues and interstitial spaces by venous circulation. As mentioned previously, the lymphatic capillaries function to remove any excess fluid left behind in the interstitial spaces. Therefore, the capillary bed is very important in maintaining the equilibrium of interstitial fluid and preventing edema.

Lymphatic System

The *lymphatic system*, an integral and complementary component of the circulatory system, is a complex vascular system composed of lymphatic capillaries, lymphatic vessels, and lymph nodes. Its primary function is to drain excess fluid and plasma proteins from bodily tissues and return them to the venous system. During circulation, more fluid leaves the capillaries than the veins can absorb. Draining excess fluid action prevents edema, which is a buildup of fluid in the interstitial

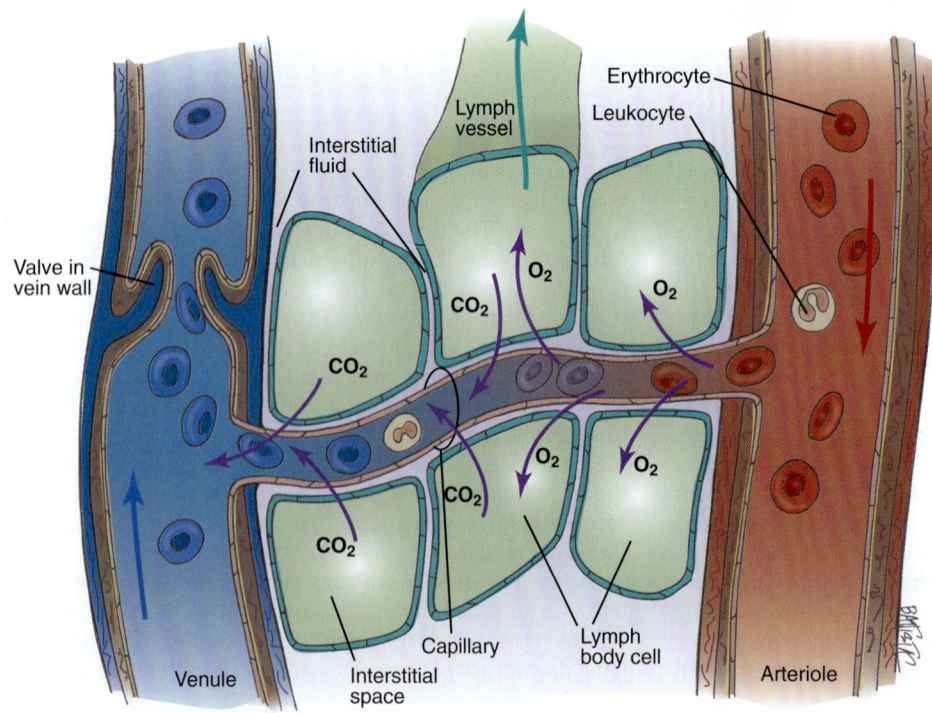

FIGURE 22-4 Normal capillary circulation ensures removal of excess fluid (edema) from the interstitial spaces as well as delivery of oxygen (O_2) and removal of carbon dioxide (CO_2).

spaces. The fluids and proteins absorbed into the lymphatic vessels by the microscopic lymphatic capillaries become lymph. These capillaries join to form larger vessels that pass through filters known as *lymph nodes*, where microorganisms, foreign materials, dead blood cells, and abnormal cells are trapped and destroyed. After the lymph is filtered, it travels to either the *right lymphatic duct*, which drains the upper right side of the body, or the *thoracic duct*, which drains the rest of the body, then back into the venous system circulation through the *subclavian veins* (Fig. 22-5).

This unique filtering feature of the lymph nodes allows the lymphatic system to perform a second function as a major part of the immune system defending the body against microorganisms. A third function of the lymphatic system is to absorb fats (lipids) from the small intestine into the bloodstream.

Lymph nodes are somewhat circular or oval. Normally they vary from very small and nonpalpable to 1 to 2 cm in diameter. Lymph nodes tend to be grouped together. They are both deep and superficial, and many are located near major joints. The superficial lymph nodes are the only lymph nodes accessible to examination. The cervical and axillary superficial lymph nodes are discussed in Chapters 15 and 20, respectively. The superficial lymph nodes of the arms and legs assessed in this

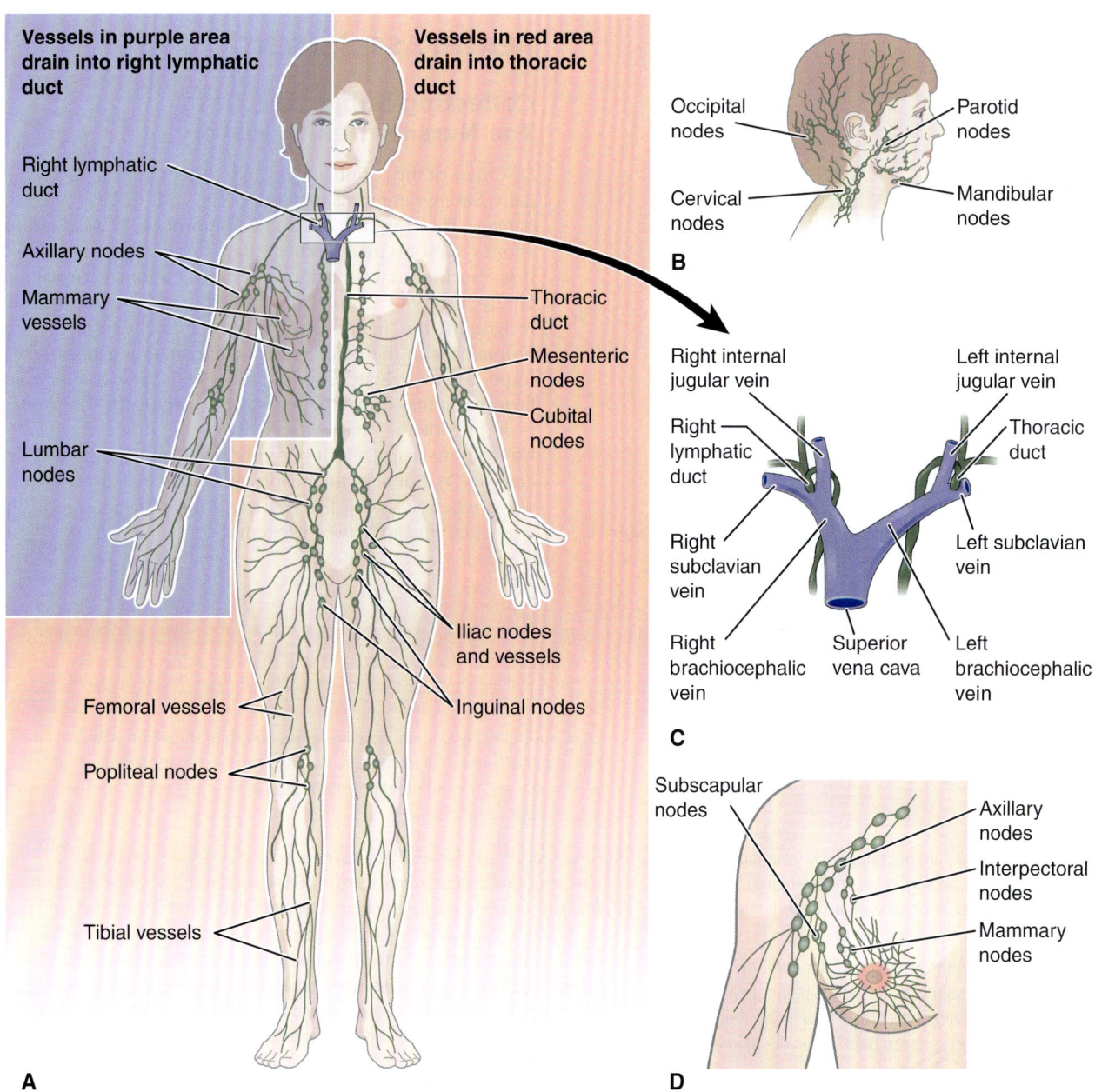

FIGURE 22-5 Lymphatic system. **A.** Lymphatic vessels drain almost every area of the body. Lymph nodes are distributed along the path of the vessels. Areas draining into the right lymphatic duct are shown in *purple;* areas draining into the thoracic duct are shown in *red.* **B.** Lymph nodes and vessels of the head. **C.** Drainage of the right lymphatic duct and thoracic duct into the subclavian veins. **D.** Lymph nodes and vessels of the breast, mammary glands, and surrounding areas (Cohen, B. J., & DePetris, A. *Medical terminology: An illustrated guide.* (2014). Philadelphia, PA: Lippincott Williams & Wilkins.)

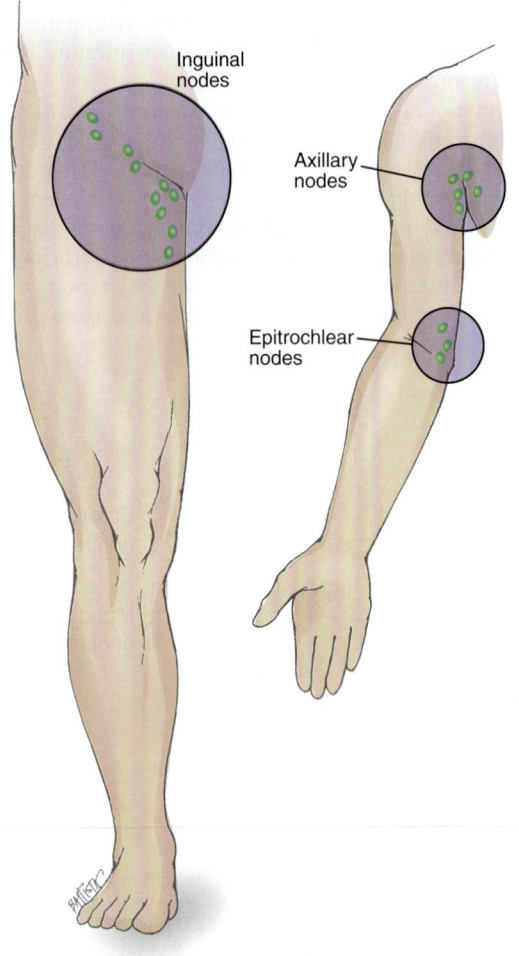

FIGURE 22-6 Superficial lymph nodes of the arms and legs.

chapter include the epitrochlear nodes and the superficial inguinal nodes.

The *epitrochlear nodes* are located approximately 3 cm above the elbow on the inner (medial) aspect of the arm. These lymph nodes drain the lower arm and hand. Lymph from the remainder of the arm and hand drains to the axillary lymph nodes. The *superficial inguinal nodes* consist of two groups: a horizontal and a vertical chain of nodes. The horizontal chain is located on the anterior thigh just under the inguinal ligament, and the vertical chain is located close to the great saphenous vein. These nodes drain the legs, external genitalia, and lower abdomen and buttocks (Fig. 22-6).

HEALTH ASSESSMENT

Collecting Subjective Data: The Nursing Health History

Disorders of the peripheral vascular system may develop gradually. Severe symptoms may not occur until there is extensive damage. Therefore, it is important for the nurse to ask questions about symptoms that the client may consider inconsequential. It is also important for the nurse to ask about personal and family history of vascular disease. This information provides insight into the client's risk for a recurrence or development of problems with the peripheral vascular system. It is especially important to evaluate aspects of the client's lifestyle and health factors that may impair peripheral vascular health. These questions provide the nurse with an avenue for discussing healthy lifestyles that can prevent or minimize peripheral vascular disease (PVD). Some of the history questions may overlap those asked when assessing the heart and the skin because of the close relationship between systems.

History of Present Health Concern

QUESTION	RATIONALE
Have you noticed any color, temperature, or texture changes in your skin?	Cold, pale, clammy skin on the extremities and thin, shiny skin with loss of hair, especially over the lower legs, are associated with arterial insufficiency. Warm skin, edema and brown pigmentation around the ankles are associated with venous insufficiency.
Do you experience pain or cramping in your legs? If so, describe the pain (aching, cramping, stabbing). How often does it occur? Does it occur with activity? Is the pain reproducible with same amount of exercise? If you have pain with walking, how far and how fast do you walk prior to the pain starting? Is the pain relieved by rest? Are you able to climb stairs? If so, how many stairs can you climb before you experience pain? Does the pain wake you from sleep?	Peripheral arterial disease (PAD) can develop over a lifetime, and often symptoms do not appear until there is a 60% blockage (Cleveland Clinic, 2016). Although many people have no symptoms with PAD, intermittent claudication is usually the first symptom and is characterized by weakness, cramping, aching, fatigue, or frank pain with activity; located in the calves, thighs, or buttocks but rarely in the feet. These symptoms are quickly relieved by rest but reproducible with same degree of exercise and may indicate PAD (Criqui & Aboyans, 2015). Additional symptoms to intermittent claudication include: • A burning or aching pain in the feet and toes while resting, especially at night while lying flat • Cool skin in the feet • Redness or other color changes of the skin • Increased occurrence of infection • Toe and foot sores that do not heal

QUESTION	RATIONALE
	Jain et al. (2012) found that a lower tolerance for stair climbing predicted a higher mortality rate in people with PAD. Leg pain that awakens a client from sleep is often associated with advanced chronic arterial occlusive disease. However, the lack of pain sensation may signal neuropathy in such disorders as diabetes. Reduced sensation or an absence of pain can result in a failure to recognize a problem or fully understand the problem's significance. **OLDER ADULT CONSIDERATIONS** Older clients with arterial disease may not have the classic symptoms of intermittent claudication, but may experience coldness, color change, numbness, and abnormal sensations. **CULTURAL CONSIDERATIONS** African Americans in the United States have higher rates than non-Hispanic whites, Hispanics, and South Asians, even accounting for the differences in risk factors, which remains unexplained (Criqui et al., 2005).
Do you experience heaviness, an aching sensation in your legs aggravated by standing or sitting for long periods, leg edema, or varicosities?	Although peripheral venous disease (PVD) is not as common as PAD, it often occurs with PAD but can occur in isolation. Symptoms of PVD include: heaviness of legs, aching sensation in legs aggravated by standing or sitting for long periods of time, leg edema, or varicosities.
Do you have any leg veins that are rope-like, bulging, or contorted?	Varicose veins are hereditary but may also develop from increased venous pressure and venous pooling (e.g., as happens during pregnancy). Standing in one place for long periods of time also increases the risk for varicosities.
Do you have any sores or open wounds on your legs? Where are they located? Are they painful?	PVD is often associated with delayed wound healing. Ulcers associated with arterial disease are usually painful and are often located on the toes, foot, or lateral ankle. Venous ulcers are usually painless and occur on the lower leg or medial ankle.
Do you have any swelling (edema) in your legs or feet? At what time of day is swelling worst? Is there any pain with swelling?	Peripheral edema (swelling) results from an obstruction of the lymphatic flow or from venous insufficiency from such conditions as incompetent valves or decreased osmotic pressure in the capillaries. It may also occur with deep vein thrombosis (DVT). Risk factors for DVT include reduced mobility, dehydration, increased viscosity of the blood, and venous stasis (Sommers, 2012). With leg or foot ulcers, edema can reduce tissue perfusion and wound oxygenation (see Evidence-Based Health Promotion and Disease Prevention 22-1).
Do you have any swollen glands or lymph nodes? If so, do they feel tender, soft, or hard?	Enlarged lymph nodes may indicate a local or systemic infection. **OLDER ADULT CONSIDERATIONS** With aging, lymphatic tissue is lost, resulting in smaller and fewer lymph nodes.
For male clients: Have you experienced a change in your usual sexual activity? Describe.	Central arterial or venous disease may be manifested early as erectile dysfunction (ED). ED may occur with decreased blood flow or an occlusion of the blood vessels in one type of PAD known as aortoiliac occlusion (Leriche syndrome) (Frederick et al., 2010). Men may be reluctant to report or discuss difficulties achieving or maintaining an erection.

Personal Health History

QUESTION	RATIONALE
Describe any problems you had in the past with the circulation in your arms and legs (e.g., blood clots, ulcers, coldness, hair loss, numbness, swelling, or poor healing).	A history of prior PVD increases a person's risk for a recurrence. Symptoms such as an absence of a prior palpable pulse; cool, pale legs; thick and opaque nails; shiny, dry skin; leg ulcerations; and reduced hair growth signal peripheral arterial occlusive disease (Sommers, 2012).
Have you had any heart or blood vessel surgeries or treatments such as coronary artery bypass grafting, repair of an aneurysm, or vein stripping?	Previous surgeries may alter the appearance of the skin and underlying tissues surrounding the blood vessels. Grafts for bypass surgeries are often taken from veins in the legs.

Continued on following page

Family History

QUESTION	RATIONALE
Do you, or does your family, have a history of DVT, diabetes, hypertension, coronary heart disease, intermittent claudication, or elevated cholesterol or triglyceride levels?	These disorders or abnormalities tend to be hereditary and cause damage to blood vessels. An essential aspect of treating PVD is to identify and then modify risk factors.

Lifestyle and Health Practices

QUESTION	RATIONALE
Do you (or did you in the past) smoke or use any other form of tobacco? How much and for how long? If you use tobacco currently, are you willing to quit?	Smoking significantly increases the risk for chronic arterial insufficiency. Furthermore, Fritschi et al. (2013) found smokers with PAD had a lower self-reported quality of life and shorter claudication pain onset when walking than nonsmokers with PAD. The risk increases according to the length of time a person smokes and the amount of tobacco smoked. If willing to quit smoking, provide resources to assist in quitting. If unwilling to quit, provide information and help identify barriers to quitting. Smoking cessation has the following benefits: reduced workload on the heart, improved respiratory function, and reduced risk for lung cancer.
Do you exercise regularly?	Regular exercise improves peripheral vascular circulation and decreases stress, pulse rate, and blood pressure, decreasing the risk for developing PVD.
For female clients: Do you use oral or transdermal (patch) contraceptives?	This is a very important question especially for smokers. Oral contraceptive pills (OCPs) are contraindicated after the age of 35 if smoking. Oral or transdermal contraceptives increase the risk for thrombophlebitis, Raynaud disease, hypertension, and edema.
Are you experiencing any stress in your life at this time?	Stress increases the heart rate and blood pressure, and can contribute to vascular disease.
How have problems with your circulation (i.e., peripheral vascular system) affected your ability to function?	Discomfort or pain associated with chronic arterial disease and the aching heaviness associated with venous disease may limit a client's ability to stand or walk for long periods. This, in turn, may affect job performance and the ability to care for a home and family or participate in social events.
Do leg ulcers or varicose veins affect how you feel about yourself?	If clients perceive the appearance of their legs as disfiguring, their body image or feelings of self-worth may be negatively influenced.
Do you regularly take medications prescribed by your physician to improve your circulation?	Drugs that inhibit platelet aggregation, such as aspirin (ASA) and/or clopidogrel (Plavix), may be prescribed to increase blood flow. Aspirin also prolongs the time it takes for blood to clot and is used to reduce the risks associated with PVD. Pentoxifylline (Trental) may be prescribed to reduce blood viscosity, improving blood flow to the tissues, thus reducing tissue hypoxia and improving symptoms. Clients who fail to take their medications regularly are at risk for developing more extensive peripheral vascular problems. These clients require teaching about their medication and the importance of taking it regularly.
Do you wear support hose to treat varicose veins?	Support stockings help to reduce venous pooling and increase blood return to the heart. There are now compression knee socks available OTC at pharmacies that are amazing! They can be easily put on by patients.

22-1 EVIDENCE-BASED HEALTH PROMOTION AND DISEASE PREVENTION: PERIPHERAL ARTERY DISEASE (PAD)

INTRODUCTION

Peripheral artery disease (PAD) is also known as peripheral vascular disease, atherosclerosis, or hardening of the arteries (Cleveland Clinic, 2016). In PAD, the arteries slowly become narrowed or blocked when plaque gradually forms inside the artery walls, which causes blood flow to organs and tissues to be reduced or stopped, resulting in damage. If left untreated, the individual is at risk for heart attack, stroke, transient ischemic attack (TIA), renal artery disease or stenosis, and amputation.

According to Hayward (2015), PAD of the lower extremities is a common cause of impaired ambulation and is a leading cause of lower extremity wounds and amputations. PAD is present in approximately 20% of adults, with 7 million Americans expected to have the disease by 2020. Criqui and Aboyans (2015) report that intermittent claudication is the most common symptom of PAD, but noninvasive measures show that PAD is several times more common in the population than is intermittent claudication. PAD prevalence and incidence are both sharply age-related, rising >10% among patients in their 60s and 70s. The disease prevalence is also associated with other diseases, such as diabetes. Mayo Clinic (2015) notes that although atherosclerosis is the primary cause, less common causes are inflammation in the arteries; injury to the limbs; unusual anatomy of ligaments or muscles; or radiation exposure.

Once the disease becomes symptomatic, the primary symptom is intermittent claudication (especially pain in the legs or arms with activity such as walking, which is relieved after a few minutes of rest). The calf is the most common location for pain.

- PAD symptoms include (Mayo Clinic, 2015):
  - Painful cramping in hip, thigh or calf muscles after certain activities, such as walking or climbing stairs (claudication)
  - Leg numbness or weakness
  - Coldness in lower leg or foot, especially when compared with the other side
  - Sores on toes, feet, or legs that won't heal
  - A change in the color of legs
  - Hair loss or slower hair growth on feet and legs
  - Slower growth of toenails
  - Shiny skin on legs
  - No pulse or a weak pulse in legs or feet
  - Erectile dysfunction in men
- If PAD progresses:
  - Pain occurs even at rest or when lying down (ischemic rest pain).
  - Pain may be intense enough to disrupt sleep.
  - Hanging legs over edge of bed or walking around room may or may not temporarily relieve pain.

As noted by the Mayo Clinic, PAD is usually an indication of more widespread atherosclerosis in other parts of the vascular system.

HEALTHY PEOPLE 2020 GOAL

Not contained in the Topics and Objectives for Healthy People 2020.

SCREENING

The U.S. Preventive Services Task Force (USPSTF, 2013) concluded that the current evidence is insufficient to assess the balance of benefits and harms of screening for PAD, and of cardiovascular disease (CVD) risk assessment with the ankle–brachial index (ABI) in adults, and recommended against routine screening for peripheral vascular disease. However, the AFP (2013) reviewed contrasting recommendations, noting a consensus of other organizations that there may be a role for screening, especially in certain high-risk populations. For example, the American Diabetes Association recommends ABI screening in all patients with diabetes who are older than 50 years; if results are normal, screening should be repeated every 5 years; patients with diabetes who are younger than 50 years should be screened if they have risk factors (e.g., smoking, hypertension, hyperlipidemia, duration of diabetes more than 10 years). Guidelines from the American College of Cardiology and American Heart Association recommend ABI screening and a directed review of symptoms in high-risk populations (e.g., persons 65 years and older; persons 50 years and older with a history of diabetes or smoking, exertional leg pain symptoms, or a nonhealing extremity wound).

Yang (2015) provides a table of recommendations for screening of PAD in adults. The recommendations of the USPSTF are contrasted with those of the American College of Preventive Medicine, American College of Cardiology/AHA, Society for Vascular Surgery, European Society of Cardiology, and the American Diabetes Association. No organization recommends routine screening of low risk or asymptomatic adults, but persons at risk who smoke or have diabetes mellitus should be screened.

The AHA (2013) responded to the USPSTF recommendation against PAD screening of asymptomatic men and women aged 65 and older by urging initial screening, noting that the benefit of identifying undiagnosed PAD is substantial.

Screening methods for PAD involve physical examination, including presence or absence of pulses in feet and legs, ABI (comparing ankle and arm blood pressures), ultrasound (including Doppler to detect blood flow through blood vessels), angiography, and blood tests for cholesterol and triglycerides (Mayo Clinic, 2015). The most common screening method is the ABI.

RISK ASSESSMENT

(Cleveland Clinic, 2016; Mayo Clinic, 2015)
- Smoking
- Diabetes
- Obesity (a body mass index over 30)
- High blood pressure
- High cholesterol
- Increasing age, especially after reaching 50 years of age
- A family history of PAD, heart disease, or stroke
- High levels of homocysteine, a protein component that helps build and maintain tissue
- African American (more than twice as likely to have as non-Hispanic whites)

People who smoke or have diabetes have the greatest risk of developing PAD due to reduced blood flow.

CLIENT EDUCATION

Teach Clients
(Mayo Clinic, 2010)
- Quit smoking if you're a smoker.
- If you have diabetes, keep your blood sugar in good control.
- Exercise regularly. Aim for 30 minutes at least three times a week after you've gotten your doctor's OK.
- Lower your cholesterol and blood pressure levels, if necessary.
- Eat a well-rounded diet and foods that are low in saturated fat.
- Maintain a healthy weight.
- Ask your health care provider about screening with an ABI measurement once you reach 50 years of age.

CASE STUDY

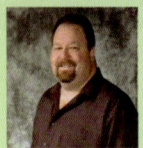

The nurse interviews Mr. Lee using specific probing questions. The client reports swelling and pain in his right lower leg. The nurse explores this health concern using the COLDSPA mnemonic.

Mnemonic	Question	Data Provided
Character	Describe the sign or symptom (feeling, appearance, sound, smell, or taste if applicable). In this case, "Describe the pain/soreness in your leg."	Mr. Lee states that he must have pulled something in his right lower leg and that now it is very sore and it hurts to walk.
Onset	When did it begin?	3 days ago.
Location	Where is it? Does it radiate? Does it occur anywhere else?	Right calf is swollen, red, warm, and tender to touch. Right calf measures 42 cm while left calf is 34.5 cm.
Duration	How long does it last? Does it recur? In this case, "Is the pain constant or intermittent?"	Pain is constant.
Severity	How bad is it? or How much does it bother you? In this case, "Rate your pain on a 0–10 point scale."	Rates pain at a 4 on a 0–10 point scale.
Pattern	What makes it better or worse? In this case, "Have you taken any medication or other treatment for the pain? Anything else that seems to make it worse/better?"	Reports increased level of pain when up walking but better when the right leg is elevated. Reports taking 1,000 mg acetaminophen 2–3 times per day to relieve pain.
Associated factors/How it **A**ffects the client	What other symptoms occur with it? How does it affect you? In this case, "Describe your activity/exercise currently and prior to 3 days ago. Are you having any shortness of breath?" (May indicate a pulmonary embolism.) Pulmonary embolism is the primary life-threatening complication of DVT (Sommers, 2012).	Sits at desk for 4–6 hours at a time. Has only limited exercise; walks several blocks for lunch, then walks back to apartment. Worries that there is something really wrong, thus has trouble concentrating on programming. Needing to elevate leg makes it difficult to work at his computer, but plans to load files on a laptop to continue to work. Denies shortness of breath or a history of clots, but states that he had a pulmonary embolus 5 years ago.

After exploring Mr. Lee's leg pain, the nurse continues with the present history. He says that he usually sits at his computer for about 4 hours, then he walks a couple of blocks to a coffee shop for lunch (a sandwich or a salad with cheese and fruit, and usually a piece of cake or pie). After lunch, Mr. Lee says he goes back to his apartment and works for another 5–6 hours. At night, he eats dinner and watches a few hours of television. Other than walking a short distance at noon, he gets no other planned exercise.

Mr. Lee's medical history includes a coronary artery bypass graft (CABG) 5 years ago for angina, complicated postoperatively by a pulmonary embolus. However, he has not had any further problems. He denies numbness, tingling, or loss of mobility in either extremity.

Collecting Objective Data: Physical Examination

The purpose of the peripheral vascular assessment is to identify any signs or symptoms of PVD including arterial insufficiency, venous insufficiency, or lymphatic involvement. This is accomplished by performing an assessment first of the arms then the legs, concentrating on skin color and temperature, major pulse sites, and major groups of lymph nodes.

Examination of the peripheral vascular system is very useful in acute care, extended care, and home health care settings. Early detection of PVD can prevent long-term complications. A complete peripheral vascular examination involves inspection, palpation, and auscultation. In addition, there are several special assessment techniques that are necessary to perform on clients with suspected peripheral vascular problems.

Compare the client's arms and legs bilaterally. Better objective data can be gained by assessing a particular feature on one extremity and then the other. For example, evaluate the strength of the dorsalis pedis pulse on the right foot and compare your findings with those of the left foot.

Preparing the Client

Ask the client to put on an examination gown and to sit upright on an examination table. Make sure that the room is a comfortable temperature (about 72°F), without drafts. This helps to prevent vasodilation or vasoconstriction. Before you begin the assessment, inform the client that it will be necessary to inspect and palpate all four extremities and that the groin will also need to be exposed for palpation of the inguinal lymph nodes as well as palpation and auscultation of the femoral arteries. Explain that the client can sit for examination of the arms but will need to lie down for examination of the legs and groin, and will need to follow your directions for several special assessment techniques toward the end of the examination. As you perform the examination, explain in detail what you are doing and answer any questions the client may have. This helps to ease any client anxiety.

Equipment

- Centimeter tape
- Stethoscope
- Doppler ultrasound device
- Conductivity gel
- Tourniquet
- Gauze or tissue
- Waterproof pen
- Blood pressure cuff

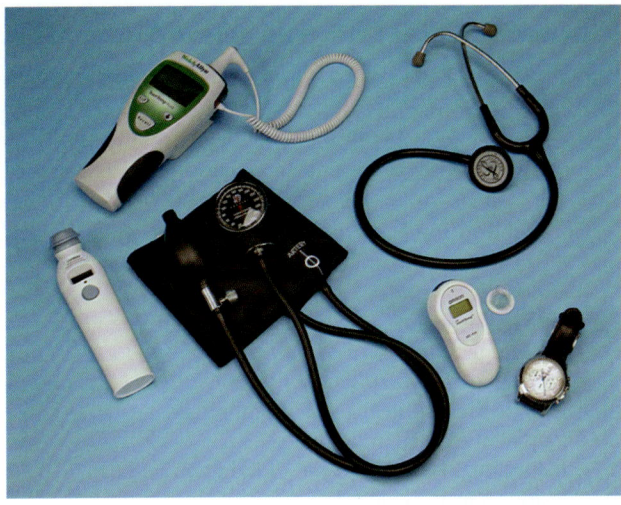

Physical Assessment

- Discuss risk factors for PVD with the client.
- Accurately inspect arms and legs for edema and venous patterning.
- Observe carefully for signs of arterial and venous insufficiency (skin color, venous pattern, hair distribution, lesions, or ulcers) and inadequate lymphatic drainage.
- Recognize characteristic clubbing.
- Palpate pulse points correctly.
- Use the Doppler ultrasound instrument correctly (Assessment Guide 22-1).

ASSESSMENT GUIDE 22-1   How to Use the Doppler Ultrasound Device

The Doppler ultrasound device transmits and receives ultrasound waves to evaluate blood flow. It works by transmitting ultra high-frequency sound waves that strike red blood cells (RBCs) in an artery or vein. The rebounding ultrasound waves produce a whooshing sound when echoing from an artery and a nonpulsating rush when echoing from a vein. The strength of the sound is determined by the velocity of the RBCs. In partially occluded vessels, RBCs pass more slowly through the vessel, thus decreasing the sound. Fully occluded vessels produce no sound. The battery-operated handheld Doppler device is used to:
- Assess unpalpable pulses in the extremities
- Determine the patency of arterial bypass grafts
- Assess tissue perfusion in an extremity

Operating the Device

When assessing peripheral circulation with a Doppler ultrasound device, first inform the patient that the assessment is painless and noninvasive. Then the test can proceed as follows:
- Apply a fingertip-sized mound of lukewarm gel over the blood vessel to be assessed.
- At a 60- to 90-degree angle, lightly place the vascular probe at the top of the mound of gel.
- Listen for a whooshing (artery) or nonpulsating, rushing (vein) sound.
- Clean the skin with a tissue.
- Clean the probe as recommended by the manufacturer.
- Mark the site with a permanent pen for easy reassessment.
- Record findings.

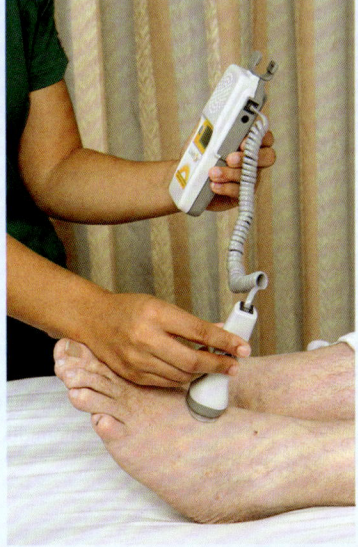

Improving Results

- A warm extremity will increase signal strength.
- Place the tube or packet of gel in warm water before use because cold gel will promote vasoconstriction and make it more difficult to detect a signal.
- Avoid pressing the probe too snugly against the skin, which may obliterate the signal.

General Routine Screening versus Focused Specialty Assessment for the Peripheral Vascular System

On a routine head-to-toe examination, the nurse would inspect the arms, hands, fingers, legs, feet, and toes for color, temperature, lesions, or ulcers. Radial, post-tibial, and dorsalis pedal pulses are also palpated to assess circulation. More advanced assessments are listed in the table below that would be performed by a nurse working in a peripheral vascular specialty or intensive care area or by a nurse practitioner to diagnose or rule out peripheral vascular insufficiency.

General Routine Screening
- Observe arm size and venous pattern; also look for edema.
- Palpate the client's fingers, hands, and arms, and note the temperature.
- Palpate to assess capillary refill time.
- Palpate the popliteal and femoral pulses.
- Palpate the radial and ulnar pulses.
- Inspect legs for distribution of hair, temperature, lesions, ulcers, or edema.
- Palpate the dorsalis pedal, and posterior tibial pulses.
- Inspect for varicosities and thrombophlebitis.

Focused Specialty Assessment
- Palpate the brachial pulses if you suspect arterial insufficiency.
- Perform the Allen test.
- Palpate the epitrochlear lymph nodes.
- Palpate the superficial inguinal lymph nodes.
- Auscultate the femoral pulses.
- Perform position change test for arterial insufficiency.
- Determine ankle–brachial index (ABI).
- Perform manual compression test if the client has varicose veins.
- Perform Trendelenburg test if client has varicose veins.

ASSESSMENT PROCEDURE	NORMAL FINDINGS	ABNORMAL FINDINGS
Arms		
INSPECTION		
Observe arm size and venous pattern; also look for edema. If there is an observable difference, measure bilaterally the circumference of the arms at the same locations with each remeasurement and record findings in centimeters. 🎯 **CLINICAL TIP** Mark locations on arms with a permanent marker to ensure the exact same locations are used with each reassessment.	Arms are bilaterally symmetric with minimal variation in size and shape. No edema or prominent venous patterning.	Lymphedema results from blocked lymphatic circulation, which may be caused by breast surgery. It usually affects one extremity, causing induration and nonpitting edema. Prominent venous patterning with edema may indicate venous obstruction (see Box 22-1). **Concept Mastery Alert** A patient with lymphedema usually presents with nonpitting edema of only one extremity, which causes induration, not ulceration, of the skin and shows no pigment changes.
Observe coloration of the hands and arms (Fig. 22-7).	Color varies depending on the client's skin tone, although color should be the same bilaterally (see Chapter 14 for more information).	Raynaud disorder is sometimes referred to as a disease, syndrome, or phenomenon (see Abnormal Findings 22-3) (National Heart, Lung, Blood Institute [NHLBI], 2014). It is a vascular disorder caused by vasoconstriction or vasospasm of the fingers or toes, characterized by rapid changes of color (pallor, cyanosis, and redness), swelling, pain, numbness, tingling, burning, throbbing, and coldness. The disorder commonly occurs bilaterally; symptoms last minutes to hours. Raynaud affects about 5% of the population and can often be controlled with minor lifestyle changes (NHLBI, 2014) (Fig. 22-8).

ASSESSMENT PROCEDURE	NORMAL FINDINGS	ABNORMAL FINDINGS
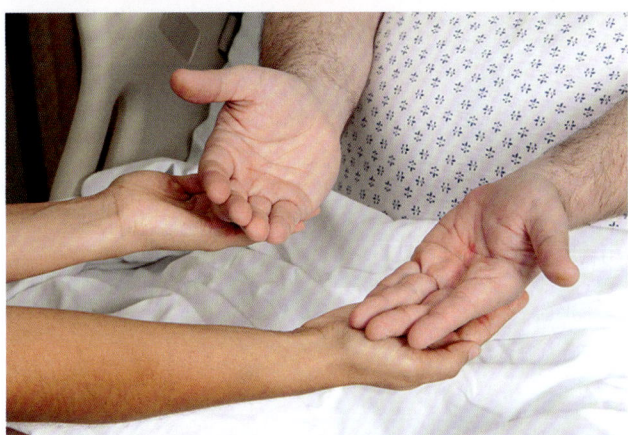 **FIGURE 22-7** Inspecting color related to circulation.	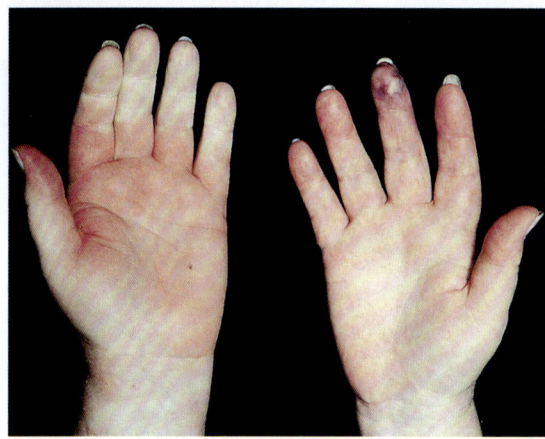 **FIGURE 22-8** Hallmarks of Raynaud disease are color changes. (Used with permission from Effeney, D. J., & Stoney, R. J. (1993). *Wylie's atlas of vascular surgery: Disorders of the extremities*. Philadelphia, PA: J. B. Lippincott.)	

PALPATION

Palpate the client's fingers, hands, and arms, and note the temperature.	Skin is warm to the touch bilaterally from fingertips to upper arms.	A cool extremity may be a sign of arterial insufficiency. Cold fingers and hands, for example, are common findings with Raynaud's.
Palpate to assess capillary refill time. Compress the nailbed until it blanches. Release the pressure and calculate the time it takes for color to return. This test indicates peripheral perfusion and reflects cardiac output. ◎ **CLINICAL TIP** Inaccurate findings may result if the room is cool, if the client has edema, has anemia, or if the client recently smoked a cigarette.	Capillary beds refill (and, therefore, color returns) in 2 seconds or less.	Capillary refill time exceeding 2 seconds may indicate vasoconstriction, decreased cardiac output, shock, arterial occlusion, or hypothermia.
Palpate the radial pulse. Gently press the radial artery against the radius (Fig. 22-9). Note elasticity and strength. ◎ **CLINICAL TIP** For difficult-to-palpate pulses, use a Doppler ultrasound device (see Evidence-Based Health Promotion and Disease Prevention 22-1).	Radial pulses are bilaterally strong (2+). Artery walls have a resilient quality (bounce).	Increased radial pulse volume indicates a hyperkinetic state (3+ or bounding pulse). Diminished (1+) or absent (0) pulse suggests partial or complete arterial occlusion (which is more common in the legs than the arms). The pulse could also be decreased from Buerger disease or scleroderma (see Box 22-2).
Palpate the ulnar pulses. Apply pressure with your first three fingertips to the medial aspects of the inner wrists. The ulnar pulses are not routinely assessed because they are located deeper than the radial pulses and are difficult to detect. Palpate the ulnar arteries if you suspect arterial insufficiency (Fig. 22-10).	The ulnar pulses may not be detectable.	Obliteration of the pulse may result from compression by external sources, as in compartment syndrome. Lack of resilience or inelasticity of the artery wall may indicate arteriosclerosis.

Continued on following page

ASSESSMENT PROCEDURE	NORMAL FINDINGS	ABNORMAL FINDINGS

Arms (Continued)

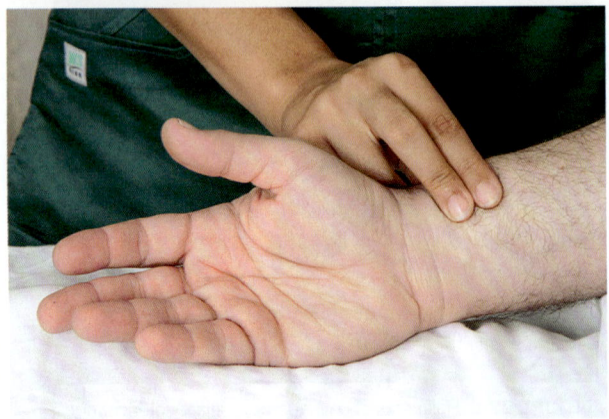

FIGURE 22-9 Palpating the radial pulse.

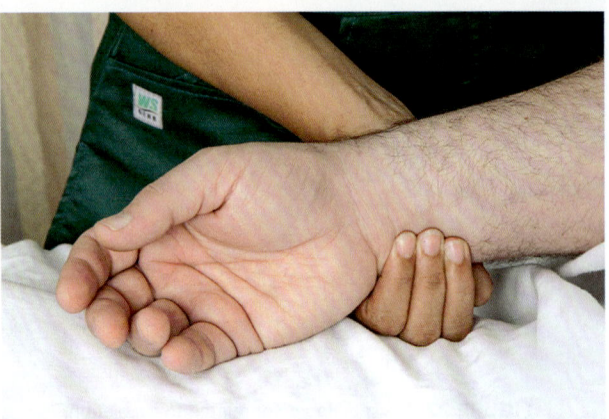

FIGURE 22-10 Palpating the ulnar pulse.

You can also palpate the brachial pulses if you suspect arterial insufficiency. Do this by placing the first three fingertips of each hand at the client's right and left medial antecubital creases. Alternatively, palpate the brachial pulse in the groove between the biceps and triceps (Fig. 22-11).	Brachial pulses have equal strength bilaterally.	Brachial pulses are increased, diminished, or absent.
Palpate the epitrochlear lymph nodes. Take the client's left hand in your right hand as if you were shaking hands. Flex the client's elbow about 90 degrees. Use your left hand to palpate behind the elbow in the groove between the biceps and triceps muscles (Fig. 22-12). If nodes are detected, evaluate for size, tenderness, and consistency. Repeat palpation on the opposite arm.	Normally, epitrochlear lymph nodes are not palpable.	Enlarged epitrochlear lymph nodes may indicate an infection in the hand or forearm, or they may occur with generalized lymphadenopathy. Enlarged lymph nodes may also occur because of a lesion in the area.

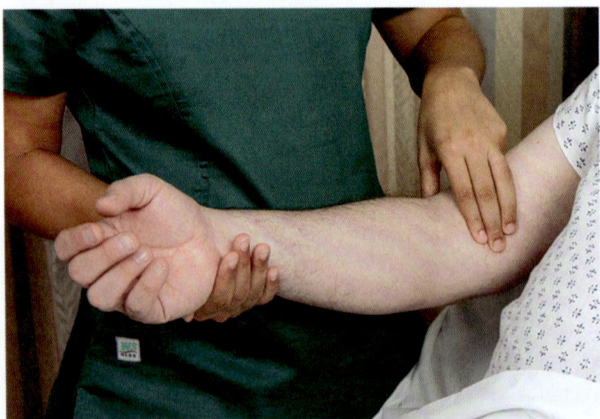

FIGURE 22-11 Palpating the brachial pulse.

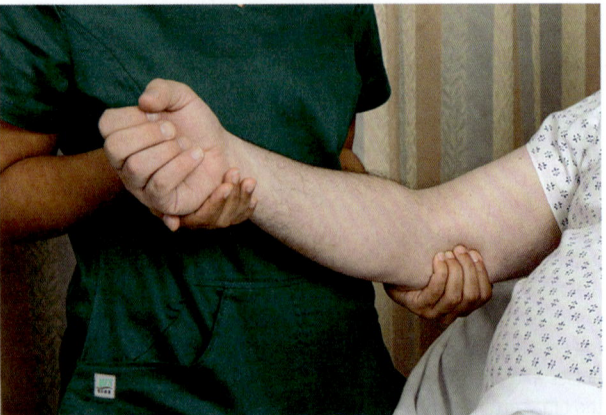

FIGURE 22-12 Palpating the epitrochlear lymph nodes located in the upper inside of the arm.

ASSESSMENT PROCEDURE	NORMAL FINDINGS	ABNORMAL FINDINGS
Perform the Allen test. The Allen test evaluates patency of the radial or ulnar arteries. An Allen test is essential before arterial sampling (arterial blood gas) or arterial line insertion/placement. It is implemented when patency is questionable or before such procedures as a radial artery puncture. The test begins by assessing ulnar patency. Have the client rest the hand palm side up on the examination table and make a fist. Then use your thumbs to occlude the radial and ulnar arteries (Fig. 22-13A). Continue pressure to keep both arteries occluded and have the client release the fist (Fig. 22-13B). Note that the palm remains pale. Release the pressure on the ulnar artery and watch for color to return to the hand. To assess radial patency, repeat the procedure as before, but at the last step, release pressure on the radial artery (Fig. 22-13C). ◎ **CLINICAL TIP** Opening the hand into exaggerated extension may cause persistent pallor (false-positive Allen test).	Pink coloration returns to the palms within 3–5 seconds if the ulnar artery is patent. Pink coloration returns within 3–5 seconds if the radial artery is patent.	With arterial insufficiency or occlusion of the ulnar artery, pallor persists. With arterial insufficiency or occlusion of the radial artery, pallor persists.

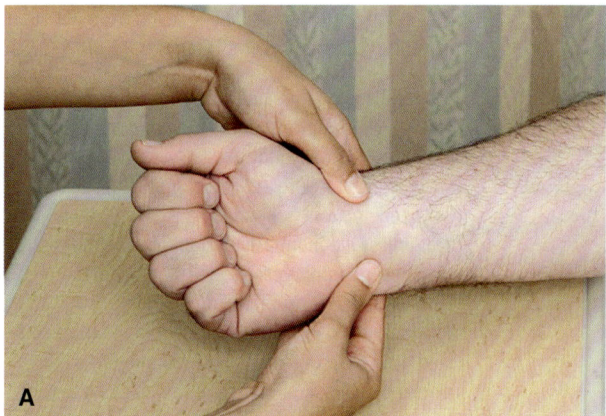
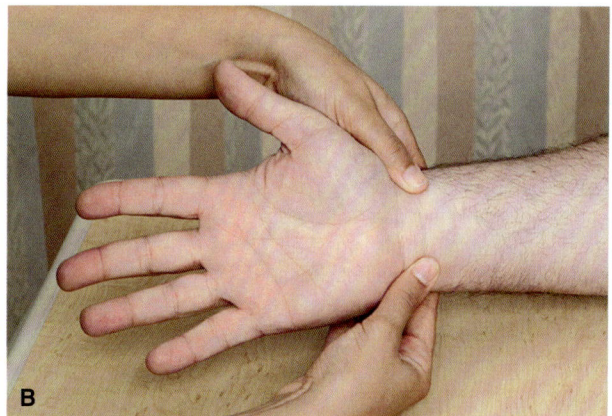
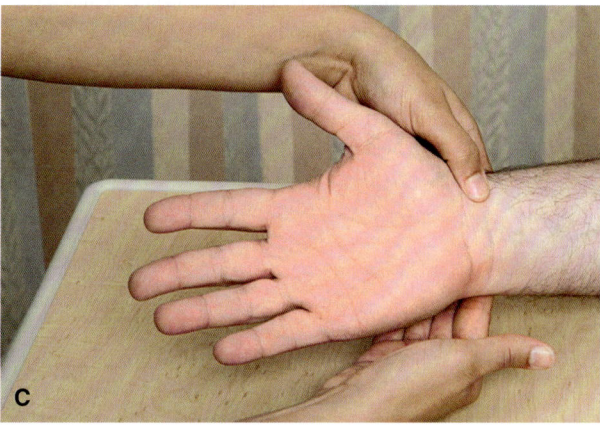

FIGURE 22-13 Performing the Allen test. **A.** Occlude radial and ulnar arteries while client makes a fist. **B.** Continue occluding arteries while client releases fist. **C.** Remove pressure on ulnar artery while observing color return to palm.

Continued on following page

ASSESSMENT PROCEDURE	NORMAL FINDINGS	ABNORMAL FINDINGS
Legs		
INSPECTION, PALPATION, AND AUSCULTATION		
Ask the client to lie supine. Then drape the groin area and place a pillow under the client's head for comfort. **Observe skin color while inspecting both legs from the toes to the groin.**	Pink color for lighter-skinned clients and pink or red tones visible under darker-pigmented skin. There should be no changes in pigmentation.	Pallor, especially when elevated, and rubor, when dependent, suggests arterial insufficiency. Dark-colored toes and blisters are seen with arterial insufficiency and gangrene (see Abnormal Findings 22-3). Gangrene is evident with ulcerations that are slow to heal, dry and shriveled skin that changes color from blue to black and eventually sloughs off, cold and numb skin; pain may or may not be present. Cyanosis when dependent suggests venous insufficiency. A rusty, ruddy, or brownish pigmentation (rubor) around the ankles indicates venous insufficiency (see Abnormal Findings 22-1).
Inspect distribution of hair on legs.	Hair covers the skin on the legs and appears on the dorsal surface of the toes. **OLDER ADULT CONSIDERATIONS** **Hair loss on the lower extremities occurs with aging and is, therefore, not an absolute sign of arterial insufficiency in the older client.**	Loss of hair on the legs suggests arterial insufficiency. Often thin, shiny skin is noted as well.
Inspect for lesions or ulcers.	Legs are free of lesions or ulcerations.	Ulcers with smooth, even margins that occur at pressure areas, such as the toes and lateral ankle, result from arterial insufficiency. Ulcers with irregular edges, bleeding, and possible bacterial infection that occur on the medial ankle result from venous insufficiency (see Abnormal Findings 22-1).
Inspect for edema. Inspect the legs for unilateral or bilateral edema. Note veins, tendons, and bony prominences. If the legs appear asymmetric, use a centimeter tape to measure in four different areas: circumference at mid-thigh, largest circumference at the calf, smallest circumference above the ankle, and across the forefoot. Compare both extremities at the same locations (Fig. 22-14).	Identical size and shape bilaterally; no swelling or atrophy.	Bilateral edema may be detected by the absence of visible veins, tendons, or bony prominences. Bilateral edema usually indicates a systemic problem, such as heart failure, or a local problem, such as lymphedema, but lymphedema is always unilateral unless elephantiasis is diagnosed (abnormal or blocked lymph vessels; see Abnormal Findings 22-4) or prolonged standing or sitting (orthostatic edema). Unilateral edema is characterized by a 1-cm difference in measurement at the ankles or a 2-cm difference at the calf, and a swollen extremity. It is usually caused by venous stasis due to insufficiency or an obstruction. It may also be caused by lymphedema (see Abnormal Findings 22-2). A difference in measurement between legs may also be due to muscular atrophy. Muscular atrophy usually results from disuse due to stroke or from being in a cast for a prolonged time.

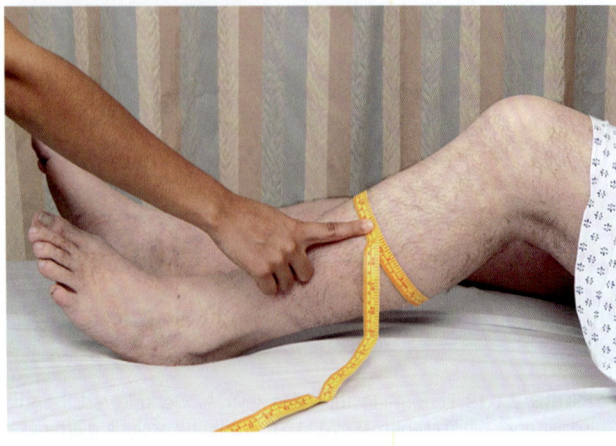

FIGURE 22-14 Measuring the calf circumference.

22 Assessing Peripheral Vascular System 479

ASSESSMENT PROCEDURE	NORMAL FINDINGS	ABNORMAL FINDINGS
CLINICAL TIP Taking a measurement in centimeters from the patella to the location to be measured can aid in getting the exact location on both legs. If additional readings are necessary, use a felt-tipped pen to ensure exact placement of the measuring tape.		
Palpate edema. If edema is noted during inspection, palpate the area to determine if it is pitting or nonpitting (see Abnormal Findings 22-2). Press the edematous area with the tips of your fingers, hold for a few seconds, then release. If the depression does not rapidly refill and the skin remains indented on release, pitting edema is present.	No edema (pitting or nonpitting) present in the legs.	Pitting edema is associated with systemic problems, such as heart failure or hepatic cirrhosis, and local causes such as venous stasis due to insufficiency or obstruction or prolonged standing or sitting (orthostatic edema). A 1+ to 4+ scale is used to grade the severity of pitting edema, with 4+ being most severe (Fig. 22-15).

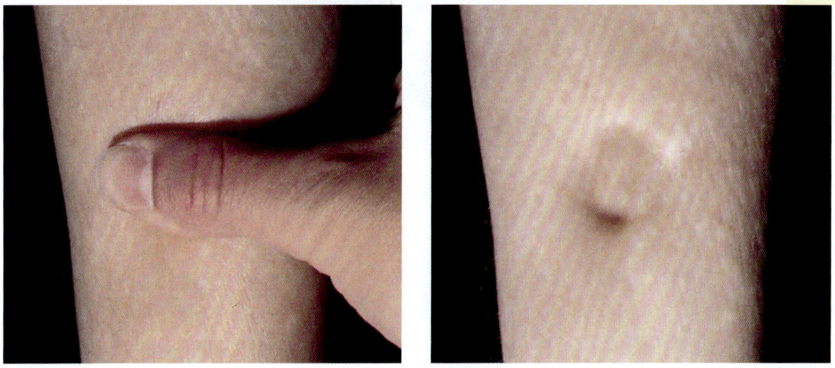

FIGURE 22-15 Pitting edema.

| **Palpate bilaterally for temperature of the feet and legs.** Use the backs of your fingers. Compare your findings in the same areas bilaterally (Fig. 22-16). Note location of any changes in temperature. | Toes, feet, and legs are equally warm bilaterally. | Generalized coolness in one leg or change in temperature from warm to cool as you move down the leg suggests arterial insufficiency. Increased warmth in the leg may be caused by superficial thrombophlebitis (see Abnormal Findings 22-4), resulting from a secondary inflammation in the tissue around the vein. |

CLINICAL TIP Bilateral coolness of the feet and legs suggests one of the following: the room is too cool, the client may have recently smoked a cigarette, the client is anemic, or the client is anxious. All of these factors cause vasoconstriction, resulting in cool skin.

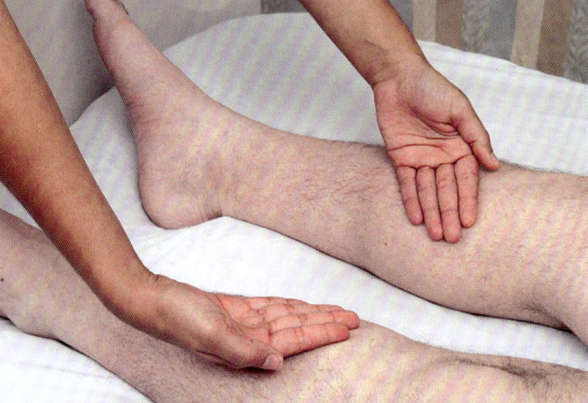

FIGURE 22-16 Palpating skin temperature.

| **Palpate the superficial inguinal lymph nodes.** First, expose the client's inguinal area, keeping the genitals draped. Feel over the upper medial thigh for the vertical and horizontal groups of superficial inguinal lymph nodes. If detected, determine size, mobility, or tenderness. Repeat palpation on the opposite thigh. | Nontender, movable lymph nodes up to 1 or even 2 cm are commonly palpated. | Lymph nodes larger than 2 cm with or without tenderness (lymphadenopathy) may be from a local infection or generalized lymphadenopathy. Fixed nodes may indicate malignancy. |

Continued on following page

ASSESSMENT PROCEDURE	NORMAL FINDINGS	ABNORMAL FINDINGS
Legs (Continued)		
Palpate the femoral pulses. Ask the client to bend the knee and move it out to the side. Press deeply and slowly below and medial to the inguinal ligament. Use two hands if necessary. Release pressure until you feel the pulse. Repeat palpation on the opposite leg. Compare amplitude bilaterally (Fig. 22-17).	Femoral pulses strong and equal bilaterally.	Weak or absent femoral pulses indicate partial or complete arterial occlusion.
Auscultate the femoral pulses. If arterial occlusion is suspected in the femoral pulse, position the stethoscope over the femoral artery and listen for bruits. Repeat for other artery (Fig. 22-18).	No sounds auscultated over the femoral arteries.	Bruits over one or both femoral arteries suggest partial obstruction of the vessel and diminished blood flow to the lower extremities.

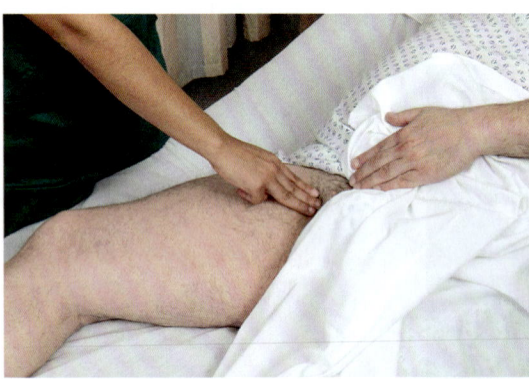

FIGURE 22-17 Palpating the femoral pulse.

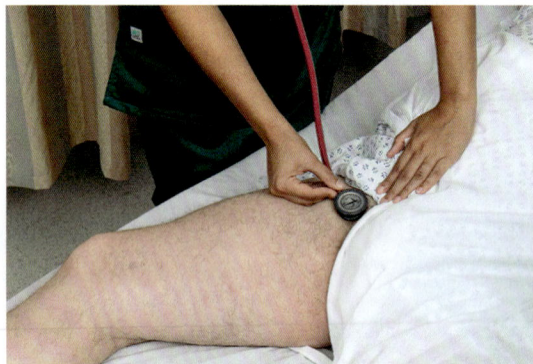

FIGURE 22-18 Auscultating the femoral pulse to detect bruits.

Palpate the popliteal pulses. Ask the client to raise (flex) the knee partially. Place your thumbs on the knee while positioning your fingers deep in the bend of the knee. Apply pressure to locate the pulse. It is usually detected lateral to the medial tendon (Fig. 22-19A). 🎯 **CLINICAL TIP** If you cannot detect a pulse, try palpating with the client in a prone position. Partially raise the leg, and place your fingers deep in the bend of the knee. Repeat palpation in opposite leg, and note amplitude bilaterally (Fig. 22-19B). Use a Doppler ultrasound to assess popliteal pulse if concerned!	It is not unusual for the popliteal pulse to be difficult or impossible to detect, and yet for circulation to be normal.	Although normal popliteal arteries may be nonpalpable, an absent pulse may also be the result of an occluded artery. Further circulatory assessment such as temperature changes, skin-color differences, edema, hair distribution variations, and dependent rubor (dusky redness) distal to the popliteal artery assists in determining the significance of an absent pulse. Cyanosis may be present yet more subtle in darker-skinned clients (Mann, 2013).

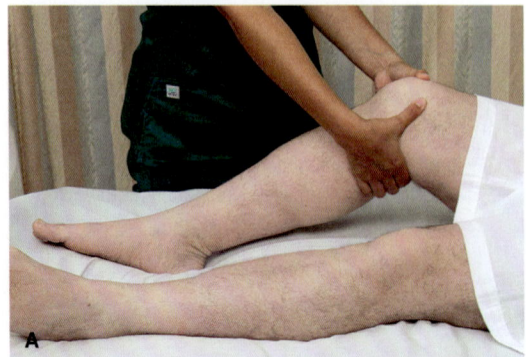
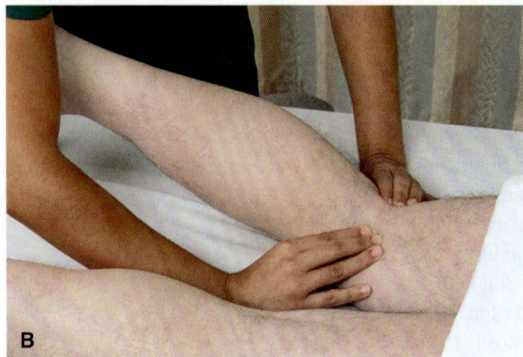

FIGURE 22-19 Palpating the popliteal pulse with the client supine (A) and prone (B).

ASSESSMENT PROCEDURE	NORMAL FINDINGS	ABNORMAL FINDINGS
Palpate the dorsalis pedis pulses. Dorsiflex the client's foot and apply light pressure lateral to and along the side of the extensor tendon of the big toe. The pulses of both feet may be assessed at the same time to aid in making comparisons. Assess amplitude bilaterally (Fig. 22-20). A Doppler ultrasound may be used if pulses are not palpable. ◎ **CLINICAL TIP** It may be difficult or impossible to palpate a pulse in an edematous foot. A Doppler ultrasound device may be useful in this situation.	Dorsalis pedis pulses are bilaterally strong. This pulse is congenitally absent in 5–10% of the population.	A weak or absent pulse may indicate impaired arterial circulation. Further circulatory assessments (temperature and color) are warranted to determine the significance of an absent pulse.
Palpate the posterior tibial pulses. Palpate behind and just below the medial malleolus (in the groove between the ankle and the Achilles tendon) (Fig. 22-21). Palpating both posterior tibial pulses at the same time aids in making comparisons. Assess amplitude bilaterally. Use a Doppler if ultrasound pulses are not palpable. ◎ **CLINICAL TIP** Edema in the ankles may make it difficult or impossible to palpate a posterior tibial pulse. In this case, Doppler ultrasound may be used to assess the pulse.	The posterior tibial pulses should be strong bilaterally. However, in about 15% of healthy clients, the posterior tibial pulses are absent.	A weak or absent pulse indicates partial or complete arterial occlusion.

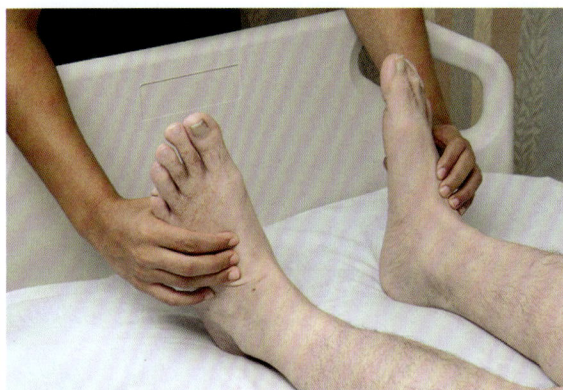

FIGURE 22-20 Palpating the dorsalis pedis pulse.

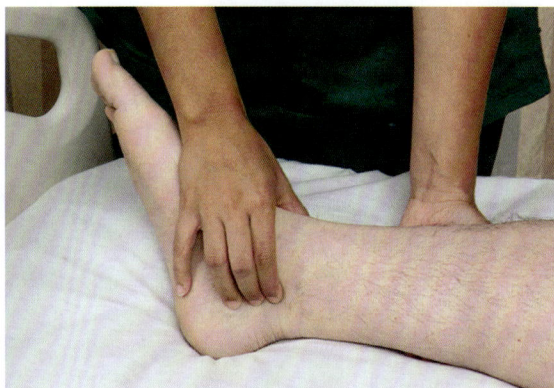

FIGURE 22-21 Palpating the posterior tibial pulse.

Inspect for varicosities and thrombophlebitis. Ask the client to stand because varicose veins may not be visible when the client is supine and not as pronounced when the client is sitting. As the client is standing, inspect for superficial vein thrombophlebitis. To fully assess for a suspected phlebitis, lightly palpate for tenderness. If superficial vein thrombophlebitis is present, note redness or discoloration on the skin surface over the vein.	Veins are flat and barely seen under the surface of the skin. 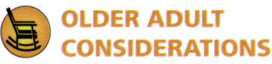 **OLDER ADULT CONSIDERATIONS** Varicosities are common in the older client.	Varicose veins may appear as distended, nodular, bulging, and tortuous, depending on severity. Varicosities are common in the anterior lateral thigh and lower leg, the posterior lateral calf, or anus (known as hemorrhoids). Varicose veins result from incompetent valves in the veins, weak vein walls, or an obstruction above the varicosity. Despite venous dilation, blood flow is decreased and venous pressure is increased. Superficial vein thrombophlebitis is marked by redness, thickening, and tenderness along the vein. Aching or cramping may occur with walking. Swelling and inflammation are often noted (see Abnormal Findings 22-4). Diagnostic testing such as venous Doppler ultrasound of the legs and referral are indicated for a definitive diagnosis.

Continued on following page

ASSESSMENT PROCEDURE	NORMAL FINDINGS	ABNORMAL FINDINGS
Special Tests for Arterial or Venous Insufficiency		
Perform position change test for arterial insufficiency. If pulses in the legs are weak, further assessment for arterial insufficiency is warranted. The client should be in a supine position. Place one forearm under both of the client's ankles and the other forearm underneath the knees. Raise the legs about 12 in above the level of the heart. As you support the client's legs, ask the client to pump the feet up and down for about a minute to drain the legs of venous blood, leaving only arterial blood to color the legs (Fig. 22-22A). At this point, ask the client to sit up and dangle legs off the side of the examination table. Note the color of both feet and the time it takes for color to return (Fig. 22-22B). ◎ **CLINICAL TIP** This assessment maneuver will not be accurate if the client has PVD of the veins with incompetent valves.	Feet pink to slightly pale in color in the light-skinned client with elevation. Inspect the soles in the dark-skinned client, although it is more difficult to see subtle color changes in darker skin. When the client sits up and dangles the legs, a pinkish color returns to the tips of the toes in 10 seconds or less. The superficial veins on top of the feet fill in 15 seconds or less. Normal responses with absent pulses suggest that an adequate collateral circulation has developed around an arterial occlusion.	Marked pallor with legs elevated is an indication of arterial insufficiency (Fig. 22-23C). Return of pink color that takes longer than 10 seconds and superficial veins that take longer than 15 seconds to fill suggest arterial insufficiency. Persistent rubor (dusky redness) of toes and feet with legs dependent also suggests arterial insufficiency (Fig. 22-23D).

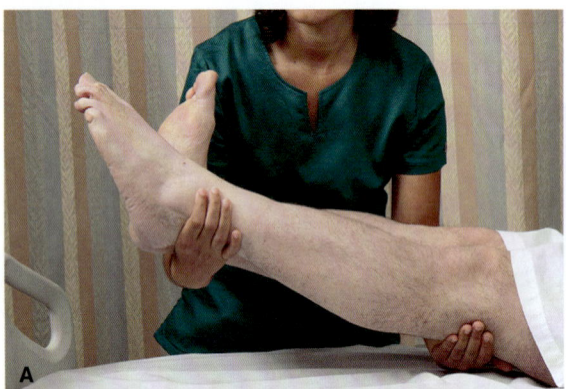
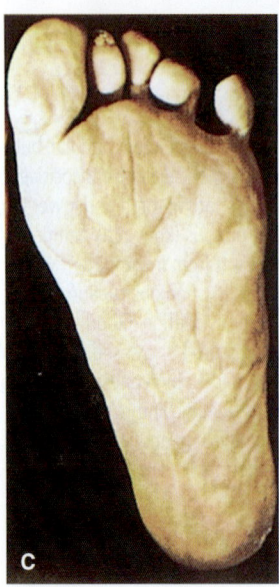
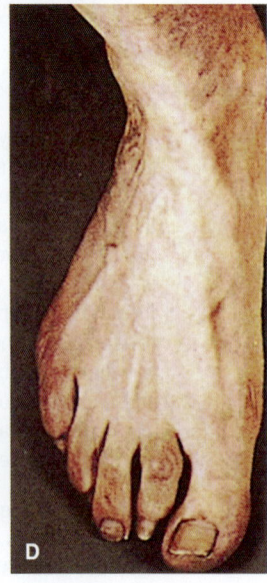
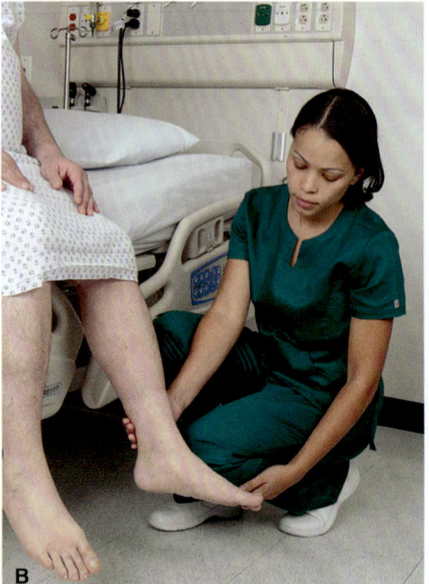

FIGURE 22-22 Testing for arterial insufficiency by elevating the legs (**A**), followed by having client dangle the legs (**B**). Marked pallor of foot when elevated seen in arterial insufficiency (**C**). Persistent rubor of dependent foot seen in arterial insufficiency (**D**). (Parts C and D from Kappert A, Winsor T. (1972). *Diagnosis of peripheral vascular disease*. Philadelphia, PA: FA Davis.)

ASSESSMENT PROCEDURE	NORMAL FINDINGS	ABNORMAL FINDINGS
Determine ankle–brachial index (ABI), also known as ankle-brachial pressure index (ABPI). Even though this **advanced skill** is most often performed in a cardiovascular center, it is important to know how the test is performed and the implications. If the client has symptoms of arterial occlusion, the ABPI should be used to compare upper- and lower-limb systolic blood pressure. The ABI is the ratio of the ankle systolic blood pressure to the arm (brachial) systolic blood pressure (see Box 22-3). The ABI is considered an accurate objective assessment for determining the degree of peripheral arterial disease. It detects decreased systolic pressure distal to the area of stenosis or arterial narrowing and allows the nurse to quantify this measurement.	Generally, the ankle pressure in a healthy person is the same or slightly higher than the brachial pressure, resulting in an ABI of approximately 1, or no arterial insufficiency.	Early recognition of cardiovascular disease even in asymptomatic people can be determined using ABI measurements (Taylor-Piliae et al., 2011). People who smoke, are physically inactive, have a body mass index >30 or are hypertensive are more likely to have an abnormal ABI, suggesting PAD (Taylor-Piliae et al., 2011). Suspect medial calcification sclerosis any time you calculate an ABPI of 1.3 or greater or measure ankle pressure at more than 300 mm Hg. This condition is associated with diabetes mellitus, chronic renal failure, and hyperparathyroidism. Medial calcific sclerosis produces falsely elevated ankle pressure by making the vessels noncompressible.
Measure ABI. Use the following steps to measure ABI: • Have the client rest in a supine position for at least 5 minutes. • Apply the blood pressure (BP) cuff to first one arm and then the other to determine the brachial pressure using the Doppler. First palpate the pulse and use the Doppler to hear the pulse. The "whooshing" sound indicates the brachial pulse. Pressures in both arms are assessed because asymptomatic stenosis in the subclavian artery can produce an abnormally low reading and should not be used in the calculations. Record the *higher reading*. • Apply the BP cuff to the right ankle, then palpate the posterior tibial pulse at the medial aspect of the ankle and the dorsalis pedis pulse on the dorsal aspect of the foot. Using the same Doppler technique as in the arms, determine and record *both* systolic pressures. Repeat this procedure on the left ankle (Fig. 22-23). If you are unable to assess these pulses, use the peroneal artery (Fig. 22-24).		In addition to abnormal ABI findings, reduced or absent pedal pulses, a cool leg unilaterally, lack of hair, and shiny skin on the leg suggests peripheral arterial occlusive disease.

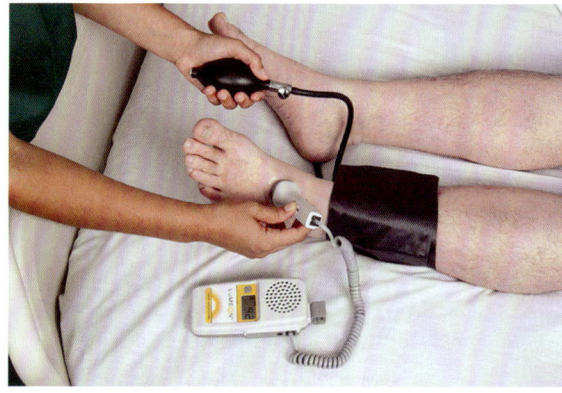

FIGURE 22-23 When measuring systolic pressure from the dorsalis pedis artery, apply the blood pressure cuff above the malleolus and the Doppler device at a 60- to 90-degree angle over the anterior tibial artery. Then, move the device downward along the length of the vessel.

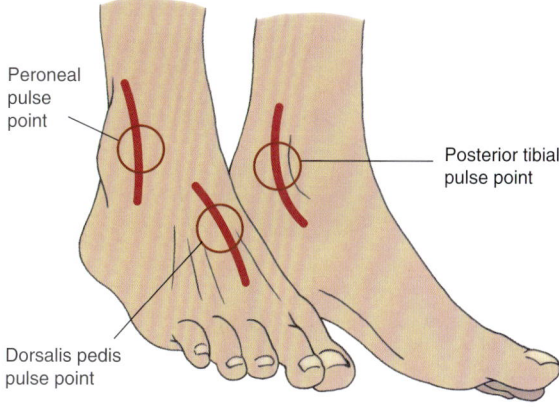

FIGURE 22-24 If you cannot measure pressure in the dorsalis pedis or posterior tibial artery, measure it in the peroneal artery, a branch of the posterior tibial artery. The blood pressure cuff can remain in place.

Continued on following page

ASSESSMENT PROCEDURE	NORMAL FINDINGS	ABNORMAL FINDINGS

Special Tests for Arterial or Venous Insufficiency (Continued)

 CLINICAL TIP

- Make sure to use a correctly sized BP cuff. The bladder of the cuff should be 20% wider than the diameter of the client's limb.
- Document BP cuff sizes used on the nursing plan of care (e.g., "12-cm BP cuff used for brachial pressure: 10-cm BP cuff used for ankle pressure"). This minimizes the risk of shift-to-shift discrepancies in ABIs.
- Inflate the BP cuff enough to ensure complete closure of the artery. Inflation should be 20–30 mmHg beyond the point at which the last arterial signal was detected.
- Avoid deflating the BP cuff too rapidly. Instead, try to maintain a deflation rate of 2–4 mmHg/sec for clients without arrhythmias and 2 mmHg/sec or slower for clients with arrhythmias. Deflating the cuff more rapidly than that may cause you to miss the client's highest pressure and record an erroneous (low) blood pressure measurement.

- Be suspicious of arterial pressure recorded at less than 40 mmHg. This may mean that the venous signal was mistaken for the arterial signal. If you measure arterial pressure, which is normally 120 mmHg at below 40 mmHg, ask a colleague to double-check your findings before you record the arterial pressure.

ABI calculation.

See Box 22-3 for the formula for calculating ABI.

Manual compression test.

If the client has varicose veins, perform manual compression to assess the competence of the vein's valves. Ask the client to stand. Firmly compress the lower portion of the varicose vein with one hand. Place your other hand 6–8 in above your first hand (Fig. 22-25). Feel for a pulsation to your fingers in the upper hand. Repeat this test in the other leg if varicosities are present.

Nexøe et al. (2012) caution about false ABI test results, which may occur in general practice settings rather than when performed in specialized vascular centers.

Inaccurate readings may also occur in people with diabetes because of artery calcification (WoundRounds, 2013).

Abnormal ABI findings, indicating PVD, are associated significantly with poorer walking endurance (McDermott et al., 2013).

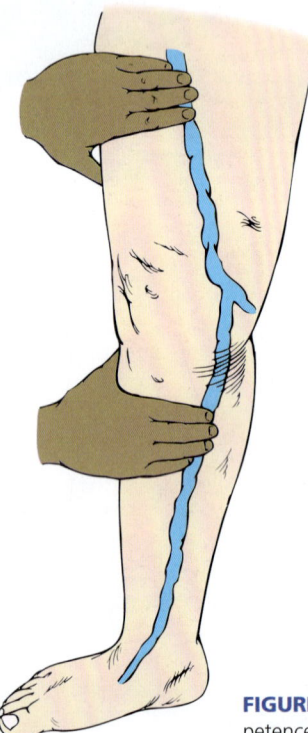

FIGURE 22-25 Performing manual compression to assess competence of venous valves in clients with varicose veins.

ASSESSMENT PROCEDURE	NORMAL FINDINGS	ABNORMAL FINDINGS
Trendelenburg test If the client has varicose veins, perform the Trendelenburg test to determine the competence of the saphenous vein valves and the retrograde (backward) filling of the superficial veins. The client should lie supine. Elevate the client's leg 90 degrees for about 15 seconds or until the veins empty. With the leg elevated, apply a tourniquet to the upper thigh. ◎ **CLINICAL TIP** Arterial blood flow is not occluded if there are arterial pulses distal to the tourniquet. Assist the client to a standing position and observe for venous filling. Remove the tourniquet after 30 seconds, and watch for sudden filling of the varicose veins from above.	No pulsation is palpated if the client has competent valves. Saphenous vein fills from below in 30 seconds. If valves are competent, there will be no rapid filling of the varicose veins from above (retrograde filling) after removal of tourniquet.	You will feel a pulsation with your upper fingers if the valves in the veins are incompetent. Filling from above with the tourniquet in place and the client standing suggests incompetent valves in the saphenous vein. Rapid filling of the superficial varicose veins from above after the tourniquet has been removed also indicates retrograde filling past incompetent valves in the veins.

BOX 22-1 STAGES OF LYMPHEDEMA

Grade	Description
Stage 0	No obvious signs or symptoms. Impaired lymph drainage is subclinical. Lymphedema (LE) may be present for months to years before progressing to later stages. Edema is not evident.
Stage I (spontaneously reversible)	Swelling is present. Affected area pits with pressure. Elevation relieves swelling. Skin texture is smooth.
Stage II (spontaneously irreversible)	Skin tissue is firmer. Skin may look tight, shiny, and tissue may have a spongy feel. Pitting may or may not be present as tissue fibrosis (hardening) begins to develop. Elevation does not completely alleviate the swelling. Hair loss or nail changes may be experienced in affected extremity. Assistance will be needed to reduce edema.
Stage III (irreversible)	LE has progressed to the lymphostatic elephantiasis stage, at which the limb is very large. Affected area is nonpitting, often with permanent eczema. Skin is firm and thick, with hard (fibrotic) underlying tissue having an unresponsive feel. Skin folds develop. At increased risk for recurrent cellulitis, infections (lymphangitis), or ulcerations. Affected limb may ooze fluid. Elevation will not alleviate symptoms.

Adapted from National Lymphedema Network (2005), Lymphedema facts. Available at http://www.lymphnet.org/lymphedemaFAQs/overview.htm

BOX 22-2 ASSESSING PULSE STRENGTH

Palpation of the pulses in the peripheral vascular examination is typically to assess amplitude or strength. Pulse amplitude is graded on a 0 to 4+ scale, with 4+ being the strongest. Elasticity of the artery wall may also be noted during the peripheral vascular examination, by palpating for a resilient (bouncy) quality rather than a more rigid arterial tone, whereas pulse rate and rhythm are best assessed during examination of the heart and neck vessels.

PULSE AMPLITUDE
Pulse amplitude is typically graded as 0 to 4+:

Rating	Description
0	Absent
1+	Weak, diminished (easy to obliterate)
2+	Normal (obliterate with moderate pressure)
3+	Strong (obliterate with firm pressure)
4+	Bounding (unable to obliterate)

BOX 22-3 CALCULATING AND INTERPRETING ANKLE–BRACHIAL INDEX (ABI)

FORMULA FOR CALCULATING ABI

Divide the higher ankle pressure for each foot by the higher brachial pressure. For example, you may have measured the highest brachial pulse as 160, the highest pulse in the right ankle as 80, and the highest pulse in the left ankle as 94. Dividing each of these ankle pressures by 160 (the highest brachial pressure; 80/160 and 94/160) will result in a right ABI of 0.5 and a left ABI of 0.59.

INTERPRETATION OF ABI VALUES

Different values obtained for the ankle–brachial index (ABI) are interpreted as follows:

- 0.00–0.40: Severe peripheral arterial disease (PAD) sufficient to cause resting pain or gangrene
- 0.41–0.90: PAD sufficient to cause claudication
- 0.91–1.30: Normal vessels
- >1.30: Noncompressible, severely calcified vessel
  Patients with an ABI less than 0.90 have a higher risk of coronary artery disease, stroke, and death and therefore should be referred to a credentialed vascular laboratory for further testing.

Source: Park, C. W. (2015). Ankle-brachial index measurement: Technique. Available at http://emedicine.medscape.com/article/1839449-overview#a3

CASE STUDY

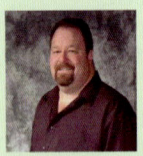

After completing the physical examination of Mr. Lee, the nurse documents the collected data.

Alert, oriented, with no shortness of breath or chest pain. T, 97.9; P, 88; R, 12; BP, 144/86. Skin warm, dry, pink, and intact. Color and temperature same bilaterally in upper extremities, with 2+ radial pulses, no edema. Capillary refill immediate bilaterally in fingers. Bilaterally 2+ femoral and popliteal pulses.

Presents with right calf swelling and is red, warm, and tender to touch as compared with left leg. Right calf measures 42 cm, while left calf is 34.5 cm. Dorsalis pedis and posterior tibial pulses 2+ and equal bilaterally. No edema in ankles or feet; warm, pink skin color with rapid capillary refill. No pain in left leg, reports a 4 rating (0–10 numeric pain scale) presently in right lower leg, no ulcerations or discoloration of skin on legs. Normal hair pattern distribution on lower extremities. No distended veins or swollen glands detected.

Validating and Documenting Findings

Validate the peripheral vascular assessment data you have collected (by asking additional questions, verifying data with another health care professional, or comparing objective with subjective findings). This is necessary to verify that the data are reliable and accurate. Documenting both normal and abnormal findings will allow for a baseline should findings change later. Following the health care facility or agency policy, document the assessment data.

CASE STUDY

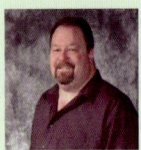

Think back to the case study. The nurse documents the following assessment of Mr. Lee.

Biologic Data: HL, 46 years old, male, Caucasian. Divorced. Working from home as a computer programmer. Awake, alert, and oriented. Appropriately asks and responds to questions.

Reason for Seeking Care: "I have pain in my right lower leg. There is soreness, some pain and swelling. It hurts more when I walk."

History of Present Health Concern: Right calf pain and swelling began 3 days ago. Reports discomfort increases when walking. Swelling and pain improves when leg is elevated. Reports no color or temperature changes in arms or left leg, no pain in left leg but reports having mild to moderate pain in right lower leg especially when he is up and moving around. States has taken acetaminophen 1,000 mg 2–3 times per day to relieve leg pain. Reports concern that he may have thrombophlebitis.

Personal Health History: Has hypertension and hyperlipidemia, both controlled by medication. Obese but otherwise no major health problems. No food or medication allergies. Has had no angina since his coronary artery bypass graft (CABG) 5 years ago. Developed pulmonary embolism following surgery. No other previous surgeries on veins or arteries. Reports having an appendectomy at age 12.

Family History: Mother has hypertension and his father's brother died from complications of diabetes. Uncertain of other family history of clotting disorders, diabetes, or history of cardiovascular disease.

Lifestyle and Health Practices: States does not smoke, and that he does manage his stress well, drinks an occasional beer 2–3 times per week with friends, no recreational drug use, and exercises by walking a few blocks most days. Lives on the second floor of an apartment building. Reports sitting for hours at computer with few breaks. Occasionally remembers to exercise feet and lower legs. States he most often takes the elevator because he becomes short of breath when takes the stairs. Tries to follow a low-fat diet to help lower cholesterol but states he finds it difficult to follow dietary restrictions. States he knows he needs to be more active and lose some weight. Has right leg pain when walking for last 3 days as described in present health concern above. Denies problems with sexual activity.

Physical Examination Findings: Alert, oriented with no shortness of breath or chest pain. T, 97.9; P, 88; R, 12; BP, 144/86. Skin warm, dry, pink, and intact. Color and temperature same bilaterally in upper extremities with 2+ radial pulses, no edema. Capillary refill rapid bilaterally in fingers. Bilaterally 2+ femoral and popliteal pulses.

Presents with right calf swelling and is red, warm, and tender to touch as compared to left leg. Right calf measures 42 cm, while left calf is 34.5 cm. Dorsalis pedis and posterior tibial pulses 2+ and equal bilaterally. No edema in ankles or feet; warm, pink skin color with rapid capillary refill. No pain in left leg, 4 rating (on a 0–10 numeric scale) presently in right lower leg, no ulcerations or discoloration of skin on legs. Normal hair pattern distribution on lower extremities. No distended veins or swollen glands detected.

ANALYSIS OF DATA: DIAGNOSTIC REASONING

After collecting subjective and objective data pertaining to the peripheral vascular assessment, identify abnormal findings and client strengths. Then cluster the data to reveal any significant patterns or abnormalities.

Selected Nursing Diagnoses

Following is a listing of selected nursing diagnoses (health promotion, risk, or actual) that may be identified when analyzing data from the peripheral vascular assessment.

Health Promotion Diagnoses

- Readiness for enhanced circulation to extremities
- Readiness for Enhanced Self-Health Management: Requests information on regular monitoring of pulse, blood pressure, cholesterol and triglyceride levels, regular exercise, smoking cessation, and weight loss.

Risk Diagnoses

- Risk for Ineffective Therapeutic Regimen Management (monitoring of pulse, blood pressure, cholesterol and triglyceride levels, and regular exercise) related to a busy lifestyle, lack of knowledge and resources to follow healthy lifestyle
- Risk for Infection related to poor circulation to and impaired skin integrity of lower extremities
- Risk for Injury related to altered sensation in lower extremities secondary to edema and/or neuropathy.
- Risk for Impaired Skin Integrity related to poor circulation to extremities secondary to arterial or venous insufficiency
- Risk for Impaired Skin Integrity related to arterial or venous insufficiency
- Risk for Activity Intolerance related to leg pain upon walking
- Risk for Ineffective Peripheral Tissue Perfusion related to poor circulation to extremities secondary to arterial or venous insufficiency
- Risk for Peripheral Neurovascular Dysfunction related to venous or arterial occlusion secondary to trauma, surgery, or mechanical compression

Actual Diagnoses

- Ineffective Tissue Perfusion (peripheral) related to arterial insufficiency
- Impaired Skin Integrity related to arterial or venous insufficiency
- Pain (acute or chronic) related to arterial or venous insufficiency
- Fear of loss of extremities related to arterial insufficiency
- Disturbed Body Image related to edema, leg ulcerations, or varicosities

Selected Collaborative Problems

After grouping the data, certain collaborative problems may become apparent. Remember that collaborative problems differ from nursing diagnoses in that they cannot be prevented through nursing interventions. However, these physiologic complications of medical conditions can be detected and monitored by the nurse. In addition, the nurse can use physician- and advanced-practice nurse-prescribed interventions to minimize the complications of these problems. The nurse may also have to refer the client in such situations for further treatment of the problem. Following is a list of collaborative problems that may be identified when obtaining a general impression. These problems are worded as Risk for Complications (RC), followed by the problem.
- RC: Thromboembolic/deep vein thrombosis
- RC: Arterial occlusion
- RC: Peripheral vascular (arterial or venous) insufficiency
- RC: Hypertension
- RC: Ischemic ulcers
- RC: Gangrene

Medical Problems

After grouping the data, it may become apparent that the client has signs and symptoms that may require medical diagnosis and treatment. Referral to a primary care provider is necessary.

CASE STUDY

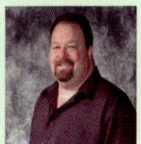

After collecting and analyzing the data for Mr. Lee, the nurse determines that the following conclusions are appropriate for this client:

Nursing Diagnoses
- Ineffective Health Maintenance r/t behaviors reflecting lack of understanding behaviors that promote wellness and prevent recurring vascular problems
- Imbalanced Nutrition: More than Body requirements r/t decreased activity and inappropriate food choices

Potential Collaborative Problems
- RC: Pulmonary embolus
- RC: Cellulitis
- RC: Deep vein thrombosis

Interdisciplinary Verbal Communication of Assessment Findings Using SBAR

SITUATION: H.L., a 46-year-old Caucasian male, thinks he "pulled something in right leg, as it is sore, swollen, and really hurts to walk." Pain is "constant" at a level of 4 (on a 0–10 point scale). Symptoms began 3 days ago which improve with leg elevation. Takes acetaminophen 1,000 mg 2–3 times per day to relieve leg pain. Concerned he may have thrombophlebitis and recounts his prior history of pulmonary embolism following surgery.

BACKGROUND PERSONAL HEALTH HISTORY: Has hypertension and hyperlipidemia controlled by medication. Coronary artery bypass graft (CABG) 5 years ago. Mother has hypertension and his father's brother died from complications of diabetes. Believes he does not manage stress well. Exercises by walking a few blocks most days. Sits at desk for 4–6 hours at a time. Has only limited exercise; walks several blocks for lunch, then walks back to apartment. Usually takes elevator because he becomes short of breath when he takes the stairs. Tries to follow a low-fat diet without much success. Aware he needs to lose weight.

ASSESSMENT: Weight: 250 lb; height: 5 ft, 9 in; T, 97.9; P, 88; R, 12; BP, 144/86. Right calf is swollen, red, warm, and tender to touch. Right calf measures 42 cm while left calf is 34.5 cm. Right calf swollen, red, warm, and tender to touch as compared to left leg. Right calf measures 42 cm, while left calf is 34.5 cm. Dorsalis pedis and posterior tibial pulses 2+ and equal bilaterally. No edema in ankles or feet; warm, pink skin color with rapid capillary refill.

RECOMMENDATION: H.L. needs to be seen by his primary health care provider to further evaluate his acute pain in right leg and to assess for potential complications of pulmonary embolus, cellulitis, or deep vein thrombosis. He has Ineffective Health Maintenance r/t lack of engaging in behaviors that promote wellness and prevention of recurring vascular problems that need to be addressed. He also needs a dietary and exercise plan for his More than Body Requirements r/t decreased activity and inappropriate food choices.

To view an algorithm depicting the process for diagnostic reasoning in this case, go to **thePoint**.

ABNORMAL FINDINGS 22-1 Characteristics of Arterial and Venous Insufficiency

ARTERIAL INSUFFICIENCY

Pain: Intermittent claudication to sharp, unrelenting, constant
Pulses: Diminished or absent
Skin characteristics: Dependent rubor
- Elevation pallor of foot
- Dry, shiny skin
- Cool-to-cold temperature
- Loss of hair over toes and dorsum of foot
- Nails thickened and ridged

Ulcer characteristics:
- Location: Tips of toes, toe webs, heel or other pressure areas if confined to bed
- Pain: Very painful
- Depth of ulcer: Deep, often involving joint space
- Shape: Circular
- Ulcer base: Pale black to dry and gangrene
- Leg edema: Minimal unless extremity kept in dependent position constantly to relieve pain

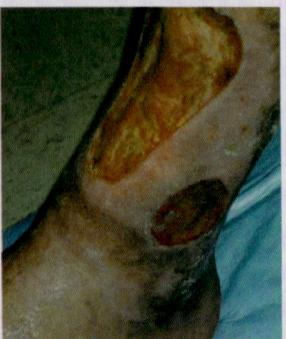

Characteristic ulcer of arterial insufficiency. (Used with permission from Berg, D. & Worzala, K. (2006). *Atlas of adult physical diagnosis*. Philadelphia, PA: Lippincott Williams & Wilkins.)

VENOUS INSUFFICIENCY

Pain: Aching, cramping
Pulses: Present but may be difficult to palpate through edema
Skin characteristics:
- Pigmentation in gaiter area (area of medial and lateral malleolus)
- Skin thickened and tough
- May be reddish-blue in color
- Frequently associated with dermatitis

Ulcer characteristics:
- Location: Medial malleolus or anterior tibial area
- Pain: If superficial, minimal pain; but may be very painful
- Depth of ulcer: Superficial
- Shape: Irregular border
- Ulcer base: Granulation tissue—beefy red to yellow fibrinous in chronic long-term ulcer
- Leg edema: Moderate to severe

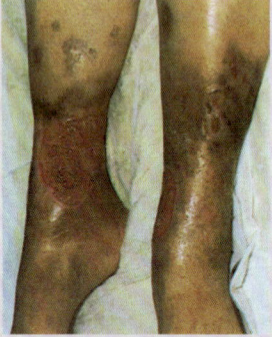

Characteristic ulcer of venous insufficiency. (Used with permission from Marks, R. (1987). *Skin disease in old age*. Philadelphia, PA: J. B. Lippincott.)

Information from Smeltzer, S. C., Bare, B. G., Hinkle, J. H., & Cheever, K. H. (2010). Brunner and Suddarth's textbook of medical surgical nursing (12th ed.). Philadelphia, PA: Lippincott Williams & Wilkins.

22 Assessing Peripheral Vascular System | 489

ABNORMAL FINDINGS 22-2 | Types of Peripheral Edema

EDEMA ASSOCIATED WITH LYMPHEDEMA

- Caused by abnormal or blocked lymph vessels
- Nonpitting
- Usually bilateral; may be unilateral
- No skin ulceration or pigmentation

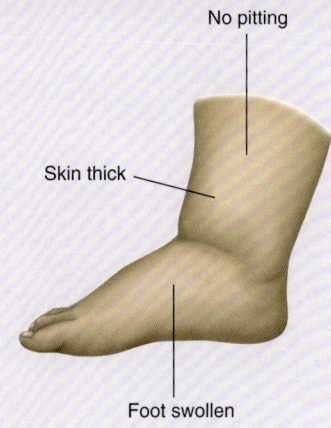

Swelling associated with lymphatic abnormality.

EDEMA ASSOCIATED WITH CHRONIC VENOUS INSUFFICIENCY

- Caused by obstruction or insufficiency of deep veins
- Pitting, documented as:
  - 1+ = slight pitting
  - 2+ = deeper than 1+
  - 3+ = noticeably deep pit; extremity looks larger
  - 4+ = very deep pit; gross edema in extremity
- Usually unilateral; may be bilateral
- Skin ulceration and pigmentation may be present

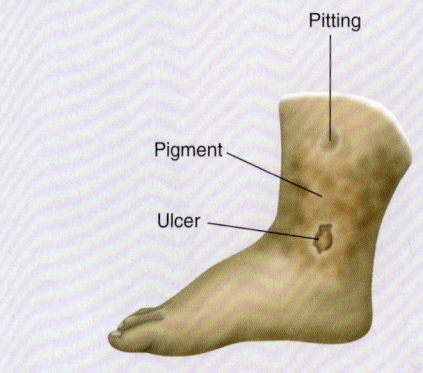

Advanced
Edema associated with chronic venous insufficiency.

ABNORMAL FINDINGS 22-3 | Abnormal Arterial Findings

NECROTIC GREAT TOE WITH BLISTERS ON TOES AND FOOT

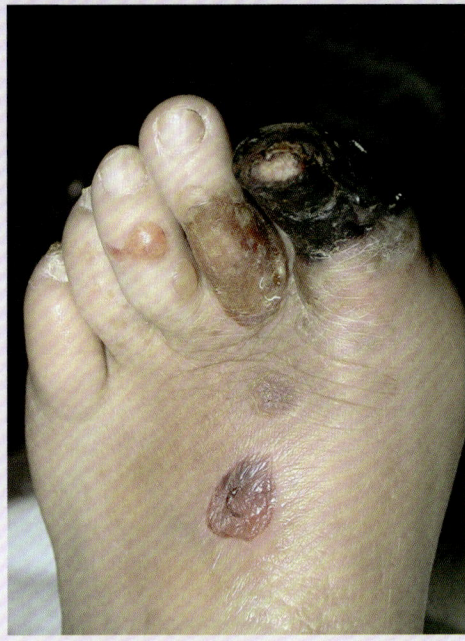

Arterial ulcer. Great toe is necrotic with blisters on the toes and foot seen in arterial insufficiency. (From Sharon Baranoski; Elizabeth Ayello, Wound Care Essentials, Wolters Kluwer Heath, 2015.)

RAYNAUD DISEASE

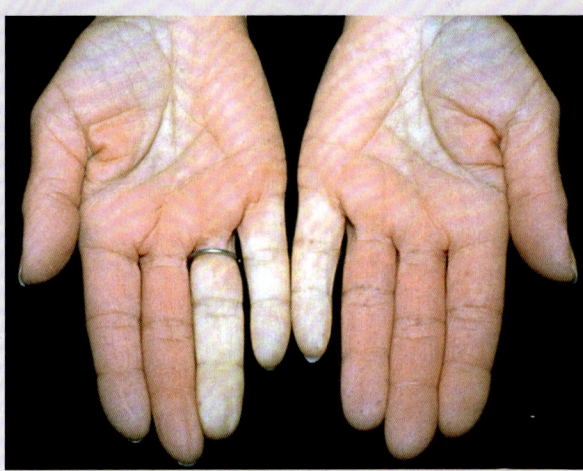

Dramatic blanching of fingers on both hands in Raynaud phenomenon. (From Noah Craft; Lindy P. Fox; Lowell A. Goldsmith; Art Papier; Ron Birnbaum; Mary G. Mercurio; Daniel Miller; Priya Rajendran; Michael Rosenblum; Emma Taylor; Paul C. Tumeh, VisualDx: Essential Adult Dermatology, Wolters Kluwer, 2015.)

490 UNIT 3 Nursing Assessment of Physical Systems

ABNORMAL FINDINGS 22-4   Abnormal Venous Findings

SUPERFICIAL THROMBOPHLEBITIS

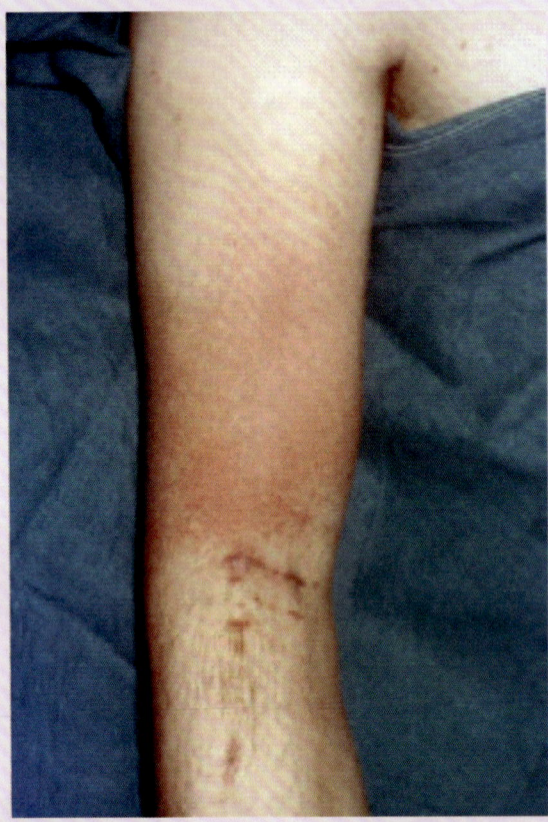

Superficial thrombophlebitis resulting from thrombus formation in the superficial veins. Often seen with unilateral localized pain, achiness, edema, redness, and warmth to touch. (From Jensen, S. (2015). *Nursing health assessment: A best practice approach.* Philadelphia, PA: Wolters Kluwer.)

LYMPHEDEMA

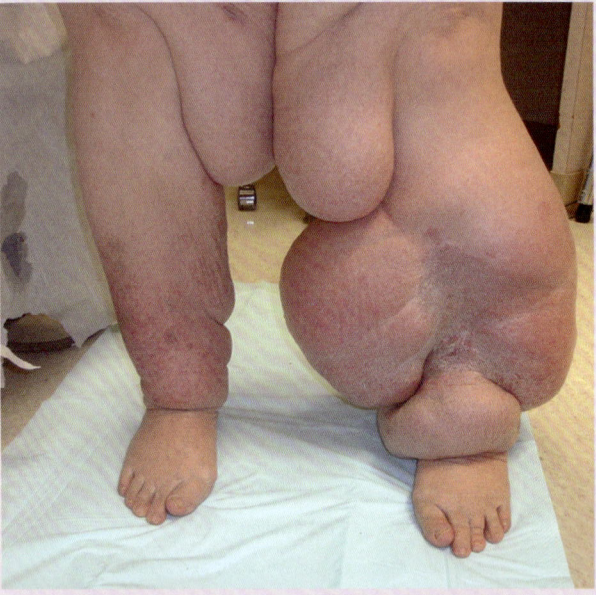

A 44-year-old female with lymphedema and massive localized lymphedema. (From Sharon Baranoski; Elizabeth Ayello, Wound Care Essentials, Wolters Kluwer Heath, 2015.)

VARICOSE VEINS

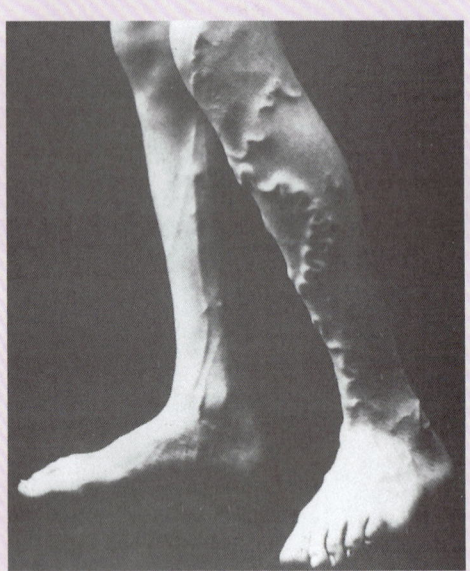

(Used with permission from Willis M. C. (2002). *Medical terminology: A programmed learning approach to the language of health care.* Baltimore, MD: Lippincott Williams & Wilkins.)

Want to know more?

A wide variety of resources to enhance your learning and understanding of this book are available on **thePoint**. Visit thePoint to access:

- NCLEX-Style Student Review Questions
- Watch and Learn Videos
- Concept in Action Animations
- And more!

References and Selected Readings

American Family Physician (AFP). (2013). Diagnosis and treatment of peripheral artery disease. Available at http://www.aafp.org/afp/2013/0901/p306.html

American Heart Association (AHA). (2013). AHA comments to USPSTF on Draft PAD Evidence Review and Recommendation 041513. Available at https://www.heart.org/idc/groups/heart-public/@wcm/@adv/documents/downloadable/ucm_451566.pdf

Cleveland Clinic. (2016). Peripheral artery disease. Available at http://my.clevelandclinic.org/services/heart/disorders/arterial-disease/peripheral-arterial-disease

Criqui, M. H., & Aboyans, V. (2015). Peripheral artery disease compendium. *Circulation Research, 116*, 1509–1526.

Criqui, M. H., Vargas, V., Denenberg, J. O., Ho, E., Allison, M., Langer, R. D., et al. (2005). Ethnicity and peripheral arterial disease: The San Diego Population Study. *Circulation*. doi: http://dx.doi.org/10.1161/CIRCULATIONAHA.105.546507

Frederick, M., Newman, J., & Kohlwes, J. (2010). Leriche syndrome. *Journal of General Internal Medicine, 25*(10), 1102–1104.

Fritschi, C., Collins, E. G., O'Connell, S., McBurney, C., Butler, J., Edwards, L. (2013). The effects of smoking status on walking ability and health-related quality of life in patients with peripheral arterial disease. *Journal of Cardiovascular Nursing, 28*(4), 380–386.

Hayward, R. (2015). Screening for lower extremity peripheral artery disease. Available at http://www.uptodate.com/contents/screening-for-lower-extremity-peripheral-artery-disease.

Jain, A., Liu, K., Ferrucci, L., Criqui, M. H., Tian, L., Guralnik, J. M., et al. (2012). The Walking Impairment Questionnaire stair-climbing score predicts mortality in men and women with peripheral arterial disease. *Journal of Vascular Surgery, 55*(6), 1662–1673.e2.

Mann, A. R. (2013). *Handbook for focus on adult health medical-surgical nursing*, Philadelphia, PA: Wolters Kluwer Health/Lippincott Williams & Wilkins.

Mayo Clinic. (2015). Peripheral artery disease (PAD). Available at http://www.mayoclinic.org/diseases-conditions/peripheral-artery-disease/symptoms-causes/dxc-20167421

McDermott, M. M., Applegate, W. B., Bonds, D. E., Buford, T. W., Church, T., Espeland, M. A., et al. (2013). Ankle brachial index values, leg symptoms, and functional performance among community-dwelling older men and women in the lifestyles interventions and independence for elders study. *Journal of the American Heart Association (JAHA), 2*(6):e000257.

National Heart, Lung, and Blood Institute (NHLBI). (2014). What is Raynauds? Available at http://www.nhlbi.nih.gov/health/health-topics/topics/raynaud

Nexøe, J., Damsbo, B., Lund, J. O., Munck, A. (2012). Measurement of blood pressure, ankle blood pressure and calculation of ankle brachial index in general practice. *The Journal of Family Practice, 29*(3):345–351.

Sommers, M. S. (2012). Pocket diseases. Philadelphia, PA: F. A. Davis.

Taylor-Piliae, R. E., Fair, J. M., Varady, A. N., Hlatky, M. A., Norton, L. C., Iribarren, C., et al. (2011). Ankle brachial index screening in asymptomatic older adults. *American Heart Journal, 161*(5), 979–985.

U.S. Preventive Services Task Force. (2013). Peripheral artery disease (PAD) and CVD in adults: Risk assessment with ankle brachial index. Available at http://www.uspreventiveservicestaskforce.org/Page/Document/UpdateSummaryFinal/peripheral-arterial-disease-pad-and-cvd-in-adults-risk-assessment-with-ankle-brachial-index

WoundRounds. (2013). False ABI in diabetic patients. Available at http://www.woundrounds.com/wound-care-technologies/false-abi-in-diabetic-patients/

Yang, E. (2015). Peripheral artery disease (PAD) guidelines. Available at http://emedicine.medscape.com/article/2500033-overview

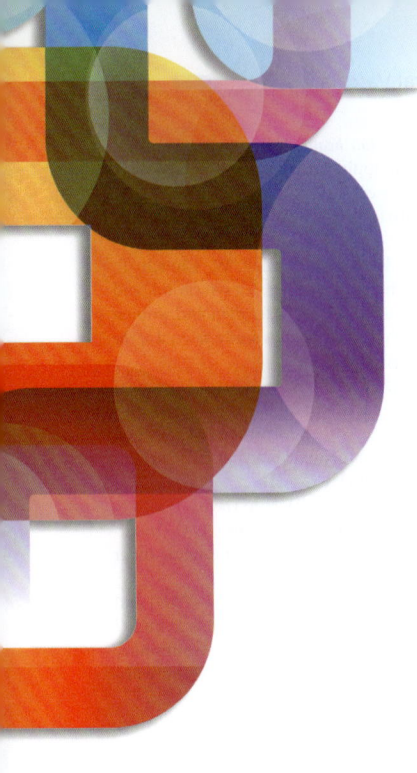

23 ASSESSING ABDOMEN

Learning Objectives

1. Describe the structure and the function of the abdomen.
2. Discuss the organs located in the four quadrants and the nine regions of the abdomen.
3. Discuss risk factors associated with diseases of abdominal organs across the cultures and ways to reduce one's risks.
4. Interview a client for an accurate nursing history of the client's abdomen and related functions of the organs within the abdomen.
5. Perform a physical assessment of the abdomen using the correct techniques.
6. Differentiate between normal and abnormal findings of the abdomen.
7. Describe the findings frequently seen with assessing the older client's abdomen.
8. Analyze the data from the interview and physical assessment of the abdomen to formulate valid nursing diagnoses, collaborative problems, and/or referrals.
9. Differentiate between general routine screening versus skills needed for focused or specialty assessment of the abdomen.
10. Document and verbally report accurate assessment findings of the abdomen.

CASE STUDY

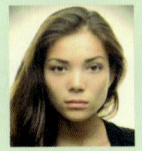

Nikki Chen, a 32-year-old graduate student, comes into the clinic reporting generalized abdominal discomfort. She states that she has not had a bowel movement in the past 4 days. She appears very nervous and fidgety and, when asked, confesses that she is very anxious about her upcoming final comprehensive examinations. She reports that she has terrible dietary habits and has not exercised in months.

STRUCTURE AND FUNCTION

The abdomen is bordered superiorly by the costal margins, inferiorly by the symphysis pubis and inguinal canals, and laterally by the flanks. It is important to understand the anatomic divisions known as the abdominal quadrants, the abdominal wall muscles, and the internal anatomy of the abdominal cavity in order to perform an adequate assessment of the abdomen.

Abdominal Quadrants

For the purposes of examination, the abdomen can be described as having four quadrants: the right upper quadrant (RUQ), right lower quadrant (RLQ), left lower quadrant (LLQ), and left upper quadrant (LUQ) as seen in Figure 23-1. The quadrants are determined by an imaginary vertical line (midline) extending from the tip of the sternum (xiphoid) through the umbilicus to the symphysis pubis. This line is bisected perpendicularly by the lateral line, which runs through the umbilicus across the abdomen. Familiarization with the organs and structures in each quadrant is essential to accurate data collection, interpretation, and documentation of findings. Another method divides the abdomen into nine regions (Fig. 23-2). Three of these regions are still commonly used to describe abdominal findings: epigastric, umbilical, and hypogastric or suprapubic. Assessment Guide 23-1 describes abdominal quadrants and regions.

Abdominal Wall Muscles

The abdominal contents are enclosed externally by the abdominal wall musculature, which includes three layers of muscle extending from the back, around the flanks, to the front. The outermost layer is the external abdominal oblique, the middle layer is the internal abdominal oblique, and the innermost layer is the transverse abdominis (Fig. 23-3). Connective tissue from these muscles extends forward to encase a vertical muscle of the anterior abdominal wall called the rectus abdominis. The fibers and connective tissue extensions of these muscles (aponeuroses) diverge in a characteristic plywood-like pattern (several thin layers arranged at right angles to each other), which provides strength to the abdominal wall. The joining of these muscle fibers and aponeuroses at the midline of the abdomen forms a white line called the linea alba, which extends vertically from the xiphoid process of the sternum to the symphysis pubis. The abdominal wall muscles protect the

23 Assessing Abdomen   493

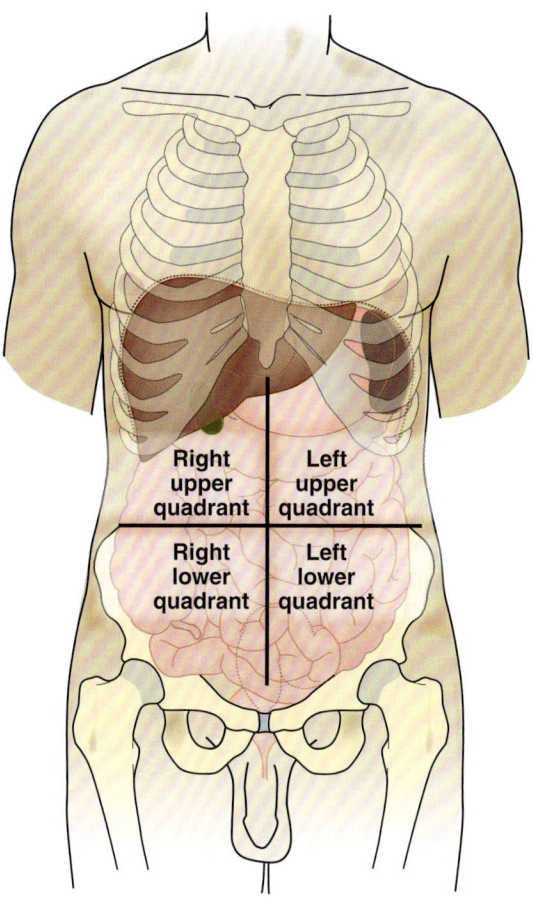

FIGURE 23-1 Abdominal quadrants.

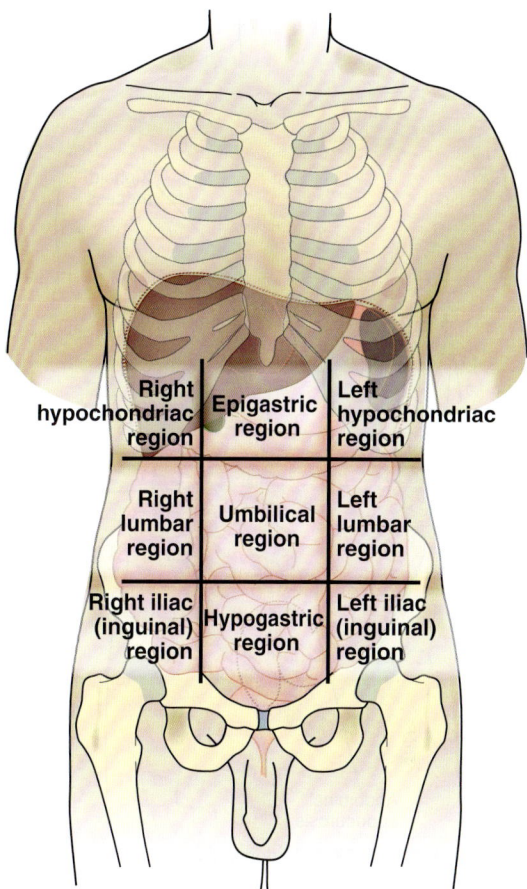

FIGURE 23-2 Abdominal regions.

internal organs and allow normal compression during functional activities such as coughing, sneezing, urination, defecation, and childbirth.

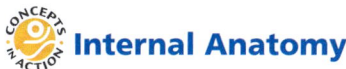 Internal Anatomy

A thin, shiny, serous membrane called the peritoneum lines the abdominal cavity (parietal peritoneum) and also provides a protective covering for most of the internal abdominal organs (visceral peritoneum). Within the abdominal cavity are structures of several different body systems: gastrointestinal, reproductive (female), lymphatic, and urinary. These structures are typically referred to as the abdominal viscera and can be divided into two types: solid viscera and hollow viscera (Fig. 23-4). Solid viscera are those organs that maintain their shape consistently: liver, pancreas, spleen, adrenal

---

ASSESSMENT GUIDE 23-1   Locating Abdominal Structures by Quadrants

Abdominal assessment findings are commonly allocated to the quadrant in which they are discovered, or their location may be described according to the nine abdominal regions that some practitioners may still use as reference marks. Quadrants and contents are listed here.

Right Upper Quadrant (RUQ)
Ascending and transverse colon
Duodenum
Gallbladder
Hepatic flexure of colon
Liver
Pancreas (head)
Pylorus (the small bowel—or ileum—traverses all quadrants)

Right adrenal gland
Right kidney (upper pole)
Right ureter

Right Lower Quadrant (RLQ)
Appendix
Ascending colon
Cecum
Right kidney (lower pole)
Right ovary and tube
Right ureter
Right spermatic cord

Left Upper Quadrant (LUQ)
Left adrenal gland
Left kidney (upper pole)
Left ureter

Pancreas (body and tail)
Spleen
Splenic flexure of colon
Stomach
Transverse descending colon

Left Lower Quadrant (LLQ)
Left kidney (lower pole)
Left ovary and tube
Left ureter
Left spermatic cord
Descending and sigmoid colon

Midline
Bladder
Uterus
Prostate gland

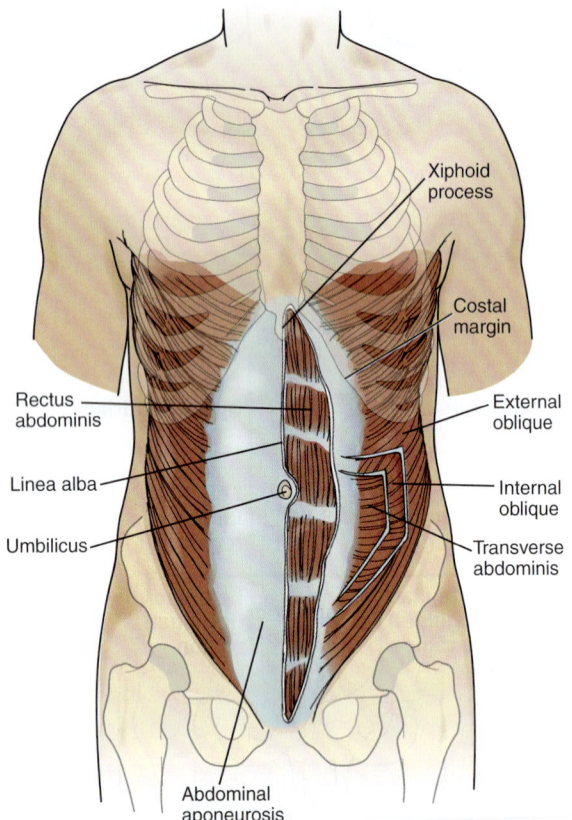

FIGURE 23-3 Abdominal wall muscles.

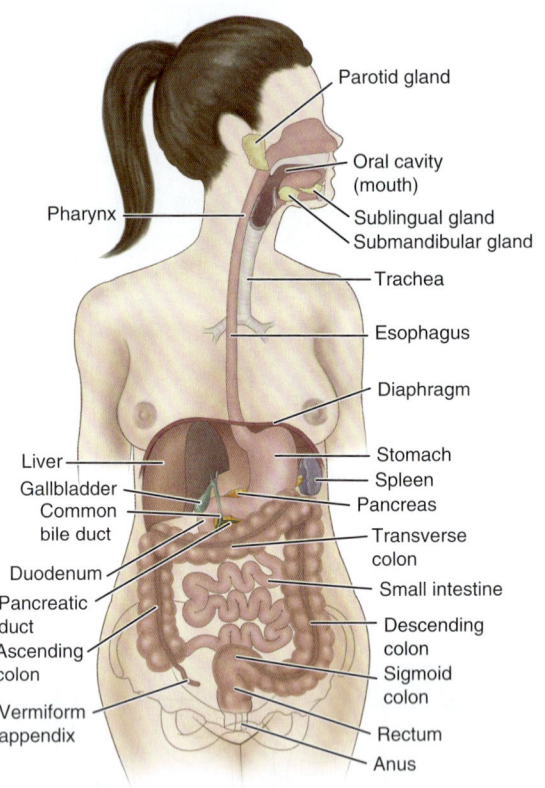

FIGURE 23-4 Abdominal viscera. (Smeltzer, S. (2010). *Brunner & Suddarth's textbook of medical-surgical nursing* (12th ed.). Philadelphia, PA: Lippincott Williams & Wilkins.)

glands, kidneys, ovaries, and uterus. The hollow viscera consist of structures that change shape depending on their contents. These include the stomach, gallbladder, small intestine, colon, and bladder.

CLINICAL TIP
Whether abdominal viscera are palpable depends on location, structural consistency, and size.

Solid Viscera

The liver is the largest solid organ in the body. It is located below the diaphragm in the RUQ of the abdomen. It is composed of four lobes that fill most of the RUQ and extend to the left midclavicular line (MCL).

CLINICAL TIP
In many people, the liver extends just below the right costal margin, where it may be palpated. If palpable, the liver has a soft consistency. The liver functions as an accessory digestive organ and has a variety of metabolic and regulatory functions as well, including glucose storage, formation of blood plasma proteins and clotting factors, urea synthesis, cholesterol production, bile formation, destruction of red blood cells, storage of iron and vitamins, and detoxification.

The pancreas, located mostly behind the stomach deep in the upper abdomen, is normally not palpable. It is a long gland extending across the abdomen from the RUQ to the LUQ. The pancreas has two functions: it is an endocrine gland and an accessory organ of digestion. The spleen is approximately 7 cm wide and is located above the left kidney just below the diaphragm at the level of the ninth, tenth, and eleventh ribs. It is posterior to the left mid-axillary line (MAL) and posterior and lateral to the stomach. This soft, flat structure is normally not palpable. In some healthy clients, the lower tip can be felt below the left costal margin.

CLINICAL TIP
When the spleen enlarges, the lower tip extends down and toward the midline.

The spleen functions primarily to filter the blood of cellular debris, to digest microorganisms, and to return the breakdown products to the liver.

The kidneys are located high and deep under the diaphragm. These glandular, bean-shaped organs measuring approximately $10 \times 5 \times 2.5$ cm are considered posterior organs and approximate with the level of the T12 to L3 vertebrae. The tops of both kidneys are protected by the posterior rib cage. Kidney tenderness is best assessed at the costovertebral angle (Fig. 23-5). The right kidney is positioned slightly lower because of the position of the liver. Therefore, in some thin clients, the bottom portion of the right kidney may be palpated anteriorly. The primary function of the kidneys is filtration and elimination of metabolic waste products. However, the kidneys also play a role in blood pressure control and maintenance of water, salt, and electrolyte balances. In addition, they function as endocrine glands by secreting hormones.

The pregnant uterus may be palpated above the level of the symphysis pubis in the midline. The ovaries are located in the

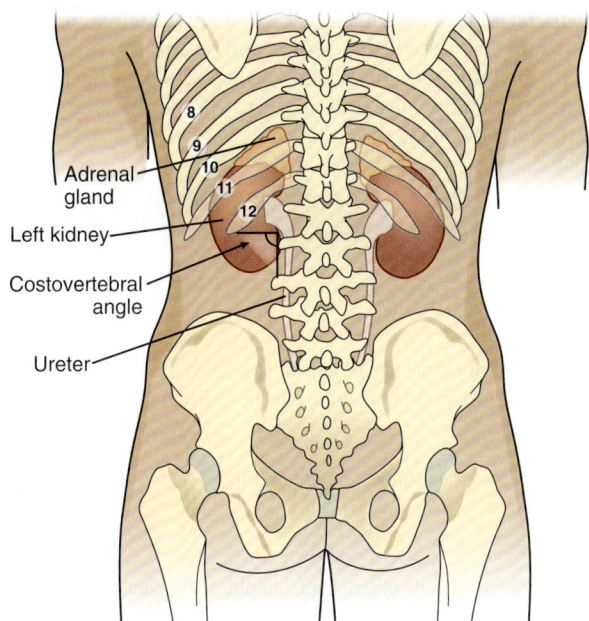

FIGURE 23-5 Position of the kidneys.

RLQ and LLQ, and are normally palpated only during a bimanual examination of the internal genitalia (see Chapter 27).

Hollow Viscera

The abdominal cavity begins with the stomach. It is a distensible, flask-like organ located in the LUQ just below the diaphragm and between the liver and spleen. The stomach is not usually palpable. The stomach's main function is to store, churn, and digest food.

The gallbladder, a muscular sac approximately 10 cm long, functions primarily to concentrate and store the bile needed to digest fat. It is located near the posterior surface of the liver lateral to the MCL. It is not normally palpated because it is difficult to distinguish between the gallbladder and the liver.

The small intestine is actually the longest portion of the digestive tract (approximately 7.0 m long) but is named for its small diameter (approximately 2.5 cm). Two major functions of the small intestine are digestion and absorption of nutrients through millions of mucosal projections lining its walls. The small intestine, which lies coiled in all four quadrants of the abdomen, is not normally palpated.

The colon, or large intestine, has a wider diameter than the small intestine (approximately 6.0 cm) and is approximately 1.4 m long. It originates in the RLQ, where it attaches to the small intestine at the ileocecal valve. The colon is composed of three major sections: ascending, transverse, and descending. The ascending colon extends up along the right side of the abdomen. At the junction of the liver in the RUQ, it flexes at a right angle and becomes the transverse colon. The transverse colon runs across the upper abdomen. In the LUQ near the spleen, the colon forms another right angle then extends downward along the left side of the abdomen as the descending colon. At this point, it curves in toward the midline to form the sigmoid colon in the LLQ. The sigmoid colon is often felt as a firm structure on palpation, whereas the cecum and ascending colon may feel softer. The transverse and descending colon may also be felt on palpation.

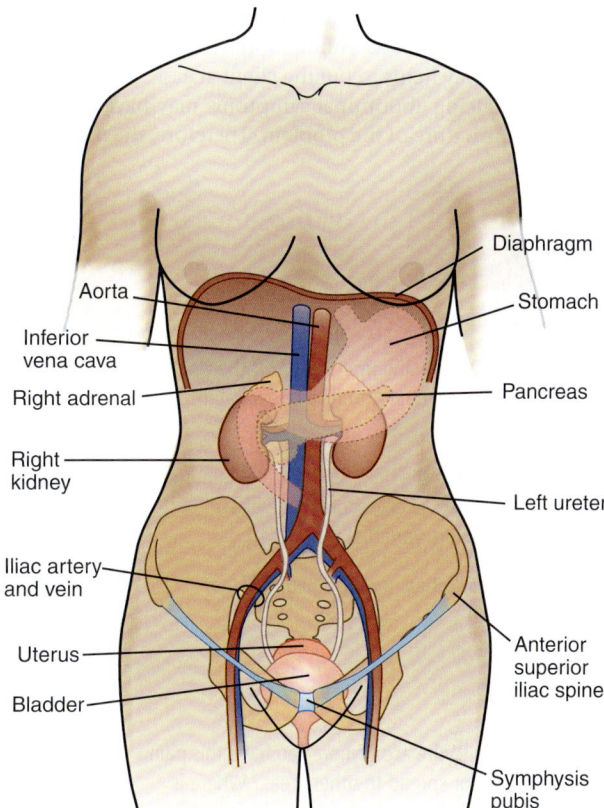

FIGURE 23-6 Abdominal and vascular structures (aorta and iliac artery and vein).

The colon functions primarily to secrete large amounts of alkaline mucus to lubricate the intestine and neutralize acids formed by the intestinal bacteria. Water is also absorbed through the large intestine, leaving waste products to be eliminated in stool.

The urinary bladder, a distensible muscular sac located behind the pubic bone in the midline of the abdomen, functions as a temporary receptacle for urine. A bladder filled with urine may be palpated in the abdomen above the symphysis pubis.

Vascular Structures

The abdominal organs are supplied with arterial blood by the abdominal aorta and its major branches (Fig. 23-6). Pulsations of the aorta are frequently visible and palpable midline in the upper abdomen. The aorta branches into the right and left iliac arteries just below the umbilicus. Pulsations of the right and left iliac arteries may be felt in the RLQ and LLQ.

HEALTH ASSESSMENT

Collecting Subjective Data: The Nursing Health History

The nurse may collect subjective data concerning the abdomen as part of a client's overall health history interview or as a focused history for a current abdominal complaint. The data focus on symptoms of particular abdominal organs and the function of the digestive system along with aspects of nutrition, usual bowel habits, and lifestyle.

Keep in mind that the client may be uncomfortable discussing certain issues such as elimination. Asking questions in a matter-of-fact way helps to put the client at ease. In addition, a client experiencing abdominal symptoms may have difficulty describing the nature of the problem. Therefore, the nurse may need to facilitate client responses and quantitative answers by encouraging descriptive terms and examples (i.e., pain as sharp or knife-like, headache as throbbing, or back pain as searing), rating scales, and accounts of effects on activities of daily living (ADLs).

History of Present Health Concern

QUESTION	RATIONALE
Abdominal Pain	
Are you experiencing abdominal pain? If the client answers yes, use COLDSPA to further explore this symptom:	Abdominal pain occurs when specific digestive organs or structures are affected by chemical or mechanical factors such as inflammation, infection, distention, stretching, pressure, obstruction, or trauma.
Character: Describe the pain (dull, aching, burning, gnawing, pressure, colicky, sharp, knife-like, stabbing, throbbing, variable).	The quality or character of the pain may suggest its origin (Box 23-1).
Onset: When did (does) the pain begin?	The onset of pain is a diagnostic clue to its origin. For example, acute pancreatitis produces sudden onset of pain, whereas the pain of pancreatic cancer may be gradual or recurrent. A client may have excessive gas after ingesting certain foods. A burning sensation in the esophagus may occur with gastric acid reflux after eating. Pain related to gastric ulcers may occur when the stomach is empty.
Location: Point to the area where you have this pain. Does it radiate or spread to other areas? Where is the pain located? Does it move or has it changed from the original location?	Location helps to determine the pain source and whether it is primary or referred (see Box 23-1). Although abdominal pain can arise from the skin and abdominal wall muscles, it may also originate from abdominal organs, including the stomach, small intestine, colon, liver, gallbladder, spleen, and pancreas. Dull or burning pain located between the breasts and umbilicus may occur with peptic ulcers.
	Pain may also be felt in the abdomen from conditions in organs that are not located in the abdominal cavity such as the lower lungs, kidneys, uterus, or ovaries. In addition, pain from organs within the abdomen may be felt in other areas outside the abdomen, for example, pancreatic inflammation may be felt in the back. This is called "referred" pain because the pain is not felt at its source.
Duration: How long does the pain last?	The duration of pain, either intermittent or prolonged, varies with different causes of the pain. For example, clients with a duodenal ulcer may have pain a few hours after eating that is relieved when they eat again.
Severity: How bad is the pain (severity) on a scale of 1 to 10, with 10 being the worst?	The client's perception of pain provides data on his or her response and tolerance to pain. Sensitivity to pain varies greatly among people.
	OLDER ADULT CONSIDERATIONS
	Sensitivity to pain may diminish with aging. Therefore, assess older adult clients carefully for acute abdominal conditions.
Pattern: When does the pain occur (timing and relation to particular events such as eating, exercise, bedtime)?	Timing and the relationship of particular events may be a clue to the origin of pain (e.g., the pain of a duodenal ulcer may awaken the client at night).
What seems to bring on the pain (precipitating factors), make it worse (exacerbating factors), or make it better (alleviating factors)?	Various factors can precipitate or exacerbate abdominal pain, such as alcohol ingestion with pancreatitis or supine position with gastroesophageal reflux disease. Lifestyle and stress factors may be implicated in certain digestive disorders, such peptic ulcer disease. Alleviating factors, such as using antacids or histamine blockers, may be a clue to origin.
Associated factors/How it **A**ffects the client: Is the pain associated with any other symptoms such as nausea, vomiting, diarrhea, constipation, gas, fever, weight loss, fatigue, or yellowing of the eyes or skin?	Associated signs and symptoms may provide diagnostic evidence to support or rule out a particular origin of pain. For example, epigastric pain accompanied by tarry stools suggests a gastric or duodenal ulcer. Abdominal pain with cramping, diarrhea, nausea, vomiting, weight loss, and lack of energy is often seen in Crohn disease.
Indigestion	
Do you experience indigestion?	Indigestion (pyrosis), often described as heartburn, may be an indication of acute or chronic gastric disorders including hyperacidity, gastroesophageal reflux disease (GERD), peptic ulcer disease, and stomach cancer.
Character: Describe how this feels.	

QUESTION	RATIONALE
Onset: When did you first experience this? When does this usually begin? **L**ocation: Point to where you usually feel indigestion. **D**uration: How long does the indigestion last? How often does it recur? **S**everity: Describe the severity of this feeling on a scale of 1–10 (10 being the worst). Does the indigestion cause you to quit any of your activities of daily living if it occurs? What activities can you not do when you have indigestion? **P**attern: Does anything in particular seem to cause or aggravate the indigestion? Have you noticed that this sensation occurs after you eat certain foods? **A**ssociated factors: Do you have other symptoms with indigestion, such as nausea, vomiting, diarrhea, or constipation?	The main symptom of GERD in adults is frequent heartburn, which is acid indigestion, a burning-type pain in the lower part of the mid-chest, behind the breast bone, and in the mid-abdomen. Some adults have GERD without heartburn, but instead may have a dry cough, asthma symptoms, or trouble swallowing (National Institute of Diabetes and Digestive and Kidney Diseases [NIDDK], 2014). Take time to determine the client's exact symptoms because many clients call indigestion gassiness, belching, bloating, and nausea (see Evidence-Based Health Promotion and Disease Prevention 23-1). Certain factors (e.g., food, drinks, alcohol, medications, stress) are known to increase gastric secretion and acidity and cause or aggravate indigestion. Indigestion accompanied by these factors indicates more than local irritation and needs further investigation. For instance, nausea and vomiting are often seen with diseases of the gastrointestinal (GI) tract, in the first trimester of pregnancy, or as an adverse effect of medications. Vomiting with blood (hematemesis) is seen with esophageal varices or duodenal ulcers. Diarrhea may be seen with food intolerances, infections, and irritable bowel.
Nausea and Vomiting	
Do you experience nausea or vomiting? Describe it. Is it triggered by any particular activities, events, or other factors (smells, eating of certain foods, riding in a car, boat, or plane, or strenuous physical exercise)?	Nausea may reflect gastric dysfunction and is also associated with many digestive disorders and diseases of the accessory organs, such as the liver and pancreas, as well as with renal failure and drug intolerance. Nausea may also be precipitated by dietary intolerance, psychological triggers, or menstruation. Nausea may also occur at particular times, such as early in the day with some pregnant clients ("morning sickness"), after meals with gastric disorders, or between meals with changes in blood glucose levels. Exertional heat related illnesses such as nausea and vomiting associated with strenuous exercise are thought to relate to dehydration, hyponatremia, heat intolerance, a vagal reaction, or gastroesophageal reflux (Nichols, 2014). Motion causes nausea and vomiting for many people when the inner ear, the eyes, and other areas of the body that detect motion perceive that the body is moving, while the other parts do not sense the motion (University of Maryland Medical Center [UMMC], 2014). Vomiting is associated with impaired gastric motility or reflex mechanisms. Description of vomitus (emesis) is a clue to the source. For example, bright hematemesis is seen with bleeding esophageal varices and ulcers of the stomach or duodenum. Certain smells and food intolerances may trigger nausea and vomiting. **CLINICAL TIP** Neuromuscular- or consciousness-impaired clients are at risk for lung aspiration with vomiting.
Appetite	
Have you noticed an increase or decrease in your appetite? Has this change affected how much you eat or your normal weight? When did it begin? Does it come and go? What other illnesses or life events were you experiencing when this occurred? Is there anything that aggravates or improves this appetite change?	Loss of appetite (anorexia) is a general complaint often associated with digestive disorders, chronic syndromes, cancers, and psychological disorders. Carefully correlate appetite changes with dietary history and weight monitoring. Significant appetite changes and food intake may adversely affect the client's weight and put the client at additional risk. **OLDER ADULT CONSIDERATIONS** Older adult clients may experience a decline in appetite from various factors such as altered metabolism, decreased taste sensation, decreased mobility, and, possibly, depression. If appetite declines, the client's risk for nutritional imbalance increases.
Bowel Elimination	
Describe your stools (how many a day and consistency and color). Have you experienced a change in bowel elimination patterns?	Changes in bowel patterns must be compared with usual patterns for the client. Normal frequency varies from 2 to 3 times per day to 3 times per week.
Do you have constipation? Describe. Do you have any accompanying symptoms?	Constipation is usually defined as a decrease in the frequency of bowel movements or the passage of hard and possibly painful stools. Signs and symptoms that accompany

Continued on following page

History of Present Health Concern (Continued)

QUESTION	RATIONALE
Bowel Elimination (Continued)	
See Rome Criteria for Constipation/Irritable Bowel Disease at: http://www.romecriteria.org/assets/pdf/19_RomeIII_apA_885–898.pdf	constipation may be a clue as to the cause of constipation, such as bleeding with malignancies or pencil-shaped stools with intestinal obstruction.
Have you experienced diarrhea? Describe. Do you have any associated symptoms? See Rome Criteria for Constipation/Irritable Bowel Disease at: http://www.romecriteria.org/assets/pdf/19_RomeIII_apA_885–898.pdf	Diarrhea is defined as frequency of bowel movements producing unformed or liquid stools. It is important to compare these stools with the client's usual bowel patterns. Bloody and mucoid stools are associated with inflammatory bowel diseases (e.g., ulcerative colitis, Crohn disease); clay-colored, fatty stools may be from malabsorption syndromes. Associated symptoms or signs may suggest the disorder's origin. For example, fever and chills may result from an infection or weight loss and fatigue may result from a chronic intestinal disorder or a cancer. **OLDER ADULT CONSIDERATIONS** Older adult clients are especially at risk for potential complications with diarrhea—such as fluid volume deficit, dehydration, and electrolyte and acid–base imbalances—because they have a higher fat-to-lean muscle ratio.
Have you experienced any yellowing of your skin or whites of your eyes, itchy skin, dark urine (yellow-brown or tea colored), or clay-colored stools?	Refer the client for evaluation of these symptoms to rule out possible liver disease.

Personal Health History

QUESTION	RATIONALE
Have you ever had any of the following gastrointestinal disorders: ulcers, gastroesophageal reflux, inflammatory or obstructive bowel disease, pancreatitis, gallbladder or liver disease, diverticulosis, or appendicitis?	Presenting clients with a list of the more common disorders may help them to identify any that they have had.
Have you had any urinary tract disease such as infections, kidney disease or nephritis, or kidney stones?	Urinary tract infections (UTIs) may become recurrent and chronic. Moreover, resistance to drugs used to treat infection must be evaluated. Chronic kidney infection may lead to permanent kidney damage. (Note that this question pertains more to the urinary system. However, it is important to ask the question here because blunt percussion over the kidneys is often performed during the abdominal examination.) **OLDER ADULT CONSIDERATIONS** Older adult clients are prone to UTIs because the activity of protective bacteria in the urinary tract declines with age.
Have you ever had viral hepatitis (type A, B, or C)? Have you ever been exposed to viral hepatitis?	Various populations (e.g., school and health care personnel) are at increased risk for exposure to hepatitis viruses. Any type of viral hepatitis may cause liver damage.
Have you ever had abdominal surgery or trauma to the abdomen?	Prior abdominal surgery or trauma may cause abdominal adhesions, thereby predisposing the client to future complications or disorders.
What prescription or over-the-counter (OTC) medications do you take? Is there a history of any of the following diseases or disorders in your family: colon, stomach, pancreatic, liver, kidney, or bladder cancer; liver disease; gallbladder disease; kidney disease?	Medications may produce side effects that adversely affect the GI tract. For example, aspirin, ibuprofen, and steroids may cause gastric bleeding. Chronic use of antacids or histamine-2 blockers may mask the symptoms of more serious stomach disorders. Overuse of laxatives may decrease intestinal tone and promote dependency. High iron intake may lead to chronic constipation.

Family History

QUESTION	RATIONALE
Has anyone in your family had any type of gastrointestinal cancer or other GI disorders?	Family history of certain disorders increases the client's risk for those disorders. Genetic testing can now identify the risk for certain cancers (colon, pancreatic, and prostate) and other diseases. Client awareness of family history can serve as a motivation for health screening and positive health promotion behaviors.

Lifestyle and Health Practices

QUESTION	RATIONALE
Do you drink alcohol? How much? How often?	Alcohol ingestion can affect the GI tract through immediate and long-term effects on such organs as the stomach, pancreas, and liver. Alcohol-related disorders include gastritis, esophageal varices, pancreatitis, and liver cirrhosis.
What types of foods and how much food do you typically consume each day? How much noncaffeinated fluid do you consume each day? How much caffeine do you think you consume each day (e.g., in tea, coffee, chocolate, and soft drinks)?	A baseline dietary and fluid survey helps to determine nutritional and fluid adequacy and risk factors for altered nutrition, constipation, diarrhea, and diseases such as cancer.
How much and how often do you exercise? Describe your activities during the day.	Regular exercise promotes peristalsis and thus regular bowel movements. In addition, exercise may help to reduce risk factors for various diseases such as cancer and hypertension (Evidence-Based Health Promotion and Disease Prevention 23-2).
What kind of stress do you have in your life? How does it affect your eating or elimination habits?	Lifestyle and associated stress and psychological factors can affect GI function through effects on secretion, tone, and motility. Some people who have high stress levels actually feel it in the gut, known informally as the "brain gut axis." Some lesser forms of stress, such as public speaking or driving in traffic, can also slow or interrupt the digestive system, resulting in abdominal pain or other GI symptoms (Harvard Medical School, 2012).
If you have a gastrointestinal disorder, how does it affect your lifestyle and how you feel about yourself?	Certain GI disorders and their effects (e.g., weight loss) or treatment (e.g., drugs, surgery) may produce physiologic or anatomic effects that affect the client's perception of self, body image, social interaction and intimacy, and life. For example, irritable bowel syndrome (IBS) can be disabling, limiting one's ability to work, attend social events, or even travel short distances (National Digestive Disease Information Clearinghouse [NDDIC], 2012).

BOX 23-1   MECHANISMS AND SOURCES OF ABDOMINAL PAIN

TYPES OF PAIN

Abdominal pain may be formally described as visceral, parietal, or referred.

- *Visceral pain* occurs when hollow abdominal organs—such as the intestines—become distended or contract forcefully, or when the capsules of solid organs such as the liver and spleen are stretched. Poorly defined or localized and intermittently timed, this type of pain is often characterized as dull, aching, burning, cramping, or colicky.
- *Parietal pain* occurs when the parietal peritoneum becomes inflamed, as in appendicitis or peritonitis. This type of pain tends to localize more to the source and is characterized as a more severe and steady pain.
- *Referred pain* occurs at distant sites that are innervated at approximately the same levels as the disrupted abdominal organ. This type of pain travels, or refers, from the primary site and becomes highly localized at the distant site. The accompanying illustrations show common clinical patterns and referents of pain.

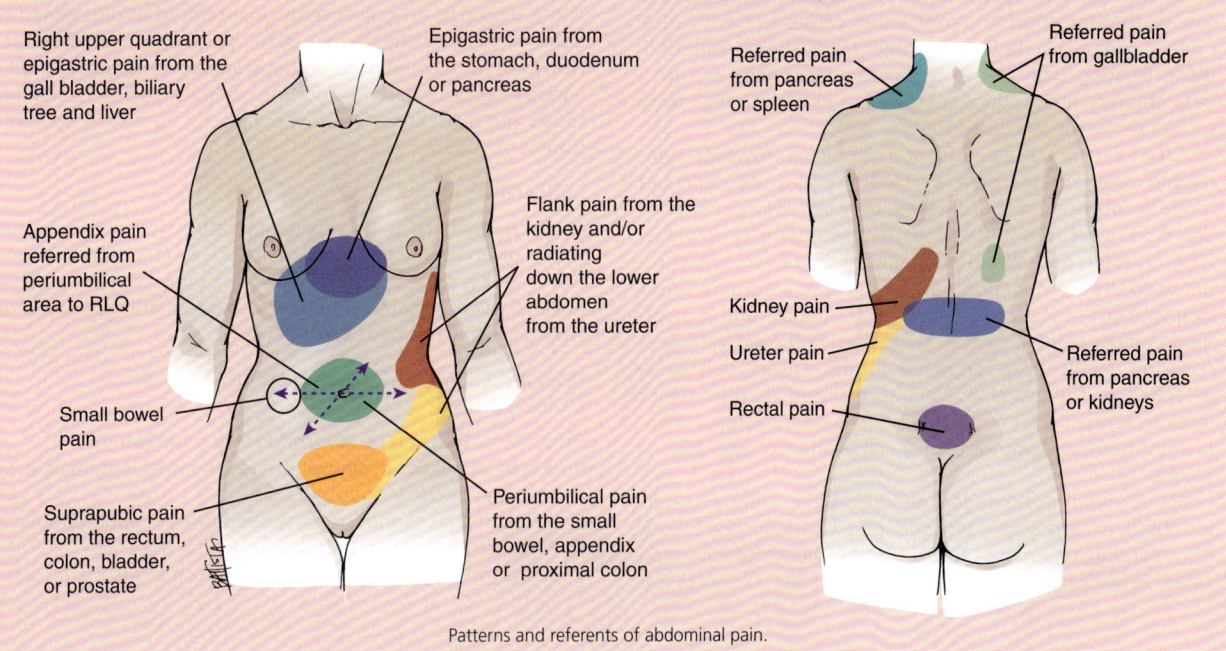

Patterns and referents of abdominal pain.

Continued on following page

BOX 23-1 MECHANISMS AND SOURCES OF ABDOMINAL PAIN (Continued)

CHARACTER OF ABDOMINAL PAIN AND IMPLICATIONS

Dull, Aching

Appendicitis
Acute hepatitis
Biliary colic
Cholecystitis
Cystitis
Dyspepsia
Glomerulonephritis
Incarcerated or strangulated hernia
Irritable bowel syndrome
Hepatocellular cancer
Pancreatitis
Pancreatic cancer
Perforated gastric or duodenal ulcer
Peritonitis
Peptic ulcer disease
Prostatitis

Burning, Gnawing

Dyspepsia
Peptic ulcer disease
Cramping ("crampy")
Acute mechanical obstruction

Appendicitis
Colitis
Diverticulitis
Gastroesophageal reflux disease (GERD)

Pressure

Benign prostatic hypertrophy
Prostate cancer
Prostatitis
Urinary retention

Colicky

Colon cancer

Sharp, Knifelike

Splenic abscess
Splenic rupture
Renal colic
Renal tumor
Ureteral colic
Vascular liver tumor

Variable

Stomach cancer

23-1 EVIDENCE-BASED HEALTH PROMOTION AND DISEASE PREVENTION: PEPTIC ULCER DISEASE

INTRODUCTION

Peptic ulcers are ulcers, or open sores, that form in the lining of the esophagus, stomach, or small intestine when acid eats away the protective mucous covering and erodes the underlying lining of these organs. (If the ulcer is in the stomach, it is known as a gastric ulcer.) A disruption of the acid and mucous balance, with increasing acid or decreasing mucous, can result in ulcer formation. Often the bacterium *Helicobacter pylori* (*H. pylori*) is active in causing the ulcer. Although usually present in the mucus, on occasion the *H. pylori* disrupt the mucous lining and inflame the organ lining. How *H. pylori* is acquired is not well understood; it may be spread from person to person, or through food or water. Other causes of peptic ulcer disease are associated with some medications, especially those treating pain (other than acetaminophen) and anti-inflammatory medications used over a long period of time, such as those for osteoarthritis.

Ulcers can be quite painful and can bleed. However, some people experience no pain until the ulcer is quite advanced. If peptic ulcers are left untreated, they can result in internal bleeding, infection, and scar tissue. Symptoms vary widely. Often there is abdominal pain, which can be felt anywhere between the sternum and navel, can cause a burning sensation that often wakes the client in the night, and is worse on an empty stomach (often temporarily relieved with acid-reducing medications or some foods). Ulcers also cause a feeling of fullness that leads to reduced fluid and food intake, hunger, an empty feeling 1–3 hours after a meal, or mild nausea. Symptoms may come and go over days or weeks.

Other symptoms may include chest pain, fatigue, weight loss, black or tarry stools, and vomiting, which may be bloody.

According to Anand (2015), the prevalence of uncomplicated peptic ulcer disease has been declining in the United States over the last 30–40 years, but the rate of complicated cases remains unchanged (thought to be due to high aspirin intake by older people). The annual U.S. rate for peptic ulcer disease is approximately 4.5 million people, with about 10% of the U.S. population having had a duodenal ulcer at some time. The gender distribution has shifted from more males to being more equally distributed between males and females, with lower rates in young males and higher rates in older females. International rates vary with the use of nonsteroidal anti-inflammatory drugs (NSAIDs) and the presence of *H. pylori*.

HEALTHY PEOPLE 2020 GOAL

There is no current objective or goal related to digestive diseases in the Healthy People 2020 topics and objectives list. However, a subcommittee on developing the Healthy People agenda has proposed the addition of digestive diseases to the topics and guidelines (HealthyPeople.gov, 2011 with no addition as of 2015).

SCREENING

At present, there is no recommendation for screening for peptic ulcer disease (Carson-DeWitt, 2015). One possibility for the future is screening for *H. pylori*, but since many people have *H. pylori* with no disease whatsoever, this approach to screening may not be cost effective.

RISK ASSESSMENT (Crowe, 2017; NDDKD, 2014; UMMC, 2015)

Risk factors that can be controlled (are modifiable):
- Use of NSAIDs or bisphosphonates (Actonel, Fosamax, etc.)
- Smoking or chewing tobacco

Risk factors that cannot be controlled (are nonmodifiable):
- Presence of *H. pylori* in gastrointestinal tract
- Stress (findings differ on whether or not stress is a factor)

- Hypersecretory condition, in which the stomach produces too much acid
- A personal or family history of ulcers (suspected genetic link)
- Radiation treatments
- Zollinger–Ellison syndrome (rare condition of a tumor in the pancreas that releases a high level of an acid-producing hormone) (National Organization of Rare Disorders, 2016).

CLIENT EDUCATION
Teach Clients
- Wash hands frequently with soap and water.
- Eat foods that have been cooked completely.
- Use all recommended cautions when taking pain relievers, such as taking as low a dose over as short a length of time as possible; take pain medications with food; avoid drinking alcohol while on pain medications.
- Avoid excessive alcohol intake (more than one drink per day for women and two drinks per day for males).
- Avoid or stop smoking and chewing tobacco.
- If medications are ordered by your primary health care provider, follow the directions carefully and report if there are continuing symptoms, symptoms worsen, or more serious symptoms occur (such as severe pain, vomiting with bleeding, tarry stools).

23-2 EVIDENCE-BASED HEALTH PROMOTION AND DISEASE PREVENTION: GASTROESOPHAGEAL REFLEX DISEASE

INTRODUCTION
Gastroesophageal reflex disease (GERD) is a digestive disease that occurs when stomach acid or contents flow back into the esophagus. The backwash (reflux) irritates the lining of the esophagus, and, if left untreated, over time chronic esophageal irritation can lead to serious complications. These complications include narrowing of the esophagus (esophageal stricture), esophageal ulcer, or Barrett esophagus, a condition involving precancerous changes in the esophagus (Mayo Clinic, 2014). When both acid reflux and heartburn occur at least twice a week, or interfere with daily life, it is recommended that a person see a healthcare provider, as permanent damage to the esophagus can result.

Symptoms of GERD include hoarseness, laryngitis, chronic dry cough, asthma or worsening of asthma symptoms, feeling as if there is a lump in the throat, sudden increase in saliva, bad breath (halitosis), earaches, and/or chest pain or discomfort (seek emergency care for chest pain) (NIDDK, 2014).

Seraq et al. (2014) note that GERD is prevalent throughout the world but the prevalence is lower than 10% in East Asia. However, the prevalence is increasing, especially in North America and East Asia.

HEALTHY PEOPLE 2020 GOAL
There is no coverage of GERD in Healthy People 2020 topics or goals.

SCREENING
The USPSTF does not address screening for GERD. Other organizations have modified their recommendations regarding the common use of endoscopy to evaluate GERD symptoms. The American College of Physicians (2013) has modified its recommendation, suggesting that upper endoscopy be limited to the following: clients who have other symptoms, such as dysphagia, bleeding, anemia, weight loss, or recurrent vomiting; clients with a history of esophageal stricture who have recurrent dysphagia symptoms; and those with severe erosive esophagitis who have completed a 2-month course of PPI therapy, to assess healing and rule out Barrett esophagus.

RISK ASSESSMENT
The Mayo Clinic (2014) and UMPC (2016) list factors that increase the chances of developing GERD:
- Obesity
- Hiatal hernia
- Pregnancy
- Smoking (weakens esophageal sphincter)
- Dry mouth
- Asthma
- Diabetes
- Delayed stomach emptying
- Connective tissue disorders, such as scleroderma
- Alcohol consumption (weakens esophageal sphincter)

CLIENT EDUCATION
Teach Clients
Teach clients the following lifestyle changes to reduce GERD (University of Pittsburgh Medical Center [UPMC], 2016):
- Avoid alcohol and tobacco intake.
- Assess foods that cause distress and avoid these foods.
- Avoid foods that cause you to swallow air, such as chewing gum, sucking hard candy, or drinking sodas (which contain air).
- Eat 5–6 small meals a day rather than 3 large ones.
- Eat slowly and chew food well.
- Do not lie down after eating. Remain upright for 2 hours
- Avoid late evening snacks.
- Avoid bending or stooping after you eat.
- Avoid lifting heavy objects.
- Avoid wearing tight clothes around waist, abdomen, or stomach.
- Lose weight if overweight.
- Raise head of bed 6–8 in.
- Try sleeping on left side.
- Take medicines exactly as prescribed.
- Tell any health care provider examining you that you have GERD.
- Keep a relaxed atmosphere when eating meals.
- Avoid the foods listed below, which increase reflux:
  - Food that is very hot or very cold
  - Fatty or fried foods
  - Peppermint or spearmint, including flavoring
  - Coffee, tea, and soft drinks that contain caffeine
  - Spicy, highly seasoned foods
  - Tomato-based dishes, such as spaghetti with sauce, chili, and pizza
  - Citrus fruits and juices, especially in the morning
  - Chocolate and sweets, if they cause symptoms

CASE STUDY

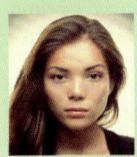

Remember Ms. Chen from the chapter opener case study? The nurse now uses COLDSPA to explore Ms. Chen's presenting concerns, then continues to interview her for GI history.

Mnemonic	Question	Data Provided
Character	Describe the sign or symptom (feeling, appearance, sound, smell, or taste if applicable).	Feeling of fullness, bloating
Onset	When did it begin?	4 days ago
Location	Where is it? Does it radiate? Does it occur anywhere else?	Abdomen with no radiation of the discomfort
Duration	How long does it last? Does it recur?	Constant
Severity	How bad is it? or How much does it bother you?	On a scale of 1–10, 4 out of 10. "I can still go to class, but I always know the discomfort is there."
Pattern	What makes it better or worse?	"Eating makes the discomfort worse. Nothing seems to make it better."
Associated factors/ How it **A**ffects the client	What other symptoms occur with it? How does it affect you?	Decreased appetite. Nausea last night. Admits to holding stool when busy at school.

After investigating Ms. Chen's complaint of abdominal discomfort, the nurse continues with the health history. Denies weight loss, ulcers, GERD, inflammatory or obstructive bowel disease, pancreatitis, gallbladder or liver disease, diverticulosis, or appendicitis. Reports routinely has 3–4 formed, brown bowel movements per week. Denies straining with bowel movement and feeling of incomplete evacuations. Reports one uncomplicated urinary tract infection 2 years ago. Denies kidney disease, nephritis or renal calculi. Reports having been immunized to hepatitis A and B. Denies exposure to hepatitis C. Denies previous abdominal surgery or trauma.

Admits to taking Alesse oral contraceptive pill one daily and a multivitamin tablet 2–3 days weekly (when she remembers). Denies allergies to medications, environment, food, or insects.

Ms. Chen denies any family history of colon, gastric, pancreatic, liver, kidney, bladder, or gallbladder disease or cancer.

Reports that she drinks two 6-oz glasses of wine 2 times weekly, usually on the weekend. Denies use of tobacco products and street drugs.

Twenty-four hour diet recall consists of the following: Breakfast—24-oz black coffee; lunch—cheeseburger and Snickers bar; dinner—bowl of Special K with 2% milk. Throughout the day drank 44-oz Diet Coke. Scant amount of noncaffeinated drink.

Recreation includes listening to music as she studies. Denies regular exercise. Walks approximately 1/4 mile to and from classes daily.

Client is very stressed about her upcoming comprehensive examinations and reports that she hardly has time to go to the grocery store and almost never cooks. Since study for comprehensive examinations began, Ms. Chen reports that she really has not paid any attention to her bowel elimination until now.

Collecting Objective Data: Physical Examination

The abdominal examination is performed for a variety of reasons: as part of a comprehensive health examination; to explore GI complaints; to assess abdominal pain, tenderness, or masses; or to monitor the client postoperatively. Assessing the abdomen can be challenging, considering the number of organs of the digestive system and the need to distinguish the source of clinical signs and symptoms.

The sequence for assessment of the abdomen differs from the typical order of assessment. Auscultate after you inspect so as not to alter the client's pattern of bowel sounds. Percussion then palpation follow auscultation. Adjust the bed level as necessary throughout the examination and approach the client from the right side. Use tangential lighting, if available, for optimal visualization of the abdomen.

The nurse needs to understand and anticipate various concerns of the client by listening and observing closely for verbal and nonverbal cues. Commonly, clients feel anxious

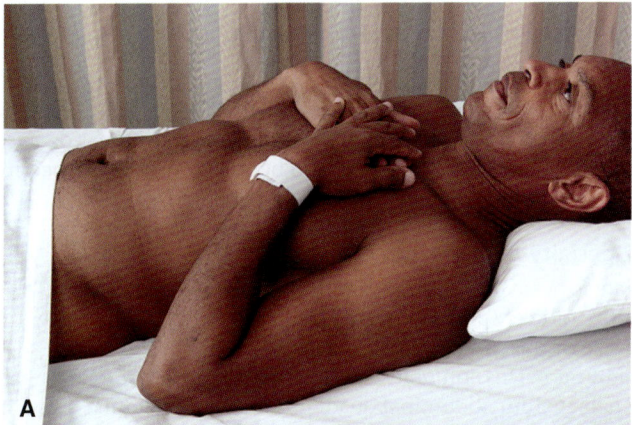 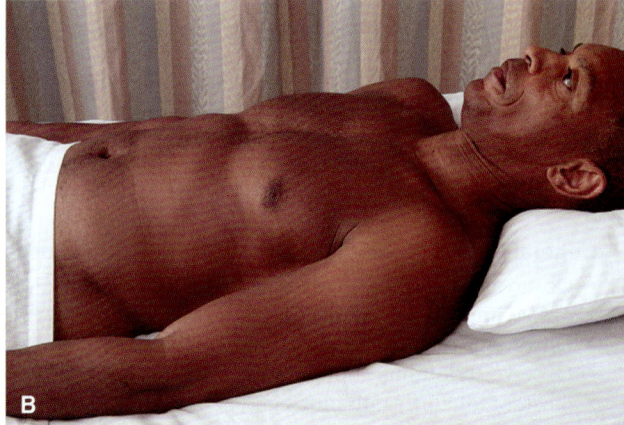

FIGURE 23-7 Two positions are appropriate for the abdominal assessment. The client may lie supine with hands resting on the center of the chest (A) or with arms resting comfortably at the sides (B). These positions best promote relaxation of the abdominal muscles.

and modest during the examination, possibly from anticipated discomfort or fear that the examiner will find something seriously wrong. As a result, the client may tense the abdominal muscles, voluntarily guarding the area. Ease anxiety by explaining each aspect of the examination, answering the client's questions, and draping the client's genital area and breasts (in women) when these are not being examined.

Another potential factor to deal with is ticklishness. A ticklish client has trouble lying still and relaxing during the hands-on parts of the examination. Try to combat this using a controlled, hands-on technique and by placing the client's hand under your own for a few moments at the beginning of palpation. Finally, warm hands are essential for the abdominal examination. Cold hands cause the client to tense the abdominal muscles. Rubbing them together or holding them under warm water just before the hands-on examination may be helpful.

Preparing the Client

Ask the client to empty the bladder before beginning the examination to eliminate bladder distention and interference with an accurate examination. Instruct the client to remove clothes and to put on a gown. Help the client to lie supine with the arms folded across the chest or resting by the sides (Fig. 23-7A, B).

> **CLINICAL TIP**
> Raising arms above the head or folding them behind the head will tense the abdominal muscles.

A flat pillow may be placed under the client's head for comfort. Slightly flex the client's legs by placing a pillow or rolled blanket under the client's knees to help relax the abdominal muscles. Drape the client with sheets so that the abdomen is visible from the lower rib cage to the pubic area.

Instruct the client to breathe through the mouth and to take slow, deep breaths. This promotes relaxation. Before touching the abdomen, ask the client about painful or tender areas. Always assess these areas at the end of the examination.

Provide reassurance that you will forewarn the client before examining these areas. Approach the client with slow, gentle, and fluid movements.

Equipment

- Small pillow or rolled blanket
- Centimeter ruler
- Stethoscope (warm the diaphragm and bell)
- Marking pen

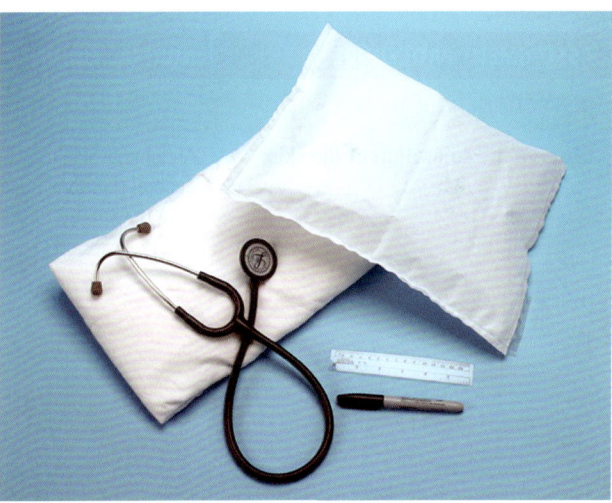

Physical Assessment

When examining the structures in the abdominal quadrants, remember to perform the examination in the following order: inspection, auscultation, percussion, and palpation.

Common abnormal findings include:

- Abdominal edema, or swelling, signifying ascites
- Abdominal masses, signifying abnormal growths or constipation
- Unusual pulsations such as those seen with an aneurysm of the abdominal aorta
- Pain associated with appendicitis.

General Routine Screening versus Focused Specialty Assessment for the Abdomen

During a routine head-to-toe examination, the nurse would inspect the abdominal skin, umbilicus, aortic pulsations, and peristaltic waves. After inspection bowel sounds are assessed by auscultation, followed by light palpation for superficial bulges or pulsations. More focused assessments, including percussion and deep palpation of the abdomen and abdominal organs, are performed in specialty areas or critical care settings where abnormalities are suspected or to be ruled out as described in the chart below.

General Routine Screening
- Observe the coloration, vascularization, scars, rashes, and lesions of the abdominal skin.
- Observe umbilicus.
- Observe abdominal contour and symmetry.
- Observe for aortic pulsations and peristaltic waves.
- Auscultate bowel sounds.
- Percuss tones over four quadrants of abdomen.
- Lightly palpate four quadrants of abdomen.

Focused Specialty Assessment
- Auscultate for vascular sounds (venous hum and/or friction rub).
- Percuss size of liver (perform scratch test if needed).
- Percuss size of spleen.
- Perform blunt percussion of liver and kidneys.
- Deeply palpate four abdominal quadrants for organs and masses.
- Palpate aorta.
- Palpate liver.
- Palpate spleen.
- Palpate kidneys.
- Palpate urinary bladder.
- Palpate for shifting, dullness.
- Perform fluid wave test.
- Assess for rebound tenderness.
- Test for referred rebound tenderness.
- Assess for psoas sign.
- Assess for obturator sign.
- Perform hypersensitivity test.
- Test for cholecystitis.

ASSESSMENT PROCEDURE	NORMAL FINDINGS	ABNORMAL FINDINGS
INSPECTION		
Observe the coloration of the skin.	Abdominal skin may be paler than the general skin tone because this skin is so seldom exposed to the natural elements.	Purple discoloration at the flanks (Grey–Turner sign) indicates bleeding within the abdominal wall, possibly from trauma to the kidneys, pancreas, or duodenum or from pancreatitis.
		The yellow hue of jaundice may be more apparent on the abdomen.
		Pale, taut skin may be seen with ascites (significant abdominal swelling indicating fluid accumulation in the abdominal cavity).
		Redness may indicate inflammation.
		Bruises or areas of local discoloration are also abnormal.
Note the vascularity of the abdominal skin.	Scattered fine veins may be visible. Blood in the veins located above the umbilicus flows toward the head; blood in the veins located below the umbilicus flows toward the lower body. **OLDER ADULT CONSIDERATIONS** Dilated superficial capillaries without a pattern may be seen in older clients. They are more visible in sunlight.	Dilated veins may be seen with cirrhosis of the liver, obstruction of the inferior vena cava, portal hypertension, or ascites. Dilated surface arterioles and capillaries with a central star (spider angioma) may be seen with liver disease or portal hypertension.

ASSESSMENT PROCEDURE	NORMAL FINDINGS	ABNORMAL FINDINGS
Note any striae (stretch marks) due to past stretching of the reticular skin layers due to fast or prolonged stretching.	New striae are pink or bluish in color; old striae are silvery, white, linear, and uneven stretch marks from past pregnancies or weight gain.	Dark bluish-pink striae are associated with Cushing syndrome. Striae may also be caused by ascites, which stretches the skin. Ascites usually results from liver failure or liver disease.
Inspect for scars. Ask about the source of a scar, and use a centimeter ruler to measure the scar's length. Document the location by quadrant and reference lines, shape, length, and any specific characteristics (e.g., 3-cm vertical scar in RLQ 4 cm below the umbilicus and 5 cm left of the midline). With experience, many examiners can estimate the length of a scar visually without a ruler.	Pale, smooth, minimally raised old scars may be seen. 🎯 **CLINICAL TIP** Scarring should be an alert for possible internal adhesions.	Nonhealing wounds, redness, inflammation. Deep, irregular scars may result from burns. 🌐 **CULTURAL CONSIDERATIONS** Keloids (excess scar tissue) result from trauma or surgery and are more common in African Americans and Asians (Fig. 23-8).
Assess for lesions and rashes.	Abdomen is free of lesions or rashes. Flat or raised brown moles, however, are normal and may be apparent.	Changes in moles including size, color, and border symmetry. Bleeding moles or petechiae (reddish or purple lesions) may also be abnormal (see Chapter 14).
Inspect the umbilicus. Note the color of the umbilical area.	Umbilical skin tones are similar to surrounding abdominal skin tones or even pinkish.	Cullen sign: A bluish or purple discoloration around the umbilicus (periumbilical ecchymosis) indicates intra-abdominal bleeding. Grey–Turner sign: bluish of purplish discoloration on the abdominal flanks.
Observe umbilical location.	Umbilicus is midline at lateral line.	A deviated umbilicus may be caused by pressure from a mass, enlarged organs, hernia, fluid, or scar tissue.
Assess contour of umbilicus.	It is recessed (inverted) or protruding no more than 0.5 cm, and is round or conical.	An everted umbilicus is seen with abdominal distention (Abnormal Findings 23-1). An enlarged, everted umbilicus suggests umbilical hernia (Abnormal Findings 23-2).
Inspect abdominal contour. Sitting at the client's side, look across the abdomen at a level slightly higher than the client's abdomen (Fig. 23-9). Inspect the area between the lower ribs and pubic bone. Measure abdominal girth as indicated in Assessment Guide 23-2.	Abdomen is flat, rounded, or scaphoid (usually seen in thin adults; Fig. 23-10). Abdomen should be evenly rounded.	A generalized protuberant or distended abdomen may be due to obesity, air (gas), or fluid accumulation (Abnormal Findings 23-1). Distention below the umbilicus may be due to a full bladder, uterine enlargement, or an ovarian tumor or cyst. Distention of the upper abdomen may be seen with masses of the pancreas or gastric dilation. 🎯 **CLINICAL TIP** The major causes of abdominal distention are sometimes referred to as the "6 Fs": Fat, feces, fetus, fibroids, flatulence, and fluid (Abnormal Findings 23-1). A scaphoid (sunken) abdomen may be seen with severe weight loss or cachexia related to starvation or terminal illness.

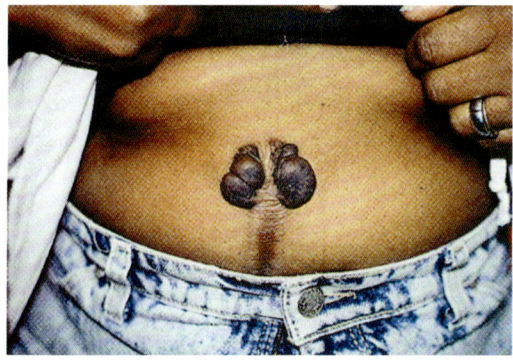

FIGURE 23-8 Keloid beyond the border of surgical scar.

Continued on following page

ASSESSMENT PROCEDURE	NORMAL FINDINGS	ABNORMAL FINDINGS

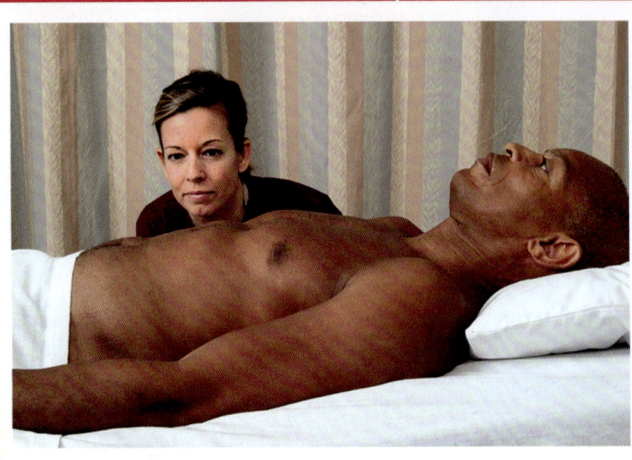

FIGURE 23-9 View abdominal contour from the client's side. Many abdomens are more or less flat; and many are round, scaphoid, or distended.

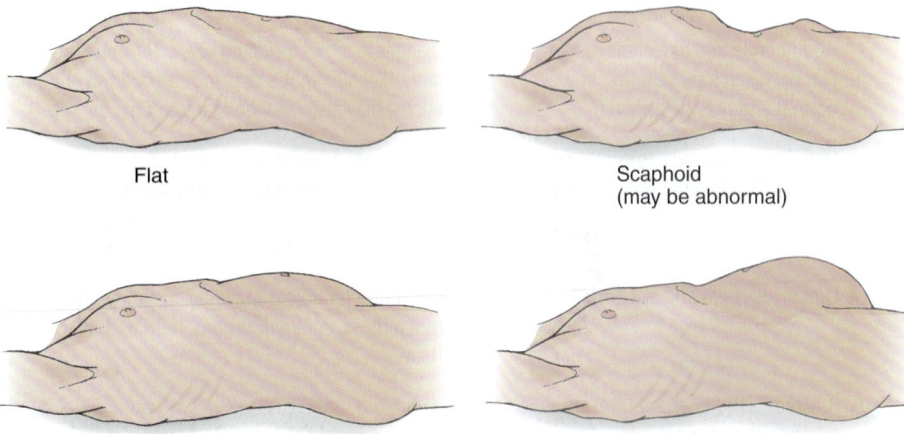

Flat

Scaphoid (may be abnormal)

Rounded

Distended/protuberant (usually abnormal)

FIGURE 23-10 Abdominal contours.

Assess abdominal symmetry. Look at the abdomen as the client lies in a relaxed supine position.	Abdomen is symmetric.	Asymmetry may be seen with organ enlargement, large masses, hernia, diastasis recti, or bowel obstruction.
Further assessment. To further assess the abdomen for herniation or diastasis recti or to differentiate a mass within the abdominal wall from one below it, ask the client to raise the head.	Abdomen does not bulge when client raises head.	A hernia (protrusion of the bowel through the abdominal wall) is seen as a bulge in the abdominal wall. Diastasis recti appears as a bulge between a vertical midline separation of the abdominis rectus muscles. This condition is of little significance. An incisional hernia may occur when a defect develops in the abdominal muscles because of a surgical incision. A mass within the abdominal wall is more prominent when the head is raised, whereas a mass below the abdominal wall is obscured (Abnormal Findings 23-2).
Inspect abdominal movement when the client breathes (respiratory movements).	Abdominal respiratory movement may be seen, especially in male clients.	Diminished abdominal respiration or change to thoracic breathing in male clients may reflect peritoneal irritation.
Observe aortic pulsations. Ultrasound has high sensitivity and specificity and is the preferred screening modality. Abdominal palpation has poor accuracy and is not recommended for screening (Agency for Healthcare Research and Quality [AHRQ], 2009)	A slight pulsation of the abdominal aorta, which is visible in the epigastrium, extends full length in thin people.	Vigorous, wide, exaggerated pulsations may be seen with abdominal aortic aneurysm.

ASSESSMENT PROCEDURE	NORMAL FINDINGS	ABNORMAL FINDINGS
OLDER ADULT CONSIDERATIONS The U.S. Preventive Services Task Force (USPSTF, 2015) recommends one-time screening for abdominal aortic aneurysm (AAA) for men between 65 and 75 years of age who have ever smoked; selectively offer screening for men 65–75 who have never smoked; and does not recommend routine screening for women.		
Observe for peristaltic waves.	Normally, peristaltic waves are not seen, although they may be visible in very thin people as slight ripples on the abdominal wall.	Peristaltic waves are increased and progress in a ripple-like fashion from the LUQ to the RLQ with intestinal obstruction (especially small intestine). In addition, abdominal distention typically is present with intestinal wall obstruction.
Auscultate for bowel sounds. Use the diaphragm of the stethoscope and make sure that it is warm before you place it on the client's abdomen. Apply light pressure or simply rest the stethoscope on a tender abdomen. Begin in the RLQ and proceed clockwise, covering all quadrants. Listen for at least 5 minutes before determining that no bowel sounds are present and that the bowels are silent.	A series of intermittent, soft clicks and gurgles are heard at a rate of 5–30 per minute. Hyperactive bowel sounds referred to as "borborygmus" may also be heard. These are the loud, prolonged gurgles characteristic of one's "stomach growling."	"Hyperactive" bowel sounds that are rushing, tinkling, and high pitched may be abnormal indicating very rapid motility heard in early bowel obstruction, gastroenteritis, diarrhea, or with use of laxatives. "Hypoactive" bowel sounds indicate diminished bowel motility. Common causes include paralytic ileus following abdominal surgery, inflammation of the peritoneum, or late bowel obstruction. May also occur in pneumonia.
CLINICAL TIP Bowel sounds may be more active over the ileocecal valve in the RLQ.	**CLINICAL TIP** Postoperatively, bowel sounds resume gradually depending on the type of surgery. The small intestine functions normally in the first few hours postoperatively; stomach emptying takes 24–48 hours to resume; and the colon requires 3–5 days to recover propulsive activity.	Decreased or absent bowel sounds signify the absence of bowel motility, which constitutes an emergency requiring immediate referral.
Confirm bowel sounds in each quadrant. Listen for up to 5 minutes (minimum of 1 minute per quadrant) to confirm the absence of bowel sounds.		Absent bowel sounds may be associated with peritonitis or paralytic ileus. High-pitched tinkling and rushes of high-pitched sounds with abdominal cramping usually indicate obstruction.
CLINICAL TIP Bowel sounds normally occur every 5–15 seconds. An easy way to remember is to equate one bowel sound to one breath sound.		
Note the intensity, pitch, and frequency of the sounds.		**CLINICAL TIP** The increasing pitch of bowel sounds is most diagnostic of obstruction because it signifies intestinal distention.
Auscultate for vascular sounds. Use the bell of the stethoscope to listen for bruits (low-pitched, murmur-like sound, pronounced BROO-ee) over the abdominal aorta and renal, iliac, and femoral arteries (Fig. 23-11).	Bruits are not normally heard over abdominal aorta or renal, iliac, or femoral arteries. However, bruits confined to systole may be normal in some clients depending on other differentiating factors.	A bruit with both systolic and diastolic components occurs when blood flow in an artery is turbulent or obstructed. This may indicate an aneurysm or renal arterial stenosis (RAS). When blood flows through a narrow vessel, it makes a whooshing sound, called a bruit. However, the absence of this sound does not exclude the possibility of RAS.

Continued on following page

ASSESSMENT PROCEDURE	NORMAL FINDINGS	ABNORMAL FINDINGS
CLINICAL TIP Auscultating for vascular sounds is especially important if the client has hypertension or if you suspect arterial insufficiency to the legs.		For a more accurate diagnosis, an ultrasound or an angiogram is needed.

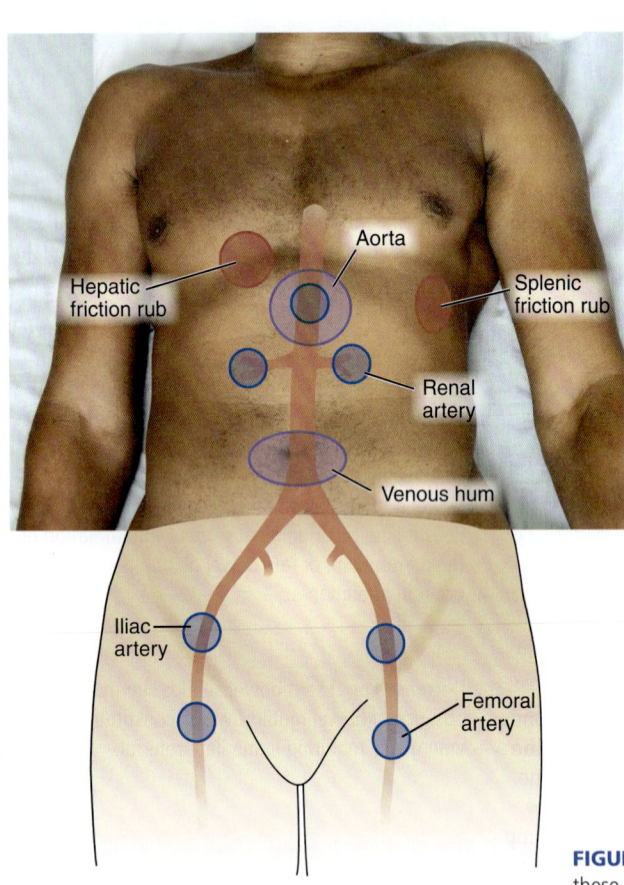

FIGURE 23-11 Vascular sounds and friction rubs can best be heard over these areas.

Listen for venous hum. Using the bell of the stethoscope, listen for a venous hum in the epigastric and umbilical areas.	Venous hum is not normally heard over the epigastric and umbilical areas.	Venous hums are rare. However, an accentuated venous hum heard in the epigastric or umbilical areas suggests increased collateral circulation between the portal and systemic venous systems, as in cirrhosis of the liver.
Auscultate for a friction rub over the liver and spleen. Listen over the right and left lower rib cage with the diaphragm of the stethoscope.	No friction rub over liver or spleen is present.	Friction rubs are rare. If heard, they have a high-pitched, rough, grating sound produced when the large surface area of the liver or spleen rubs the peritoneum. They are heard in association with respiration. A friction rub heard over the lower right costal area is associated with hepatic abscess or metastases. A rub heard at the anterior axillary line in the lower left costal area is associated with splenic infarction, abscess, infection, or tumor.
Percuss for tone. Lightly and systematically percuss all quadrants, as seen in Figure 23-12.	Generalized tympany predominates over the abdomen because of air in the stomach and intestines. Dullness is heard over the liver and spleen.	Accentuated tympany or hyperresonance is heard over a gaseous distended abdomen.

ASSESSMENT PROCEDURE	NORMAL FINDINGS	ABNORMAL FINDINGS
	Dullness may also be elicited over a non-evacuated descending colon (Fig. 22-13).	An enlarged area of dullness is heard over an enlarged liver or spleen.
		Abnormal dullness is heard over a distended bladder, large masses, or ascites.
		If you suspect ascites, perform the shifting dullness and fluid wave tests. These special techniques are described later.

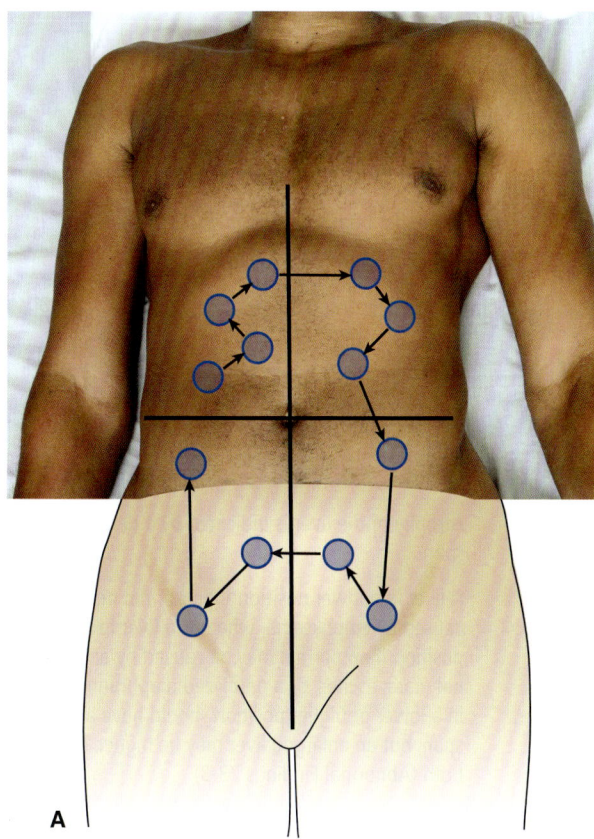

A Abdominal percussion pattern

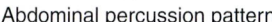

B Abdominal percussion technique

FIGURE 23-12 Abdominal percussion sequences may proceed clockwise or up and down over the abdomen.

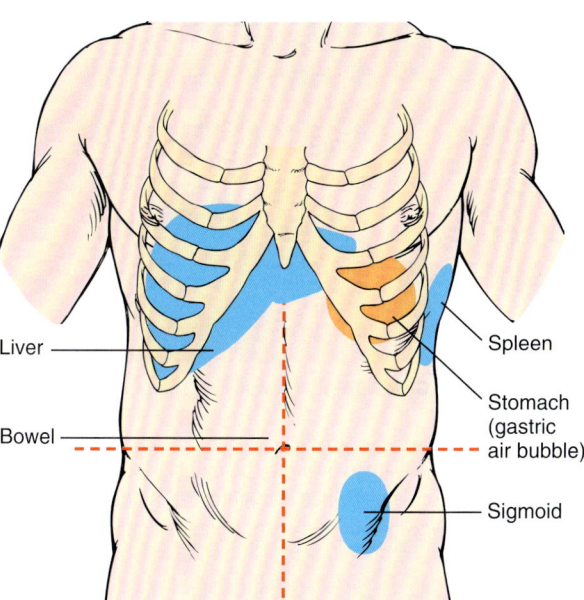

FIGURE 23-13 Normal percussion findings. *Blue* indicates dullness. *Orange* indicates tympany.

Continued on following page

ASSESSMENT PROCEDURE	NORMAL FINDINGS	ABNORMAL FINDINGS
Percuss the span or height of the liver by determining its lower and upper borders.	The lower border of liver dullness is located at the costal margin to 1–2 cm below.	🎯 **CLINICAL TIP** If you cannot find the lower border of the liver, keep in mind that the lower border of liver dullness may be difficult to estimate when obscured by intestinal gas.
To assess the lower border, begin in the RLQ at the mid-clavicular line (MCL) and percuss upward (Fig. 23-14). Note the change from tympany to dullness. Mark this point: It is the lower border of liver dullness. To assess the descent of the liver, ask the client to take a deep breath and hold; then repeat the procedure. Remind the client to exhale after percussing.	On deep inspiration, the lower border of liver dullness may descend from 1 to 4 cm below the costal margin.	
To assess the upper border, percuss over the upper right chest at the MCL and percuss downward, noting the change from lung resonance to liver dullness. Mark this point: It is the upper border of liver dullness.	The upper border of liver dullness is located between the left fifth and seventh intercostal spaces.	The upper border of liver dullness may be difficult to estimate if obscured by pleural fluid of lung consolidation.
Measure the distance between the two marks: this is the span of the liver (Fig. 23-15)	The normal liver span at the MCL is 6–12 cm (greater in men and taller clients, less in shorter clients). 🎯 **CLINICAL TIP** Normally, liver size decreases after age 50.	Hepatomegaly, a liver span that exceeds normal limits (enlarged), is characteristic of liver tumors, cirrhosis, abscess, and vascular engorgement. Atrophy of the liver is indicated by a decreased span. A liver in a lower position than normal may be caused by emphysema, whereas a liver in a higher position than normal may be caused by an abdominal mass, ascites, or a paralyzed diaphragm. A liver in a lower or higher position should have a normal span, but an enlarged liver may be higher, lower, or both (Abnormal Findings 23-3).

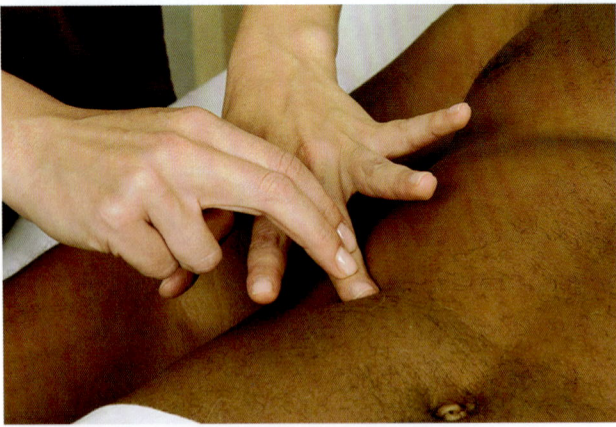

FIGURE 23-14 Begin liver percussion in the RLQ and percuss upward toward the chest.

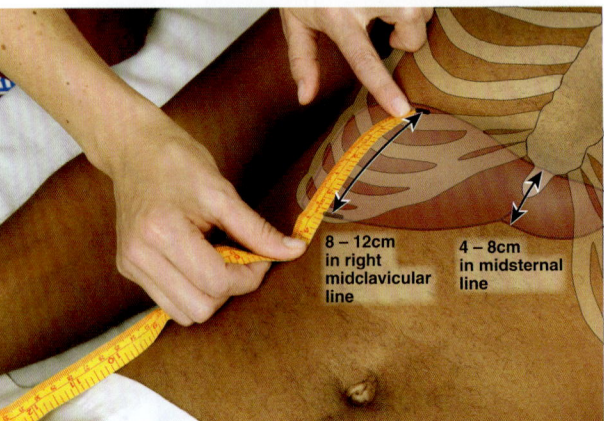

FIGURE 23-15 Normal liver span.

Repeat percussion of the liver at the midsternal line (MSL).	The normal liver span at the MSL is 4–8 cm.	An enlarged liver may be roughly estimated (not accurately) when more intense sounds outline a liver span or borders outside the normal range.

ASSESSMENT PROCEDURE	NORMAL FINDINGS	ABNORMAL FINDINGS
The scratch test is a technique that can be used to ascertain the location and size of the liver and spleen. This test can be particularly useful if the abdomen is tense (rigid or guarded), distended, obese, or too tender to palpate. (Gupta et al., 2013). To perform the scratch test, place the diaphragm of your stethoscope at the second to last intercostal space, MCL. (see Fig. 23-16). Use one finger to very lightly stroke the skin horizontally, starting at the umbilicus. Continue to stroke the skin, moving toward the lower costal margin. The sound will suddenly be transmitted through the stethoscope and increase in intensity. This indicates the lower border of the liver.	The normal liver span at the MSL is 4–8 cm.	An enlarged liver may be roughly estimated (not accurately) when more intense sounds outline a liver span or borders outside the normal range.

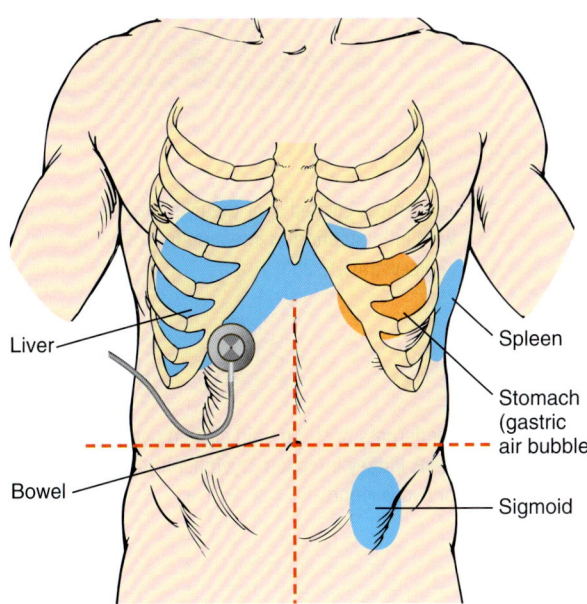

FIGURE 23-16 Scratch test.

🎯 **CLINICAL TIP**
The scratch test has been found to have high reproducibility but methods vary and additional research is needed.

Percuss the spleen. Begin posterior to the left mid-axillary line (MAL), and percuss downward, noting the change from lung resonance to splenic dullness.	The spleen is an oval area of dullness approximately 7 cm wide near the left tenth rib and slightly posterior to the MAL.	Splenomegaly is characterized by an area of dullness greater than 7 cm wide. The enlargement may result from traumatic injury, portal hypertension, and mononucleosis.

🎯 **CLINICAL TIP**
Results of splenic percussion may be obscured by air in the stomach or bowel.

Continued on following page

ASSESSMENT PROCEDURE	NORMAL FINDINGS	ABNORMAL FINDINGS
A second method for detecting splenic enlargement is to percuss the last left interspace at the anterior axillary line (AAL) while the client takes a deep breath (Fig. 23-17).	Normally, tympany (or resonance) is heard at the last left interspace.	On inspiration, dullness at the last left interspace at the AAL suggests an enlarged spleen (Abnormal Findings 23-3). **CLINICAL TIP** Other sources of dullness (e.g., full stomach or feces in the colon) must be ruled out before confirming splenomegaly.

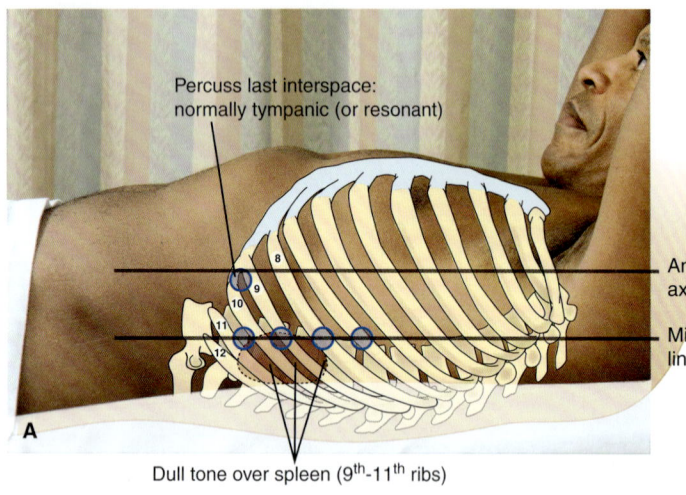
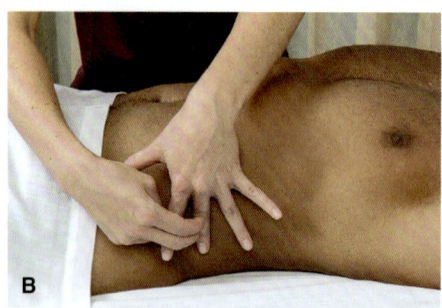

FIGURE 23-17 Last left interspace at the anterior axillary line.

ASSESSMENT PROCEDURE	NORMAL FINDINGS	ABNORMAL FINDINGS
Perform blunt percussion on the liver and the kidneys. This is to assess for tenderness in difficult-to-palpate structures. Percuss the liver by placing your left hand flat against the lower right anterior rib cage. Use the ulnar side of your right fist to strike your left hand.	Normally, no tenderness is elicited.	Tenderness elicited over the liver may be associated with inflammation or infection (e.g., hepatitis or cholecystitis).
Perform blunt percussion on the kidneys at the costovertebral angles (CVA) over the twelfth rib (Fig. 23-18).	Normally, no tenderness or pain is elicited or reported by the client. The examiner senses only a dull thud.	Tenderness or sharp pain elicited over the CVA suggests kidney infection (pyelonephritis), renal calculi, or hydronephrosis.

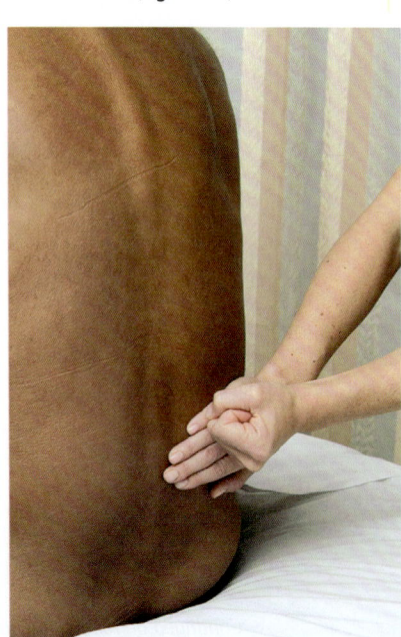

FIGURE 23-18 Performing blunt percussion over the kidney.

23 Assessing Abdomen   513

ASSESSMENT PROCEDURE	NORMAL FINDINGS	ABNORMAL FINDINGS
CLINICAL TIP This technique requires that the client sit with his or her back to you. Therefore, it may be best to incorporate blunt percussion of the kidneys with your thoracic assessment because the client will already be in this position.		
Perform light palpation. Box 23-2 provides considerations for palpation. Light palpation is used to identify areas of tenderness and muscular resistance. Using the fingertips, begin palpation in a nontender quadrant, and compress to a depth of 1 cm in a dipping motion. Then gently lift the fingers and move to the next area (Fig. 23-19). For techniques to minimize the client's voluntary guarding (a tensing or rigidity of the abdominal muscles usually involving the entire abdomen), see Box 23-2. Keep in mind that the rectus abdominis muscle relaxes on expiration.	Abdomen is nontender and soft. There is no guarding.	Involuntary reflex guarding is serious and reflects peritoneal irritation. The abdomen is rigid and the rectus muscle fails to relax with palpation when the client exhales. It can involve all or part of the abdomen but is usually seen on the side (i.e., right vs. left rather than upper or lower) because of nerve tract patterns. Right-sided guarding may be due to cholecystitis. **Concept Mastery Alert** The nurse suspects a hernia if a protrusion appears on the client's abdomen when the nurse asks the client to cough or bear down. Involuntary reflex guarding is a sign of peritoneal irritation and the client should be assessed further for possible infection.
Deeply palpate all quadrants to delineate abdominal organs and detect subtle masses. Using the palmar surface of the fingers, compress to a maximum depth (5–6 cm). Perform bimanual palpation if you encounter resistance or to assess deeper structures (Fig. 23-20).	Normal (mild) tenderness is possible over the xiphoid, aorta, cecum, sigmoid colon, and ovaries with deep palpation. Figure 23-21 illustrates normally palpable structures in the abdomen.	Severe tenderness or pain may be related to trauma, peritonitis, infection, tumors, or enlarged or diseased organs.

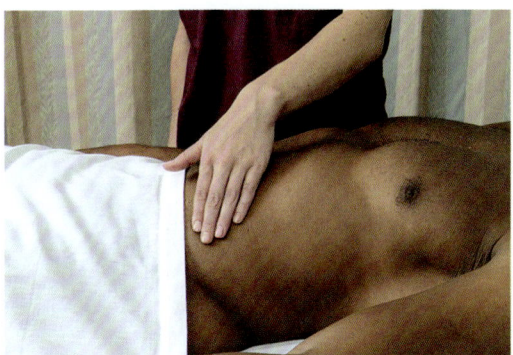

FIGURE 23-19 Performing light palpation.

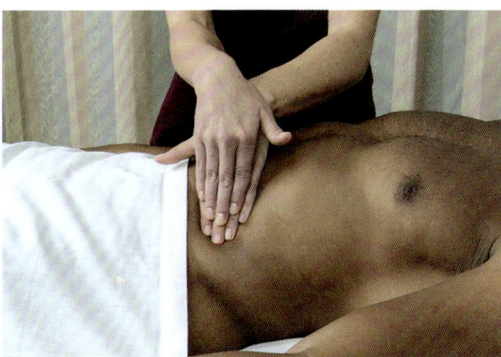

FIGURE 23-20 Performing deep bimanual palpation.

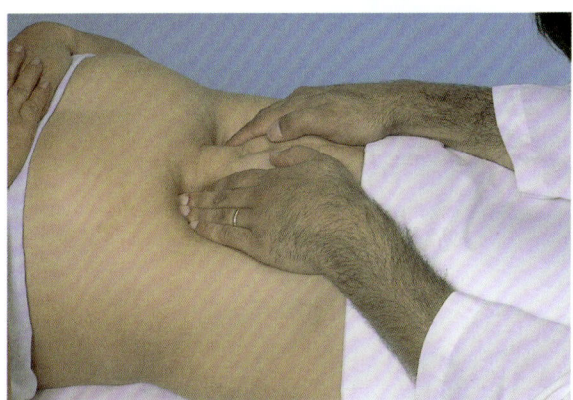

FIGURE 23-21 Normally palpable structures in the abdomen.

Continued on following page

ASSESSMENT PROCEDURE	NORMAL FINDINGS	ABNORMAL FINDINGS
Palpate for masses. Note their location, size (cm), shape, consistency, demarcation, pulsatility, tenderness, and mobility. Do not confuse a mass with an organ or structure.	No palpable masses are present.	A mass detected in any quadrant may be due to a tumor, cyst, abscess, enlarged organ, aneurysm, or adhesions.
Palpate the umbilicus and surrounding area for swellings, bulges, or masses.	Umbilicus and surrounding area are free of swellings, bulges, or masses.	A soft center of the umbilicus can be a potential for herniation. Palpation of a hard nodule in or around the umbilicus may indicate metastatic nodes from an occult gastrointestinal cancer.
Palpate the aorta. Use your thumb and first finger or use two hands and palpate deeply in the epigastrium, slightly to the left of midline (Fig. 23-22). Assess the pulsation of the abdominal aorta. **OLDER ADULT CONSIDERATIONS** If the client is older than age 50 or has hypertension, assess the width of the aorta.	The aorta is approximately 2.5–3.0 cm wide with a moderately strong and regular pulse. Possibly mild tenderness may be elicited.	A wide, bounding pulse may be felt with an abdominal aortic aneurysm. A prominent, laterally pulsating mass above the umbilicus with an accompanying audible bruit strongly suggests an aortic aneurysm (Abnormal Findings 23-3). **CLINICAL TIP** Do not palpate a pulsating midline mass; it may be a dissecting aneurysm that can rupture from the pressure of palpation. Also avoid deep palpation over tender organs as in the case of polycystic kidneys, Wilms tumor, transplantation, or suspected splenic trauma.
Palpate the liver. Note consistency and tenderness. To palpate *bimanually,* stand at the client's right side and place your left hand under the client's back at the level of the eleventh to twelfth ribs. Lay your right hand parallel to the right costal margin (your fingertips should point toward the client's head). Ask the client to inhale, then compress upward and inward with your fingers. Have the client exhale and hold your hand in place as the client inhales a second time. With deep inhalation the edge of the liver is more easily palpated. (Fig. 23-23.)	The liver is usually not palpable, although it may be felt in some thin clients. If the lower edge is felt, it should be firm, smooth, and even. Mild tenderness may be normal.	A hard, firm liver may indicate cancer. Nodularity may occur with tumors, metastatic cancer, late cirrhosis, or syphilis. Tenderness may be from vascular engorgement (e.g., congestive heart failure), acute hepatitis, or abscess. A liver more than 1–3 cm below the costal margin is considered enlarged (unless displaced by the diaphragm).

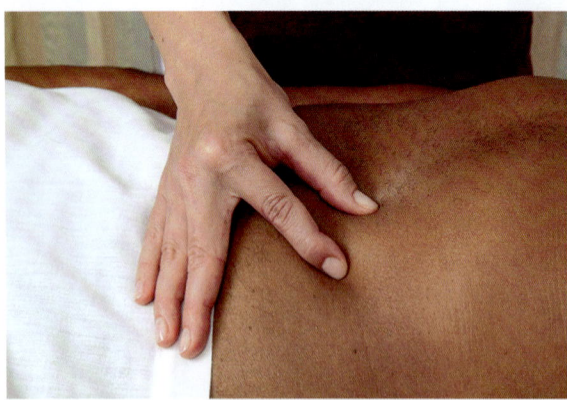

FIGURE 23-22 Palpating the aorta.

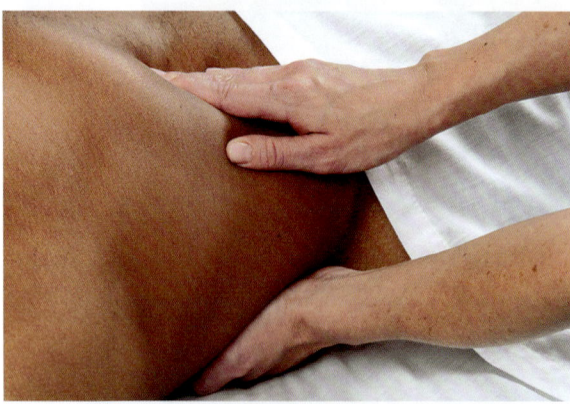

FIGURE 23-23 Bimanual technique for liver palpation.

To palpate by *hooking,* stand to the right of the client's chest. Curl (hook) the fingers of both hands over the edge of the right costal margin. Ask the client to take a deep breath and gently but firmly pull inward and upward with your fingers (Fig. 23-24).		Enlargement may be due to hepatitis, liver tumors, cirrhosis, and vascular engorgement.

23 Assessing Abdomen 515

ASSESSMENT PROCEDURE	NORMAL FINDINGS	ABNORMAL FINDINGS

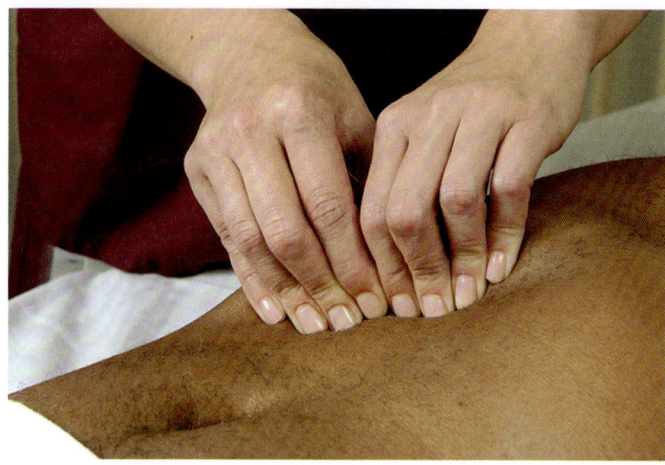

FIGURE 23-24 Hooking technique for liver palpation.

Palpate the spleen. Stand at the client's right side, reach over the abdomen with your left arm, and place your hand under the posterior lower ribs. Pull up gently. Place your right hand below the left costal margin with the fingers pointing toward the client's head. Ask the client to inhale and press inward and upward as you provide support with your other hand (Fig. 23-25).

Alternatively, asking the client to turn onto the right side may facilitate splenic palpation by moving the spleen downward and forward (Fig. 23-26). Document the size of the spleen in centimeters below the left costal margin. Also note consistency and tenderness.

The spleen is seldom palpable at the left costal margin. Rarely, the tip is palpable in the presence of a low, flat diaphragm (e.g., chronic obstructive lung disease) or with deep diaphragmatic descent on inspiration. If the edge of the spleen can be palpated, it should be soft and nontender.

A palpable spleen suggests enlargement (up to three times the normal size), which may result from infections, trauma, mononucleosis, chronic blood disorders, and cancers. The splenic notch may be felt, which is an indication of splenic enlargement. Splenic enlargement may not always be pathologic.

SAFETY TIP *Caution: To avoid traumatizing and possibly rupturing the organ, be gentle when palpating an enlarged spleen.*

The spleen feels soft with a rounded edge when it is enlarged from infection. It feels firm with a sharp edge when it is enlarged from chronic disease.

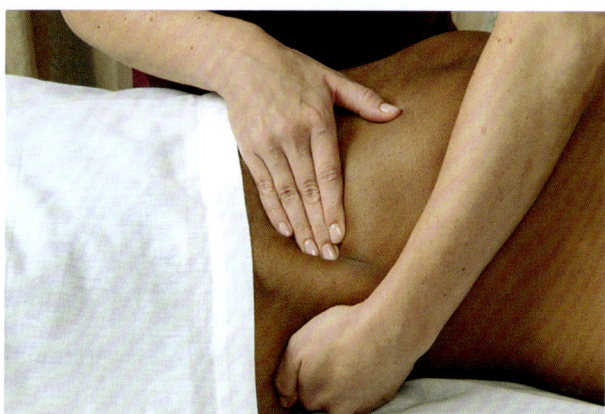

FIGURE 23-25 Palpating the spleen.

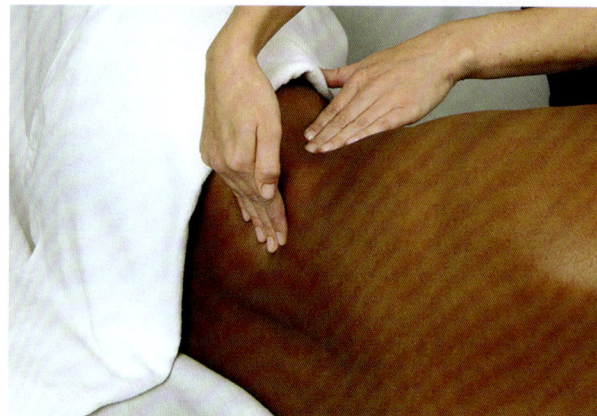

FIGURE 23-26 Palpating the spleen with the client in side-lying position.

CLINICAL TIP
Be sure to palpate with your fingers below the costal margin so you do not miss the lower edge of an enlarged spleen.

Tenderness accompanied by peritoneal inflammation or capsular stretching is associated with splenic enlargement.

Continued on following page

ASSESSMENT PROCEDURE	NORMAL FINDINGS	ABNORMAL FINDINGS
Palpate the kidneys. To palpate the right kidney, support the right posterior flank with your left hand and place your right hand in the RUQ just below the costal margin at the MCL. To capture the kidney, ask the client to inhale. Then compress your fingers deeply during peak inspiration. Ask the client to exhale and hold the breath briefly. Gradually release the pressure of your right hand. If you have captured the kidney, you will feel it slip beneath your fingers. To palpate the left kidney, reverse the procedure (Fig. 23-27).	The kidneys are usually not palpable. Sometimes the lower pole of the right kidney may be palpable by the capture method because of its lower position. If palpated, it should feel firm, smooth, and rounded. The kidney may or may not be slightly tender.	An enlarged kidney may be due to a cyst, tumor, or hydronephrosis. It can be differentiated from splenomegaly by its smooth rather than sharp edge, absence of a notch, and overlying tympany on percussion (Abnormal Findings 23-3).
Palpate the urinary bladder. Palpate for a distended bladder when the client's history or other findings warrant (e.g., dull percussion noted over the symphysis pubis). Begin at the symphysis pubis and move upward and outward to estimate bladder borders (Fig. 23-28).	An empty bladder is neither palpable nor tender.	A distended bladder is palpated as a smooth, round, and somewhat firm mass extending as far as the umbilicus. It may be further validated by dull percussion tones.

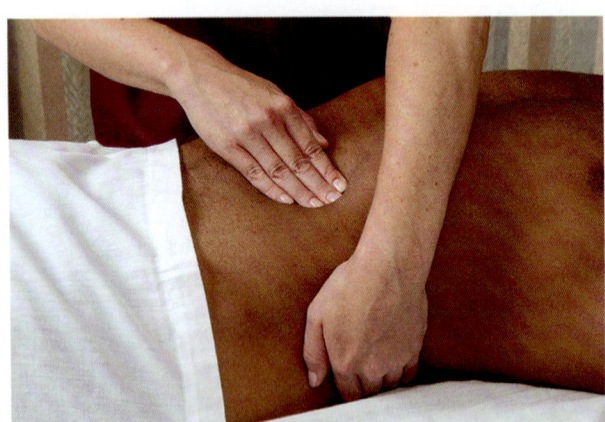

FIGURE 23-27 Palpating the kidney.

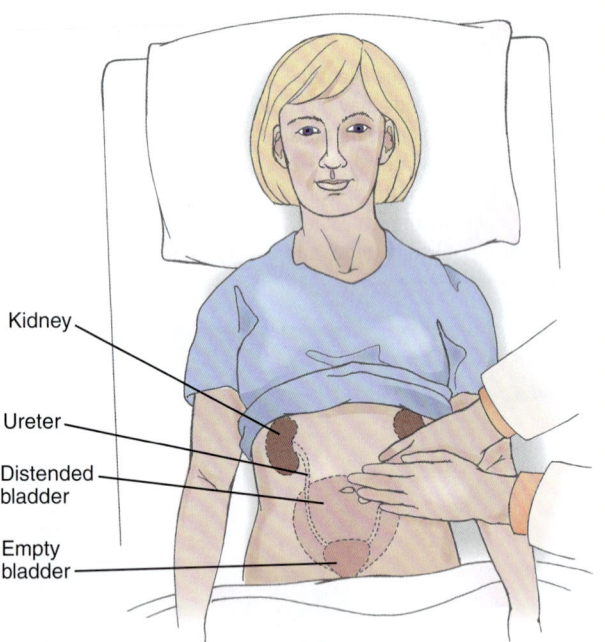

FIGURE 23-28 Palpating distended bladder (*larger dotted line* is area of distention).

TESTS FOR ASCITES

Test for shifting dullness. If you suspect that the client has ascites because of a distended abdomen or bulging flanks, perform this special percussion technique. The client should remain supine. Percuss the flanks from the bed upward toward the umbilicus.	The borders between tympany and dullness remain relatively constant throughout position changes.	When ascites is present and the client is supine, the fluid assumes a dependent position and produces a dull percussion tone around the flanks. Air rises to the top and tympany is percussed around the umbilicus. When the client turns onto one side and ascites is present, the fluid assumes a dependent position and air rises to the top.

ASSESSMENT PROCEDURE	NORMAL FINDINGS	ABNORMAL FINDINGS
Note the change from dullness to tympany and mark this point. Now help the client turn onto the side. Percuss the abdomen from the bed upward. Mark the level where dullness changes to tympany (Fig. 23-29).		There is a marked increase in the height of the dullness. This test is not always reliable, thus definitive testing by ultrasound is necessary. Ascites often is a sign of severe liver disease due to portal hypertension (high pressure in the blood vessels of the liver and low albumin levels (Cesario et al., 2013).
Perform the fluid wave test. A second special technique to detect ascites is the fluid wave test. The client should remain supine. You will need assistance with this test. Ask the client or an assistant to place the ulnar side of the hand and the lateral side of the forearm firmly along the midline of the abdomen. Firmly place the palmar surface of your fingers and hand against one side of the client's abdomen. Use your other hand to tap the opposite side of the abdominal wall (Fig. 23-30).	No fluid wave is transmitted.	Movement of a fluid wave against the resting hand suggests large amounts of fluid are present (ascites). Because this test is not completely reliable, definitive testing by ultrasound is needed.

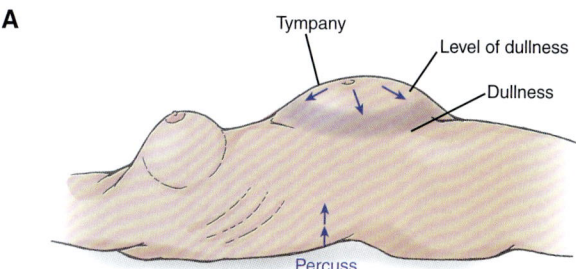
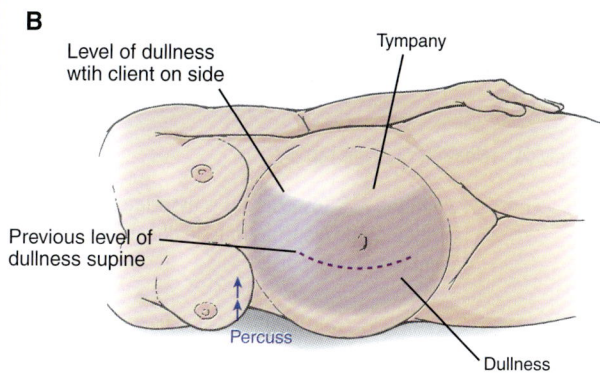
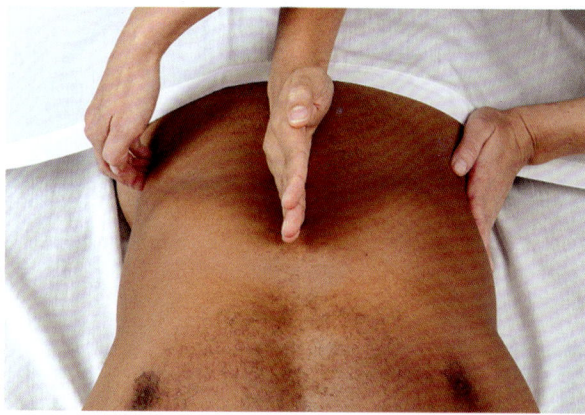

FIGURE 23-29 Percussing for level of dullness with client supine (A) and lying on the side (B).

FIGURE 23-30 Performing fluid wave test.

TESTS FOR APPENDICITIS/PERITONEAL IRRITATION

(See Assessment Guide 23-3 to differentiate various signs of Appendicitis and Peritoneal Irritation.)		
Assess for rebound tenderness. If the client has abdominal pain or tenderness, test for rebound tenderness by palpating deeply at 90 degrees into the abdomen halfway between the umbilicus and the anterior iliac crest (McBurney point)	No rebound tenderness is present.	The client has rebound tenderness when the client perceives sharp, stabbing pain as the examiner releases pressure from the abdomen (Blumberg sign). It suggests peritoneal irritation (as from appendicitis).

Continued on following page

ASSESSMENT PROCEDURE	NORMAL FINDINGS	ABNORMAL FINDINGS
Then suddenly release pressure. Listen and watch for the client's expression of pain. Ask the client to describe which hurt more—the pressing in or the releasing—and where on the abdomen the pain occurred. 🎯 **CLINICAL TIP** Test for rebound tenderness should always be performed at the end of the examination because a positive response produces pain and muscle spasm that can interfere with the remaining examination.		If the client feels pain at an area other than where you were assessing for rebound tenderness, consider that area as the source of the pain (see test for referred rebound tenderness, below).
Test for referred rebound tenderness. Palpate deeply in the LLQ and quickly release pressure (Fig. 23-31).	No rebound pain is elicited.	Pain in the RLQ during pressure in the LLQ is a positive Rovsing sign. It suggests acute appendicitis. **SAFETY TIP** *Avoid continued palpation when test findings are positive for appendicitis because of the danger of rupturing the appendix.*

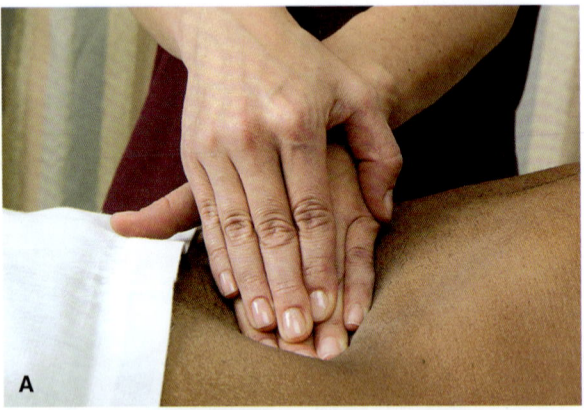 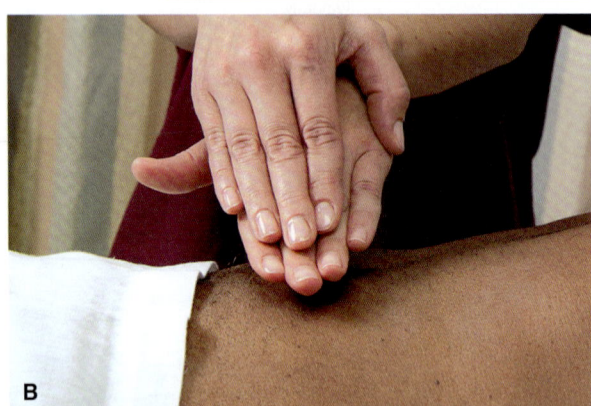

FIGURE 23-31 Assessing for Rovsing sign: palpating deeply (**A**); releasing pressure rapidly (**B**).

Assess for psoas sign. Ask the client to lie on the left side. Hyperextend the client's right leg. (Fig. 23-32.)	No abdominal pain is present.	Pain in the RLQ (psoas sign) is associated with irritation of the iliopsoas muscle due to appendicitis (an inflamed appendix).

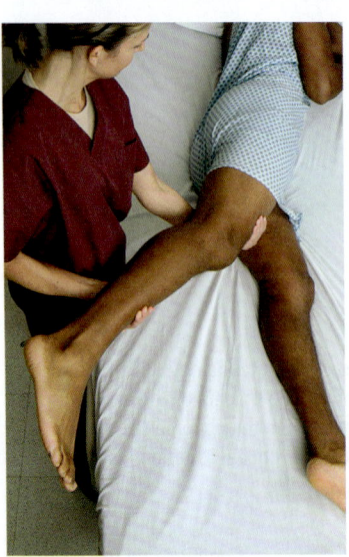

FIGURE 23-32 Testing for psoas sign.

ASSESSMENT PROCEDURE	NORMAL FINDINGS	ABNORMAL FINDINGS
Assess for obturator sign. Support the client's right knee and ankle. Flex the hip and knee, and rotate the leg internally and externally (Fig. 23-33).	No abdominal pain is present.	Pain in the RLQ indicates irritation of the obturator muscle due to appendicitis or a perforated appendix.

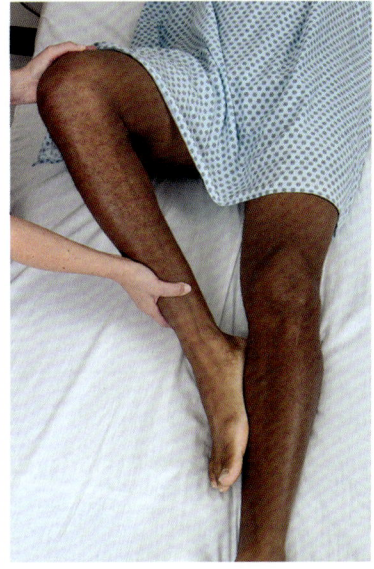

FIGURE 23-33 Testing for obturator sign.

ASSESSMENT PROCEDURE	NORMAL FINDINGS	ABNORMAL FINDINGS
Perform hypersensitivity test. Stroke the abdomen with a sharp object (e.g., broken cotton tipped applicator or tongue blade) or grasp a fold of skin with your thumb and index finger and quickly let go. Do this several times along the abdominal wall.	The client feels no pain and no exaggerated sensation.	Pain or an exaggerated sensation felt in the RLQ is a positive skin hypersensitivity test and may indicate appendicitis.

TEST FOR CHOLECYSTITIS

Assess RUQ pain or tenderness, which may signal cholecystitis (inflammation of the gallbladder). Press your fingertips under the liver border at the right costal margin and ask the client to inhale deeply.	No increase in pain is present.	Accentuated sharp pain that causes the client to hold his or her breath (inspiratory arrest) is a positive Murphy sign and is associated with acute cholecystitis.

ASSESSMENT GUIDE 23-2 Measuring Abdominal Girth

In clients with abdominal distention, abdominal girth (circumference) should be assessed periodically (daily in hospital, during a doctor's office visit, with home nursing visits) to evaluate the progress or treatment of distention. Waist circumference measurement is also recommended in screening for cardiovascular risk factors.* To facilitate accurate assessment and interpretation, the following guidelines are recommended:

1. Measure abdominal girth at the same time of day, ideally in the morning just after voiding, or at a designated time for bedridden clients or those with indwelling catheters.
2. The ideal position for the client is standing; otherwise, the client should be in the supine position. The client's head may be slightly elevated (for orthopneic clients). The client should be in the same position for all measurements.
3. Use a disposable or easily cleaned tape measure. If a tape measure is not available, use a strip of cloth or gauze, then measure the gauze with a cloth tape measure or yardstick.
4. Place the tape measure behind the client and measure at the umbilicus. *Use the umbilicus as a starting point when measuring abdominal girth, especially when distention is apparent.*
5. Record the distance in designated units (inches or centimeters).
6. Take all future measurements from the same location. Marking the abdomen with a ballpoint pen can help you identify the measuring site. As a courtesy, the nurse needs to explain the purpose of the marking pen and ask the client not to wash the mark off until it is no longer needed.

*Central obesity risk is defined as a waist circumference greater than 40 in (102 cm) in men and greater than 35 in (88 cm) in women. Central obesity is correlated with metabolic syndrome and increased risk for coronary heart disease (Phillips & Prins, 2008).

BOX 23-2 CONSIDERATIONS FOR PALPATING THE ABDOMEN

- Avoid touching tender or painful areas until last, and reassure the client of your intentions.
- Perform light palpation before deep palpation to detect tenderness and superficial masses.
- Keep in mind that the normal abdomen may be tender, especially in the areas over the xiphoid process, liver, aorta, lower pole of the kidney, gas-filled cecum, sigmoid colon, and ovaries.
- Overcome ticklishness and minimize voluntary guarding by asking the client to perform self-palpation. Place your hands over the client's. After a while, let your fingers glide slowly onto the abdomen while still resting mostly on the client's fingers. The same can be done by using a warm stethoscope as a palpating instrument—again letting your fingers drift over the edge of the diaphragm—and palpate without promoting a ticklish response.
- Work with the client to promote relaxation and minimize voluntary guarding. Use the following techniques:
  - Place a pillow under the client's knees.
  - Ask the client to take slow, deep breaths through the mouth.
  - Apply light pressure over the client's sternum with your left hand while palpating with the right. This encourages the client to relax the abdominal muscles during breathing against sternal resistance.

ASSESSMENT GUIDE 23-3 Abdominal Signs

Name	Description	Cause
Psoas sign	Pain in RLQ when leg is hyperextended	Irritation of the iliopsoas muscle due to appendicitis (an inflamed appendix).
Obturator sign	Pain in the RLQ when hip and knee are flexed and leg is rotated internally and externally	Irritation of the obturator muscle due to appendicitis or a perforated appendix.
Murphy sign	Pain elicited when pressure is applied under the liver border at the right costal margin and client inhales deeply.	Inflammation of the gallbladder
Rovsing sign	Pain in the RLQ during pressure in the LLQ	Acute appendicitis
Blumberg sign	Abdominal pain or tenderness experienced when examiner, tests for rebound tenderness by palpating deeply at 90 degrees into the abdomen one-halfway between the umbilicus and the anterior iliac crest (McBurney point)	Peritoneal irritation

CASE STUDY

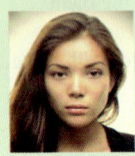

The chapter case study is now used to demonstrate the physical examination of Ms. Chen's abdomen.

Abdominal skin is pale pink, free of striae, scars, lesions, or rashes. Umbilicus is midline and recessed, with no bulges. Abdomen is round, distended, symmetric, and without bulges or lumps. No diastasis recti noted with neck flexion. No respiratory movement, peristaltic waves, or aortic pulsations noted. Bowel sounds (10 per minute) present with moderate gurgles × 4 quadrants. No bruits, venous hums, or friction rubs auscultated.

Percussion reveals generalized tympany with dullness over the liver, spleen, and descending colon. Liver span is 8 cm at the MCL and 6 cm at the MSL. No tenderness with blunt percussion over the liver or kidneys. No abdominal tenderness or guarding with light palpation. Mild tenderness over the xiphoid, aorta, cecum, and sigmoid colon with deep palpation. No rebound tenderness. Palpable firm mass noted in LLQ. Liver, spleen, kidneys, and urinary bladder not palpable. No evidence of fluid wave or shifting dullness. No ballotable masses. Negative psoas sign, obturator sign, Rovsing sign, and Murphy sign.

Validating and Documenting Findings

Validate the abdominal assessment data you have collected. This is necessary to verify that the data are reliable and accurate. Document the assessment data following the health care facility or agency policy.

CASE STUDY

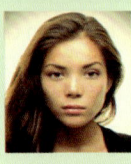

The clinic nurse documented the following subjective and objective assessment findings of Ms. Chen's abdominal evaluation.

Biographical Data: NC, 32 years old. Korean American. Employed as a graduate assistant in the Chemistry department of the local university. Awake, alert, and oriented. Asks and answers questions appropriately.

Chief Complaint: "I haven't had a bowel movement in 4 days and I cannot get my pants buttoned."

History of Present Health Concern: Abdominal discomfort has escalated over the past 4 days as client has not had a bowel movement. Reports increased stress and extremely poor eating habits since beginning study for comprehensive examinations. Rates pain as

4 out of 10 on scale of 1–10 and describes it as dull and constant. Reports decreased appetite over the past week. States had episode of nausea last night lasting approximately 2 hours. Admits to holding stool when she is busy at school. Denies melena, hematochezia, or hematemesis.

Past Health History: Denies weight loss, ulcers, GERD, inflammatory or obstructive bowel disease, pancreatitis, gallbladder or liver disease, diverticulosis, or appendicitis. Reports routinely has 3–4 formed, brown bowel movements per week. Denies straining with bowel movement and feeling of incomplete evacuations. Reports one uncomplicated urinary tract infection 2 years ago. Denies kidney disease, nephritis, or renal calculi. Reports having been immunized to hepatitis A and B. Denies exposure to hepatitis C. Denies previous abdominal surgery or trauma.

Admits to taking Alesse oral contraceptive pill one daily and a multivitamin tablet 2–3 days weekly (when she remembers). Denies allergies to medications, environment, food, or insects.

Family History: Denies any family history of colon, gastric, pancreatic, liver, kidney, bladder, gallbladder disease or cancer.

Lifestyle and Health Practices: Reports that she drinks two 6-oz glasses of wine 2 times weekly, usually on the weekend. Denies use of tobacco products and street drugs.

Twenty-four hour diet recall consists of the following: Breakfast—24-oz black coffee; lunch—cheeseburger and Snickers bar; dinner—bowl of Special K with 2% milk. Throughout the day drank 44-oz Diet Coke. Scant amount of noncaffeinated drink.

Recreation includes listening to music as she studies. Denies regular exercise. Walks approximately ¼ mile to and from classes daily.

Client is very stressed about her upcoming comprehensive examinations, and reports that she hardly has time to go to the grocery store and almost never cooks. Since study for comprehensive examinations began, Ms. Chen reports that she really has not paid any attention to her bowel elimination. States that she would like help with handling her diet, fluid intake, and stress when under so much pressure.

Physical Examination Findings: Abdominal skin is tan, free of striae, scars, lesions, or rashes. Umbilicus is midline and recessed with no bulges. Abdomen is round, distended, symmetric, and without bulges or lumps. No diastasis recti noted with neck flexion. No respiratory movement, peristaltic waves, or aortic pulsations noted. Bowel sounds (10 per minute) present with moderately pitched gurgles × 4 quadrants. No bruits, venous hums, or friction rubs auscultated.

Percussion reveals generalized tympany with dullness over the liver, spleen, and descending colon. Liver span is 8 cm at the MCL and 6 cm at the MSL.

No tenderness with blunt percussion over the liver or kidneys. No abdominal tenderness or guarding with light palpation. Mild tenderness over the xiphoid, aorta, cecum, and sigmoid colon with deep palpation. No rebound tenderness. Palpable firm mass noted in LLQ. Liver, spleen, kidneys, and urinary bladder not palpable. No evidence of fluid wave or shifting dullness. No ballotable masses. Negative psoas sign, obturator sign, Rovsing sign and Murphy sign.

ANALYSIS OF DATA: DIAGNOSTIC REASONING

After collecting assessment data, you will need to analyze it using diagnostic reasoning skills. Following are some possible conclusions that may be drawn after assessment of the client's abdomen.

Selected Nursing Diagnoses

After collecting subjective and objective data pertaining to the abdomen, you will need to identify abnormal findings and cluster the data to reveal any significant patterns or abnormalities. These data will then be used to make clinical judgments (nursing diagnoses: health promotion, risk, or actual) about the status of the client's abdomen. Following is a listing of selected nursing diagnoses that you may identify when analyzing data for this part of the assessment.

Health Promotion Diagnoses

- Readiness for Enhanced Health Management: Requests information on ways to improve nutritional status

Risk Diagnoses

- Risk for Fluid Volume Deficit related to excessive nausea and vomiting or diarrhea
- Risk for Impaired Skin Integrity related to fluid volume deficit secondary to decreased fluid intake, nausea, vomiting, diarrhea, fecal or urinary incontinence, or ostomy drainage
- Risk for Impaired Oral Mucous Membranes related to fluid volume deficit secondary to nausea, vomiting, diarrhea, or gastrointestinal intubation
- Risk for Urinary Retention related to urinary stasis and decreased fluid intake
- Risk for Imbalanced Nutrition: Less Than Body Requirements related to lack of dietary information or inadequate intake of nutrients secondary to values or religious beliefs or eating disorders
- Risk for dysfunctional gastrointestinal motility

Actual Diagnoses

- Diarrhea related to dietary intolerances
- Constipation related to insufficient physical activity and fluid intake

- Imbalanced Nutrition: Less Than Body Requirements related to malabsorption, decreased appetite, frequent nausea, and vomiting
- Imbalanced Nutrition: More Than Body Requirements related to intake that exceeds caloric needs
- Ineffective Sexuality Pattern related to fear of rejection by partner secondary to offensive odor and drainage from colostomy or ileostomy
- Grieving related to change in manner of bowel elimination
- Disturbed Body Image related to change in abdominal appearance secondary to presence of stoma
- Diarrhea related to malabsorption and chronic irritable bowel syndrome or medications
- Constipation related to decreased fluid intake, decreased dietary fiber, decreased physical activity, bedrest, or medications
- Perceived Constipation related to decrease in usual pattern and frequency of bowel elimination
- Bowel Incontinence related to muscular or neurologic dysfunction secondary to age, disease, or trauma
- Ineffective Health Maintenance related to chronic or inappropriate use of laxatives or enemas
- Activity Intolerance related to fecal or urinary incontinence
- Anxiety related to fear of fecal or urinary incontinence
- Social Isolation related to anxiety and fear of fecal or urinary incontinence
- Pain: Abdominal (referred, distention, or surgical incision)
- Impaired Urinary Elimination related to catheterization secondary to obstruction, trauma, infection, neurologic disorders, or surgical intervention
- Urinary Retention related to obstruction of part of the urinary tract or malfunctioning of drainage devices (catheters) and need to learn bladder emptying techniques
- Impaired Urinary Elimination related to pain of bladder infection
- Functional Incontinence related to age-related urgency and inability to reach toilet in time secondary to decreased bladder tone and inability to recognize "need-to-void cues"
- Reflex Urinary Incontinence related to lack of knowledge of ways to trigger a more predictable voiding schedule
- Stress Incontinence related to knowledge deficit of pelvic floor muscle exercises
- Total Incontinence related to need for bladder retraining program
- Urge Incontinence related to need for knowledge of preventive measures secondary to infection, trauma, or neurogenic problems

Selected Collaborative Problems

After grouping the data, certain collaborative problems may emerge. Remember that collaborative problems differ from nursing diagnoses in that they cannot be prevented by nursing interventions. However, these physiologic complications of medical conditions can be detected and monitored by the nurse. In addition, the nurse can use physician- and nurse-prescribed interventions to minimize the complications of these problems. The nurse may also have to refer the client for further treatment of the problem. Following is a list of collaborative problems that may be identified when assessing the abdomen. These problems are worded as Risk for Complications (RC), followed by the problem.

- RC: Peritonitis
- RC: Ileus
- RC: Afferent loop syndrome
- RC: Early dumping syndrome
- RC: Late dumping syndrome
- RC: Malabsorption syndrome
- RC: Intestinal bleeding
- RC: Renal calculi
- RC: Abscess formation
- RC: Bowel obstruction
- RC: Toxic megacolon
- RC: Mesenteric thrombosis
- RC: Obstruction of bile flow
- RC: Fistula formation
- RC: Hyponatremia/hypernatremia
- RC: Hypokalemia/hyperkalemia
- RC: Hypoglycemia/hyperglycemia
- RC: Hypocalcemia/hypercalcemia
- RC: Metabolic acidosis
- RC: Uremic syndrome
- RC: Urinary obstruction
- RC: Hypertension
- RC: Gastroesophageal reflux disease
- RC: Peptic ulcer disease
- RC: Hepatic failure
- RC: Pancreatitis

Medical Problems

After grouping the data, it may become apparent that the client has signs and symptoms that may require medical diagnosis and treatment. Referral to a primary care provider is necessary.

CASE STUDY

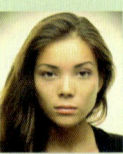

After collecting and analyzing the data for Ms. Chen, the nurse determines that the following conclusions are appropriate:

- Constipation r/t body tension, lack of exercise and inadequate water intake.
- Ineffective Individual Coping r/t increased life stress and lack of knowledge of appropriate management strategies.
- Ineffective Health Maintenance r/t knowledge deficit and possibly lack of motivation to change unhealthful behaviors.
- Readiness for Enhanced Self-health Management of stress and eating behaviors.

Because there is no medical diagnosis, there are no collaborative problems at this time.

Interdisciplinary Verbal Communication of Assessment Findings Using SBAR

SITUATION: N.C., a 32-year-old female Korean American graduate student, has generalized dull, constant abdominal pain (4 out of 10 on scale of 1–10). Has not had a bowel movement for 4 days, and can't button pants. Anxious due to upcoming final examination. Abdominal discomfort has escalated over past 4 days. Decreased appetite over the past week with 2-hour episode of nausea last night. Holds stool when she is busy at school.

BACKGROUND: Routinely has 3–4 formed, brown bowel movements per week. Diet last 24 hours; High carbohydrates and fat. Eats fast foods and does not cook. Denies regular exercise. Requests help to improve her diet, fluid intake, and stress when under so much pressure.

PHYSICAL EXAMINATION FINDINGS: Abdomen is round, distended, symmetric, and without bulges or lumps. No diastasis recti noted with neck flexion. Bowel sounds (10 per minute) present with moderately pitched gurgles × 4 quadrants. Percussion reveals generalized tympany with dullness over the liver, spleen, and descending colon. Liver span is 8 cm at the MCL and 6 cm at the MSL. No abdominal tenderness or guarding with light palpation. Mild tenderness over the xiphoid, aorta, cecum, and sigmoid colon with deep palpation. No rebound tenderness. Palpable firm mass noted in LLQ.

RECOMMENDATION: N.C. has constipation r/t body tension, lack of exercise and inadequate water intake. She also has Readiness for Enhanced Health Management of stress and eating behaviors as evidenced by request for help with diet, fluid intake, and dealing with stress. She also presents with Ineffective Individual Coping r/t increased life stress and lack of knowledge of appropriate management strategies. She needs to work with a dietitian to develop a dietary plan including fiber and adequate fluids. Assistance with an exercise regimen and stress management plan also needs to be established with the appropriate health care practitioners.

To view an algorithm depicting the process of diagnostic reasoning for this case, go to thePoint.

ABNORMAL FINDINGS 23-1 | Abdominal Distention

With the exception of pregnancy, abdominal distention is usually considered an abnormal finding. Percussion may help determine the cause.

PREGNANCY (NORMAL FINDING)

Pregnancy is included here so that the examiner may differentiate it from abnormal findings.

It causes a generalized protuberant abdomen, protuberant umbilicus, a fetal heart beat that can be heard on auscultation, percussible tympany over the intestines, and dullness over the uterus.

FAT

Obesity accounts for most uniformly protuberant abdomens. The abdominal wall is thick, and tympany is the percussion tone elicited. The umbilicus usually appears sunken.

FECES

Hard stools in the colon appear as a localized distention. Percussion over the area discloses dullness.

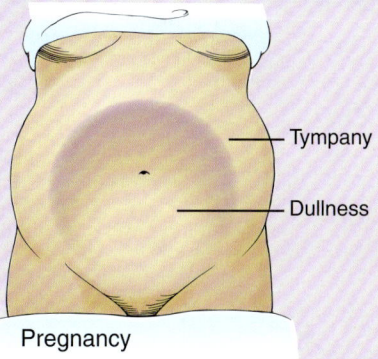
Pregnancy

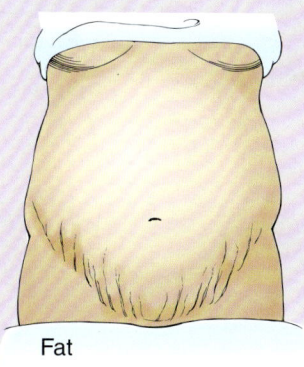
Fat

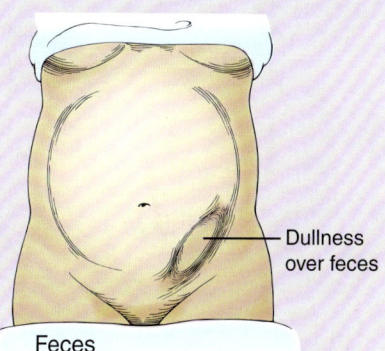
Feces

Continued on following page

524 UNIT 3 Nursing Assessment of Physical Systems

ABNORMAL FINDING 23-1 Abdominal Distention (Continued)

FIBROIDS AND OTHER MASSES

A large ovarian cyst or fibroid tumor appears as generalized distention in the lower abdomen. The mass displaces bowel, thus the percussion tone over the distended area is dullness, with tympany at the periphery. The umbilicus may be everted.

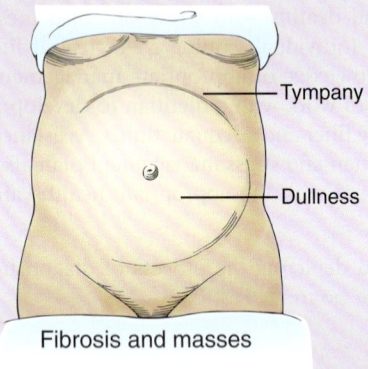
Fibrosis and masses

FLATUS

The abdomen distended with gas may appear as a generalized protuberance (as shown), or it may appear more localized. Tympany is the percussion tone over the area.

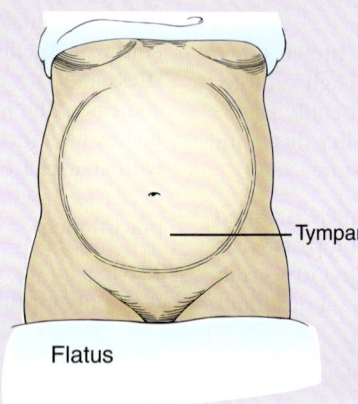
Flatus

ASCITIC FLUID

Fluid in the abdomen causes generalized protuberance, bulging flanks, and an everted umbilicus. Percussion reveals dullness over fluid (bottom of abdomen and flanks) and tympany over intestines (top of abdomen).

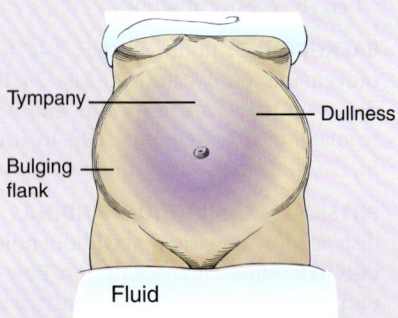

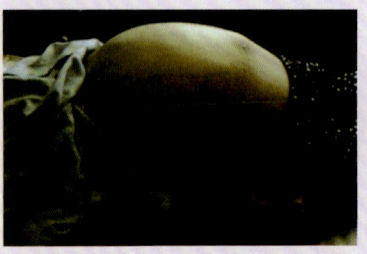

ABNORMAL FINDINGS 23-2 Abdominal Bulges

UMBILICAL HERNIA

An umbilical hernia results from the bowel protruding through a weakness in the umbilical ring. This condition occurs more frequently in infants, but also occurs in adults.

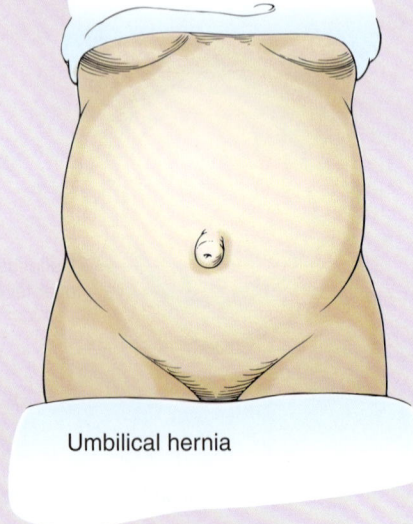
Umbilical hernia

EPIGASTRIC HERNIA

An epigastric hernia occurs when the bowel protrudes through a weakness in the linea alba. The small bulge appears midline between the xiphoid process and the umbilicus. It may be discovered only on palpation.

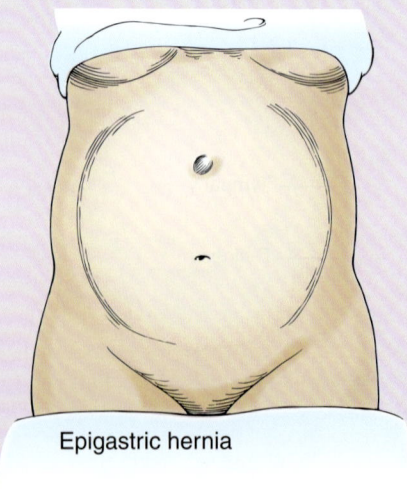
Epigastric hernia

DIASTASIS RECTI

Diastasis recti occurs when the bowel protrudes through a separation between the two rectus abdominis muscles. It appears as a midline ridge. The bulge may appear only when the client raises the head or coughs. The condition is of little significance.

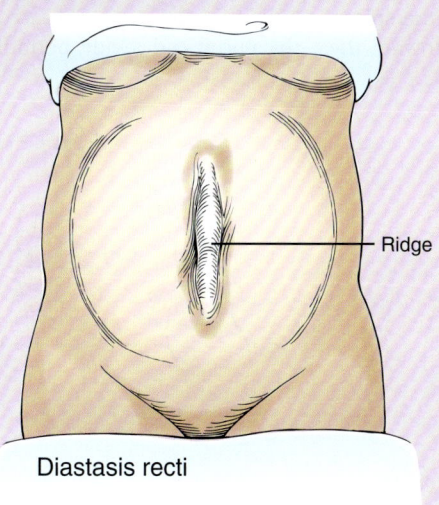

Diastasis recti

INCISIONAL HERNIA

An incisional hernia occurs when the bowel protrudes through a defect or weakness resulting from a surgical incision. It appears as a bulge near a surgical scar on the abdomen.

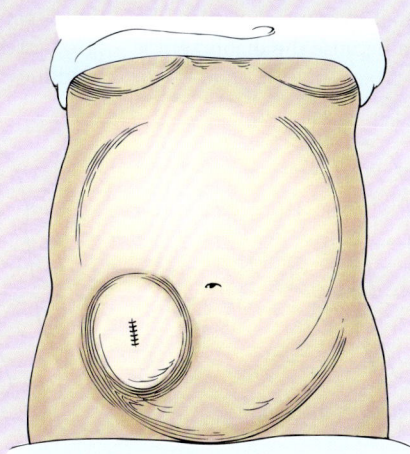

Incisional hernia

ABNORMAL FINDINGS 23-3 — Enlarged Abdominal Organs and Other Abnormalities

ENLARGED LIVER

An enlarged liver (hepatomegaly) is defined as a span greater than 12 cm at the midclavicular line (MCL) and greater than 8 cm at the midsternal line (MSL). An enlarged nontender liver suggests cirrhosis. An enlarged tender liver suggests congestive heart failure, acute hepatitis, or abscess.

ENLARGED NODULAR LIVER

An enlarged firm, hard, nodular liver suggests cancer. Other causes may be late cirrhosis or syphilis.

LIVER HIGHER THAN NORMAL

A liver that is in a higher position than normal span may be caused by an abdominal mass, ascites, or a paralyzed diaphragm.

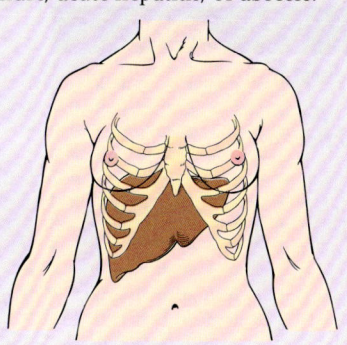

Enlarged liver.

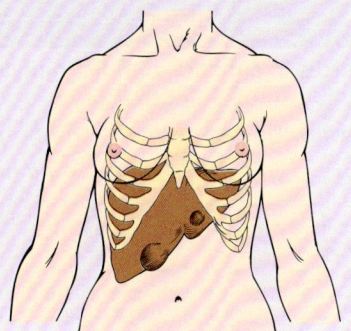

Enlarged nodular liver.

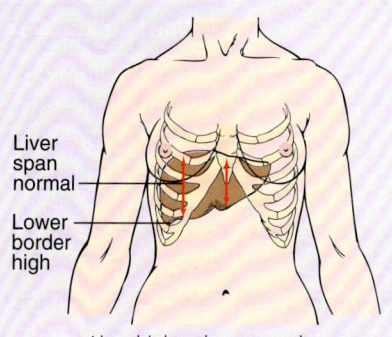

Liver higher than normal.

Continued on following page

ABNORMAL FINDINGS 23-3: Enlarged Abdominal Organs and Other Abnormalities (Continued)

LIVER LOWER THAN NORMAL

A liver in a lower position than normal with a normal span may be caused by emphysema because the diaphragm is low.

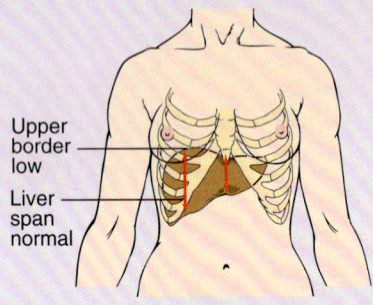

Liver lower than normal.

ENLARGED SPLEEN

An enlarged spleen (splenomegaly) is defined by an area of dullness exceeding 7 cm. When enlarged, the spleen progresses downward and toward the midline.

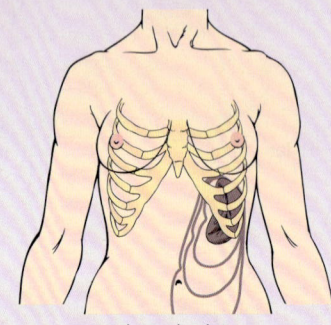

Enlarged spleen.

AORTIC ANEURYSM

A prominent, laterally pulsating mass above the umbilicus strongly suggests an aortic aneurysm. It is accompanied by a bruit and a wide, bounding pulse.

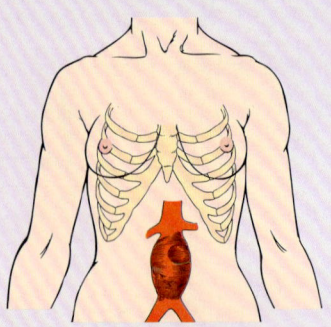

Aortic aneurysm.

ENLARGED KIDNEY

An enlarged kidney may be due to a cyst, tumor, or hydronephrosis. It may be differentiated from an enlarged spleen by its smooth rather than sharp edge, the absence of a notch, and tympany on percussion.

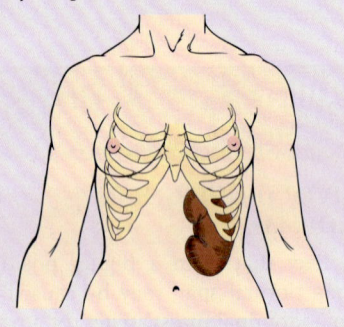

Enlarged kidney.

ENLARGED GALLBLADDER

An extremely tender, enlarged gallbladder suggests acute cholecystitis. A positive finding is Murphy sign (sharp pain that causes the client to hold the breath).

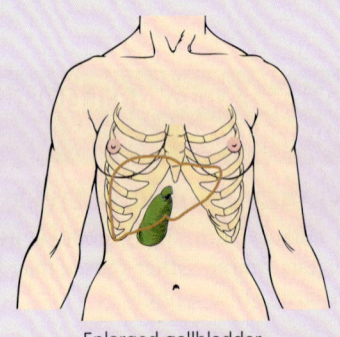

Enlarged gallbladder.

Want to know more?

A wide variety of resources to enhance your learning and understanding of this book are available on thePoint. Visit thePoint to access:

- NCLEX-Style Student Review Questions
- Watch and Learn Videos
- Concept in Action Animations
- And more!

References and Selected Readings

Agency for Healthcare Research and Quality (AHRQ). (2009). *Who should be screened for abdominal aortic aneurysm? Clinical fact sheet.* Rockville, MD: AHRQ. Available at http://www.ahrq.gov/clinic/cvd/aaaprovider.htm

American College of Physicians. (2013). ACP publishes recommendations on upper endoscopy for gastroesophageal reflux disease. *American Family Physician, 88*(12), 865. Available at http://www.aafp.org/afp/2013/1215/p865.html

Anand, B. (2015). Peptic ulcer disease: Epidemiology. Available at http://emedicine.medscape.com/article/181753-overview#a7

Carson-DeWitt, R. (2015). Screening for peptic ulcer disease. Available at http://health.cvs.com/GetContent.aspx?token=f75979d3-9c7c-4b16-af56-3e122a3f19e3&chunkiid=19988

Cesario, K., Choure, A., & Carey, W. (2013). Cirrhotic ascites. Available at http://www.clevelandclinicmeded.com/medicalpubs/diseasemanagement/hepatology/complications-of-cirrhosis-ascites/

Crowe, S. (2017). Patient education: Peptic ulcer disease (Beyond the basics). Available at https://www.uptodate.com/contents/peptic-ulcer-disease-beyond-the-basics

Gupta, K., Dhawan, A., Abel, C., Talley, N., & Attia, J. (2013). A re-evaluation of the scratch test for locating the liver edge. *BMC Gastroenterology, 13*, 35. doi: 10.1186/1471-230X-13-35. Available at http://bmcgastroenterol.biomedcentral.com/articles/10.1186/1471-230X-13-35

Harvard Medical School. (2012). The gut-brain connections. Available at http://www.health.harvard.edu/healthbeat/the-gut-brain-connection

Healthy People 2020 (2015). Topics and objectives. Available at http://www.healthypeople.gov/2020/topics-objectives

HealthyPeople.gov. (2011). About Healthy People: Secretary's advisory committee. Available at http://healthypeople.gov/2020/about/advisory/FACA11Minutes.aspx?page=4

Mayo Clinic. (2014). GERD. Available at http://www.mayoclinic.org/diseases-conditions/gerd/basics/definition/con-20025201

National Digestive Disease Information Clearinghouse (NDDIC). (2012). Irritable bowel syndrome. Available at http://digestive.niddk.nih.gov/ddiseases/pubs/ibs/

National Institute of Diabetes and Digestive and Kidney Diseases (NIDDK). (2014). Smoking and the digestive system. Available at http://www.niddk.nih.gov/health-information/health-topics/digestive-diseases/smoking/Pages/facts.aspx

National Institute of Diabetes and Digestive and Kidney Diseases (NIDDK). (2014). Symptoms and causes of GER and GERD. Available at http://www.niddk.nih.gov/health-information/health-topics/digestive-diseases/ger-and-gerd-in-adults/Pages/symptoms-causes.aspx

National Organization of Rare Disorders. (2016). Zollinger-Ellison syndrome. Available at https://rarediseases.org/rare-diseases/zollinger-ellison-syndrome/

Nichols, A. (2014). Heat-related illness in sports and exercise. *Current Review in Musculoskeletal Medicine, 7*(4), 355–365.

Phillips, L., & Prins, J. (2008). The link between abdominal obesity and the metabolic syndrome. *Current Hypertension Reports, 10*(2), 156–164. Available at http://www.ncbi.nlm.nih.gov/pubmed/18474184

Seraq, H., Sweet, S., Winchester, C., & Dent. J. (2014). Update on the epidemiology of gastro-oesogeal reflux disease: A systematic review. *Gut, 63*(6), 871–880.

University of Maryland Medical Center (UMMC). (2014). Motion sickness. Available at http://umm.edu/health/medical/altmed/condition/motion-sickness

University of Maryland Medical Center (UMMC). (2015). Peptic ulcer. Available at http://www.umm.edu/health/medical/altmed/condition/peptic-ulcer

University of Pittsburgh Medical Center (UPMC). (2016). GERD: Gastroesophageal reflux disease. Available at http://www.upmc.com/patients-visitors/education/gastro/pages/gerd.aspx

U.S. Preventive Services Task Force (USPSTF). (2015). Abdominal aortic aneurysm: Screening. Available at http://www.uspreventiveservicestaskforce.org/Page/Document/UpdateSummaryFinal/abdominal-aortic-aneurysm-screening

24 ASSESSING MUSCULOSKELETAL SYSTEM

Learning Objectives

1. Describe the structure and the function of the musculoskeletal system.
2. Interview a client for an accurate nursing history of the musculoskeletal system.
3. Perform a physical assessment of the musculoskeletal system using the correct techniques.
4. Differentiate between normal and abnormal findings of the musculoskeletal system.
5. Describe the findings frequently seen with assessing the older client's musculoskeletal system.
6. Analyze the data from the interview and physical assessment of the musculoskeletal system to formulate valid nursing diagnoses, collaborative problems, and/or referrals.
7. Differentiate between general routine screening versus skills needed for focused or specialty assessment of the musculoskeletal system.
8. Document and verbally report accurate assessment findings of the musculoskeletal system.

CASE STUDY

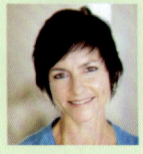

Frances Funstead, a 55-year-old Caucasian woman, presents to the occupational health nurse asking for help with her back pain. She works on an assembly line and believes her back pain may be related to her job.

STRUCTURE AND FUNCTION

The body's bones, muscles, and joints compose the musculoskeletal system. Controlled and innervated by the nervous system, the musculoskeletal system's overall purpose is to provide structure and movement for body parts.

Bones

Bones provide structure and protection, serve as levers, store calcium, and produce blood cells. A total of 206 bones make up the *axial skeleton* (head and trunk) and the *appendicular skeleton* (extremities, shoulders, and hips; Fig. 24-1).

Composed of osseous tissue, bones can be divided into two types: *compact bone*, which is hard and dense and makes up the shaft and outer layers; and *spongy bone*, which contains numerous spaces and makes up the ends and centers of the bones. Bone tissue is formed by active cells called *osteoblasts* and degraded by cells referred to as *osteoclasts*. Bones contain red marrow that produces blood cells and yellow marrow composed mostly of fat.

The *periosteum* covers the bones; it contains osteoblasts and blood vessels that promote nourishment and formation of new bone tissues. Bone shapes vary and include short bones (e.g., carpals), long bones (e.g., humerus, femur), flat bones (e.g., sternum, ribs), and bones with an irregular shape (e.g., hips, vertebrae).

Skeletal Muscles

The body consists of three types of *muscles:* skeletal, smooth, and cardiac. The musculoskeletal system is made up of 650 *skeletal (voluntary) muscles,* which are under conscious control (Fig. 24-2), and are made up of long muscle fibers (fasciculi) arranged together in bundles and joined by connective tissue. Skeletal muscles attach to bones by way of strong, fibrous cords called *tendons. These muscles* assist with posture, produce body heat, and allow the body to move. Skeletal muscle movements (illustrated in Box 24-1) include:

- Abduction: Moving away from midline of the body
- Adduction: Moving toward midline of the body
- Circumduction: Circular motion
- Inversion: Moving inward
- Eversion: Moving outward
- Extension: Straightening the extremity at the joint and increasing the angle of the joint
  - Hyperextension: Joint bends greater than 180 degrees

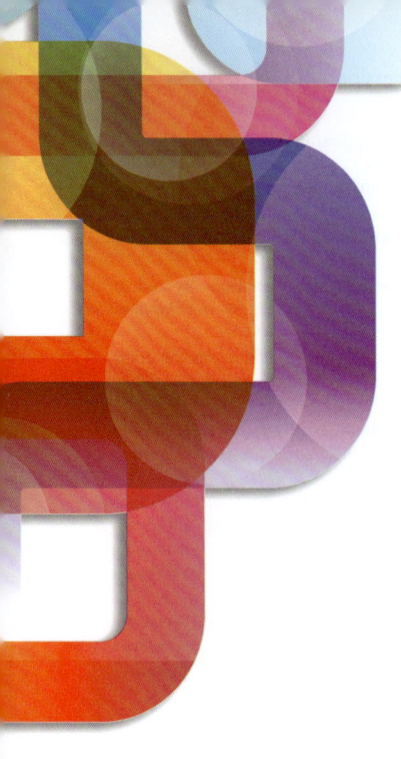

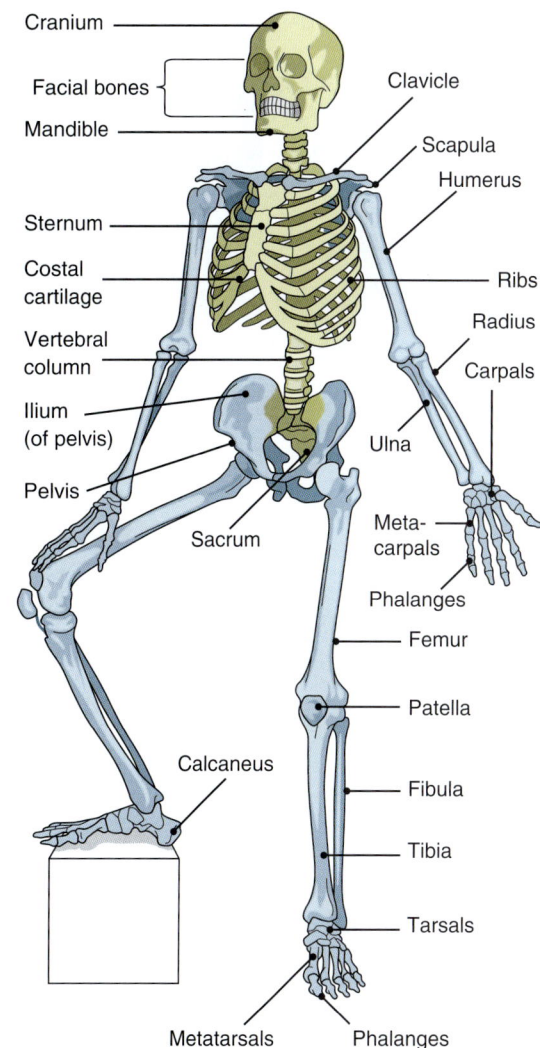

FIGURE 24-1 Major bones of the skeleton. The axial skeleton is shown in *yellow;* the appendicular skeleton is shown in *blue.*

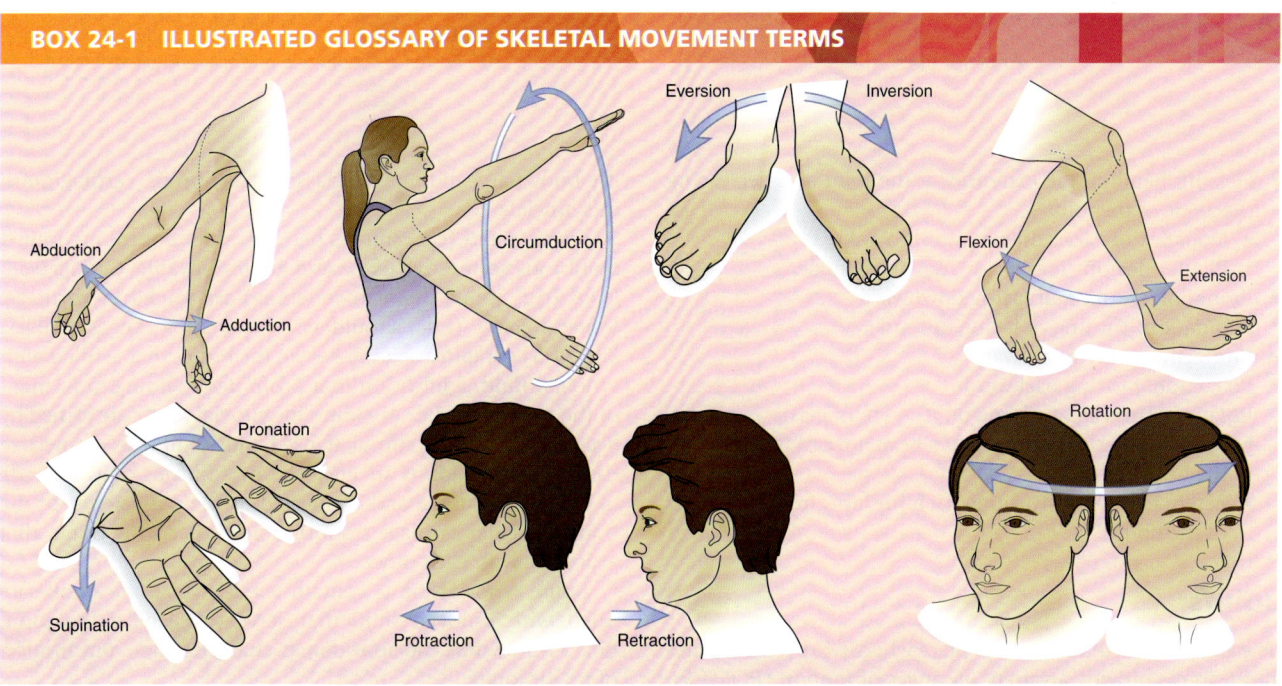

BOX 24-1   ILLUSTRATED GLOSSARY OF SKELETAL MOVEMENT TERMS

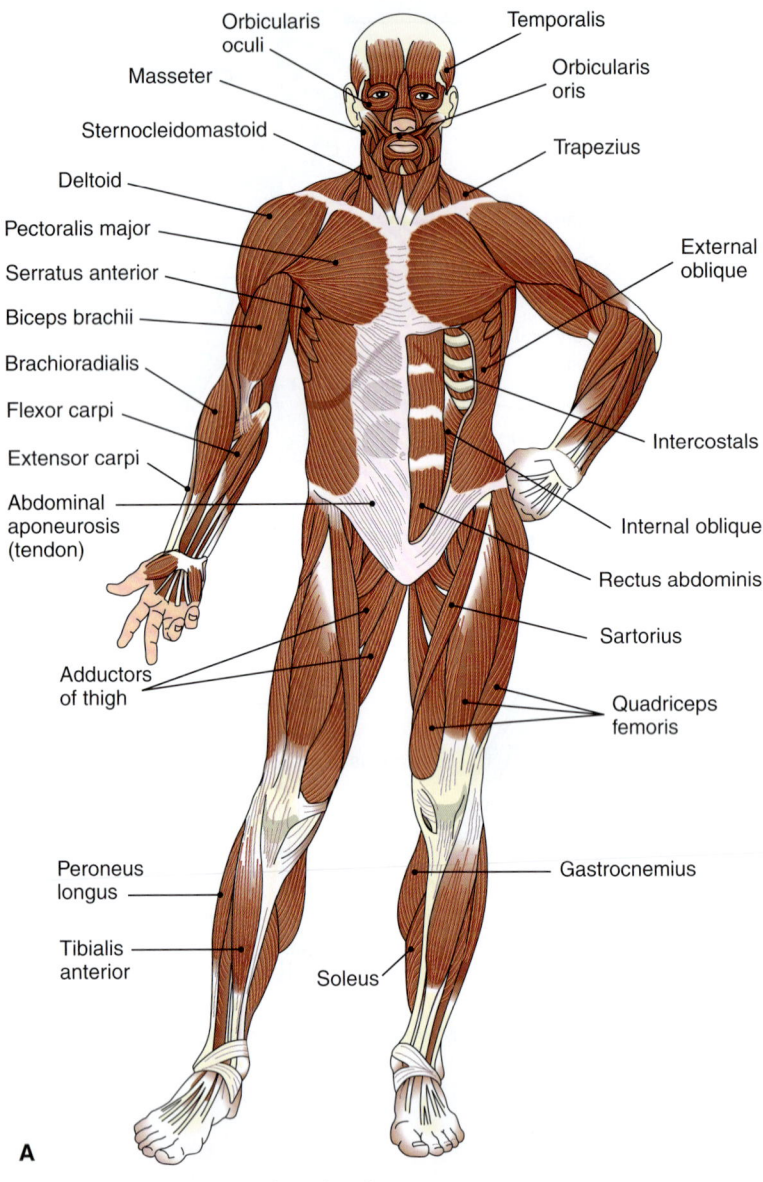

FIGURE 24-2 Muscles of the body: (A) anterior; (B) posterior. (*continued on following page*)

- Flexion: Bending the extremity at the joint and decreasing the angle of the joint
  - Dorsiflexion: Toes draw upward to ankle
  - Plantar flexion: Toes point away from ankle
- Pronation: Turning or facing downward
- Supination: Turning or facing upward
- Protraction: Moving forward
- Retraction: Moving backward
- Rotation: Turning of a bone on its own long axis
  - Internal rotation: Turning of a bone toward the center of the body
  - External rotation: Turning of a bone away from the center of the body

Joints

The *joint* (or articulation) is the place where two or more bones meet. Joints provide a variety of ranges of motion (ROM) for the body parts and may be classified as fibrous, cartilaginous, or synovial.

Fibrous joints (e.g., sutures between skull bones) are joined by fibrous connective tissue and are immovable. *Cartilaginous joints* (e.g., joints between vertebrae) are joined by cartilage. *Synovial joints* (e.g., shoulders, wrists, hips, knees, ankles; Fig. 24-3) contain a space between the bones that is filled with synovial fluid, a lubricant that promotes a sliding movement of the ends of the bones. Bones in synovial joints are joined by *ligaments*, which are strong, dense bands of fibrous connective tissue. Synovial joints are enclosed by a fibrous capsule made of connective tissue and connected to the periosteum of the bone. Articular cartilage smooths and protects the bones that articulate with each other.

Some synovial joints contain *bursae*, which are small sacs filled with synovial fluid that serve to cushion the joint. Box 24-2 reviews the appearance, characteristics, and motion of major joints.

24 Assessing Musculoskeletal System 531

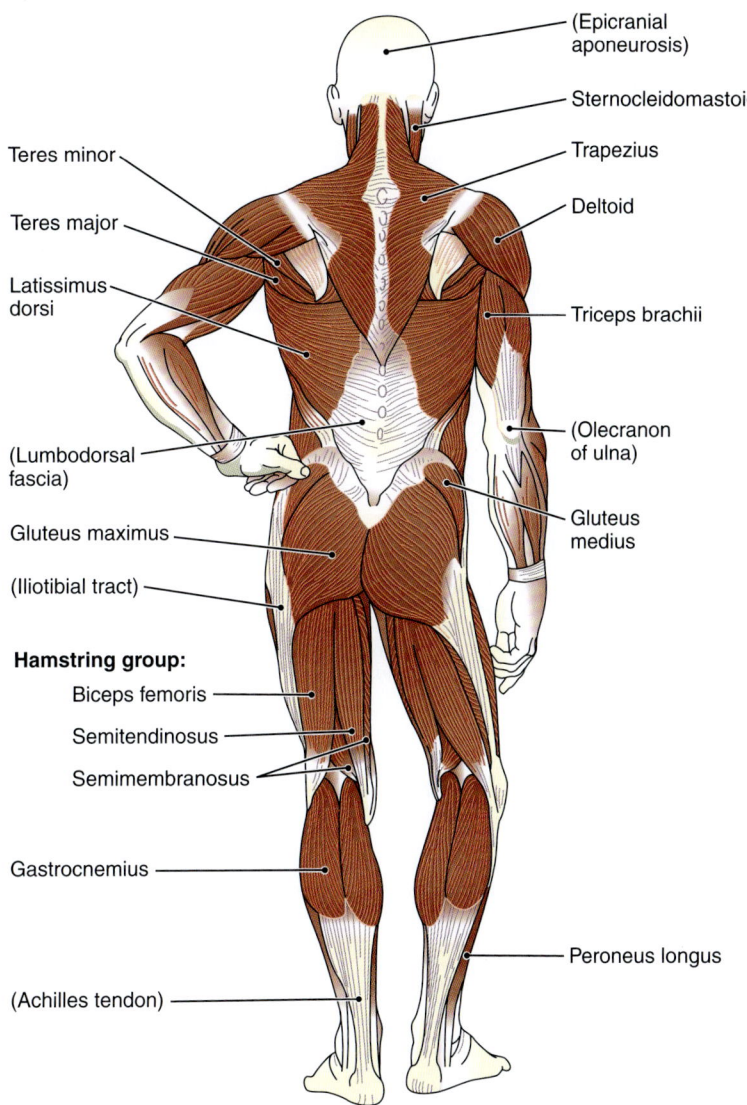

FIGURE 24-2 (Continued) B Posterior view

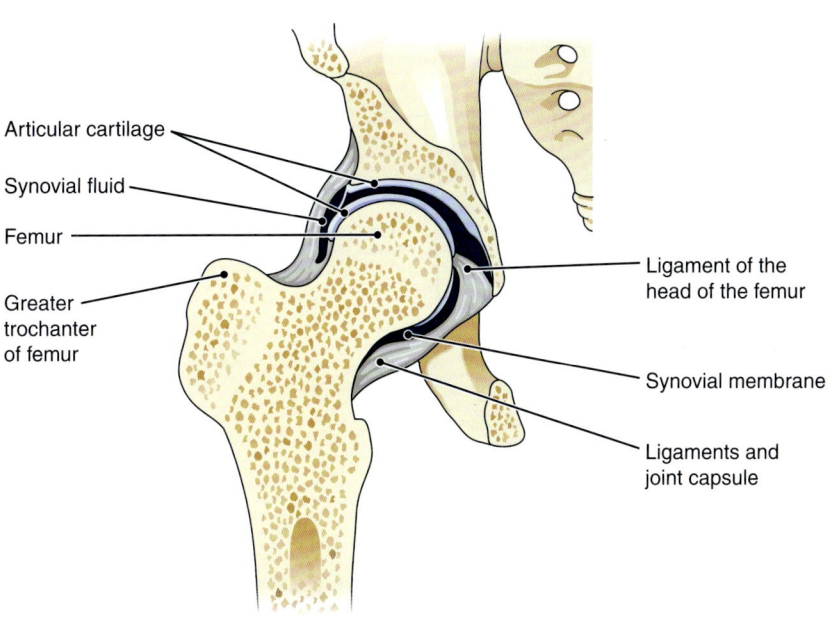

FIGURE 24-3 Components of synovial joints (right hip joint).

BOX 24-2 UNDERSTANDING MAJOR JOINTS

TEMPOROMANDIBULAR
Articulation between the temporal bone and mandible. Motion:
- Opens and closes mouth.
- Projects and retracts jaw.
- Moves jaw from side to side.

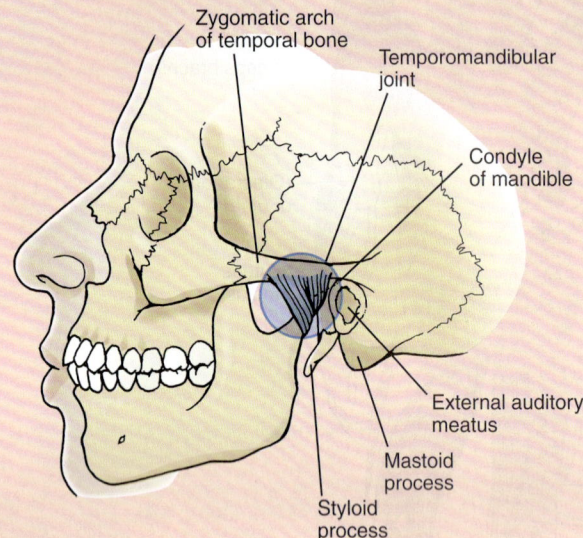

ELBOW
Articulation between the ulna and radius of the lower arm and the humerus of the upper arm; contains a synovial membrane and several bursae. Motion:
- Flexion and extension of the forearm
- Supination and pronation of the forearm

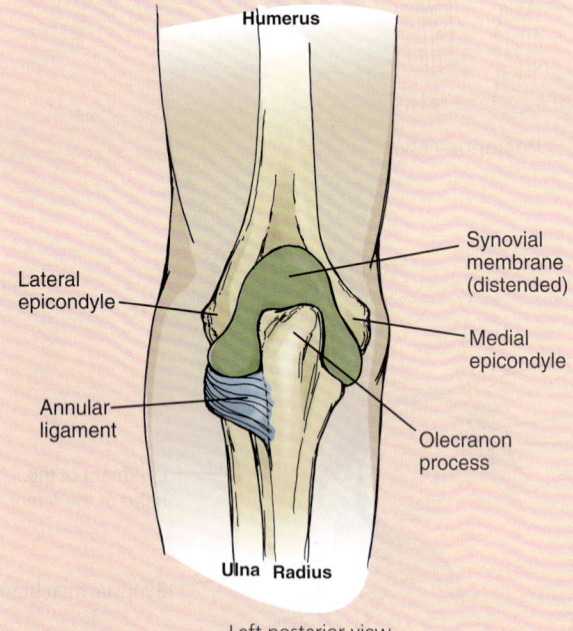

Left posterior view.

STERNOCLAVICULAR
Junction between the manubrium of the sternum and the clavicle; has no obvious movements.

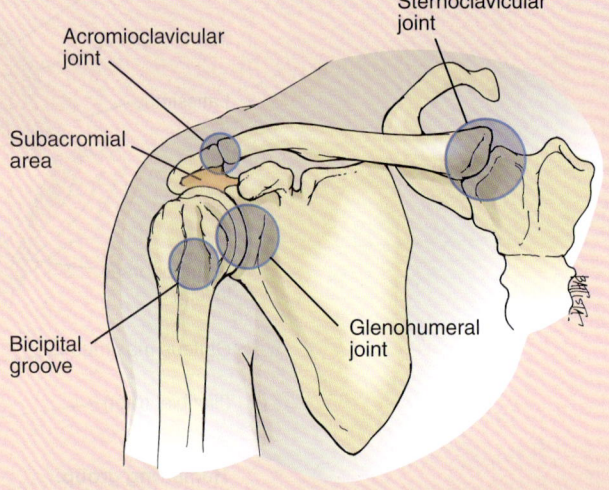

SHOULDER
Articulation of the head of the humerus in the glenoid cavity of the scapula. The acromioclavicular joint includes the clavicle and acromion process of the scapula. It contains the subacromial and subscapular bursae. Motion:
- Flexion and extension
- Abduction and adduction
- Circumduction
- Rotation (internal and external)

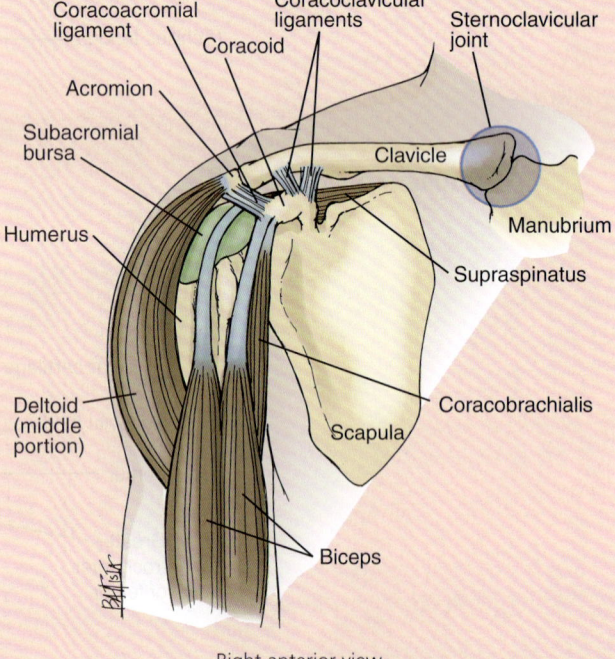

Right anterior view.

WRIST, FINGERS, THUMB

Articulation between the distal radius, ulnar bone, carpals, and metacarpals. Contains ligaments and is lined with a synovial membrane. Motion:
- Wrists: Flexion, extension, hyperextension, adduction, radial and ulnar deviation
- Fingers: Flexion, extension, hyperextension, abduction, and circumduction
- Thumb: Flexion, extension, and opposition

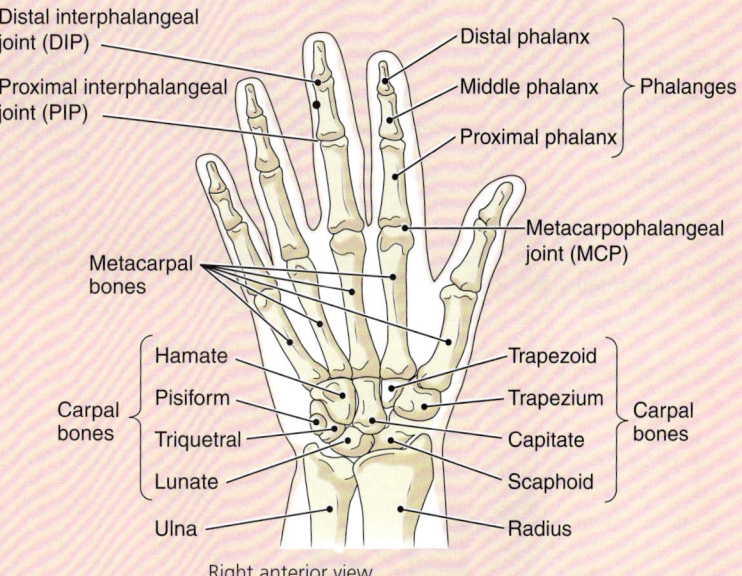

Right anterior view.

VERTEBRAE (LATERAL VIEW)

Thirty-three bones: 7 concave-shaped cervical (C); 12 convex-shaped thoracic (T); 5 concave-shaped lumbar (L); 5 sacral (S); and 3–4 coccygeal, connected in a vertical column. Bones are cushioned by elastic fibrocartilaginous plates (intervertebral discs) that provide flexibility and posture to the spine. Paravertebral muscles are positioned on both sides of vertebrae. Motion:
- Flexion
- Hyperextension
- Lateral bending
- Rotation

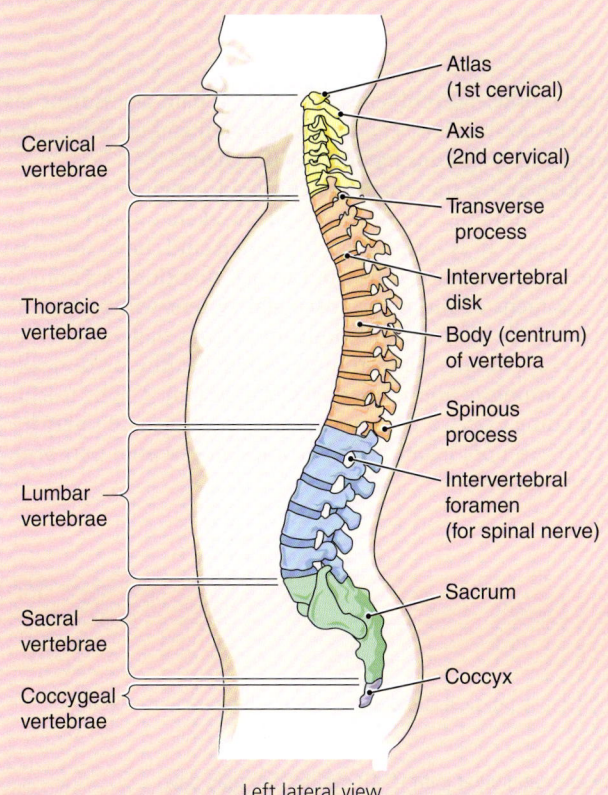

Left lateral view.

HIP

Articulation between the head of the femur and the acetabulum. Contains a fibrous capsule. Motion:
- Flexion with knee flexed and with knee extended
- Extension and hyperextension
- Circumduction
- Rotation (internal and external)
- Abduction
- Adduction

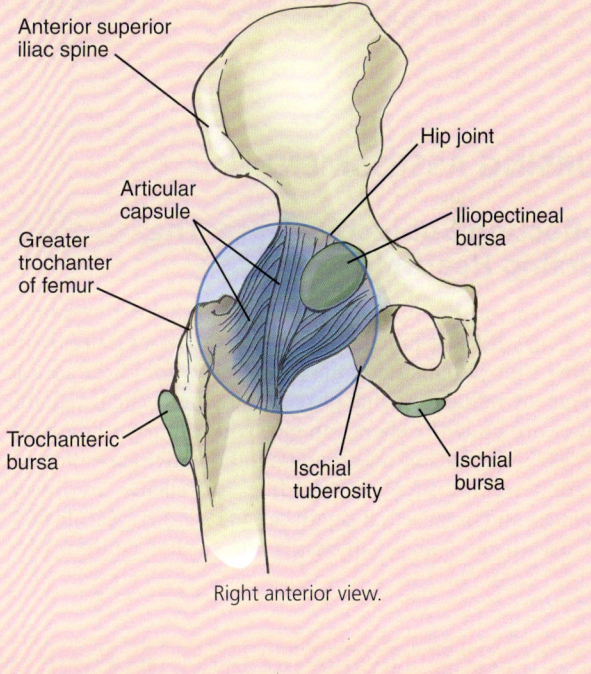

Right anterior view.

Continued on following page

BOX 24-2 UNDERSTANDING MAJOR JOINTS (Continued)

KNEE
Articulation of the femur, tibia, and patella; contains fibrocartilaginous discs (medial and lateral menisci) and many bursae. Motion:
- Flexion
- Extension

ANKLE AND FOOT
Articulation between the talus (large posterior foot tarsal), tibia, and fibula. The talus also articulates with the navicular bones. The heel (calcaneus bone) is connected to the tibia and fibula by ligaments. Motion:
- Ankle: Plantar flexion and dorsiflexion
- Foot: Inversion and eversion
- Toes: Flexion, extension, abduction, adduction

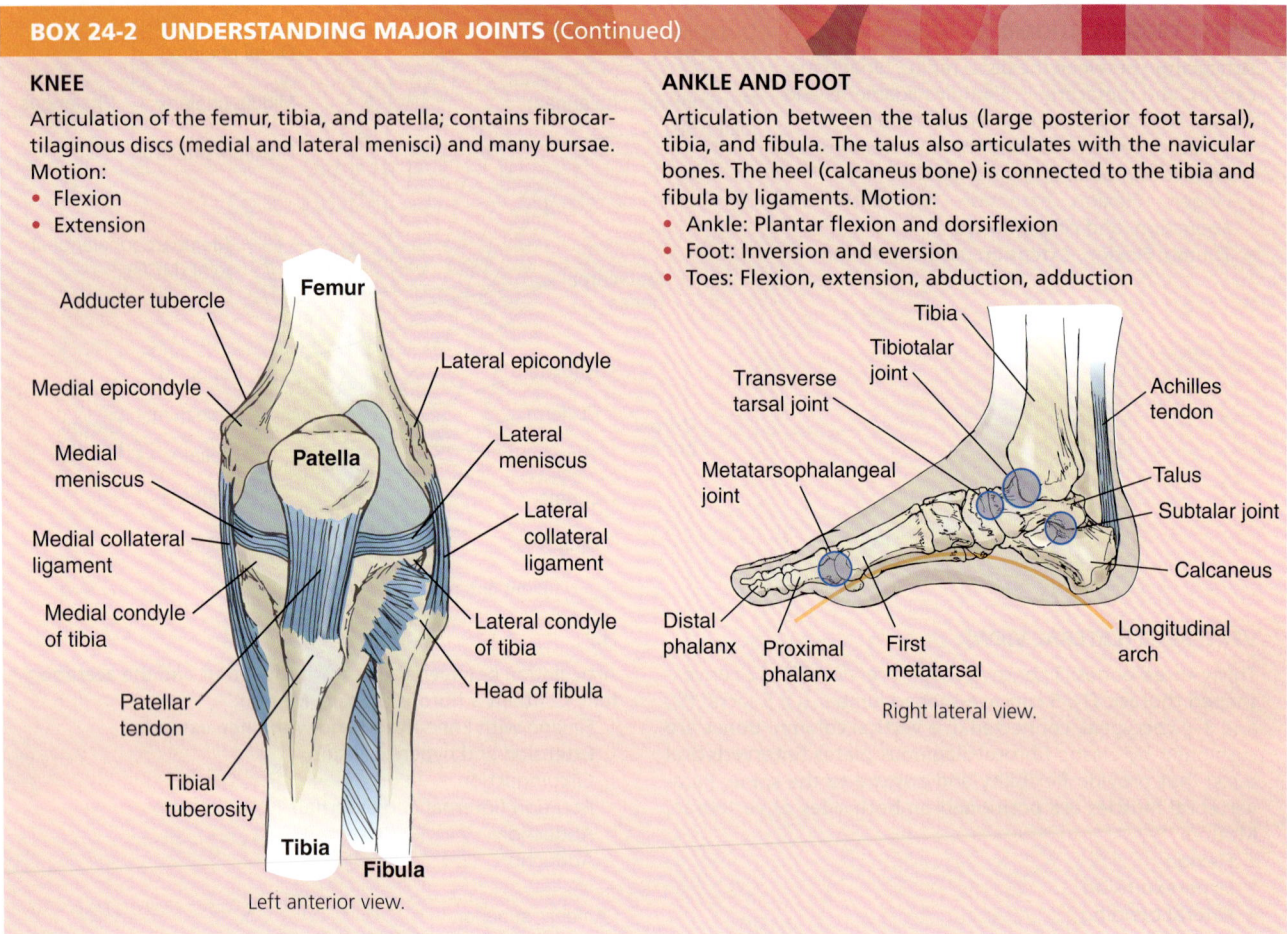

NURSING ASSESSMENT

Collecting Subjective Data: The Nursing Health History

Assessment of the musculoskeletal system helps to evaluate the client's level of functioning with activities of daily living (ADLs). This system affects the entire body, from head to toe, and greatly influences what physical activities a client can and cannot do. Only the client can give you data regarding pain, stiffness, and levels of movement and how ADLs are affected. In addition, information regarding the client's nutrition, activities, and exercise is a significant part of the musculoskeletal assessment. Pain or stiffness is often a chief concern with musculoskeletal problems; therefore, a pain assessment may also be needed. It is very important to remember to investigate signs and symptoms reported by the client.

Remember, too, that the neurologic system is responsible for coordinating the functions of the skeleton and muscles. Therefore, it is important to understand how these systems relate to each other and to ask questions accordingly. Assessment of the musculoskeletal system will provide the nurse with information about the client's daily activity and exercise patterns that promote either healthy or unhealthy functioning of the musculoskeletal system. Client teaching regarding exercise, diet, positioning, posture, and safety habits to promote health thus becomes an essential part of this examination.

History of Present Health Concern

QUESTION	RATIONALE
Have you had any recent weight gain?	Weight gain can increase physical stress and strain on the musculoskeletal system.
Describe any difficulty that you have chewing. Is it associated with tenderness or pain?	Clients with temporomandibular joint (TMJ) dysfunction may have difficulty chewing and may describe their jaws as "getting locked or stuck." Jaw tenderness, pain, or a clicking sound may also be present with TMJ.

QUESTION	RATIONALE
Describe any joint, muscle, or bone pain you have. Where is the pain? What does the pain feel like (stab, ache)? When did the pain start? When does it occur? How long does it last? Any stiffness, swelling, limitation of movement?	Bone pain is often dull, deep, and throbbing. Joint or muscle pain is described as aching, but has been differentiated between mechanical- and inflammatory-type pains (Harris et al., 2012). Sharp, knife-like pain occurs with most fractures and increases with motion of the affected body part. Osteoarthritis pain usually begins in one set of joints and on one side of the body, with a feeling of pain deep in the joint, improving with rest but worsening with rainy weather, perhaps a sensation of bones grating together, with stiffness early in the morning improving with movement. Rheumatoid arthritis pain is varied and may feel burning, throbbing, occurs on both sides of the body, worsens after sitting for long periods, has inconsistent pattern of worse and less pain, and with a feeling of heat and soreness in joints (Rodriguez, 2015). Fibromyalgia, a disorder characterized by widespread musculoskeletal pain accompanied by fatigue, sleep, memory, and mood changes, or cognitive disorders, is hard to diagnose (Mayo Clinic, 2015). Causes seem to be genetic or from triggers such as infections or physical or emotional trauma. Females, those with family history, or those having a rheumatic disease are at risk. Diagnosis no longer includes specific pressure points for pain, but only the history of widespread pain for 3 months with no underlying cause for the pain. Although nonspecific, blood tests for CBC, sedimentation rate, and thyroid function are often performed.

Personal Health History

QUESTION	RATIONALE
Describe any past problems or injuries you have had to your joints, muscles, or bones. What treatment was given? Do you have any aftereffects from the injury or problem?	This information provides baseline data for the physical examination. Past injuries may affect the client's current ROM and level of function in affected joints and extremities. A history of recurrent fractures may be seen with osteomalacia but should also raise the question of possible physical abuse. **OLDER ADULT CONSIDERATIONS** **Bones lose their density with age, putting the older client at risk for bone fractures, especially of the wrists, hips, and vertebrae. Older clients who have osteomalacia or osteoporosis are at an even greater risk for fractures.**
When were your last tetanus and polio immunizations?	Joint stiffening and other musculoskeletal symptoms may be a transient effect of the tetanus, whooping cough, diphtheria, or polio vaccines (Centers for Disease Control and Prevention [CDC], 2015). **OLDER ADULT CONSIDERATIONS** **Joint-stiffening conditions may be misdiagnosed as arthritis, especially in the older adult.**
Have you ever been diagnosed with diabetes mellitus, sickle cell anemia, systemic lupus erythematosus (SLE), or osteoporosis?	Having diabetes mellitus, sickle cell anemia, or SLE places the client at risk for development of musculoskeletal problems such as osteoporosis and osteomyelitis. Type 1 diabetes increases risk of low bone density, and may increase fracture risk, but fractures may be related to poor vision and nerve damage, which are likely to produce falls. Although clients with type 2 diabetes often have increased body weight and thereby increased bone density, they too are likely to have an increased risk of fractures due to vision and nerve damage (National Institutes of Health Osteoporosis and Related Bone Diseases National Resource Center [NIH ORBDNRC], 2015). Clients who are immobile or have a reduced intake of calcium and vitamin D are especially prone to develop osteoporosis. **OLDER ADULT CONSIDERATIONS** **Osteoporosis is more common as a person ages because that is when bone resorption increases, calcium absorption decreases, and production of osteoblasts decreases.**
For middle-aged women: Have you started menopause? Are you taking estrogen or hormone replacement therapy?	Women who begin menarche late or begin menopause early are at greater risk for development of osteoporosis because of decreased estrogen levels, which tend to decrease the density of bone mass (Li & Zhu, 2005).

Continued on following page

Family History

QUESTION	RATIONALE
Do you have a family history of rheumatoid arthritis, gout, or osteoporosis?	These conditions tend to be familial and can increase the client's risk for development of these diseases.

Lifestyle and Health Practices

QUESTION	RATIONALE
What activities do you engage in to promote the health of your muscles and bones (e.g., exercise, diet, weight reduction)?	This question provides the examiner with knowledge of how much the client understands and actively participates in activities to promote the health of the musculoskeletal system.
What medications are you taking?	Some medications can affect musculoskeletal function. Diuretics, for example, can alter electrolyte levels, leading to muscle weakness. Steroids can deplete bone mass, thereby contributing to osteoporosis. Adverse reactions to HMG-CoA reductase inhibitors (statins) can include myopathy, which can cause muscle pain, soreness, tiredness, or weakness (U.S. Food and Drug Administration [USFDA], 2015).
Do you smoke tobacco? How much and how often?	Smoking increases the risk of osteoporosis (see Evidence-Based Health Promotion and Disease Prevention 24-1).
Do you drink alcohol or caffeinated beverages? How much and how often?	Excessive consumption of alcohol or caffeine can increase the risk of osteoporosis.
Describe your typical 24-hour diet. Are you able to consume milk or milk-containing products? Do you take any calcium supplements?	Adequate protein in the diet promotes muscle tone and bone growth; vitamin C promotes healing of tissues and bones. A calcium deficiency increases the risk of osteoporosis. Vitamin D intake via sun exposure, dietary sources and/or supplement is required to absorb calcium (Usual recommendations vary between 400 IU and 1,000 IU per day, varying with age. The Institute of Medicine notes that a safe upper limit for vitamin D intake is 4,000 IU daily for most adults [National Osteoporosis Foundation, 2016]). A diet high in purine (e.g., meat, liver, sardines) and alcohol can trigger gouty arthritis. **CULTURAL CONSIDERATIONS** Lactose intolerance (a deficiency of the lactase enzyme) affects up 65% of adult humans (and animals) due to decreased production of the lactase enzyme at weaning. Between 80% and 100% of Asians and Native Americans are lactose intolerant. Most of the world's population is between 50% and 90% intolerant. Only those of Northern European descent have only a 5–20% intolerance (Lactose Intolerance by Ethnicity and Region, 2010).
Describe your activities during a typical day. How much time do you spend in the sunlight?	A sedentary lifestyle increases the risk of osteoporosis. Prolonged immobility leads to muscle atrophy. Exposure to 20 minutes of sunlight per day promotes the production of vitamin D in the body. Vitamin D deficiency can cause osteomalacia and limit calcium absorption.
Describe any routine exercise that you do.	Regular exercise promotes flexibility, muscle tone, and strength, while weight-bearing exercises are the only exercises that can promote bone density. Regular exercise can also help to slow the usual musculoskeletal changes, progressive loss of total bone mass (osteopenia/osteoporosis), and degeneration of skeletal muscle fibers (sarcopenia) that occur with aging. Improper body positioning in contact sports results in injury to the bones, joints, or muscles.
Describe your occupation.	Certain job-related activities increase the risk for development of musculoskeletal problems. For example, incorrect body mechanics, heavy lifting, or poor posture can contribute to back problems; consistent, repetitive wrist and hand movements can lead to the development of carpal tunnel syndrome.
Describe your posture at work and at leisure. What type of shoes do you usually wear? Do you use any special footwear (i.e., orthotics)?	Poor posture, prolonged forward bending (as in sitting) or backward leaning (as in working overhead), or long-term carrying of heavy objects on the shoulders can result in back problems. Contracture of the Achilles tendon can occur with prolonged use of high-heeled shoes.

QUESTION	RATIONALE
Do you have difficulty performing normal activities of daily living (bathing, dressing, grooming, eating)? Do you use assistive devices (e.g., walker, cane, braces) to promote your mobility and activities of daily living?	Impairment of the musculoskeletal system may impair the client's ability to perform normal ADLs. Correct use of assistive devices can promote safety and independence. Some clients may feel embarrassed and not use their prescribed or needed assistive device.
How have your musculoskeletal problems interfered with your ability to interact or socialize with others? Have they interfered with your usual sexual activity?	Musculoskeletal problems, especially chronic ones, can disable and cripple the client, which may impair socialization and prevent the client from performing the same roles as in the past. Back problems, joint pain, or muscle stiffness may interfere with sexual activities.
How did you view yourself before you had this musculoskeletal problem, and how do you view yourself now?	Body image disturbances and chronic low self-esteem may occur with a disabling or crippling problem.
Has your musculoskeletal problem added stress to your life? Describe.	Musculoskeletal problems often greatly affect ADLs and role performance, resulting in changed relationships and increased stress.
Have you ever had a bone density screening? When was your last one?	The U.S. Preventive Services Task Force (USPSTF, 2011) recommends that women younger than age 60 get bone density scans if they have risk factors for osteoporosis, including a history of fractured bones, being Caucasian, smoking, alcohol abuse, or a slender frame. Bone density screening is recommended for all women at age 60.
Ask clients to complete the online interactive International Osteoporosis Foundation (IOF) One-Minute Osteoporosis Risk Test (http://www.iofbonehealth.org/iof-one-minute-osteoporosis-risk-test) and to discuss the results with their health care provider.	Answering "yes" to any of these questions does not mean one has osteoporosis. However, positive answers indicate that the client has risk factors that may lead to osteoporosis and fractures.

24-1 EVIDENCE-BASED HEALTH PROMOTION AND DISEASE PREVENTION: OSTEOPOROSIS

INTRODUCTION

Osteoporosis is a disease in which bones demineralize and become porous and fragile, making them susceptible to fractures. The bone loss occurs silently and progressively, and often no symptoms are noted until the first fracture occurs. Normally, bones are densest during the early 20s, but aging causes the bone remodeling process (bone resorption and bone formation) to change, leading to lower bone mass and osteoporosis, when bone resorption outpaces reformation (The International Osteoporosis Foundation [IOF], 2015a). Osteoporosis fractures most commonly occur in the spine, wrist, and hip. Spinal fractures lead to loss in height and development of a curved upper back (often called a Dowager hump).

As of 2014, the National Osteoporosis Foundation (NOF) reported that 54 million Americans aged 50 and older are affected by osteoporosis (10.2 million) or low bone mass (43.4 million). According to the IOF (2015b), osteoporosis affects 200 million women worldwide—approximately one tenth of women aged 60, one fifth of women aged 70, two fifths of women aged 80 and two thirds of women aged 90. One in 3 women and 1 in 5 men will have a fractured bone, with hip, forearm, and vertebral fractures predominating. Europeans and Americans accounted for 51% of osteoporosis-related fractures in the year 2000, followed by people from the Western Pacific and Southeast Asia. Osteoporosis is lowest in black males and highest in white females (Andrews & Boyle, 2016, p. 92). The Bosham Clinic Medical (2014, p. 1) states that osteoporosis is a global health problem and the great majority of persons at high risk of hip fracture (as high as 80%) have already had at least one osteoporotic fracture that has neither been identified nor treated.

HEALTHY PEOPLE 2020 GOAL

Healthy People 2020 (2016) has a topic category for arthritis, osteoporosis, and chronic back conditions. Osteoporosis is described as a disease that is "marked by reduced bone strength leading to an increased risk of fractures (broken bones)."

GOAL (for all 3 conditions)

Prevent illness and disability related to arthritis and other rheumatic conditions, osteoporosis, and chronic back conditions.

OBJECTIVES (OSTEOPOROSIS)

- Reduce the proportion of adults with osteoporosis by 10%, from 5.9% of adults aged 50 years and older in 2005–2008, to 5.3%.
- Reduce the number of hip fractures in adults aged 65 years and older by 10% (both females and males).

Continued on following page

24-1 EVIDENCE-BASED HEALTH PROMOTION AND DISEASE PREVENTION: OSTEOPOROSIS (Continued)

SCREENING

The U.S. Preventive Services Task Force (USPSTF, 2011) recommends screening for osteoporosis in women aged 65 years or older and in younger women whose fracture risk is equal to or greater than that of a 65-year-old Caucasian woman who has no additional risk factors. The USPSTF concludes that the current evidence is insufficient to assess the balance of benefits and harms of screening for osteoporosis in men. The inclusion of women under 65 years of age (and as young as 50) who have risk for fracture is a new recommendation. The risk factors these younger women must have to indicate screening include, "having parents who fractured bones, being white, a history of smoking, alcohol abuse, or a slender frame" (Goodman, 2011). The recommended screening is for a bone density scan. A simple, easy to take 1-minute osteoporosis risk assessment test can be recommended by any health care provider, either to be administered or for clients to take themselves (IOF, 2015c).

RISK ASSESSMENT

Assess for the following risk factors for *osteoporosis* (IOF, 2015a):

Fixed risk factors:
- Age
- Female gender
- Family history of osteoporosis
- Previous fracture
- Ethnicity
- Menopause/hysterectomy
- Long-term glucocorticoid therapy
- Rheumatoid arthritis
- Primary/secondary hypogonadism in men

Modifiable risk factors (for osteoporosis and for fractures):
- Alcohol (greater than 2 drinks a day)
- Smoking (past or current history)
- Low body mass index (<20 kg/m^2)
- Poor nutrition (low calcium intake and low protein intake)
- Vitamin D deficiency
- Eating disorders (leading to nutrition deficiencies)
- Low dietary calcium intake
- Insufficient exercise (especially sedentary lifestyle)
- Frequent falls

Assess for the following risk factors for *fracture* (for questions to ask clients, see Osteoporosis Canada, 2017):
- Age 65 or older
- Vertebral compression fracture
- Fracture with minimal trauma after age 40
- Family history of osteoporotic fracture (especially parental hip fracture)
- Long-term (more than 3 months continuously) use of glucocorticoid therapy such as prednisone
- Medical conditions (such as celiac disease, Crohn disease) that inhibit absorption of nutrients
- Primary hyperparathyroidism
- Tendency to fall
- Spinal fracture apparent on x-ray
- Hypogonadism (low testosterone in men, loss of menstrual periods in younger women)
- Early menopause (before age 45)
- Rheumatoid arthritis
- Hyperthyroidism
- Low body weight (<60 kg)
- If present weight is more than 10% below weight at age 25
- Low calcium intake
- Excess alcohol (consistently more than 2 drinks a day)
- Smoking
- Low bone mineral density (BMD)

Risk factors are additive, meaning that the more risk factors a person has, the greater the risk of developing osteoporosis.

CLIENT EDUCATION (IOF, 2015A)

Teach Parents of Children and Adolescents to Help Their Children
- Ensure a nutritious diet with adequate calcium intake.
- Avoid protein malnutrition and undernutrition.
- Maintain an adequate supply of vitamin D.
- Participate in regular physical activity.
- Avoid the effects of second-hand smoke.

Teach Clients to Prevent Bone Loss
- Ensure a nutritious diet and adequate calcium intake.
- Avoid undernutrition, particularly the effects of severe weight-loss diets and eating disorders.
- Maintain an adequate supply of vitamin D.
- Participate in regular weight-bearing activity.
- Avoid smoking and second-hand smoking.
- Avoid heavy drinking.

CASE STUDY

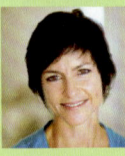

The case study introduced at the beginning of the chapter is now used to demonstrate how a nurse would use the COLDSPA mnemonic to explore Ms. Funstead's presenting concerns of back pain.

Mnemonic	Question	Data Provided
Character	Describe the sign or symptom (feeling, appearance, sound, smell, or taste if applicable).	"I have a dull, achy pain in my lower back. My back feels stiff and painful when I try to move certain ways."
Onset	When did it begin?	"I first noticed the pain about 2 weeks ago. It has gotten worse over the past 2 or 3 days."

Mnemonic	Question	Data Provided
Location	Where is it? Does it radiate? Does it occur anywhere else?	"It's in my lower back, just below my waist." Client denies radiation of pain, numbness, or paresthesias in the lower extremities.
Duration	How long does it last? Does it recur?	"I usually notice it in the morning when I first get up. It gets worse on days I have to work, getting in and out of the car, bending over, and sometimes just when I change positions. I have noticed that standing for long periods of time makes it really bad."
Severity	How bad is it? or How much does it bother you?	"It's bad enough that I have had to ask my supervisor for breaks after standing for a couple hours. After work, I go home and lie down. I haven't been cooking or cleaning for the past week." Client rates pain as 7 on scale of 0–10 prior to taking ibuprofen. An hour after taking ibuprofen, rates pain as 3–4 on a scale of 0–10.
Pattern	What makes it better or worse?	"Ibuprofen has helped some, but it seems to wear off before the next dose is due. I've tried resting and stretching too. Resting and stretching help some, but the pain never goes away completely."
Associated factors/How it Affects the client	What other symptoms occur with it? How does it affect you?	Client denies bowel or bladder incontinence. "I haven't been able to walk with my friends after work for the past 2 weeks. Also, I haven't been able to have sexual relations with my husband. I am tired of hurting."

After investigating Frances Funstead's concerns regarding back pain, the nurse continues with the health history.

Ms. Funstead denies any recent weight gain. She denies any past problems with joints, muscles, or bones. She reports that her immunizations are up to date. Denies diabetes, sickle cell anemia, SLE, or osteoporosis. Ms. Funstead reports that she is postmenopausal and not taking any estrogen replacement therapy.

Ms. Funstead denies family history of rheumatoid arthritis, gout, or osteoporosis.

Ms. Funstead reports that she tries to walk 30 minutes three times weekly and is usually successful. Client denies issues with weight gain or loss, but does feel as if she needs to lose weight. Ms. Funstead's medications include: Calcium with vitamin D supplement two times daily, ibuprofen 400 mg every 8 hours as needed.

Client denies use of tobacco or alcohol. She admits to drinking 3–4 cups of coffee each morning and 32 oz of diet cola throughout the day. Her 24-hour diet recall includes: Breakfast—cereal bar and coffee; lunch—low-calorie frozen meal, yogurt, apple, diet cola; dinner—chicken noodle soup, salad, fruit smoothie, 8-oz glass of 2% milk. Activities in a typical day include: Awakens at 5:30 AM and gets ready for work. Works from 7 AM to 3 PM. Walks after work with friends. Goes home, prepares dinner, does household chores, watches TV; in bed by 10:30 PM.

Ms. Funstead works at a local factory on an assembly line. She picks up small parts and places them in a motor. She twists from side to side throughout the work day. She has one 15-minute break in the morning, 30 minutes for lunch, and one 15-minute break in the afternoon. She stands while at work and is required to wear steel-toed shoes. She denies difficulty performing ADLs until this back problem developed. She does not require the use of assistive devices for mobility. Client denies any change in body image or self-esteem.

Collecting Objective Data: Physical Examination

Physical assessment of the musculoskeletal system provides data regarding the client's posture, gait, bone structure, muscle strength, and joint mobility, as well as the client's ability to perform ADLs.

The physical assessment includes inspecting and palpating the joints, muscles, and bones, testing ROM, and assessing muscle strength. See Assessment Guide 24-1 for guidelines to use when performing the musculoskeletal assessment.

Preparing the Client

Because this examination is lengthy, be sure that the room is at a comfortable temperature and provide rest periods as necessary. Provide adequate draping to avoid unnecessary exposure of the client yet adequate visualization of the part being examined. Explain that you will ask the client frequently to change positions and to move various body parts against resistance and gravity. Clear, simple directions need to be given throughout the examination to help the client understand how to move body parts to allow you to assess the musculoskeletal system. Demonstrating to the client how to move the various body parts and providing verbal directions facilitate examination.

OLDER ADULT CONSIDERATIONS
Some positions required for this examination may be very uncomfortable for the older client who may have decreased flexibility. Be sensitive to the client's needs and adapt your technique as necessary.

ASSESSMENT GUIDE 24-1 Assessing Joints and Muscles

The following are guidelines for assessing joints and muscle strength:

Joints

1. Inspect size, shape, color, and symmetry. Note any masses, deformities, or muscle atrophy. Compare bilateral joint findings.
2. Palpate for edema, heat, tenderness, pain, nodules, or crepitus. Compare bilateral joint findings.
3. Test each joint's range of motion (ROM). Demonstrate how to move each joint through its normal ROM, then ask the client to actively move the joint through the same motions. Compare bilateral joint findings.

OLDER ADULT CONSIDERATIONS

Older clients usually have slower movements, reduced flexibility, and decreased muscle strength because of age-related muscle fiber and joint degeneration, reduced elasticity of the tendons, and joint capsule calcification.

If you identify a limitation in ROM, measure ROM with a goniometer (a device that measures movement in degrees). To do so, move the arms of the goniometer to match the angle of the joint being assessed. Then describe the limited motion of the joint in degrees: for example, "elbow flexes from 45 degrees to 90 degrees."

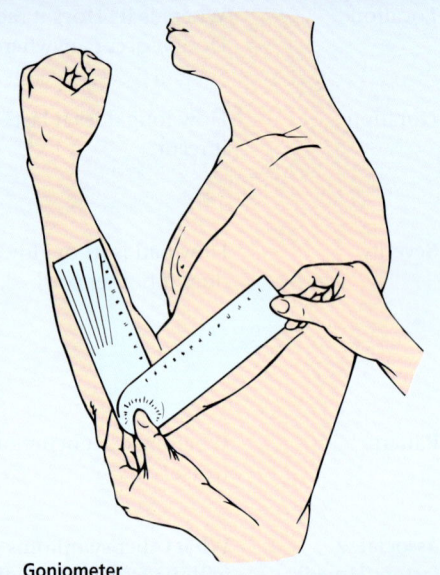

Goniometer

Muscles

1. Test muscle strength by asking the client to move each extremity through its full ROM against resistance. Do this by applying some resistance against the part being moved. Document muscle strength by using a standard scale (see the following Rating Scale for Muscle Strength). If the client cannot move the part against your resistance, ask the client to move the part against gravity. If this is not possible, then attempt to move the part passively through its full ROM. If this is not possible, then inspect and feel for a palpable contraction of the muscle while the client attempts to move it. Compare bilateral joint findings.

CLINICAL TIP

Do not force the part beyond its normal range. Stop passive motion if the client expresses discomfort or pain. Be especially cautious with the older client when testing ROM. When comparing bilateral strength, keep in mind that the client's dominant side will tend to be the stronger side.

2. Rate muscle strength in accord with the following strength table.

Rating	Explanation	Strength Classification
5	Active motion against full resistance	Normal
4	Active motion against some resistance	Slight weakness
3	Active motion against gravity	Average weakness
2	Passive ROM (gravity removed and assisted by examiner)	Poor ROM
1	Slight flicker of contraction	Severe weakness
0	No muscular contraction	Paralysis

Equipment

- Tape measure
- Goniometer (optional)
- Skin marking pen (optional)

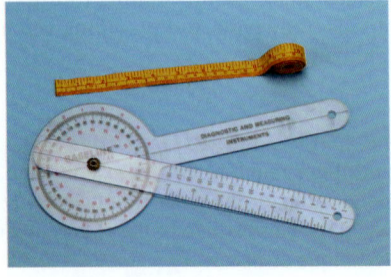

Physical Assessment

- Observe gait and posture.
- Inspect joints, muscles, and extremities for size, symmetry, and color.
- Palpate joints, muscles, and extremities for tenderness, edema, heat, nodules, or crepitus.
- Test muscle strength and ROM of joints.
- Compare bilateral findings of joints and muscles.
- Perform special tests for carpal tunnel syndrome.
- Perform the "bulge," "ballottement," and McMurray knee tests.

General Routine Screening versus Focused Specialty Assessment for the Musculoskeletal System

The nurse routinely observes the client's posture, gait, and movements, along with activities of daily living. However, if the client describes the inability or limited ability to move a joint or extremity or describes pain in a joint or muscle, a more complete assessment is required. This would include inspection of symmetry, color, range of motion, and strength. In addition, the nurse would palpate the joint, bone, or muscles for tenderness, heat, swelling, or nodules. More advanced or specialty tests include testing for carpal tunnel, the bulge test, and the ballottement test. A total head-to-toe musculoskeletal examination would more likely be performed by a physical therapist or a primary care provider.

General Routine Screening
- Observe posture and gait.
- Inspect the following for symmetry, color and mobility:
  - Temporomandibular joint (TMJ)
  - Sternoclavicular joint
  - Cervical, thoracic, and lumbar spine
  - Shoulders, arms, and elbows
  - Wrists, hands, and fingers
  - Hips, knees, ankles, and feet
- Palpate the following for tenderness, heat, swelling, or nodules:
  - Temporomandibular joint (TMJ)
  - Sternoclavicular joint
  - Cervical, thoracic, and lumbar spine
  - Shoulders, arms, and elbows
  - Wrists, hands, and fingers
  - Hips, knees, ankles, and feet

Focused Specialty Assessment
- Measure the ROM with a goniometer of each of the following:
  - Temporomandibular joint (TMJ)
  - Cervical and lumbar spine
  - Shoulders
  - Elbows, wrists, and fingers
  - Hips, knees, ankles, and toes
- Palpate the anatomic snuffbox
- Test for carpal tunnel syndrome.
- Test for thumb weakness.
- Observe for the "flick" signal.
- Perform "squeeze test" of hand and foot.
- Measure leg length.
- Perform the bulge test.
- Perform the ballottement test.

ASSESSMENT PROCEDURE	NORMAL FINDINGS	ABNORMAL FINDINGS
Posture and Gait		
INSPECTION		
Observe posture. Observe the client's posture while standing with the feet together, noting alignment of the head, trunk, pelvis, and extremities. Also observe client's posture while sitting.	Posture is erect and comfortable for age.	Slumped shoulders may result from poor posture (especially while seated) or from depression. Abnormal curvatures of the spine include lordosis, scoliosis, or kyphosis (see abnormal spinal curvatures in Abnormal Findings 24-1).
Observe gait. Observe the client's gait as the client enters and walks around the room. Note: • Base of support • Weight-bearing stability • Foot position • Stride and length and cadence of stride • Arm swing • Posture	Evenly distributed weight. Client able to stand on heels and toes. Toes point straight ahead. Equal on both sides. Posture erect, movements coordinated and rhythmic, arms swing in opposition, stride length appropriate.	Uneven weight bearing is evident. Client cannot stand on heels or toes. Toes point in or out. Client limps, shuffles, propels forward, or has wide-based gait. (See Chapter 25, Assessing Neurologic System, for specific abnormal gait findings.)
Assess for the risk of falling backward in the older or handicapped client by performing the "nudge test." Stand behind the client and put your arms around the client while you gently nudge the sternum.	Client does not fall backward.	Falling backward easily is seen with cervical spondylosis and Parkinson disease.

OLDER ADULT CONSIDERATIONS
Some older clients have an impaired sense of position in space, which may contribute to the risk of falling.

Continued on following page

542 UNIT 3 Nursing Assessment of Physical Systems

ASSESSMENT PROCEDURE	NORMAL FINDINGS	ABNORMAL FINDINGS

Temporomandibular Joint (TMJ)

INSPECTION AND PALPATION

Inspect and palpate the TMJ. Have the client sit; put your index and middle fingers just anterior to the external ear opening (Fig. 24-4A). Ask the client to open the mouth as widely as possible. (The tips of your fingers should drop into the joint spaces as the mouth opens.) • Move the jaw from side to side (Fig. 24-4B). • Protrude (push out) and retract (pull in) jaw (Fig. 24-4C).	Snapping and clicking may be felt and heard in the normal client. Mouth opens 1–2 in (distance between upper and lower teeth). The client's mouth opens and closes smoothly. Jaw moves laterally 1–2 cm. Jaw protrudes and retracts easily.	Decreased ROM, swelling, tenderness, or crepitus may be seen in arthritis. Decreased muscle strength with muscle and joint disease. Decreased ROM, and a clicking, popping, or grating sound may be noted with TMJ dysfunction.

 Concept Mastery Alert

A client with arthritis in the jaw has decreased range of motion of the jaw, and crepitus is felt when the jaw is palpated. A grating sound may be heard in a client with temporomandibular joint (TMJ) dysfunction.

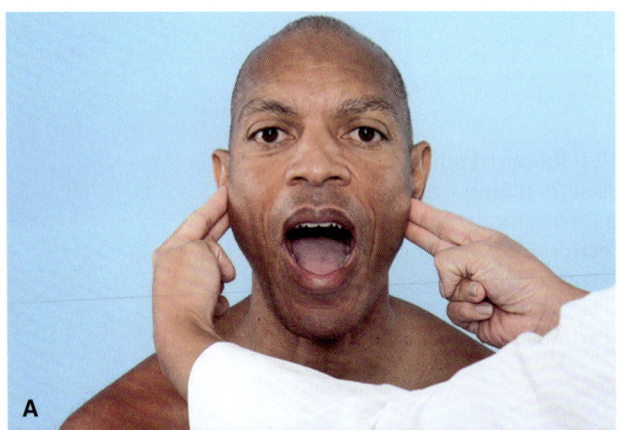

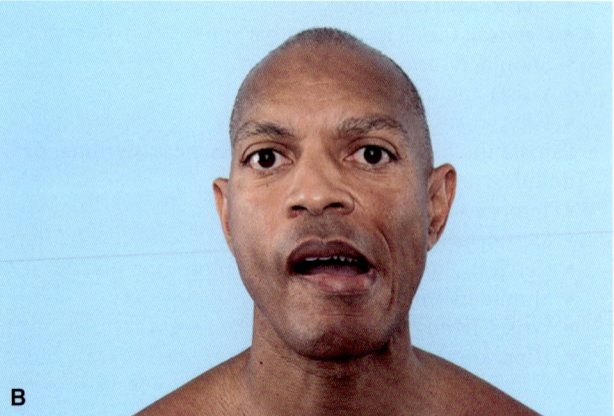

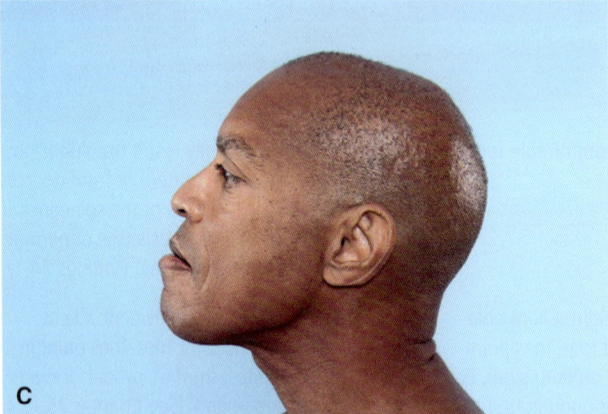

FIGURE 24-4 Inspecting and palpating the temporomandibular joint. (**A**) Put your index and middle fingers just anterior to the external ear opening and have the client open the mouth. (**B**) Move the jaw from side to side. (**C**) Protrude (push out) and retract (pull in) jaw.

Test ROM. Ask the client to open the mouth and move the jaw laterally against resistance. Next, as the client clenches the teeth, feel for the contraction of the temporal and masseter muscles to test the integrity of cranial nerve V (trigeminal nerve).	Jaw has full ROM against resistance. Contraction palpated with no pain or spasms.	Lack of full contraction with cranial nerve V lesion. Pain or spasms occur with myofascial pain syndrome.

Sternoclavicular Joint

INSPECTION AND PALPATION

With client sitting, inspect the sternoclavicular joint for location in midline, color, swelling, and masses. Then palpate for tenderness or pain.	There is no visible bony overgrowth, swelling, or redness; joint is nontender.	Swollen, red, or enlarged joint or tender, painful joint is seen with inflammation of the joint.

ASSESSMENT PROCEDURE	NORMAL FINDINGS	ABNORMAL FINDINGS

Cervical, Thoracic, and Lumbar Spine

INSPECTION AND PALPATION

Observe the cervical, thoracic, and lumbar curves from the side, then from behind. Have the client standing erect with the gown positioned to allow an adequate view of the spine (Fig. 24-5). Observe for symmetry, noting differences in height of the shoulders, iliac crests, and buttock creases.

Cervical and lumbar spines are concave; thoracic spine is convex. Spine is straight (when observed from behind).

 OLDER ADULT CONSIDERATIONS
An exaggerated thoracic curve (kyphosis) is common with aging.

 CULTURAL CONSIDERATIONS
Some findings that appear to be abnormalities are, in fact, variations related to culture or sex. For example, some African Americans have a large gluteal prominence, making the spine appear to have lumbar lordosis. In addition, the number of vertebrae may differ. Racial and sex variations from the usual 23 chromosomes found in 85–93% of all people include 11% of African American women with 24, and 12% of Eskimo and Native American men with 25 (Andrews & Boyle, 2016)

A flattened lumbar curvature may be seen with a herniated lumbar disc or ankylosing spondylitis. Lateral curvature of the thoracic spine with an increase in the convexity on the curved side is seen in scoliosis. An exaggerated lumbar curve (lordosis) is often seen in pregnancy or obesity (Abnormal Findings 24-1). Unequal heights of the hips suggest unequal leg lengths.

Palpate the spinous processes and the paravertebral muscles on both sides of the spine for tenderness or pain.

Nontender spinous processes; well-developed, firm and smooth, nontender paravertebral muscles. No muscle spasm.

Compression fractures and lumbosacral muscle strain can cause pain and tenderness of the spinal processes and paravertebral muscles.

Test ROM of the cervical spine. Test ROM of the cervical spine by asking the client to touch the chin to the chest (flexion) and to look up at the ceiling (hyperextension) (Fig. 24-6).

Flexion of the cervical spine is 45 degrees. Extension of the cervical spine is 45 degrees.

Cervical strain is the most common cause of neck pain. It is characterized by impaired ROM and neck pain from abnormalities of the soft tissue (muscles, ligaments, and nerves) due to straining or injuring the neck. Causes of strains can include sleeping in the wrong position, carrying a heavy suitcase, or being in an automobile crash.

Cervical disc degenerative disease and spinal cord tumors are associated with impaired ROM and pain that radiates to the back,

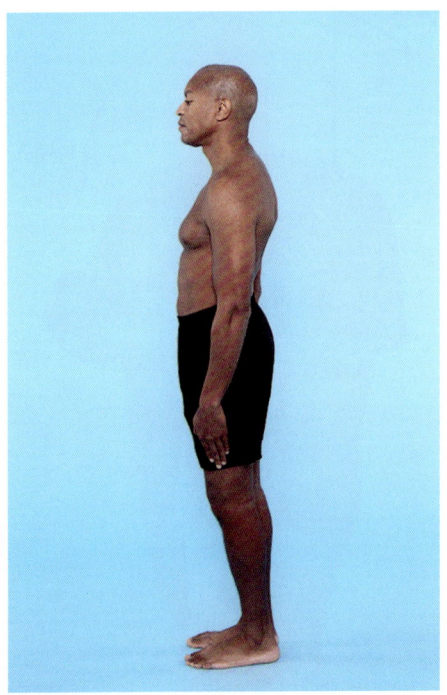

FIGURE 24-5 Normal curve of the spine.

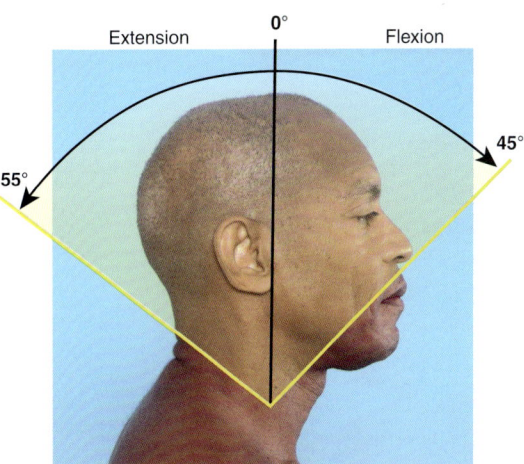

FIGURE 24-6 Normal range of motion of the cervical spine: hyperextension-flexion.

Continued on following page

ASSESSMENT PROCEDURE	NORMAL FINDINGS	ABNORMAL FINDINGS
Cervical, Thoracic, and Lumbar Spine (Continued)		
		shoulder, or arms. Neck pain with a loss of sensation in the legs may occur with cervical spinal cord compression. **CLINICAL TIP** Impaired ROM and neck pain associated with fever, chills, and headache could be indicative of a serious infection such as meningitis.
Test lateral bending. Ask the client to touch each ear to the shoulder on that side (Fig. 24-7).	Normally the client can bend 40 degrees to the left side and 40 degrees to the right side.	Limited ROM is seen with neck injuries, osteoarthritis, spondylosis, or with disc degeneration.
Evaluate rotation. Ask the client to turn the head to the right and left (Fig. 24-8).	About 70 degrees of rotation is normal.	Limited ROM is seen with neck injuries, osteoarthritis, spondylosis, or with disc degeneration.
Ask the client to repeat the cervical ROM movements against resistance.	Client has full ROM against resistance. Strength 5/5.	Decreased ROM against resistance is seen with joint or muscle disease.
Test ROM of the lumbar spine. Ask the client to bend forward and touch the toes (flexion; Fig. 24-9). Observe for symmetry of the shoulders, scapula, and hips. **OLDER ADULT CONSIDERATIONS** Similarly, ask an older client to bend forward but do not insist that he or she touch toes unless the client is comfortable with the movement.	Flexion of 75–90 degrees, smooth movement, lumbar concavity flattens out, and the spinal processes are in alignment.	Lateral curvature disappears in functional scoliosis; unilateral exaggerated thoracic convexity increases in structural scoliosis. Spinal processes are out of alignment. See Figure 24-1

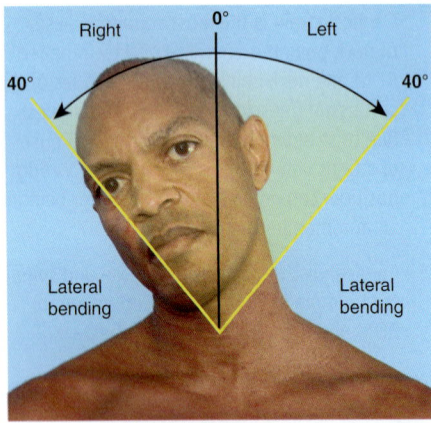

FIGURE 24-7 Normal range of motion of the cervical spine: lateral bending.

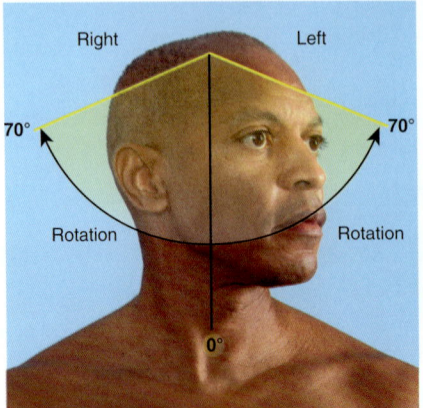

FIGURE 24-8 Normal range of motion of the cervical spine: rotation.

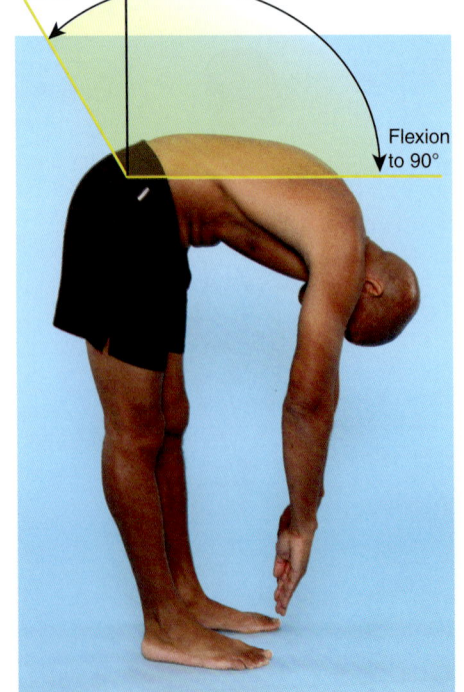

FIGURE 24-9 Thoracic and lumbar spines: flexion.

ASSESSMENT PROCEDURE	NORMAL FINDINGS	ABNORMAL FINDINGS
Sit down behind the client, stabilize the client's pelvis with your hands, and ask the client to bend sideways (lateral bending), bend backward toward you (hyperextension), and twist the shoulders one way then the other (rotation).	Lateral bending capacity of the thoracic and lumbar spines should be about 35 degrees (Fig. 24-10A); hyperextension about 30 degrees; and rotation about 30 degrees (Fig. 24-10B).	Low back strain from injury to soft tissues is a common cause of impaired ROM and pain in the lumbar and thoracic regions. Other causes of impaired ROM in the lumbar and thoracic areas include osteoarthritis, ankylosing spondylitis, and congenital abnormalities that may affect the spinal vertebral spacing and mobility.

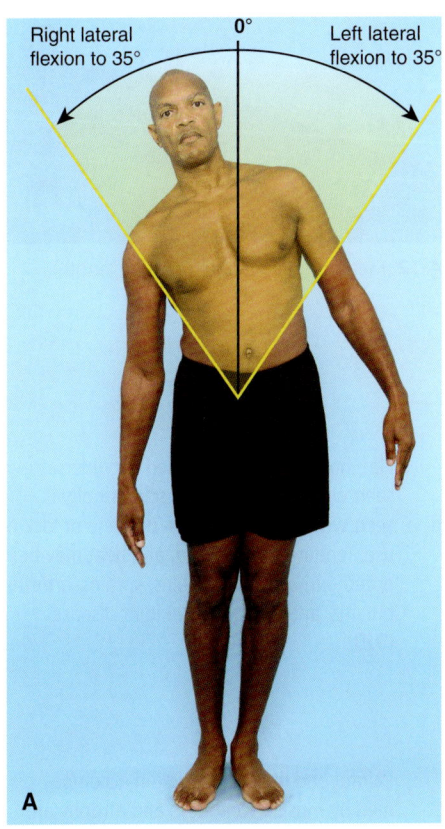
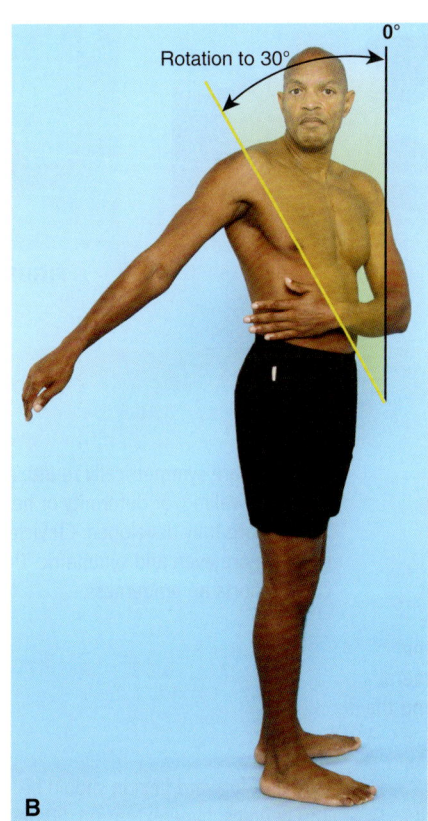

FIGURE 24-10 Thoracic and lumbar spines: (**A**) lateral bending; (**B**) rotation.

Test for back and leg pain. If the client has low back pain that radiates down the back, perform the straight leg test to check for a herniated nucleus pulposus. Ask the client to lie flat and raise each relaxed leg independently to the point of pain. At the point of pain, dorsiflex the client's foot (Fig. 24-11). Note the degree of elevation when pain occurs, the distribution and character of the pain, and the results from dorsiflexion of the foot.

Measure leg length. If you suspect that the client has one leg longer than the other, measure them. Ask the client to lie down with legs extended. With a measuring tape, measure the distance between the anterior superior iliac spine and the medial malleolus, crossing the tape on the medial side of the knee (true leg length; Fig. 24-12).	Measurements are equal or within 1 cm. If the legs still look unequal, assess the apparent leg length by measuring from a nonfixed point (the umbilicus) to a fixed point (medial malleolus) on each leg.	Unequal leg lengths are associated with scoliosis. Equal true leg lengths but unequal apparent leg lengths are seen with abnormalities in the structure or position of the hips and pelvis.

Continued on following page

ASSESSMENT PROCEDURE	NORMAL FINDINGS	ABNORMAL FINDINGS

Cervical, Thoracic, and Lumbar Spine (Continued)

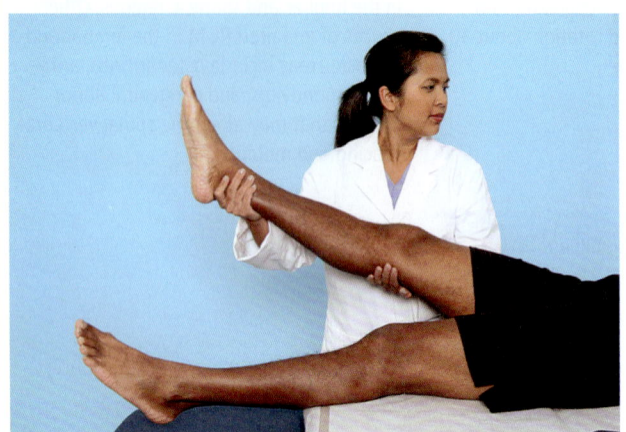

FIGURE 24-11 Performing the straight leg test.

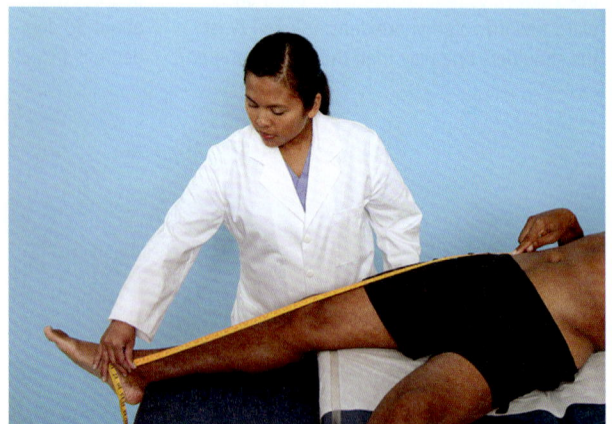

FIGURE 24-12 Measuring leg length (true leg length).

Shoulders, Arms, and Elbows

INSPECTION AND PALPATION

Inspect and palpate shoulders and arms. With the client standing or sitting, inspect anteriorly and posteriorly for symmetry, color, swelling, and masses. Palpate for tenderness, swelling, or heat. Anteriorly palpate the clavicle, acromioclavicular joint, subacromial area, and the biceps. Posteriorly palpate the glenohumeral joint, coracoid area, trapezius muscle, and the scapular area.	Shoulders are symmetrically round; no redness, swelling, or deformity or heat. Muscles are fully developed. Clavicles and scapulae are even and symmetric. The client reports no tenderness.	Flat, hollow, or less-rounded shoulders are seen with dislocation. Muscle atrophy is seen with nerve or muscle damage or lack of use. Tenderness, swelling, and heat may be noted with shoulder strains, sprains, arthritis, bursitis, and degenerative joint disease (DJD).
Test ROM. Explain to the client that you will be assessing ROM (consisting of flexion, extension, adduction, abduction, and motion against resistance). Ask client to stand with both arms straight down at the sides. Next, ask the client to move the arms forward (flexion), then backward with elbows straight (Fig. 24-13).	Extent of forward flexion should be 180 degrees; hyperextension, 50 degrees; adduction, 50 degrees; and abduction 180 degrees.	Painful and limited abduction accompanied by muscle weakness and atrophy are seen with a rotator cuff tear. Client has sharp catches of pain when bringing hands overhead with rotator cuff tendinitis. Chronic pain and severe limitation of all shoulder motions are seen with calcified tendinitis.
Then have the client bring both hands together overhead, elbows straight, followed by moving both hands in front of the body past the midline with elbows straight (this tests adduction and abduction) (Fig. 24-14).		
In a continuous motion, have the client bring the hands together behind the head with elbows flexed (this tests external rotation; Fig. 24-15A) and behind the back (internal rotation; Fig. 24-15B). Repeat these maneuvers against resistance.	Extent of external and internal rotation should be about 90 degrees, respectively. The client can flex, extend, adduct, abduct, rotate, and shrug shoulders against resistance.	Inability to shrug shoulders against resistance is seen with a lesion of cranial nerve XI (spinal accessory). Decreased muscle strength is seen with muscle or joint disease.

24 Assessing Musculoskeletal System 547

ASSESSMENT PROCEDURE	NORMAL FINDINGS	ABNORMAL FINDINGS

Shoulders, Arms, and Elbows (Continued)

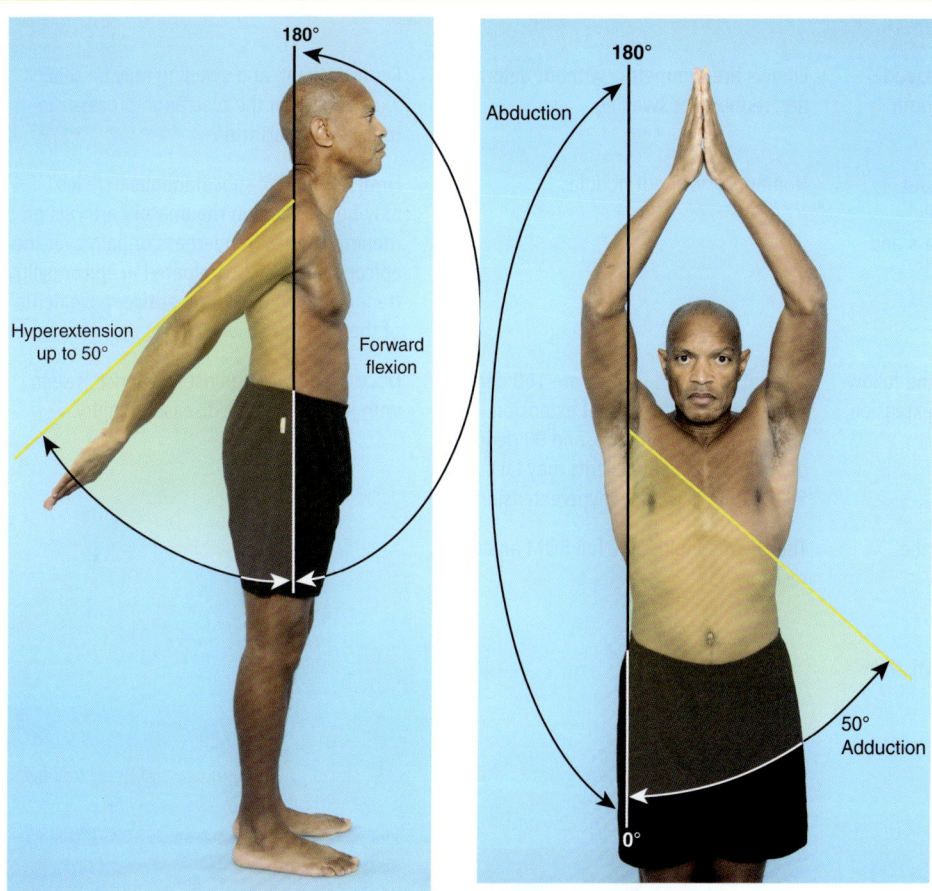

FIGURE 24-13 Normal range of motion of the shoulder: flexion/extension.

FIGURE 24-14 Normal range of motion of the shoulder: adduction/abduction.

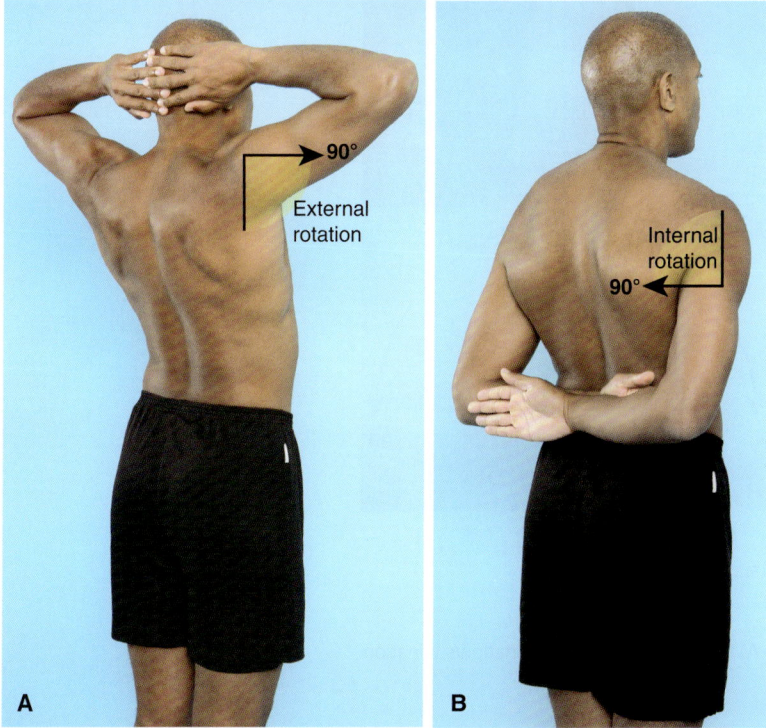

FIGURE 24-15 Normal range of motion of the shoulder: (A) external rotation; (B) internal rotation.

Continued on following page

ASSESSMENT PROCEDURE	NORMAL FINDINGS	ABNORMAL FINDINGS
Elbows		
INSPECTION AND PALPATION		
Inspect for size, shape, deformities, redness, or swelling. Inspect elbows in both flexed and extended positions.	Elbows are symmetric, without deformities, redness, or swelling.	Redness, heat, and swelling may be seen with bursitis of the olecranon process due to trauma or arthritis.
With the elbow relaxed and flexed about 70 degrees, use your thumb and middle fingers to palpate the olecranon process and epicondyles.	Nontender; without nodules.	Firm, nontender, subcutaneous nodules may be palpated in rheumatoid arthritis or rheumatic fever. Tenderness or pain over the epicondyles may be palpated in epicondylitis (tennis elbow) due to repetitive movements of the forearm or wrists.
Test ROM. Ask the client to perform the following movements to test ROM, flexion, extension, pronation, and supination.	Normal ranges of motion are 160 degrees of flexion, 180 degrees of extension, 90 degrees of pronation, and 90 degrees of supination. Some clients may lack 5–10 degrees or have hyperextension.	Decreased ROM against resistance is seen with joint or muscle disease or injury.
Flex the elbow and bring the hand to the forehead (Fig. 24-16A).	The client should have full ROM against resistance.	
Straighten the elbow.		
Then hold arm out, turn the palm down, then turn the palm up (Fig. 24-16B).		
Last, have the client repeat the movements against your resistance.		

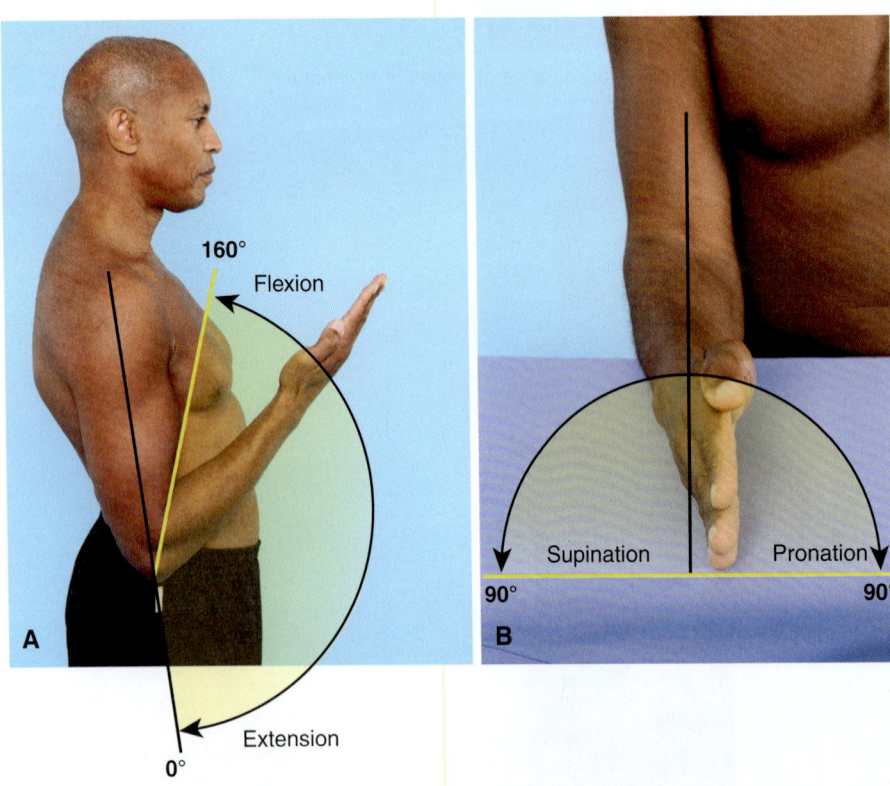

FIGURE 24-16 Normal range of motion of the elbow: (**A**) flexion/extension; (**B**) pronation/supination.

ASSESSMENT PROCEDURE	NORMAL FINDINGS	ABNORMAL FINDINGS

Wrists

INSPECTION AND PALPATION

Inspect wrist size, shape, symmetry, color, and swelling. Then palpate for tenderness and nodules (Fig. 24-17).	Wrists are symmetric, without redness, or swelling. They are nontender and free of nodules.	Swelling is seen with rheumatoid arthritis. Tenderness and nodules may be seen with rheumatoid arthritis. A nontender, round, enlarged, swollen, fluid-filled cyst (ganglion) may be noted on the wrists (Abnormal Findings 24-2). Signs of a wrist fracture include pain, tenderness, swelling, and inability to hold a grip; as well as pain that goes away and then returns as a deep, dull ache. Extreme tenderness occurs when pressure is applied on the side of the hand between the two tendons leading to the thumb (UCSF Medical Center, 2016).

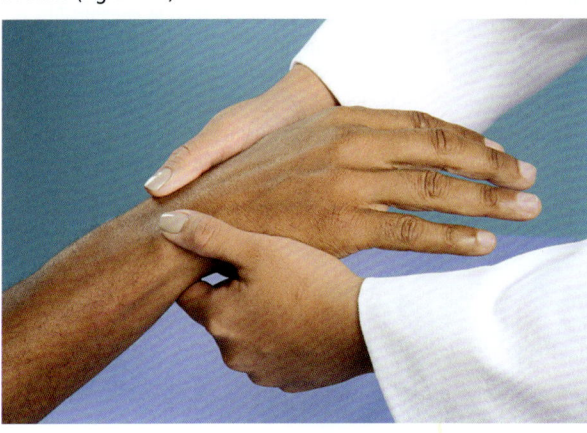

FIGURE 24-17 Palpating the wrists.

Perform the squeeze test by squeezing the client's hand across the knuckle joints as shown (Fig. 24-18).	Client tolerates test without extreme pain	Extreme pain may indicate rheumatoid arthritis and psoriatic arthritis of the hand (Arthritis Research UK, 2013).

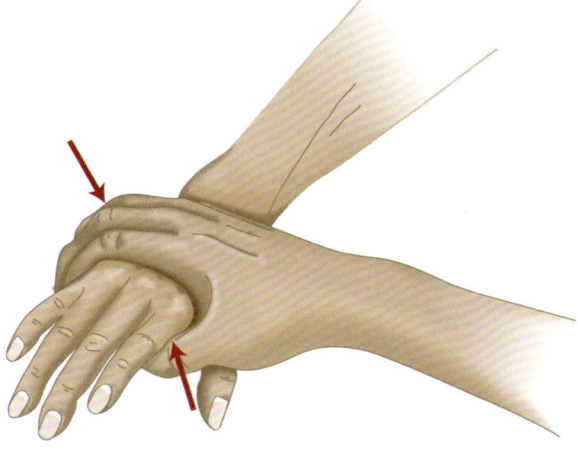

FIGURE 24-18 Squeeze test on the hand.

Palpate the anatomic snuffbox (the hollow area on the back of the wrist at the base of the fully extended thumb; Fig. 24-19).	No tenderness palpated in anatomic snuffbox.	Snuffbox tenderness may indicate a scaphoid fracture, which is often the result of falling on an outstretched hand.

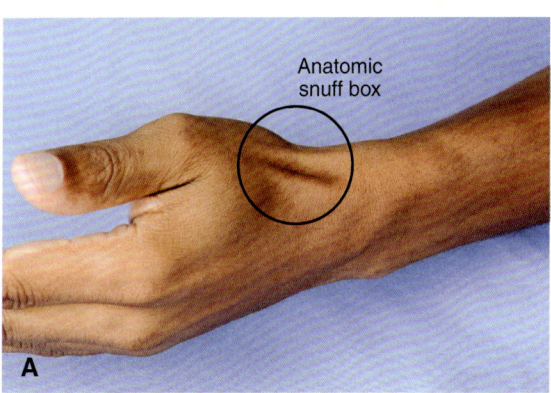 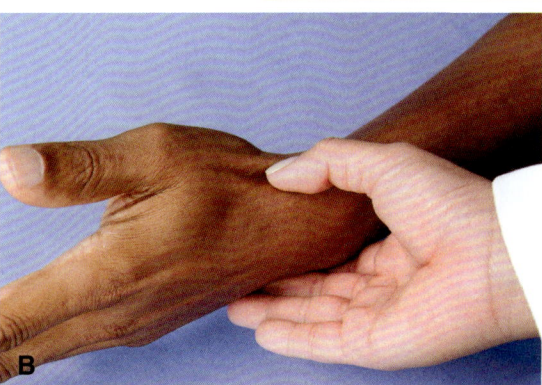

FIGURE 24-19 (A) Anatomic snuffbox. (B) Palpating the anatomic snuffbox.

Continued on following page

UNIT 3 Nursing Assessment of Physical Systems

ASSESSMENT PROCEDURE	NORMAL FINDINGS	ABNORMAL FINDINGS

Wrists (Continued)

Test ROM. Ask the client to bend the wrist down and back (flexion and extension; Fig. 24-20A).

Next have the client hold the wrist straight and move the hand outward and inward (deviation; Fig. 24-20B). Repeat these maneuvers against resistance.

Normal ranges of motion are 90 degrees of flexion, 70 degrees of hyperextension, 55 degrees of ulnar deviation, and 20 degrees of radial deviation. Client should have full ROM against resistance.

🌐 CULTURAL CONSIDERATIONS
Unequal lengths of the ulna and radius have been found in some ethnic groups (e.g., Swedes and Chinese) (Andrews & Boyle, 2016)

Ulnar deviation of the wrist and fingers with limited ROM is often seen in rheumatoid arthritis.

Increased pain with extension of the wrist against resistance is seen in epicondylitis of the lateral side of the elbow. Increased pain with flexion of the wrist against resistance is seen in epicondylitis of the medial side of the elbow. Decreased muscle strength is noted with muscle and joint disease.

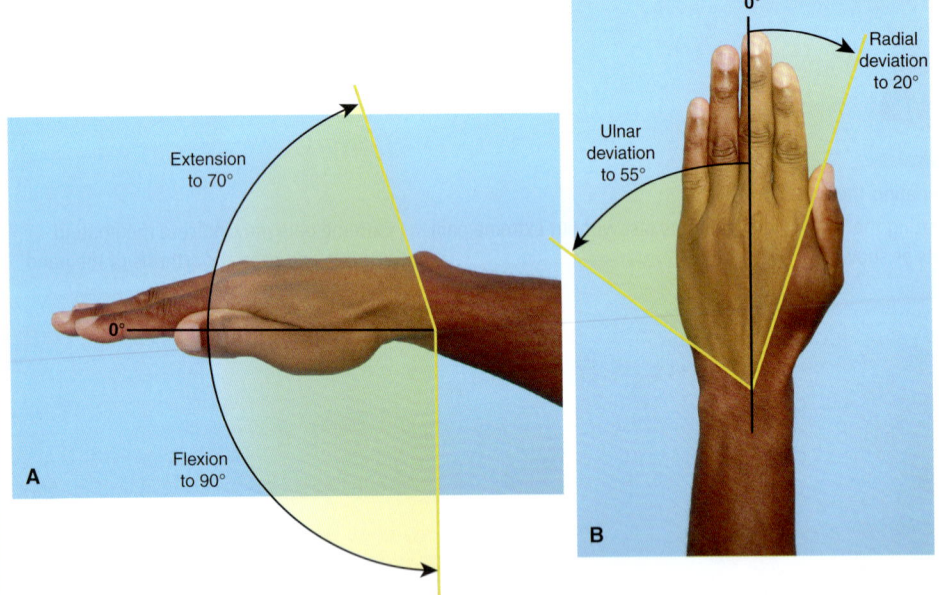

FIGURE 24-20 Range of motion of the wrists: (A) flexion/hyperextension; (B) radial–ulnar deviation.

Tests for carpal tunnel syndrome (CTS).

Perform Phalen test.

Ask the client to place the backs of both hands against each other while flexing the wrists 90 degrees with fingers pointed downward and wrists dangling (Fig. 24-21A). Have the client hold this position for 60 seconds.

No tingling, numbness, burning, or pain result from Phalen test.

If symptoms (tingling, numbness, burning, or pain) develop within a minute with Phalen test, carpal tunnel syndrome is suspected. Client may report tingling, numbness, and pain with carpal tunnel syndrome.

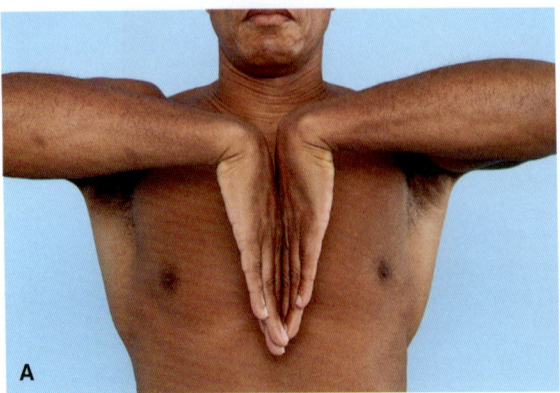
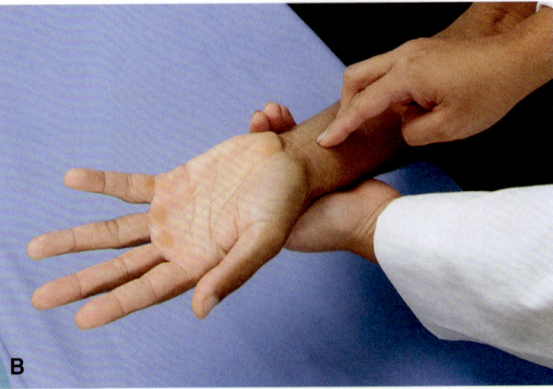

FIGURE 24-21 Tests for carpal tunnel syndrome: (A) Phalen test; (B) Tinel test.

ASSESSMENT PROCEDURE	NORMAL FINDINGS	ABNORMAL FINDINGS
Phalen test is positive in about 70% of cases and has a false-positive rate of about 30% (Carpal-Tunnel.net, 2011).		However, if the test lasts longer than a minute, pain and tingling may occur even in clients without carpal tunnel syndrome.
Perform test for Tinel sign: Use your finger to percuss lightly over the median nerve (located on the inner aspect of the wrist; Fig. 24-21B). Compared to other tests, Tinel sign may be very unreliable to diagnose CTS with anything up to 50% false-positive and false-negative rates—essentially no better than tossing a coin (East Kent Hospitals University, 2011).	No tingling or shocking sensation experienced with test for Tinel sign.	Tingling or shocking sensation experienced with test for Tinel sign. Median nerve entrapped in the carpal tunnel results in pain, numbness, and impaired function of the hand and fingers (Fig. 24-22).

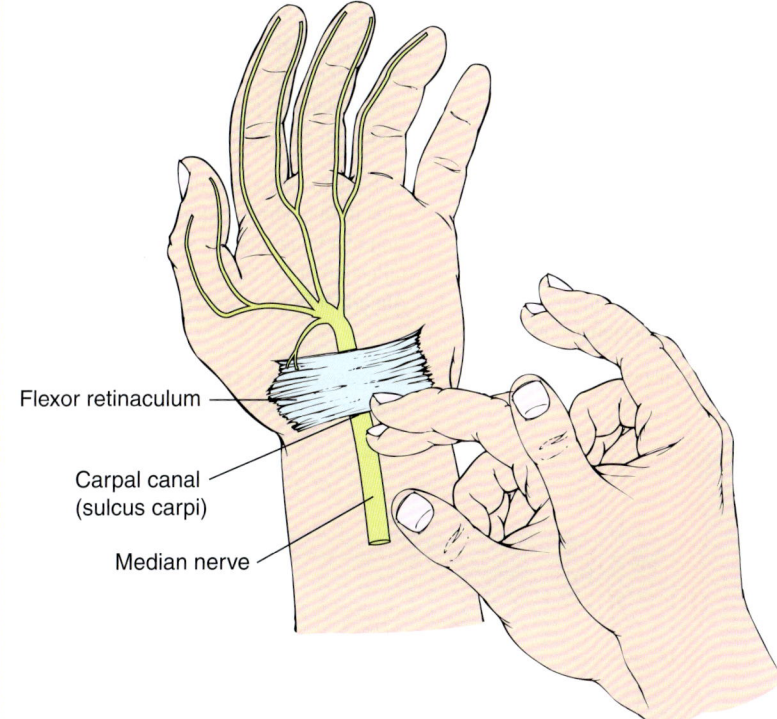

FIGURE 24-22 Median nerves entrapped in the carpal tunnel results in pain, numbness, and impaired function of the hand and fingers.

ASSESSMENT PROCEDURE	NORMAL FINDINGS	ABNORMAL FINDINGS
Observe for the flick signal. Ask the client, "What do you do when your symptoms are worse?"	Client will not shake or flick wrist when asked this question.	If the patient responds with a motion that resembles shaking a thermometer (flick signal), carpal tunnel may be suspected. However, the Flick signal was originally claimed to be 93% sensitive and 95% specific for carpal tunnel syndrome (CTS), but subsequent investigations have found it performs less well (Carpal-tunnel.net, 2011).
Test for thumb weakness: • Ask the client to raise thumb up from the plane of the palm. • Ask the client to stretch the thumb so that its pad rests on the pad of the little finger pad.	Client can raise thumb up from the plane and stretch the thumb finger pad to the little finger pad.	Client cannot raise the thumb up from the plane and stretch the thumb pad to the little finger pad. This indicates thumb weakness in carpal tunnel syndrome.

Continued on following page

ASSESSMENT PROCEDURE	NORMAL FINDINGS	ABNORMAL FINDINGS

Hands and Fingers

INSPECTION AND PALPATION

Inspect size, shape, symmetry, swelling, and color. Palpate the fingers from the distal end proximally, noting tenderness, swelling, bony prominences, nodules, or crepitus of each interphalangeal joint. Assess the metacarpophalangeal joints by squeezing the hand from each side between your thumb and fingers. Palpate each metacarpal of the hand, noting tenderness and swelling.	Hands and fingers are symmetric, non-tender, and without nodules. Fingers lie in straight line. No swelling or deformities. Rounded protuberance noted next to the thumb over the thenar prominence. Smaller protuberance seen adjacent to the small finger.	Pain, tenderness, swelling, shortened finger, depressed knuckle, finger crossing over adjacent finger when making a fist, or inability to move the finger may be seen with finger fractures (UCSF Medical Center, 2016).
		Swollen, stiff, tender finger joints are seen in acute rheumatoid arthritis. Boutonnière deformity and swan-neck deformity are seen in long-term rheumatoid arthritis (see Abnormal Findings 24-2). Atrophy of the thenar prominence may be evident in carpal tunnel syndrome.
		In osteoarthritis, hard, painless nodules may be seen over the distal interphalangeal joints (Heberden nodes) and over the proximal interphalangeal joints (Bouchard nodes) (see Abnormal Findings 24-2).
Test ROM (Fig. 24-23). Ask the client to (A) spread the fingers apart (abduction), (B) make a fist (adduction), (C) bend the fingers down (flexion) and then up (hyperextension), (D) move the thumb away from other fingers, and then (E) touch the thumb to the base of the small finger.	Normal ranges are 20 degrees of abduction, full adduction of fingers (touching), 90 degrees of flexion, and 30 degrees of hyperextension. The thumb should easily move away from other fingers and 50 degrees of thumb flexion is normal.	Inability to extend the ring and little fingers is seen in Dupuytren contracture. Painful extension of a finger may be seen in tenosynovitis (infection of the flexor tendon sheathes; see Abnormal Findings 24-2).
Repeat these maneuvers against resistance.	The client normally has full ROM against resistance.	Decreased muscle strength against resistance is associated with muscle and joint disease.

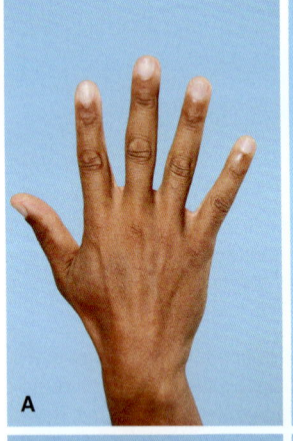
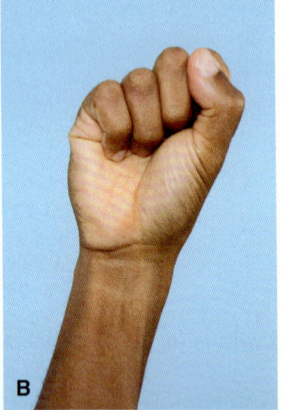
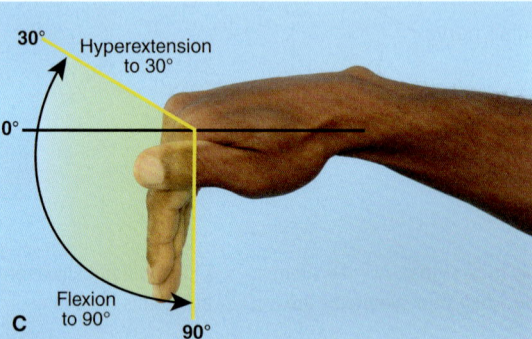
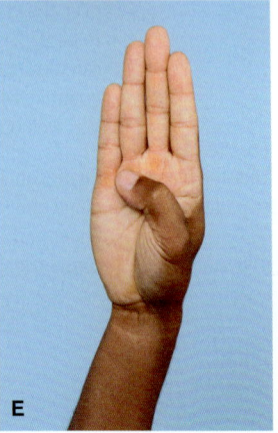

FIGURE 24-23 Normal range of motion of the fingers: (**A**) abduction; (**B**) adduction; (**C**) flexion–hyperextension; (**D**) thumb away from fingers; (**E**) thumb touching base of small finger.

24 Assessing Musculoskeletal System   553

ASSESSMENT PROCEDURE	NORMAL FINDINGS	ABNORMAL FINDINGS
Hips		
INSPECTION AND PALPATION		

With the client standing, inspect symmetry and shape of the hips (Fig. 24-24). Observe for convex thoracic curve and concave lumbar curve. Palpate for stability, tenderness, and crepitus. 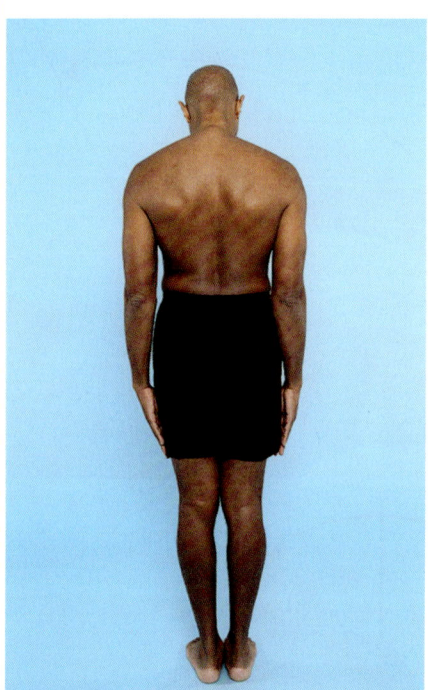	Buttocks are equally sized; iliac crests are symmetric in height. Hips are stable, nontender, and without crepitus. **FIGURE 24-24** Inspecting the hips and buttocks.	Instability, inability to stand, and/or a deformed hip area are indicative of a fractured hip. Tenderness, edema, decreased ROM, and crepitus are seen in hip inflammation and DJD. The most common injuries of the hip and groin region in athletes are groin pulls and hamstring strains (Hong, 2015). Strains, a stretch or tear of muscle or tendons, often occur in the lower back and the hamstring muscle.
Test ROM (Fig. 24-25). **SAFETY TIP** *If the client has had a total hip replacement, do not test ROM unless the physician gives permission to do so, due to the risk of dislocating the hip prosthesis.* With the client supine, ask the client to: • Raise extended leg (Fig. 24-25A). • Flex knee up to chest while keeping other leg extended (Fig. 24-25B). • Move extended leg (Fig. 24-25C) away from midline of body as far as possible and then toward midline of body as far as possible (abduction and adduction). • Bend knee and turn leg (Fig. 24-25D) inward (rotation) and then outward (rotation). • Ask the client to lie prone (Fig. 24–25E) and lift extended leg off table. Alternatively, ask the client to stand and swing extended leg backward.	Normal ROM: 90 degrees of hip flexion with the knee straight and 120 degrees of hip flexion with the knee bent and the other leg remaining straight. Normal ROM: • 45–50 degrees of abduction • 20–30 degrees of adduction • 40 degrees internal hip rotation • 45 degrees external hip rotation. • 15 degrees hip hyperextension.	Inability to abduct the hip is a common sign of hip disease. Pain and a decrease in internal hip rotation may be a sign of osteoarthritis or femoral neck stress fracture. Pain on palpation of the greater trochanter and pain as the client moves from standing to lying down may indicate bursitis of the hip.
Repeat these maneuvers against resistance.	Full ROM against resistance. Strength 5/5.	Decreased muscle strength against resistance is seen in muscle and joint disease.

Continued on following page

554   UNIT 3 Nursing Assessment of Physical Systems

ASSESSMENT PROCEDURE	NORMAL FINDINGS	ABNORMAL FINDINGS

Hips (Continued)

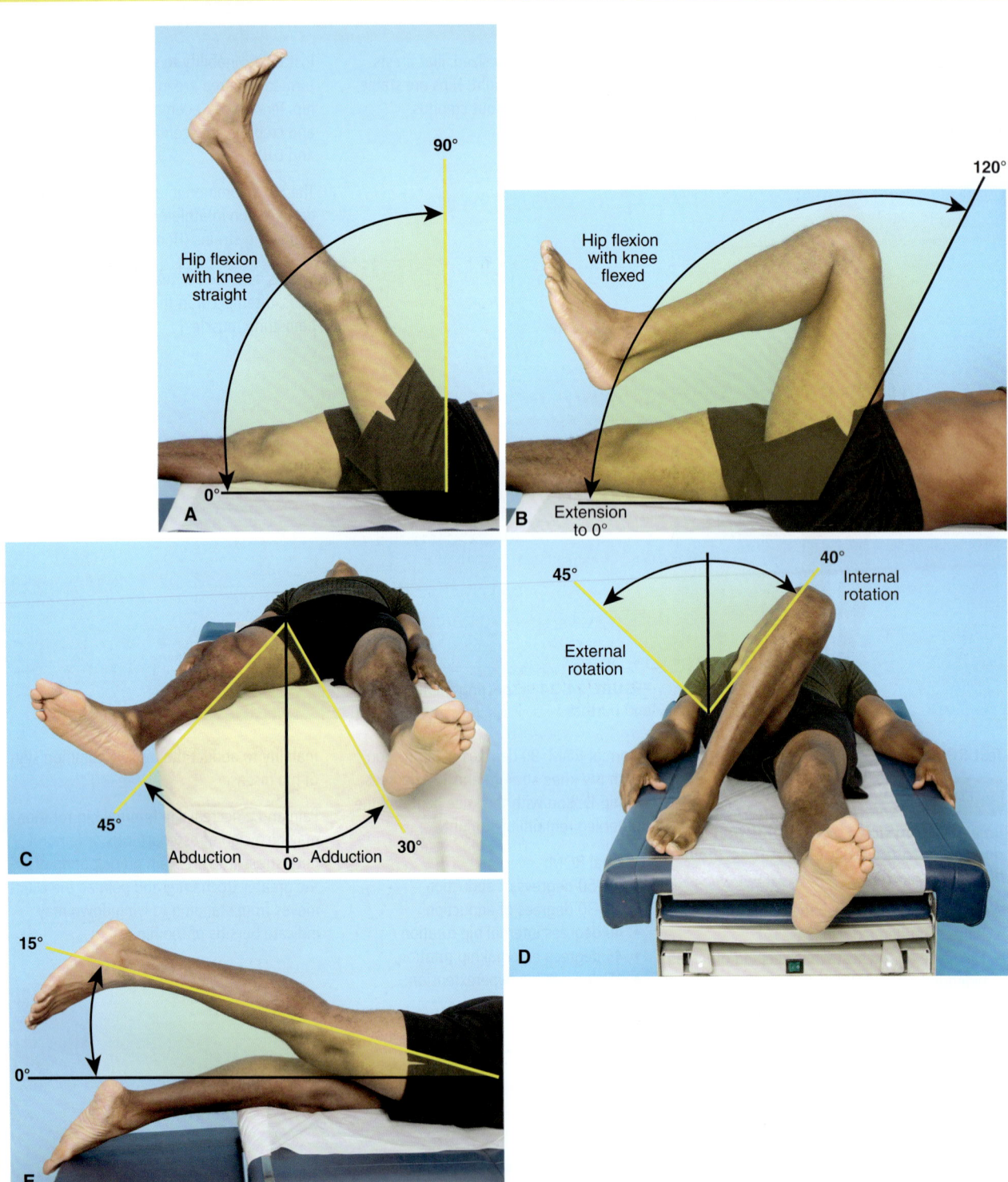

FIGURE 24-25 Normal range of motion of the hips: (A) hip flexion with extended knee straight; (B) hip flexion with knee bent; (C) abduction/adduction; (D) internal and external rotation; (E) hyperextension.

24 Assessing Musculoskeletal System 555

ASSESSMENT PROCEDURE	NORMAL FINDINGS	ABNORMAL FINDINGS

Knees

INSPECTION AND PALPATION

With the client supine then sitting with knees dangling, inspect for size, shape, symmetry, swelling, deformities, and alignment. Observe for quadriceps muscle atrophy.	Knees symmetric, hollows present on both sides of the patella, no swelling or deformities. Lower leg in alignment with the upper leg.	Knees turn in with knock knees (genu valgum) and turn out with bowed legs (genu varum). Swelling above or next to the patella may indicate fluid in the knee joint or thickening of the synovial membrane.
Palpate for tenderness, warmth, consistency, and nodules. Begin palpation 10 cm above the patella, using your fingers and thumb to move downward toward the knee (Fig. 24-26).	Nontender and cool. Muscles firm. No nodules. **OLDER ADULT CONSIDERATIONS** Some older clients may have a bow-legged appearance because of decreased muscle control.	Tenderness and warmth with a boggy consistency may be symptoms of synovitis. Asymmetric muscular development in the quadriceps may indicate atrophy.
Perform the bulge test if swelling is present. If you notice swelling, perform the bulge test to determine if the swelling is due to accumulation of fluid or soft-tissue swelling. The bulge test helps to detect small amounts of fluid in the knee. With the client in a supine position, use the ball of your hand firmly to stroke the medial side of the knee upward, three to four times, to displace any accumulated fluid (Fig. 24-27A).	No bulge of fluid appears on medial side of knee.	Bulge of fluid appears on medial side of knee, with a small amount of joint effusion.
Then press on the lateral side of the knee and look for a bulge on the medial side of the knee (Fig. 24-27B).		

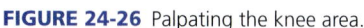

FIGURE 24-26 Palpating the knee area.

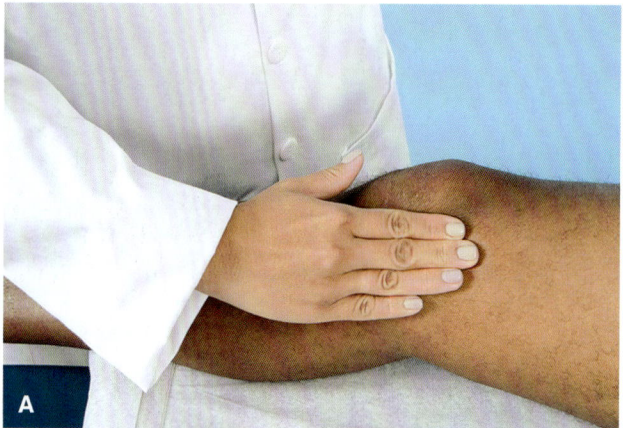
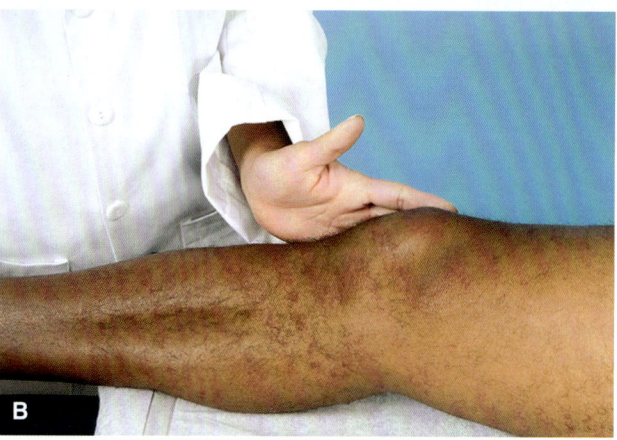

FIGURE 24-27 Performing the "bulge" knee test: (A) stroking the knee; (B) observing the medial side for bulging.

Continued on following page

ASSESSMENT PROCEDURE	NORMAL FINDINGS	ABNORMAL FINDINGS
Knees (Continued)		
Perform the ballottement test. This test helps to detect large amounts of fluid in the knee. With the client in a supine position, firmly press your nondominant thumb and index finger on each side of the patella. This displaces fluid in the suprapatellar bursa, located between the femur and patella. Then with your dominant fingers, push the patella down on the femur (Fig. 24-28). Feel for a fluid wave or a click.	No movement of the patella is noted. Patella rests firmly over the femur.	Fluid wave or click palpated, with large amounts of joint effusion. A positive ballottement test may be present with meniscal tears.
Palpate the tibiofemoral space. As you compress the patella, slide it distally against the underlying femur. Note crepitus or pain.	There is no pain on examination. Crepitus may be present.	A patellofemoral disorder may be suspected if both crepitus and pain are present on examination.
Test ROM (Fig. 24-29). Ask the client to: • Bend each knee up (flexion) toward buttocks or back. • Straighten the knee (extension/hyperextension). • Walk normally.	Normal ranges: 120–130 degrees of flexion; 0 degrees of extension to 15 degrees of hyperextension.	Osteoarthritis is characterized by a decreased ROM with synovial thickening and crepitation. Flexion contractures of the knee are characterized by an inability to extend knee fully.
Repeat these maneuvers against resistance.	Client should have full ROM against resistance.	Decreased muscle strength against resistance is seen in muscle and joint disease.

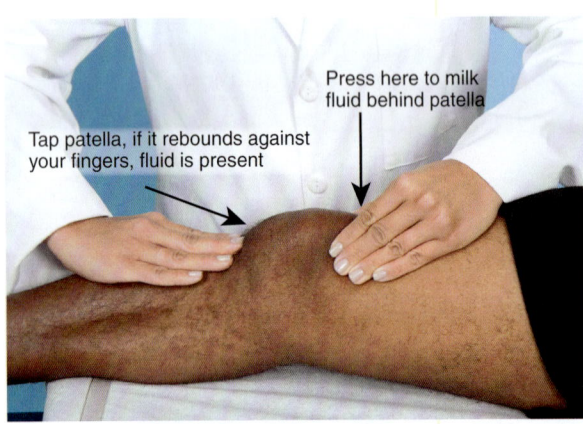

FIGURE 24-28 Performing the "ballottement" knee test.

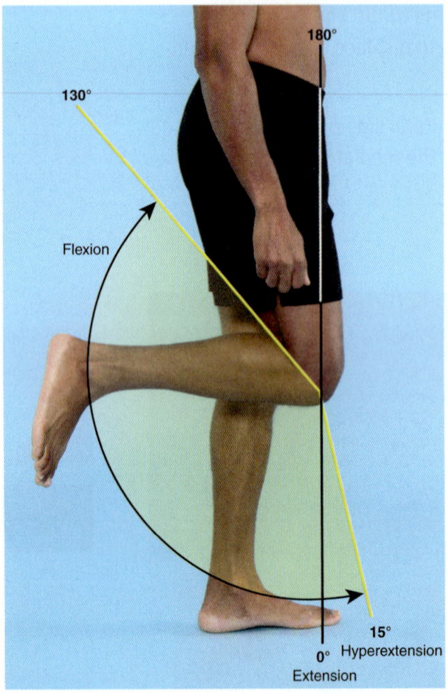

FIGURE 24-29 Normal range of motion of the knee.

Test for pain and injury. If the client complains of a "giving in" or "locking" of the knee, perform McMurray test (Fig. 24-30). With the client in the supine position, ask the client to flex one knee and hip. Then place your thumb and index finger of one hand on either side of the knee. Use your other hand to hold the heel of the foot up. Rotate the lower leg and foot laterally. Slowly extend the knee, noting pain or clicking. Repeat, rotating lower leg and foot medially. Again, note pain or clicking.	No pain or clicking noted.	Pain or clicking is indicative of a torn meniscus of the knee. There are a number of provocative knee tests for knee and ligament injuries, which can be seen in Budoff and Nirschl (2013).

ASSESSMENT PROCEDURE	NORMAL FINDINGS	ABNORMAL FINDINGS

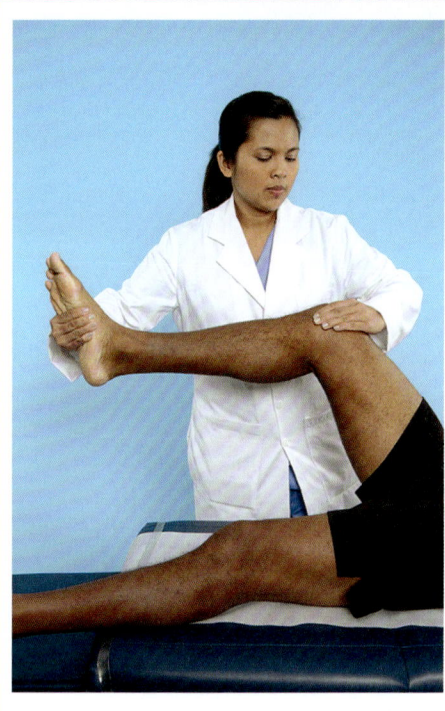

FIGURE 24-30 Performing McMurray test.

Ankles and Feet

INSPECTION AND PALPATION

With the client sitting, standing, and walking, inspect position, alignment, shape, and skin.	Toes usually point forward and lie flat; however, they may point in (pes varus) or point out (pes valgus). Toes and feet are in alignment with the lower leg. Smooth, rounded medial malleolar prominences with prominent heels and metatarsophalangeal joints. Skin is smooth and free of corns and calluses. Longitudinal arch; most of the weight bearing is on the foot midline.	A laterally deviated great toe with possible overlapping of the second toe and possible formation of an enlarged, painful, inflamed bursa (bunion) on the medial side is seen with hallux valgus. Common abnormalities include feet with no arches (pes planus or "flat feet"), feet with high arches (pes cavus); painful thickening of the skin over bony prominences and at pressure points (corns); nonpainful thickened skin that occurs at pressure points (calluses); and painful warts (verruca vulgaris) that often occur under a callus (plantar warts; Abnormal Findings 24-3).
Palpate ankles and feet for tenderness, heat, swelling, or nodules (Fig. 24-31). Palpate the toes from the distal end proximally, noting tenderness, swelling, bony prominences, nodules, or crepitus of each interphalangeal joint.	No pain, heat, swelling, or nodules are noted.	Ankles are the most common site of sprains, which occur with stretched or torn ligaments (tough bands of fibrous tissue connecting bones in a joint (National Institute of Arthritis and Musculoskeletal and Skin Diseases [NIAMS], 2014). Tender, painful, reddened, hot, and swollen metatarsophalangeal joint of the great toe is seen in gouty arthritis. Nodules of the posterior ankle may be palpated with rheumatoid arthritis.

Continued on following page

ASSESSMENT PROCEDURE	NORMAL FINDINGS	ABNORMAL FINDINGS

Ankles and Feet (Continued)

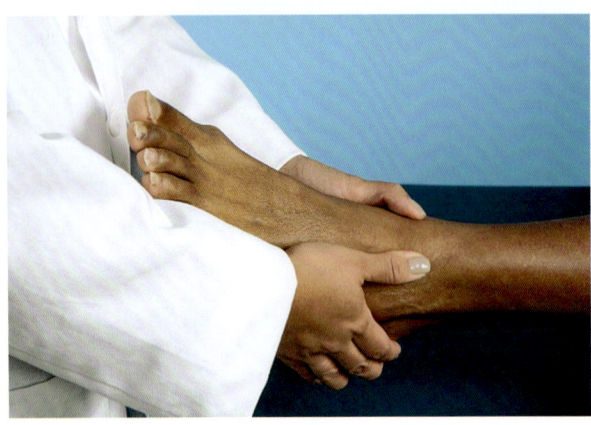

FIGURE 24-31 Palpating the ankles and feet.

Assess the metatarsophalangeal joints by squeezing the foot from each side with your thumb and fingers. Palpate each metatarsal, noting swelling or tenderness. Palpate the plantar area (bottom) of the foot, noting pain or swelling.

Pain and tenderness of the metatarsophalangeal joints are seen in inflammation of the joints, rheumatoid arthritis, and DJD. Tenderness of the calcaneus of the bottom of the foot may indicate plantar fasciitis. Plantar fasciitis is the most common cause of heel pain, which occurs when the strong supportive band of tissue in the arch of the foot becomes irritated and inflamed (Goff & Crawford, 2011).

Use the Ottawa ankle and foot rules (Box 24-3) to determine need for x-ray referral (Tiemstra, 2012).

Perform the squeeze test by squeezing the middle of the foot with your hand across top of foot as shown (Fig. 24-32).

Client tolerates squeeze test without extreme pain.

Extreme pain may indicate rheumatoid arthritis and psoriatic arthritis of the foot.

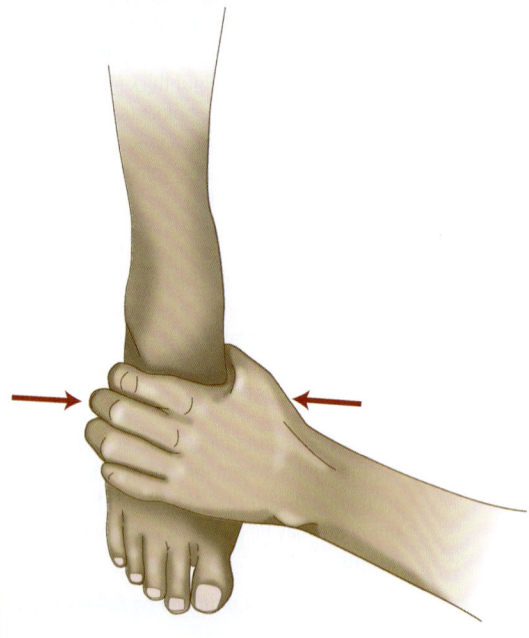

FIGURE 24-32 Squeeze test on the foot.

ASSESSMENT PROCEDURE	NORMAL FINDINGS	ABNORMAL FINDINGS
Test ROM (Fig. 24-33). Ask the client to: • Point toes upward (dorsiflexion) and then downward (plantarflexion, Fig. 24-33A). • Turn soles outward (eversion) and then inward (inversion, Fig. 24-33B). • Rotate foot outward (abduction) and then inward (adduction, Fig. 24-33C). • Turn toes under foot (flexion) and then upward (extension).	Normal ranges: • 20 degrees dorsiflexion of ankle and foot and 45 degrees plantarflexion of ankle and foot. • 20 degrees of eversion and 30 degrees of inversion. • 10 degrees of abduction and 20 degrees of adduction. • 40 degrees of flexion and 40 degrees of extension.	Decreased strength against resistance is seen in muscle and joint disease. Hyperextension of the metatarsophalangeal joint and flexion of the proximal interphalangeal joint is apparent in hammer toe (see Abnormal Findings 24-3).

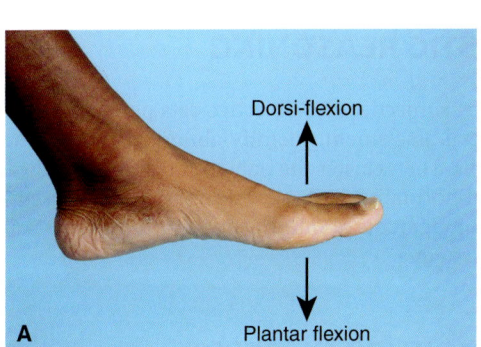
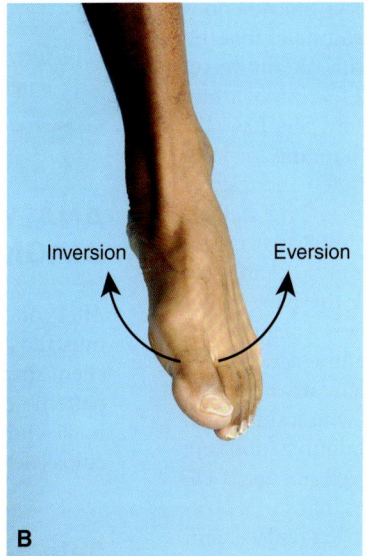
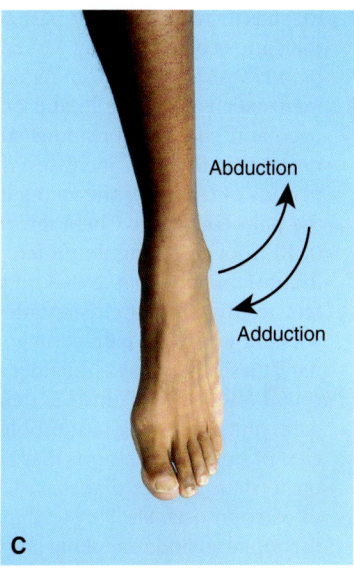

FIGURE 24-33 Normal range of motion of the feet and ankles: (**A**) dorsiflexion–plantarflexion; (**B**) eversion–inversion; (**C**) abduction–adduction.

Repeat these maneuvers against resistance.	Client has full ROM against resistance.	Decreased strength against resistance is common in muscle and joint disease.

CASE STUDY

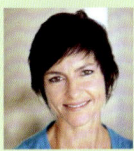

The chapter case study is now used to demonstrate the physical examination of Frances Funstead's back.
Inspection: Posture erect. Movement is coordinated and rhythmic. Arms swing in opposition. Able to stand on heels and toes. Cervical and lumbar spines are concave. Thoracic spine is convex.
Palpation: Cervical, thoracic, and lumbar spinous processes nontender. Lumbar paravertebral muscles are firm, taut, and tender bilaterally. Lumbar spine: Flexion is decreased at 60 degrees; lateral bending is decreased at 25 degrees and guarded bilaterally; hyperextension is normal at 30 degrees; rotation decreased at 20 degrees bilaterally and elicits discomfort. The straight leg test is negative. Leg length is equal.

BOX 24-3 OTTAWA ANKLE RULES FOR X-RAY REFERRAL

ANKLE X-RAY INDICATORS
Malleolar-area pain and bone tenderness at the tips of 6-cm edges of the lateral malleolus or medial malleolus, or the inability to bear weight immediately or during examination indicate the need for an ankle x-ray.

FOOT X-RAY INDICATORS
Pain in the midfoot area and bone tenderness at the base of the fifth metatarsal or the navicular bone area, or the inability to bear weight immediately or during examination, indicate the need for a foot x-ray (Tiemstra, 2012).

Validating and Documenting Findings

Validate the musculoskeletal assessment data you have collected. This is necessary to verify that the data are reliable and accurate.

CASE STUDY

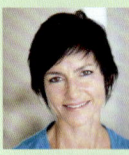

Think back to the case study. The occupational health nurse documented the following subjective and objective assessment findings of Frances Funstead's back examination.

Biographic Data: Ms. Funstead, 55-year-old Caucasian woman. Alert and oriented. Asks and answers questions appropriately.

Reason for Seeking Health Care: "I have pain and stiffness in my lower back."

History of Present Health Concern: The client reports that 2 weeks ago she developed low back pain and stiffness that has increased over the past 2–3 days. She describes the pain as dull and achy. Ms. Funstead states that the pain is worse in the morning and with certain movements such as getting in and out of the car, bending over, and changing positions suddenly. She has also noted that the pain increases after standing for long periods of time. Despite taking ibuprofen and resting, the pain continues. Client rates pain as 7 on scale of 0–10 prior to taking ibuprofen. An hour after taking ibuprofen, rates pain as 3–4 on scale of 0–10. Ibuprofen, resting, and stretching alleviate the pain somewhat; however, the pain never goes away. Client denies paresthesias and bowel/bladder incontinence.

Personal History: Ms. Funstead denies any recent weight gain. She denies any past problems with joints, muscles, or bones. She reports that her immunizations are up to date. Denies diabetes, sickle cell anemia, SLE, or osteoporosis. Ms. Funstead reports that she is postmenopausal and not taking any estrogen replacement therapy.

Family History: Ms. Funstead denies family history of rheumatoid arthritis, gout, or osteoporosis.

Lifestyle and Health Practices: Ms. Funstead reports that she tries to walk 30 minutes three times weekly and is usually successful. Client denies issues with weight gain or loss, but does feel as if she needs to lose weight. Ms. Funstead's medications include: Calcium with vitamin D supplement two times daily, ibuprofen 400 mg every 8 hours as needed.

Client denies use of tobacco or alcohol. She admits to drinking 3–4 cups of coffee each morning and 32 oz of diet cola throughout the day. Her 24-hour diet recall includes: Breakfast–cereal bar and coffee; lunch—low-calorie frozen meal, yogurt, apple, diet cola; dinner—chicken noodle soup, salad, fruit smoothie, 8-oz glass of 2% milk. Activities in a typical day include: Awakens at 5:30 AM and gets ready for work. Works from 7 AM to 3 PM. Walks after work with friends. Goes homes, prepares dinner, does household chores, watches TV; in bed by 10:30 PM.

Ms. Funstead works at a local factory on an assembly line. She picks up small parts and places them in a motor. She twists from side to side throughout the work day. She has one 15-minute break in the morning, 30 minutes for lunch, and one 15-minute break in the afternoon. She stands while at work and is required to wear steel-toed shoes. She denies difficulty performing ADLs. She does not require the use of assistive devices for mobility. Client denies any change in body image or self-esteem.

Physical Examination Findings

Inspection: Posture erect. Movement is coordinated and rhythmic. Arms swing in opposition. Able to stand on heels and toes. Cervical and lumbar spines are concave. Thoracic spine is convex.

Palpation: Cervical, thoracic, and lumbar spinous processes nontender. Lumbar paravertebral muscles are firm, taut, and tender bilaterally.

Lumbar spine: Flexion is decreased at 60 degrees; lateral bending is decreased at 25 degrees and guarded bilaterally; hyperextension is normal at 30 degrees; rotation decreased at 20 degrees bilaterally and elicits discomfort. Lasègue test (straight leg test) is negative. Leg length is equal.

ANALYSIS OF DATA: DIAGNOSTIC REASONING

After collecting subjective and objective data pertaining to the musculoskeletal assessment, identify abnormal findings and client strengths. Then cluster the data to reveal any significant patterns or abnormalities. These data may then be used to make clinical judgments about the status of the client's musculoskeletal system.

Selected Nursing Diagnoses

Following is a list of selected nursing diagnoses (health promotion, risk, or actual) that you may identify when analyzing the cue clusters.

Health Promotion Diagnoses

- Readiness for Enhanced Health Management: activity and exercise patterns related to expressed desire to improve status

Risk Diagnoses

- Risk for Trauma related to repetitive movements of wrists or elbows with recreation or occupation
- Risk for Injury: Pathologic fractures related to osteoporosis
- Risk for Injury to joints, muscles, or bones related to environmental hazards
- Risk for Disuse Syndrome
- Risk for Urinary Retention related to urine stasis secondary to immobility

Actual Diagnoses

- Impaired Physical Mobility related to impaired joint movement, decreased muscle strength, or fractured bone
- Activity Intolerance related to muscle weakness or joint pain
- Constipation related to decreased gastric motility and muscle tone secondary to immobility
- Ineffective Sexuality Pattern related to lower back pain
- Acute (or Chronic) Pain related to joint, muscle, or bone problems

- Impaired Skin Integrity related to prolonged pressure on the skin secondary to immobility
- Impaired Social Interaction related to depression or immobility
- Disturbed Body Image related to skeletal deformities

Selected Collaborative Problems

After grouping the data, certain collaborative problems may become apparent. Remember that collaborative problems differ from nursing diagnoses in that they cannot be prevented by nursing interventions alone. However, these physiologic complications of medical conditions can be detected and monitored by the nurse. In addition, the nurse can use physician- and nurse-prescribed interventions to minimize the complications of these problems. The nurse may also have to refer the client in such situations for further treatment of the problem.

Following is a list of collaborative problems that may be identified when obtaining a general impression. These problems are worded as Risk for Complications (RC), followed by the problem:
- RC: Osteoporosis
- RC: Joint dislocation
- RC: Compartmental syndrome
- RC: Pathologic fractures

Medical Problems

After grouping the data, it may become apparent that the client's signs and symptoms clearly require medical diagnosis and treatment. Referral to a primary care provider is necessary.

CASE STUDY

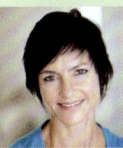

After collecting and analyzing the data for Frances Funstead, the nurse determines that the following conclusions are appropriate:

Nursing Diagnoses
- Acute pain: lower back r/t possible work pattern strain on back muscles
- Readiness for Enhanced Health Management r/t seeking help from occupational health nurse
- Impaired Home Maintenance r/t limitations on ability to care for home
- Risk for Interrupted Family Processes r/t inability to participate in sexual relations with husband, and to fulfill usual home maintenance role

Potential Collaborative Problems
- RC: Nerve damage, vertebral or sciatic
- RC: Slipped or herniated disc
- RC: Emotional depression
- RC: Leg muscle paralysis

Interdisciplinary Verbal Communication of Assessment Findings Using SBAR

SITUATION: Ms. Funstead, a 55-year-old Caucasian woman, has dull, achy lower back pain, rated a 7 (scale 1–10), which for the last 2 weeks has hurt more with movement and extended standing and has increased over last 2–3 days. Believes this is related to her assembly line job, during which she needs frequent breaks from standing, and also needs to lie down after work. Resting and stretching relieve pain a little. Reports ibuprofen decreases pain to level 4 but pain increases before next dose is due. Has interfered with her ability to walk for exercise and to have sexual relations with husband. Denies paresthesias and bowel/bladder incontinence.

BACKGROUND: Works at a local factory on an assembly line where she picks up small parts and places them in a motor, twisting from side to side. Has 15-minute breaks in the morning and afternoon and 30-minute lunch break. She stands while at work and is required to wear steel-toed shoes.

ASSESSMENT: Posture erect and gait is coordinated and rhythmic. Arms swing in opposition. Able to stand on heels and toes. Cervical and lumbar spines are concave. Thoracic spine is convex. Cervical, thoracic, and lumbar spinous processes nontender. Lumbar paravertebral muscles are firm, taut, and tender bilaterally. Lumbar spine: Flexion is decreased at 60 degrees; lateral bending is decreased at 25 degrees and guarded bilaterally; hyperextension is normal at 30 degrees; rotation decreased at 20 degrees bilaterally and elicits discomfort. The straight leg test is negative. Leg length is equal.

RECOMMENDATION: Ms. Funstead has acute pain: lower back r/t possible work pattern strain on back muscles. She is ready for Enhanced Health Management r/t seeking help from occupational health nurse. In addition, she is at Risk for Interrupted Family Processes r/t inability to participate in sexual relations with husband, and to fulfill usual home maintenance role. She needs to be assessed by her primary care provider for the potential complications of nerve damage, vertebral or sciatic, and a slipped or herniated disc. She also needs to receive physical therapy for her back pain and assistance to be able to return to her usual activities of daily living (working, walking, caring for home, and sexual relations with her husband).

To view an algorithm depicting the process of diagnostic reasoning for this case, go to thePoint.

ABNORMAL FINDINGS   24-1   **Abnormal Spinal Curvatures**

THORACIC KYPHOSIS, LORDOSIS, AND SCOLIOSIS

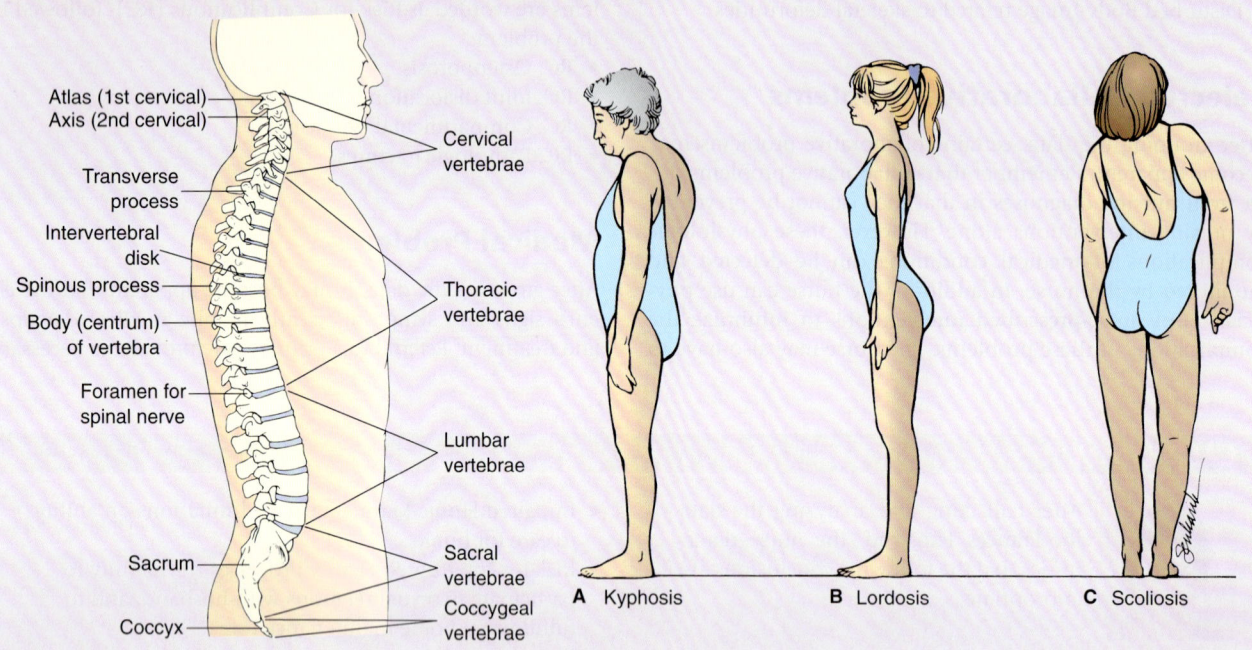

A Kyphosis   B Lordosis   C Scoliosis

FLATTENING OF THE LUMBAR CURVATURE

Flattening of the lumbar curvature may be seen with a herniated lumbar disc or ankylosing spondylitis.

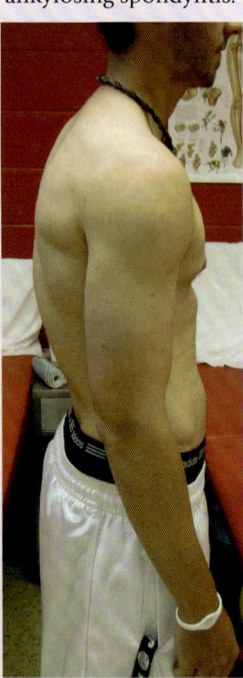

LUMBAR HYPERLORDOSIS

Hip flexion contracture and hip extensor weakness drive the lumbar spine into increasing lordosis to balance head over pelvis. Note the use of the hands for stability.

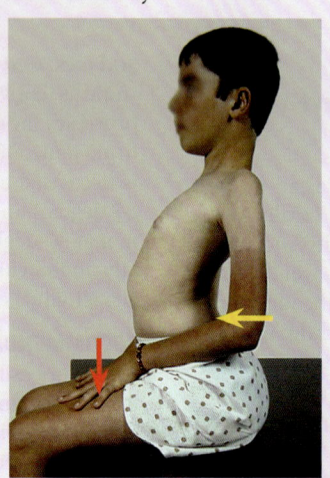

KYPHOSIS

A rounded thoracic convexity (kyphosis).

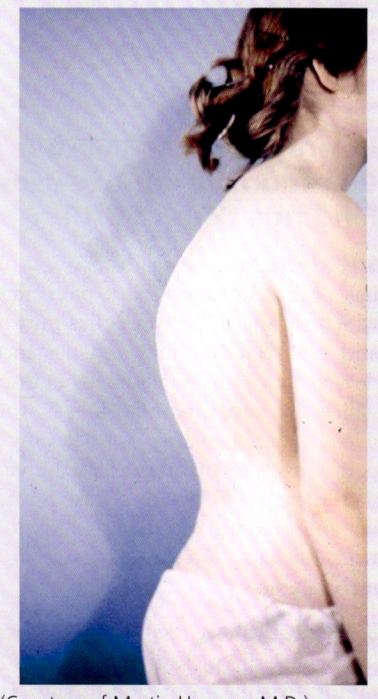

(Courtesy of Martin Herman, M.D.)

SCOLIOSIS

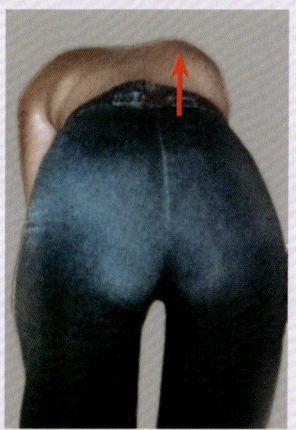

A lateral curvature of the spine with an increase in convexity on the side that is curved is seen in scoliosis.

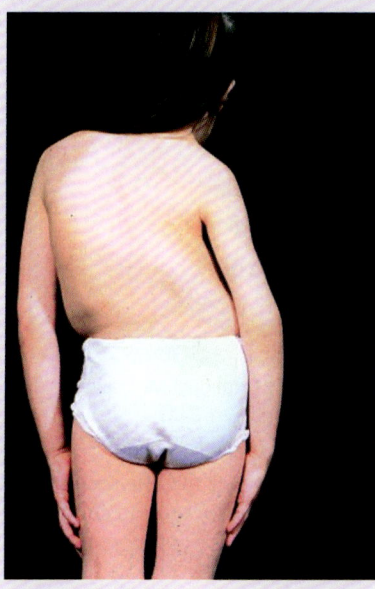

(Used with permission from SIU/Biomedical Communications/Custom Medical Stock Photography.)

ANKYLOSING SPONDYLITIS

Clinical manifestations of ankylosing spondylitis

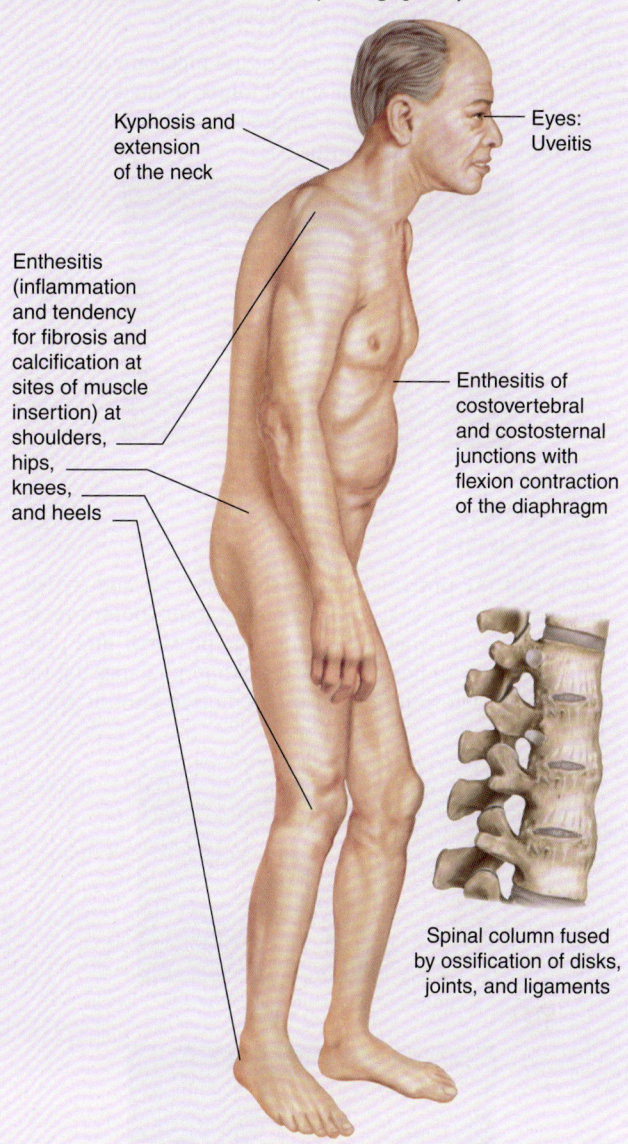

Kyphosis and extension of the neck

Eyes: Uveitis

Enthesitis (inflammation and tendency for fibrosis and calcification at sites of muscle insertion) at shoulders, hips, knees, and heels

Enthesitis of costovertebral and costosternal junctions with flexion contraction of the diaphragm

Spinal column fused by ossification of disks, joints, and ligaments

---

ABNORMAL FINDINGS 24-2 | Abnormalities Affecting the Wrists, Hands, and Fingers

The following abnormalities are commonly associated with the upper extremities. Early detection is important because early intervention may help to preserve dexterity and daily function.

ACUTE RHEUMATOID ARTHRITIS

Tender, painful, swollen, stiff joints are seen in acute rheumatoid arthritis.

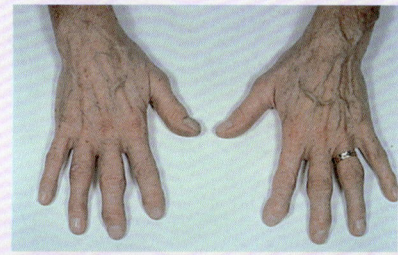

(© 1991 National Medical Slide Bank/CMSP.)

Continued on following page

ABNORMAL FINDINGS 24-2　Abnormalities Affecting the Wrists, Hands, and Fingers (Continued)

CHRONIC RHEUMATOID ARTHRITIS
Chronic swelling and thickening of the metacarpophalangeal and proximal interphalangeal joints, limited range of motion, and finger deviation toward the ulnar side are seen in chronic rheumatoid arthritis.

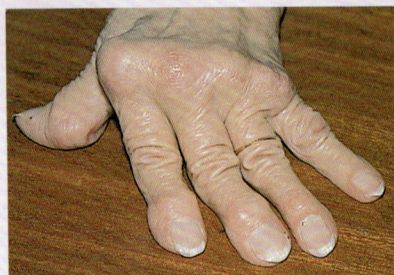
(© 1995 Science Photo Library.)

BOUTONNIÈRE AND SWAN-NECK DEFORMITIES
Flexion of the proximal interphalangeal joint and hyperextension of the distal interphalangeal joint (boutonnière deformity) and hyperextension of the proximal interphalangeal joint with flexion of the distal interphalangeal joint (swan-neck deformity) are also common in chronic rheumatoid arthritis.

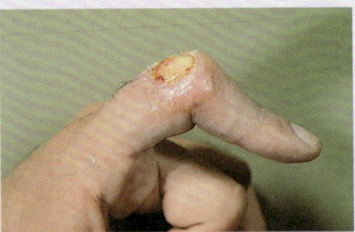
Boutonnière deformity (© 1990 CMSP).

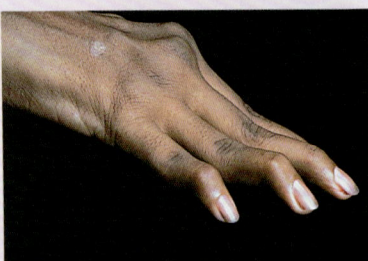
Swan-neck deformity (© 1991 National Medical Slide Bank/CMSP).

GANGLION
Nontender, round, enlarged, swollen, fluid-filled cyst (ganglion) is commonly seen at the dorsum of the wrist.

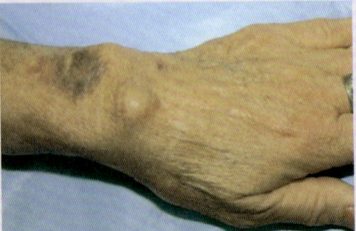

OSTEOARTHRITIS
Osteoarthritis (degenerative joint disease) nodules on the dorsolateral aspects of the distal interphalangeal joints (Heberden nodes) are due to the bony overgrowth of osteoarthritis. Usually hard and painless, they may affect middle-aged or older adults and often, although not always, are associated with arthritic changes in other joints. Flexion and deviation deformities may develop.

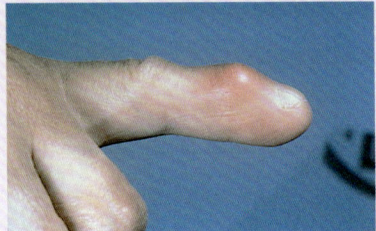
Heberden nodes (© 1991 National Medical Slide Bank/CMSP).

Similar nodules on the proximal interphalangeal joints (Bouchard nodes) are less common. The metacarpophalangeal joints are spared.

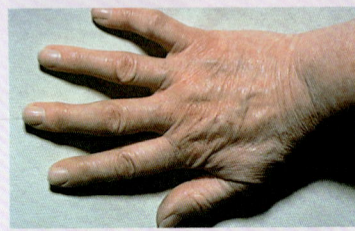
Bouchard nodes (© 1991 National Medical Slide Bank/CMSP).

TENOSYNOVITIS
Painful extension of a finger may be seen in acute tenosynovitis (infection of the flexor tendon sheaths).

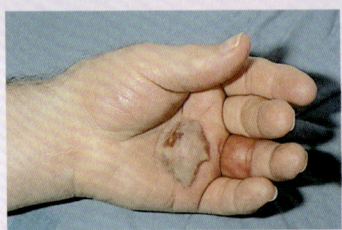
(© 1995 Michael English, M.D./CMSP.)

THENAR ATROPHY
Atrophy of the thenar prominence due to pressure on the median nerve is seen in carpal tunnel syndrome.

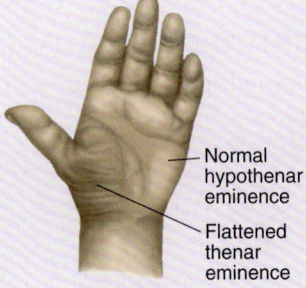
– Normal hypothenar eminence
– Flattened thenar eminence

(Used with permission from Bickley, L. S., & Szilagyi, P. (2003). *Bates' guide to physical examination and history taking* (8th ed.). Philadelphia, PA: Lippincott Williams & Wilkins.)

ABNORMAL FINDINGS 24-3 Abnormalities of the Feet and Toes

The following abnormalities affect the feet and toes, typically causing discomfort and impeding mobility. Early detection and treatment can help to restore or maximize function.

ACUTE GOUTY ARTHRITIS

In gouty arthritis, the metatarsophalangeal joint of the great toe is tender, painful, reddened, hot, and swollen.

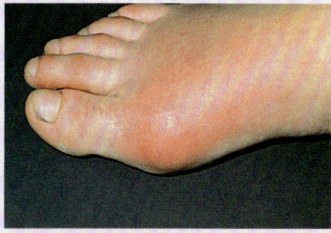

FLAT FEET

A flat foot (pes planus) has no arch and may cause pain and swelling of the foot surface.

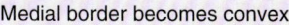

Medial border becomes convex

Sole touches floor

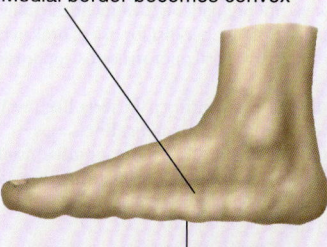

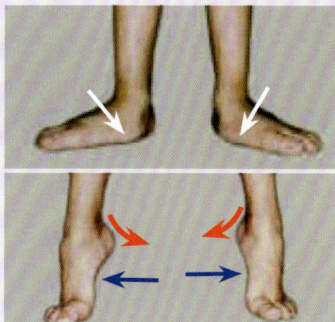

Examining flexibility of the flat foot.

CALLUS

Calluses are nonpainful, thickened skin that occurs at pressure points.

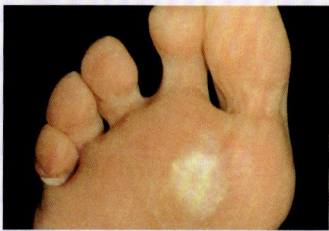

HALLUX VALGUS

Hallux valgus is an abnormality in which the great toe is deviated laterally and may overlap the second toe. An enlarged, painful, inflamed bursa (bunion) may form on the medial side.

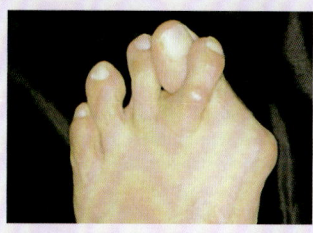

CORN

Corns are painful thickenings of the skin that occur over bony prominences and at pressure points. The circular, central, translucent core resembles a kernel of corn.

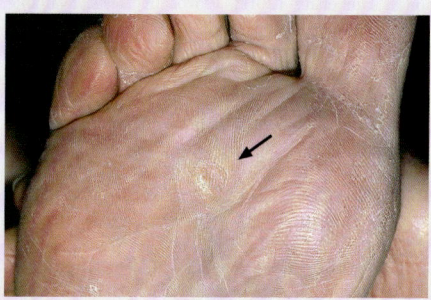

HAMMER TOE

Hyperextension at the metatarsophalangeal joint with flexion at the proximal interphalangeal joint (hammer toe) commonly occurs with the second toe.

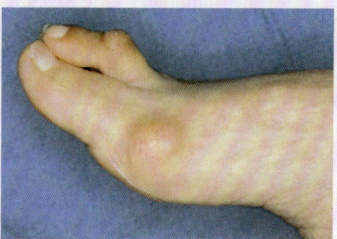

PLANTAR WART

Plantar warts are painful warts (verruca vulgaris) that often occur under a callus, appearing as tiny dark spots.

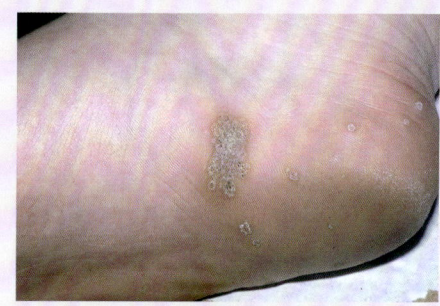

Image credits: Gouty arthritis, © 1995 Science Photo Library/CMSP; Flat feet, from Bickley, L. S., & Szilagyi, P. (2003). *Bates' guide to physical examination and history taking* (8th ed.). Philadelphia, PA: Lippincott Williams & Wilkins; Examining flat feet, Diab, M., Staheli, L.T. (2015). *Practice of paediatric orthopaedics* (3rd ed.). Philadelphia, PA: Wolters Kluwer l Lippincott Williams & Wilkins; Corn and Plantar wart, from Goodheart, H. P. (2003). *Goodheart's photoguide of common skin disorders* (2nd ed.). Philadelphia, PA: Lippincott Williams & Wilkins).

Want to know more?

A wide variety of resources to enhance your learning and understanding of this book are available on thePoint. Visit thePoint to access:

NCLEX-Style Student Review Questions
Watch and Learn Videos
Concept in Action Animations
And more!

References and Selected Readings

Andrews, M., & Boyle, J. (2016). *Transcultural concepts in nursing care* (7th ed.). Philadelphia, PA: Lippincott Williams & Wilkins.

Arthritis Research UK. (2013). Step 1 – Recognizing symptoms before seeking help. Available at http://www.arthritisresearchuk.org/arthritis-information/inflammatory-arthritis-pathway/step-one.aspx

Budoff, J., & Nirschl, R. (2013). Knee problems: Diagnostic tests for knee and ligament injuries. *Consultant*, 53(9), 629–632. Available at http://www.consultant360.com/articles/knee-problems-diagnostic-tests-ligament-injuries

Carpal-Tunnel.net. (2011). Provocative tests. Available at http://www.carpaltunnel.net/diagnosing/provocative

Centers for Disease Control and Prevention (CDC). (2015). Tdap (tetanus, diphtheria, pertussis) VIS. Available at http://www.cdc.gov/vaccines/hcp/vis/vis-statements/tdap.html

East Kent Hospitals University. (2011). Provocative tests. Available at http://www.carpal-tunnel.net/diagnosing/provocative

Goff, J., & Crawford, R. (2011). Diagnosis and treatment of plantar fasciitis. *American Family Physician*, 84(6), 676–692. Available at http://www.aafp.org/afp/2011/0915/p676.html

Goodman, B. (2011). New recommendations for osteoporosis screening. Available at http://www.webmd.com/osteoporosis/news/20110119/new-recommendations-osteoporosis-screening

Harris, C., Gurden, S., Martindale, J., & Jeffries, C. (2012). Differentiating mechanical and inflammatory back pain. Available at file:///C:/Users/Jane Kelley-PC/Downloads/ibp-module%20(1).pdf

Healthy People 2020. (2016). Arthritis, osteoporosis, and chronic back pain conditions. Available at http://www.healthypeople.gov/2020/topics-objectives/topic/Arthritis-Osteoporosis-and-Chronic-Back-Conditions

Hong, E. (2015). Hip and groin injuries in the athlete. Available at http://www.philly.com/philly/blogs/sportsdoc/Hip-and-groin-injuries-in-the-athlete.html

International Osteoporosis Foundation (IOF). (2015a). Osteoporosis & musculoskeletal disorders. Available at http://www.iofbonehealth.org/osteoporosis-musculoskeletal-disorders

International Osteoporosis Foundation (IOF). (2015b). Osteoporosis: Facts & statistics. Available at http://www.iofbonehealth.org/facts-statistics

International Osteoporosis Foundation (IOF). (2015c). The new interactive IOF one-minute osteoporosis risk test. Available at http://www.iofbonehealth.org/iof-one-minute-osteoporosis-risk-test

"Lactose Intolerance by Ethnicity and Region". (2010). Available at http://milk.procon.org/view.resource.php?resourceID=000661

Li, H., & Zhu, H. (2005). Relationship between the age of menarche, menopause and other factors and postmenopause osteoporosis. *Zhonghua Fu Chan KeZaZhi*, 40(12), 796–798. Available at http://www.ncbi.nlm.nih.gov/pubmed/16412321

Mayo Clinic. (2015). Fibromyalgia. Available at http://www.mayoclinic.org/diseases-conditions/fibromyalgia/basics/complications/con-20019243

National Institute of Arthritis and Musculoskeletal and Skin Diseases (NIAMS). (2014). What are sprains and strains? Available at http://www.niams.nih.gov/health_info/Sprains_Strains/sprains_and_strains_ff.asp#c

National Institutes of Health Osteoporosis and Related Bone Diseases National Resource Center (NIH ORBDNRC). (2015). What people with diabetes need to know about osteoporosis. Available at http://www.niams.nih.gov/health_info/bone/Osteoporosis/Conditions_Behaviors/diabetes.asp

National Osteoporosis Foundation (NOF). (2014). 54 million Americans affected by osteoporosis or low bone mass. Available at http://nof.org/news/2948

National Osteoporosis Foundation (NOF). (2016). Calcium/vitamin D. Available at https://www.nof.org/patients/treatment/calciumvitamin-d/

Osteoporosis Canada. (2017). Checklist for risk of broken bones and osteoporosis. Available at http://www.osteoporosis.ca/osteoporosis-and-you/diagnosis/risk-factors/

Rodriguez, D. (2015). What arthritis pain feels like. Available at http://www.everydayhealth.com/arthritis/pain-and-stiffness.aspx

The Bosham Clinic Medical. (2014). Osteoporosis. Available at http://www.theboshamclinic.co.uk/medical/treatments/osteoporosis

Tiemstra, J. (2012). Update on acute ankle sprains. American Family Physician, 85(12), 1170–1176.

UCSF Medical Center. (2016). Hand and wrist fractures. Available at https://www.ucsfhealth.org/conditions/hand_and_wrist_fractures/

U.S. Food and Drug Administration (USFDA). (2015). FDA expands advice on statin risks. Available at http://www.fda.gov/ForConsumers/ConsumerUpdates/ucm293330.htm

U.S. Preventive Services Task Force (USPSTF). (2011). Screening for osteoporosis. Available at http://www.uspreventiveservicestaskforce.org/uspstf10/osteoporosis/osteors.htm

25 ASSESSING NEUROLOGIC SYSTEM

Learning Objectives

1. Describe the structure and the function of the central and peripheral nervous systems.
2. Discuss risk factors associated with a cerebral vascular accident (CVA), commonly known as stroke, across the cultures and ways to reduce one's risks.
3. Interview a client for an accurate nursing history of the neurologic system.
4. Perform a physical assessment of the neurologic system using the correct techniques.
5. Differentiate between normal and abnormal findings of the neurologic system.
6. Describe the findings frequently seen with assessing the older client's neurologic system.
7. Analyze the data from the interview and physical assessment of the neurologic system to formulate valid nursing diagnoses, collaborative problems, and/or referrals.
8. Differentiate between general routine screening versus skills needed for focused or specialty assessment of the neurologic system.
9. Document and verbally report accurate assessment findings of the neurologic system.

CASE STUDY

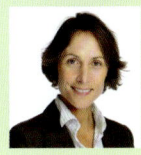

Linda Hutchison, a 49-year-old Caucasian high school teacher, has had multiple sclerosis (MS) for over 20 years. She has been very tired lately, has had trouble maintaining urinary continence, is experiencing weakness, and describes a "pins and needles" feeling in her legs. Also, muscle spasms at night are affecting her ability to sleep. She is concerned about an exacerbation of her MS and arrives at her scheduled appointment to discuss ways to prevent this from happening.

 ## STRUCTURE AND FUNCTION

The very complex neurologic system is responsible for coordinating and regulating all body functions. It consists of two structural components: the central nervous system (CNS) and the peripheral nervous system.

Central Nervous System

The CNS encompasses the brain and spinal cord, which are covered by meninges, three layers of connective tissue that protect and nourish the CNS. The subarachnoid space surrounds the brain and spinal cord. The subarachnoid space is filled with cerebrospinal fluid (CSF), which is formed in the ventricles of the brain and flows through the ventricles into the space. This fluid-filled space cushions the brain and spinal cords, nourishes the CNS, and removes waste materials. Electrical activity of the CNS is governed by neurons located throughout the sensory and motor neural pathways. The CNS contains upper motor neurons that influence lower motor neurons, located mostly in the peripheral nervous system.

Brain

Located in the cranial cavity, the brain has four major divisions: the cerebrum, the diencephalon, the brain stem, and the cerebellum (Fig. 25-1).

Cerebrum

The cerebrum is divided into the right and left cerebral hemispheres, which are joined by the corpus callosum—a bundle of nerve fibers responsible for communication between the hemispheres. Each hemisphere sends and receives impulses from the opposite sides of the body and consists of four lobes (frontal, parietal, temporal, and occipital). The lobes are composed of a substance known as gray matter, which mediates higher-level functions such as memory, perception, communication, and initiation of voluntary movements. Consisting of aggregations of neuronal cell bodies, gray matter rims the surfaces of the cerebral hemispheres, forming the cerebral cortex.

Table 25-1 describes the specific functions of each lobe. Damage to a lobe results in impairment of the specific function directed by that lobe.

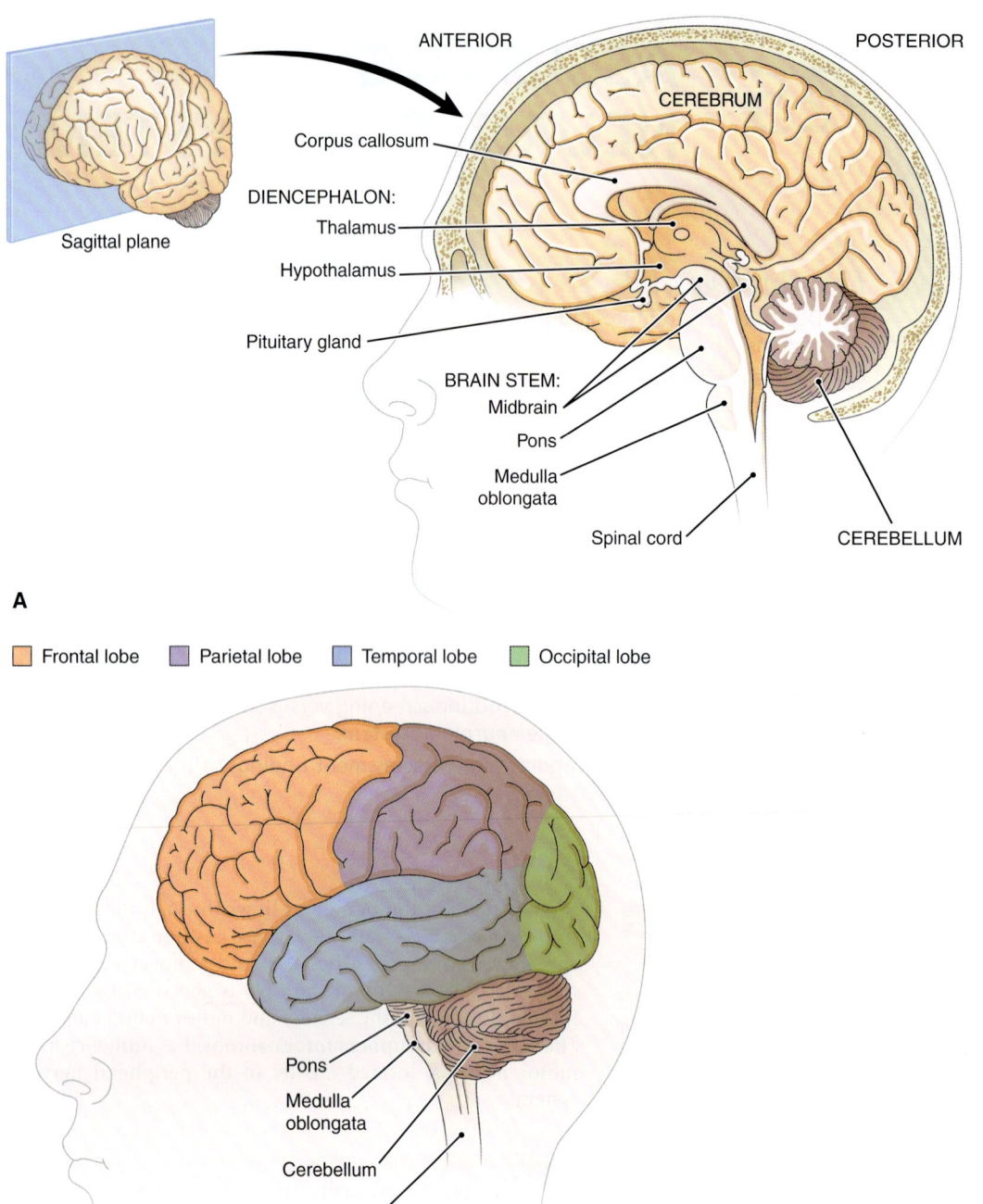

FIGURE 25-1 (**A**) Structures of the brain (sagittal section). (**B**) Lobes of the brain.

TABLE 25-1	Lobes of the Cerebral Hemispheres and Their Function
Lobe	Function
Frontal	Directs voluntary, skeletal actions (left side of lobe controls right side of body and right side of lobe controls left side of body). Also influences communication (talking and writing), emotions, intellect, reasoning ability, judgment, and behavior. Contains Broca area, which is responsible for speech.
Parietal	Interprets tactile sensations, including touch, pain, temperature, shapes, and two-point discrimination.
Occipital	Influences the ability to read with understanding and is the primary visual receptor center.
Temporal	Receives and interprets impulses from the ear. Contains Wernicke area, which is responsible for interpreting auditory stimuli.

25 Assessing Neurologic System   569

cerebellum to the cerebrum and the midbrain to the medulla. It is responsible for various reflex actions. The medulla oblongata contains the nuclei for cranial nerves, and has centers that control and regulate respiratory function, heart rate and force, and blood pressure.

Cerebellum

The cerebellum, located behind the brain stem and under the cerebrum, also has two hemispheres. Although the cerebellum does not initiate movement, its primary functions include coordination and smoothing of voluntary movements, maintenance of equilibrium, and maintenance of muscle tone.

Spinal Cord

The spinal cord (Fig. 25-2) is located in the vertebral canal and extends from the medulla oblongata to the first lumbar vertebra. (Note that the spinal cord is not as long as the vertebral canal.) The inner part of the cord has an H-shaped appearance and is made up of two pairs of columns (dorsal and ventral) consisting of gray matter. The outer part is made up of white matter and surrounds the gray matter (Fig. 25-3). The spinal cord conducts sensory impulses up ascending tracts to the brain, conducts motor impulses down descending tracts to neurons that stimulate glands and muscles throughout the body, and is responsible for simple reflex activity. Reflex activity involves various neural structures. For example, the stretch reflex—the simplest type of reflex arc—involves one sensory neuron (afferent), one motor neuron (efferent), and one synapse. An example of this is the knee jerk, which is elicited by tapping the patellar tendon. More complex reflexes involve three or more neurons.

Neural Pathways

Sensory impulses travel to the brain by way of two ascending neural pathways (the spinothalamic tract and posterior columns; Fig. 25-4). These impulses originate in the afferent fibers of the peripheral nerves and are carried through the posterior (dorsal) root into the spinal cord. Sensations of pain, temperature, and crude and light touch travel by way of the spinothalamic tract; sensations of position, vibration, and fine touch travel by way of the posterior columns. Motor impulses are conducted to the muscles by two descending

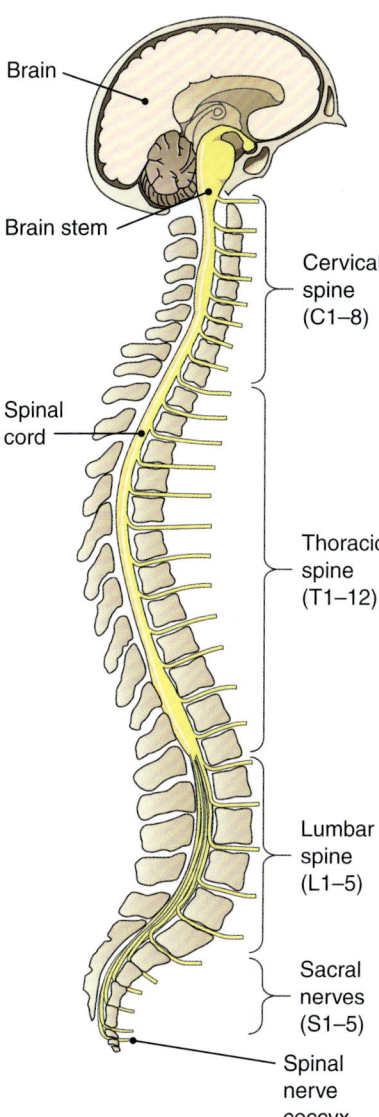

FIGURE 25-2 Spinal cord.

Diencephalon

The diencephalon lies beneath the cerebral hemispheres and consists of the thalamus and hypothalamus. Most sensory impulses travel through the gray matter of the thalamus, which is responsible for screening and directing the impulses to specific areas in the cerebral cortex. The hypothalamus (part of the autonomic nervous system, which is a part of the peripheral nervous system) is responsible for regulating many body functions, including water balance, appetite, vital signs (temperature, blood pressure, pulse, and respiratory rate), sleep cycles, pain perception, and emotional status.

Brain Stem

Located between the cerebral cortex and the spinal cord, the brain stem consists of mostly nerve fibers and has three parts: the midbrain, pons, and medulla oblongata. The midbrain serves as a relay center for ear and eye reflexes, and relays impulses between the higher cerebral centers and the lower pons, medulla, cerebellum, and spinal cord. The pons links the

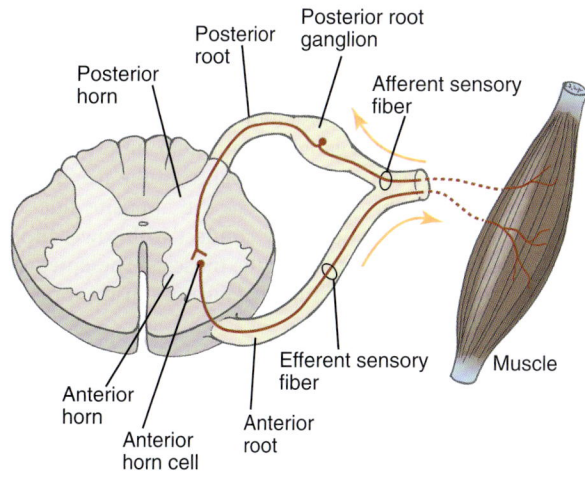

FIGURE 25-3 Cross-section of the spinal cord.

570 UNIT 3 Nursing Assessment of Physical Systems

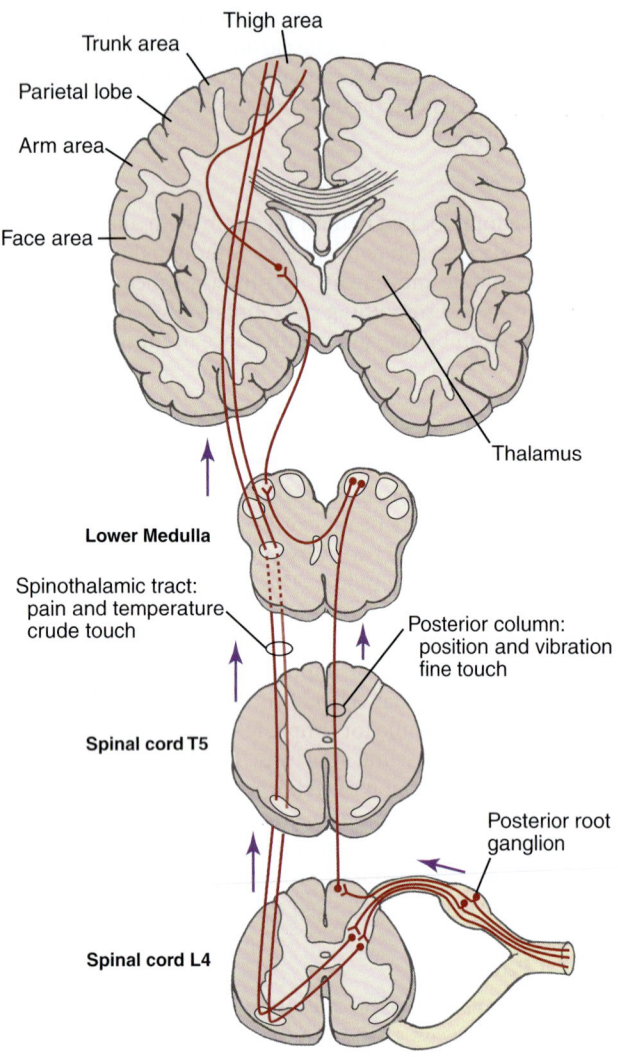

FIGURE 25-4 Sensory (ascending) neural pathways.

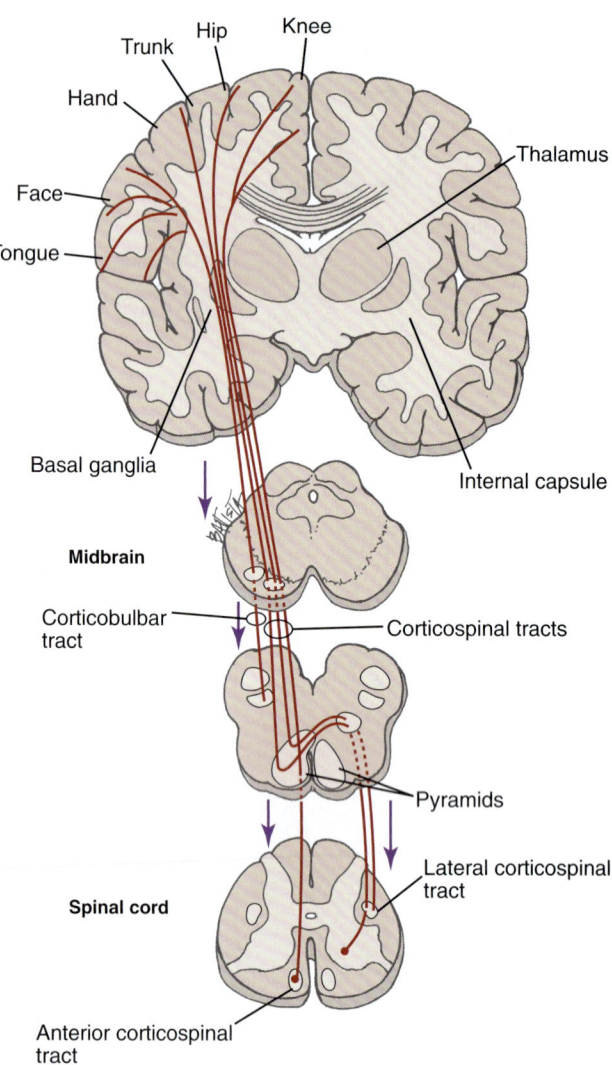

FIGURE 25-5 Motor (descending) neural pathways.

neural pathways: the pyramidal (corticospinal) tract and extrapyramidal tract (Fig. 25-5). The motor neurons of the pyramidal tract originate in the motor cortex and travel down to the medulla, where they cross over to the opposite side then travel down the spinal cord, where they synapse with a lower motor neuron in the anterior horn of the spinal cord. These impulses are carried to muscles and produce voluntary movements that involve skill and purpose. The extrapyramidal tract motor neurons consist of those motor neurons that originate in the motor cortex, basal ganglia, brain stem, and spinal cord outside the pyramidal tract. They travel from the frontal lobe to the pons, where they cross over to the opposite side and down the spinal cord, where they connect with lower motor neurons that conduct impulses to the muscles. These neurons conduct impulses related to maintenance of muscle tone and body control.

Peripheral Nervous System

Carrying information to and from the CNS, the peripheral nervous system consists of 12 pairs of cranial nerves and 31 pairs of spinal nerves. These nerves are categorized as two types of fibers: somatic and autonomic. Somatic fibers carry CNS impulses to voluntary skeletal muscles; autonomic fibers carry CNS impulses to smooth, involuntary muscles (in the heart and glands). The somatic nervous system mediates conscious, or voluntary, activities; the autonomic nervous system mediates unconscious, or involuntary, activities.

Cranial Nerves

Twelve pairs of cranial nerves evolve from the brain or brain stem (Fig. 25-6) and transmit motor or sensory messages. The nurse needs to remember the names of these 12 cranial nerves when assessing the client. A useful mnemonic for the 12 cranial nerves in Table 25-2 is "On Old Olympus' Towering Tops, A Finn and German Viewed Some Hops." To recall the type of impulse each nerve carries, listed in column 2 of this table, another useful mnemonic is "Some Say Marry Money, But My Brother Says Bad Business Marries Money." The third column in the table provides the primary function of each cranial nerve.

Spinal Nerves

Comprising 8 cervical, 12 thoracic, 5 lumbar, 5 sacral, and 1 coccygeal nerves, the 31 pairs of spinal nerves are named after

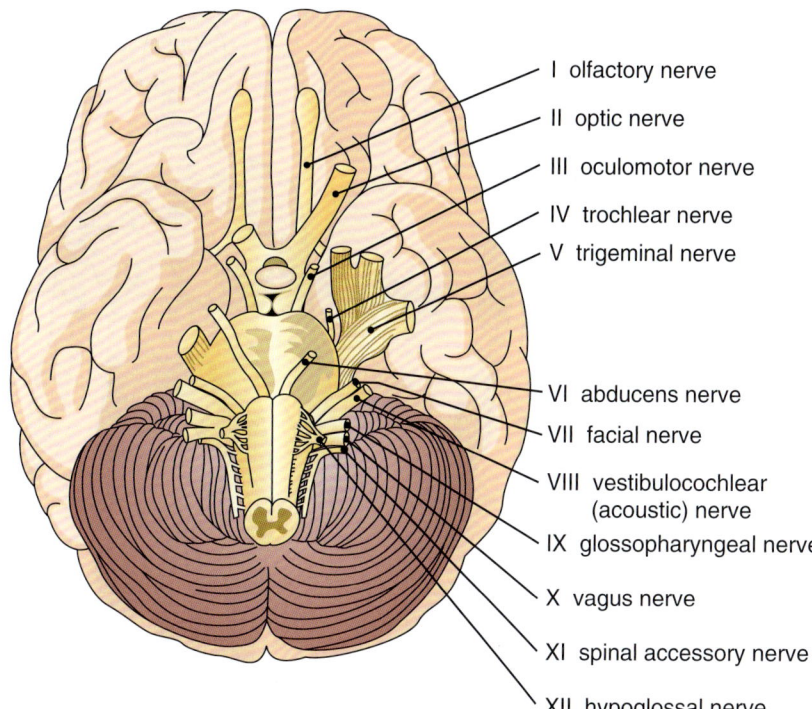

FIGURE 25-6 Cranial nerves, inferior view.

TABLE 25-2 Cranial Nerves: Type and Function

Cranial Nerve (Name)	Type of Impulse	Function
I (olfactory)	Sensory	Carries smell impulses from nasal mucous membrane to brain.
II (optic)	Sensory	Carries visual impulses from eye to brain.
III (oculomotor)	Motor	Contracts eye muscles to control eye movements (interior lateral, medial, and superior), constricts pupils, and elevates eyelids.
IV (trochlear)	Motor	Contracts one eye muscle to control inferomedial eye movement.
V (trigeminal)	Sensory motor	Carries sensory impulses of pain, touch, and temperature from the face to the brain. Influences clenching and lateral jaw movements (biting, chewing).
VI (abducens)	Motor	Controls lateral eye movements.
VII (facial)	Sensory	Contains sensory fibers for taste on anterior two thirds of tongue, and stimulates secretions from salivary glands (submaxillary and sublingual) and tears from lacrimal glands.
	Motor	Supplies the facial muscles and affects facial expressions (smiling, frowning, closing eyes).
VIII (acoustic, vestibulocochlear)	Sensory	Contains sensory fibers for hearing and balance.
IX (glossopharyngeal)	Sensory	Contains sensory fibers for taste on posterior third of tongue and sensory fibers of the pharynx that result in the gag reflex when stimulated.
	Motor	Provides secretory fibers to the parotid salivary glands; promotes swallowing movements.
X (vagus)	Sensory motor	Carries sensations from the throat, larynx, heart, lungs, bronchi, gastrointestinal tract, and abdominal viscera. Promotes swallowing, talking, and production of digestive juices.
XI (spinal accessory)	Motor	Innervates neck muscles (sternocleidomastoid and trapezius) that promote movement of the shoulders and head rotation. Also promotes some movement of the larynx.
XII (hypoglossal)	Motor	Innervates tongue muscles that promote the movement of food and talking.

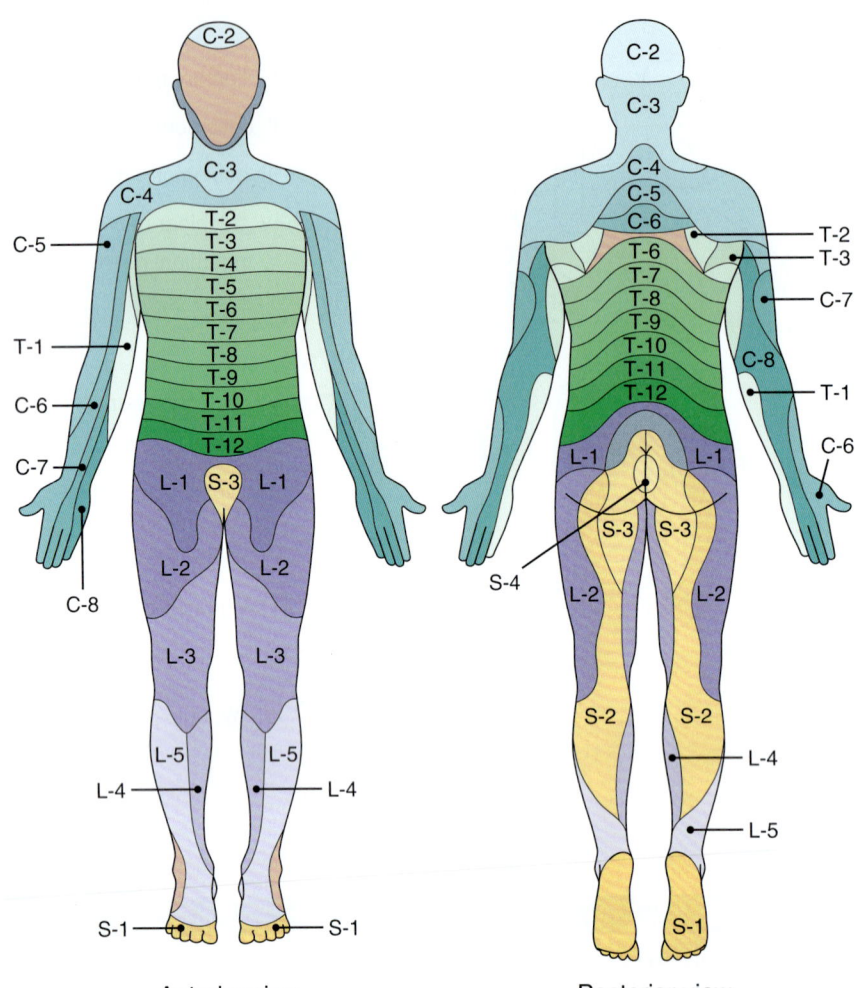

FIGURE 25-7 Anterior and posterior dermatomes (areas of skin innervated by spinal nerves).

the vertebrae below each one's exit point along the spinal cord (see Fig. 25-2). Each nerve is attached to the spinal cord by two nerve roots. The sensory (afferent) fiber enters through the dorsal (posterior) roots of the cord; the motor (efferent) fiber exits through the ventral (anterior) roots of the cord. The sensory root of each spinal nerve innervates an area of the skin called a dermatome (Fig. 25-7).

Autonomic Nervous System

Some peripheral nerves have a special function associated with automatic activities; they are referred to as the autonomic nervous system. Autonomic nervous system impulses are carried by both cranial and spinal nerves. These impulses are carried from the CNS to the involuntary, smooth muscles that make up the walls of the heart and glands. The autonomic nervous system, which maintains the internal homeostasis of the body, incorporates the sympathetic and parasympathetic nervous systems. The sympathetic nervous system ("fight-or-flight" system) is activated during stress and elicits responses such as decreased gastric secretions, bronchiole dilatation, increased pulse rate, and pupil dilatation. These sympathetic fibers arise from the thoracolumbar level (T1 to L2) of the spinal cord. The parasympathetic nervous system functions to restore and maintain normal body functions, for example, by decreasing heart rate. The parasympathetic fibers arise from the craniosacral regions (S1 to S4 and cranial nerves III, VI, IX, and X).

HEALTH ASSESSMENT

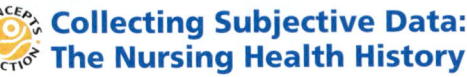

Collecting Subjective Data: The Nursing Health History

Problems with other body systems may affect the neurologic system, and neurologic system disorders can affect all other body systems. Regardless of the source of the neurologic problem, the client's total lifestyle and level of functioning are often affected. Because of their subjective nature, neurologic problems related to activities of daily living (ADLs) are typically detected through an in-depth nursing history. For example, problems with loss of concentration, loss of sensation, or dizziness are usually identified only through precise questioning during the interview with the client.

Clients who are experiencing symptoms associated with the neurologic system (such as headaches or memory loss) may be very fearful that they have a serious condition such as a metastatic brain tumor or a difficult-to-treat disease such as Alzheimer's. Fear of losing control and independence, along with threatened self-esteem or role performance, are common. The examiner needs to be sensitive to these fears and concerns because the client may decline to share important information with the examiner if these fears and concerns are not addressed.

History of Present Health Concerns

QUESTION	RATIONALE
Headaches	
Do you experience headaches? Use COLDSPA to further explore: • **C**haracter: Describe the character of the pain. • **O**nset: When do they occur? • **L**ocation: Point to the location of your head in which you feel the headache. • **D**uration: How long does it last? • **S**everity: Does it interfere with your activities of daily living? • **P**attern: What relieves the headache? What makes it worse? • **A**ssociated factors/How it affects the client: Do you have any other associated symptoms (nausea, vomiting, dizziness)?	See Chapter 15 for a description of various types of headaches. Morning headaches that subside after arising may be an early sign of increased intracranial pressure such as with a brain tumor.
Seizures	
Do you experience seizures (altered or loss of consciousness that occurs with involuntary muscle movements and sensory disturbances)?	Seizures occur with epilepsy, metabolic disorders, head injuries, and high fevers.
Describe what happens before you have the seizure and where on your body the seizure starts. Does anything seem to initiate a seizure? Do you lose control of your bladder during the seizure? How often? How do you feel afterward? Do you take medications for the seizures? Do you wear medical identification to alert others that you have seizures? Do you take safety precautions regarding driving or operating dangerous machinery?	In some cases, an aura (an auditory, visual, or motor sensation) forewarns the client that a seizure is about to occur. Where the seizure starts and what occurs before and after can aid in determining the type of seizure (e.g., generalized seizure, formerly known as grand mal and affecting both hemispheres of the brain, or absence seizure, also known as petit mal) and its treatment. Clients with generalized seizures often experience bladder incontinence during the seizure. Antiepileptic medications (anticonvulsants) must be distributed at a therapeutic level in the blood to be effective. **SAFETY TIP** *Wearing a medical identification tag, such as a MedicAlert bracelet, as well as the client's knowledge of the medication regimen and the importance of safety measures, provide information on the client's willingness to be involved in and adhere to the treatment plan.*
Dizziness	
Do you experience dizziness or lightheadedness or problems with balance or coordination? If so, how often? When does it occur? Does it occur with activity? Have you had any falls with the lightheadedness or dizziness? Do you have any clumsy movement(s)?	Dizziness or lightheadedness may be related to carotid artery disease, cerebellar abscess, Ménière disease, or inner ear infection. Imbalance and difficulty coordinating or controlling movements are seen in neurologic diseases involving the cerebellum, basal ganglia, extrapyramidal tracts, or the vestibular part of cranial nerve VIII (acoustic). Diminished cerebral blood flow and vestibular response may increase the risk of falls.
Numbness, Tingling/Prickling (Paresthesias)	
Do you experience any numbness or tingling? If yes, use COLDSPA to further assess: • **C**haracter: Describe the sensations (e.g., Pins and needles? Burning? Sand running over skin?) • **O**nset: When does this begin and when does it occur? Do you have numbness or tingling? • **L**ocation: Where do you have this sensation? • **D**uration: How long does this last? Is it continuous? • **S**everity: Does it interfere with your ability to perform any activities? • **P**attern: Does anything relieve or make it worse (activities, rest)? • **A**ssociated factors/How it affects the client: Does it occur with other symptoms?	Loss of sensation, tingling, or burning (paresthesia) may occur with damage to the brain, spinal cord, or peripheral nerves (see Abnormal Findings 25-3).

Continued on following page

History of Present Health Concerns (Continued)

QUESTION	RATIONALE
Senses	
Have you noticed a decrease in your ability to smell or to taste?	A decrease in the ability to smell may be related to a dysfunction of cranial nerve I (olfactory) or a brain tumor. A decrease in the ability to taste may be related to dysfunction of cranial nerves VII (facial) or IX (glossopharyngeal). **OLDER ADULT CONSIDERATIONS** Decreased taste and scent sensation occurs normally in older adults.
Have you experienced any ringing in your ears (tinnitus) or hearing loss?	Ringing in the ears and decreased ability to hear may occur with dysfunction of cranial nerve VIII (acoustic). **OLDER ADULT CONSIDERATIONS** There is a normal decrease in the older person's ability to hear.
Have you noticed any change in your vision?	Changes in vision may occur with dysfunction of cranial nerve II (optic), increased intracranial pressure, or brain tumors. Damage to cranial nerves III (oculomotor), IV (trochlear), or VI (abducens) may cause double or blurred vision. Transient blind spots may be an early sign of a cerebrovascular accident (CVA). **OLDER ADULT CONSIDERATIONS** There is a normal decrease in the older person's ability to see.
Difficulty Speaking	
Do you have difficulty understanding when people are talking to you? Do you have difficulty making others understand you? Do you have difficulty forming words (dysarthria) or comprehending and expressing your thoughts (dysphasia)?	Injury to the cerebral cortex can impair the ability to speak or understand verbal language.
Difficulty Swallowing (Dysphagia)	
Do you experience difficulty swallowing?	Difficulty swallowing may relate to CVA, Parkinson disease, myasthenia gravis, Guillain–Barré syndrome, or dysfunction of cranial nerves IX (glossopharyngeal), X (vagus), or XII (hypoglossal).
Muscle Control	
Have you lost bowel or bladder control or do you retain urine?	Loss of bowel control or urinary retention and bladder distention are seen with spinal cord injury or tumors.
Do you have muscle weakness? Do you have any loss of movements? If so, where?	Unilateral weakness or paralysis (loss of motor function from lesion[s] in the neurologic or muscular systems) may result from CVA, compression of the spinal cord, or nerve injury. Progressive weakness is a symptom of several nervous system diseases.
Do you experience any repetitive involuntary trembling, quivering, shaking, or other movements? Describe.	*Fasciculations* (continuous, rapid twitching of resting muscles) may be seen in lower motor neuron disease. *Tremors* (involuntary contraction of opposing groups of muscles) are typical in degenerative neurologic disorders, such as Parkinson disease (3–6 per second while muscles are at rest or "pin rolling" between thumb and opposing finger), or in cerebellar disease and multiple sclerosis (variable rate, and especially with intentional movement). *Tics* (involuntary repetitive twitching movements) may be seen in Tourette syndrome, habit psychogenic tics, or tardive dyskinesias. *Myoclonus* (sudden jerks of arms or legs) may occur normally when falling asleep as a single jerk. However, severe jerking is often seen with grand mal seizures. *Chorea* (sudden rapid, jerky voluntary and involuntary movements of limbs, trunk or face) is seen in Huntington disease and Sydenham chorea). *Athetosis* (twisting, writhing, slow continuous movements) is seen in cerebral palsy (see Abnormal Findings 25-2).

QUESTION	RATIONALE
	OLDER ADULT CONSIDERATIONS Older adults may experience intentional tremors (tremors that occur with intentional movements). This may be seen with extending the hands, head nodding for "yes or no," or extending one's tongue, which may protrude back and forth. Such tremors are not associated with disease, but they may cause embarrassment or emotional distress.

Memory Loss

Do you experience any memory loss?	Recent memory (24-hour memory) is often impaired in amnesic disorders, Korsakoff syndrome, delirium, and dementia. Remote memory (past dates and historical accounts) may be impaired in cerebral cortex disorders.

Past Health History

QUESTION	RATIONALE
Have you ever had any type of head injury with or without loss of consciousness (e.g., sports injury, auto accident, fall)? If so, describe any physical or mental changes that have occurred as a result. What type of treatment did you receive?	Head injuries, even if minor, can produce long-term neurologic deficits and affect the client's level of functioning.
Have you ever had meningitis, encephalitis, injury to the spinal cord, or a stroke? If so, describe any physical or mental changes that have occurred as a result. What type of treatment did you receive?	These disorders can affect the long-term physical and mental status of the client.

Family History

QUESTION	RATIONALE
Do you have a family history of high blood pressure, stroke, Alzheimer disease, dementia, epilepsy, brain cancer, or Huntington chorea?	These disorders may be genetic. Some tend to run in families.

Lifestyle and Health Practices

Do you take any prescription or nonprescription medications? How much alcohol do you drink? Do you use recreational drugs such as marijuana, tranquilizers, barbiturates, or cocaine?	Prescription and nonprescription drugs can cause various neurologic symptoms such as tremors or dizziness, altered level of consciousness, decreased response times, and changes in mood and temperament.
Do you smoke?	Nicotine, which is found in cigarettes, constricts the blood vessels, which decreases blood flow to the brain. Cigarette smoking is a risk factor for CVA (Evidence-Based Health Promotion and Disease Prevention 25-1).
Do you wear your seatbelt when riding in vehicles? Do you wear protective headgear when riding a bicycle or playing sports?	Seatbelts and protective headgear can prevent head injury.
Describe your usual daily 24-hour diet recall.	Peripheral neuropathy can result from a deficiency in niacin, folic acid, or vitamin B_{12}.
Have you ever had prolonged exposure to lead, insecticides, pollutants, or other chemicals?	Prolonged exposure to these substances can alter neurologic status.
Do you frequently lift heavy objects or perform repetitive motions?	Intervertebral disc injuries may result when heavy objects are lifted improperly. Peripheral nerve injuries can occur from repetitive movements.
Can you perform your normal IADLs (independent activities of daily living)?	Neurologic symptoms and disorders often negatively affect the ability to perform IADLs.
Has your neurologic problem changed the way you view yourself? Describe.	Low self-esteem and body image problems may lead to depression and changes in role functions.
Has your neurologic problem added much stress to your life? Describe.	Neurologic problems can impair ability to fulfill role responsibilities, greatly increasing stress. Stress can increase existing neurologic symptoms.

CASE STUDY

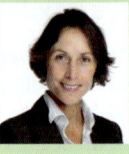

The case study introduced at the beginning of the chapter is now used to demonstrate how a nurse would use the COLDSPA mnemonic to explore Ms. Hutchison's presenting concerns.

Mnemonic	Question	Data Provided
Character	Describe the sign or symptom (feeling, appearance, sound, smell, or taste if applicable).	"I am very tired by the end of the week. I am also experiencing weakness, urinary incontinence, and a 'pins and needles' feeling in my legs. Leg spasms at night are preventing me from sleeping."
Onset	When did it begin?	"The symptoms began with my recent job change from office manager to teacher."
Location	Where is it? Does it radiate? Does it occur anywhere else?	"My whole body is affected by the fatigue. The weakness, 'pins and needles' feeling, and cramps are localized in my legs. Thankfully, I am not experiencing any problems with my vision."
Duration	How long does it last? Does it recur?	The symptoms get worse as the week continues. If I rest over the weekend, I am OK again by Monday morning. The last severe exacerbation of my MS occurred while I was going through my divorce. The exacerbation lasted 6 months before I went into remission."
Severity	How bad is it? or How much does it bother you?	"By Friday, the symptoms are so bad that all I can do is rest all weekend."
Pattern	What makes it better or worse?	"Activity and work make it worse and rest makes it better."
Associated factors/How it **A**ffects the client	What other symptoms occur with it? How does it affect you?	"I have no social life as I have to rest all weekend after a week at work."

After investigating Linda Hutchison's report of increasing tiredness, weakness, urinary incontinence, and a "pins and needles" feeling in her legs, the nurse continues with the health history.

Ms. Hutchison denies numbness, seizures, or dizziness. She has not noticed a change in sensations of taste or smell, hearing, or vision. Client denies difficulty speaking or swallowing. She denies loss of bowel control but describes bladder incontinence. Client denies recent or remote memory loss.

Client denies head injury, meningitis, encephalitis, spinal cord injury, or stroke.

Ms. Hutchison reports that her mother has hypertension and migraine headaches. Her father and two sisters are in excellent health. Maternal grandmother has hypertension and obesity. Maternal grandfather died as a result of an automobile accident at age 35. Paternal grandmother has rheumatoid arthritis. Paternal grandfather has coronary artery disease, hypertension, and diabetes type 2. Ms. Hutchinson denies a family history of cerebrovascular disease, epilepsy, brain cancer, or Huntington chorea.

Lifestyle and health practices: Takes oxybutynin (Ditropan) as prescribed for MS. Takes multivitamin daily. Denies use of tobacco or recreational drugs. Reports drinking two to three glasses of wine every 2 to 3 months. Reports wearing a seatbelt at all times. Denies participation in any activities requiring protective headgear. 24-hour diet recall: Breakfast—cereal with 2% milk and 1 cup of coffee; lunch—plain ham and cheese sandwich, 1 small bag plain potato chips, and an apple with unsweetened iced tea; dinner—petite filet mignon, loaded baked potato, salad, water.

Denies exposure to lead, insecticides, pollutants, or other chemicals. Denies frequent heavy lifting or repetitive motions. Reports that she is able to perform ADLs independently. Denies any change in self-esteem or body image.

Collecting Objective Data: Physical Examination

A complete neurologic examination consists of evaluating the following five areas:
- Mental status (discussed in Chapter 6)
- Cranial nerves
- Motor and cerebellar systems
- Sensory system
- Reflexes

Perform the examinations in an order that moves from a level of higher cerebral integration to a lower level of reflex activity.

Mental status examinations provide information about cerebral cortex function. Cerebral abnormalities disturb the client's intellectual ability, communication ability, or emotional behaviors. A mental status examination is often performed at the beginning of

25-1 EVIDENCE-BASED HEALTH PROMOTION AND DISEASE PREVENTION: CEREBROVASCULAR ACCIDENT (STROKE)

INTRODUCTION

Cerebrovascular accident, better known as stroke and sometimes as brain attack, happens when blood flow to a portion of the brain is interrupted or stops, depriving the brain cells of oxygen. If the blood flow is blocked for more than a few seconds, brain cells begin to die and permanent damage may result. There are several types of strokes: hemorrhagic, ischemic, and TIA (or transient ischemic attack). The National Stroke Association (2016b) describes hemorrhagic and ischemic strokes. Hemorrhagic strokes result when a brain aneurysm bursts or a weakened blood vessel in the brain leaks. Hemorrhagic strokes are less common (about 15% of strokes) but account for 40% of stroke deaths. Ischemic strokes occur when a blood vessel carrying blood to the brain is blocked by a clot. These clots can be embolic (move through the vessel) or thrombotic (develop within the vessel). A mini-stroke that causes no damage but indicates stroke risk is called a transient ischemic attack (TIA). Stroke symptoms of a TIA usually last for a short time but may last up to 24 hours before symptoms disappear.

The National Stroke Association (2016a) reports that stroke is the fifth leading cause of death in the United States, and is a leading cause of disability. There are many myths associated with stroke:

Myth	Fact
Stroke cannot be prevented.	Up to 80% of strokes are preventable.
There is no treatment for stroke.	At any sign of stroke call 9-1-1 immediately. Treatment may be available.
Stroke only affects the elderly.	Stroke can happen to anyone at any time.
Stroke happens in the heart.	Stroke is a "brain attack."
Stroke recovery only happens for the first few months after a stroke.	Stroke recovery is a lifelong process.
Strokes are rare.	In the United States, there are nearly 7 million stroke survivors. Stroke is the fifth leading cause of death in the United States.
Strokes are not hereditary.	Family history of stroke increases your chance for stroke.
If stroke symptoms go away, you don't have to see a doctor.	Temporary stroke symptoms are called transient ischemic attacks (TIA). They are warning signs before actual stroke and need to be taken seriously.

Adapted from National Stroke Association. (2016a). *Myth vs fact: Stroke facts*. Available at http://www.stroke.org/understand-stroke/what-stroke/stroke-facts.

CLINICAL TIP

Stroke is an emergency. Recognize the signs and symptoms and act fast! (National Stroke Association, 2016b.)

Signs and symptoms:
- Sudden numbness or weakness of face, arm, or leg, especially on one side of the body
- Sudden confusion, trouble speaking or understanding
- Sudden trouble seeing in one or both eyes
- Sudden trouble walking, dizziness, loss of balance, or coordination
- Sudden severe headache with no known cause

Act FAST. Use FAST to remember the warning signs of a stroke:
- FACE: Ask the person to smile. Does one side of the face droop?
- ARMS: Ask the person to raise both arms. Does one arm drift downward?
- SPEECH: Ask the person to repeat a simple phrase. Is speech slurred or strange?
- TIME: If you observe any of these signs, call 9-1-1 immediately.

HEALTHY PEOPLE 2020 GOAL

Healthy People 2020 (2016) addresses stroke along with heart attack as part of seeking to improve cardiovascular health.

GOAL

Improve cardiovascular health and quality of life through prevention, detection, and treatment of risk factors for heart attack and stroke; early identification and treatment of heart attacks and strokes; and prevention of repeat cardiovascular events.

OBJECTIVES

- Reduce stroke deaths by 20%.
- Increase the proportion of adults who have had their blood pressure measured within the preceding 2 years and can state whether their blood pressure was normal or high by 2% to 92.6%.
- Reduce the proportion of people in the population with hypertension by 10% (adults to 26.9%; children and adolescents to 3.2%).
- (Developmental) Increase the proportion of adults with prehypertension who meet the recommended guidelines.
- (Developmental) Increase the proportion of adults with hypertension who meet the recommended guidelines.
- Increase the proportion of adults with hypertension who are taking the prescribed medications to lower their blood pressure.
- Increase the proportion of adults with hypertension whose blood pressure is under control.
- (Developmental) Increase the proportion of adults aged 20 years and older who are aware of and respond to early warning symptoms and signs of a stroke.
- Other objectives are included that refer to blood cholesterol levels, aspirin use, and timely artery-opening therapy.

SCREENING

The U.S. Preventive Services Task Force (USPSTF, 2015) only addresses the efficacy of using aspirin as a preventative for cardiovascular disease and cancer, without addressing the potential harms from its use. The USPSTF used the ACC/AHA Risk Calculator (Husten, 2014) with reservations, as the calculator

Continued on following page

25-1 EVIDENCE-BASED HEALTH PROMOTION AND DISEASE PREVENTION: CEREBROVASCULAR ACCIDENT (STROKE) (Continued)

was thought to overpredict risk. Husten (2014) reviewed studies of the ACC/AHA calculator and found even more issues, so does not recommend the calculator as a screening tool.

Goldstein et al. (2011) review evidence and newer guidelines for stroke assessment, concluding, "Extensive evidence identifies a variety of specific factors that increase the risk of a first stroke and that provide strategies for reducing that risk."

Screening for risk factors is essential and useful for all clients. However, the new guidelines recommend against more invasive screening using ultrasound or MRI unless reasonable risk is established (Goldstein et al., 2011).

A list of stroke screening tools, for prehospital use, acute status, functional assessment, outcome assessment, and other diagnostic screening tests is available online from the Internet Stroke Center (2016).

RISK ASSESSMENT

Major risk factors for stroke (National Heart, Lung, Blood Institute [NHLBI], 2015):

- Hypertension—the main risk factor (at or above 140/90 millimeters of mercury [mmHg] over time; or with diabetes or chronic kidney disease, high blood pressure is defined as 130/80 mmHg or higher)
- Diabetes mellitus
- Heart disease (coronary heart disease, cardiomyopathy, heart failure, and atrial fibrillation)
- Smoking (as well as exposure to secondhand smoke)
- Age and gender (risk increases with age; men more likely to have stroke at younger age; women more likely to die of stroke; women who take birth control pills at slightly higher risk)
- Race and ethnicity (more strokes in African Americans, Native Americans, and Alaska Natives than in white, Hispanic, or Asian Americans)
- Personal or family history of stroke or TIA
- Brain aneurysms or arteriovenous malformations (AVMs)

Other stroke risk factors, many of which can be controlled:

- Alcohol and illegal drug use
- Certain medical conditions such as sickle cell disease, vasculitis, or bleeding disorders
- Lack of physical activity
- Overweight and obesity
- Stress and depression
- Unhealthy cholesterol levels
- Unhealthy diet
- Use (especially prolonged use) of NSAID medications, such as ibuprofen and naproxen, but not aspirin

Note that stroke can occur in persons who have no known risk factors for stroke.

CLIENT EDUCATION

Teach Clients

- Do not smoke. If you do smoke, quit.
- Control your cholesterol through diet, exercise, and medicines, if needed.
- Control high blood pressure through diet, exercise, and medicines, if needed.
- Control diabetes through diet, exercise, and medicines, if needed.
- Exercise at least 30 minutes a day.
- Maintain a healthy weight by eating healthy foods, eating less, and joining a weight loss program, if needed.
  - Choose a diet rich in fruits, vegetables, and whole grains.
  - Choose lean proteins, such as chicken, fish, beans, and legumes.
  - Choose low-fat dairy products, such as 1% milk and other low-fat items.
  - Avoid sodium (salt) and fats found in fried foods, processed foods, and baked goods.
  - Eat fewer animal products and foods that contain cheese, cream, or eggs.
  - Read labels, and stay away from saturated fat and anything that contains partially hydrogenated or hydrogenated fats. These products are usually loaded with unhealthy fats.
- Limit how much alcohol you drink. This means 1 drink a day for women and 2 a day for men.
- Avoid cocaine and other illegal drugs.
- Talk to your doctor about the risk of taking birth control pills.
- Your doctor may suggest taking aspirin or another drug called clopidogrel (Plavix) to help prevent blood clots from forming. DO NOT take aspirin without talking to your doctor first.

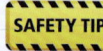 **SAFETY TIP** *If you are taking these drugs or other blood thinners, you should take steps to prevent yourself from falling or tripping.*

KNOW THE WARNING SIGNS OF STROKE (National Stroke Association, 2016b)

Teach clients to recognize stroke if experiencing the symptoms or if another person is experiencing these symptoms.

Stroke is a medical emergency. Seek help immediately because treatment is time limited.

Don't wait for the symptoms to improve or worsen. If you believe you are having a stroke—or someone you know is having a stroke—call 9-1-1 immediately. Making the decision to call for medical help can make the difference in avoiding a lifelong disability. Act FAST!

Symptoms of stroke are:

- Sudden numbness or weakness of the face, arm, or leg (especially on one side of the body)
- Sudden confusion, trouble speaking, or understanding speech
- Sudden trouble seeing in one or both eyes
- Sudden trouble walking, dizziness, loss of balance, or coordination
- Sudden severe headache with no known cause

Act FAST. Use FAST to remember the warning signs of a stroke:

- FACE: Ask the person to smile. Does one side of the face droop?
- ARMS: Ask the person to raise both arms. Does one arm drift downward?
- SPEECH: Ask the person to repeat a simple phrase. Is speech slurred or strange?
- TIME: If you observe any of these signs, call 9-1-1 immediately.

the head-to-toe examination because it provides clues regarding the validity of the subjective information provided by the client. For example, if the nurse finds that the client's thought processes are distorted and memory is impaired, another means of obtaining necessary subjective data must be identified (see Chapter 6).

The *cranial nerve evaluation* provides information regarding the transmission of motor and sensory messages, primarily to the head and neck. Many of the cranial nerves are evaluated during the head, neck, eye, and ear examinations.

The *motor and cerebellar systems* are assessed to determine functioning of the pyramidal and extrapyramidal tracts. The cerebellar system is assessed to determine the client's level of balance and coordination. The motor system examination is usually performed during the musculoskeletal examination.

Examining the *sensory system* provides information regarding the integrity of the spinothalamic tract, posterior columns of the spinal cord, and parietal lobes of the brain, whereas testing *reflexes* provides clues to the integrity of deep and superficial reflexes. Deep reflexes depend on an intact sensory nerve, a functional synapse in the spinal cord, an intact motor nerve, a neuromuscular junction, and competent muscles. Superficial reflexes depend on skin receptors rather than muscles.

If meningitis is suspected, the examiner may try to elicit Brudzinski sign and Kernig sign (see the Physical Assessment section), which are characteristic of meningeal irritation. Sometimes, a complete neurologic examination is unnecessary. In such cases, the nurse performs a "neuro check"—a brief screening of the client's neurologic status. A neuro check includes the following assessment points:
- Level of consciousness
- Pupillary checks
- Movement and strength of extremities
- Sensation in extremities
- Vital signs

A neuro check is useful in an emergency situation and when frequent assessments are needed during an acute phase of illness to detect rapid changes in neurologic status. It is also useful for a client who has already had a complete neurologic examination but needs to be rechecked for changes related to therapy or other conditions.

Preparing the Client

Prepare the client for the neurologic examination by asking that he or she remove all clothing and jewelry and put on an examination gown. Initially have the client sit comfortably on the examination table or bed, but explain that several different position changes will be necessary throughout the different parts of the examination. Assure the client that each position will be explained before the start of the particular examination.

Explain also that the examination will take a considerable amount of time to perform and that you will provide rest periods as needed. If the client is older or physically weak, divide the examination into parts, to be performed over two different time periods. Explain that actions the client will be asked to perform, such as counting backward or hopping on one foot, may seem unusual but that these activities are parts of a comprehensive neurologic evaluation.

◎ **CLINICAL TIP**
Demonstrate what you want the client to do, especially during the cerebellar examination, when the client will need to perform several different coordinated movements.

Equipment

General
- Examination gloves

Cranial Nerve Examination
- Cotton-tipped applicators
- Newsprint to read
- Ophthalmoscope
- Paper clip
- Penlight
- Snellen chart
- Sterile cotton ball
- Substances to smell or taste such as soap, coffee, vanilla, salt, sugar, lemon juice
- Tongue depressor
- Tuning fork

Motor and Cerebellar Examination
- Tape measure

Sensory Examination
- Cotton ball
- Objects to feel such as a quarter or key
- Paper clip
- Test tubes containing hot and cold water
- Tuning fork (low-pitched)

Reflex Examination
- Cotton-tipped applicator
- Reflex (percussion) hammer

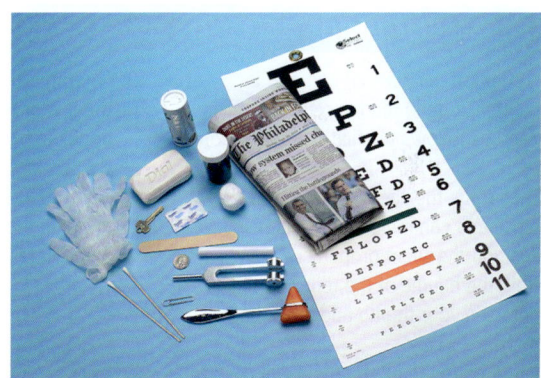

Physical Assessment

Prior to the physical examination, review these key points:
- Understand what is meant by mental status and level of consciousness (see Chapter 6).
- Know how to correctly apply and interpret mental status examinations and how to use the Glasgow Coma Scale (GCS; see Chapter 6).
- Identify the 12 cranial nerves and their sensory and motor functions.
- Know how to thoroughly assess movement, balance, coordination, sensation, and reflexes.
- Know how to use a reflex hammer (Assessment Guide 25-1).
- Coordinate patient education—particularly in regard to risks related to stroke—with the health interview and physical examination.

General Routine Screening versus Focused Specialty Assessment for the Neurologic System

Typically, the nurse would not do a complete neurologic examination, which consists of six parts: mental status (covered in Chapter 6), cranial nerves, motor and cerebellar systems, sensory system, and reflexes. However, the nurse needs to know how to perform all parts of this examination, regardless of where she practices nursing. Parts of this long examination will be used in everyday practice in all specialty areas as problems are detected and further assessment is needed. For example, if the client is showing signs of impending stroke, it would be important to know how to test the motor and sensory systems as appropriate. If a client is having trouble swallowing, the nurse would want to test cranial nerves IX and X. There are also times it is necessary to check specific reflexes if the client reports numbness or immobility of a limb. Nurses working in intensive care units and neurologic specialty areas perform all of these assessments frequently as needed.

General Routine Screening
- Assess level of consciousness.
- Observe behavior and affect.
- Observe dress, grooming, hygiene.
- Observe facial expressions.
- Observe speech.
- Assess mood feelings, expressions.
- Assess cranial nerve II.
- Evaluate posture, gait, balance, involuntary movements.
- Assess light touch, pain.

Focused Specialty Assessment
- Assess thought processes and perceptions.
- Assess orientation, concentration, recent and remote memory, use of memory to learn, abstract reasoning, judgment, SLUMS test, visual, perceptual and constructional ability (Chapter 6).
- Comprehensive testing of cranial nerves I through XII.
- Perform the Romberg test.
- Assess coordination.
- Assess rapid alternating movements.
- Assess light touch, pain, and temperature sensations.
- Test vibratory sensation, sensitivity to position, tactile discrimination, point localization, graphesthesia, extinction.
- Test superficial and deep tendon reflexes.
- Test for meningeal irritation (Brudzinski sign and Kernig sign).

ASSESSMENT GUIDE 25-1 How to Use the Reflex Hammer

The reflex (or percussion) hammer is used to elicit deep tendon reflexes. Proceed as follows to elicit a deep tendon reflex:

1. Encourage the client to relax because tenseness can inhibit a normal response.
2. Position the client properly.
3. Hold the handle of the reflex hammer between your thumb and index finger so it swings freely.
4. Palpate the tendon that you will need to strike to elicit the reflex.
5. Using a rapid wrist movement, briskly strike the tendon. Observe the response. Avoid a slow or weak movement for striking.
6. Compare the response of one side with the other.
7. To prevent pain, use the pointed end to strike a small area, and the wider, blunt (flat) end to strike a wider or more tender area.
8. Use a reinforcement technique, which causes other muscles to contract and thus increases reflex activity, to assist in eliciting a response if no response can be elicited.
9. For arm reflexes, ask the client to clench the jaw or to squeeze one thigh with the opposite hand, then immediately strike the tendon. For leg reflexes, ask the client to lock the fingers of both hands and pull them against each other, then immediately strike the tendon.

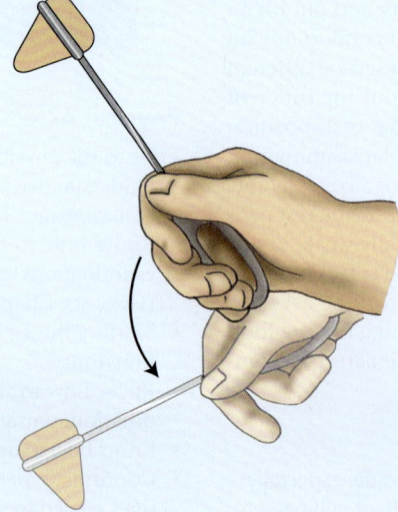

10. Rate and document reflexes using the following scale and figure.
    - Grade 4+ Hyperactive, very brisk, rhythmic oscillations (clonus); abnormal and indicative of disorder
    - Grade 3+ More brisk or active than normal, but not indicative of a disorder

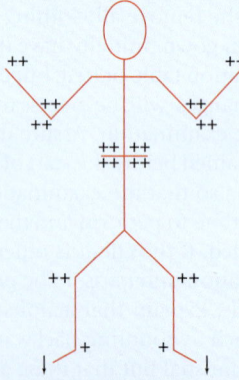

   - Grade 2+ Normal, usual response
   - Grade 1+ Decreased, less active than normal
   - Grade 0 No response

ASSESSMENT PROCEDURE	NORMAL FINDINGS	ABNORMAL FINDINGS
Cranial Nerves (CN)		
Test CN I (olfactory). For all assessments of the cranial nerves, have client sit in a comfortable position at your eye level. Ask the client to clear the nose to remove any mucus, then to close eyes, occlude one nostril, and identify a scented object that you are holding such as soap, coffee, or vanilla (Fig. 25-8). Repeat procedure for the other nostril.	Client correctly identifies scent presented to each nostril. **SOME OLDER CLIENTS' SENSE OF SMELL MAY BE DECREASED.**	Inability to smell (neurogenic anosmia) or identify the correct scent may indicate olfactory tract lesion or tumor or lesion of the frontal lobe. Loss of smell may also be congenital or due to other causes such as nasal or sinus problems. It may also be caused by injury of nerve tissue at the top of the nose or the higher smell pathways in the brain due to viral upper respiratory infection. Smoking and use of cocaine may also impair one's sense of smell.
Test CN II (optic). Use a Snellen chart to assess vision in each eye (see Chapter 16 for additional information).	Client has 20/20 vision OD (right eye) and OS (left eye).	Abnormal findings include difficulty reading Snellen chart, missing letters, and squinting.
Ask the client to read a newspaper or magazine paragraph to assess near vision.	Client reads print at 14 in without difficulty.	Client reads print by holding closer than 14 in or holds print farther away as in presbyopia, which occurs with aging.
Assess visual fields of each eye by confrontation.	Full visual fields (see Chapter 16).	Loss of visual fields may be seen in retinal damage or detachment, with lesions of the optic nerve, or with lesions of the parietal cortex (see Chapter 16).
Use an ophthalmoscope to view the retina and optic disc of each eye.	Round red reflex is present, optic disc is 1.5 mm, round or slightly oval, well-defined margins, creamy pink with paler physiologic cup. Retina is pink (see Chapter 16).	Papilledema (swelling of the optic nerve) results in blurred optic disc margins and dilated, pulsating veins. Papilledema occurs with increased intracranial pressure from intracranial hemorrhage or a brain tumor. Optic atrophy occurs with brain tumors (see Chapter 16).
Assess CN III (oculomotor), IV (trochlear), and VI (abducens). Inspect margins of the eyelids of each eye.	Eyelid covers about 2 mm of the iris.	Ptosis (drooping of the eyelid) is seen with weak eye muscles such as in myasthenia gravis (Fig. 25-9).

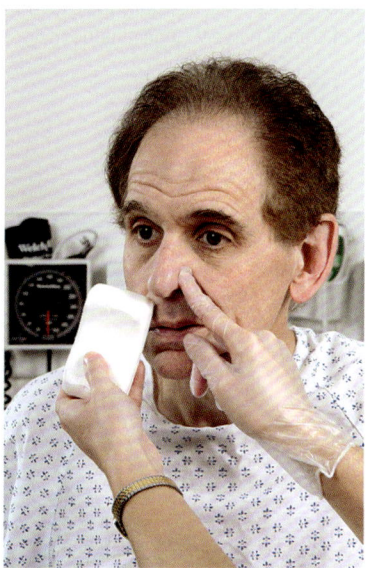

FIGURE 25-8 Asking client to identify smell of soap bar with eyes closed to test cranial nerve I.

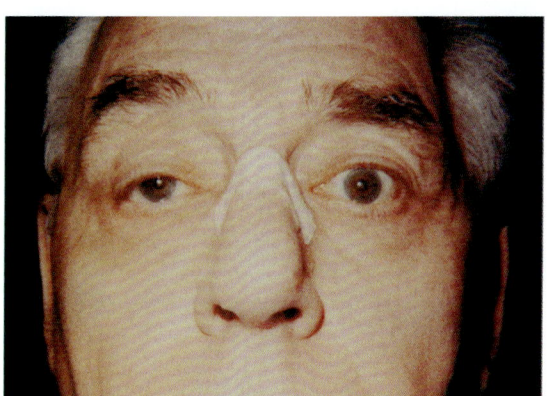

FIGURE 25-9 Muscular eye weakness seen in myasthenia gravis. (Used with permission from Tasman, W., & Jaeger, E. (2009). The Wills Eye Hospital atlas of clinical ophthalmology (2nd ed.). Philadelphia, PA: Lippincott Williams & Wilkins.)

Continued on following page

ASSESSMENT PROCEDURE	NORMAL FINDINGS	ABNORMAL FINDINGS
Cranial Nerves (CN) (Continued)		
Assess extraocular movements. If nystagmus is noted, determine the direction of the fast and slow phases of movement (see Chapter 16).	Eyes move in a smooth, coordinated motion in all directions (the six cardinal fields).	Some abnormal eye movements and possible causes follow: • Nystagmus (rhythmic oscillation of the eyes): *cerebellar disorders.* • Limited eye movement through the six cardinal fields of gaze: *increased intracranial pressure.* • Paralytic strabismus: *paralysis of the oculomotor, trochlear, or abducens nerves* (see Chapter 16).
Assess pupillary response to light (direct and indirect) and accommodation in both eyes (see Chapter 16).	Bilateral illuminated pupils constrict simultaneously. Pupil opposite the one illuminated constricts simultaneously.	Some abnormalities and their implications follow: • Dilated pupil (6–7 mm): *oculomotor nerve paralysis.* • Argyll Robertson pupils: *CNS syphilis, meningitis, brain tumor, alcoholism.* • Constricted, fixed pupils: *narcotics abuse or damage to the pons.* • Unilaterally dilated pupil unresponsive to light or accommodation: *damage to cranial nerve III (oculomotor).* • Constricted pupil unresponsive to light or accommodation: *lesions of the sympathetic nervous system.*
Assess CN V (trigeminal). Test motor function. Ask the client to clench the teeth while you palpate the temporal and masseter muscles for contraction (Fig. 25-10). 🎯 **CLINICAL TIP** This test may be difficult to perform and evaluate in the client without teeth.	Temporal and masseter muscles contract bilaterally.	Decreased contraction in one of both sides. Asymmetric strength in moving the jaw may be seen with lesion or injury of the 5th cranial nerve. Pain occurs with clenching of the teeth. Bilateral muscle weakness is seen with peripheral or central nervous system dysfunction. Unilateral muscle weakness may indicate a lesion of cranial nerve V (trigeminal).

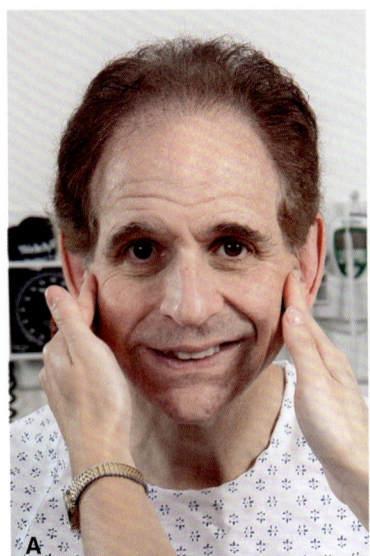
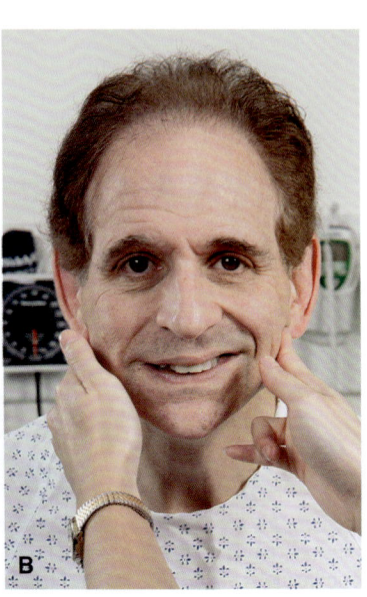

FIGURE 25-10 Testing motor function of cranial nerve V. **A.** Palpating temporal muscles. **B.** Palpating masseter muscles.

ASSESSMENT PROCEDURE	NORMAL FINDINGS	ABNORMAL FINDINGS
Test sensory function. Tell the client: "I am going to touch your forehead, cheeks, and chin with the sharp or dull side of this paper clip. Please close your eyes and tell me if you feel a sharp or dull sensation. Also tell me where you feel it" (Fig. 25-11). Vary the sharp and dull stimulus in the facial areas and compare sides. Repeat test for light touch with a wisp of cotton. **SAFETY TIP** *To avoid transmitting infection, use a new object with each client. Avoid "stabbing" the client with the object's sharp side.*	The client correctly identifies sharp and dull stimuli and light touch to the forehead, cheeks, and chin.	Inability to feel and correctly identify facial stimuli occurs with lesions of the trigeminal nerve or lesions in the spinothalamic tract or posterior columns.
Test corneal reflex. Ask the client to look away and up while you lightly touch the cornea with a fine wisp of cotton (Fig. 25-12). Repeat on the other side. **CLINICAL TIP** This reflex may be absent or reduced in clients who wear contact lenses.	Eyelids blink bilaterally.	An absent corneal reflex may be noted with lesions of the trigeminal nerve or lesions of the motor part of cranial nerve VII (facial).

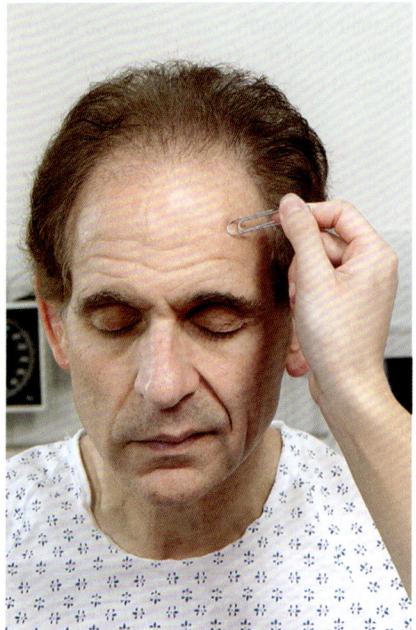

FIGURE 25-11 Testing sensory function of cranial nerve V: dull stimulus using a paper clip.

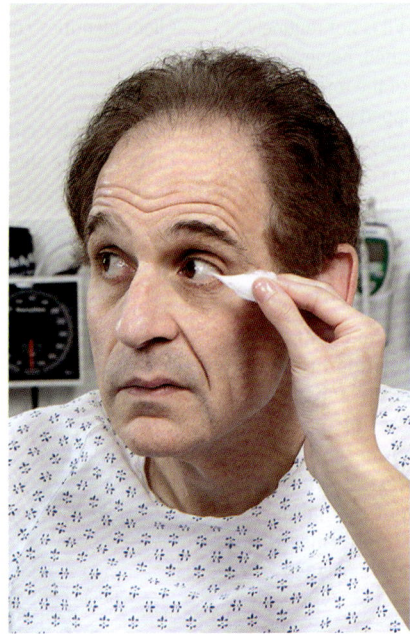

FIGURE 25-12 Testing corneal reflex.

Test CN VII (facial). Test motor function. Ask the client to: • Smile • Frown and wrinkle forehead (Fig. 25-13A) • Show teeth • Puff out cheeks (Fig. 25-13B) • Purse lips • Raise eyebrows • Close eyes tightly against resistance	Client smiles, frowns, wrinkles forehead, shows teeth, puffs out cheeks, purses lips, raises eyebrows, and closes eyes against resistance. Movements are symmetric.	Inability to close eyes, wrinkle forehead, or raise forehead along with paralysis of the lower part of the face on the affected side is seen with Bell palsy (a peripheral injury to cranial nerve VII [facial]). Paralysis of the lower part of the face on the opposite side affected may be seen with a central lesion that affects the upper motor neurons, such as from stroke.

Continued on following page

ASSESSMENT PROCEDURE	NORMAL FINDINGS	ABNORMAL FINDINGS

Cranial Nerves (CN) (Continued)

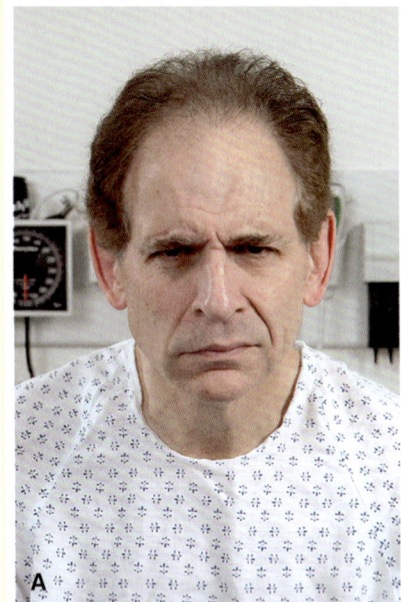
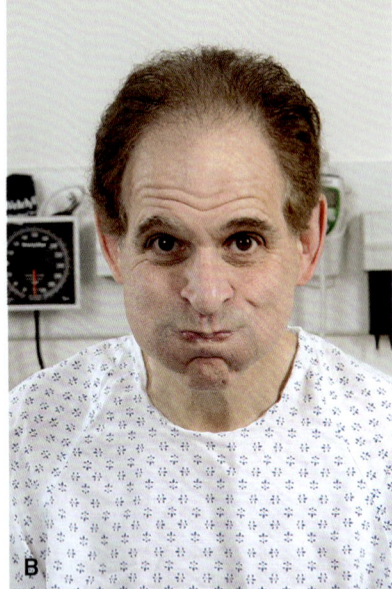

FIGURE 25-13 Testing cranial nerve VII. **A.** Frowning and wrinkling forehead. **B.** Puffing out cheeks.

Sensory function of CN VII is not routinely tested. If testing is indicated, however, touch the anterior two thirds of the tongue with a moistened applicator dipped in salt, sugar, or lemon juice. Ask the client to identify the flavor. If the client is unsuccessful, repeat the test using one of the other solutions. If needed, repeat the test using the remaining solution.	Client identifies correct flavor. **OLDER ADULT CONSIDERATIONS** In some older clients, the sense of taste may be decreased.	Inability to identify correct flavor on anterior two thirds of the tongue suggests impairment of cranial nerve VII (facial). *Concept Mastery Alert* Damage to cranial nerve VII (facial) results in the client's inability to close the eyes and wrinkle or raise the forehead. Loss of visual fields and drooping of eyelids is seen in damage to cranial nerve II (ocular).

> **CLINICAL TIP**
> Make sure that the client leaves the tongue protruded to identify the flavor. Otherwise, the substance may move to the posterior third of the tongue (vagus nerve innervation). The posterior portion is tested similarly to evaluate functioning of cranial nerves IX and X. The client should rinse the mouth with water between each taste test.

Test CN VIII (acoustic/vestibulocochlear). Test the client's hearing ability in each ear and perform the Weber and Rinne tests to assess the cochlear (auditory) component of cranial nerve VIII (see Chapter 17 for detailed procedures).	Client hears whispered words from 1 to 2 ft. *Weber test:* Vibration heard equally well in both ears. *Rinne test:* AC > BC (air conduction is twice as long as bone conduction).	Vibratory sound lateralizes to good ear in sensorineural loss. Air conduction is longer than bone conduction, but not twice as long, in a sensorineural loss (see Chapter 17).

> **CLINICAL TIP**
> The vestibular component, responsible for equilibrium, is not routinely tested. In comatose clients, the test is used to determine integrity of the vestibular system. (See a neurology textbook for detailed testing procedures.)

ASSESSMENT PROCEDURE	NORMAL FINDINGS	ABNORMAL FINDINGS
Test CN IX (glossopharyngeal) and X (vagus).		
Test motor function. Ask the client to open mouth wide and say "ah" while you use a tongue depressor on the client's tongue (Fig. 25-14).	Uvula and soft palate rise bilaterally and symmetrically on phonation.	Soft palate does not rise with bilateral lesions of cranial nerve X (vagus). Unilateral rising of the soft palate and deviation of the uvula to the normal side are seen with a unilateral lesion of cranial nerve X (vagus).
Test the gag reflex by touching the posterior pharynx with the tongue depressor. ◎ **CLINICAL TIP** Warn the client that you are going to do this and that the test may feel a little uncomfortable.	Gag reflex intact. Some normal clients may have a reduced or absent gag reflex.	An absent gag reflex may be seen with lesions of cranial nerve IX (glossopharyngeal) or X (vagus).
Check the client's ability to swallow by giving the client a drink of water. Also note the client's voice quality.	Client swallows without difficulty. No hoarseness noted.	Dysphagia or hoarseness may indicate a lesion of cranial nerve IX (glossopharyngeal) or X (vagus) or other neurologic disorder.
Test CN XI (spinal accessory). Ask the client to shrug the shoulders against resistance to assess the trapezius muscles (Fig. 25-15).	There is symmetric, strong contraction of the trapezius muscles.	Asymmetric muscle contraction or drooping of the shoulder may be seen with paralysis or muscle weakness due to neck injury or torticollis.

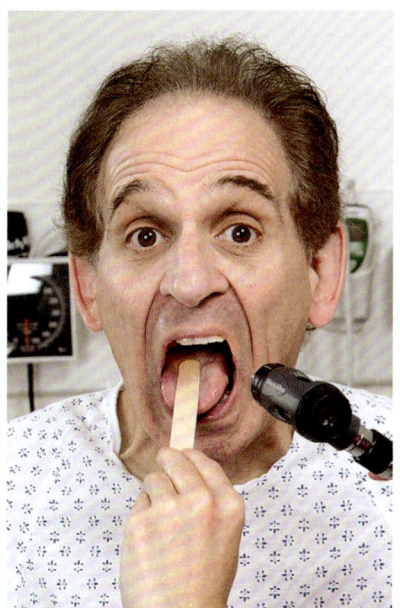

FIGURE 25-14 Testing cranial nerves IX and X: checking uvula rise and gag reflex.

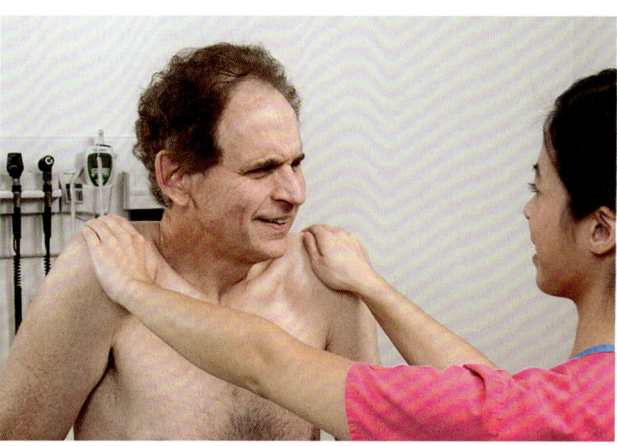

FIGURE 25-15 Testing cranial nerve XI: assessing strength of the trapezius muscle.

Ask the client to turn the head against resistance, first to the right then to the left, to assess the sternocleidomastoid muscles (Fig. 25-16).	There is strong contraction of sternocleidomastoid muscle on the side opposite the turned face.	Atrophy with fasciculations may be seen with peripheral nerve disease.
Test CN XII (hypoglossal). To assess strength and mobility of the tongue, ask the client to protrude tongue, move it to each side against the resistance of a tongue depressor, and then put it back in the mouth.	Tongue movement is symmetric and smooth, and bilateral strength is apparent.	Fasciculations and atrophy of the tongue may be seen with peripheral nerve disease. Deviation to the affected side is seen with a unilateral lesion.

Continued on following page

| ASSESSMENT PROCEDURE | NORMAL FINDINGS | ABNORMAL FINDINGS |
|---|---|---|//

Cranial Nerves (CN) (Continued)

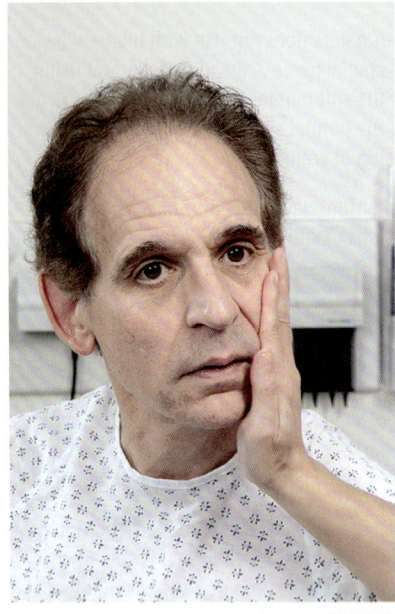

FIGURE 25-16 Testing cranial nerve XI: assessing strength of the sternocleidomastoid muscle.

Motor and Cerebellar Systems

ASSESSMENT PROCEDURE	NORMAL FINDINGS	ABNORMAL FINDINGS
Assess condition and movement of muscles. Assess the size and symmetry of all muscle groups (see Chapter 24 for detailed procedures).	Muscles are fully developed and symmetric in size (bilateral sides may vary 1 cm from each other). **OLDER ADULT CONSIDERATIONS** Some older clients may have reduced muscle mass from degeneration of muscle fibers.	Muscle atrophy may be seen in diseases of the lower motor neurons or muscle disorders (see Chapter 24 and Abnormal Findings 25-1). Injury of the central spinal cord is associated with extremity weakness. Loss of motor function, pain and temperature seen in anterior cord syndrome. Loss of proprioception seen in posterior cord syndrome. A loss of strength, proprioception, pain and temperature is seen in Brown–Séquard syndrome.
Assess the strength and tone of all muscle groups (see Chapter 24).	Relaxed muscles contract voluntarily and show mild, smooth resistance to passive movement. All muscle groups are equally strong against resistance, without flaccidity, spasticity, or rigidity.	Soft, limp, flaccid muscles are seen with lower motor neuron involvement. Spastic muscle tone is noted with involvement of the corticospinal motor tract. Rigid muscles that resist passive movement are seen with abnormalities of the extrapyramidal tract.
Note any unusual involuntary movements such as fasciculations, tics, or tremors.	No fasciculations, tics, or tremors are noted. **OLDER ADULT CONSIDERATIONS** Some older clients may normally have hand or head tremors or dyskinesia (repetitive movements of the lips, jaw, or tongue).	See Abnormal Findings 25-2. Fasciculation (rapid twitching of resting muscle) seen in lower motor neuron disease or fatigue. Tic (twitch of the face, head, or shoulder) from stress or neurologic disorder. Unusual, bizarre face, tongue, jaw, or lip movements from chronic psychosis or long-term use of psychotropic drugs. Tremors (rhythmic, oscillating movements) from Parkinson disease, cerebellar disease, multiple sclerosis (with movement), hyperthyroidism, or anxiety.

ASSESSMENT PROCEDURE	NORMAL FINDINGS	ABNORMAL FINDINGS
Evaluate gait and balance. To assess gait and balance, ask the client to walk naturally across the room. Note posture, freedom of movement, symmetry, rhythm, and balance. ◎ **CLINICAL TIP** It is best to assess gait when the client is not aware that you are directly observing the gait. Ask the client to walk in heel-to-toe fashion (tandem walking; Fig. 25-17), next on the heels, then on the toes. Demonstrate the walk first; then stand close by in case the client loses balance. 🪑 **OLDER ADULT CONSIDERATIONS** For some older clients, this examination may be very difficult. **Perform the Romberg test.** Ask the client to stand erect with arms at side and feet together. Note any unsteadiness or swaying. Then with the client in the same body position, ask the client to close the eyes for 20 seconds. Again note any imbalance or swaying (Fig. 25-18). **SAFETY TIP** *Stand near the client to prevent a fall should the client lose balance.*	Gait is steady; opposite arm swings. 🪑 **OLDER ADULT CONSIDERATIONS** Some older clients may have a slow and uncertain gait. The base may become wider and shorter and the hips and knees may be flexed for a bent-forward appearance. Client maintains balance with tandem walking. Walks on heels and toes with little difficulty. Client stands erect with minimal swaying, with eyes both open and closed.	Slow, twisting movements in the extremities and face from cerebral palsy. Brief, rapid, irregular, jerky movements (at rest) from Huntington chorea. Slower twisting movements associated with spasticity (athetosis) seen with cerebral palsy. Gait and balance can be affected by disorders of the motor, sensory, vestibular, and cerebellar systems. Therefore, a thorough examination of all systems is necessary when an uneven or unsteady gait is noted (see Abnormal Findings 25-3). An uncoordinated or unsteady gait that did not appear with the client's normal walking may become apparent with tandem walking or when walking on heels and toes. Positive Romberg test: Swaying and moving feet apart to prevent fall is seen with disease of the posterior columns, vestibular dysfunction, or cerebellar disorders.

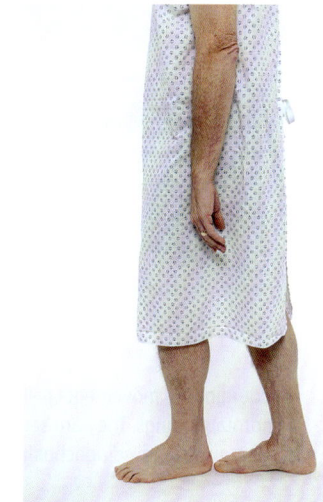

FIGURE 25-17 Testing balance: tandem walking.

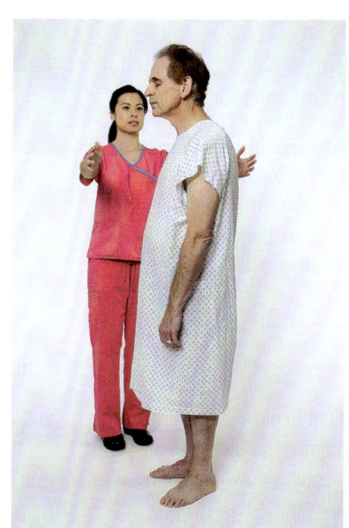

FIGURE 25-18 Performing the Romberg test.

Continued on following page

ASSESSMENT PROCEDURE	NORMAL FINDINGS	ABNORMAL FINDINGS
Motor and Cerebellar Systems (Continued)		
Now ask the client to stand on one foot and to bend the knee of the leg the client is standing on (Fig. 25-19). Then ask the client to hop on that foot. Repeat on the other foot. 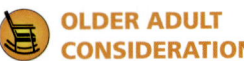 **OLDER ADULT CONSIDERATIONS** This test is often impossible for the older adult to perform because of decreased flexibility and strength. Moreover, it is not usual to perform this test with the older adult because it puts the client at risk.	Bends knee while standing on one foot; hops on each foot without losing balance.	Inability to stand or hop on one foot is seen with muscle weakness or disease of the cerebellum.
Assess coordination. Demonstrate the finger-to-nose test to assess accuracy of movements, then ask the client to extend and hold arms out to the side with eyes open. Next, say, "Touch the tip of your nose first with your right index finger, then with your left index finger. Repeat this three times" (Fig. 25-20). Next, ask the client to repeat these movements with eyes closed.	Client touches finger to nose with smooth, accurate movements, with little hesitation. ◎ **CLINICAL TIP** When assessing coordination of movements, bear in mind that normally the client's dominant side may be more coordinated than the nondominant side.	Uncoordinated, jerky movements and inability to touch the nose may be seen with cerebellar disease.

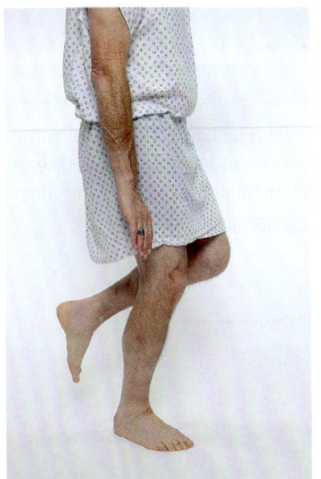

FIGURE 25-19 Tandem balance: standing and hopping on one foot.

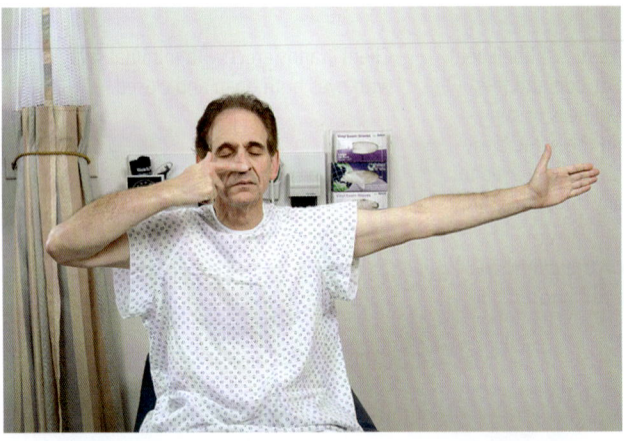

FIGURE 25-20 Testing coordination: the finger-to-nose test.

Assess rapid alternating movements. Have the client sit down. First, ask the client to touch each finger to the thumb and to increase the speed as the client progresses. Repeat with the other side.	Client touches each finger to the thumb rapidly. **OLDER ADULT CONSIDERATIONS** For some older clients, rapid alternating movements are difficult because of decreased reaction time and flexibility.	Inability to perform rapid alternating movements may be seen with cerebellar disease, upper motor neuron weakness, or extrapyramidal disease.
Next, ask the client to put the palms of both hands down on both legs, then turn the palms up, then turn the palms down again (Fig. 25-21). Ask the client to increase the speed.	Client rapidly turns palms up and down.	Uncoordinated movements or tremors are abnormal findings. They are seen with cerebellar disease (dysdiadochokinesia).
Perform the heel-to-shin test. Ask the client to lie down (supine position) and to slide the heel of the right foot down the left shin (Fig. 25-22). Repeat with the other heel and shin.	Client is able to run each heel smoothly down each shin.	Deviation of heel to one side or the other may be seen in cerebellar disease.

25 Assessing Neurologic System 589

ASSESSMENT PROCEDURE	NORMAL FINDINGS	ABNORMAL FINDINGS

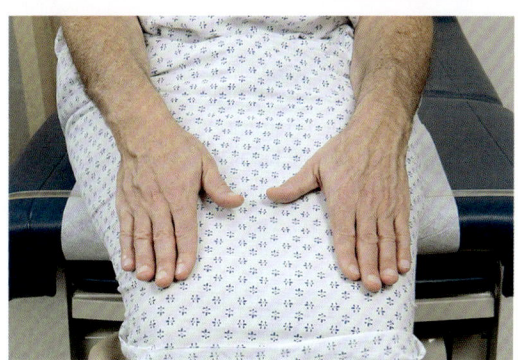

FIGURE 25-21 Testing rapid alternating movements: palms.

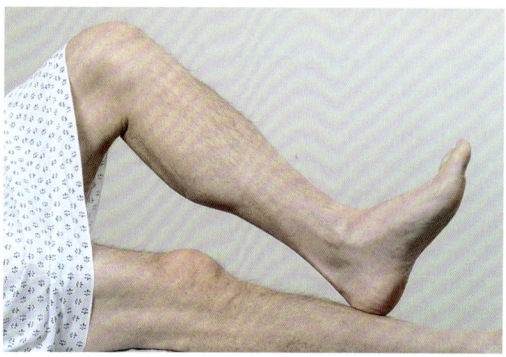

FIGURE 25-22 Performing the heel-to-shin test.

If the client is unconscious note his or her posture.

Primitive posturing is seen in unconscious states due to loss of motor control. (A) Decorticate posturing occurs when cortical loss is present. (B) Decerebrate posturing occurs when the midbrain is involved. (For illustrations of A and B, see Abnormal Findings 25-4.)

Sensory System

Assess light touch, pain, and temperature sensations. For each test, ask clients to close both eyes and tell you what they feel and where they feel it. Scatter stimuli over the distal and proximal parts of all extremities and the trunk to cover most of the dermatomes. It is not necessary to cover the entire body surface unless you identify abnormal symptoms such as pain, numbness, or tingling.

To test light touch sensation, use a wisp of cotton to touch the client (Fig. 25-23).

To test pain sensation, use the blunt (Fig. 25-24A) and sharp ends (Fig. 25-24B) of a safety pin or paper clip.

Client correctly identifies light touch.

🪑 **OLDER ADULT CONSIDERATIONS**
In some older clients, light touch and pain sensations may be decreased.

Client correctly differentiates between dull and sharp sensations and hot and cold temperatures over various body parts.

Many disorders can alter a person's ability to perceive sensations correctly. These include peripheral neuropathies (due to diabetes mellitus, folic acid deficiencies, and alcoholism) and lesions of the ascending spinal cord, brain stem, cranial nerves, and cerebral cortex. See Abnormal Findings 25-1.

Client reports:
- Anesthesia (absence of touch sensation)
- Hypesthesia (decreased sensitivity to touch)

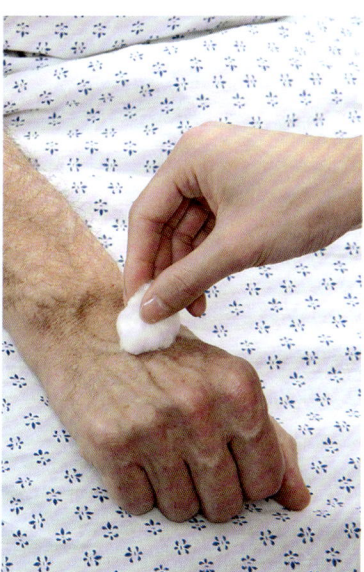

FIGURE 25-23 Testing light touch sensation.

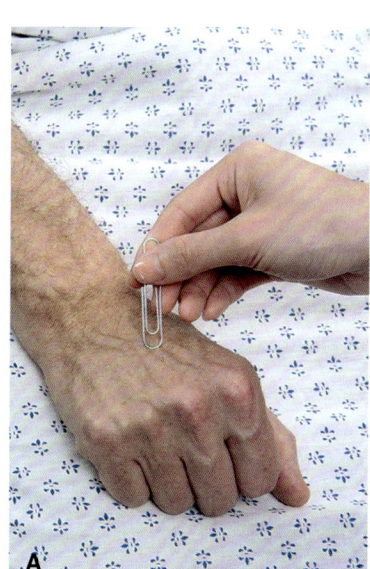 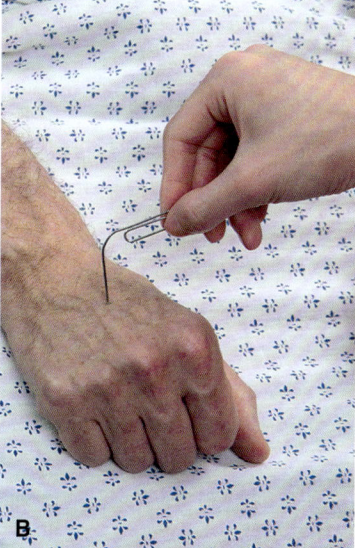

FIGURE 25-24 Testing pain sensation. **A.** Dull stimulus. **B.** Sharp stimulus.

Continued on following page

ASSESSMENT PROCEDURE	NORMAL FINDINGS	ABNORMAL FINDINGS
Sensory System (Continued)		
To test temperature sensation, use test tubes filled with hot and cold water. 🎯 **CLINICAL TIP** Test temperature sensation only if abnormalities are found in the client's ability to perceive light touch and pain sensations. Temperature and pain sensations travel in the lateral spinothalamic tract, thus temperature need not be tested if pain sensation is intact.		• Hyperesthesia (increased sensitivity to touch) • Analgesia (absence of pain sensation) • Hypalgesia (decreased sensitivity to pain) • Hyperalgesia (increased sensitivity to pain)
Test vibratory sensation. Strike a low-pitched tuning fork on the heel of your hand and hold the base on the distal radius (Fig. 25-25A), forefinger tip (Fig. 25-25B), medial malleolus (Fig. 25-25C), and, last, the tip of the great toe (Fig. 25-25D). Ask the client to indicate what he or she feels. Repeat on the other side.	Client correctly identifies sensation. 🪑 **OLDER ADULT CONSIDERATIONS** Vibratory sensation at the ankles may decrease after age 70 (Willacy, 2011), but vibration sense is more likely to be absent at the great toe and preserved at the ankle bones (Gilman, 2002).	Inability to sense vibrations may be seen in posterior column disease or peripheral neuropathy (e.g., as seen with diabetes or chronic alcohol abuse).

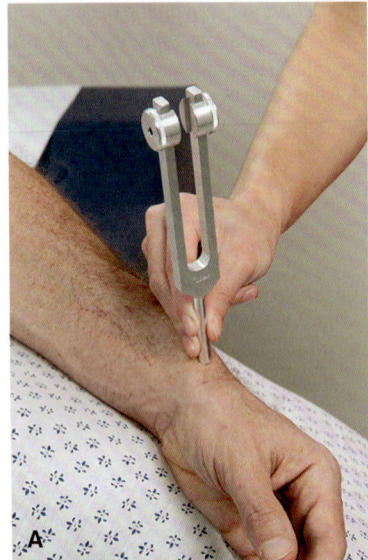
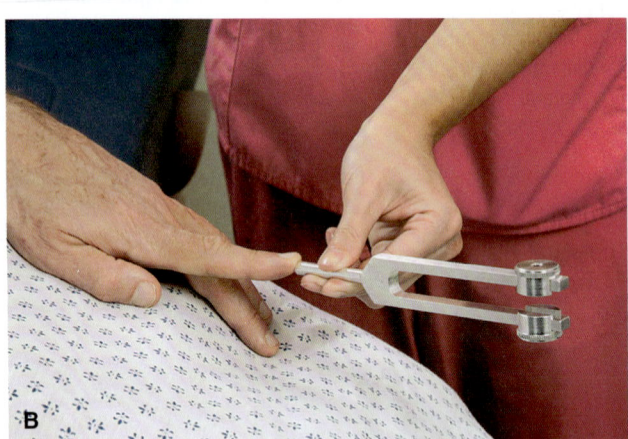
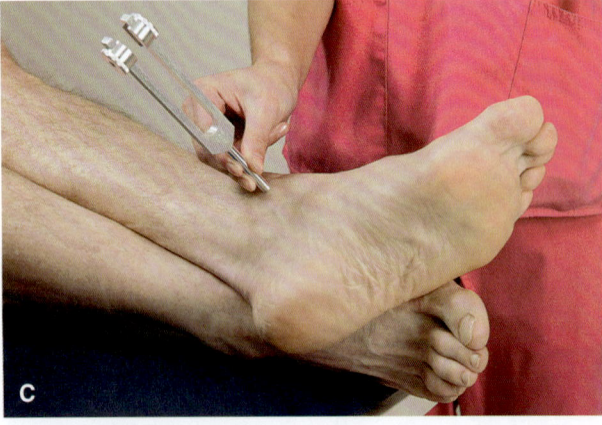
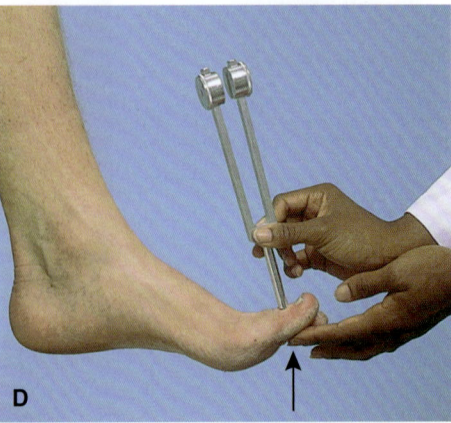

FIGURE 25-25 Testing vibratory sensation. Strike a low-pitched tuning fork on the heel of your hand and hold the base on the distal radius **(A)**, distal (DIP) joint of the index finger **(B)**, medial malleolus **(C)**, and, last, distal (DIP) joint of the great toe **(D)**.

ASSESSMENT PROCEDURE	NORMAL FINDINGS	ABNORMAL FINDINGS
CLINICAL TIP If vibratory sensation is intact distally, then it is intact proximally.		
Test sensitivity to position. Ask the client to close both eyes. Then hold the client's toe or a finger on the lateral sides and move it up or down (Fig. 25-26). Ask the client to tell you the direction it is moved. Repeat on the other side.	Client correctly identifies directions of movements. **OLDER ADULT CONSIDERATIONS** In some older clients, the sense of position of the great toe may be reduced.	Inability to identify the directions of the movements may be seen in posterior column disease or peripheral neuropathy (e.g., as seen with diabetes or chronic alcohol abuse).
CLINICAL TIP If position sense is intact distally, then it is intact proximally.		
Assess tactile discrimination (fine touch). Remember that the client should have eyes closed. To test stereognosis, place a familiar object such as a quarter, paper clip, or key in the client's hand and ask the client to identify it (Fig. 25-27). Repeat with another object in the other hand.	Client correctly identifies object.	Inability to correctly identify objects (astereognosis), area touched, number written in hand; to discriminate between two points; or identify areas simultaneously touched may be seen in lesions of the sensory cortex.

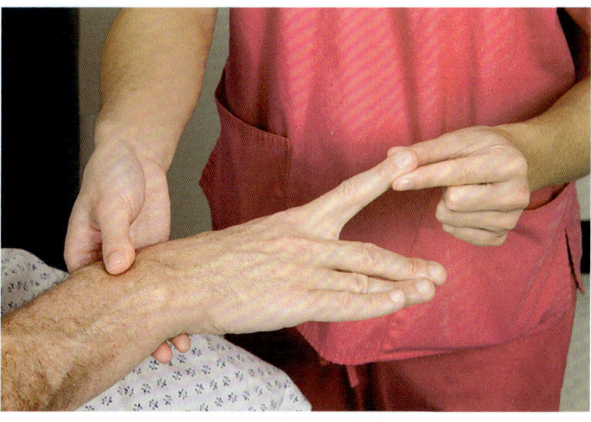

FIGURE 25-26 Testing position sense.

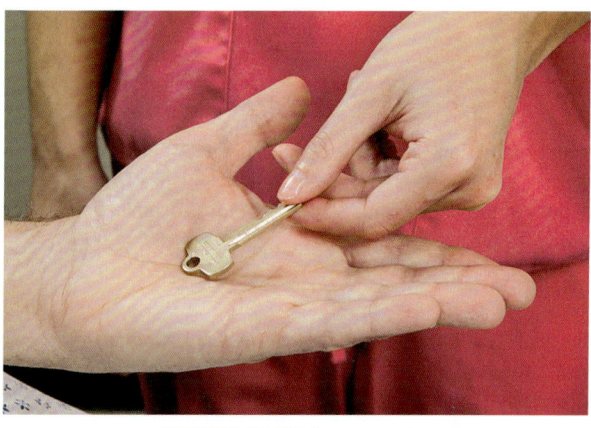

FIGURE 25-27 Stereognosis.

To test point localization, briefly touch the client and ask the client to identify the points touched.	Client correctly identifies area touched.	Same as above.
To test graphesthesia, use a blunt instrument to write a number, such as 2, 3, or 5, on the palm of the client's hand (Fig. 25-28). Ask the client to identify the number. Repeat with another number on the other hand.	Client correctly identifies number written.	Same as above.

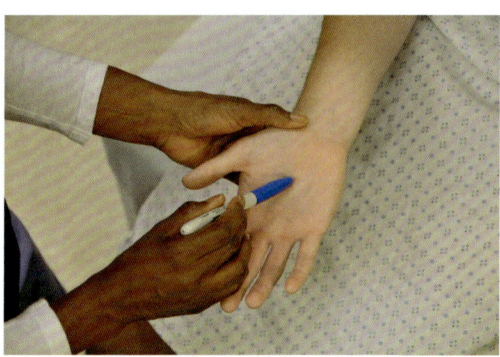

FIGURE 25-28 Graphesthesia.

Continued on following page

ASSESSMENT PROCEDURE	NORMAL FINDINGS	ABNORMAL FINDINGS
Sensory System (Continued)		
Two-point discrimination can be determined on the fingertips, forearm, dorsal hands, back, or thighs. Ask the client to identify the number of points (one or two) felt when touched with the EKG calibers. Measure the distance between the two points when the client can no longer distinguish the two points as separate (client states only one point is felt) (Fig. 25-29).	Client identifies two points on: • Fingertips at 2–5 mm apart • Forearm at 40 mm apart • Dorsal hands at 20–30 mm apart • Back at 40 mm apart • Thighs at 70 mm apart	Same as above.

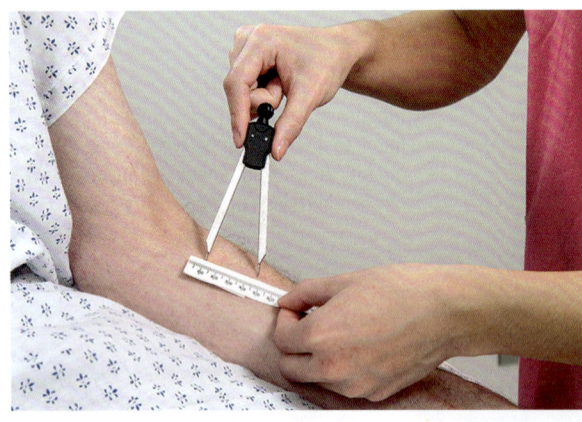

FIGURE 25-29 Two-point discrimination.

To test extinction, simultaneously touch the client in the same area on both sides of the body at the same point. Ask the client to identify the area touched.	Client correctly identifies points touched. See Table 25-3 for normal two-point discrimination findings.	Same as above.
Reflexes		
Test deep tendon reflexes. Position client in a comfortable sitting position. Use the reflex hammer to elicit reflexes (see Assessment Guide 25-1). **CLINICAL TIP** If deep tendon reflexes are diminished or absent, two reinforcement techniques may be used to enhance their response. When testing the arm reflexes, have the client clench the teeth. When testing the leg reflexes, have the client interlock the hands. **OLDER ADULT CONSIDERATIONS** Reinforcement techniques may also help the older client who has difficulty relaxing.	Normal reflex scores range from 1+ (present but decreased) to 2+ (normal) to 3+ (increased or brisk, but not pathologic). **OLDER ADULT CONSIDERATIONS** Older clients usually have deep tendon reflexes intact, although a decrease in reaction time may slow the response (Lim et al., 2009; Sirven & Malamut, 2008).	Absent or markedly decreased (hyporeflexia) deep tendon reflexes (rated 0) occur when a component of the lower motor neurons or reflex arc is impaired; this may be seen with spinal cord injuries. Markedly hyperactive (hyperreflexia) deep tendon reflexes (rated 4+) may be seen with lesions of the upper motor neurons and when the higher cortical levels are impaired. **OLDER ADULT CONSIDERATIONS** Some older clients may have decreased deep tendon reflexes and unstable balance due to peripheral neuropathy, which also causes disturbed proprioception, loss of vibratory and temperature sense, and possible pain, tingling, and distal weakness (Yeager, 2016).
Test biceps reflex. Ask the client to partially bend the arm at the elbow with palm up. Place your thumb over the biceps tendon and strike your thumb with the pointed side of the reflex hammer (Fig. 25-30). Repeat on the other side. (This evaluates the function of spinal levels C5 and C6.)	Elbow flexes and contraction of the biceps muscle is seen or felt. Ranges from 1+ to 3+. Forearm flexes and supinates. Ranges from 1+ to 3+.	No response or an exaggerated response is abnormal.

ASSESSMENT PROCEDURE	NORMAL FINDINGS	ABNORMAL FINDINGS
Assess brachioradialis reflex. Ask the client to flex elbow with palm down and hand resting on the abdomen or lap. Use the flat side of the reflex hammer to tap the tendon at the radius about 2 in above the wrist (Fig. 25-31). Repeat on the other side. (This evaluates the function of spinal levels C5 and C6.)	Flexion and supination of forearm.	No response or an exaggerated response is abnormal.

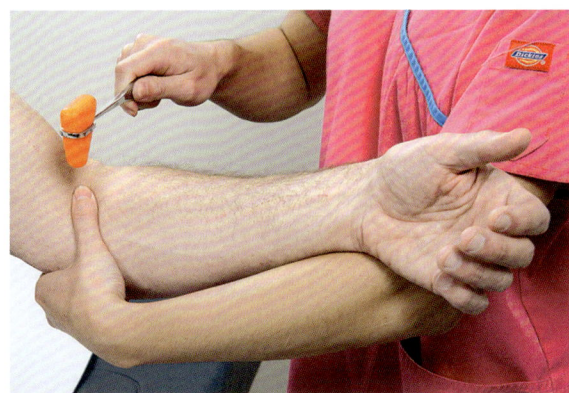

FIGURE 25-30 Eliciting the biceps reflex.

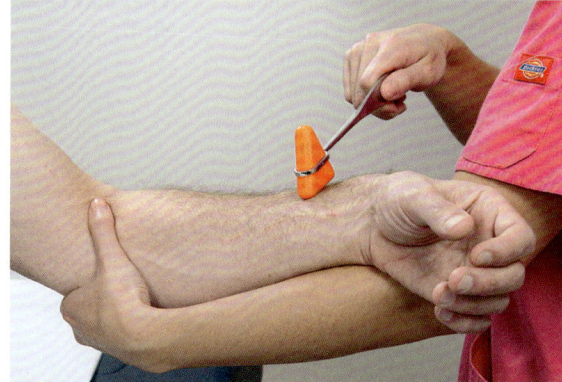

FIGURE 25-31 Eliciting the brachioradialis reflex.

Test triceps reflex. Ask the client to hang the arm freely ("limp, like it is hanging from a clothesline to dry") while you support it with your nondominant hand. With the elbow flexed, use the flat side of the reflex hammer to tap the tendon above the olecranon process (Fig. 25-32). Repeat on the other side. This evaluates the function of spinal levels C6, C7, and C8.	Elbow extends, triceps contracts. Ranges from 1+ to 3+.	No response or exaggerated response.

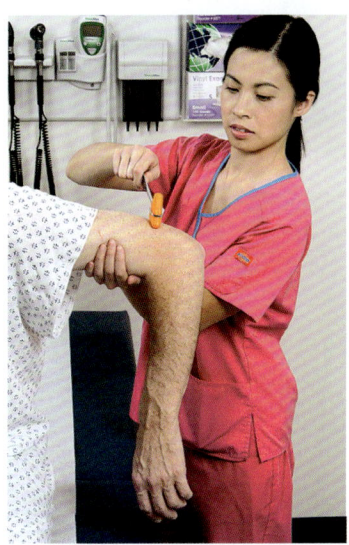

FIGURE 25-32 Eliciting the triceps reflex.

Assess patellar reflex. Ask the client to let both legs hang freely off the side of the examination table. Using the flat side of the reflex hammer, tap the patellar tendon, which is located just below the patella (Fig. 25-33A). Repeat on the other side. For the client who cannot sit up, gently flex the knee and strike the patella (Fig. 25-33B). This evaluates the function of spinal levels L2, L3, and L4.	Knee extends, quadriceps muscle contracts. Ranges from 1+ to 3+.	No response or an exaggerated response is abnormal.

Continued on following page

UNIT 3 Nursing Assessment of Physical Systems

ASSESSMENT PROCEDURE	NORMAL FINDINGS	ABNORMAL FINDINGS
Reflexes (Continued)		
Test Achilles reflex. With the client's leg still hanging freely, dorsiflex the foot. Tap the Achilles tendon with the flat side of the reflex hammer (Fig. 25-34A). Repeat on the other side. For assessing the reflex in the client who cannot sit up, have the client flex one knee and support that leg against the other leg. Dorsiflex the foot and tap the tendon using the flat side of the reflex hammer (Fig. 25-34B). This evaluates the function of spinal levels S1 and S2.	Normal response is plantarflexion of the foot. Ranges from 1+ to 3+. **OLDER ADULT CONSIDERATIONS** **In some older clients, the Achilles reflex may be absent or difficult to elicit.**	No response or an exaggerated response is abnormal.

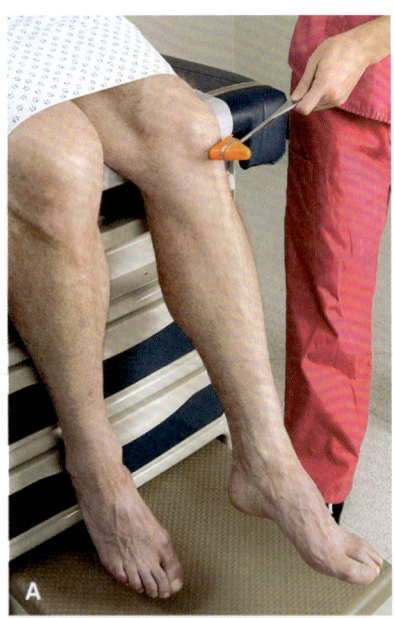
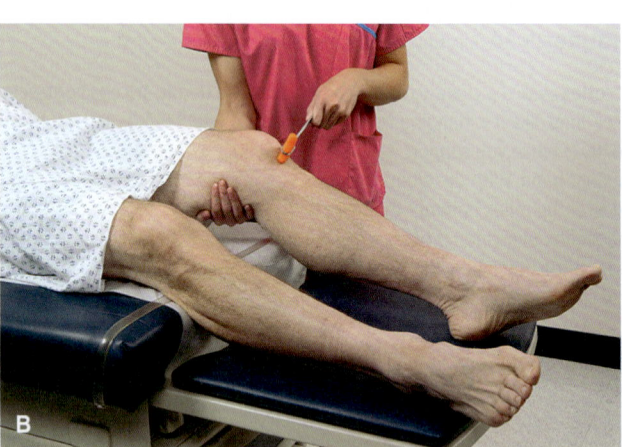

FIGURE 25-33 Eliciting the patellar reflex (**A**) and the patellar reflex in the supine position (**B**).

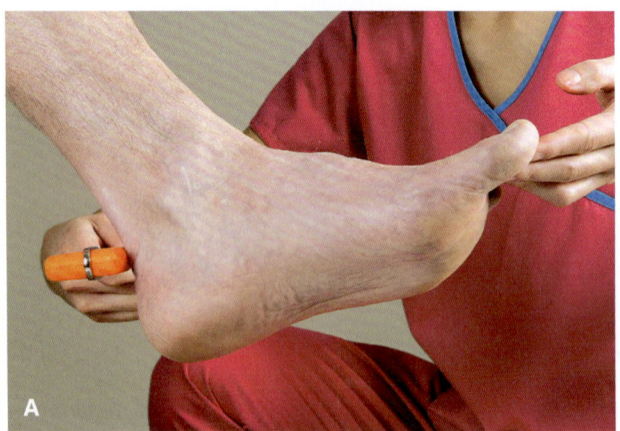
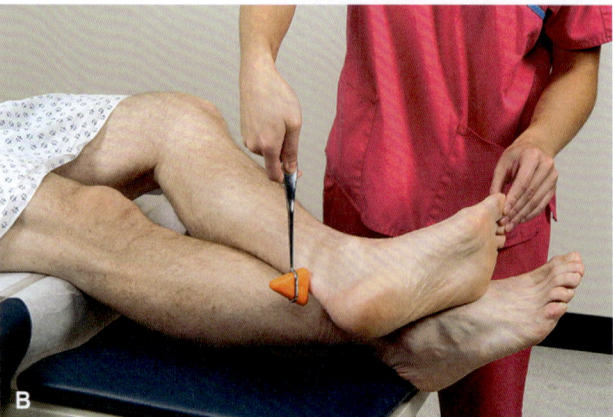

FIGURE 25-34 Eliciting the Achilles reflex (**A**) and the Achilles reflex in the supine position (**B**).

Test ankle clonus when the other reflexes tested have been hyperactive. Place one hand under the knee to support the leg, then briskly dorsiflex the foot toward the client's head (Fig. 25-35). Repeat on the other side.	No rapid contractions or oscillations (clonus) of the ankle are elicited.	Repeated rapid contractions or oscillations of the ankle and calf muscle are seen with lesions of the upper motor neurons.

ASSESSMENT PROCEDURE	NORMAL FINDINGS	ABNORMAL FINDINGS

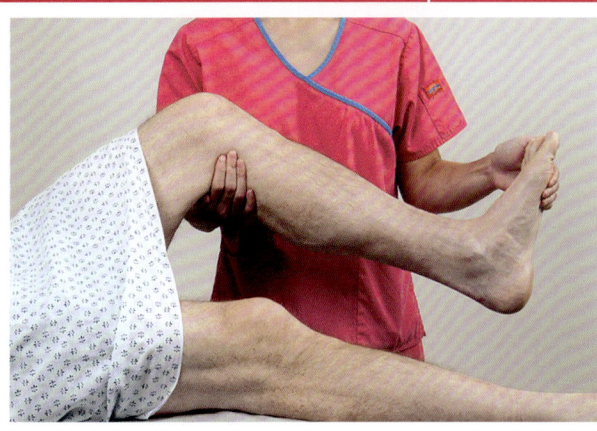

FIGURE 25-35 Testing for ankle clonus.

Test superficial reflexes.

Assess plantar reflex.

> 🎯 **CLINICAL TIP**
> Use the handle end of the reflex hammer to elicit superficial reflexes, whose receptors are in the skin rather than the muscles.

With the end of the reflex hammer or tongue blade, stroke the lateral aspect of the sole from the heel to the ball of the foot, curving medially across the ball (Fig. 25-36A). Repeat on the other side. This evaluates the function of spinal levels L4, L5, S1, and S2.

Flexion of the toes occurs (plantar response; Fig. 25-36A).

 OLDER ADULT CONSIDERATIONS
In some older adult clients, flexion of the toes may be difficult to elicit and may be absent.

The toes will fan out for abnormal response (positive Babinski response).

Except in infancy, extension (dorsiflexion) of the big toe and fanning of all toes (positive Babinski response) are seen with lesions of upper motor neurons. Unconscious states resulting from drug and alcohol intoxication, brain injury, or subsequent to an epileptic seizure may also cause it.

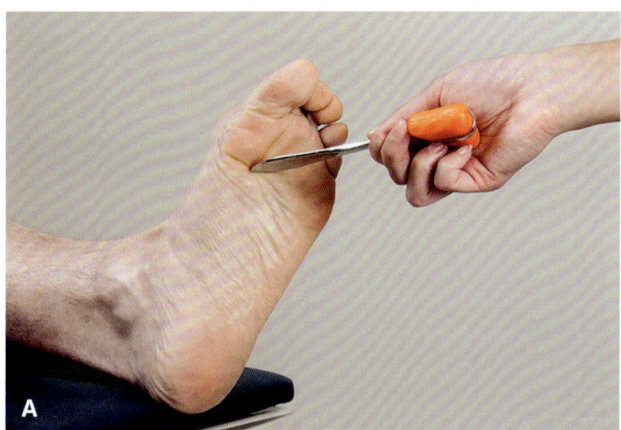 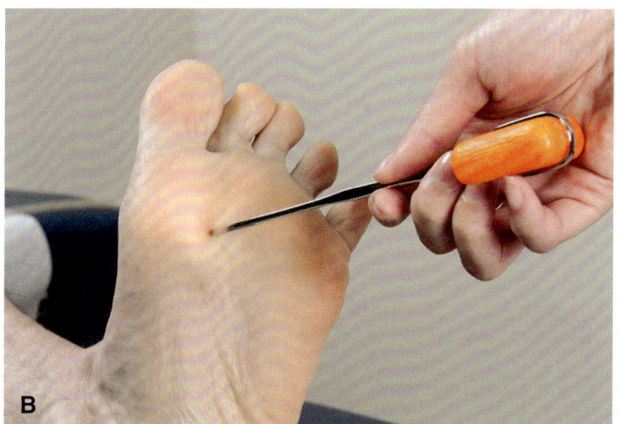

FIGURE 25-36 Eliciting a normal plantar response (**A**) and a positive Babinski sign (**B**).

Test abdominal reflex. Lightly stroke the abdomen on each side, above and below the umbilicus. This evaluates the function of spinal levels T8, T9, and T10 with the upper abdominal reflex and spinal levels T10, T11, and T12 with the lower abdominal reflex.

Abdominal muscles contract; the umbilicus deviates toward the side being stimulated (Fig. 25-37).

> 🎯 **CLINICAL TIP**
> The abdominal reflex may be concealed because of obesity or muscular stretching from pregnancies. This is not an abnormality.

Superficial reflexes may be absent with lower or upper motor neuron lesions.

Test cremasteric reflex in male clients. Lightly stroke the inner aspect of the upper thigh. This evaluates the function of spinal levels T12, L1, and L2.

Scrotum elevates on stimulated side (see Fig. 25-37).

Absence of reflex may indicate motor neuron disorder.

Continued on following page

ASSESSMENT PROCEDURE	NORMAL FINDINGS	ABNORMAL FINDINGS

Reflexes (Continued)

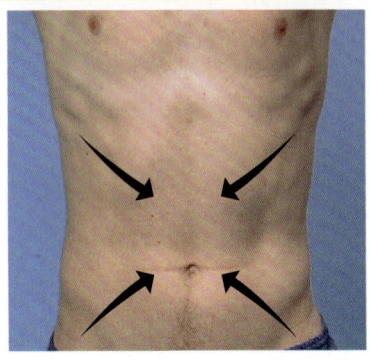

FIGURE 25-37 Abdominal and cremasteric reflexes.

Tests for Meningeal Irritation or Inflammation

If you suspect that the client has meningeal irritation or inflammation from infection or subarachnoid hemorrhage, assess the client's neck mobility. First, make sure that there is no injury to the cervical vertebrae or cervical cord. Then, with the client supine, place your hands behind the patient's head and flex the neck forward until the chin touches the chest if possible.	Neck is supple; client can easily bend head and neck forward.	Pain in the neck and resistance to flexion can arise from meningeal inflammation, arthritis, or neck injury.
Test for Brudzinski sign. As you flex the neck, watch the hips and knees in reaction to your maneuver.	Hips and knees remain relaxed and motionless.	Pain and flexion of the hips and knees are positive Brudzinski signs, suggesting meningeal inflammation.
Test for Kernig sign. Flex the client's leg at both the hip and the knee, then straighten the knee.	No pain is felt. Discomfort behind the knee during full extension occurs in many normal people.	Pain and increased resistance to extending the knee are positive Kernig signs. When Kernig sign is bilateral, the examiner suspects meningeal irritation.

CASE STUDY

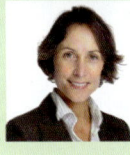

The chapter case study is now used to demonstrate a physical assessment of Linda Hutchison's nervous system.

Alert, thin, middle-aged woman with mildly elevated blood pressure and pulse rate (136/92 and 98). According to her chart, Ms. Hutchison's blood pressure is normally 100/70.

CN I: Able to correctly identify scents bilaterally.

CN II: Vision 20/20 right eye, left eye, and both eyes. Visual fields intact. Red reflex present bilaterally. No other internal structures visualized by examiner.

CN III, IV, VI: Extraocular movements intact. No ptosis noted bilaterally. Slight nystagmus noted when eyes are in extreme lateral positions. Pupils 5 mm, constricting to 3 mm bilaterally. Pupils reactive to light and accommodation.

CN V: Temporal and masseter muscles contract bilaterally. Able to identify light touch to forehead, cheek, and chin. Corneal light reflex symmetric.

CN VII: Able to smile, frown, wrinkle forehead, show teeth, puff out cheeks, purse lips, raise eyebrows, and close eyes against resistance.

CN VIII: Able to hear whispers from 3 ft bilaterally. Weber test with equal lateralization. Rinne test AC > BC.

CN IX, X: Uvula and soft palate rise symmetrically with phonation. Gag reflex present. Swallows without difficulty.

CN XI: Equal shoulder shrug with resistance bilaterally. Turns head in both directions with resistance.

CN XII: Tongue midline without tremor. Strength of tongue intact.

Motor function: No atrophy of muscles noted. Slight tremors and weakness of leg muscles noted. Full range of motion of all extremities. No fasciculations or tics noted. Unable to walk heel-to-toe without some loss of balance. Romberg sign is negative. Rapid alternating and finger-to-nose movements smooth and intact. Heel-to-shin movement smooth and intact.

Sensory: Identifies light, sharp, and dull sensation to extremities and trunk. Vibratory sensation, stereognosis, graphesthesia, and two-point discrimination are intact.

Reflexes: 2+ bilateral brachioradialis, bicep, triceps. 4+ patellar. Achilles and plantar reflexes with mild clonus. Abdominal reflex present. Babinski with toe flexion.

TABLE 25-3	Two-Point Discrimination Findings	
Two-Point Discrimination	Right	Left
Measurements in mm		
Fingertips	6	6
Dorsal hand	15	15
Chest	45	49
Forearm	39	35
Back	45	45
Upper arm	40	45
Reflexes		
Biceps	2+	2+
Triceps	2+	2+
Patellar	3+	3+
Achilles	2+	2+
Abdominal	1+	1+
Babinski	Negative	Negative

Validating and Documenting Findings

Validate the neurologic assessment data you have collected. This is necessary to verify that the data are reliable and accurate. Document the data following the health care facility or agency policy. The Summary Sheet of International Standards (Fig. 25-38) may used to document the summary of sensory and motor function changes resulting from spinal cord injuries.

CLINICAL TIP
When documenting your assessment findings, it is better to describe the client's response than to label the behavior.

CASE STUDY

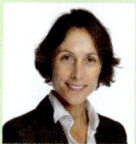

Think back to the case study. The clinic nurse documented the following subjective and objective assessment findings of Angela Hutchison's neurologic examination.

Biographical Data: LH, 49-year-old Caucasian woman. Alert and oriented. Asks and answers questions appropriately. Had been working as an office manager at the local high school, but recently began teaching (her first love) language classes (French and German); she is also responsible for teaching two physical education (PE) classes a week.

Reason for Seeking Health Care: "I have been so tired and weak lately, and have been having trouble with urinary continence and a 'pins and needles' feeling in my legs. Leg spasms at night are keeping me awake. I am anxious that I will have an exacerbation of my MS."

History of Present Health Concern: The current symptoms began after she recently changed jobs. "I get so tired by the end of the week. If I rest all weekend, I am OK by Monday morning." Ms. Hutchison has had MS for 20 years, but has managed to function at a near-normal level for most of that time. "I had one severe exacerbation during my divorce, but I went into remission after about 6 months."

Personal Health History: Ms. Hutchison denies numbness, seizures, or dizziness. She has not noticed a change in sensations of taste or smell, hearing, or vision. Client denies difficulty speaking or swallowing. She denies loss of bowel control. Client denies

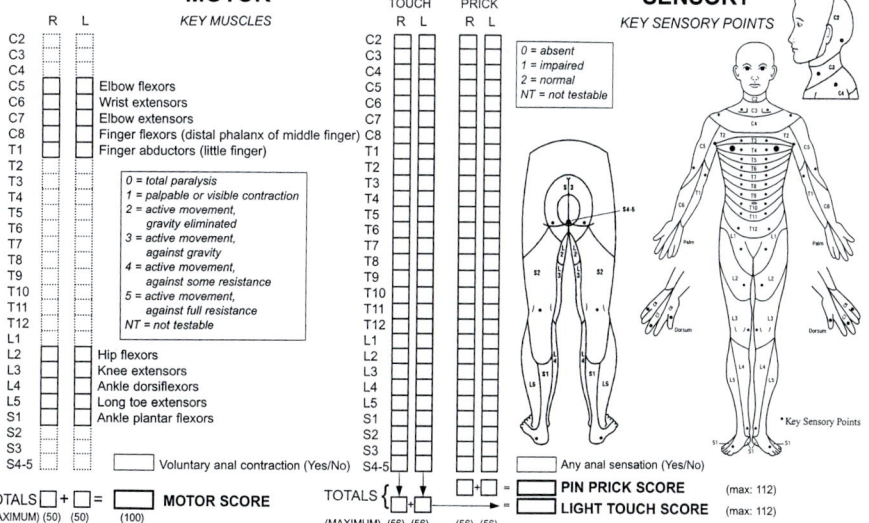

FIGURE 25-38 Summary sheet of International Standards for Neurological and Functional Classification of Spinal Cord Injury. (Used with permission of the American Spinal Injury Association. (1996). International standards for neurological and functional classification of spinal cord injury. Chicago: American Spinal Injury Association.)

recent or remote memory loss. Client denies head injury, meningitis, encephalitis, spinal cord injury, or stroke.

Family History: Ms. Hutchison reports that her mother has hypertension and migraine headaches. Her father and two sisters are in excellent health. Maternal grandmother has hypertension and obesity. Maternal grandfather died as a result of an automobile accident at age 35. Paternal grandmother has rheumatoid arthritis. Paternal grandfather has coronary artery disease, hypertension, and diabetes type 2. Ms. Hutchinson denies a family history of cerebrovascular disease, epilepsy, brain cancer, or Huntington chorea.

Lifestyle and Health Practices: Takes oxybutynin (Ditropan) as prescribed for MS. Takes multivitamin daily. Denies use of tobacco or recreational drugs. Reports drinking two to three glasses of wine every 2 to 3 months. Reports wearing a seatbelt at all times. Denies participation in any activities requiring protective headgear. 24-hour diet recall: Breakfast—cereal with 2% milk and 1 cup of coffee; lunch—plain ham and cheese sandwich, 1 small bag plain potato chips, and an apple, with unsweetened iced tea; dinner—petite filet mignon, loaded baked potato, salad, water.

Denies exposure to lead, insecticides, pollutants, or other chemicals. Denies frequent heavy lifting or repetitive motions. Reports that she is able to perform ADLs independently. Denies any change in self-esteem or body image.

Physical Examination Findings: Alert, thin, middle-aged woman with mildly elevated blood pressure and pulse rate (136/92 and 98). According to her chart, Ms. Hutchison's blood pressure is normally 100/70.

CN I: Able to correctly identify scents bilaterally.

CN II: Vision 20/20 right eye, left eye, and both eyes. Visual fields intact. Red reflex present bilaterally. No other internal structures visualized by examiner.

CN III, IV, VI: Extraocular movements intact. No ptosis noted bilaterally. Slight nystagmus noted when eyes are in extreme lateral positions. Pupils 5 mm, constricting to 3 mm bilaterally. Pupils reactive to light and accommodation.

CN V: Temporal and masseter muscles contract bilaterally. Able to identify light touch to forehead, cheek, and chin. Corneal light reflex symmetric.

CN VII: Able to smile, frown, wrinkle forehead, show teeth, puff out cheeks, purse lips, raise eyebrows, and close eyes against resistance.

CN VIII: Able to hear whispers from 3 ft bilaterally. Weber test with equal lateralization. Rinne test AC > BC.

CN IX, X: Uvula and soft palate rise symmetrically with phonation. Gag reflex present. Swallows without difficulty.

CN XI: Equal shoulder shrug with resistance bilaterally. Turns head in both directions with resistance.

CN XII: Tongue midline without tremor. Strength of tongue intact.

Motor function: No atrophy of muscles noted. Slight tremors and weakness of leg muscles noted. Full range of motion of all extremities. No fasciculations or tics noted. Unable to walk heel-to-toe without some loss of balance. Romberg sign is negative. Rapid alternating movements and finger-to-nose movements smooth and intact. Heel-to-shin movement smooth and intact.

Sensory: Identifies light, sharp, and dull sensation to extremities and trunk. Vibratory sensation, stereognosis, graphesthesia, and two-point discrimination are intact.

Reflexes: 2+ bilateral brachioradialis, bicep, triceps. 4+ patellar. Achilles and plantar reflexes with mild clonus. Abdominal reflex present. Babinski with toe flexion.

ANALYSIS OF DATA: DIAGNOSTIC REASONING

After collecting subjective and objective data pertaining to the neurologic assessment, identify abnormal findings and client strengths. Then cluster the data to reveal any significant patterns or abnormalities. These data may then be used to make clinical judgments about the status of the client's neurologic health.

Selected Nursing Diagnoses

Following is a listing of selected nursing diagnoses (health promotion, risk, or actual) that you may identify when analyzing the cue clusters.

Health Promotion Diagnoses

- Readiness for Enhanced Communication
- Readiness for Enhanced Spiritual Well-Being

Risk Diagnoses

- Risk for Injury related to disturbed sensory-perceptual patterns
- Risk for Aspiration related to impaired gag reflex
- Risk for Self-Directed Violence, related to depression, suicidal tendencies, developmental crisis, lack of support systems, loss of significant others, poor coping mechanisms, and behaviors

Actual Diagnoses

- Impaired Verbal Communication related to aphasia, psychological impairment, or organic brain disorder
- Acute or Chronic Confusion related to dementia, head injury, stroke, or alcohol or drug abuse
- Impaired Memory related to dementia, stroke, head injury, or alcohol or drug abuse
- Ineffective Impulse Control related to substance abuse, co-dependency, developmental disorder, or organic brain disorders
- Impaired Swallowing related to absent gag reflex or decreased muscle strength for mastication, or facial paralysis

- Sexual Dysfunction related to peripheral neuropathy
- Impaired Environmental Interpretation Syndrome related to dementia, depression, or alcoholism
- Self-Care Deficit (bathing, hygiene, toileting, or feeding) related to paralysis, weakness, or confusion
- Reflex Urinary Incontinence related to spinal cord or brain damage
- Unilateral Neglect related to poor vision on one side, trauma, or neurologic disorder
- Activity Intolerance related to fatigue, confusion, paralysis, weakness

Selected Collaborative Problems

After grouping the data, certain collaborative problems may become apparent. Remember that collaborative problems differ from nursing diagnoses in that they cannot be prevented with nursing interventions alone. However, these physiologic complications of medical conditions can be detected and monitored by the nurse. In addition, the nurse can use physician- and nurse-prescribed interventions to minimize the complications of these problems. The nurse may also have to refer the client in such situations for further treatment of the problem. Following is a list of collaborative problems that may be identified when assessing the neurologic system. These problems are worded as Risk for Complications (RC), followed by the problem.

- RC: Increased intracranial pressure
- RC: Stroke
- RC: Seizures
- RC: Spinal cord compression
- RC: Meningitis
- RC: Cranial nerve impairment
- RC: Paralysis
- RC: Peripheral nerve impairment
- RC: Increased intraocular pressure
- RC: Corneal ulceration
- RC: Neuropathies

Medical Problems

After grouping the data, the client's signs and symptoms may require medical diagnosis and treatment. Referral to a primary care provider is necessary.

CASE STUDY

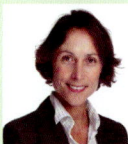

After collecting and analyzing the data for Linda Hutchison, the nurse determines that the following conclusions are appropriate:

Nursing Diagnoses
- Activity Intolerance r/t fatigue secondary to MS in remission and increased physical demands of new position at work.
- Anxiety r/t possible loss of teaching position secondary to acceleration of illness symptoms.
- Risk for Loneliness r/t difficulty maintaining social contacts and attending social events due to fatigue

Collaborative Problems
- RC: Hypertension
- RC: Urinary incontinence
- RC: Active multiple sclerosis

Refer Ms. Hutchison to a neurologist for evaluation of her treatment regimen.

To view an algorithm depicting the process of diagnostic reasoning for this case, go to thePoint.

Interdisciplinary Verbal Communication of Assessment Findings Using SBAR

SITUATION: LH, an alert and thin 49-year-old Caucasian female high school teacher who has had MS for 20 years, presents with weakness and extreme fatigue, urinary incontinence, a "pins and needles" feeling in her legs, and nocturnal muscle spasms that decrease her sleep. She is requesting ways to prevent an exacerbation of MS, which she fears is happening. Takes oxybutynin (Ditropan) as prescribed for MS.

BACKGROUND: Symptoms began after she recently changed jobs. Has had MS for 20 years, but has managed ADLs to function at a near-normal level except for one severe 6-month exacerbation during her divorce. Mother has hypertension and migraine headaches.

ASSESSMENT: Alert, thin, elevated blood pressure and pulse rate (136/92 and 98: usually 100/70). 24-hour dietary recall high in calories and fat. Full range of motion of all extremities. Slight tremors and weakness of leg muscles noted. No fasciculations or tics noted. Some loss of balance noted when walking heel-to-toe. Rest of neurologic examination shows no abnormalities. Achilles and plantar reflexes with mild clonus.

RECOMMENDATION: L.H. has Activity Intolerance r/t fatigue secondary to MS in remission and increased physical demands of new position at work. She is experiencing Anxiety r/t possible loss of teaching position secondary to acceleration of illness symptoms. She is at risk for Loneliness r/t difficulty maintaining social contacts and attending social events due to fatigue. Collaborative Problems include hypertension, urinary incontinence, and active multiple sclerosis for which she needs to be seen by her primary care provider for evaluation of her current treatment regimen.

ABNORMAL FINDINGS 25-1 Abnormal Motor and Sensory Findings in Spinal Cord Injuries

DESCRIPTION	DIAGRAM
Cross-section of the spinal cord demonstrating the major tracts of the spinal cord. (Used with permission from Frymoyer, J. W., Wiesel, S. W., et al. (2004). *The adult and pediatric spine*. Philadelphia, PA: Lippincott Williams & Wilkins.)	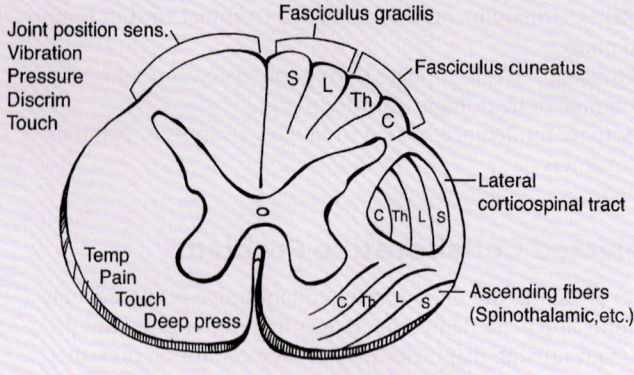
Brown-Séquard syndrome. A hemisection of the spinal cord resulting in ipsilateral loss of strength and proprioception and contralateral loss of pain and temperature. (Used with permission from Frymoyer, J. W., Wiesel, S. W., et al. (2004). *The adult and pediatric spine*. Philadelphia, PA: Lippincott Williams & Wilkins.)	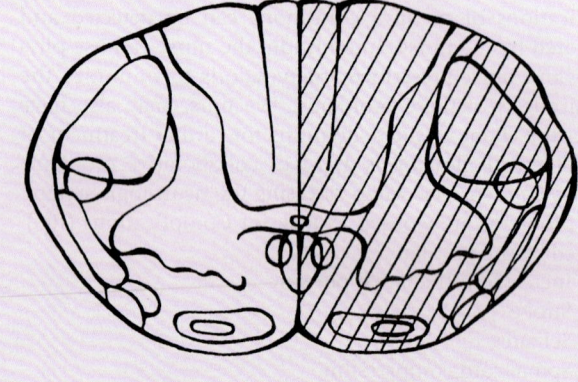
Central cord syndrome. Injury results in sacral sparing and preferentially upper- more than lower-extremity weakness. (Used with permission from Frymoyer, J. W., Wiesel, S. W., et al. (2004). *The adult and pediatric spine*. Philadelphia, PA: Lippincott Williams & Wilkins.)	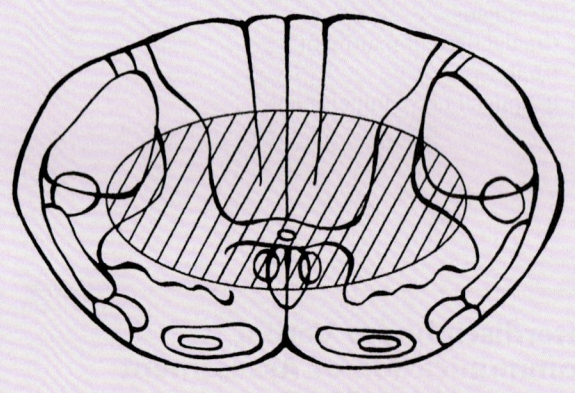
Anterior cord syndrome. Injury results in variable loss of motor function as well as pain and temperature. Proprioception is preserved. (Used with permission from Frymoyer, J. W., Wiesel, S. W., et al. (2004). *The adult and pediatric spine*. Philadelphia, PA: Lippincott Williams & Wilkins.)	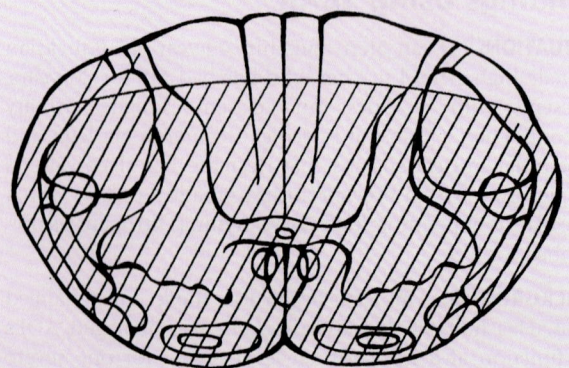

DESCRIPTION

Posterior cord syndrome. Injury results in loss of proprioception and variable preservation of motor function and pain and temperature sensation. (Used with permission from Frymoyer, J. W., Wiesel, S. W., et al. (2004). *The adult and pediatric spine.* Philadelphia, PA: Lippincott Williams & Wilkins.)

DIAGRAM

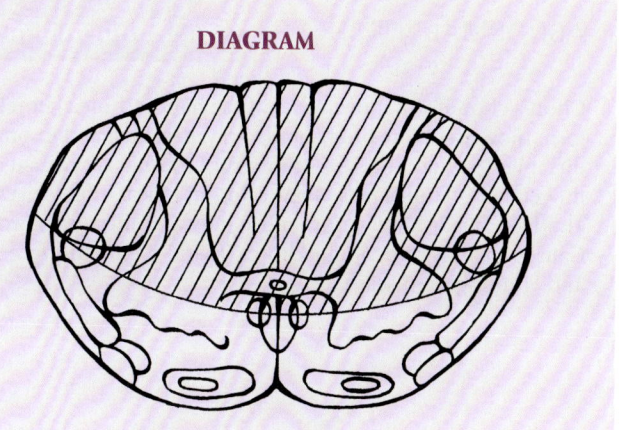

ABNORMAL FINDING 25-2 — Abnormal Muscle Movements

Atrophy and fasciculations of the tongue in a patient with amyotrophic lateral sclerosis.

Pathway of tremor impulse down the arm of a male figure.

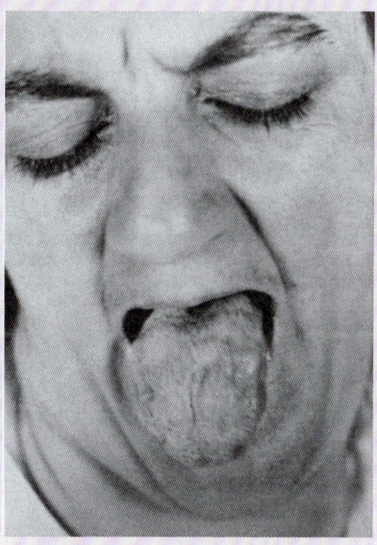

Eye tic. Tics are brief, repetitive, stereotyped, coordinated movements occurring at irregular intervals. Examples include repetitive winking, grimacing, and shoulder shrugging. Causes include Tourette syndrome and drugs such as phenothiazines and amphetamines.

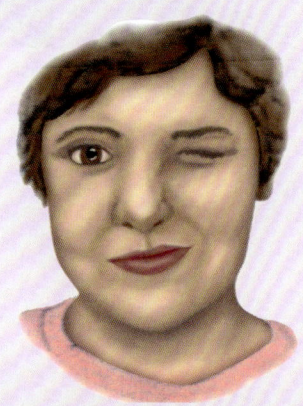

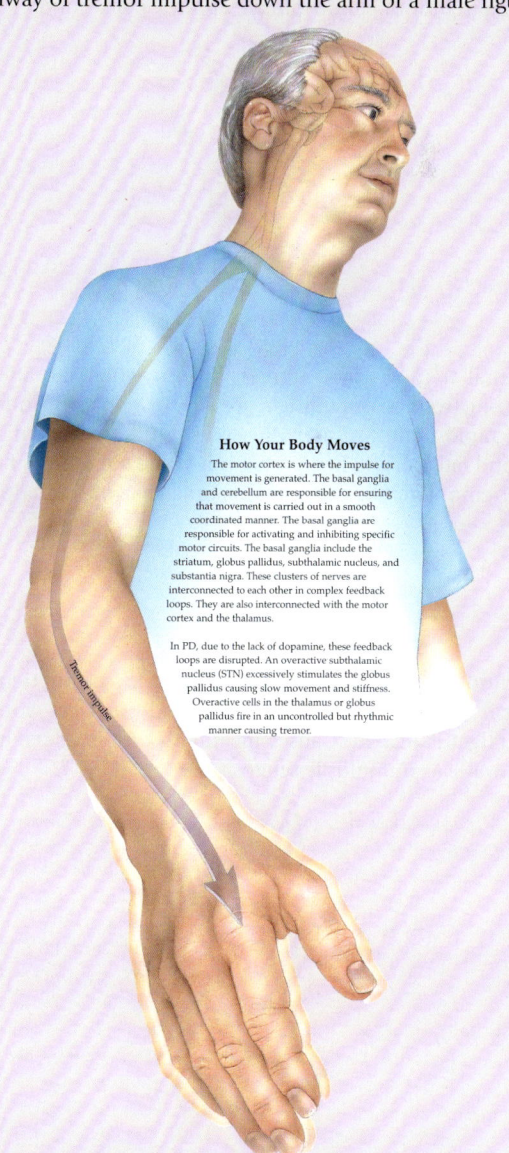

How Your Body Moves

The motor cortex is where the impulse for movement is generated. The basal ganglia and cerebellum are responsible for ensuring that movement is carried out in a smooth coordinated manner. The basal ganglia are responsible for activating and inhibiting specific motor circuits. The basal ganglia include the striatum, globus pallidus, subthalamic nucleus, and substantia nigra. These clusters of nerves are interconnected to each other in complex feedback loops. They are also interconnected with the motor cortex and the thalamus.

In PD, due to the lack of dopamine, these feedback loops are disrupted. An overactive subthalamic nucleus (STN) excessively stimulates the globus pallidus causing slow movement and stiffness. Overactive cells in the thalamus or globus pallidus fire in an uncontrolled but rhythmic manner causing tremor.

Continued on following page

| ABNORMAL FINDINGS | 25-2 | **Abnormal Muscle Movements** (Continued) |

Chorea choreiform movements of the hand. Chorea choreiform movements are brief, rapid, jerky, irregular, and unpredictable. They occur at rest or interrupt normal coordinated movements. Unlike tics, they seldom repeat themselves. The face, head, lower arms, and hands are often involved. Causes include Sydenham chorea (with rheumatic fever) and Huntington disease.

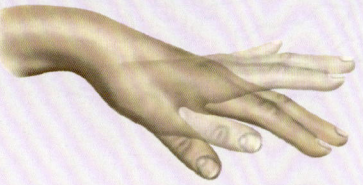

Athetosis. Athetoid movements are slower and more twisting and writhing than choreiform movements, and have a larger amplitude. They most commonly involve the face and the distal extremities. Athetosis is often associated with spasticity. Causes include cerebral palsy.

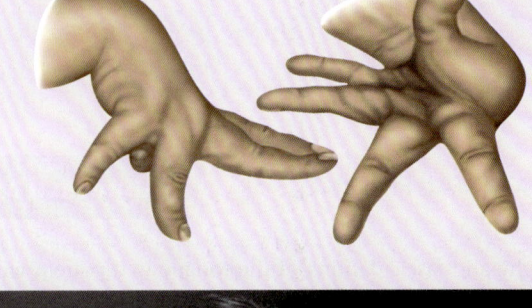

Resting (static) tremors. These tremors are most prominent at rest, and may decrease or disappear with voluntary movement. Illustrated is the common, relatively slow, fine, pill-rolling tremor of parkinsonism, about 5 per second.

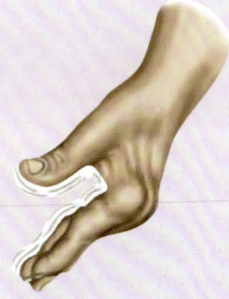

Postural tremor. These tremors appear when the affected part is actively maintaining a posture. Examples include the fine, rapid tremor of hyperthyroidism, the tremors of anxiety and fatigue, and benign essential (and sometimes familial) tremor. Tremor may worsen somewhat with intention.

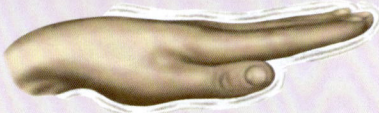

Intention tremor of a pointed finger. Intention tremors, absent at rest, appear with activity and often get worse as the target is neared. Causes include disorders of cerebellar pathways, as in multiple sclerosis.

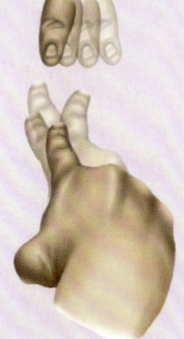

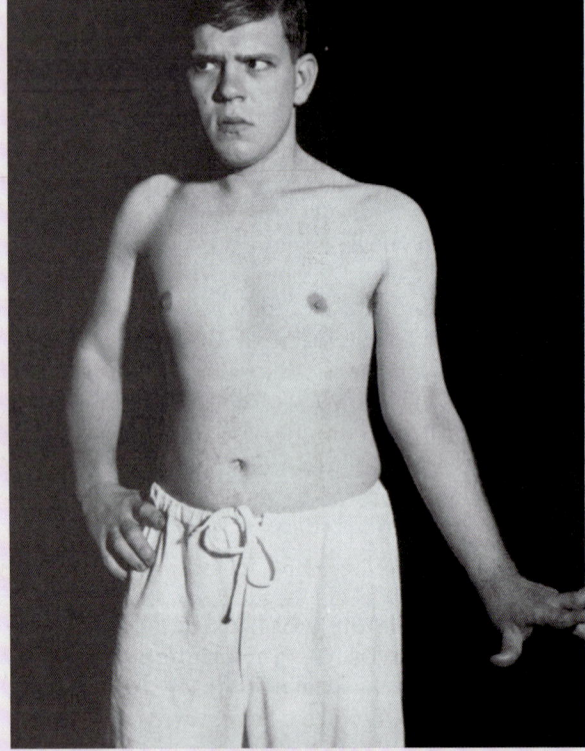

A patient with congenital unilateral athetosis.

Image credits: Atrophy and fasciculations of the tongue, Eye tic, Choreiform movements of the hand, Resting tremors, Postural tremors, Intention tremor, Athetosis: *From Bickley, L. S., & Szilagyi, P. (2003). Bates' guide to physical examination and history taking (8th ed.). Philadelphia, PA: Lippincott Williams & Wilkins;* Pathway of tremor impulse: Anatomical Chart Company.

ABNORMAL FINDINGS 25-3 Abnormal Gaits

An individual normally walks a little bit differently from everyone else, but sometimes a person's gait is distinctively abnormal, suggesting that the person has a neurologic problem. Some common abnormal gaits and their causes follow:

CEREBELLAR ATAXIA
- Wide-based, staggering, unsteady gait.
- Romberg test results are positive (client cannot stand with feet together).
- Seen with cerebellar diseases or alcohol or drug intoxication.

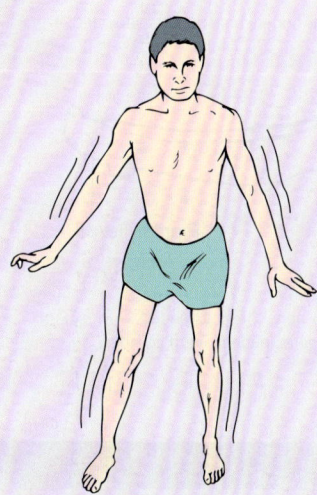
Cerebellar ataxia.

PARKINSONIAN GAIT
- Shuffling gait, turns accomplished in very stiff manner.
- Stooped-over posture with flexed hips and knees.
- Typically seen in Parkinson disease *and drug-induced parkinsonian* because of effects on the basal ganglia.

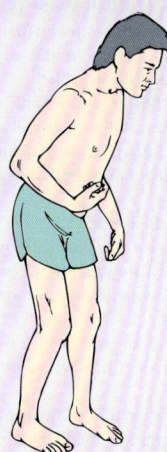
Parkinsonian gait.

SCISSORS GAIT
- Stiff, short gait; thighs overlap each other with each step.
- Seen with partial paralysis of the legs.

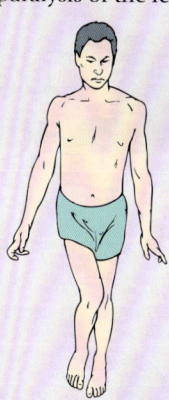
Scissors gait.

SPASTIC HEMIPARESIS
- Flexed arm held close to body while client drags toe of leg or circles it stiffly outward and forward.
- Seen with lesions of the upper motor neurons in the cortical spinal tract, such as occurs in stroke.

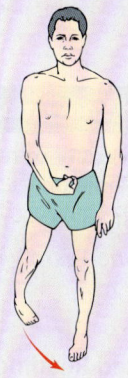
Spastic hemiparesis.

FOOTDROP
- Client lifts foot and knee high with each step, then slaps the foot down hard on the ground.
- Client cannot walk on heels.
- Characteristic of diseases of the lower motor neurons.

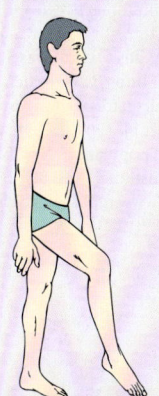
Footdrop (steppage) gait.

ABNORMAL FINDINGS 25-4 — Abnormal Postures in Unconscious Clients

Primitive posturing in an unconscious patients results from loss of motor control.

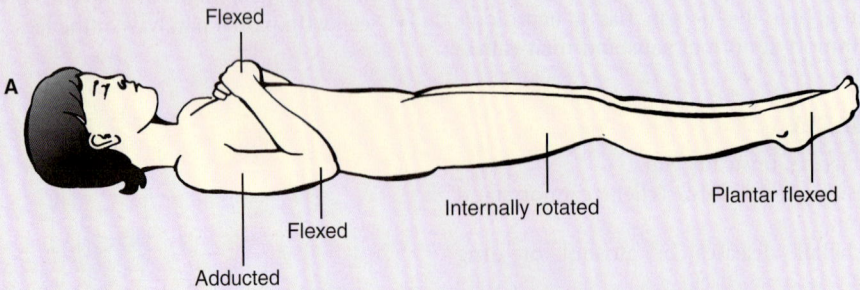

Decorticate posturing. Occurs with lesions of cerebral cortex. Arms, wrists, and fingers flexed; arms adducted; lower extremities extended, internally rotated, with plantar flexion of feet.

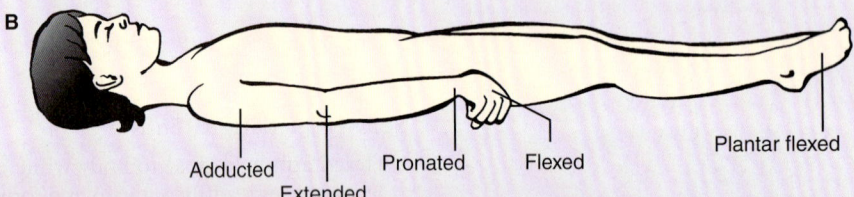

Decerebrate posturing. Occurs with lesions of brain stem at midbrain or upper pons. Arms extended, adducted, internally rotated, and wrists pronated, and fingers flexed. Back hyperextended. Teeth clinched. Legs extended with plantar flexion.

Want to know more?

A wide variety of resources to enhance your learning and understanding of this book are available on thePoint. Visit thePoint to access:

NCLEX-Style Student Review Questions
Watch and Learn Videos
Concepts in Action Animations
And more!

References and Selected Readings

Gilman, S. (2002). Joint position sense and vibration sense: Anatomical organisation and assessment. *Journal of Neurology, Neurosurgery, & Psychiatry, 73,* 473–477.

Goldstein, L., Bushnell, C., Adams, R., et al. (2011). Guidelines for the primary prevention of stroke: A guideline for healthcare professionals from the American Heart Association/American Stroke Association. *Stroke, 42,* 517–584. Available at http://stroke.ahajournals.org/content/42/2/517.full.pdf

Healthy People 2020. (2016). Heart disease and stroke. Available at https://www.healthypeople.gov/2020/topics-objectives/topic/heart-disease-and-stroke/objectives

Husten, L. (2014). ACC/AHA Risk Cardiovascular Risk Calculator questioned again. Available at http://www.jwatch.org/fw109392/2014/10/08/acc-aha-cardiovascular-risk-calculator-again-questioned

Lim, K. S., Bong, Y., Chaw, Y., et al. (2009). Wide range of normality in deep tendon reflexes in the normal population. *Neurology Asia, 14,* 21–25.

National Heart, Lung, Blood Institute (NHLBI). (2015). Who is at risk for a stroke? Available at https://www.nhlbi.nih.gov/health/health-topics/topics/stroke/atrisk

National Stroke Association. (2016a). Myths vs facts: Stroke facts. Available at http://www.stroke.org/understand-stroke/what-stroke/stroke-facts

National Stroke Association. (2016b). What is a stroke? Available at http://www.stroke.org/understand-stroke/what-stroke

Sirven, J., & Malamut, B. (2008). *Clinical neurology of the older adult* (2nd ed.). Philadelphia, PA: Lippincott, Williams & Wilkins.

The Internet Stroke Center. (2016). Stroke assessment scales. Available at http://www.strokecenter.org/professionals/stroke-diagnosis/stroke-assessment-scales/

U.S. Preventive Services Task Force (USPSTF). (2015). Draft recommendation statement: Aspirin to prevent cardiovascular disease and cancer. Available at http://www.uspreventiveservicestaskforce.org/Page/Document/draft-recommendation-statement/aspirin-to-prevent-cardiovascular-disease-and-cancer

Willacy, H. (2011). Neurological examination of the lower limbs. Available at http://www.patient.co.uk/doctor/Neurological-Examination-of-the-Lower-Limbs.htm

Yeager, D. (2016). Diagnosing peripheral neuropathy. *Aging Well, 5*(4),14. Available at http://www.todaysgeriatricmedicine.com/archive/070912p14.shtml

26 ASSESSING MALE GENITALIA AND RECTUM

Learning Objectives

1. Describe the structure and the function of male genitalia, anus, rectum, and prostate.
2. Discuss risk factors associated with HIV/AIDS, prostate and testicular cancer across the cultures and ways to reduce one's risks.
3. Interview a client for an accurate nursing history of the male genitalia, anus, rectum, and prostate.
4. Perform a physical assessment of male genitalia, anus, rectum, and prostate using the correct techniques.
5. Differentiate between normal and abnormal findings of male genitalia, anus, rectum, and prostate.
6. Explain the correct method for teaching a client how to perform testicular self-examination.
7. Describe the findings frequently seen with assessing the older male client's genitalia, anus, rectum, and prostate.
8. Analyze the data from the interview and physical assessment of the male genitalia, anus, rectum, and prostate to formulate valid nursing diagnoses, collaborative problems, and/or referrals.
9. Differentiate between general routine screening versus skills needed for focused or specialty assessment of the male genitalia, anus, rectum, and prostate.
10. Document and verbally report accurate assessment findings of the male genitalia, anus, rectum, and prostate.

CASE STUDY

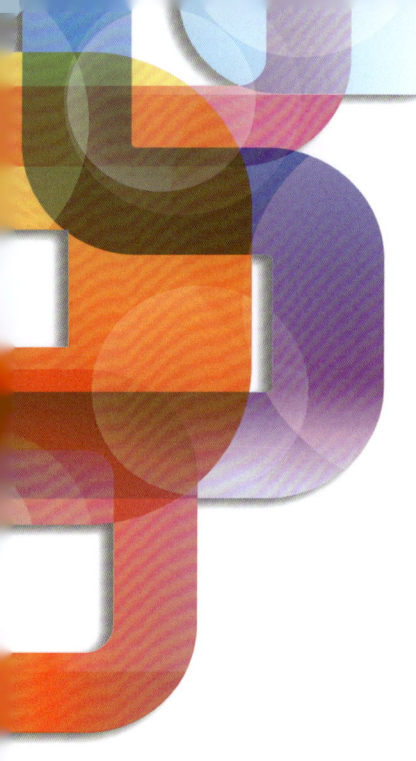

Carl Weeks is a 52-year-old African American man who has been receiving diabetes education from the occupational health nurse at work since his diagnosis of diabetes. His diabetic status is currently stable but he complains today of fever, chills, and malaise. He states that he has to urinate frequently and when he goes, it burns and is painful. He states that he is "peeing often in little dribbles." He also complains that it hurts when he defecates or tries to have sexual intercourse with his wife.

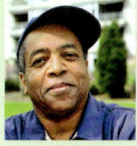

STRUCTURE AND FUNCTION

To assess the external and internal male genitalia, anus, rectum, and prostate, a basic understanding of the normal structures and functions of these areas is necessary. This understanding helps to guide the physical examination and readily assists the examiner in identifying abnormalities. In addition to an understanding of the genitalia, anus, rectum, and prostate, the nurse needs to be familiar with the inguinal (or groin) structures because hernias are common in this area.

External Genitalia

The external genitalia consist of the penis and the scrotum (Fig. 26-1).

Penis

The penis is the male reproductive organ. Attached to the pubic arch by ligaments, the penis is freely movable. The shaft of the penis is composed of three cylindrical masses of vascular erectile tissue that are bound together by fibrous tissue—two corpora cavernosa on the dorsal side and the corpus spongiosum on the ventral side. The corpus spongiosum extends distally to form the acorn-shaped glans. The base of the glans, or corona, is somewhat larger as compared with the shaft of the penis. If the man has not been circumcised, a hood-like fold of skin called the foreskin or prepuce covers the glans. In the center of the corpus spongiosum is the urethra, which travels through the shaft and opens as a slit at the tip of the glans as the urethral meatus. A fold of foreskin that extends ventrally from the urethral meatus is called the frenulum. The penis has a role in both reproduction and urination.

605

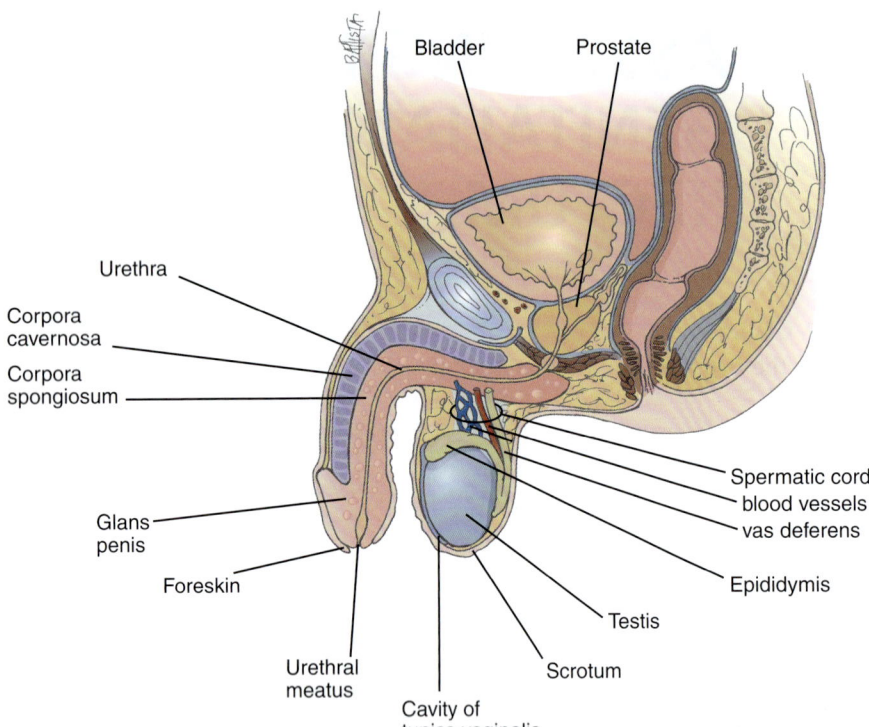

FIGURE 26-1 External and internal male genitalia.

Scrotum

The scrotum is a thin-walled sac that is suspended below the pubic bone, posterior to the penis. This darkly pigmented structure contains sweat and sebaceous glands and consists of folds of skin (rugae) and the cremaster muscle. The scrotum functions as a protective covering for the testes, epididymis, and vas deferens and helps to maintain the cooler-than-body temperature necessary for production of sperm (less than 37°C). The scrotum can maintain temperature control because the cremaster muscle is sensitive to changes in temperature. The muscle contracts when too cold, raising the scrotum and testes upward toward the body for warmth (cremasteric reflex). This accounts for the wrinkled appearance of the scrotal skin. When the temperature is warm, the muscle relaxes, lowering the scrotum and testes away from the heat of the body. When the cremaster muscle relaxes, the scrotal skin appears smooth.

Internal Genitalia

Testes

Internally the scrotal sac is divided into two portions by a septum, each portion containing one testis (testicle; see Fig. 26-1). The testes are a pair of ovoid-shaped organs, similar to the ovaries in the woman, that are approximately 3.7 to 5 cm long, 2.5 cm wide, and 2.5 cm deep. Each testis is covered by a serous membrane called the tunica vaginalis, which separates the testis from the scrotal wall. The tunica vaginalis is double layered and lubricated to protect the testes from injury. The function of the testes is to produce spermatozoa and the male sex hormone testosterone.

Spermatic Cord

The testes are suspended in the scrotum by a spermatic cord. The spermatic cord contains blood vessels, lymphatic vessels, nerves, and the vas deferens (or ductus deferens), which transports spermatozoa away from the testis. The spermatic cord on the left side is usually longer; thus the left testis hangs lower than the right testis.

The epididymis is a comma-shaped, coiled, tubular structure that curves up over the upper and posterior surface of the testis. It is within the epididymis that the spermatozoa mature.

> **CLINICAL TIP**
> While the epididymis is usually located over the posterior surface of the testes, it is located anteriorly in about 6% to 7% of the male population.

The vas deferens is a firm, muscular tube that is continuous with the lower portion of the epididymis (see Fig. 26-1). It travels up within the spermatic cord through the inguinal canal into the abdominal cavity. At this point, it separates from the spermatic cord and curves behind the bladder. It joins with the duct of the seminal vesicle (this will be further discussed in the section on structure and function of the prostate) and forms the ejaculatory duct. Finally, the ejaculatory duct empties into the urethra within the prostate gland.

The vas deferens provides the passage for transporting sperm from the testes to the urethra for ejaculation. Along the way, secretions from the vas deferens, seminal vesicles, prostate gland, and Cowper's (or bulbourethral) glands mix with the sperm and form semen.

Inguinal Area

When assessing the male genitalia, the nurse needs to be familiar with structures of the inguinal or groin area because hernias (protrusion of loops of bowel through weak areas of the musculature) are common in this location (Fig. 26-2).

26 Assessing Male Genitalia and Rectum   607

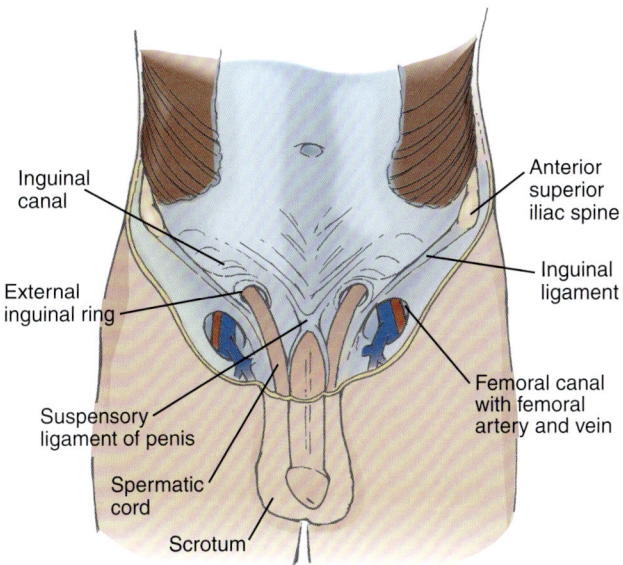

FIGURE 26-2 Inguinal area.

The inguinal area is contained between the anterior superior iliac spine laterally and the symphysis pubis medially.

Running diagonally between these two landmarks, just above and parallel with the inguinal ligament, is the inguinal canal. The inguinal canal is a tube-like structure (4 to 5 cm or 1.5 to 2 in long in an adult) through which the vas deferens travels as it passes through the lower abdomen.

The external inguinal ring is the exterior opening of the inguinal canal, which can be palpated above and lateral to the symphysis pubis. It feels triangular and slit-like. The internal inguinal ring is the internal opening of the inguinal canal. It is located 1 to 2 cm above the midpoint of the inguinal ligament and cannot be palpated. The femoral canal is another potential spot for a hernia. The femoral canal is located posterior to the inguinal canal and medial to and running parallel with the femoral artery and vein.

Anus and Rectum

The *anal canal* is the final segment of the digestive system. It begins at the anal sphincter and ends at the anorectal junction (also known as the pectinate line, mucocutaneous junction, or dentate line). It measures from 2.5 to 4 cm long. It is lined with skin that contains no hair or sebaceous glands but does contain many somatic sensory nerves, making it susceptible to painful stimuli. The *anal opening* (or anal verge) can be distinguished from the perianal skin by its hairless, moist appearance. The anal verge extends interiorly, overlying the external anal sphincter.

Within the anus are the two sphincters that normally hold the anal canal closed except when passing gas and feces. The *external sphincter* is composed of skeletal muscle and is under voluntary control. The *internal sphincter* is composed of smooth muscle and is under involuntary control by the autonomic nervous system. Dividing the two sphincters is the palpable intersphincteric groove. The anal canal proceeds upward toward the umbilicus. Just above the internal sphincter is the *anorectal junction*, the dividing point of the anal canal and the rectum. The rectum is lined with folds of mucosa, known as the columns of Morgagni. The anorectal junction is not palpable, but may be visualized during internal examination. The folds contain a network of arteries, veins, and visceral nerves. Between the columns are recessed areas known as anal crypts; there are 8 to 12 anal crypts and 5 to 8 papillae. If the veins in these folds undergo chronic pressure, they may become engorged with blood, forming hemorrhoids (Fig. 26-3).

The *rectum* is the lowest portion of the large intestine and is approximately 12 cm long, extending from the end of the *sigmoid colon* to the anorectal junction. It enlarges above the anorectal junction and proceeds in a posterior direction toward the hollow of the sacrum and coccyx, forming the rectal

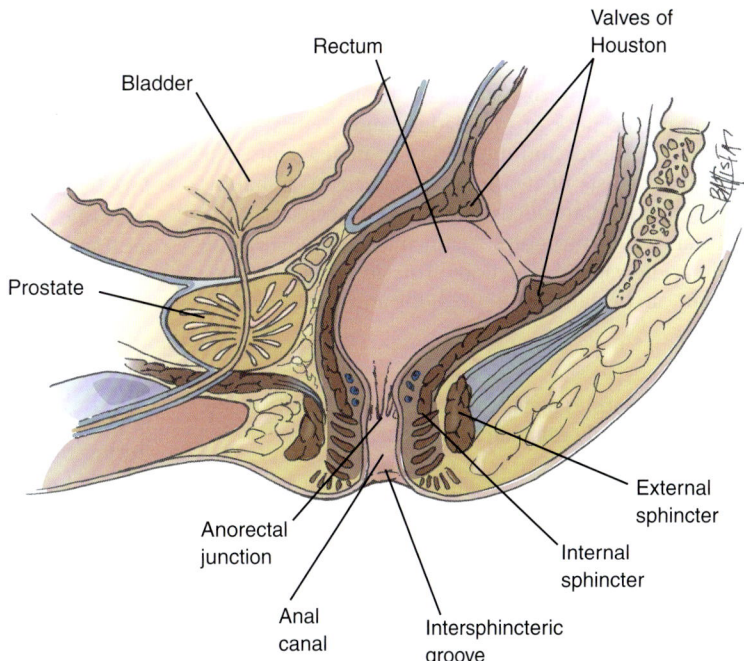

FIGURE 26-3 Anal and rectal structures.

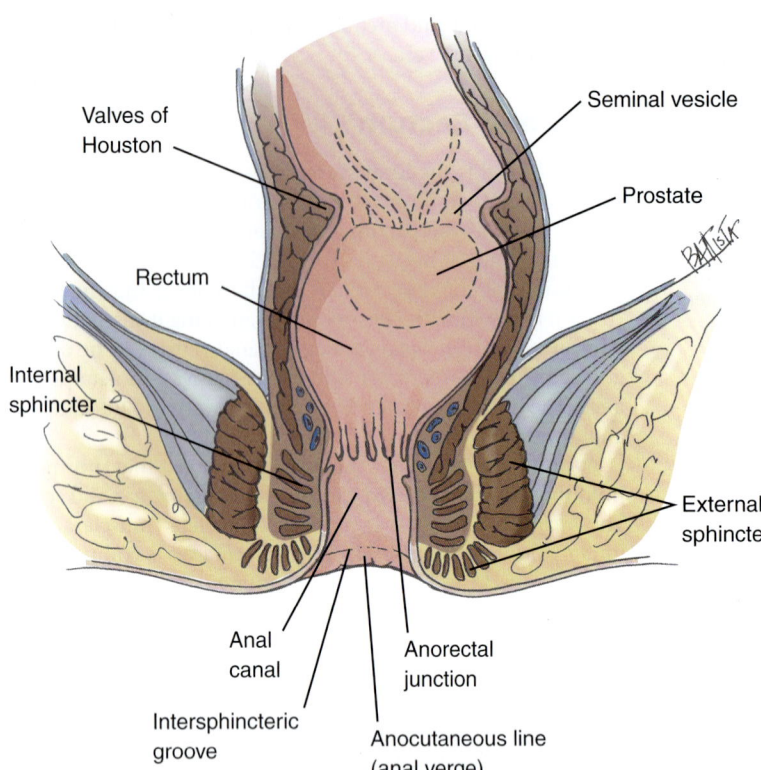

FIGURE 26-4 Prostate gland and nearby structures.

ampulla. The anal canal and rectum are at approximately right angles to each other. The inside of the rectum contains three inward foldings called the valves of Houston. The function of the valves of Houston is unclear. The lowest valve may be felt, usually on the client's left side.

The *peritoneum* lines the upper two thirds of the anterior rectum and dips down enough so that it may be palpated where it forms the *rectovesical pouch* in men and the *rectouterine pouch* in women.

Prostate

The *prostate gland* is approximately 2.5 to 4 cm in diameter, surrounding the neck of the bladder and urethra; it lies between these structures and the rectum in male clients. The prostate gland consists of two lobes separated by a shallow groove called the median sulcus (Fig. 26-4). It secretes a thin, milky substance that promotes sperm motility and neutralizes female acidic vaginal secretions. This chestnut- or heart-shaped organ can be palpated through the anterior wall of the rectum.

CLINICAL TIP
Prostatic hyperplasia, enlargement of the prostate gland, has become increasingly common in men over age 40.

Located on either side of and above the prostate gland are the *seminal vesicles*. These are rabbit-ear–shaped structures that produce the ejaculate that nourishes and protects sperm. They are not normally palpable. The *Cowper's (or bulbourethral) glands* are mucus-producing, pea-sized organs located posterior to the prostate gland. These glands surround and empty into the urethra. They are not normally palpable either.

HEALTH ASSESSMENT

Collecting Subjective Data: The Nursing Health History

When interviewing the male client for information regarding his genitalia, anus, rectum, and prostate, keep in mind that this may be a very sensitive topic and can prove to be embarrassing for both the client and the examiner. Moreover, the examiner should be aware of his or her own feelings regarding body image, fear of cancer, and sexuality. Western culture emphasizes the importance of the male sex role function. Self-esteem and body image are entwined with the male sex role. Anxiety, embarrassment, and fear may influence the client's ability to discuss problems and ask questions. Therefore, it is important to ease the client's anxiety as much as possible. Ask the questions in a straightforward manner, and let the client voice any concerns throughout the assessment. In some cultural groups, only nurses of the same gender will be considered acceptable assessors of intimate body areas.

A trusting relationship is key to a successful interview. Keep in mind that serious or life-threatening problems may be present. Testicular cancer, for example, carries a high mortality rate, especially if not detected early. The information gathered during this portion of the health history interview provides a basis for teaching about important health screening issues such as testicular self-examination. It also is a good time to teach the client about risk factors related to diseases, such as HIV, colorectal or prostate cancer, and about ways to decrease those risk factors. Additionally, explore in some depth with a symptom analysis any symptoms that the client reports or hints about.

History of Present Health Concern

QUESTION	RATIONALE
Pain	
Do you have pain in your penis, scrotum, testes, or groin?	Complaints of pain in these areas may indicate a hernia or an inflammatory process, such as epididymitis. Other etiologies may include pyronies, herpes, prostitis, other STIs, muscle strain, testicular torsion, varicocele, UTI, diabetic neuropathy, orchitis, hydrocele, or malignancy.
Itching	
Do you have any itching in your pubic hair area?	Perineal itching is seen with crab lice (*Pediculosis pubis*)
Lesions	
Have you noticed any lesions on your penis or genital area? If so, do the lesions itch, burn, or sting? Please describe the lesions.	Lesions may be a sign of a sexually transmitted infection (STI) or cancer.
Discharge	
Have you noticed any discharge from your penis? If so, how much? What color is it? What type of odor does it have?	Discharge may indicate an infection.
Lumps, Swelling, Masses	
Do you have any lumps, swelling, or masses in your scrotum, genital, or groin area? Have you noticed a change in the size of the scrotum?	Lumps, swelling, or masses found in the scrotum, genital, or groin area may indicate infection, hernia, or cancer. Enlargement of the scrotum may indicate hydrocele, hematocele, hernia, or cancer. **OLDER ADULT CONSIDERATIONS** The scrotum also enlarges with aging.
Do you have a heavy, dragging feeling in your scrotum?	A testicular tumor or scrotal hernia may cause a feeling of heaviness in the scrotum.
Urination	
Do you experience difficulty urinating (i.e., urgency, hesitancy, frequency, or difficulty starting or maintaining a stream)? How many times do you urinate during the night?	Difficulty urinating may indicate an infection or blockage, including prostatic enlargement.
Have you started taking any new medications?	Urinating more than one time during the night may indicate prostate abnormalities. Excessive intake of fluids and some medications, such as diuretics, may also cause nocturia.
Have you noticed any change in the color, odor, or amount of your urine?	Changes in urine color or odor may indicate an infection. Blood in the urine (hematuria) should be referred for medical investigation because this may indicate infection, kidney stones, benign prostatic hypertrophy (BPH), or cancer. A decrease in amount of voided urine may indicate prostate enlargement or kidney problems.
Do you experience any pain or burning when you urinate?	Painful urination may be a sign of urinary tract infection (UTI), prostatitis, or an STI.
Do you ever experience urinary incontinence or dribbling?	Incontinence may occur after prostatectomy. Dribbling may be a sign of overflow incontinence. Other causes of incontinence after prostatectomy are related to age, enlarged prostate or prior benign prostate surgery, diabetes or neurologic diseases, smoking, excessive blood loss during surgery, size or stage of prostate tumor, or radiation after surgery (Jaffe, 2014).
Sexual Dysfunction	
Have you recently had a change in your pattern of sexual activity or sexual desire?	A change in sexual activity or sexual desire (libido) needs to be investigated to determine the cause.

Continued on following page

History of Present Health Concern (Continued)

QUESTION	RATIONALE
Do you have difficulty attaining or maintaining an erection? Do you have any problem with ejaculation? Do you have pain with ejaculation?	Erectile dysfunction (ED) occurs frequently in adult males and may be attributed to various factors or disorders (e.g., alcohol use, diabetes, depression, antihypertensive medications). Pain with ejaculation may indicate epididymitis **OLDER ADULT CONSIDERATIONS** ED increases in frequency with age.
Do you have or have you had any trouble with fertility?	A male factor is solely responsible in about 20% of infertile couples and contributory in another 30% to 40% (University of Wisconsin School of Medicine and Public Health, 2012).

Bowel Patterns

What is your usual bowel pattern? Have you noticed any recent change in the pattern? Any pain while passing a bowel movement?	A change in bowel pattern is associated with many disorders and is one of the warning signs of cancer. A more thorough evaluation, including laboratory tests and colonoscopy, may be necessary.
Do you experience constipation?	Constipation may indicate a bowel obstruction, irritable bowel syndrome (IBS) or colon cancer, or the need for dietary counseling.
Do you experience diarrhea? Is the diarrhea associated with any nausea or vomiting?	Diarrhea may signal impaction, gastroenteritis, medication side effect, IBS, IBD, colitis, or indicate the need for dietary counseling.
Do you have trouble controlling your bowels?	Fecal incontinence occurs with neurologic disorders and some gastrointestinal infections.

Stool

What is the color of your stool? Hard or soft? Have you noticed any blood on or in your stool? If so, how much?	Black stools may indicate gastrointestinal bleeding or the use of iron supplements or Pepto-Bismol. Red blood in the stool is found with hemorrhoids, polyps, cancer, or colitis. Clay-colored stools result from a lack of bile pigment.
Have you noticed any mucus in your stool? Have you noticed that your stools are oily, greasy, or bulky, or that they float?	Large amounts of mucus that occur on a regular basis, associated with diarrhea, may be caused by some intestinal infections. Bloody mucus in stool, or mucus with abdominal pain, may be seen in Crohn disease, ulcerative colitis, and even cancer. Steatorrhea (fats in the stool) causes stools that appear oily or greasy and are bulky and float, as a result of impaired digestion and/or absorption of fats. Steatorrhea may be seen in pancreatitis (acute or chronic), pancreatic cancer, pancreatic enzyme deficiency (exocrine insufficiency), gallstones, particularly bile duct stones, sclerosing cholangitis, and Zollinger–Ellison syndrome.

Itching and Pain

Do you experience any itching or pain in the rectal area?	STIs, hemorrhoids, pinworms, or anal trauma may cause itching or pain.

Past Health History

QUESTION	RATIONALE
Describe any prior medical problems you have had, how they were treated, and the results.	Prior problems directly affect the physical assessment findings. For example, if cancer was present in the past, it may recur. Diabetes and some antihypertensive medications may cause impotence.
When was the last time you had a testicular examination by your primary health care provider? What was the result?	Most physicians agree that an examination of a man's testicles should be part of the general physical examination. The American Cancer Society (ACS) recommends a testicular exam as part of a routine cancer-related check-up.
Have you ever been tested for human immunodeficiency virus (HIV), human papilloma virus	In 2015, the CDC reported that three reportable STIs (chlamydia, gonorrhea, and syphilis) have increased in the United States for the first time since 2006 (CDC, 2015a). About 20 million new cases of these STIs occur each year in the United States, half of these among young people (HPV),

QUESTION	RATIONALE
herpes simplex virus (HSV), chlamydia, gonorrhea, and/or trichomoniasis, hepatitis, and syphilis? What were the results? Why were you tested?	(CDC, 2016b). A variety of other STIs are also prevalent, such as hepatitis B virus (HBV), herpes simplex virus type 2 (HSV-2), HIV, HPV, and trichomoniasis. See Evidence-Based Health Promotion and Disease Prevention 26-1.
Have you ever had anal or rectal trauma or surgery? Were you born with any congenital deformities of the anus or rectum? Have you had prostate surgery? Have you had hemorrhoids or surgery for hemorrhoids?	Past conditions influence the findings of physical assessment. Congenital deformities, such as imperforate anus, are often surgically repaired when the client is very young.
When was the last time you had a stool test to detect blood?	The ACS recommends a stool test every year after age 50 to detect occult blood (ACS, 2016a). Additional tests recommended are a yearly fecal immunochemical test (FIT), and a stool DNA test every 5 years.
Have you ever had a sigmoidoscopy? Colonoscopy?	A flexible sigmoidoscopy examination is recommended every 5 years after the age of 50 and a colonoscopy every 10 years. Any test with positive findings should be followed by a colonoscopy (ACS, 2016a). A controversy exists between the recommendations from the U.S. scientific community, about colonoscopy being the gold standard of colon cancer screening, and those of the Canadian Task Force on Preventive Health Care (Canada's equivalent of the USPSTF). See the discussion in Cassels (2016).
When was the last time you had a digital rectal examination (DRE)? What was the result?	The DRE may also be done as a part of screening for prostate cancer. It is less effective than the PSA blood test to detect prostate cancer, but may find cancers in men with normal PSA levels. Thus it should be included as a part of prostate cancer screening (ACS, 2015a). See Evidence-Based Health Promotion and Disease Prevention 26-2.
Have you ever had blood taken for a prostate screening, which measures the level of prostate-specific antigen (PSA) in your blood? When was the test performed and what was the result?	Men age 50 or more should talk to a health care provider about the pros and cons of PSA testing so that they can make an informed decision regarding testing. African American men or men who have a father or brother who had prostate cancer before age 65 should have this discussion beginning at age 45. Men at higher risk (first degree relative with prostate cancer at an early age) should begin testing at 40 years of age. If a man decides to be tested, he should have a PSA blood test with or without a rectal examination. Repeat testing is dependent on the PSA level (ACS, 2015a).

Family History

QUESTION	RATIONALE
Is there a history of polyps or colon, rectal, or prostate cancer in your family?	Colorectal cancer risk is increased by a family history of colorectal cancer and/or polyps. Genetic studies also suggest that a strong family history may be responsible for 5% to 10% of prostate cancers (ACS, 2016b).

Lifestyle and Health Practices

QUESTION	RATIONALE
How many sexual partners do you have?	A client with multiple sexual partners increases his risk of contracting an STI or HIV (see Evidence-Based Health Promotion and Disease Prevention 26-1).
What kind of birth control method do you use, if any?	Currently, men have five birth control options, which include: abstinence, condoms, outercourse, vasectomy, and withdrawal. Practicing fertility awareness–based methods may also prevent pregnancy. Using a condom reduces the risk of STIs (CDC, 2013). Scientific work is being done to develop effective and easy to use male contraceptives (Tarico, 2013).
Are you satisfied with your current level of physical and sexual activity and sexual functioning?	Pain or heaviness due to hernias may limit the ability to work or perform regular exercise. Infection may limit a client's ability to engage in sexual activity. ED impedes sexual intercourse. Incontinence may affect the client's ability to work or engage in social activities.

Continued on following page

Lifestyle and Health Practices (Continued)

QUESTION	RATIONALE
Do you have concerns about fertility? If you experience fertility troubles, how has this affected your relationship?	Concerns about fertility can increase stress and can have a negative impact on relationships.
Do you have an intimate partner or someone you consider to be a significant other? Are you comfortable with expression of your sexuality? Are you satisfied with your sexual relationship? If no, would you like to explain further?	These questions communicate the importance of sexual relationships and give the client permission to discuss the topic. Further data may be obtained from these questions, which assist the nurse in focusing on additional questions and referring the client to a health care practitioner as needed.
Do you have any fears related to sex? Can you identify any stress in your current relationship that relates to sex?	Fear can cause inhibition and decrease sexual satisfaction. Stress can prevent satisfactory sexual performance.
Do you feel comfortable communicating with your partner about your sexual likes and dislikes?	Lack of open communication can cause problems with relationships and lead to feelings of guilt and depression.
What do you know about STIs and their prevention?	The client's knowledge of STIs and their prevention provides a basis for health education in this area.
Are you currently exposed to chemicals or radiation? Have you been exposed in the past?	Exposure to radiation and certain chemicals increases the risk of developing cancer.
Describe the activity you perform in a typical day. Do you do any heavy lifting?	Strenuous activity and heavy lifting may predispose the client to development of an inguinal hernia.
Do you perform testicular self-examinations? When was the last time you performed this examination?	Male clients who do not perform testicular self-examinations need to be informed about the connection between self-examination and early interventions for abnormalities (Testicular Cancer Foundation, 2017). Male clients should be aware of the need for a monthly testicular self-examination and its importance in the early diagnosis and treatment of testicular cancer (Box 26-1).
Do you use any laxatives, stool softeners, enemas, or other bowel movement–enhancing medications?	Frequent use of certain laxatives over a period of weeks or months can decrease the colon's natural ability to contract and actually worsen constipation (GI Society, 2015).
Do you engage in anal sex?	It is possible for either sex partner to become infected with HIV during anal sex. HIV can be found in the blood, semen, preseminal fluid, or vaginal fluid of a person infected with the virus (see Evidence-Based Health Promotion and Disease Prevention 26-1). In general, the person receiving the semen is at greater risk of getting HIV because the lining of the rectum is thin and may allow the virus to enter the body during anal sex. However, a person who inserts his penis into an infected partner also is at risk because HIV can enter through the urethra (the opening at the tip of the penis) or through small cuts, abrasions, or open sores on the penis (CDC, 2015c). Anal sex may also cause fissures, rectal prolapse, and hemorrhoid formation.
Do you take any medications for your prostate?	Men with benign prostatic hypertrophy (BPH) with "voiding symptoms," such as urinary urgency, may take an alpha-adrenergic blocker such as terazosin (Hytrin), 5-alpha reductase inhibitors such as dutasteride (Avodart) or finasteride (Proscar) that may reduce the size of the prostate, or a combination of both types of medication. Phosphodiesterase-5 (PDE-5) inhibitors (used for erection problems) such as tadalafil (Cialis) may help reduce BPH symptoms whether or not the client has erection problems (Urology Care Foundation, 2017).
How much high-fiber food and roughage do you consume every day? Do you eat foods high in saturated fat?	Fiber adds bulk to the digestive system and shortens the time that wastes, which often contain carcinogens, travel through the colon, thus decreasing the chance for intestinal cells to be affected (Zeng et al., 2014). High-fat diets have been implicated in colon cancer and in prostate cancer. High-fat diets can produce more intestinal stem cells, or cause other cells to behave like stem cells, which may give rise to intestinal tumors (Beyaz et al., 2016).

QUESTION	RATIONALE
Do you engage in regular exercise?	The links between diet, weight, and exercise and colorectal cancer are some of the strongest for any type of cancer. If you are not physically active, you have a greater chance of developing colorectal cancer. Increasing physical activity may reduce your risk (ACS, 2016b). See Evidence-Based Health Promotion and Disease Prevention 27-3: Colorectal Cancer.
Have any anal or rectal problems affected your normal activities of daily living (working or engaging in recreation)?	Some problems, such as hemorrhoids or bowel incontinence, may affect a client's ability to work or interact socially.

26-1 EVIDENCE-BASED HEALTH PROMOTION AND DISEASE PREVENTION: HIV/AIDS

INTRODUCTION

The 2014 UNAIDS reported in a press release of July16 that there were 35 million people living with HIV worldwide, and of those, 19 million were unaware of their having the virus. Of those who found out they were HIV positive, 90% went for antiretroviral treatment (ART). In sub-Saharan Africa, 76% of people on ART achieved viral suppression, whereby they are unlikely to transmit the virus to their sexual partners; and for every 10% increase in treatment coverage there was a 1% decline in the percentage of new infections among people living with HIV.

The CDC (2015a) reported that at the end of 2012 (the last year for data) 1.2 million people in the United States were living with HIV, and of those, 12.8% were unaware that they were infected. The distribution of new infections varied by ethnicity: African Americans (44%), Whites (31%); Hispanic/Latinos 21%. HIV infection varied by transmission as well: Men having sex with men (MSM, 63%); heterosexual contact (23%); injection drug use 8%; and MSM and intravenous drug use combined (3%). MSM are only 2% of the population but account for the 65% of the HIV infections. HIV infection varies by age as well: ages 13 to 24 constitute 16% of population, but 26% of HIV infections; but 72% of those are MSM between the ages of 13 and 24.

The CDC (2015b) reports that in the United States, persons 50 and older accounted for 21% of those infected with HIV (especially those aged 50 to 54). Nurses are often reluctant to discuss sexually related behaviors with older adults, but it is a necessary professional role.

HEALTHY PEOPLE 2020 GOAL

Overview

AIDS is a disease caused by the human immunodeficiency virus (HIV). The HIV virus is transmitted from person to person in a variety of ways: via exchange of body fluids, usually through sexual transmission, but also through contact with infected blood (e.g., blood transfusions, infected needles); by mother to child during pregnancy, childbirth, or breastfeeding; by intravenous drug users; and by other mechanisms of body fluid transfer. The highest incidence of HIV in the United States still occurs in MSM, followed by intravenous drug users.

HIV damages the immune system by destroying CD4 white blood cells (helper T cells) and prevents the body from defending itself against other organisms, allowing development of opportunistic infections such as tuberculosis, cancer, and pneumonia (National Institutes of Health [NIH], 2017). The time from infection with HIV to development of AIDS (acquired immunodeficiency disease syndrome) may be years. At present, there is no cure for AIDS, but medications help to suppress the virus in most people who have access to these very expensive treatments. Although the incidence of AIDS has been reduced by use of this medication in some nations, the organization AVERT (Averting HIV and AIDS) (2015) noted that the populations of many countries in Africa, Asia, and the country of Haiti in the Americas are still being decimated by the disease.

Primary or acute HIV infection may last a few weeks and have symptoms (noticeable or mild, even unnoticed) of fever, muscle aches and joint pain, rash, headache, sore throat, swollen lymph glands (mainly on the neck, and a first sign of infection), diarrhea, weight loss, oral yeast infection (thrush), and/or shingles (herpes zoster). With chronic HIV infection, no further symptoms other than those revealed through blood work are noted. Without treatment, HIV will progress to AIDS in about 10 years, and the immune system is severely damaged, allowing opportunistic infections. Once HIV infection progresses to AIDS, in about 10 years, additional symptoms are: soaking night sweats; recurring fevers; chronic diarrhea; persistent white spots or unusual lesions on tongue or in mouth; persistent unexplained fatigue; weight loss; and skin rashes or bumps (Mayo Clinic, 2015a). These symptoms may be indicative of a number of illnesses. During this phase, the viral load is particularly high, which accounts for the ease of transmission during this early stage. Swollen lymph nodes may persist and over time other symptoms may appear, such as fatigue, weight loss, and shortness of breath.

Definitive diagnosis that HIV infection has progressed to AIDS is confirmed by a CD4 count under 200 cells/mm^3 (AIDS.gov, 2015). Opportunistic infections (OIs) are signs of a declining immune system. Most life-threatening OIs occur when the *CD4 count* is below 200 cells/mm^3. OIs are the most common cause of death for people with HIV/AIDS. A CD4 of between 500 and 200 cells/mm^3 tends to allow for *Candida albicans* (thrush) and Kaposi sarcoma. A CD4 between 200 and 100 cells/mm^3 tends to allow for *Pneumocystis jirovecii* pneumonia, histoplasmosis, coccidioidomycosis, and progressive multifocal leukoencephalopathy (PML). A CD4 count below 100 cells/mm^3 allows for toxoplasmosis, cryptosporidiosis, cytomegalovirus, and other infections. AIDS.gov (2013) noted that tuberculosis is the leading cause of death for people living with HIV worldwide.

It is important to note that HIV is a preventable disease. Effective HIV prevention interventions have been proven to reduce HIV transmission. People who get tested for HIV and learn that they are infected can make significant behavior changes to improve their health and reduce the risk of transmitting HIV to their sex or drug-using partners.

Goal

Prevent HIV infection and its related illness and death.

Continued on following page

26-1 EVIDENCE-BASED HEALTH PROMOTION AND DISEASE PREVENTION: HIV/AIDS (Continued)

Objectives
Healthy People 2020 (2014) has 23 objectives for HIV. These objectives relate to the 2010 White House AIDS Strategy goals:
1. Reducing the number of people who become infected with HIV.
2. Increasing access to care and improving health outcomes for people living with HIV.
3. Reducing HIV-related health disparities.

The specific objectives and associated recommendations for the 23 HIV objectives are too cumbersome to include here. Please access the Healthy People 2020 website for these details. The objectives demonstrate an aggressive effort to increase the use of resources and reduce the acquisition of HIV and AIDS.

Other Organization Targets
AVERT (2015) provides a review of targets set by various organizations. For example, the most aggressive is the UN Fast Track strategy, launched in 2014, that aims to greatly step up the HIV response in low- and middle-income countries to end the epidemic by 2030.

SCREENING
The U.S. Preventive Services Task Force (USPSTF, 2015a) strongly recommends that clinicians screen for HIV in all adolescents and adults aged 15 to 65, and for younger adolescents or older adults at increased risk for HIV infection. The USPSTF recommends that clinicians screen all pregnant women for HIV, including those who present in labor who are untested and whose HIV status is unknown.

RISK ASSESSMENT
Because HIV is preventable, knowing risks and practicing risk-reducing behaviors will help to stem the epidemic of this infection.
Risks include:
- Unprotected sex (especially male-on-male anal intercourse)
- Presence of another STI
- Use of intravenous drugs, especially sharing needles
- Being an uncircumcised male
- Being the fetus of an HIV-positive mother
- Mother–infant transmission during pregnancy or delivery
- Exchange of blood or body fluids through blood transfusions, needle sticks, breast-feeding by HIV-infected mother, body piercing with nonsterilized instruments

CLIENT EDUCATION
Teach Clients
Use precautions to decrease transfer of body fluids:
- Avoid unprotected sex (use a new condom every time you have sex) or practice sexual abstinence (CDC, 2013)
- Avoid having multiple sex partners.
- Avoid anal sex.
- Avoid intravenous drug use.
- Avoid mixing sex and alcohol or drugs.
- If you take medications requiring needle use, use a new, sterile needle each time.
- Consider circumcision, if uncircumcised and lifestyle is risky.
- Follow guidelines for handling body secretions, objects that touch bodily secretions, or contaminated items.
- Openly discuss HIV risk behavior history with partner and use above precautions.

If you already have HIV/AIDS:
- Eat healthy, well-rounded diet.
- Avoid food and drink that may easily transmit foodborne illness (e.g., raw eggs, unpasteurized dairy products, raw seafood, undercooked meat (cook well done).
- Get immunizations against other illnesses if allowed by physician.
- Be aware that companion animals may harbor parasites that can cause infections.
- Tell your sex partner right away if you are HIV positive.
- If pregnant, seek medical care right away.
- Seek support from support group to deal with your emotions.
- Obtain and stay on antiretroviral protocol, if available.

26-2 EVIDENCE-BASED HEALTH PROMOTION AND DISEASE PREVENTION: PROSTATE CANCER

INTRODUCTION
According to the Centers for Disease Control and Prevention (2016), prostate cancer is the second most common cancer (after nonmelanoma skin cancer) and one of the leading causes of cancer death in men in the United States (lung cancer is first). The incidence and mortality trends of prostate cancer in the United States declined between 2002 and 2011. Prostate cancer is slow-growing and can be readily treated if found early. There is no sure way to prevent prostate cancer, but diet and lifestyle behaviors are thought to help with prevention. A common problem in almost all men as they grow older is an enlarged prostate (benign prostatic hyperplasia, or BPH). Some symptoms of BPH and prostate cancer are the same. Having BPH does not raise your risk of prostate cancer.

HEALTHY PEOPLE 2020 GOAL
Overview
Healthy People 2020 (2016) addresses the topic of prostate cancer as one of the many cancers but includes a goal and an objective specific to prostate cancer.

Goal
Reduce the number of new cancer cases, as well as the illness, disability, and death caused by cancer. Reduce the death rate from cancer of the prostate.

Objectives
- Reduce the rate of prostate cancer deaths from 24.2 per 100,000 males in 2007 to 21.8 per 100,000.

SCREENING
U.S. Preventive Services Task Force Recommendation Statement (USPSTF, 2015b) has concluded that the benefits do not outweigh the risks when routine screening is done for prostate cancer. Therefore, currently the USPSTF recommends against routine screening with a prostate-specific antigen (PSA) test for men in the United States.

The National Cancer Institute (2015) notes that the PSA test to detect prostate cancer is nonspecific, as the PSA level may be elevated in benign prostate hypertrophy or with infection or inflammation of the prostate. If a prostate biopsy is done and is negative, then an additional test (this one of urine) may be done for the PCA3 gene for prostate cancer. The effectiveness of combining PSA level and digital rectal examination (DRE) is being studied.

The American Association of Family Physicians (AAFP, 2015) provides a comparison of several organizations' recommendations for prostate screening:

AAFP: Do not routinely screen for prostate cancer using a PSA test or DRE.
American College of Preventive Medicine: Do not routinely perform PSA-based screening for prostate cancer.
American Geriatric Society: Do not screen for prostate cancer (with the PSA test) without considering life expectancy and the risks of testing, overdiagnosis, and overtreatment.
American Society for Clinical Oncology: Do not perform PSA testing for prostate cancer in men with no symptoms of the disease when they are expected to live for less than 10 years.
American Urological Society: Offer PSA screening for prostate cancer only after engaging in shared decision making.

In summary, the PSA is available but is unreliable, and men between 50 and 70 years of age who are expected to live at least 10 years should have the risks and benefits of screening explained to them by their health care provider.

The Canadian Task Force on Preventive Health Care (2014) recommends not using the PSA test to screen for prostate cancer. Cancer Research UK (2014) reports that there is no prostate cancer screening program in the United Kingdom. This is due to the unreliability of the PSA and other screening methods.

RISK ASSESSMENT

According to ACS (2015b), risk factors for prostate cancer are:
- Age: rare in men under 40, rises rapidly after age 50
- Race/ethnicity: highest for African American or Caribbean males of African origin; occurs less often in Asian, Hispanic/Latino men than in whites
- Geography: most common in North America, northwestern Europe, Australia, and on Caribbean islands; less common in Asia, Africa, Central America, and South America.
- Family history: having a father or brother with prostate cancer
- Certain gene changes
- Exposure to agent orange
- Excessive alcohol consumption
- Working on a farm, in a tire plant, with paint, with cadmium or firefighters exposed to toxic chemicals.
- Diet: unclear, but slightly higher risk for those who eat a diet high in red meat or high fat daily, and fewer vegetables. High calcium intake may be a factor. *Note that prostate cancer is less common in people who do not eat meat (vegetarians).*
- Low melatonin levels (sleeping with even small light source; shift work) (Florida Atlantic University, n.d.)

Studies with unclear or ambivalent findings, or only slight risk suggested:
- Obesity has not been found to be a factor but obese men have a lower risk of getting the less dangerous form of the disease.
- Prostatitis
- STIs
- Vasectomy
- Smoking (more related to small increased risk of dying with prostate cancer vs. getting it)

CLIENT EDUCATION
Teach Clients
Behaviors found to lower risk of prostate cancer:
- Frequent ejaculation (Harvard Medical School, 2011)
- Eating a diet high in fruits and vegetables (at least 2½ cups of a variety of vegetables and fruits daily), staying physically active (exercise most days of the week), and maintaining a healthy weight (ACS, 2015b)
- Taking vitamin E and selenium (ambivalent study results)
- Possible preventive effect from medications for benign prostatic hypertrophy; aspirin (unclear results)
- Sleeping in a completely dark room
- Avoiding shift work that requires daytime sleep
- Drink green tea daily (Doheny, 2012).

Observe for the following symptoms (which may or may not be present, but are likely in more advanced stages) and report any you experience to a health care provider (Mayo Clinic, 2015b):
- Trouble urinating
- Decreased force in the stream of urine
- Blood in the semen
- Swelling in the legs
- Bone pain
- Erectile dysfunction

BOX 26-1   SELF-ASSESSMENT: TESTICULAR SELF-EXAMINATION

Testicular self-examination (TSE) should be performed once a month; it is neither difficult nor time consuming. A convenient time is often after a warm bath or shower when the scrotum is more relaxed.
1. Stand in front of a mirror and check for scrotal swelling.
2. Use both hands to palpate the testis; the normal testicle is smooth and uniform in consistency.
3. With the index and middle fingers under the testis and the thumb on top, roll the testis gently in a horizontal plane between the thumb and fingers (A).
4. Feel for any evidence of a small lump or abnormality.
5. Follow the same procedure and palpate upward along the testis (B).
6. Locate the epididymis (C), a cord-like structure on the top and back of the testicle that stores and transports sperm.
7. Repeat the examination for the other testis. It is normal to find that one testis is larger than the other.
8. If you find any evidence of a small, pea-like lump, consult your physician. It may be due to an infection or a tumor growth.

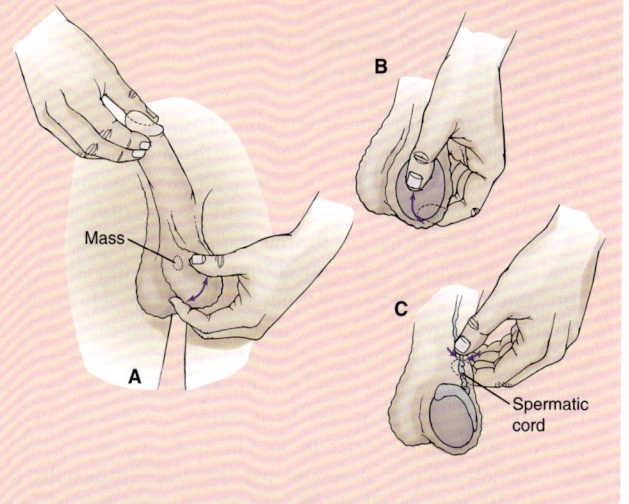

CASE STUDY

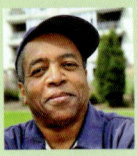

The case study of Carl Weeks that was introduced at the beginning of the chapter will now be used to demonstrate how a nurse would use the COLDSPA mnemonic to organize the client's presenting concerns and continue to interview the client for his health history.

Mnemonic	Question	Data Provided
Character	Describe the sign or symptom (feeling, appearance, sound, smell, or taste if applicable).	"I have burning and pain when I pee. I feel like I am peeing often but in little dribbles. It also hurts when I have a bowel movement or try to have sex with my wife."
Onset	When did it begin?	"Suddenly, started last night."
Location	Where is it? Does it radiate? Does it occur anywhere else?	"The pain seems to start in my lower back and goes all the way down to my bottom and around the front of my hips."
Duration	How long does it last? Does it recur?	"It has been constant since last night."
Severity	How bad is it? Or, How much does it bother you? How would you rate your pain on a scale of 0–10?	"I feel miserable— neither I nor my wife got any sleep last night because I was up every hour." Rates pain as a "9."
Pattern	What makes it better or worse?	"The more I drink, the more I am going to the bathroom. I took some Aleve and that seemed to help a little."
Associated factors/How it Affects the client	What other symptoms occur with it? How does it affect you?	"I have to strain to get my urine out and my stream is weak. I am tired because I couldn't sleep."

After investigating Mr. Weeks' complaint of recent painful urination and pain with defecation and sexual intercourse, the nurse continues with the health history.

Client states that since last night he has had pain with urination, also complains of hesitancy, a decreased stream, and painful ejaculation. Denies urethral discharge, urethral meatal itching, hematuria, or incontinence. Has been married for 30 years and has only had one sex partner during that time. Has never been diagnosed with an STI. Has had fever "off and on" for the last 24 hours. States that he has some pain with defecation. His normal bowel pattern is daily with formed, brown stool. Denies any recent history of blood or changes in his bowel. Denies any family history of genitalia or rectal cancer. Reports that he does not drink alcoholic beverages. Currently does not smoke cigarettes; has not smoked for 10 years. However, he did smoke 1 pack per day for 20 years. Had first colonoscopy at age 50; states results were normal. He is scheduled through his PCP to have yearly physical and labs drawn, and will have a PSA at that time.

Collecting Objective Data: Physical Examination

The purpose of examining the male genitalia is to detect abnormalities that may range from life-threatening diseases to painful conditions that interfere with normal function. Abnormalities should be detected as early as possible so that the client can be referred for further testing or treatment. The physical assessment is also a good time to allow the client to demonstrate the proper techniques for testicular self-examination and to provide teaching if necessary (see Box 26-1). A DRE may also be performed as part of the examination. This is important because some conditions, such as cancerous tumors, may be asymptomatic. Early detection of a problem is one way to promote early treatment and a more positive outcome. The examiner may also use this time (especially if the examination is a well examination) to integrate teaching about ways to reduce risk factors for diseases and disorders of the anus, rectum, and prostate.

The hands-on physical examination of the male genitalia, anus, rectum, and prostate may create anxiety, embarrassment, and nervousness about exposing these body parts and about what might be discovered. Ease client anxiety by explaining in detail what is going to occur. Throughout the examination, explain the significance of each portion of the examination; this encourages relaxation. Remember to preserve the client's modesty. It is also helpful to encourage the client to ask questions during the examination. If the examination is being performed as part of the comprehensive physical, perform it at the end of the genitalia examination. Make sure to always have a chaperone present in the room with you while performing the examination. The role of a chaperone is predominantly to comfort and protect the client, but he or she also serves a secondary role to protect doctors from false allegations (Wai et al., 2008).

26 Assessing Male Genitalia and Rectum   617

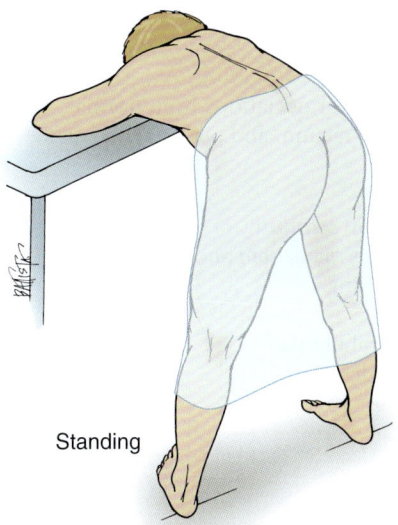
Standing

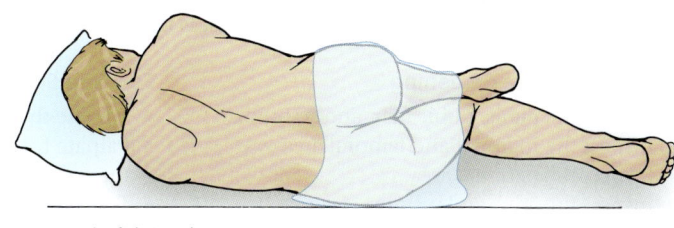
Left lateral

FIGURE 26-5 Selected positions for anorectal examination.

CLINICAL TIP
Examiners and the client are often worried that the male client will have an erection during the hands-on examination. Usually the client is too nervous for this to occur. If it does occur, reassure the client that it is not unusual and continue the examination in an unhurried and calm manner.

Preparing the Client
Before the examination, instruct the client to empty his bladder so that he will be comfortable. If a urine specimen is necessary, provide the client with a container. If the client is not wearing an examination gown for a total physical examination, provide a drape and ask him to lower his pants and underwear. Explain to the client that he will be asked to stand (if able) for most of the examination of the genitalia. The most frequently used position for inspection and palpation of the anus, rectum, and prostate is the left lateral position. This position allows adequate inspection and palpation of the anus, rectum, and prostate (in men) and is usually more comfortable for the client. The client's torso and legs can be draped during the examination, which helps to lessen the feeling of vulnerability. To help the client into this position, ask him to lie on the left side, with the buttocks as close to the edge of the examining table as possible, and to bend the right knee. However, some examiners find it easiest to perform the male anus, rectum, and prostate examination while the client stands and bends over the examining table with his hips flexed.

Whichever position the examiner decides would be best for the particular client and examination, it is important to determine if the client is as comfortable as possible in that position (Fig. 26-5). In addition, no matter which position is chosen, the examiner must realize that he or she will only be able to examine to a certain point up in the rectum using the finger. If an examination of the upper rectum and sigmoid colon is necessary, a sigmoidoscopy should be performed.

Equipment
- Stool
- Gown
- Disposable non-latex gloves
- Flashlight (for possible transillumination)
- Stethoscope (for possible auscultation)
- Water soluble lubricant
- Specimen card

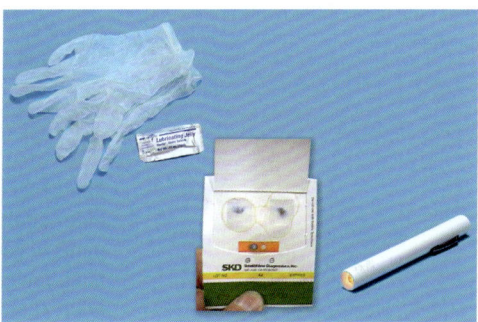

Physical Assessment
During the examination of the client, remember these key points:
- Wear disposable gloves.
- Prepare the client thoroughly for the physical examination to put the client at the greatest ease.
- Perform the examination professionally and preserve the client's modesty.
- Preserve client's privacy.
- Inspect and palpate penis, scrotum, and inguinal area for inflammation, infestations, rashes, lesions, and lumps.
- During the testicular examination, describe the importance of testicular self-examination and explain how to perform the examination as you are performing it.
- Understand the structures and functions of the anorectal region.
- Make sure to have a chaperone in the room while performing the examination.

SAFETY TIP *Wear gloves for every step of the examination to ensure safety for the nurse and the patient, and to prevent contamination.*

618 UNIT 3 Nursing Assessment of Physical Systems

> ### General Routine Screening versus Focused Specialty Assessment for the Male Genitalia, Anus, Rectum, and Prostate
>
> The main role of the registered nurse in assessment of the male genitalia is inspection for deviations from normal. In more advanced practices palpation is also used to assess the status of the male genitals, anus, rectum, and prostate.
>
> **General Routine Screening**
> - Inspect the penis, pubic hair, and scrotum.
> - Inspect the inguinal and femoral areas.
> - Inspect the perianal area.
> - Inspect the anus and rectum.
> - Inspect stool.
>
> **Focused Specialty Assessment**
> - Palpate the pubic hair, penis, and scrotum.
> - Palpate for urethral discharge, *spermatic cord* and vas deferens from the epididymis to the inguinal ring.
> - Transilluminate the scrotum.
> - Palpate for inguinal and femoral hernia.
> - Palpate for inguinal lymph nodes.
> - Palpate the anus and rectum

ASSESSMENT PROCEDURE	NORMAL FINDINGS	ABNORMAL FINDINGS
Penis		
INSPECTION AND PALPATION		
Inspect the base of the penis and pubic hair. Sit on a stool with the client facing you and standing (Fig. 26-6). Ask the client to raise his gown or drape. Note pubic hair growth pattern and any excoriation, erythema, or infestation at the base of the penis and within the pubic hair.	Pubic hair is coarser than scalp hair. The normal pubic hair pattern in adults is hair covering the entire groin area, extending to the medial thighs and up the abdomen toward the umbilicus. The base of the penis and the pubic hair are free of excoriation, erythema, and infestation (Fig. 26-7). **OLDER ADULT CONSIDERATIONS** Pubic hair may be gray and sparse in older adult clients. In addition, the penis becomes smaller and the testes hang lower in the scrotum in older adult clients.	Absence or scarcity of pubic hair may be seen in clients receiving chemotherapy. Lice or nit (eggs) infestation at the base of the penis or pubic hair is known as pediculosis pubis. This is commonly referred to as "crabs."

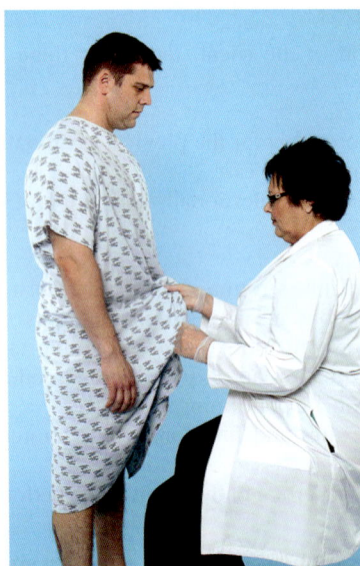

FIGURE 26-6 In positioning the male client for a genital examination, the examiner sits and the client stands.

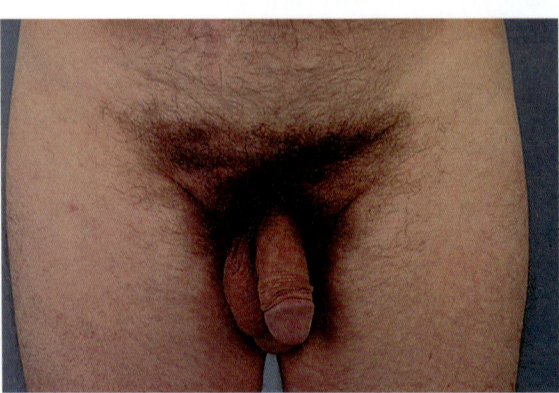

FIGURE 26-7 Normal appearance of external male genitalia (© B. Proud).

ASSESSMENT PROCEDURE	NORMAL FINDINGS	ABNORMAL FINDINGS
Inspect the skin of the shaft. Observe for rashes, lesions, or lumps.	The skin of the penis is wrinkled and hairless and is normally free of rashes, lesions, or lumps. Genital piercing is becoming more common, and nurses may see male clients with one or more piercings of the penis. **CULTURAL CONSIDERATIONS** **Pubertal rites in some cultures include (among many genital mutilations) slitting the penile shaft (penile subincision), leaving an opening that may extend the entire length of the shaft (Project Gutenberg, 2016).**	Rashes, lesions, or lumps may indicate STI or cancer (see Abnormal Findings 26-1). Drainage around piercings indicates infection.
Palpate the shaft. Palpate any abnormalities noted during inspection. Also note any hardened or tender areas.	The penis in a nonerect state is usually soft, flaccid, and nontender.	Tenderness may indicate inflammation or infection.
Inspect the foreskin. Observe for color, location, and integrity of the foreskin in uncircumcised men.	The foreskin, which covers the glans in an uncircumcised male client, is intact and uniform in color with the penis.	Discoloration of the foreskin may indicate scarring or infection.
Inspect the glans. Observe for size, shape, and lesions or redness.	The glans size and shape vary, appearing rounded, broad, or even pointed. The surface of the glans is normally smooth, free of lesions and redness.	Chancres (red, oval ulcerations) from syphilis, genital warts, and pimple-like lesions from herpes are sometimes detected on the glans.
If the client is not circumcised, ask him to retract his foreskin (if the client is unable to do so, the nurse may retract it) to allow observation of the glans. This may be painful.	The foreskin retracts easily. A small amount of whitish material, called smegma, normally accumulates under the foreskin.	A tight foreskin that cannot be retracted is called *phimosis*. A foreskin that, once retracted, cannot be returned to cover the glans is called *paraphimosis*. Chancres (red, oval ulcerations) from syphilis and genital warts are sometimes detected under the foreskin (see Abnormal Findings 26-1).
Note the location of the urinary meatus on the glans.	The urinary meatus is slit-like and normally found in the center of the glans. **CULTURAL CONSIDERATIONS** **If pubertal mutilation has occurred, actual discharge of urine and semen will occur at the location of the shaft opening.**	*Hypospadias* is displacement of the urinary meatus to the ventral surface of the penis. *Epispadias* is displacement of the urinary meatus to the dorsal surface of the penis (see Abnormal Findings 26-1).
Palpate for urethral discharge. Gently squeeze the glans between your index finger and thumb (Fig. 26-8).	The urinary meatus is normally free of discharge.	A yellow discharge is usually associated with gonorrhea. A clear or white discharge is usually associated with urethritis. Any discharge should be cultured.

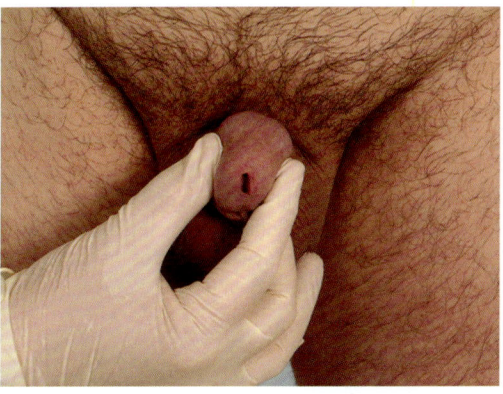

FIGURE 26-8 Palpating for urethral discharge (© B. Proud).

Continued on following page

ASSESSMENT PROCEDURE	NORMAL FINDINGS	ABNORMAL FINDINGS

Scrotum

INSPECTION

Inspect the size, shape, and position of the scrotum. Ask the client to hold his penis out of the way. Observe for swelling, lumps, or bulges.

The scrotum varies in size (according to temperature) and shape. The scrotal sac hangs below or at the level of the penis. The left side of the scrotal sac usually hangs lower than the right side.

 OLDER ADULT CONSIDERATIONS
The scrotal sac appears to droop more in older men.

An enlarged scrotal sac may result from fluid (hydrocele), blood (hematocele), bowel (hernia), or tumor (cancer). A varicocele is an enlargement of the **veins** within the **scrotum, which may cause** low sperm production and decreased sperm quality, which can cause infertility. (Abnormal Findings 26-2).

Inspect the scrotal skin. Observe color, integrity, and lesions or rashes. To perform an accurate inspection, you must spread out the scrotal folds (rugae) of skin (Fig. 26-9). Lift the scrotal sac to inspect the posterior skin.

Scrotal skin is thin and rugated, (crinkled) with little hair dispersion. Its color is slightly darker than that of the penis. Lesions and rashes are not normally present. However, sebaceous cysts (small, yellowish, firm, nontender, benign nodules) are a normal finding.

 OLDER ADULT CONSIDERATIONS
The skin of the scrotal sac in older men has fewer rugae.

Rashes, lesions, and inflammation are abnormal findings (Fig. 26-10).

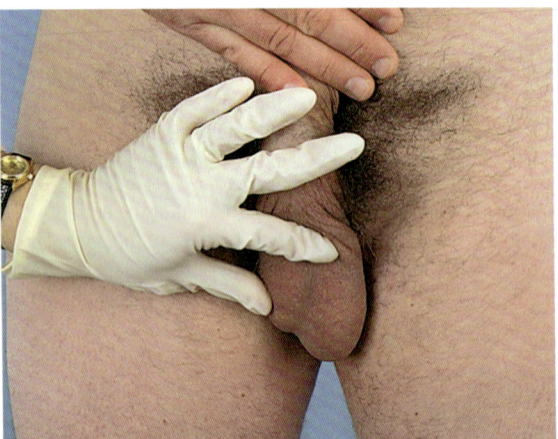

FIGURE 26-9 When inspecting the scrotal skin, have the client hold the penis aside while the examiner inspects (© B. Proud).

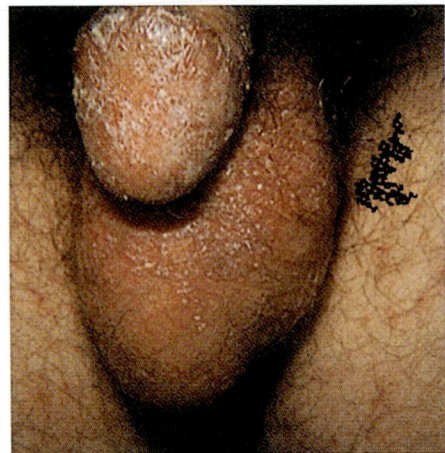

FIGURE 26-10 Inflammation of the penis and scrotum may be seen in Reiter syndrome, an idiopathic inflammatory disorder affecting the skin, joints, and mucous membranes. (Used with permission from Goodheart, H. P. (1999). *A photoguide of common skin disorders*. Baltimore, MD: Lippincott Williams & Wilkins.)

PALPATION

Palpate the scrotal contents. Palpate each *testis* and *epididymis* between your thumb and first two fingers (Fig. 26-11). Note size, shape, consistency, nodules, masses, and tenderness.

⊙ **CLINICAL TIP**
Do not apply too much pressure to the testes because this will cause pain.

Testes are ovoid, approximately 3.5 to 5 cm long, 2.5 cm wide, and 2.5 cm deep, and equal bilaterally in size and shape. They are smooth, firm, rubbery, mobile, free of nodules, and rather tender to pressure. The epididymis is nontender, smooth, and softer than the testes.

 OLDER ADULT CONSIDERATIONS
Testes may be smaller and feel softer to palpation in older men.

Absence of a testis suggests *cryptorchidism* (an undescended testicle). Painless nodules may indicate cancer. Tenderness and swelling may indicate acute orchitis, torsion of the spermatic cord, a strangulated hernia, or epididymitis (see Abnormal Findings 26-2). If the client has epididymitis, passive elevation of the testes may relieve the scrotal pain (Prehn sign).

ASSESSMENT PROCEDURE	NORMAL FINDINGS	ABNORMAL FINDINGS
Palpate each *spermatic cord* and vas deferens from the epididymis to the inguinal ring. The spermatic cord will lie between your thumb and finger (Fig. 26-12). Note any nodules, swelling, or tenderness.	The spermatic cord and vas deferens should feel uniform on both sides. The cord is smooth, nontender, and rope-like.	Palpable, tortuous veins suggest varicocele. A beaded or thickened cord indicates infection or cysts. A cyst suggests hydrocele of the spermatic cord.

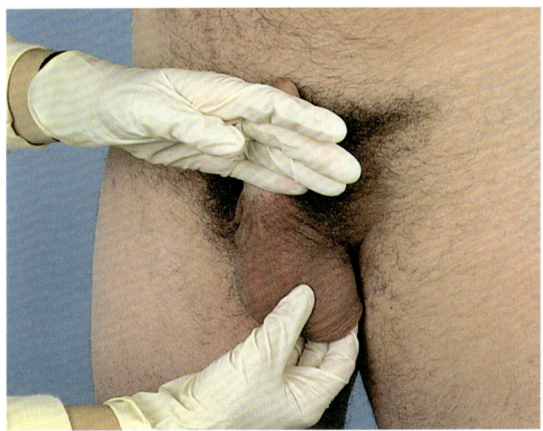

FIGURE 26-11 Palpating the scrotal contents (© B. Proud).

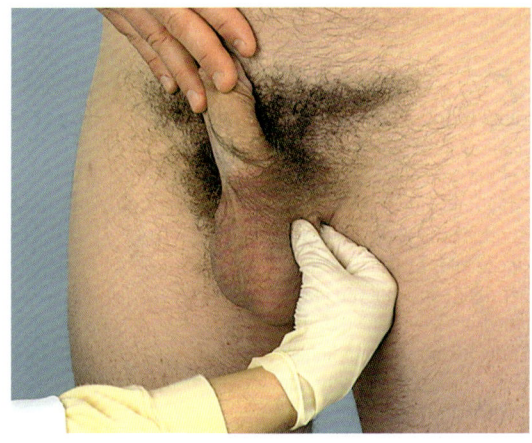

FIGURE 26-12 When palpating the spermatic cord, have the client hold the penis aside (© B. Proud).

Assessment of scrotal mass found during examination.		
If an abnormal mass or swelling was noted during inspection and palpation of the scrotum, **perform transillumination.** Darken the room and shine a light from the back of the scrotum through the mass. Look for a red glow.	Normally scrotal contents do not transilluminate.	Swellings or masses that contain serous fluid—hydrocele, spermatocele—light up with a red glow. Swellings or masses that are solid or filled with blood—tumor, hernias, or varicocele—do not light up with a red glow.
If during inspection and palpation of the scrotal contents, you palpated a scrotal mass, ask the client to lie down. Note whether the mass disappears. If it remains, **auscultate it for bowel sounds.** Finally, gently palpate the mass and try to push it upward into the abdomen. **CLINICAL TIP** If the client complains of extreme tenderness or nausea, do not try to push the mass up into the abdomen.	Normal findings are not expected.	If the bulge disappears, no scrotal hernia is present, but the mass may result from something else. Refer the client for further evaluation. A mass on or around the scrotum should be considered malignant until testing proves otherwise. If the mass remains, place your fingers above the scrotal mass. If you can get your fingers above the mass, suspect hydrocele (see Abnormal Findings 26-2). Bowel sounds auscultated over the mass indicate the presence of bowel and thus a scrotal hernia. Bowel sounds will not be heard over a hydrocele. If you cannot push the mass into the abdomen, suspect an *incarcerated hernia.* A hernia is *strangulated* when its blood supply is cut off. The client typically complains of extreme tenderness and nausea. If you suspect that the client has a strangulated hernia, refer the client immediately to the physician and prepare him for surgery.

Continued on following page

ASSESSMENT PROCEDURE	NORMAL FINDINGS	ABNORMAL FINDINGS
Inguinal Area		
INSPECTION		
Inspect for inguinal and femoral hernia. Inspect the inguinal and femoral areas for bulges. Ask the client to turn head and cough or to bear down as if having a bowel movement, and continue to inspect the areas.	The inguinal and femoral areas are normally free from bulges.	Bulges that appear at the external inguinal ring or at the femoral canal when the client bears down may signal a hernia (Abnormal Findings 26-3).
PALPATION		
Palpate for inguinal hernia and inguinal nodes. Ask the client to shift his weight to the left for palpation of the right inguinal canal and vice versa. Place your right index finger into the client's right scrotum and press upward, invaginating the loose folds of skin (Fig. 26-13). Palpate up the spermatic cord until you reach the triangular-shaped, slit-like opening of the external inguinal ring. Try to push your finger through the opening and, if possible, continue palpating up the inguinal canal. When your finger is in the canal or at the external inguinal ring, ask the client to bear down or cough. Feel for any bulges against your finger. Then, repeat the procedure on the opposite side.	Bulging or masses are not normally palpated.	A bulge or mass may indicate a hernia.

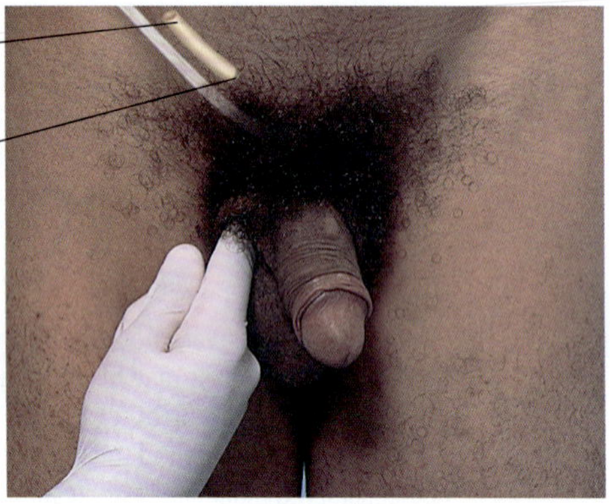

FIGURE 26-13 Palpating for an inguinal hernia (© B. Proud).

Palpate inguinal lymph nodes. If nodes are palpable, note size, consistency, mobility, or tenderness.	No enlargement or tenderness is normal.	Enlarged or tender lymph nodes may indicate an inflammatory process or infection of the penis or scrotum.
Palpate for femoral hernia. Palpate on the front of the thigh in the femoral canal area. Ask the client to bear down or cough. Feel for bulges. Repeat on the opposite thigh.	Bulges or masses are not normally palpated.	Bulge or mass palpated as client bears down or coughs.
Anus and Rectum		
INSPECTION		
Inspect the perianal area. Spread the client's buttocks and inspect the anal opening and surrounding area (Fig. 26-14) for the following: • Lumps • Ulcers	The anal opening should appear hairless, moist, and tightly closed. The skin around the anal opening is coarser and more darkly pigmented. The surrounding perianal area should be free of redness, lumps, ulcers, lesions, and rashes.	Lesions may indicate STIs, cancer, or hemorrhoids. A thrombosed external hemorrhoid appears swollen. It is itchy, painful, and bleeds when the client passes stool. A previously thrombosed hemorrhoid appears as a skin tag that protrudes from the anus.

ASSESSMENT PROCEDURE	NORMAL FINDINGS	ABNORMAL FINDINGS
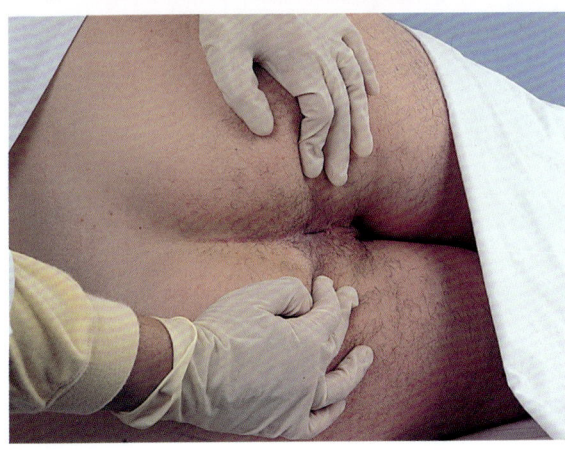 FIGURE 26-14 Inspecting the perianal area.		
• Lesions • Rashes • Redness • Fissures • Thickening of the epithelium		A painful mass that is hardened and reddened suggests a perianal abscess. A swollen skin tag on the anal margin may indicate a fissure in the anal canal. Redness and excoriation may be from scratching an area infected by fungi or pinworms. A small opening in the skin that surrounds the anal opening may be an anorectal fistula (Abnormal Findings 26-4). Thickening of the epithelium suggests repeated trauma from anal intercourse.
Ask the client to perform Valsalva's maneuver by straining or bearing down. Inspect the anal opening for any bulges or lesions. 🎯 **CLINICAL TIP** Document any abnormalities by noting position in relation to a face of a clock.	No bulging or lesions appear.	Bulges of red mucous membrane may indicate a rectal prolapse. Hemorrhoids or an anal fissure may also be seen (see Abnormal Findings 26-4).
Inspect the sacrococcygeal area. Inspect this area for any signs of swelling, redness, dimpling, or hair.	Area is normally smooth, and free of redness and hair.	A reddened, swollen, or dimpled area covered by a small tuft of hair located midline on the lower sacrum suggests a pilonidal cyst (see Abnormal Findings 26-4).
PALPATION		
Palpate the anus. Inform the client that you are going to perform the internal examination at this point. Explain that it may feel like his bowels are going to move but that this will not happen. Lubricate your gloved index finger; ask the client to bear down. As the client bears down, place the pad of your index finger on the anal opening and apply slight pressure; this will cause relaxation of the sphincter. 🎯 **CLINICAL TIP** Never use your fingertip—this causes the sphincter to tighten and, if forced into the rectum, may cause pain.	Client's sphincter relaxes, permitting entry.	Sphincter tightens, making further examination unrealistic.

Continued on following page

ASSESSMENT PROCEDURE	NORMAL FINDINGS	ABNORMAL FINDINGS
Anus and Rectum (Continued)		
When you feel the sphincter relax, insert your finger gently with the pad facing down (Fig. 26-15 and Fig. 26-16). 🎯 **CLINICAL TIP** **If severe pain prevents your entrance to the anus, do not force the examination.** If the sphincter does not relax and the client reports severe pain, spread the gluteal folds with your hands in close approximation to the anus and attempt to visualize a lesion that may be causing the pain. If tension is maintained on the gluteal folds for 60 seconds, the anus will dilate normally.	Examination finger enters anus.	Examination finger cannot enter the anus.
Ask the client to tighten the external sphincter; note the tone.	The client can normally close the sphincter around the gloved finger.	Poor sphincter tone may be the result of a spinal cord injury, previous surgery, trauma, or a prolapsed rectum. Tightened sphincter tone may indicate anxiety, scarring, or inflammation.
Rotate finger to examine the muscular anal ring. Palpate for tenderness, nodules, and hardness.	The anus is normally smooth, nontender, and free of nodules and hardness.	Tenderness may indicate hemorrhoids, fistula, or fissure. Nodules may indicate polyps or cancer. Hardness may indicate scarring or cancer.
Palpate the rectum. Insert your finger further into the rectum as far as possible (Fig. 26-17). Next, turn your hand clockwise then counterclockwise. This allows palpation of as much rectal surface as possible. Note tenderness, irregularities, nodules, and hardness.	The rectal mucosa is normally soft, smooth, nontender, and free of nodules.	Hardness and irregularities may be from scarring or cancer. Nodules may indicate polyps or cancer (see Abnormal Findings 26-4).

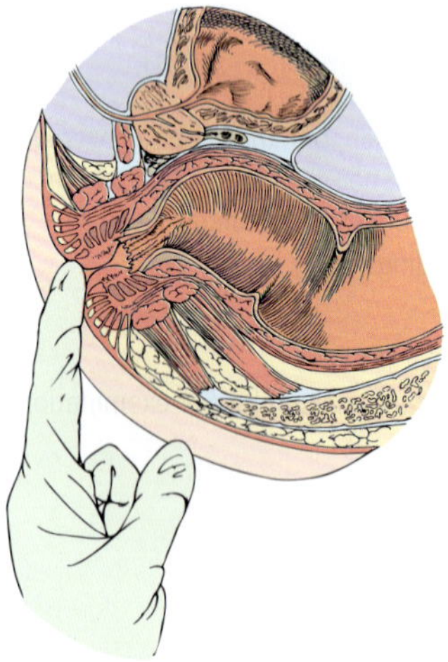

FIGURE 26-15 Relaxing the anal sphincter.

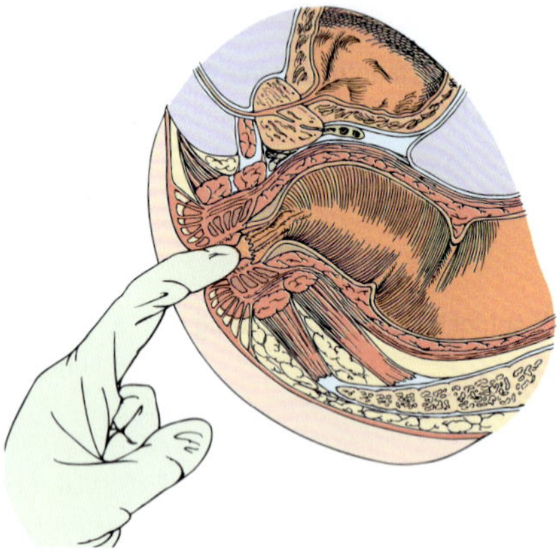

FIGURE 26-16 Palpating the anus.

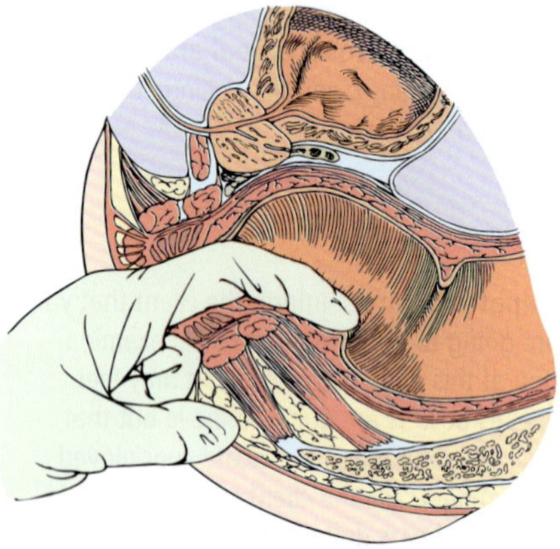

FIGURE 26-17 Palpating the rectal wall.

Palpate the peritoneal cavity. This area may be palpated in men above the prostate gland in the area of the seminal vesicles on the anterior surface of the rectum. Note tenderness or nodules.	This area is normally smooth and nontender.	A peritoneal protrusion into the rectum, called a *rectal shelf* (see Abnormal Findings 26-4) may indicate a cancerous lesion or peritoneal metastasis. Tenderness may indicate peritoneal inflammation.

ASSESSMENT PROCEDURE	NORMAL FINDINGS	ABNORMAL FINDINGS

Prostate Gland

PALPATION

The prostate can be palpated on the anterior surface of the rectum by turning the hand fully counterclockwise so that the pad of your index finger faces toward the client's umbilicus (Fig. 26-18).

> **CLINICAL TIP**
> You may need to move your body away from the client to achieve the proper angle for examination.

Tell the client that he may feel an urge to urinate but that he will not. Move the pad of your index finger over the prostate gland, trying to feel the sulcus between the lateral lobes. Note the size, shape, and consistency of the prostate, and identify any nodules or tenderness.

The prostate is normally nontender and rubbery. It has two lateral lobes that are divided by a median sulcus. The lobes are normally smooth, 2.5 cm long, and heart-shaped.

A swollen, tender prostate may indicate acute prostatitis. An enlarged smooth, firm, slightly elastic prostate that may not have a median sulcus suggests benign prostatic hypertrophy (BPH). A hard area on the prostate or hard, fixed, irregular nodules on the prostate suggest cancer (Abnormal Findings 26-5).

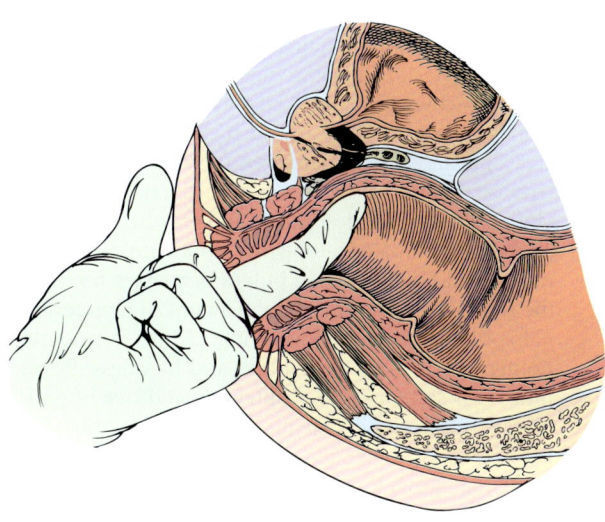

FIGURE 26-18 Palpating the prostate gland.

> **SAFETY TIP** Palpating the prostate gland prior to drawing a prostate-specific antigen (PSA) will likely raise the PSA level.

CHECK STOOL

Inspect the stool. Withdraw your gloved finger. Inspect any fecal matter on your glove. Assess the color, and test the feces for occult blood. Provide the client with a towel to wipe the anorectal area.

Stool is normally semi-solid, brown, and free of blood.

Black stool may indicate upper gastrointestinal bleeding, gray or tan stool results from the lack of bile pigment, and yellow stool suggests steatorrhea (increased fat content). Blood detected in the stool may indicate cancer of the rectum or colon. Refer the client for an endoscopic examination of the colon.

CASE STUDY

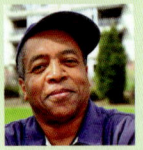

The chapter case study is now used to demonstrate the physical examination of Mr. Weeks' genitalia, anus, rectum, and prostate.

Visual inspection discloses normal adult male pubic hair growth. Pubic hair and base of penis are free of excoriation and infestation. Circumcised penis is free of rashes, lesions. Glans is rounded and free of lesions. No masses or swelling noted in the scrotum, left side hangs slightly lower than the right side. Skin is free of lesions and appears rugated and darkly pigmented. Client's anal opening is hairless and closed tightly. No bulging or lesions appear when client performs Valsalva maneuver. The anus and perianal area are free of redness, lumps, ulcers, and rash. The sacrococcygeal area appears smooth and free from redness and hair. Upon palpation, the penis is soft, flaccid, and nontender. Both testes descended and free from masses; no masses palpated along the epididymis or spermatic cord bilaterally. No bulges or masses noted to the inguinal or femoral canal. Client can close external sphincter around gloved finger. Anus is smooth, nontender, and free of nodules and hardness. Rectal mucosa is soft, smooth, nontender, and free of nodules. Peritoneal cavity area is smooth and nontender. Prostate gland is tender, warm, swollen, and boggy. Fecal matter on gloved finger reveals semi-soft, brown stool.

Validating and Documenting Findings

Validate the male genitalia, anus, rectum, and prostate assessment data that you have collected. This is necessary to verify that the data are reliable and accurate. Document the assessment data in accord with the health care facility or agency policy.

CASE STUDY

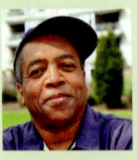

Think back to the case study. The nurse documented the following subjective and objective assessment findings of the evaluation of Mr. Weeks.

Biographical Data: 52-year-old African American male lives at home with wife.

Reason for Seeking Care: Frequent urination that burns and is painful, also pain with defecation or with the act of sexual intercourse.

History of Present Health Concern (pertinent to male genitalia, anus, rectum, and prostate): States that since last night he has had pain with urination, also complains of hesitancy, a decreased stream, and painful ejaculation. Denies urethral discharge, urethral meatal itching, hematuria, or incontinence. Rates pain as a 9 out of 10 on a scale of 0–10.

Personal History: Is married 30 years and has only had one sex partner during that time. Has never been diagnosed with an STI. States that he has some pain with defecation. His normal bowel pattern is daily with formed, brown stool. Denies any recent history of blood or changes in his bowel, denies laxative use.

Family History: Denies any family history of genitalia, rectal, or prostate cancer.

Lifestyle and Health Practices: Reports that he does not drink alcoholic beverages. Currently does not smoke cigarettes; has not smoked for 10 years. However, he did smoke 1 pack per day for 20 years. Had first colonoscopy at age 50, states results were normal. He is scheduled through his PCP to have yearly physical and labs drawn and will have a PSA at that time.

Physical Examination Findings: Visual inspection discloses normal adult male pubic hair growth. Pubic hair and base of penis are free of excoriation and infestation. Circumcised penis is free of rashes, lesions. Glans is rounded and free from lesions. Scrotal skin is free of lesions and appears rugated and darkly pigmented. No masses or swelling noted in the scrotum, left side hangs slightly lower than the right side. Client's anal opening is hairless and closed tightly. No bulging or lesions appear when client performs Valsalva maneuver. The anus and perianal area are free of redness, lumps, ulcers, and rash. The sacrococcygeal area appears smooth and free of redness and hair. Upon palpation, the penis is soft, flaccid, and nontender. Both testes descended and free from masses, no masses palpated along the epididymis or spermatic cord bilaterally. No bulges or masses noted to the inguinal or femoral canal. Client can close external sphincter around gloved finger. Anus is smooth, nontender, and free of nodules and hardness. Rectal mucosa is soft, smooth, nontender, and free of nodules. Peritoneal cavity area is smooth and nontender. Prostate gland is tender, warm, swollen, and boggy. Fecal matter on gloved finger reveals semi-soft, brown stool.

Analysis of Data: Diagnostic Reasoning

After collecting subjective and objective data pertaining to the male genitalia, anus, rectum, and prostate, identify abnormal findings and client strengths. Then cluster the data to reveal any significant patterns or abnormalities. These data may then be used to make clinical judgments about the status of the male client's genitalia, anal, rectal, and prostatic health.

Selected Nursing Diagnoses

Following is a listing of selected nursing diagnoses (health promotion, risk, or actual) that the nurse may identify when analyzing the cue clusters.

Health Promotion Diagnoses

- Readiness for Enhanced Health Management of reproductive system
- Readiness for Enhanced Health Management
  - Requests information on testicular self-examination (TSE)
  - Requests information on ways to prevent an STI
  - Requests information on birth control
  - Requests information on proper lifting techniques to prevent hernia formation
  - Requests information on purpose and need for colorectal examination

Risk Diagnoses

- Risk for Ineffective Health Maintenance (monthly testicular self-examination, TSE) related to lack of knowledge of the importance of TSE
- Risk for Injury related to poor lifting techniques
- Risk for Infection related to unprotected sexual intercourse
- Risk for Ineffective Sexuality Pattern related to impending surgery
- Risk for Ineffective Health Maintenance related to lack of knowledge of need for recommended colorectal and prostate examinations
- Risk for Impaired Skin Integrity in rectal area related to chronic irritation secondary to diarrhea

Actual Diagnoses

- Fear of testicular cancer related to existing risk factors
- Disturbed Body Image related to hernia repair
- Pain: Dysuria related to gonorrhea, infection, or genital reproductive surgery
- Acute Pain: Rectal
- Ineffective Health Maintenance related to lack of knowledge of testicular self-examination
- Sexual Dysfunction related to decreased libido secondary to fear of urinary incontinence, pain in surgical site, anxiety, or fear
- Sexual Dysfunction related to erectile dysfunction secondary to psychological or physiologic factors
- Sexual Dysfunction related to lack of ejaculation secondary to surgical removal of seminal vesicles and transection of the vas deferens
- Ineffective Sexuality Patterns related to feelings of loss of masculinity and sexual attractiveness secondary to chronic diarrhea or pain
- Anxiety related to impending genital reproductive surgery and lack of knowledge of outcome of surgery
- Diarrhea related to chronic inflammatory bowel disease
- Situational Low Self-Esteem related to loss of control over bowel elimination

Selected Collaborative Problems

After grouping the data, certain collaborative problems may become apparent. Remember that collaborative problems differ from nursing diagnoses in that they cannot be prevented by nursing interventions. However, these physiologic complications of medical conditions can be detected and monitored by a nurse. In addition, the nurse can use physician- and nurse-prescribed interventions to minimize the complications of these problems. The nurse may also have to refer the client in such situations for further treatment of the problem. Following is a list of collaborative problems that may be identified when assessing the male genitalia, anus, rectum, and prostate. These problems are worded as Risk for Complications (RC), followed by the problem.

- RC: Gonorrhea
- RC: Syphilis
- RC: Genital warts
- RC: Erectile dysfunction
- RC: Inability to ejaculate
- RC: Hernia
- RC: Hemorrhage
- RC: Urinary incontinence
- RC: Urinary retention
- RC: Prostatic hypertrophy
- RC: Fistula
- RC: Fissure
- RC: Hemorrhoids
- RC: Rectal bleeding
- RC: Rectal abscess

Medical Problems

After grouping the data, the client's signs and symptoms may clearly require referral to a primary care provider for medical diagnoses (i.e., testicular cancer).

CASE STUDY

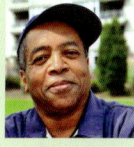

After collecting and analyzing the data for Carl Weeks, the nurse determines that the following conclusions are appropriate:

Nursing Diagnoses
- Impaired Urinary Elimination r/t unknown etiology, possible enlarged prostate and urinary tract infection
- Risk for Urinary Retention r/t unknown etiology, possible enlarged prostate
- Risk for Urge Urinary Incontinence r/t burning on urination and frequency

Potential Collaborative Problems
- RC: Sepsis
- RC: Urinary retention
- RC: Bladder stones
- RC: Hydronephrosis
- RC: Atonic bladder

To view an algorithm depicting the process of diagnostic reasoning for this case, go to thePoint.

Interdisciplinary Verbal Communication of Assessment Findings Using SBAR

SITUATION: CW, a 52-year-old African American man, presents with fever, chills, and malaise. Has frequent burning, painful dribbling urination with hesitancy that began last night. Has constant lower back pain (9 on scale of 10) that goes to bottom of buttocks and around the front of his hips since last night. Received some relief with Aleve. Also reports pain with defecation and painful ejaculation with intercourse.

BACKGROUND: Sexual partner wife of 30 years. No history of STDs.

ASSESSMENT: Visual inspection of pubic hair, circumcised penis, scrotum and perianal area nonsignificant. Anal opening hairless and closed tightly. Upon palpation, the penis is soft, flaccid, and nontender. Both testes descended and free from masses. No masses palpated along the epididymis or spermatic cord, nor inguinal or femoral canal. Client can close external sphincter around gloved finger. Anus and rectal mucosa nonsignificant. Prostate gland tender, warm, swollen, and boggy. Fecal matter on gloved finger reveals semi-soft, brown stool.

RECOMMENDATION: Client has Impaired Urinary Elimination r/t unknown etiology, possible enlarged prostate and urinary tract infection. He is at risk for Urinary Retention r/t unknown etiology, possible enlarged prostate and for Urge Urinary Incontinence r/t burning on urination and frequency. He needs to be seen by his primary care provider for further evaluation of sepsis, urinary retention, bladder stones, hydronephrosis, and atonic bladder.

ABNORMAL FINDINGS 26-1 Abnormalities of the Penis

SYPHILITIC CHANCRE
- Initially a small, silvery-white papule that develops a red, oval ulceration.
- Painless.
- A sign of primary syphilis (a sexually transmitted infection [STI]) that spontaneously regresses.
- May be misdiagnosed as herpes.

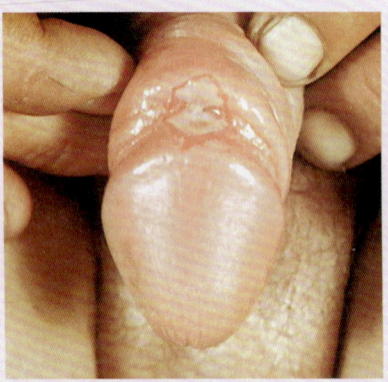

GENITAL WARTS
- Single or multiple, moist, fleshy papules.
- Painless.
- STI caused by the human papillomavirus.

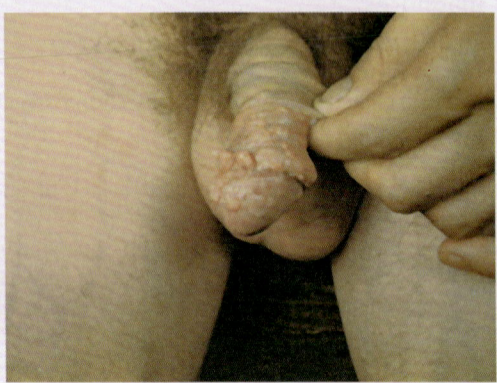

HERPES PROGENITALIS
- Clusters of pimple-like, clear vesicles that erupt and become ulcers.
- Painful.
- Initial lesions of this STI—typically caused by HSV-1 or HSV-2—disappear, and the infection remains dormant for varying periods of time. Recurrences can be frequent or minimally episodic.

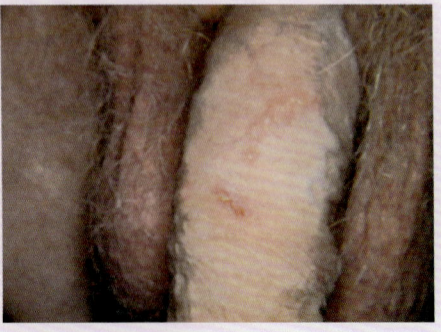

CANCER OF THE GLANS PENIS
- Appears as hardened nodule or ulcer on the glans.
- Painless.
- Occurs primarily in uncircumcised men.

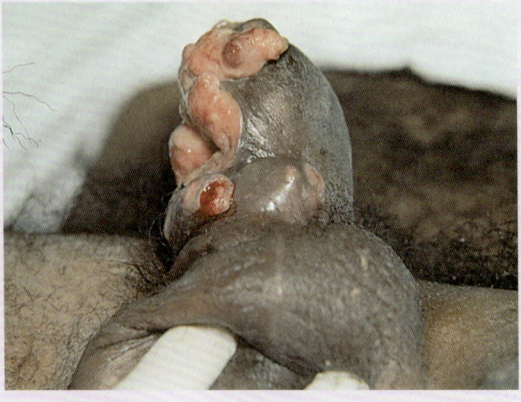

PHIMOSIS

With phimosis, the foreskin cannot be retracted over the penis tip.

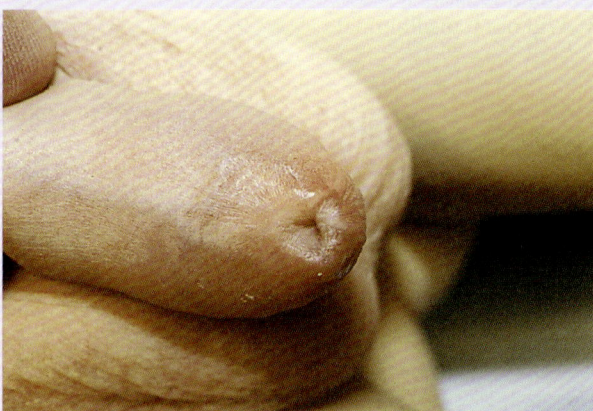

PARAPHIMOSIS

A foreskin that is left in a retracted position leads to venous congestion and edema of the foreskin.

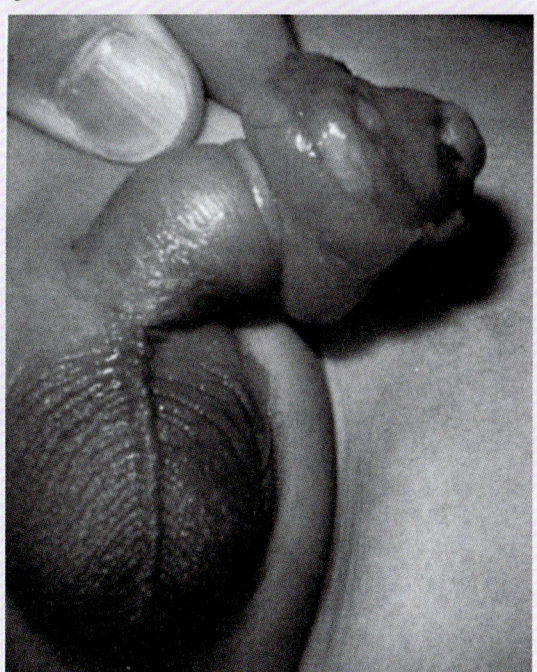

HYPOSPADIAS

- Urethral meatus is located underneath the glans (ventral side).
- This condition is a congenital defect.
- A groove extends from the meatus to the normal location of the urethral meatus.

A ventral view (A) shows the urethra opening on the underside of the penis. In this photo of a baby with hypospadias (B), the urethral opening is on the scrotum.

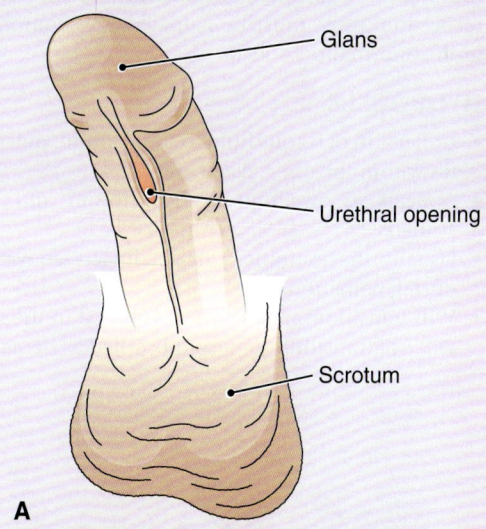

A

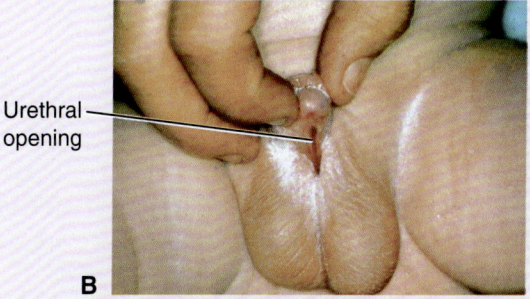

B

EPISPADIAS

- The urethral meatus is located on the top of the glans (dorsal side); occurs rarely.
- This condition is a congenital defect.

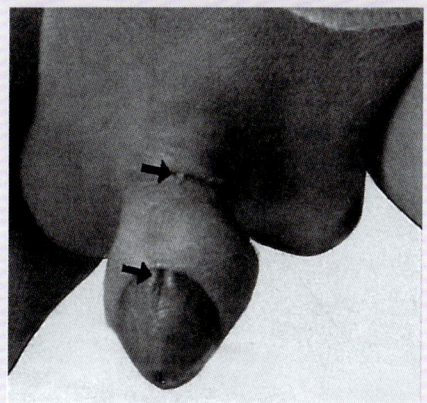

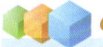 **Concept Mastery Alert**

When the urinary meatus is displaced in a male on the ventral side of the penis, it is known as hypospadias. (The prefix hypo- means "under, beneath, or below.") When it is displaced on the dorsal side of the penis, it is known as epispadias. (The prefix epi- means "on, upon, or beside.")

630 UNIT 3 Nursing Assessment of Physical Systems

ABNORMAL FINDINGS 26-2 Abnormalities of the Scrotum

Although some scrotal abnormalities can be seen by visual inspection, most must be palpated. Descriptions of common abnormalities follow.

HYDROCELE
- Collection of serous fluid in the scrotum, outside the testes within the tunica vaginalis.
- Appears as swelling in the scrotum and is usually painless.
- Usually the examiner can get fingers above this mass during palpation.
- Will transilluminate (if there is blood in the scrotum, it will not transilluminate and is called a "hematocele").

- When palpated, the testis feels enlarged and smooth—tumor replaces testis.
- Will not transilluminate.

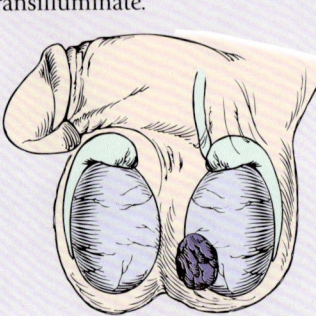
A. Early.

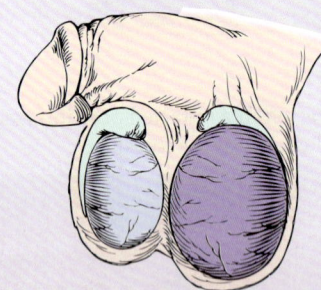
B. Late.

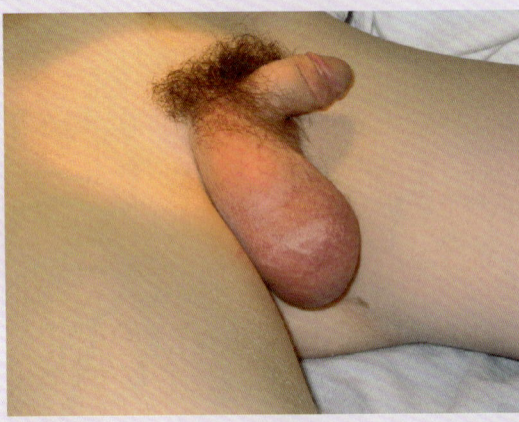

SCROTAL HERNIA
- A loop of bowel protrudes into the scrotum to create what is known as an indirect inguinal hernia.
- Hernia appears as swelling in the scrotum.
- Palpable as a soft mass and fingers cannot get above the mass.

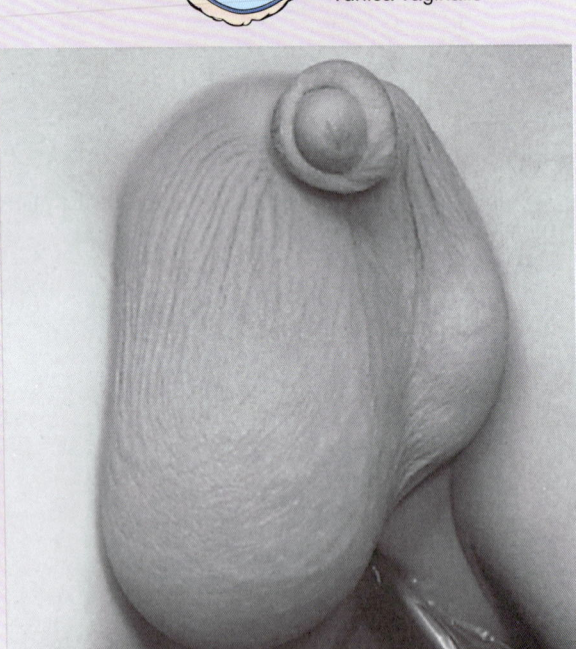

TESTICULAR TUMOR
- Initially a small, firm, nontender nodule on the testis.
- As the tumor grows, the scrotum appears enlarged and the client complains of a heavy feeling.

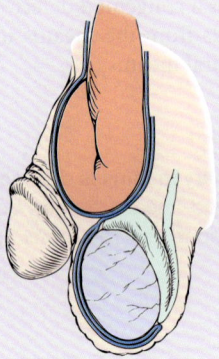

CRYPTORCHIDISM
- Failure of one or both testicles to descend into scrotum.
- Scrotum appears undeveloped and testis cannot be palpated.
- Causes increased risk of testicular cancer.

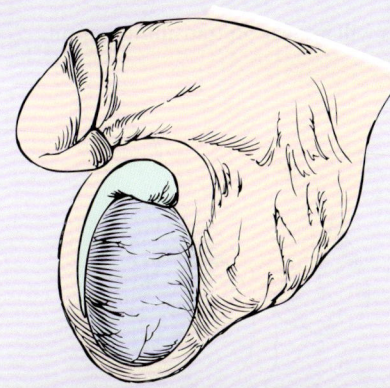

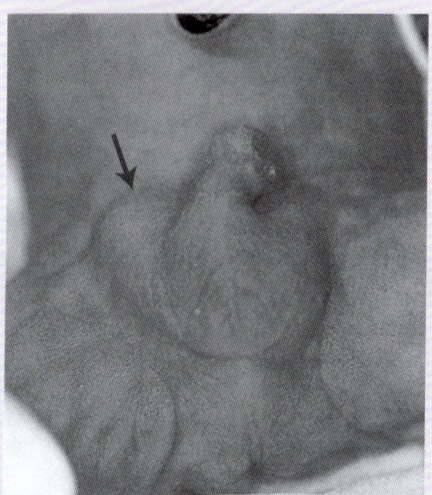

EPIDIDYMITIS
- Infection of the epididymis.
- Client usually complains of sudden pain.
- Scrotum appears enlarged, reddened, and swollen; tender epididymis is palpated.
- Usually associated with prostatitis or bacterial infection.

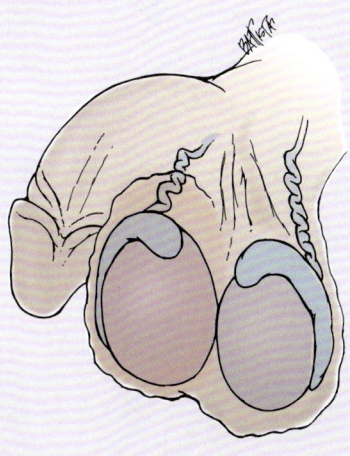

ORCHITIS
- Inflammation of the testes, associated frequently with mumps.
- Client complains of pain, heaviness, and fever.
- Scrotum appears enlarged and reddened.
- Swollen, tender testis is palpated. The examiner may have difficulty differentiating between testis and epididymis.

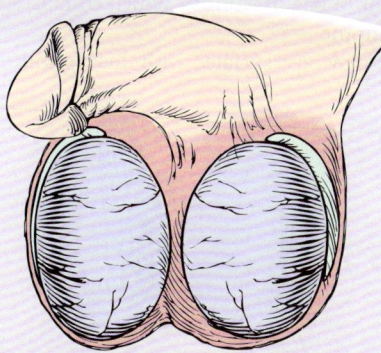

SMALL TESTES
- Small (less than 3.5 cm long), soft testes indicate atrophy. Atrophy may result from cirrhosis, hypopituitarism, estrogen administration, extended illness, or the disorder may occur after orchitis.
- Small (less than 2 cm long), firm testes may indicate Klinefelter syndrome.

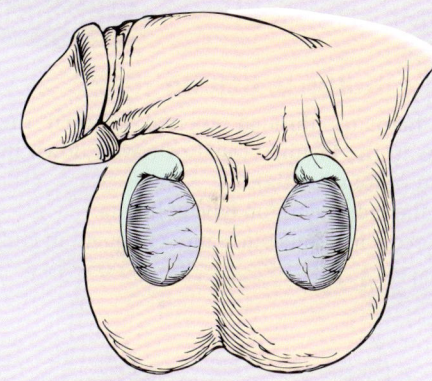

TORSION OF SPERMATIC CORD
- Very painful condition caused by twisting of spermatic cord.
- Scrotum appears enlarged and reddened.
- Palpation reveals thickened cord and swollen, tender testis that may be higher in scrotum than normal.
- This condition requires immediate referral for surgery because circulation is obstructed.

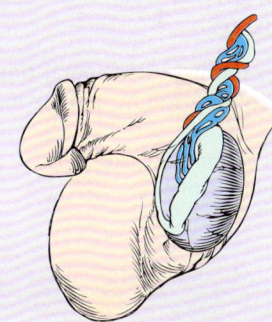

Continued on following page

ABNORMAL FINDINGS 26-2 — Abnormalities of the Scrotum (Continued)

VARICOCELE
- Abnormal dilation of veins in the spermatic cord.
- Client may complain of discomfort and testicular heaviness.
- Tortuous veins are palpable and feel like a soft, irregular mass or "a bag of worms," which collapses when the client is supine.
- Infertility may be associated with this condition.

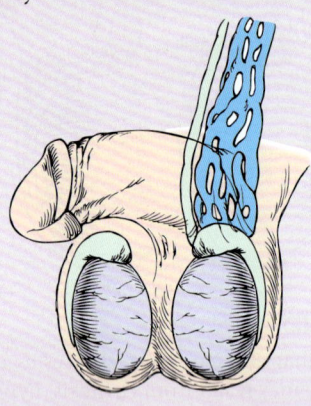

SPERMATOCELE
- Sperm-filled cystic mass located on epididymis.
- Palpable as small and nontender, and movable above the testis.
- This mass will appear on transillumination.

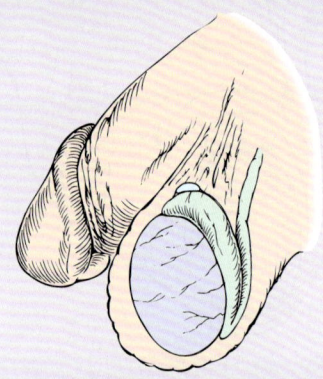

ABNORMAL FINDINGS 26-3 — Inguinal and Femoral Hernias

INDIRECT INGUINAL HERNIA
- Bowel herniates through internal inguinal ring and remains in the inguinal canal or travels down into the scrotum (scrotal hernia).
- This is the most common type of hernia.
- It may occur in adults but is more frequent in children.

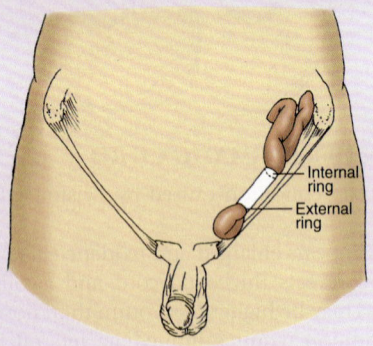

DIRECT INGUINAL HERNIA
- Bowel herniates from behind and through the external inguinal ring. It rarely travels down into the scrotum.
- This type of hernia is less common than an indirect hernia.
- It occurs mostly in adult men older than age 40.

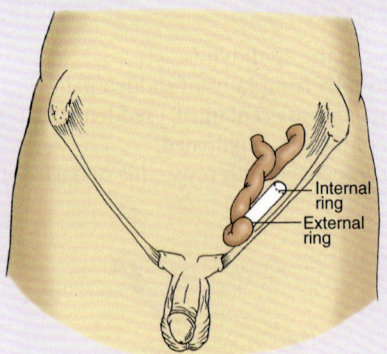

FEMORAL HERNIA
- Bowel herniates through the femoral ring and canal. It never travels into the scrotum, and the inguinal canal is empty.
- This is the least common type of hernia.
- It occurs mostly in women.

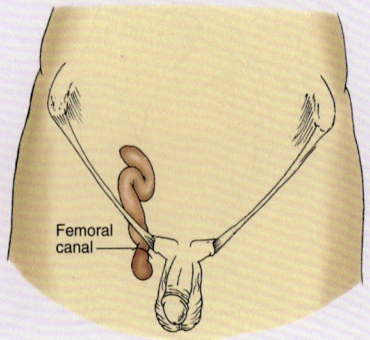

ABNORMAL FINDINGS 26-4 Abnormalities of the Anus and Rectum

EXTERNAL HEMORRHOID

Hemorrhoids are usually painless papules caused by varicose veins. They can be internal or external (above or below the anorectal junction). This external hemorrhoid has become thrombosed—it contains clotted blood, is very painful and swollen, and itches and bleeds with bowel movements.

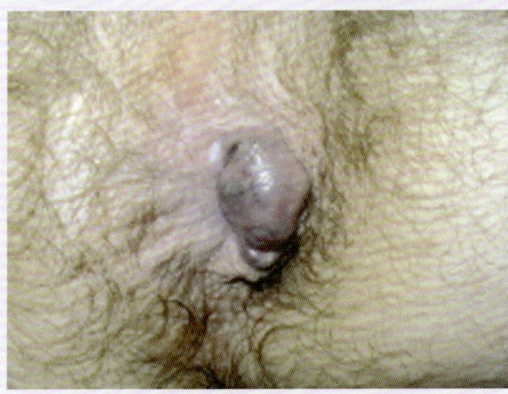

PERIANAL ABSCESS

Perianal abscess is a cavity of pus, caused by infection in the skin around the anal opening. It causes throbbing pain and is red, swollen, hard, and tender.

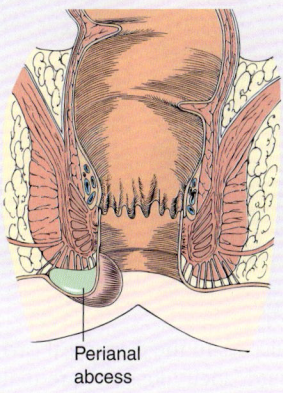

ANAL FISSURE

These splits in the tissue of the anal canal are caused by trauma. A swollen skin tag ("sentinel tag") is often present below the fissure on the anal margin. They cause intense pain, itching, and bleeding.

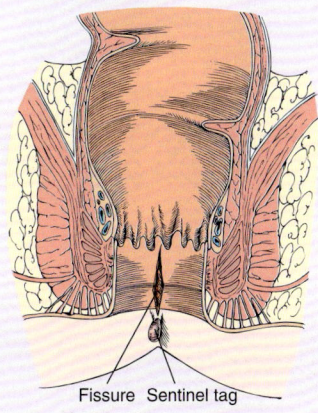

ANORECTAL FISTULA

This is evidenced by a small, round opening in the skin that surrounds the anal opening. It suggests an inflammatory tract from the anus or rectum out to the skin. A previous abscess may have preceded the fistula.

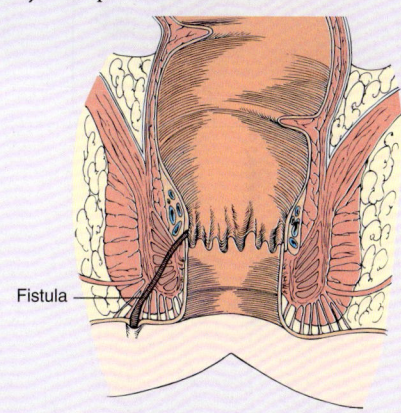

With an anoscope inserted in the anal canal, an anal fissure can be seen in the posterior midline of the squamous epithelium of the anal canal. A sentinel skin tag can be seen on the distal end of the fissure on the anal verge.

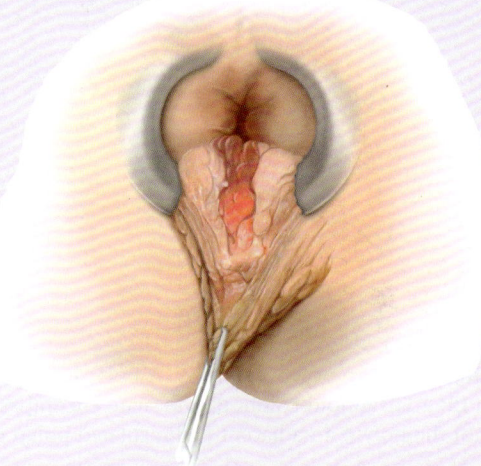

RECTAL PROLAPSE

This occurs when the mucosa of the rectum protrudes out through the anal opening. It may involve only the mucosa or the mucosa and the rectal wall. It appears as a red, doughnut-like mass with radiating folds.

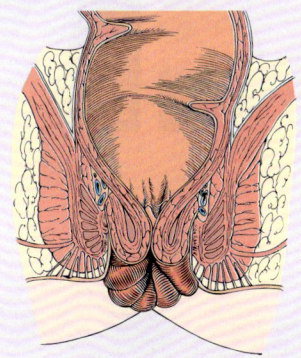

Continued on following page

ABNORMAL FINDINGS 26-4 Abnormalities of the Anus and Rectum (Continued)

PILONIDAL CYST

This congenital disorder is characterized by a small dimple or cyst/sinus that contains hair. It is located midline in the sacrococcygeal area and has a palpable sinus tract.

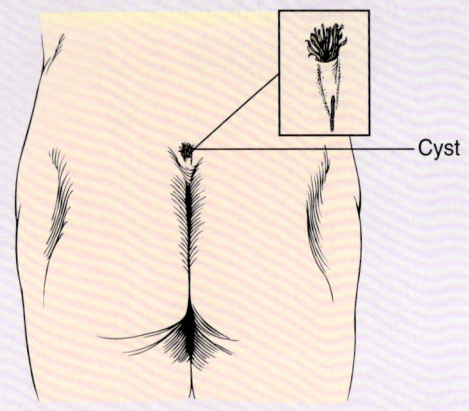

RECTAL POLYPS

These soft structures are rather common and occur in varying sizes and numbers. There are two types: pedunculated (on a stalk) and sessile (on the mucosal surface).

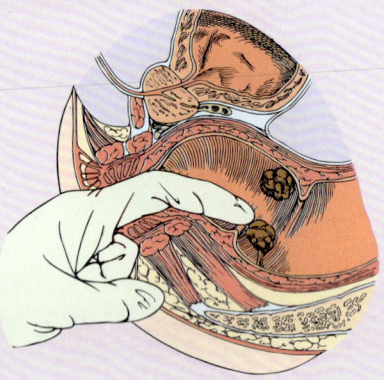

Technique of snare polypectomy. A: A polyp on a stalk is seen in the midsigmoid colon. B: The snare encompasses the head of the polyp; an adjacent pedunculated polyp can be seen.

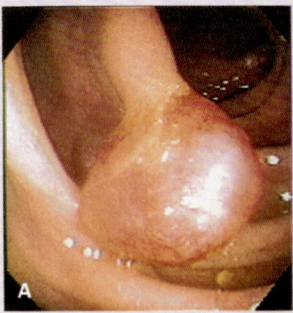 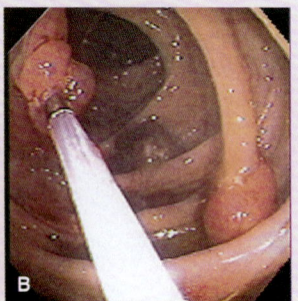

RECTAL CANCER

A rectal carcinoma is usually asymptomatic until it is quite advanced. Thus, routine rectal palpation is essential. A cancer of the rectum may feel like a firm nodule, an ulcerated nodule with rolled edges, or, as it grows, a large, irregularly shaped, fixed, hard nodule.

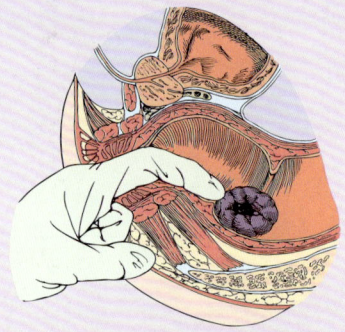

Rectal cancer before (left) and after (right) neoadjuvant chemoradiation. This patient had a good response to treatment.

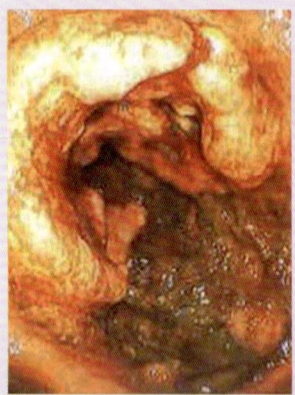 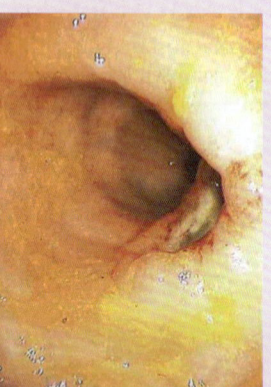

RECTAL SHELF

If cancer metastasizes to the peritoneal cavity, it may be felt as a nodular, hard, shelf-like structure that protrudes onto the anterior surface of the rectum in the area of the seminal vesicles in men and in the area of the rectouterine pouch in women.

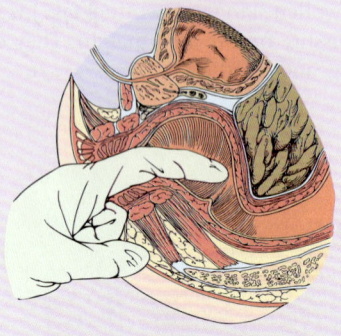

ABNORMAL FINDINGS 26-5 Abnormalities of the Prostate Gland

ACUTE PROSTATITIS
The prostate is swollen, tender, firm, and warm to the touch. Prostatitis is caused by a bacterial infection.

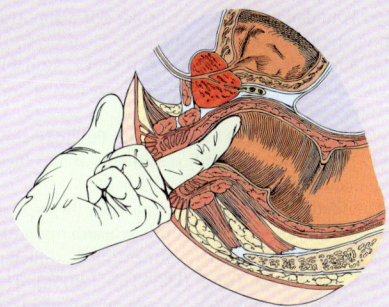

Swelling and inflammation characteristic of acute prostatitis.

BENIGN PROSTATIC HYPERTROPHY
The prostate is enlarged, smooth, firm, and slightly elastic. The median sulcus may not be palpable. It is common in men older than 50 years.

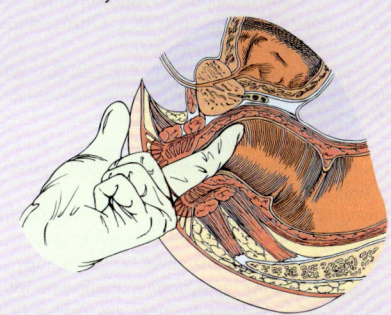

Enlargement characteristic of benign prostatic hypertrophy.

CANCER OF THE PROSTATE
A hard area on the prostate or hard, fixed, irregular nodules on the prostate suggest cancer. The median sulcus may not be palpable.

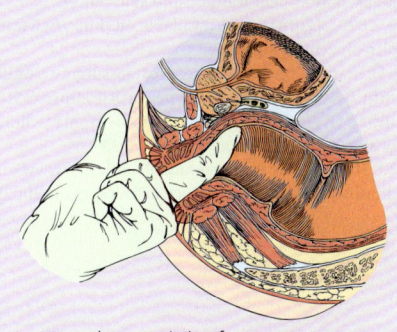

Mass characteristic of prostate cancer.

Want to know more?

A wide variety of resources to enhance your learning and understanding of this book are available on **thePoint**. Visit thePoint to access:

- NCLEX-Style Student Review Questions
- Watch and Learn Videos
- Concepts in Action Animations
- And more!

References and Selected Readings

AIDS.gov. (2013). Tuberculosis and HIV. Available at https://www.aids.gov/hiv-aids-basics/staying-healthy-with-hiv-aids/potential-related-health-problems/tuberculosis/

AIDS.gov. (2015). CD4 count. Available at https://www.aids.gov/hiv-aids-basics/just-diagnosed-with-hiv-aids/understand-your-test-results/cd4-count/

American Association of Family Physicians (AAFP). (2015). Prostate cancer screening. Available at http://www.aafp.org/afp/2015/1015/p683.html

American Cancer Society (ACS). (2015a). American Cancer Society recommendations for prostate cancer early detection. Available at http://www.cancer.org/cancer/prostatecancer/moreinformation/prostatecancerearlydetection/prostate-cancer-early-detection-acs-recommendations

American Cancer Society (ACS). (2015b). What are the risk factors for prostate cancer? Available at http://www.cancer.org/cancer/prostatecancer/detailedguide/prostate-cancer-risk-factors

American Cancer Society (ACS). (2016a). American Cancer Society recommendations for colorectal cancer early detection. Available at http://www.cancer.org/cancer/colonandrectumcancer/moreinformation/colonandrectumcancerearlydetection/colorectal-cancer-early-detection-acs-recommendations

American Cancer Society (ACS). (2016b). Colorectal cancer risk factors. Available at http://www.cancer.org/cancer/colonandrectumcancer/detailedguide/colorectal-cancer-risk-factors

AVERT. (2015). Global HIV targets. Available at http://www.avert.org/professionals/hiv-around-world/global-response/targets

Beyaz, S., Mana, M., Roper, J., et al. (2016). High-fat diet enhances stemness and tumorigenity of intestinal progenitors. *Nature*, 531, 55–58.

Canadian Task Force on Preventive Health Care. (2014). Screening for prostate cancer (2014). Available at http://canadiantaskforce.ca/ctfphc-guidelines/2014-prostate-cancer/

Cancer Research UK. (2014). Screening for prostate cancer. Available at http://www.cancerresearchuk.org/about-cancer/type/prostate-cancer/about/screening-for-prostate-cancer

Cassels, A. (2016, February 26). Colonoscopies: America's gold standard, while Canada says they are not justified. Available at http://www.healthnewsreview.org/2016/02/americas-closed-information-border-news-of-canadian-colon-cancer-screening-guidelines-denied-entry/

Centers for Disease Control and Prevention (CDC). (2013). Condom fact sheet in brief. Available at http://www.cdc.gov/condomeffectiveness/brief.html

Centers for Disease Control and Prevention (CDC). (2014). Reported STDs in the United States. Available at http://www.cdc.gov/std/stats14/std-trends-508.pdf

Centers for Disease Control and Prevention (CDC). (2015a). HIV/AIDS basic statistics. Available at http://www.cdc.gov/hiv/basics/statistics.html

Centers for Disease Control and Prevention (CDC). (2015b). HIV among people aged 50 and over. Available at http://www.cdc.gov/hiv/group/age/olderamericans/index.html

Centers for Disease Control and Prevention (CDC). (2015c). HIV transmission. Available at http://www.cdc.gov/hiv/basics/transmission.html

Centers for Disease Control and Prevention (CDC). (2016a). Prostate cancer. Available at http://www.cdc.gov/cancer/prostate/

Centers for Disease Control and Prevention (CDC). (2016b). Sexually transmitted diseases (STDs): Diseases and related conditions. Available at https://www.cdc.gov/std/general/default.htm

Doheny, K. (2012). Green tea and cancer prevention: New clues. Available at http://www.webmd.com/prostate-cancer/news/20121018/green-tea-cancer-prevention-new-clues

Florida Atlantic University. (n.d.). Lights at night and prostate cancer risks in men. Available at http://physics.fau.edu/observatory/lightpol-prostate.html

GI Society. (2015). Treating constipation with laxatives. Available at http://www.badgut.org/information-centre/a-z-digestive-topics/treating-constipation-with-laxatives/

Harvard Medical School. (2011). Does frequent ejaculation help ward off prostate cancer? Available at http://www.harvardprostateknowledge.org/does-frequent-ejaculation-help-ward-off-prostate-cancer

Healthy People 2020. (2014). HIV. Available at http://www.healthypeople.gov/2020/topics-objectives/topic/hiv

Jaffe, W. (2014). Urinary incontinence after prostate surgery & radiation surgery. Available at http://www.oncolink.org/types/article.cfm?c=1518&id=7039

Mayo Clinic. (2015a). HIV/AIDS. Available at http://www.mayoclinic.org/diseases-conditions/hiv-aids/basics/definition/con-20013732

Mayo Clinic. (2015b). Prostate cancer. Available at http://www.mayoclinic.org/diseases-conditions/prostate-cancer/basics/definition/con-20029597

National Cancer Institute (NCI). (2015). Prostate cancer. Available at http://www.cancer.gov/types/prostate/patient/prostate-screening-pdq#section/_13

National Health Institutes (NIH). (2017). AIDSinfo. Available at https://aidsinfo.nih.gov/

Project Gutenberg. (2016). Male genital mutilation. Available at http://www.gutenberg.us/articles/male_genital_mutilation#Infibulation

Tarico, V. (2013). Better birth control for men: 8 promising possibilities. Available at http://rhrealitycheck.org/article/2013/10/02/better-birth-control-for-men-8-promising-possibilities/\

Testicular Cancer Foundation. (2017). Testicular self-exam. Available at https://testicularcancer.org/testicular-self-exam/

UNAIDS. (2014). Press release: UNAIDS report shows. Available at http://www.unaids.org/en/resources/presscentre/pressreleaseandstatementarchive/2014/july/20140716prgapreport

University of Wisconsin School of Medicine and Public Health: Department of Urology. (2012). Male factor infertility. Available at http://www.urology.wisc.edu/search?q=male+factor+infertility

Urology Care Foundation. (2017). Benign prostatic hyperplasia (BPH): Medical therapies. Available at http://www.urologyhealth.org/urologic-conditions/benign-prostatic-hyperplasia-(bph)/treatment/medical-therapies

U.S. Preventive Services Task Force (USPSTF). (2015a). Human immunodeficiency virus (HIV) infection: Screening. Available at http://www.uspreventiveservicestaskforce.org/Page/Document/UpdateSummaryFinal/human-immunodeficiency-virus-hiv-infection-screening

U.S. Preventive Services Task Force (USPSTF). (2015b). Screening for prostate cancer. Available at http://www.uspreventiveservicestaskforce.org/Page/Document/UpdateSummaryFinal/prostate-cancer-screening

Wai, D., Katsaris, M., & Singhal, R. (2008). Chaperones: Are we protecting patients? *The British Journal of General Practice, 58*(546), 54–57.

Zeng, H., Lazarova, D., & Bordonaro, M. (2014). Mechanisms linking dietary fiber, gut microbiota and colon cancer prevention. *World Journal of Gastrointestinal Oncology, 6*(2), 41–51.

27 ASSESSING FEMALE GENITALIA, ANUS, AND RECTUM

Learning Objectives

1. Describe the structure and the function of the female genitalia, anus, and rectum.
2. Discuss risk factors associated with cervical cancer across the cultures and ways to reduce one's risks.
3. Interview a client for an accurate nursing history of the female genitalia, anus, and rectum.
4. Perform a physical assessment of the female genitalia, anus, and rectum, using the correct techniques.
5. Differentiate between normal and abnormal findings of female genitalia, anus, and rectum.
6. Describe the findings frequently seen with assessing the older client's female genitalia, anus, and rectum.
7. Analyze the data from the interview and physical assessment of the female genitalia, anus, and rectum to formulate valid nursing diagnoses, collaborative problems, and/or referrals.
8. Differentiate between general routine screening versus skills needed for focused or specialty assessment of the female genitalia, anus, and rectum.
9. Document and verbally report accurate assessment findings of the female genitalia, anus, and rectum.

CASE STUDY

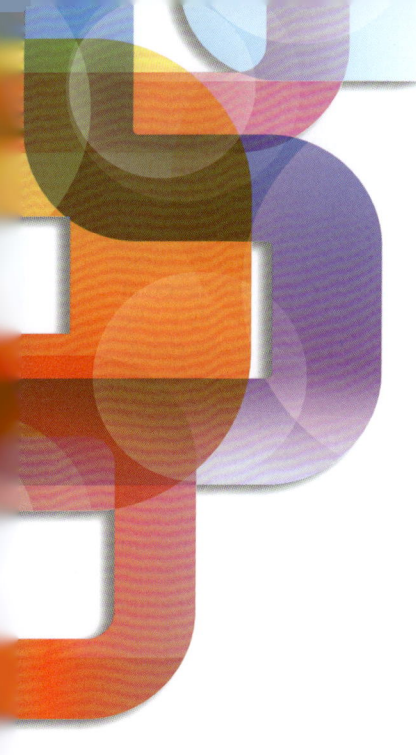

Melinda Carlisle is a 22-year-old college student who comes into the college nurse-managed clinic. She complains, "I feel like I have the flu—no energy, a headache, and fever." She reports a recent outbreak of genital lesions after a sexual encounter 10 days ago ("first and only") with a fellow student she only recently met. She denies the use of any protection or birth control, stating, "He refused to use anything and I didn't insist." She took her temperature at home, and states it was 100.6°F. When questioned, she confirms that she has a great deal of itching and pain in the vaginal area and that "urinating and having a bowel movement hurts a lot."

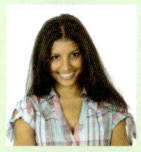

STRUCTURE AND FUNCTION

In order to perform an adequate assessment of the female genitalia, anus, and rectum, the examiner must have a knowledge base of the structure and function of the female genitalia (external and internal structures) and the anus and rectum.

External Genitalia

The external genitalia include those structures that can be readily identified through inspection (Fig. 27-1). The area is sometimes referred to as the *vulva* or *pudendum* and extends from the mons pubis to the anal opening. The *mons pubis* is the fat pad located over the symphysis pubis. The normal adult mons pubis is covered with pubic hair in a triangular pattern. It functions to absorb force and to protect the *symphysis pubis* during *coitus* (sexual intercourse). The *labia majora* are two folds of skin that extend posteriorly and inferiorly from the mons pubis to the perineum. The skin folds are composed of adipose tissue, sebaceous glands, and sweat glands. The outer surface of the *labia majora* is covered with pubic hair in the adult, whereas the inner surface is pink, smooth, and moist.

Inside the labia majora are the thinner skin folds of the *labia minora*. These folds join anteriorly at the clitoris and form a *prepuce* or hood; posteriorly the two folds join to form the *frenulum*. Compared with the labia majora, the labia minora are hairless and usually darker pink. They contain numerous sebaceous glands that promote lubrication and maintain a moist environment in the vaginal area. The *clitoris* is located at the anterior end of the labia minora. It is a small, cylindrical mass of erectile tissue and nerves with three parts: the *glans,* the *corpus,* and the *crura.* The glans is the visible rounded portion of

637

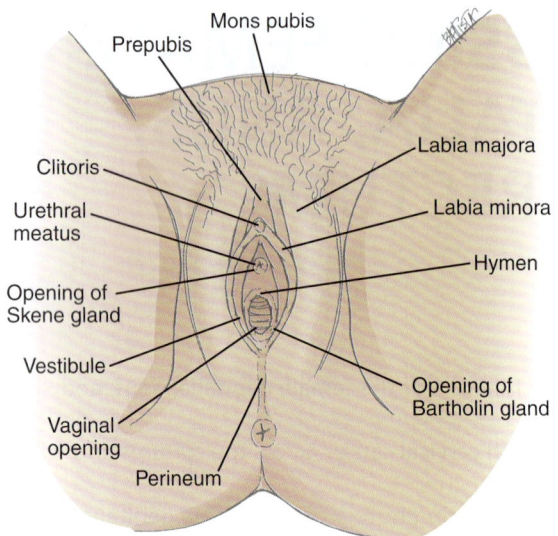

FIGURE 27-1 External genitalia.

the clitoris. The corpus is the body, and the crura are two bands of fibrous tissue that attach the clitoris to the pelvic bone. The clitoris is similar to the male penis and contains many blood vessels that become engorged during sexual arousal.

The skin folds of the labia majora and labia minora form a boat-shaped area (or fossa) called the *vestibule*. The vestibule contains several openings. Located between the clitoris and the vaginal orifice is the *urethral meatus*. The openings of *Skene glands* are located on either side of the urethral opening and are usually not visible. Skene glands secrete mucus that lubricates and maintains a moist vaginal environment. These small glands are often referred to as the *lesser vestibular glands*. Below the urethral meatus is the *vaginal orifice*. This is the external opening of the vagina and has either a slit-like or irregular circular structure, depending on the configuration of a *hymen*. The hymen is a fold of membranous tissue that covers part of the vagina. On either side of and slightly posterior to the vaginal orifice (between the vaginal orifice and the labia minora) are the openings to *Bartholin glands*. These glands secrete mucus, which lubricates the area during sexual intercourse. These small glands, which are not visible to the naked eye, are often referred to as the *greater vestibular glands*.

Internal Genitalia

The internal genital structures function as the female reproductive organs (Fig. 27-2). They include the vagina, the cervix, the uterus, the fallopian tubes, and the ovaries. The *vagina*, a muscular, tubular organ, extends up and slightly back toward the rectum from the vaginal orifice (external opening) to the cervix. It lies between the rectum posteriorly and the urethra and bladder anteriorly, and is approximately 10 cm long. The vagina performs many functions. It allows the passage of menstrual flow, receives the penis during sexual intercourse, and serves as the lower portion of the birth canal during delivery.

The *vaginal wall* comprises four layers. The outer layer is composed of pink squamous epithelium and connective tissue. It is under the direct influence of the hormone estrogen and contains many mucus-producing cells. This outer layer of epithelium lies in transverse folds called *rugae*. These transverse folds allow the vagina to expand during intercourse; they also facilitate vaginal delivery of a fetus. The second layer is the submucosal layer. It contains the blood vessels, nerves, and lymphatic channels. The third layer is composed of smooth muscle, and the fourth layer consists of connective tissue and the vascular network. The normal vaginal environment is acidic (pH of 3.8–4.2). This environment is maintained because the vaginal flora is composed of Döderlein bacilli, and the bacilli act on glycogen to produce lactic acid. This acidic environment helps to prevent vaginal infection.

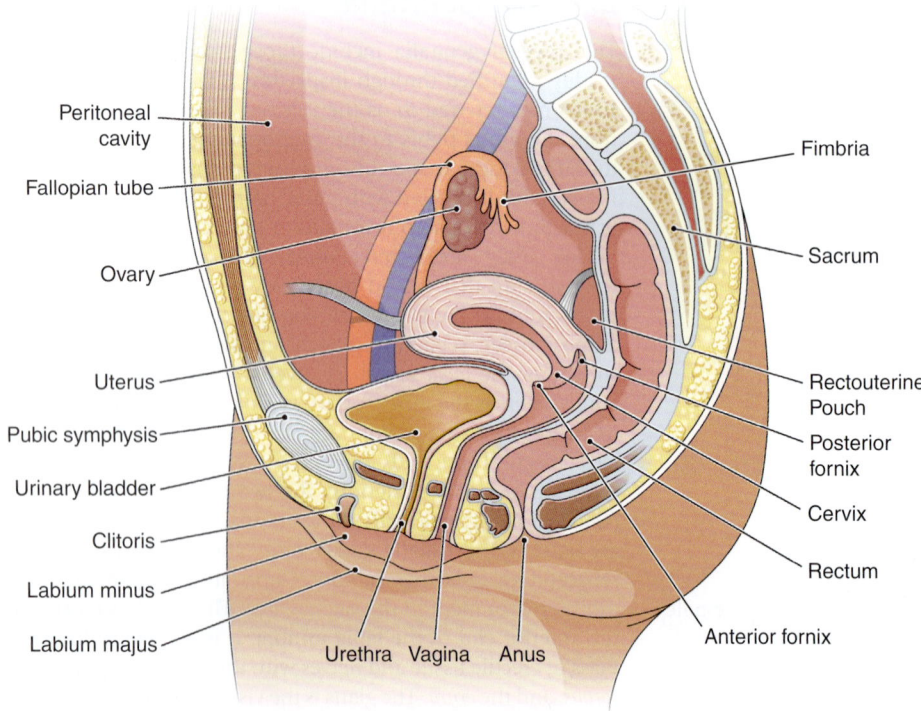

FIGURE 27-2 Female reproductive system (*sagittal section*). This view shows the relationship of the reproductive organs to each other and to other organs.

In the upper end of the vagina, the *cervix* dips down and forms a circular recess that gives rise to areas known as the anterior and posterior fornices. The cervix (or neck of the uterus) separates the upper end of the vagina from the isthmus of the uterus. The junction of the isthmus and the cervix forms the *internal os;* the junction of the cervix and the vagina forms the *external os* or ectocervix. The "os" refers to the opening in the center of the cervix.

◎ CLINICAL TIP
The external os of a woman who is nulliparous (having borne no offspring) will appear as a small, round depression on examination. The external os of a woman who has given birth will appear slit-like due to dilation of the cervix.

The cervix is composed of smooth muscle, muscle fibers, and connective tissue. Two types of epithelium cover the external os or ectocervix—pink squamous epithelium (which lines the vaginal walls) and red, rough-looking columnar epithelium (which lines the endocervical canal). The columnar epithelium may be visible around the os. The point where the two types of epithelium meet is called the *squamocolumnar junction.* The squamocolumnar junction migrates toward the cervical os with maturation or with increased estrogen levels. This migration creates an area known as the transformational zone. The transformational zone is important:

1. 90% of the neoplasms of the lower genital tract originate in this area.
2. This is the area from which cells are obtained for cervical cytology or the Papanicolaou smear (Pap test).

The cervix functions to allow the entrance of sperm into the uterus and to allow the passage of menstrual flow. It also secretes mucus and prevents the entrance of vaginal bacteria. During childbirth, the cervix stretches (dilates) to allow the passage of the fetus.

The *uterus* is a pear-shaped muscular organ that has two components: the *corpus,* or body, and the cervix, or neck (discussed previously). The corpus of the uterus is divided into the fundus (upper portion), the body (central portion), and the isthmus (narrow lower portion). The uterus is usually situated in a forward position above the bladder at approximately a 45-degree angle to the vagina when standing (anteverted and anteflexed positions; see Fig. 27-2). The normal-sized uterus is approximately 7.5 cm long, 5 cm wide, and 2.5 cm thick. The uterus is movable.

The *endometrium,* the *myometrium,* and the *peritoneum* are the three layers of the uterine wall. The endometrium is the inner mucosal layer. The endometrium is composed of epithelium, connective tissue, and a vascular network. Estrogen and progesterone influence the thickness of this tissue. Uterine glands contained within the endometrium secrete an alkaline substance that keeps the uterine cavity moist. A portion of the endometrium sheds during menses and childbirth. The myometrium is the middle layer of the uterus. It is composed of three layers of smooth muscle fibers that surround blood vessels. This layer functions to expel the products of conception. The peritoneum is the outer uterine layer that covers the uterus and separates it from the abdominal cavity. The peritoneum forms anterior and posterior pouches around the uterus. The posterior pouch is called the *recto-uterine pouch* or the *cul-de-sac of Douglas.*

The *ovaries* are a pair of small, oval-shaped organs, each of which is situated on a lateral aspect of the pelvic cavity. Each is approximately 3 cm long, 2 cm wide, and 1 cm deep. The ovaries are connected to the uterus by the ovarian ligament. The ovary functions to develop and release ova and to produce hormones such as estrogen, progesterone, and testosterone. The *ovum* travels from the ovary to the uterus through the *fallopian tubes.* These 8- to 12-cm long tubes begin near the ovaries and enter the uterus just beneath the fundus. The end of the tube near the ovary has fringe-like extensions called *fimbriae.* The ovaries, fallopian tubes, and supporting ovarian ligaments are referred to as the *adnexa* (Latin for appendages).

Anus and Rectum

The *anal canal* is the final segment of the digestive system; it begins at the anal sphincter and ends at the anorectal junction (also known as the pectinate line, mucocutaneous junction, or dentate line). It measures from 2.5 to 4 cm long. It is lined with skin that contains no hair or sebaceous glands but does contain many somatic sensory nerves, making it susceptible to painful stimuli. The *anal opening,* or anal verge, can be distinguished from the perianal skin by its hairless, moist appearance. The anal verge extends interiorly, overlying the external anal sphincter.

Within the anus are the two sphincters that normally hold the anal canal closed except when passing gas and feces. The *external sphincter* is composed of skeletal muscle and is under voluntary control. The *internal sphincter* is composed of smooth muscle and is under involuntary control by the autonomic nervous system. Dividing the two sphincters is the palpable intersphincteric groove. The anal canal proceeds upward toward the umbilicus. Just above the internal sphincter is the *anorectal junction,* the dividing point of the anal canal and the rectum. The rectum is lined with folds of mucosa, known as the columns of Morgagni. The anorectal junction is not palpable, but may be visualized during internal examination. The folds contain a network of arteries, veins, and visceral nerves. Between the columns are recessed areas known as anal crypts; there are 8 to 12 anal crypts and 5 to 8 papillae. If the veins in these folds undergo chronic pressure, they may become engorged with blood, forming hemorrhoids (Fig. 27-3).

The *rectum* is the lowest portion of the large intestine and is approximately 12 cm long, extending from the end of the *sigmoid colon* to the anorectal junction. It enlarges above the anorectal junction and proceeds in a posterior direction toward the hollow of the sacrum and coccyx, forming the rectal ampulla. The anal canal and rectum are at approximately right angles to each other. The inside of the rectum contains three inward foldings called the valves of Houston. The function of the valves of Houston is unclear. The lowest valve may be felt, usually on the client's left side.

The peritoneum lines the upper two thirds of the anterior rectum and dips down enough so that it may be palpated where it forms the *rectovesical pouch* in men and the *rectouterine pouch* in women.

NURSING ASSESSMENT

Collecting Subjective Data: The Nursing Health History

When interviewing the client about genital, reproductive, anal, and rectal health, keep in mind the sensitivities of the client as

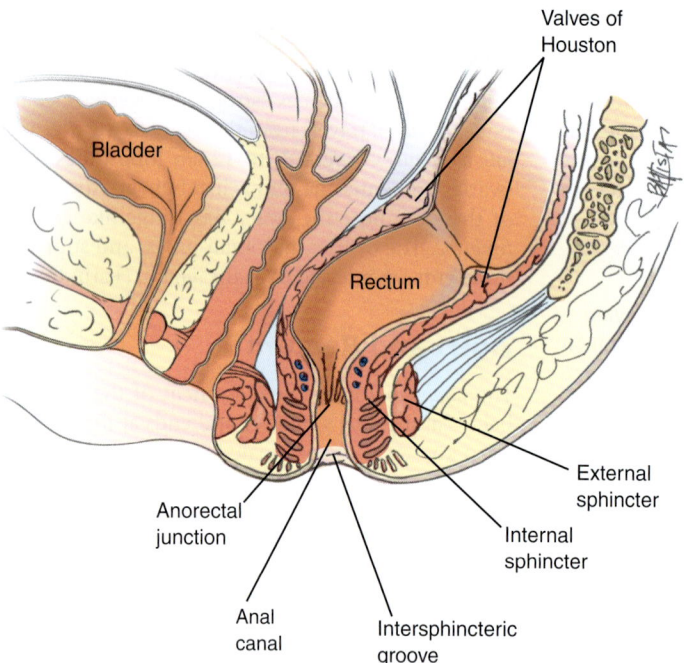

FIGURE 27-3 Anal and rectal structures.

well as your own feelings regarding body image, fear of cancer, sexuality, and the like. Ask the questions in a straightforward manner, and let the client voice any concerns throughout the assessment.

CULTURAL CONSIDERATIONS
Clients from some cultures (e.g., Islam) may insist on having a female nurse for both the nursing history and physical assessment of the female genitalia, anus, and rectum.

Western culture tends to emphasize the importance of a woman's reproductive ability, thereby entwining self-esteem and body image with the female sex role. Anxiety, embarrassment, and fear may affect the client's ability to discuss problems and ask questions. Because some problems can be serious or even life-threatening, it is important to establish a trusting relationship with the client because the information gathered during the subjective examination may suggest a problem or point to the possibility of a problem developing. Cancer of the cervix, for example, is associated with a high mortality rate. However, related risk factors are highly modifiable and cure rates are high in disease that is discovered early.

History of Present Health Concern

QUESTION	RATIONALE
Menstrual Cycle	
What was the date of your last menstrual period? Do your menstrual cycles occur on a regular schedule? How long do they last? Describe the typical amount of blood flow you have with your periods. Any clotting?	A normal menstrual cycle usually occurs approximately every 18 to 45 days. The average length of menstrual blood flow is 3 to 7 days. The absence of menstruation, excessive bleeding, or a marked change in menstrual pattern indicates a need to collect more information.
What other symptoms do you experience before or during your period (cramps, bloating, moodiness, breast tenderness)?	Headache, weight gain, mood swings, abdominal cramping, and bloating are common complaints before or during the menstrual period. Some women experience premenstrual syndrome (PMS), in which the symptoms become severe enough to impair the woman's ability to function.
How old were you when you started your period? **CULTURAL CONSIDERATIONS** Menarche (beginning of menstruation) tends to begin earlier in women living in developed countries and later in women who live in undeveloped countries.	In the United States, ages of menarche range from 10.5 to 15.5 years of age. It occurs at about 17% body fat, and 22% body fat is needed to maintain menstruation (Neinstein, 2013).
Have you stopped menstruating or have your periods become irregular? Are you currently taking any contraceptives containing estrogen or progesterone? Do you have any spotting between periods? What symptoms have you experienced?	Irregularities or amenorrhea may be due to pregnancy, depression, ovarian tumors, ovarian cysts, autoimmune disease nutritional and hormonal imbalances, and medications. Cessation of menstruation that is not related to hormonal therapy is termed *menopause* (see next rationale).

QUESTION	RATIONALE
Menopause	
Are you still having periods? Have your periods changed?	Menopause (absence of menses for 12 months) is a normal physiologic process that occurs in women between the ages of 40 to 58 years, with a mean age of 50. Menopause occurring before age 30 is termed *premature menopause;* menopause between ages 31 and 40 is considered early; menopause occurring in women older than age 58 years is termed *delayed menopause.* Premature and delayed menopause may be due to genetic predisposition, an endocrine disorder, or gynecologic dysfunction. Artificial or surgical menopause occurs in women who have dysfunctional ovaries or who have had their ovaries removed surgically. During the perimenopausal period, hormone levels may fluctuate, resulting in menstrual irregularities. Periods may be heavier or may become scant. 🌐 **CULTURAL CONSIDERATIONS** Lifelong poverty and lower educational level are associated with earlier menopause across the world (Velez, Alvarado, Lord, & Zunzunegui, 2010).
Are you experiencing any symptoms of menopause?	Hormone fluctuations impact vasomotor instability, resulting in symptoms. About 60% of menopausal women experience hot flashes and night sweats. Mood swings, irritability, decreased appetite, vaginal dryness, spotting, and irregular vaginal bleeding may also occur.
Are you on a hormone-replacement therapy (HRT) regimen? If so, what type, and dosage? Are you satisfied with HRT?	It is important to discuss and explain the risk versus benefits of HRT with the client. For a woman posthysterectomy (does not have a uterus), taking estrogen alone sometimes alleviates the symptoms of menopause. However, estrogen has been linked to some types of cancer (e.g., breast, endometrial) and it increases the glycogen content in vaginal secretions, predisposing clients to yeast infections. Progestin therapy is only needed if the woman is posthysterectomy. There are a few newer reports of the benefits of progesterone for women without a uterus, to balance various physiologic functions (Paoletti, 2010). Studies have shown that in women who use estrogen therapy (ET) alone, there does not seem to be any effect on the risk of colorectal cancer. The American Cancer Society (ACS) (2015) describes findings of studies of women who use estrogen–progestin combination therapy (EPT) and the relationship to colorectal cancer. There is a lower risk of getting colorectal cancer at all, but of those who do get colorectal cancer, the cancers were more advanced (more likely to have spread to lymph nodes or distant sites) than those in the women not taking hormones.
Are you continuing to have any symptoms of menopause while taking HRT?	If vasomotor symptoms continue, the client may need to have her dosage of HRT adjusted or she may need to take a different type of HRT.
What are your concerns about going through menopause?	Menopause is a normal stage in a woman's life. Some women have mixed feelings about experiencing menopause. Some may grieve their loss of child-bearing capabilities; others may welcome this new phase of life, as they feel relieved no longer having to be concerned about pregnancy.
Vaginal Discharge, Pain, Masses	
Are you experiencing vaginal discharge that is unusual in terms of color, amount, or odor?	Vaginal discharge may be normal or from an infection.

Continued on following page

History of Present Health Concern (Continued)

QUESTION	RATIONALE
Vaginal Discharge, Pain, Masses (Continued)	
Do you experience pain or itching in your genital or groin area?	Complaints of pain in the area of the vulva, vagina, uterus, cervix, or ovaries may indicate infection. Itching may indicate infection or infestation. **OLDER ADULT CONSIDERATIONS** **The older client is more susceptible to vaginal infection because of atrophy of the vaginal mucosa associated with aging. Women with vaginal atrophy have a greater chance of chronic vaginal infections and urinary function problems. It can also make sexual intercourse painful (Rice, 2015).**
Do you have any lumps, swelling, or masses in your genital area?	These findings may indicate infection, lymphedema, or cancer. Past occurrences should be monitored for recurrence.
Sexual Dysfunction	
Do you have any problems with your sexual performance?	A broad opening question about sex allows the client to focus the interview to areas where she has concerns. Some women have difficulty achieving orgasm and may believe there is something wrong with them. **OLDER ADULT CONSIDERATIONS** **As women age, their estrogen production decreases, causing atrophy of the vaginal mucosa. These women may experience dyspareunia and may need to use lubrication to increase comfort during intercourse. Women experiencing surgical menopause, symptoms of which occur more abruptly, may also benefit from lubrication.**
Have you recently had a change in your sexual activity pattern or libido?	A change in sexual activity or libido needs to be investigated for the cause. A woman who is dissatisfied with her sexual performance may experience a decreased libido.
Do you experience (or have you experienced) problems with fertility?	Infertility is the failure to conceive (regardless of cause) after 1 year of unprotected intercourse. Approximately 35% of infertility cases are related to female fertility factors from a variety of causes (Puscheck & Lucidi, 2012).
Urination	
Do you have any difficulty urinating? Do you have any burning or pain with urination? Has your urine changed color or developed an odor? Have you noticed any blood in your urine?	Urinary frequency, burning, or pain (dysuria) are signs of infection (urinary tract or sexually transmitted infections [STIs]), whereas hesitancy or straining could indicate blockage. Change in color and development of an abnormal odor could indicate infection or renal insufficiency/failure.
Do you have difficulty controlling your urine?	Difficulty controlling urine (incontinence) may indicate urge incontinence (incontinence related to the inability to hold urine beyond the time of mental awareness of the need to urinate) or stress incontinence (increased intra-abdominal pressure). During sneezing or coughing, increased abdominal pressure causes spontaneous urination. **OLDER ADULT CONSIDERATIONS** **Urinary incontinence may develop in older women from muscle weakness or loss of urethral elasticity.**
Bowel Patterns	
What is your usual bowel pattern? Have you noticed any recent change in the pattern? Any pain while passing a bowel movement?	A change in bowel pattern is associated with many disorders and is one of the warning signs of cancer. A more thorough evaluation, including laboratory tests, may be necessary.

QUESTION	RATIONALE
Do you experience constipation?	Constipation may indicate a bowel obstruction or the need for dietary counseling.
Do you experience diarrhea? Is the diarrhea associated with any nausea or vomiting?	Diarrhea may signal impaction or indicate the need for dietary counseling.
Do you have trouble controlling your bowels?	Fecal incontinence occurs with neurologic disorders and some gastrointestinal infections.

Stool

What is the color of your stool? Hard or soft? Have you noticed any blood on or in your stool? If so, how much?	Black stools may indicate gastrointestinal bleeding or the use of iron supplements or Pepto-Bismol. Red blood in the stool is found with hemorrhoids, polyps, cancer, or colitis. Clay-colored stools result from a lack of bile pigment.
Have you noticed any mucus in your stool?	Mucus in the stool may indicate steatorrhea (excessive fat in the stool). Mucus in the stool (sometimes call mucoid stool) is normal if in small amounts. Excessive mucus may be a manifestation of irritable bowel syndrome or irritable bowel disorder.

Itching and Pain

Do you experience any itching or pain in the rectal area?	STIs, hemorrhoids, pinworms, candida, or anal trauma may cause itching (see Evidence-Based Health Promotion and Disease Prevention 27-1). STI, hemorrhoids, fissure, or trauma may cause pain.

Personal Health History

QUESTION	RATIONALE
Describe any prior gynecologic problems you have had and the results of any treatment.	Some problems, such as bacterial vaginosis or cancer, may recur. Prior problems directly affect the physical assessment.
When was your last pelvic or rectovaginal examination by a health care provider? Was a Pap test performed? What was the result?	Pelvic and rectal examinations are used to detect masses, ovarian tenderness, or organ enlargement. The Pap smear test is a screening test for cervical cancer. The American Congress of Obstetricians and Gynecologists (ACOG, 2016) recommends that an annual Pap test and pelvic examinations should be done at age 21 (not before). The Pap test may be performed less frequently at the discretion of the health care provider (see Evidence-Based Health Promotion and Disease Prevention 27-2 for guidelines for age 21 and older).
Have you ever been diagnosed with an STI? If so, what? How was it treated?	STIs can increase the client's risk of pelvic inflammatory disease (PID), which leads to scarring and adhesions on the fallopian tubes. Scarred fallopian tubes increase the risk for infertility and ectopic pregnancy.
Have you ever been pregnant? How many times? How many children do you have? Is there any chance that you might be pregnant now? Any miscarriages or abortions?	The female client's ability to become impregnated and carry a fetus to term is important baseline information. It is important to know if the client is pregnant in case medications or x-ray tests need to be prescribed, as certain medications or x-ray tests might be contraindicated during pregnancy.
Have you ever been diagnosed with diabetes?	Diabetes predisposes women to vaginal yeast infections.
Have you ever had anal or rectal trauma or surgery? Were you born with any congenital deformities of the anus or rectum? Have you had hemorrhoids or surgery for hemorrhoids?	Past conditions influence the findings of physical assessment. Congenital deformities, such as imperforate anus, are often surgically repaired when the client is very young.
Have you ever had a fecal occult blood test (FOBT)? When? Guaiac or Hemoccult?	The ACS (2016a) recommends a stool test every year after age 50 to detect occult blood or other signs of cancer. See Evidence-Based Health Promotion and Disease Prevention 27-3 for further guidelines.

Continued on following page

Personal Health History (Continued)

QUESTION	RATIONALE
Have you ever had a sigmoidoscopy?	A sigmoidoscopy examination is recommended every 5 years after age 50 (ACS, 2016a).
Have you had a colonoscopy? When was your last one?	The U.S. Preventive Services Task Force (USPSTF) recommends screening for colorectal cancer starting at age 50 years and continuing until age 75 years. Colonoscopy is recommended only every 10 years due to small gains versus risks from this invasive test (USPSTF, 2016). The USPSTF recommends against routine screening for colorectal cancer in adults ages 76 to 85 years, except for individual who have never been screened before and are likely to benefit (healthy enough to undergo treatment if colorectal cancer is detected, and who do not have comorbid conditions that would significantly limit life expectance. The USPSTF recommends against any screening for adults over 85 years.

Lifestyle and Health Practices

Do you smoke?	The risk for cervical cancer increases in clients who smoke and who are infected with human papillomavirus (HPV, a type of STI).
How many sexual partners have you had in your lifetime? In the last 6 months? Currently?	A client who has multiple sexual partners increases her risk of contracting STIs.
Do you use contraceptives? What kind? How often? If you take oral contraceptives, do you experience side effects?	Failure to use any type of contraceptive increases the risk of becoming pregnant.
	Failure to use a barrier type of contraceptive (male or female condom) may increase the risk of STIs and human immunodeficiency virus (HIV) infection.
	Minor side effects of oral contraceptives (e.g., weight gain, breast tenderness, headaches, nausea) might develop, which usually subside after the third cycle. Oral contraceptives increase the glycogen content of vaginal secretions, which increases the risk of vaginal yeast infections.
	Major side effects of oral contraceptives include thromboembolic disorders, cerebrovascular accident (CVA), and myocardial infarction (MI).
Have genital problems affected the way in which you normally function?	Diseases or disorders of the genitalia may cause pain and discomfort that affect a client's ability to work, to perform normal household duties, or to care for family. In addition, normal sexual activity may be affected because of pain, embarrassment, or decreased libido.
What do you call your intimate partner or someone you consider to be a significant other? What is your sexual preference? Are you sexually active with males, females, or both? Do you have questions or concerns about your sexual orientation, sexual desires, or sexuality?	Inform client of the confidentiality of the sexual history. An overall average of 3.8% of Americans identify themselves as LGBT (lesbian, gay, bisexual, or transgender), far below the average of 23% that the American public estimated the population to be (Gallup, 2015). Use gender-neutral terms for sexual orientation until the client reveals the terms to use. Once identified, the nurse should use the same terms as the client such as "lesbian," "gay," or "homosexual." It is important to assess the needs of sexual minorities. To assess the client's risk, distinguish sexual identity from sexual behaviors. An awareness of the client's sexual preference allows the examiner to focus the examination. If the client is homosexual, she may not have the same concerns as a heterosexual woman. If she engages in oral sex, she will need to take precautions to prevent orovaginal transmission of infection. Note suggestions for improving care for LBGT clients (Gay and Lesbian Medical Association, 2016).
Do you engage in anal sex?	Anal sex increases the risk for STIs, infection by HIV, HPV, fissures, rectal prolapse, and hemorrhoid formation.
Do you feel comfortable communicating with your partner about your sexual likes and dislikes?	Sexual relationships are enhanced through open communication. Lack of open communication can cause problems with relationships and lead to feelings of guilt and depression.

QUESTION	RATIONALE
Do you have any fears related to sex? Can you identify any stress in your current relationship that relates to sex?	Fear can inhibit performance and decrease sexual satisfaction. Stress can prevent satisfactory sex role performance.
Do you have concerns about fertility? If you have trouble with fertility, how has this affected your relationship with your partner or extended family?	Women often feel responsible for infertility and need to discuss their feelings. Concerns about fertility can increase stress. Problems with fertility can have a negative impact on relationships with the partner and can cause tension within an extended family, especially when other women in the family have children.
Do you perform monthly genital self-examinations?	Each female client should be aware of the need for monthly genital self-examination and its importance in early diagnosis and treatment of problems (Crooks & Baur, 2017).
How do you anticipate going through menopause? Or How do you feel about going through menopause if currently experiencing it?	Menopause is a normal development of aging. However, in some women the process induces fear, anxiety, or even grief. The nurse can assist the client to resolve some of these feelings.
Have you ever been tested for HIV? What was the result? Why were you tested?	HIV increases the client's risk for any other infection. A high-risk exposure may require serial testing. The Centers for Disease Control and Prevention (CDC) (2015) recommends that all adolescents and adults ages 15 to 65 years be screened for HIV.
What do you know about toxic shock syndrome?	Toxic shock syndrome (TSS) is a life-threatening infection. TSS was initially found to be associated with using high-absorbency tampons, especially prolonged, continual use of these, but TSS has occurred in other circumstances. An association has been found for TSS and the use of menstrual cups (thought to be an alternative to tampons). TSS has also been found in nonmenstruating women (and, surprisingly, in men) (Mitchell et al., 2015).
What do you know about STIs and their prevention?	The client's knowledge of STIs and prevention provides a basis for health education in this area.
Do you wear cotton underwear and avoid tight jeans?	Cotton allows air to circulate. Nylon and tight-fitting jeans create a moist environment, which promotes vaginal yeast infections.
After a bowel movement or urination, do you wipe from front to back?	The vaginal and urethral openings are close to the anus and are easily contaminated by *Escherichia coli* and other bacteria if care is not taken to wipe from front to back.
Do you douche frequently?	Frequent douching changes the natural flora of the vagina, predisposing the vagina to yeast infections.
Do you use any laxatives, stool softeners, enemas, or other bowel movement–enhancing medications?	Long-term use of these agents can alter the body's ability to regulate bowel function. Short-term use may indicate the need for dietary counseling.
How much high-fiber food and roughage do you consume every day? Do you eat foods high in saturated fat?	Although high fat diets have been implicated in colon cancer (see Evidence-Based Health Promotion and Disease Prevention 27-3), eating a diet high in dietary fiber, especially cereal fiber and whole grains, has been shown to reduce the risk of colorectal cancer (Klatt, 2015). Women need 25 to 26 g of fiber and men need 38 g of fiber per day (Turner & Lupton, 2011, Table 1).
Do you engage in regular exercise?	Sedentary lifestyle has been linked to the development of colorectal cancer, and physical activity has been associated with a reduction in risk. The amount of exercise needed has not been established.
Do you use calcium supplements?	Some observational studies indicate that the colon cancer risk drops as calcium intake increases; others do not reflect any effect. The National Cancer Institute (2009), therefore, does not recommend the use of calcium supplements in the effort to prevent colorectal cancer.

Continued on following page

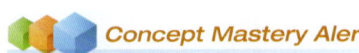

Concept Mastery Alert

In general, untreated sexually transmitted infections (STIs) lead frequently to pelvic inflammatory disease. One particular STI (human papilloma virus) may lead to cervical cancer.

27-1 EVIDENCE-BASED HEALTH PROMOTION AND DISEASE PREVENTION: HEMORRHOIDS

INTRODUCTION

Hemorrhoids, also called piles, are swollen and inflamed veins in the lower rectum and anus (Mayo Clinic, 2013a). They may be located inside the rectum (internal hemorrhoids) or under the skin around the anus (external hemorrhoids). Causes for hemorrhoids include straining during a bowel movement, pregnancy, sitting for long periods on the toilet, chronic constipation or diarrhea, obesity, anal intercourse, low fiber diet, and other conditions that increased pressure on the veins due to intra-abdominal pressure. Symptoms of hemorrhoids include painless bleeding during bowel movements; itching or irritation, pain, discomfort, or swelling in the anal region; lump near the anus, which may be sensitive or painful; and leakage of feces. Although hemorrhoids are usually uncomplicated, they may be pushed out of the anus and protrude, or they may become prolapsed outside the anus, or become thrombosed or strangulated, which occurs when the blood supply to an internal hemorrhoid is cut off. This causes extreme pain and may lead to gangrene. Anemia is the other potential consequence of hemorrhoids if the rectal bleeding is substantial.

CLINICAL TIP

Hemorrhoids often cause a small amount of bright red blood with bowel movements, although occasionally larger amounts of blood may be passed. However, rectal bleeding can occur with other diseases, including colorectal and anal cancer.

A health care provider's evaluation is needed if severe pain develops or if hemorrhoid symptoms began along with a marked change in bowel habits, with the passing of black, tarry or maroon stools, blood clots, or blood mixed in with the stool. These types of stools can signal more extensive bleeding elsewhere in the digestive tract.

Hemorrhoids are more likely to occur as a person ages, as the tissues that support the veins in the rectum and anus can weaken and stretch with aging. Symptomatic hemorrhoids have an estimated prevalence of 4.4% in the worldwide general population; and in the United States, 10 million people per year seek medical treatment for this condition (Thornton, 2015). There is no difference in rates by gender except for females during pregnancy. Thornton reports that rates increase with age through middle age, with the peak between 45 and 65 years of age. About half of all adults in the United States have itching, discomfort, and bleeding that may be associated with hemorrhoids (Mayo Clinic, 2013a). Hemorrhoids are more likely in Caucasians, people of higher socioeconomic status, and those who live in rural areas.

SCREENING

Neither Healthy People 2020 nor the U.S. Preventive Services Task Force addresses hemorrhoids.

RISK ASSESSMENT (Mayo Clinic, 2013a; Thornton, 2015)

- Straining at bowel movements
- Prolonged sitting on the toilet
- Obesity
- Pregnancy
- Anal intercourse
- Familial tendency
- Lack of erect posture
- Higher socioeconomic status
- Chronic diarrhea or constipation
- Colon cancer
- Liver disease
- Anything causing elevated anal resting pressure
- Spinal cord injury
- Loss of rectal muscle tone
- Rectal surgery
- Episiotomy
- Inflammatory bowel disease (ulcerative colitis, Crohn disease)

CLIENT EDUCATION

Hemorrhoids are a normal condition unless complications develop.

Teach Clients

- See your health care provider if you have rectal bleeding, which can indicate other diseases such as rectal cancer.
- Seek emergency care if you experience large amounts of rectal bleeding, lightheadedness, dizziness, or faintness, or extreme pain.
- Avoid straining with bowel movements.
- Avoid standing or sitting for prolonged periods, especially sitting on the toilet.
- Attempt to have a bowel movement as soon as the feeling occurs.
- Avoid anal intercourse.
- Avoid rubbing or cleaning too hard around the anus, which may make symptoms, such as itching and irritation, worse.
- Eat a diet high in fiber, especially cereal fiber and whole grains (consider a fiber supplement if you experience constipation).
- Drink 6 to 8 glasses of water or nonalcoholic fluids per day.
- Get regular exercise (and exercise to lose weight if obese).
- Avoid long periods of sitting.
- If you have hemorrhoids: (Mayo Clinic, 2013a)
  - Use over-the-counter creams or soothing pads.
  - Soak your anal area in plain warm water 10 to 15 minutes 2 to 3 times a day.
  - Bathe (preferably) or shower daily to cleanse the skin around your anus gently with warm water. Soap is not necessary and may aggravate the problem. Gently dry the area with a hair dryer after bathing.
  - Do not use dry toilet paper.
  - Apply ice packs or cold compresses on your anus to relieve swelling.
  - If not contraindicated, an over-the-counter pain medication can be used.

27-2 EVIDENCE-BASED HEALTH PROMOTION AND DISEASE PREVENTION: CERVICAL CANCER

INTRODUCTION

Cervical cancer originates in the uterine cervix, the narrow neck at the lower part of the uterus, connecting the uterus to the vagina (ACS, 2017a). Approximately 8 out of 10 cervical cancers originate in surface cells lining the cervix (squamous cell carcinomas). This is a slow developing cancer and it is preceded by a precancerous stage of dysplasia, which is easily diagnosed with a Pap smear test. Dysplasia is 100% treatable. When dysplastic cells become cancerous (malignant), the first detectable stage is *carcinoma in situ* (CIS)—a noninvasive cervical cancer. As cancer cells multiply, some may invade the lining of the cervix, spread to nearby tissue, and enter the bloodstream or lymphatic system. When this happens, it can spread to other parts of the body.

According to the CDC (2015), cervical cancer used to be the leading cause of cancer death for women in the United States. However, in the past 40 years, the number of cases of cervical cancer and the number of deaths from cervical cancer have decreased significantly. This decline largely is the result of many women getting regular Pap tests, which can find cervical precancer before it turns into cancer. ACS, 2017a notes that the incidence of cervical cancer in the United States has decreased by more than 50% in the past 30 years because of widespread screening with cervical cytology, including the Pap test (Pap smear). New technologies, including HPV testing, continue to evolve, as do guidelines for managing abnormal results. The WHO (2016a) reports that cervical cancer rates are highest in high-income countries (as are the rates for all cancers). The lowest cervical cancer rates are found in Eastern Mediterranean countries. However, an unusually high rate of cervical cancer was found in the African region where income levels tend to be low.

The WHO (2015) notes that virtually all cases of cervical cancer are caused by human papillomavirus (HPV), and just two types of HPV, 16 and 18, are responsible for 70% of all cases. HPV is acquired through intercourse with an infected partner.

HEALTHY PEOPLE 2020 GOAL

Overview
Healthy People 2020 (2016) addresses the topic of cervical cancer as one of many cancers, but includes a goal and an objective specific to cervical cancer. Also, there is a category for Immunization and Infectious Diseases that has a goal for HPV (Healthy People 2020, 2016).

Goal
Reduce the number of new cancer cases, as well as the illness, disability, and death caused by cancer. Reduce invasive cervical cancer.

Objectives
- Reduce the rate of invasive uterine cervical cancer by 10% to 7.2 per 100,000 women
- Increase the proportion of women who receive a cervical cancer screening by 10% to 93%.
- Increase the proportion of women who were counseled by their provider about Pap tests by 10% to 66.2%.
- Increase the proportion of cancer survivors who are living 5 years or longer after diagnosis by 10% to 71.7%.
- Increase the vaccination coverage level of three doses of human papillomavirus vaccine for males and females 13 to 15 years of age.

SCREENING

The U.S. Preventive Services Task Force (USPSTF, 2012; being updated with a date of 2018) recommends a variety of screening protocols based on age and a combination of cervical cancer and HPV screenings. Recommendations include:
- Screening for cervical cancer in women ages 21 to 65 years with cytology (Pap smear) every 3 years
- Screening with a combination of cytology and HPV testing every 5 years for women ages 30 to 65 years who want to lengthen the screening interval

USPSTF recommends against screening for:
- Cervical cancer in women younger than age 21 years
- Cervical cancer in women older than age 65 years who have had adequate prior screening and are not otherwise at high risk for cervical cancer
- Cervical cancer in women who have had a hysterectomy with removal of the cervix and who do not have a history of a high-grade precancerous lesion (i.e., cervical intraepithelial neoplasia [CIN] grade 2 or 3) or cervical cancer
- Cervical cancer with HPV testing, alone or in combination with cytology, in women younger than age 30 years

RISK ASSESSMENT

According to ACS (2016d), risk factors for cervical cancer (and HPV) are:
- Human papilloma virus (HPV) infection
- Smoking
- Immunosuppression
- Chlamydia infection
- Diet low in fruits and vegetables
- Being overweight
- Intrauterine device use
- Having multiple full-term pregnancies
- Being younger than 17 at first full-term pregnancy
- Poverty
- Having a mother who took diethylstilbestrol (DES) while pregnant
- Family history of cervical cancer

CLIENT EDUCATION

Because lifestyle, especially related to sexual practices, has such an important effect on the development and prevention of cervical cancer, it is essential to teach ways to modify the risk of developing disease.

Teach Clients
- Avoid risky sexual practices: do not have sex at an early age; do not have multiple partners; avoid high-risk sexual activities and partners who participate in these.
- Consult with a health care professional about having an HPV vaccination for boys and girls as early as 9 years old and up to 26 years old, but especially between 10 and 11 years of age (ACOG, 2015).
- Follow the USPSTF guidelines for routine Pap smears.
- If your mother took DES to prevent miscarriage, maintain a careful preventive screening schedule.
- Eat nutritious food and have routine care for illnesses that weaken your immune system.
- Talk to your partner about your expectations of sexual health before becoming intimate.

27-3 EVIDENCE-BASED HEALTH PROMOTION AND DISEASE PREVENTION: COLORECTAL CANCER

INTRODUCTION
Excluding skin cancers, colorectal cancer (CRC) is the third most common cancer diagnosis in the United States (ACS, 2017b). The ACS estimates that there will be 95,520 new cases of colon cancer and 39,910 cases of rectal cancer in the United States in 2017. The lifetime risk for CRC is 1 in 21 men and 1 in 23 women. CRC is also the third leading cause of cancer-related death in the United States when men and women are considered separately and the second leading cause of death when men and women are considered together.

CRC originates in the large intestine or rectum as opposed to other cancers that may affect the colon, such as, for example, lymphoma, sarcoma, or melanoma (ACS, 2017b). Most CRCs begin as a polyp on the inner lining of the colon or rectum. Some types of polyps, but not all, can change to cancer over the course of several years. Another type of precancer, dysplasia, is an area in a polyp or in the lining of the colon or rectum where the cells look abnormal, but not like true cancer cells. Because cancer found early is readily treatable, early diagnosis is essential before the cancer has spread to deeper tissues.

HEALTHY PEOPLE 2020 GOAL
Overview
Healthy People 2020 (2014/16) address the topic of CRC as one of the many cancers but includes a goal and an objective specific to CRC.

Goal
Reduce the number of new cancer cases, as well as the illness, disability, and death caused by cancer. Reduce invasive CRC.

Objectives
- Reduce the number of invasive CRC cases to 39.9 new cases per 100,000 population.
- Increase the proportion of adults who receive colorectal screening based on the newest guidelines to 70.5%.
- Increase the proportion of cancer survivors who are living 5 years or longer after diagnosis by 10% to 71.7%.

SCREENING
The U.S. Preventive Services Task Force (USPSTF, 2016) recommends screening for CRC starting at age 50 years and continuing until age 75 (using fecal occult blood testing, sigmoidoscopy, or colonoscopy). The risks and benefits of the screening methods vary. The USPSTF recommends against routine screening for CRC in adults ages 76 to 85 years, except for individuals who have never been screened before and are likely to benefit (healthy enough to undergo treatment if CRC is detected, and who do not have comorbid conditions that would significantly limit life expectancy). The USPSTF recommends against any screening for adults over 85 years. The Task Force also concludes that the evidence is insufficient to assess the benefits and harms of computed tomographic colonography and fecal DNA testing as screening modalities for CRC.

The ACS (2016a) recommends that starting at age 50, an individual at average risk for CRC be screened by one of the following: a flexible sigmoidoscopy every 5 years, a colonoscopy every 10 years (should be done if other tests are positive in any case), a double contrast barium enema every 5 years, or a CT colonography every 5 years. In addition other tests recommended are a guaiac-based fecal blood test every year, a fecal immunochemical (FIT) test every year, or a stool DNA every 3 years. A rectal examination is not recommended as a standalone test. More elaborate testing is recommended for those persons with a history or polyps or others at high risk.

RISK ASSESSMENT
According to the ACS (2016b), the following risk factors for colorectal cancer cannot be changed:
- Older age, especially after 50
- African American or eastern European descent, especially Ashkenazi Jews
- Having cancer elsewhere in the body
- Having inflammatory bowel disease (either Crohn's or ulcerative colitis)
- Having a personal history of colorectal polyps or CRC
- Having a family history of colorectal polyps or CRC
- Having a personal history of breast cancer
- Having certain genetic syndromes: familial adenomatous polyposis (FAP) or hereditary nonpolyposis colorectal cancer (HNPCC), also known as Lynch syndrome
- Having diabetes mellitus type 2

Risk factors that can be changed:
- Being obese
- Physical inactivity
- Diet high in red meat and processed meat; cooking meat at high temperature (frying, broiling, grilling)
- Diet low in vegetables, fruits, and whole grains
- Smoking
- Alcohol use of more than 2 drinks a day for men and 1 drink a day for women.
- Human papilloma virus (about 95% of anal cancers are caused by HPV) (WHO, 2015)

CLIENT EDUCATION
Because lifestyle has such an important effect on the development and prevention of CRC, it is essential to teach ways to modify the risk of developing disease.

Teach Clients
- Call your health care provider if you notice any of the following symptoms: black, tarry stools, blood during a bowel movement, change in bowel habits, or unexplained weight loss.
- Follow preventive screening schedules as recommended by the USPSTF (2016) if you are between 50 and 75 years of age.
- If you are of African American or Eastern European descent, or if you have a family history of colon cancer or colon polyps, or if you have a history of inflammatory bowel syndromes or a history of breast cancer or other cancer, inform your health care provider and follow recommended screening protocols.
- Avoid a diet high in red and processed meat, high fat, or low in fiber.
- Avoid smoking cigarettes and keep alcohol intake to a minimum.

CASE STUDY

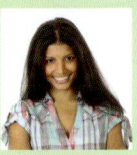

The case study of Ms. Carlisle that was introduced at the beginning of the chapter will now be used to demonstrate how a nurse would utilize the COLDSPA mnemonic to organize the client's presenting concerns and continue to interview the client for her gynecologic history.

Mnemonic	Question	Data Provided
Character	Describe the sign or symptom (feeling, appearance, sound, smell, or taste if applicable).	"I have pain and itching in and around my vagina and anus and burning when I urinate and have a bowel movement."
Onset	When did it begin?	"Started a few days after I slept with a man about 10 days ago. Then I broke out with some lesions and the pain, itching, and burning started."
Location	Where is it? Does it radiate? Does it occur anywhere else?	"The pain is right where my urine and stool come out. Sometimes the burning goes up my back and it hurts to sit on my bottom; it cramps right above my pubic area."
Duration	How long does it last? Does it recur?	"It has not gone away since it started, but it hurts even more when I go to the bathroom."
Severity	How bad is it? or How much does it bother you? What is your pain on a scale of 0–10?	"I can't do anything, it hurts so bad. On a scale of 0–10, I rate it as an 8."
Pattern	What makes it better or worse?	"I went to the pharmacy last night and bought pain reliever and that seemed to make it somewhat better."
Associated factors/How it **A**ffects the client	What other symptoms occur with it? How does it affect you?	"I stayed home from school today because I am so miserable."

After investigating Ms. Carlisle's complaint of recent outbreak of genital lesions and burning upon urination and defecation, the nurse continues with the health history.

Client states that her menstrual cycle is regular, occurring every 28 days. Last menstrual period was 2 weeks ago, beginning on the 10th and ending on the 13th. Experiences bloating and mild cramping with period. Denies abdominal discomfort. Appetite good. Has one bowel movement daily that is brown, soft, and formed. Denies constipation. No history of hemorrhoids. Denies vaginal discharge, lumps, swelling, or masses. Reports pain and itching in genitalia and anus. No loss of bowel or bladder control. However, she states that urine seems to burn her genital and anal area. Denies any prior gynecologic or rectal abnormalities.

Denies any family history of reproductive, gynecologic, or rectal cancer. Reports that she drinks one to two alcoholic beverages on the weekends only, but does not drink and drive. Denies cigarette smoking or use of illicit drugs. Denies texting and driving. States that her immunizations are up to date, including vaccination for HPV. Has had one sexual encounter; reports attempt at anal intercourse that was not successful. Denies condom use or any form of birth control. States, "I have always been healthy—I don't know why I behaved so stupidly and put my health at risk." Denies performance of monthly vulvar self-examination. Reports awareness of toxic shock syndrome and wears tampons only during heavy flow days, changing them every few hours. States has never had a Pap test.

Collecting Objective Data: Physical Examination

The physical examination of the female genitalia, anus, and rectum may create client anxiety. The client may be very embarrassed about exposing her genitalia and nervous that an infection or disorder will be discovered. Be sure to explain in detail what you will be doing throughout the examination and to explain the significance of each portion of the examination. Encourage the client to ask questions. Begin by sitting on a stool at the end of the examination table and draping the client so that only the vulva is exposed. This helps to preserve the client's modesty. Shine the light source so that it illuminates the genital area, allowing full visualization of all structures.

A digital rectal exam (DRE) may also be performed as part of the examination. Detecting problems with the anus and rectum is the primary objective of this examination. This is important because some conditions, such as cancerous tumors, may be asymptomatic. Early detection of a problem is one way to promote early treatment and a more positive outcome. Use this time (especially if the examination is a well examination) to integrate teaching about ways to reduce risk factors for diseases and disorders of the anus and rectum.

Proceed slowly and explain all steps of the examination as you proceed. When performing the examination of the anus and rectum, use gentle movements with your finger and make sure you use adequate lubrication. Listen to and watch the client for signs of discomfort or tensing muscles. Encourage relaxation and explain each step of the examination along the way. If the examination is being performed as part of the comprehensive physical examination, perform the examination of the anus and rectum at the end of the genitalia examination.

Preparing the Client

Tell the client before she comes in for the examination (at least 4 to 5 days ahead of time) not to douche, which is never recommended (Office on Women's Health, U.S. Department of Health and Human Services [USDHHS], 2015). Inform her not to use vaginal creams, jellies, medicines, or spermicidal foams for 2 to 3 days before a gynecologic examination, all of which can interfere with cervical cells. Also inform client not to have sex within 24 hours of the examination, as it can cause tissue inflammation (Johns Hopkins Medicine, n.d.).

When the client arrives, ask her to urinate before the examination so that she does not experience bladder discomfort. If a clean-catch urine specimen is needed, provide a container and vaginal wipes. When the client is in the examining room, ask her to remove her underwear and bra and to put on a gown with the opening in the back. If she is also having a breast examination at this time, suggest that she leave the opening in the front—a sheet can be used for draping. Tell her that she can leave her socks on if desired because the stirrups on the examination table are metal and may be cool. Leave the room while the client changes.

After the client has changed, enter the room with a chaperone and assist the client into the dorsal lithotomy position. This is a supine position with the feet in stirrups. Position the client's hips toward the bottom of the examination table so that the feet can rest comfortably in the stirrups. Ask the client not to put her hands over her head because this tightens the abdominal muscles. She should relax her arms at her sides. If possible, elevate the client's head and shoulders. This allows the nurse to maintain eye contact with the client during the examination and enables the client to see what the nurse is doing. Another technique is to offer the client a mirror so that she can view the examination (Fig. 27-4). This is a good way to teach normal anatomy and to get the client more involved and interested in maintaining or improving her genital health.

It is most logical for the female client to stay in the lithotomy position after the vaginal examination for the

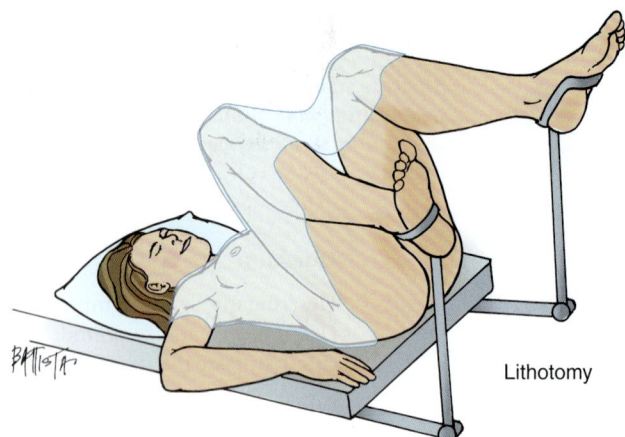

FIGURE 27-5 Lithotomy position for female anorectal examination.

anus and rectum examination (Fig. 27-5). See Figure 26-5 for additional positions that may be used for the anorectal examination.

No matter which position is chosen, the examiner must realize that he or she will only be able to examine to a certain point up in the rectum using the finger. If an examination of the upper rectum and sigmoid colon is necessary, a sigmoidoscopy should be arranged with her health care provider.

Equipment

Some of the following equipment is depicted in Figure 27-6:
- Stool
- Light
- Vaginal speculum
- Water-soluble lubricant
- Large swabs for vaginal examination
- Specimen container
- Gloves (nonsterile)
- Bifid spatula
- Endocervical broom
- pH paper
- Feminine napkins
- Hand-held mirror

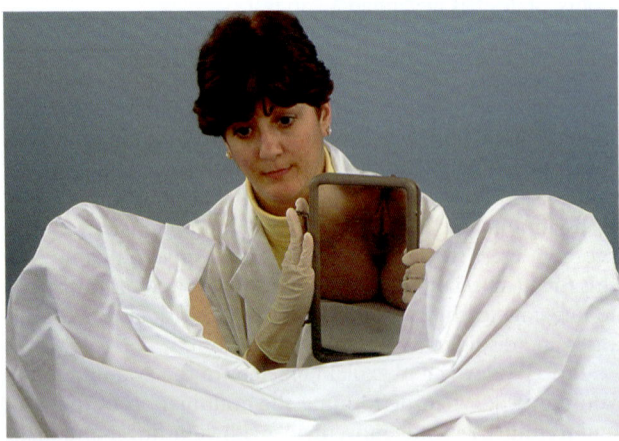

FIGURE 27-4 Mirror image of the examination promotes interest in gynecologic health (© B. Proud).

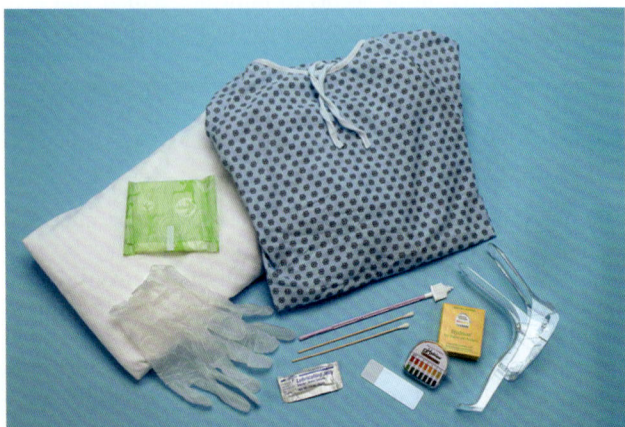

FIGURE 27-6 Some of the equipment needed for examining female genitalia, anus, and rectum include disposable gloves, speculums, slides and special solutions, spatulas, endocervical brooms, and other devices.

Physical Assessment

During the examination of the client, remember these key points:
- Respect the client's privacy.
- Perform the examination professionally and preserve the client's modesty.
- Prepare the client thoroughly for the physical examination to put the client at the greatest ease.
- Have a chaperone in the room with you when examining the female genitalia, rectum, and anus.
- Wash hands, wear gloves, and make sure equipment is between room temperature and body temperature.
- Inspect and palpate female external and internal structures correctly.
- Understand the structures and functions of the anorectal region.
- Use examination and laboratory equipment properly.
- Understand the difference between common variations and abnormal findings.

General Routine Screening versus Focused Specialty Assessment for the Female Genitalia, Anus, and Rectum

On a routine head-to-toe assessment the registered nurse would not typically need to inspect the external genitalia unless an alert client presents with problems or voices concerns with the female genitalia. Yet the nurse would inspect the external genitalia when performing procedures such as bathing clients who could not bathe themselves or when inserting a urinary catheter. The nurse would also want to inspect the vaginal area when irritation occurs from incontinence or immobility. Vaginal yeast infections are common in these situations and also with antibiotic therapy. Further inspection and palpation of the cervix and internal vagina, rectal examination, and Pap smear are performed by nurse practitioners or physicians.

General Routine Screening
- Inspect the mons pubis, labia majora, and perineum.
- Inspect the labia minora, clitoris, urethral meatus, and vaginal opening.
- Inspect the perianal area and sacrococcygeal area.

Focused Specialty Assessment
- Palpate Bartholin glands and urethra.
- Inspect the size of the vaginal opening and the angle of the vagina.
- Inspect the vaginal musculature.
- Inspect the cervix, vagina, and vaginal walls.
- Palpate the vaginal wall, cervix, uterus, and ovaries.
- Palpate the rectum and rectal sphincter.
- Perform the rectovaginal examination.
- Palpate the cervix through the anterior rectal wall.

ASSESSMENT PROCEDURE	NORMAL FINDINGS	ABNORMAL FINDINGS
External Genitalia		
Inspect the mons pubis. Wash your hands and put on gloves. As you begin the examination, note the distribution of pubic hair. Also be alert for signs of infestation.	Pubic hair is distributed in an inverted triangular pattern and there are no signs of infestation. **OLDER ADULT CONSIDERATIONS** Older clients may have gray, thinning pubic hair. Some clients may have piercing of the genital area.	Women's removal of or trimming of pubic hair has become normal. This practice varies with age, and razor shaving was by far the most popular removal method, with fewer than 5% of women engaging in waxing, electrolysis, or laser hair removal (Castleman, 2015). Lice or nits (eggs) at the base of the pubic hairs indicate infestation with pediculosis pubis. This condition, commonly referred to as "crabs," is most often transmitted by sexual contact.
Observe and palpate inguinal lymph nodes.	There should be no enlargement or swelling of the lymph nodes.	Enlarged inguinal nodes may indicate a vaginal infection or may be the result of irritation from hair removal.
Inspect the labia majora and perineum. Observe the labia majora	The labia majora are equal in size and free of lesions, swelling, and excoriation. A healed tear or episiotomy scar may be visible on the perineum if the client has given birth. The perineum should be smooth.	Lesions may be from an infectious disease, such as herpes or syphilis (see Abnormal Findings 27-1).

Continued on following page

ASSESSMENT PROCEDURE	NORMAL FINDINGS	ABNORMAL FINDINGS
External Genitalia (Continued)		
and perineum for lesions, swelling, and excoriation (Fig. 27-7).	Keep in mind the woman's childbearing status during inspection. For example, the labia of a woman who has not delivered offspring vaginally will meet in the middle. The labia of a woman who has delivered vaginally will not meet in the middle and may appear shriveled. **CULTURAL CONSIDERATIONS** In pubertal rites in some cultures, the clitoris is surgically removed and the labia are sutured, leaving only a small opening for menstrual flow. Once married, the woman undergoes surgery to reopen the labia (WHO, 2016b). It is increasingly common to find piercings of the female genitalia.	Excoriation and swelling may be from scratching or self-treatment of the lesions. Evaluate all lesions and refer the client to a primary care provider for treatment.
Inspect the labia minora, clitoris, urethral meatus, and vaginal opening. Use your gloved hand to separate the labia majora and inspect for lesions, excoriation, swelling, and/or discharge (Fig. 27-8).	The labia minora appear symmetric, dark pink, and moist. The clitoris is a small mound of erectile tissue, sensitive to touch. The normal size of the clitoris varies. The urethral meatus is small and slit-like. The vaginal opening is positioned below the urethral meatus. Its size depends on sexual activity or vaginal delivery. A hymen may cover the vaginal opening partially or completely.	Asymmetric labia may indicate abscess. Lesions, swelling, bulging in the vaginal opening, and discharge are abnormal findings (see Abnormal Findings 27-1). Excoriation may result from the client scratching or self-treating a perineal irritation.

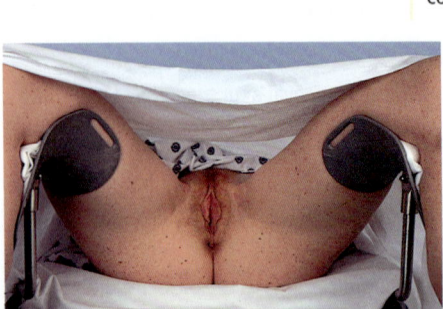

FIGURE 27-7 Inspecting the pubic hair, labia majora, and perineum (© B. Proud).

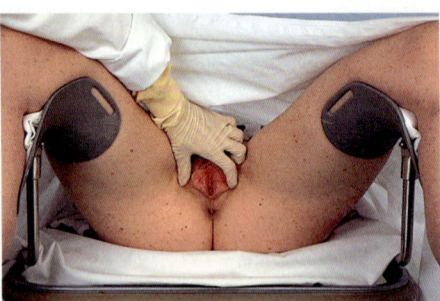

FIGURE 27-8 Inspecting the labia minora, clitoris, urethral orifice, and vaginal opening.

Palpate Bartholin glands. If the client has labial swelling or a history of it, palpate Bartholin glands for swelling, tenderness, and discharge (Fig. 27-9). Place your index finger in the vaginal opening and your thumb on the labia majora. With a gentle pinching motion, palpate from the inferior portion of the posterior labia majora to the anterior portion. Repeat on the opposite side.	Bartholin glands are usually soft, nontender, and drainage free.	Swelling, pain, and discharge may result from infection and abscess (Fig. 27-10). If you detect a discharge, obtain a specimen to send to the laboratory for culture.

ASSESSMENT PROCEDURE	NORMAL FINDINGS	ABNORMAL FINDINGS
Palpate the urethra. If the client reports urethral symptoms or urethritis, or if you suspect inflammation of Skene glands, insert your gloved index finger into the superior portion of the vagina and milk the urethra from the inside, pushing up and out (Fig. 27-11).	No drainage should be noted from the urethral meatus. The area is normally soft and nontender.	Drainage from the urethra indicates possible urethritis. Any discharge should be cultured. Urethritis may occur with infection with *Neisseria gonorrhoeae* or *Chlamydia trachomatis*.

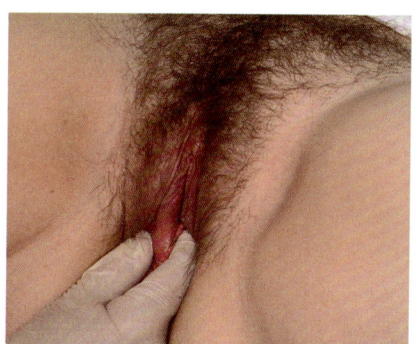

FIGURE 27-9 Technique for palpating Bartholin gland.

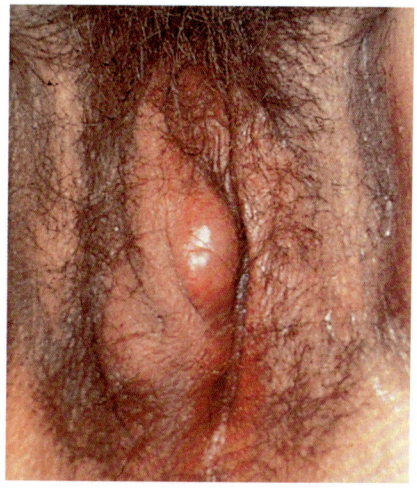

FIGURE 27-10 Abscess of Bartholin gland, a painful condition and common sign of *Neisseria gonorrhoeae* infection (© 1992, National Medical Slide Bureau, CMSP).

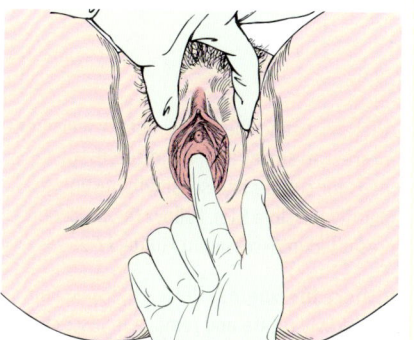

FIGURE 27-11 Milking the urethra.

Internal Genitalia

ASSESSMENT PROCEDURE	NORMAL FINDINGS	ABNORMAL FINDINGS
Inspect the size of the vaginal opening and the angle of the vagina. Insert your gloved index finger into the vagina, noting the size of the opening and whether the lining of the vagina is thinning or feels dry. Then attempt to touch the cervix. This will help you establish the size of the speculum you need to use for the examination and the angle at which to insert it. Next, while maintaining tension, gently pull the labia majora outward. Note hymenal configuration and transections or injury.	The normal vaginal opening varies in size according to the client's age, sexual history, and whether she has given birth vaginally. The vagina is typically tilted posteriorly at a 45-degree angle and should feel moist.	A condition in which the vagina becomes thinner and dryer is vaginal atrophy. This occurs when the body lacks estrogen. Some causes may include: menopause, breast feeding, surgical removal of the ovaries, and radiation or chemotherapy treatments for cancer or as a side effect of breast cancer hormone treatment. The risk increases if the client smokes, has not had a vaginal birth, or rarely has sexual activity, which increases blood flow to tissues (Mayo Clinic, 2013b). In children, any loss of hymenal tissue between the 3 o'clock position and the 9 o'clock position indicates trauma (penetration by digits, penis or foreign objects). See Chapter 31 for more information about sexual abuse in children. This finding is not as relevant in adults.
Inspect the vaginal musculature. Keep your index finger inserted in the client's vaginal opening. Ask the client to squeeze around your finger. Use your middle and index fingers to separate the labia minora. Ask the client to bear down.	The client should be able to squeeze around the examiner's finger. Typically, the nulliparous woman can squeeze tighter than the multiparous woman. No bulging and no urinary discharge.	Absent or decreased ability to squeeze the examiner's finger indicates decreased muscle tone. Decreased tone may decrease sexual satisfaction. Bulging of the anterior wall may indicate a cystocele. Bulging of the posterior wall may indicate a rectocele. If the cervix or uterus protrudes down, the client may have uterine prolapse (see Abnormal Findings 27-1). If urine leaks out, the client may have stress incontinence.

Continued on following page

ASSESSMENT PROCEDURE	NORMAL FINDINGS	ABNORMAL FINDINGS

Internal Genitalia (Continued)

Inspect the cervix. Follow the guidelines for using a speculum in Assessment Guide 27-1. With the speculum inserted in position to visualize the cervix, observe cervical color, size, and position. Also observe the surface and the appearance of the os. Look for discharge and lesions.	The surface of the cervix is normally smooth, pink, and even. Normally, it is midline in position and projects 1 to 3 cm into the vagina. In pregnant clients, the cervix appears blue (Chadwick sign). 🪑 **OLDER ADULT CONSIDERATIONS** **In older women, the cervix appears pale after menopause (Box 27-1).** The cervical os normally appears as a small, round opening in nulliparous women and appears slit-like in parous women (Fig. 27-12).	In a nonpregnant woman, a bluish cervix may indicate cyanosis; in a nonmenopausal woman, a pale cervix may indicate anemia. Redness may be from inflammation. Asymmetric, reddened areas, strawberry spots, and white patches are also abnormal. Cervical lesions may result from polyps, cancer, or infection. Cervical enlargement or projection into the vagina more than 3 cm may be from prolapse or tumor, and further evaluation is needed.
After inspecting the cervix, obtain specimens for the Pap smear and, if indicated, specimens for culture and sensitivity testing to identify possible STIs. Follow the procedure presented in Assessment Guide 27-2.	Cervical secretions are normally clear or white and without unpleasant odor. Secretions may vary according to timing within the menstrual cycle.	Colored, malodorous, or irritating discharge is abnormal; a specimen should be obtained for culture.
Inspect the vagina. Unlock the speculum and slowly rotate and remove it. Inspect the vagina as you remove the speculum. Note the vaginal color, surface, consistency, and any discharge. If you are preparing a wet mount slide, use a cotton swab to collect the specimen of vaginal secretions from the anterior vaginal fornix or the lateral vaginal walls before you collect the specimens for the Pap or other test. Avoid the posterior fornix, which is contaminated with cervical secretions. Use part of the wet mount sample to test the pH of the vaginal secretions.	The vagina should appear pink, moist, smooth, and free of lesions and irritation. It should also be free of any colored or malodorous discharge.	Reddened areas, lesions, and colored, malodorous discharge are abnormal and may indicate vaginal infections, STIs, or cancer (Abnormal Findings 27-2 and 27-3). Altered pH may indicate infection.

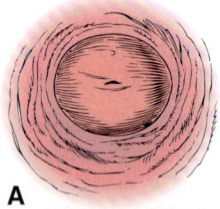 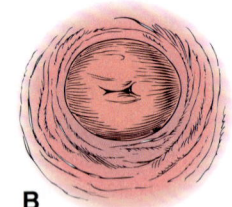

A   B

FIGURE 27-12 The cervical os in nulliparous women (A) and in parous women (B).

Bimanual Examination

Palpate the vaginal wall. Tell the client that you are going to do a manual examination and explain its purpose. Apply water-soluble lubricant to the gloved index and middle fingers of your dominant hand. Then stand and approach the client at the correct angle. Placing your nondominant hand on the client's lower abdomen, insert your index and middle fingers into the vaginal opening. Apply pressure to the posterior wall, and wait for the vaginal opening to relax before palpating the vaginal walls for texture and tenderness (Fig. 27-13).	The vaginal wall should feel smooth, and the client should not report any tenderness.	Tenderness or lesions may indicate infection.

ASSESSMENT PROCEDURE	NORMAL FINDINGS	ABNORMAL FINDINGS
Palpate the cervix. Advance your fingers until they touch the cervix and run fingers around the circumference. Palpate for: • Contour • Consistency • Mobility • Tenderness	The cervix should feel firm and soft (like the tip of your nose). It is rounded, and can be moved somewhat from side to side without eliciting tenderness.	A hard, immobile cervix may indicate cancer. Pain with movement of the cervix (cervical motion tenderness, CMT) may indicate infection (Chandelier sign).
Palpate the uterus. Move your fingers intravaginally into the opening above the cervix and gently press the hand resting on the abdomen downward, squeezing the uterus between the two hands (Fig. 27-14). Note uterine size, position, shape, and consistency.	The fundus, the large, upper end of the uterus, is normally round, firm, and smooth. In most women, it is at the level of the pubis; the cervix is aimed posteriorly (anteverted position). However, several other positions are considered normal (Box 27-2).	An enlarged uterus above the level of the pubis is abnormal; an irregular shape suggests abnormalities such as myomas (fibroid tumors) or endometriosis.
Attempt to bounce the uterus between your two hands to assess mobility and tenderness.	The normal uterus moves freely and is not tender.	A fixed or tender uterus may indicate fibroids, infection, or masses (see Abnormal Findings 27-4).
Palpate the ovaries. Slide your intravaginal fingers toward the left ovary in the left lateral fornix and place your abdominal hand on the left lower abdominal quadrant. Press your abdominal hand toward your intravaginal fingers and attempt to palpate the ovary (Fig. 27-15).	Ovaries are approximately 3 × 2 × 1 cm (or the size of a walnut) and almond-shaped.	Enlarged size, masses, immobility, and extreme tenderness are abnormal and should be evaluated (Abnormal Findings 27-5).

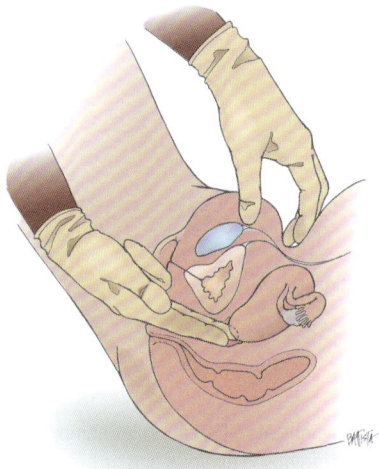

FIGURE 27-13 Palpating the vaginal walls.

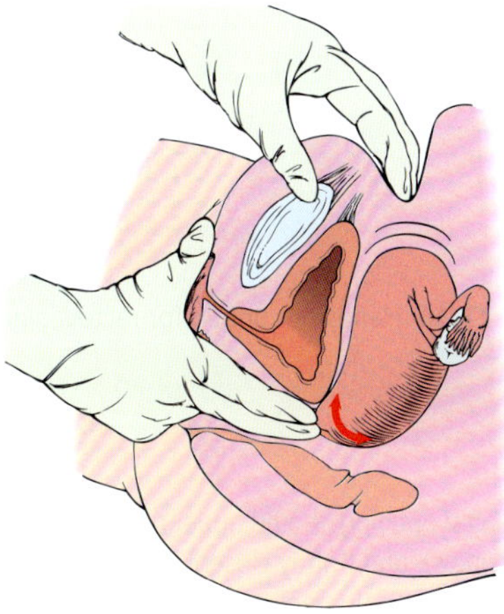

FIGURE 27-14 Palpating the uterus, bimanual examination.

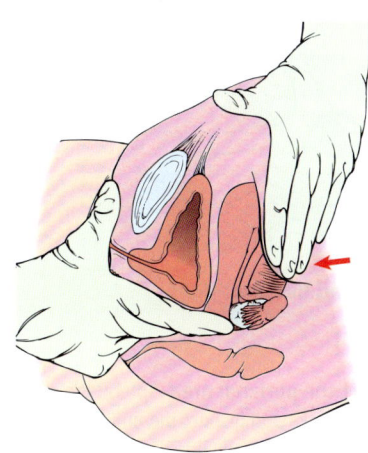

FIGURE 27-15 Palpating the ovaries.

Slide your intravaginal fingers to the right lateral fornix and attempt to palpate the right ovary. Note size, shape, consistency, mobility, and tenderness.

Withdraw your intravaginal hand and inspect the glove for secretions.

🎯 **CLINICAL TIP**
It is normal for the ovaries to be difficult or impossible to palpate in obese women, in postmenopausal women because the ovaries atrophy, and in women who are tense during the examination.

Ovaries are firm, smooth, mobile, and somewhat tender on palpation.

A clear, minimal amount of drainage appearing on the glove from the vagina is normal.

Large amounts of colorful, frothy, or malodorous secretions are abnormal. Ovaries that are palpable 3 to 5 years after menopause are also abnormal.

Continued on following page

ASSESSMENT PROCEDURE	NORMAL FINDINGS	ABNORMAL FINDINGS
Rectovaginal Examination		
Explain that you are going to perform a rectovaginal examination and explain its purpose. Forewarn the client that she may feel uncomfortable as if she wants to move her bowels but that she will not. Encourage her to relax. **Change the glove** on your dominant hand and lubricate your index and middle fingers with a water-soluble lubricant.		
Ask the client to bear down to promote relaxation of the sphincter and insert your index finger into the vaginal orifice and your middle finger into the rectum. While pushing down on the abdominal wall with your other hand, palpate the internal reproductive structures through the anterior rectal wall (Fig. 27-16). Pay particular attention to the area behind the cervix, the rectovaginal septum, the cul-de-sac, and the posterior uterine wall. Withdraw your vaginal finger and continue with the rectal examination.	The rectovaginal septum is normally smooth, thin, movable, and firm. The posterior uterine wall is normally smooth, firm, round, movable, and nontender.	Masses, thickened structures, immobility, and tenderness are abnormal.

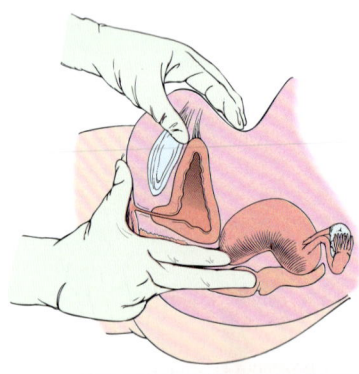

FIGURE 27-16 Hands positioned for rectovaginal examination.

Anus and Rectum

INSPECTION

Inspect the perianal area. Spread the client's buttocks and inspect the anal opening and surrounding area (Fig. 27-17) for the following: • Lumps • Ulcers	The anal opening should appear hairless, moist, and tightly closed. The skin around the anal opening is coarser and more darkly pigmented. The surrounding perianal area should be free of redness, lumps, ulcers, lesions, and rashes.	Lesions may indicate STIs, cancer, or hemorrhoids. A thrombosed external hemorrhoid appears swollen. It is itchy, painful, and bleeds when the client passes stool. A previously thrombosed hemorrhoid appears as a skin tag that protrudes from the anus. A painful mass that is hardened and reddened suggests a perianal abscess. A swollen skin tag on the anal margin may indicate a fissure in the anal canal. Redness and excoriation may be from scratching an area infected by fungi or pinworms.

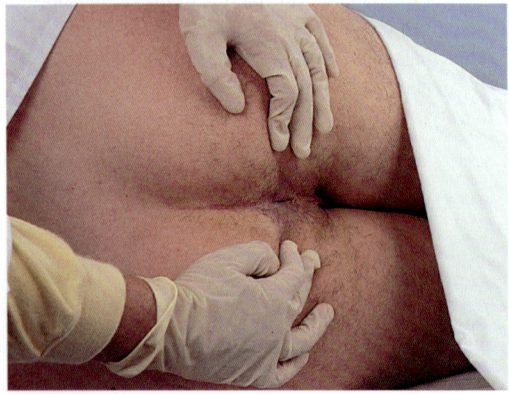

FIGURE 27-17 Inspecting the perianal area.

ASSESSMENT PROCEDURE	NORMAL FINDINGS	ABNORMAL FINDINGS
• Lesions • Rashes • Redness • Fissures Thickening of the epithelium		A small opening in the skin that surrounds the anal opening may be an anorectal fistula (see Abnormal Findings 26-4). Thickening of the epithelium suggests repeated trauma from anal intercourse.
Ask the client to perform Valsalva maneuver by straining or bearing down. Inspect the anal opening for any bulges or lesions. **CLINICAL TIP** Document any abnormalities by noting position in relation to a face of a clock.	No bulging or lesions appear.	Bulges of red mucous membrane may indicate a rectal prolapse. Hemorrhoids or an anal fissure may also be seen (see Abnormal Findings 26-4).
Inspect the sacrococcygeal area. Inspect this area for any signs of swelling, redness, dimpling, or hair.	Area is normally smooth, and free of redness and hair.	A reddened, swollen, or dimpled area covered by a small tuft of hair located midline on the lower sacrum suggests a pilonidal cyst (see Abnormal Findings 26-4).

PALPATION

Palpate the anus. Inform the client that you are going to perform the internal examination at this point. Explain that it may feel like her bowels are going to move but that this will not happen. Lubricate your gloved index finger; ask the client to bear down. As the client bears down, place the pad of your index finger on the anal opening and apply slight pressure; this will cause relaxation of the sphincter. **SAFETY TIP** *Never use your fingertip— this causes the sphincter to tighten and, if forced into the rectum, may cause pain.*	Client's sphincter relaxes, permitting entry.	Sphincter tightens, making further examination unrealistic.
When you feel the sphincter relax, insert your finger gently with the pad facing down (Figs. 27-18 and 27-19). **SAFETY TIP** *If severe pain prevents your entrance to the anus, do not force the examination.*	Examination finger enters anus.	Examination finger cannot enter the anus.

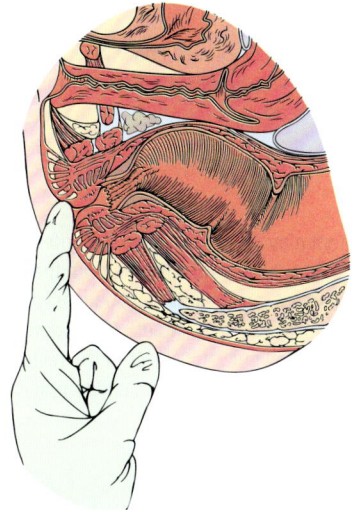

FIGURE 27-18 Relaxing the anal sphincter.

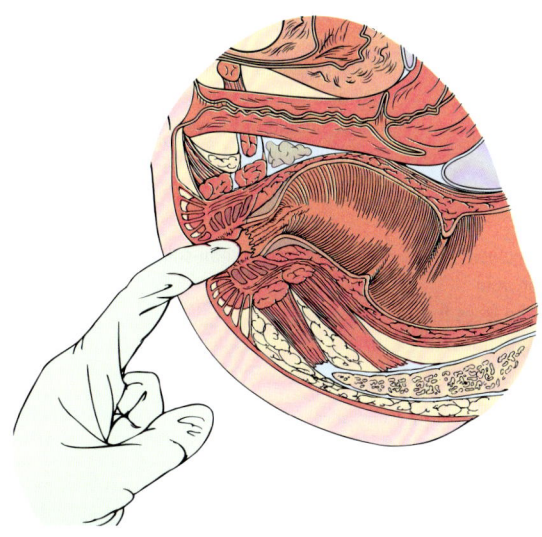

FIGURE 27-19 Palpating the anus.

Continued on following page

ASSESSMENT PROCEDURE	NORMAL FINDINGS	ABNORMAL FINDINGS
Anus and Rectum (Continued)		
If the sphincter does not relax and the client reports severe pain, spread the gluteal folds with your hands in close approximation to the anus and attempt to visualize a lesion that may be causing the pain. If tension is maintained on the gluteal folds for 60 seconds, the anus will dilate normally.		
Ask the client to tighten the external sphincter; note the tone.	The client can normally close the sphincter around the gloved finger.	Poor sphincter tone may be the result of a spinal cord injury, previous surgery, trauma, or a prolapsed rectum. Tightened sphincter tone may indicate anxiety, scarring, or inflammation.
Rotate finger to examine the muscular anal ring. Palpate for tenderness, nodules, and hardness.	The anus is normally smooth, nontender, and free of nodules and hardness.	Tenderness may indicate hemorrhoids, fistula, or fissure. Nodules may indicate polyps or cancer. Hardness may indicate scarring or cancer.
Palpate the rectum. Insert your finger further into the rectum as far as possible (Fig. 27-20). Next, turn your hand clockwise then counterclockwise. This allows palpation of as much rectal surface as possible. Note tenderness, irregularities, nodules, and hardness.	The rectal mucosa is normally soft, smooth, nontender, and free of nodules.	Hardness and irregularities may be from scarring or cancer. Nodules may indicate polyps or cancer (see Abnormal Findings 26-4).

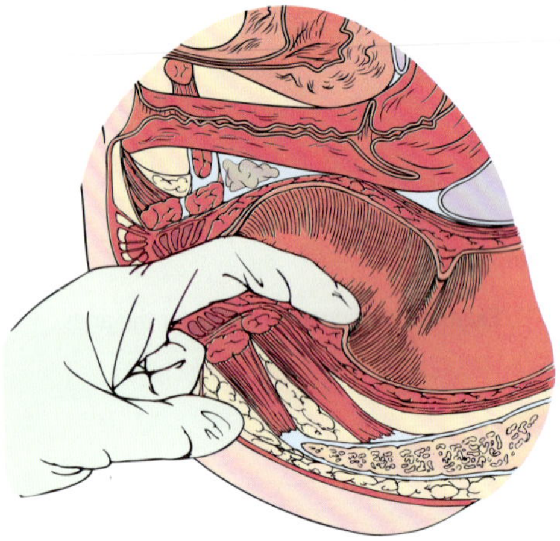

FIGURE 27-20 Palpating the rectal wall.

Palpate the cervix through the anterior rectal wall.	Cervix palpated as small round mass. May also palpate tampon or retroverted uterus. Should not have any bright red blood when gloved finger is removed.	Bright red blood on gloved finger when removed. Large mass palpated. Do not mistake tampon for mass.

CHECK STOOL

Inspect the stool. Withdraw your gloved finger. Inspect any fecal matter on your glove. Assess the color, and test the feces for occult blood. Provide the client with a towel to wipe the anorectal area.	Stool is normally semi-solid, brown, and free of blood.	Black stool may indicate upper gastrointestinal bleeding, gray or tan stool results from the lack of bile pigment, and yellow stool suggests steatorrhea (increased fat content). Blood detected in the stool may indicate cancer of the rectum or colon. Refer the client for an endoscopic examination of the colon.

ASSESSMENT GUIDE 27-1 Using a Speculum

1. Before using the speculum, choose the instrument that is the correct size for the client. Vaginal speculums come in two basic types:
   - *Graves speculum*—appropriate for most adult women and available in various lengths and widths.
   - *Pederson speculum*—appropriate for virgins and some postmenopausal women who have a narrow vaginal orifice. Speculums can be metal with a thumbscrew that is tightened to lock the blades in place or plastic with a clip that is locked to keep the blades in place. (Plastic speculums are shown in Fig. A.)

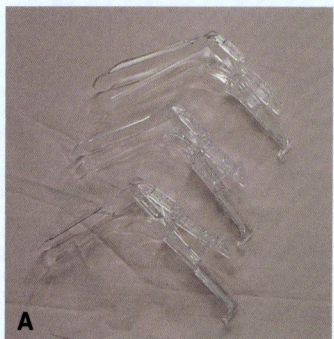

A

2. Encourage the client to take deep breaths and to maintain her feet in the stirrups with her knees resting in an open, relaxed fashion.
3. Place two fingers of your gloved nondominant hand against the posterior vaginal wall and wait for relaxation to occur.
4. Insert the fingers of your gloved nondominant hand about 2.5 cm into the vagina and spread them slightly while pushing down against the posterior vagina.
5. Lubricate the blades of the speculum with vaginal secretions from the client. Do not use commercial lubricants on the speculum. Lubricants are typically bacteriostatic and will alter vaginal pH and the cell specimens collected for cytologic, bacterial, and viral analysis.
6. Hold the speculum with two fingers around the blades and the thumb under the screw or lock. This is important for keeping the blades closed. Position the speculum so that the blades are vertical.
7. Insert the speculum between your fingers into the posterior portion of the vaginal orifice at a 45-degree angle downward. When the blades pass your fingers inside the vagina, rotate the closed speculum so that the blades are in a horizontal position (Fig. B).

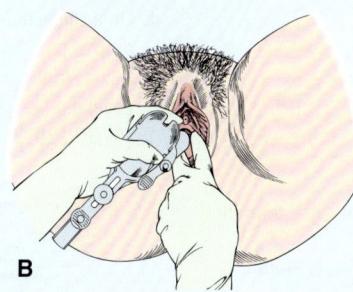

B

CLINICAL TIP
Be careful during the speculum insertion not to pinch the labia or pull the pubic hair. If the vaginal orifice seems tight or you are having trouble inserting the speculum, ask the client to bear down. This may help relax the muscles of the perineum and promote opening of the orifice.

8. Continue inserting the speculum until the base touches the fingertips inside the vagina.
9. Remove the fingers of your gloved nondominant hand from the client's posterior vagina.
10. Press handles together (Fig. C) to open blades and allow visualization of the cervix.

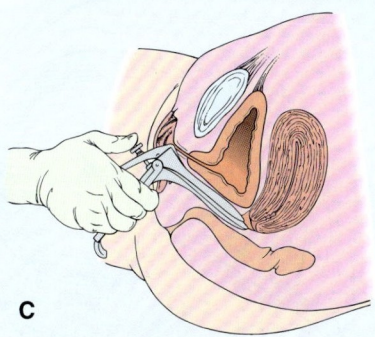

C

11. Secure the speculum in place by tightening the thumbscrew or locking the plastic clip (Fig. D).

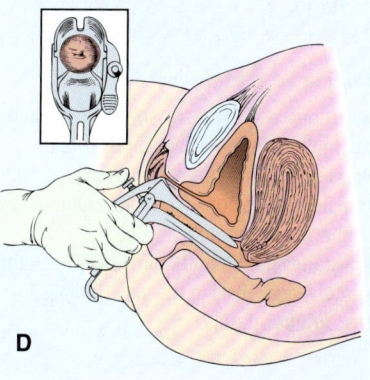

D

ASSESSMENT GUIDE 27-2 Obtaining Tissue Specimens for Analysis

Various laboratory tests are based on an analysis of cells obtained from tissue specimens and prepared on culture media or on slides for microscopic examination. For women especially, such tests are life-saving tools that can detect disease in early treatable stages. Some methods for obtaining tissue specimens follow.

Papanicolaou (Pap) Smear

The new standard of care for the Pap smear is liquid-based technology. The traditional Pap smear is estimated to be 80% accurate in detection of low- and high-grade lesions of the cervix. The thin prep, or liquid-based, technology has improved accuracy of findings by about 54%. The specimen for the Pap smear is obtained in the same way, using a wooden spatula, cotton swab, or brush; but the specimen is placed in the preservative solution rather than on a slide (Lab Tests Online, 2012). This solution may be used to test for human papilloma virus (HPV) and to determine HPV type.

Obtaining an Ectocervical and Endocervical Specimen

The procedure for gathering endocervical and ectocervical specimens is performed on nonpregnant clients. This combined procedure uses a special cytobroom to collect both endocervical and ectocervical cells.

1. Insert the cytobroom into the cervical os (Fig. A).
2. Rotate the cytobroom in a full circle five times, collecting cell specimens from the squamocolumnar junction and the cervical surface.

Continued on following page

ASSESSMENT GUIDE 27-2   Obtaining Tissue Specimens for Analysis (Continued)

3. Withdraw the cytobroom.
4. Swish the broom in the preservative solution by pushing the broom into the bottom of the vial 10 times, forcing the bristles apart. Swirl the broom vigorously to further release material.
5. Discard the cytobroom.
6. Tighten the cap on the preservative. This solution is sent to the laboratory.

7. Record client's name and date on the vial.
8. Send the vial to laboratory.

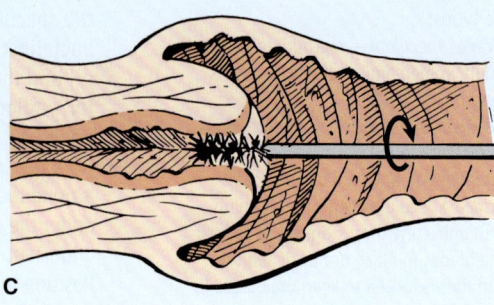
C

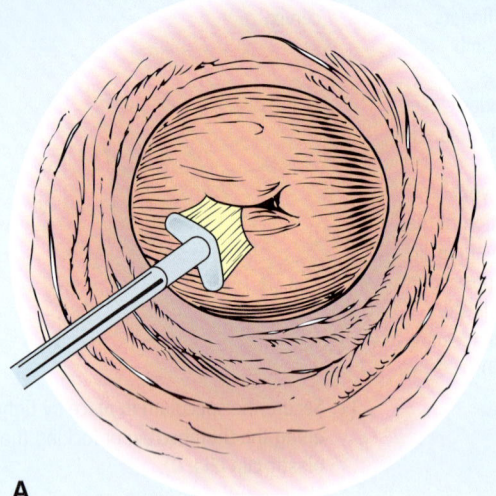
A

Obtaining an Ectocervical Specimen

1. Insert one end of plastic spatula (i.e., longer on the ends than in the middle) into the cervical os (Fig. B).
2. Press down and rotate the spatula, scraping the cervix and the transformation zone (squamocolumnar junction) in a full circle.
3. Withdraw the spatula.
4. Rinse the spatula in the preservative solution by swishing the spatula vigorously in the vial 10 times.
5. Discard the spatula.

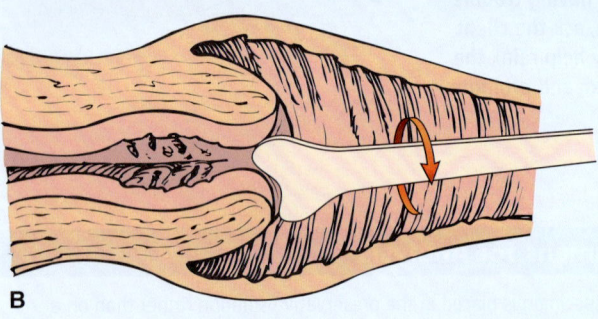
B

Obtaining an Endocervical Specimen

1. Insert the endocervical brush into the cervical os. Use the endocervical brush to increase the number of cells obtained for analysis.
2. Rotate the brush one half-turn in one direction (Fig. C) very gently to minimize possible bleeding.
3. Withdraw the brush.
4. Rinse the brush in the preservative solution by rotating the device in the solution 10 times while pushing against the vial wall. Swirl the brush vigorously to further release material.
5. Discard the brush.
6. Tighten the cap on the solution.

Vaginal Specimen

1. Select appropriately sized speculum; warm speculum and test it on the patient's leg for comfortable temperature.
2. Insert speculum at a 45-degree angle, then rotate and open when completely inserted.
3. Obtain a specimen of vaginal fluid from the posterior fornix (see Fig. 27-2, p. 638).
4. On a single glass slide, place a drop of sodium chloride (NaCl) and a drop of potassium hydroxide (KOH) on separate ends of the slide.
5. Mix a small amount of vaginal fluid with each solution and apply coverslip (Association of Professors of Gynecology and Obstetrics [APGO], 2008).

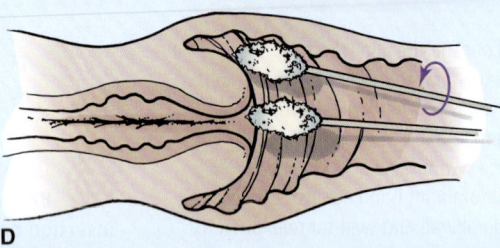
D

CLINICAL TIP
Do not apply great pressure when transferring the specimens onto the glass slides. Too much pressure may alter or destroy the cell structure. In addition, if you will be obtaining a specimen with the endocervical brush, do so after you obtain a tissue specimen with a spatula because bleeding may follow use of the brush.

Culture Specimens: Gonorrhea and Chlamydia

Specimens for gonorrhea or *Chlamydia* cultures are obtained if you suspect the client has these STIs. The exact procedures for gathering and preparing the specimens vary according to each laboratory's policy. General guidelines follow.

1. Insert a cotton-tipped applicator into the cervical os and rotate it in a full circle.
2. Leave the applicator in place for approximately 20 seconds to make sure it becomes saturated with specimen.
3. Withdraw the applicator.
4. For *Neisseria gonorrhoeae* cultures: Spread the specimen onto a special culture plate (Thayer-Martin) in a "Z" pattern while rotating the applicator, or put in a liquid medium for transport and send to the laboratory.
5. For *Chlamydia trachomatis* cultures: Immerse a special swab (provided with test medium) in a liquid medium and refrigerate the sample until it is transported to the laboratory.

BOX 27-1 COMMON VARIATIONS OF THE CERVIX

Certain cervical variations are common. Such variations include cervical eversion, Nabothian cysts, differently shaped cervical os (in nulliparous women and parous women), and various lacerations.

CERVICAL EVERSION

This is a normal finding in many women and usually occurs after vaginal birth or when the woman takes oral contraceptives. The columnar epithelium from within the endocervical canal is everted and appears as a deep red, rough ring around the cervical os, surrounded by the normal pink color of the cervix.

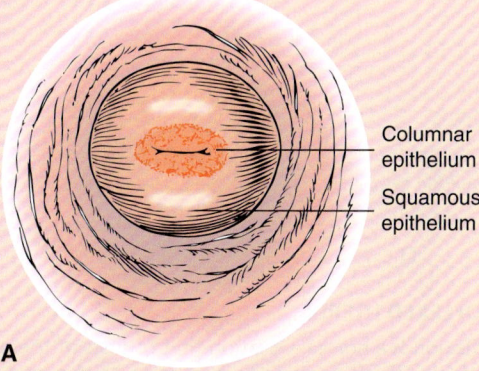

Columnar epithelium
Squamous epithelium

A

NABOTHIAN (RETENTION) CYSTS

Nabothian (retention) cysts (normal findings after childbirth) are small (less than 1 cm), yellow, translucent nodules on the cervical surface. Normal odorless and nonirritating secretions may be present on pink, healthy tissue. (Irritating secretions would appear on reddened tissue.) The viscosity of these secretions ranges from thin to thick; their appearance ranges from clear to cloudy, depending on the phase of the menstrual cycle.

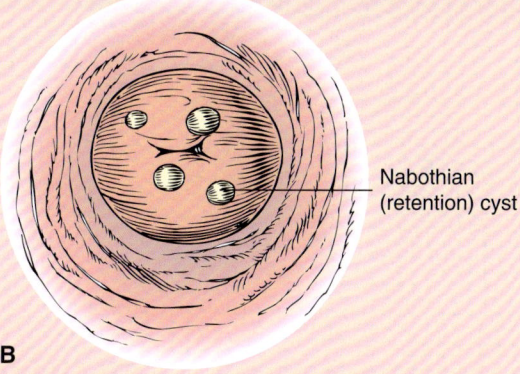

Nabothian (retention) cyst

B

Nabothian cysts may occur when the everted columnar epithelium spontaneously transforms into squamous epithelium, a process called *squamous metaplasia*. Occasionally the tissue blocks endocervical glands and cysts develop.

BILATERAL TRANSVERSE LACERATION

This drawing illustrates a type of healed laceration that may be seen in a woman who has given birth vaginally.

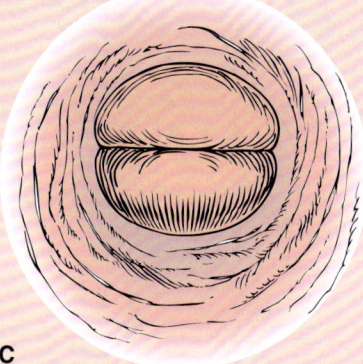

C

UNILATERAL TRANSVERSE LACERATION

Vaginal birth may cause trauma to the cervix and produce tears or lacerations. Therefore, healed lacerations may be seen as a normal variation. This drawing illustrates a unilateral transverse laceration.

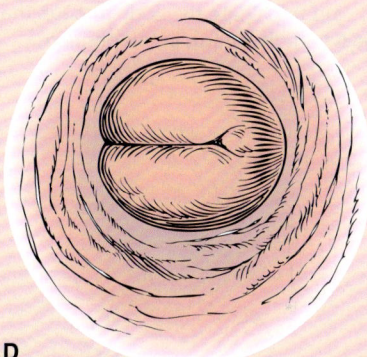

D

STELLATE LACERATION

This drawing illustrates a type of healed laceration that may be seen in a woman who has given birth vaginally.

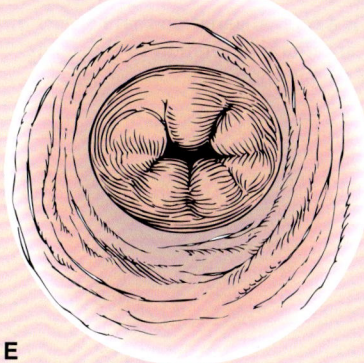

E

BOX 27-2 COMMON VARIATIONS IN POSITIONS OF THE UTERUS

ANTEVERTED
This is the most typical position of the uterus. The cervix is pointed posteriorly, and the body of the uterus is at the level of the pubis over the bladder.

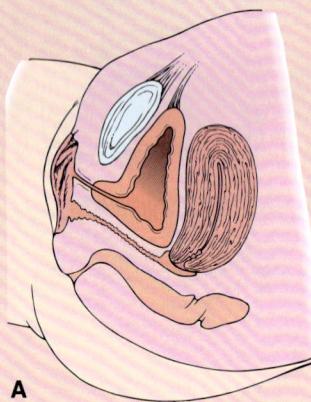

A

MIDPOSITION
This is a normal variation. The cervix is pointed slightly more anteriorly (compared with the anteverted position), and the body of the uterus is positioned more posteriorly than the anteverted position, midway between the bladder and the rectum. It may be difficult to palpate the body through the abdominal and rectal walls with the uterus in this position.

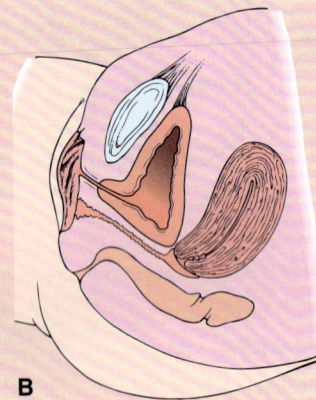

B

ANTEFLEXED
Anteflexion is a normal variation that consists of the uterine body flexed anteriorly in relation to the cervix. The position of the cervix remains normal.

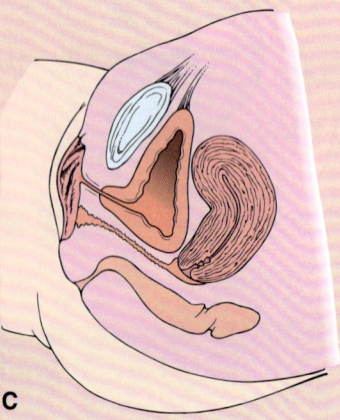

C

RETROVERTED UTERUS
Retroversion is a normal variation that consists of the cervix and body of the uterus tilting backward. The uterine wall may not be palpable through the abdominal wall or the rectal wall in moderate retroversion. However, if the uterus is prominently retroverted, the wall may be felt through the posterior fornix or the rectal wall.

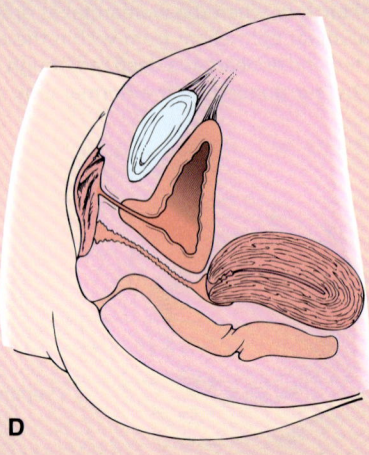

D

RETROFLEXED UTERUS
Retroflexion is a normal variation that consists of the uterine body being flexed posteriorly in relation to the cervix. The position of the cervix remains normal. The body of the uterus may be felt through the posterior fornix or the rectal wall.

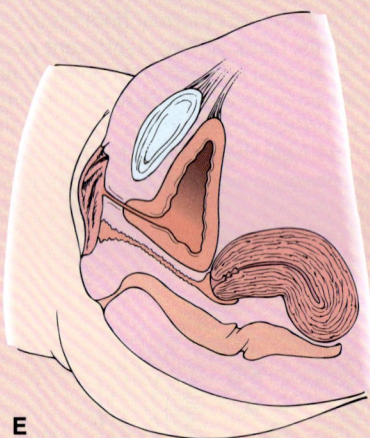

E

CASE STUDY

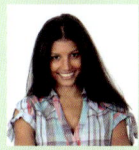

The chapter case study is now used to demonstrate the physical examination of Ms. Carlisle's external and internal genitalia, and the anus and rectum.

Visual inspection discloses normal hair distribution of the mons pubis, with lesions present as vesicles. Ulcerations noted as well. Labia majora with mild erythema and vesicular lesions along with mild excoriation. Labia minora dark pink, moist, and free of lesions or excoriation. Vesicles and ulcerations extend into the perianal area. Visual inspection of the anus reveals multiple vesicular lesions noted around the anal opening. Upon palpation of the inguinal area and external genitalia, no masses or edema were noted to the inguinal lymph nodes bilaterally. Mild edema noted to the labia majora. Labia minora free from edema and discharge. Bartholin glands soft, nontender, and free from discharge. No bulging at vaginal orifice. No discharge from urethral opening. Routine Pap smear performed. Vaginal walls smooth and pink. Cervix slightly anterior, pink, smooth in appearance, slit-like os, without lesions or discharge present. Bimanual examination indicates cervix mobile, nontender, and firm, with no masses or nodules detected. Firm fundus located anteriorly at level of symphysis pubis, without tenderness, lesions, or nodules. Smooth, firm, almond-shaped, mobile ovaries approximately 3 cm in size palpated bilaterally, no excessive tenderness or masses noted. No malodorous, colored vaginal discharge on gloved fingers. Firm, smooth, nontender, movable posterior uterine wall and firm, smooth, thin, movable rectovaginal septum palpated during rectovaginal examination. Good sphincter tone noted with the anus, noted to be smooth, nontender, and free of nodules and hardness. Fecal matter on gloved finger reveals semi-soft, brown stool.

Validating and Documenting Findings

Validate the female genitalia, anus, and rectum assessment data that you have collected. This is necessary to verify that the data are reliable and accurate. Document the assessment data following the health care facility or agency policy.

CASE STUDY

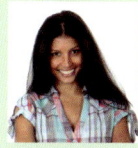

Think back to the case study. The nurse documented the following subjective and objective assessment findings of the evaluation of Ms. Carlisle.

Biographical Data: MD, born January 26, 1990. Caucasian female. Full-time student, history major.

Reason for Seeking Care: "I feel like I have the flu—no energy, a headache, and fever; also, urinating and having a bowel movement hurts a lot." Temperature taken at home was 100.6°F.

History of Present Health Concern (pertinent to the female genitalia): Vaginal area discomfort that began with a recent outbreak of genital lesions after a sexual encounter 10 days ago with a fellow male student. This was her first and only sexual experience. Rates pain as an 8 out of 10 on a scale of 0–10 and describes it as sharp and burning. Denies the use of any protection or birth control, stating that he refused to use anything and she didn't insist.

Personal History: Regular menstrual cycle occurring every 28 days. Last menstrual period was 2 weeks ago, beginning on the 10th and ending on the 13th. Experiences bloating and mild cramping with period. Appetite good. Has one bowel movement daily that is brown, soft, and formed. Denies constipation. No history of hemorrhoids. Denies vaginal discharge, lumps, swelling, or masses. Reports pain and itching in genitalia and anus. Denies loss of bowel or bladder. States, however, that her urine seems to burn her genital and anal area. Denies any prior gynecologic abnormalities.

Family History: Denies any family history of reproductive or gynecologic cancer.

Lifestyle and Health Practices: Reports that she drinks one to two alcoholic beverages on the weekends only, but does not drink and drive. Denies cigarette smoking or use of illicit drugs. Denies texting and driving. States that her immunizations are up to date, including the vaccination for HPV. Has had one sexual encounter, denies condom use or any form of birth control. States, "I have always been healthy—I don't know why I behaved so stupidly and put my health at risk." Denies performance of monthly vulvar self-examination. Reports awareness of toxic shock syndrome and wears tampons only during heavy flow days, changing them every few hours. States has never had a Pap test.

Physical Examination Findings: Visual inspection discloses normal hair distribution of the mons pubis, with lesions present as vesicles. Ulcerations noted as well. Labia majora with mild erythema and vesicular lesions along with mild excoriation. Labia minora dark pink, moist, and free of lesions or excoriation. Vesicles and ulcerations extend into the perianal area. Visual inspection of the anus reveals multiple vesicular lesions noted around the anal opening. Upon palpation of the inguinal area and external genitalia, no masses or edema were noted to the inguinal lymph nodes bilaterally. Mild edema noted to the labia majora. Labia minora free from edema and discharge. Bartholin glands soft, nontender, and free from discharge. No bulging at vaginal orifice. No discharge from urethral opening. Routine Pap smear performed. Vaginal walls smooth and pink. Cervix slightly anterior, pink, smooth in appearance, slit-like os, without lesions or discharge present. Bimanual examination indicates cervix mobile, nontender and firm, with no masses or nodules

> detected. Firm fundus located anteriorly at level of symphysis pubis, without tenderness, lesions, or nodules. Smooth, firm, almond-shaped, mobile ovaries approximately 3 cm in size palpated bilaterally, no excessive tenderness or masses noted. No malodorous, colored vaginal discharge on gloved fingers. Firm, smooth, nontender, movable posterior uterine wall and firm, smooth, thin, movable rectovaginal septum palpated during rectovaginal examination. Good sphincter tone noted with the anus noted to be smooth, nontender, and free of nodules and hardness. Fecal matter on gloved finger reveals semi-soft, brown stool.

ANALYSIS OF DATA: DIAGNOSTIC REASONING

After collecting subjective and objective data pertaining to the female genitalia, anus and rectum, identify abnormal findings and client strengths. Then cluster the data to reveal any significant patterns or abnormalities; these data may be used to make clinical judgments about the status of the client's genitalia, anal, and rectal health.

Selected Nursing Diagnoses

Following is a listing of selected nursing diagnoses (health promotion, risk, or actual) that the nurse may identify when analyzing the cue clusters.

Health Promotion Diagnoses

- Readiness for Enhanced Health Management: Requests information on external genitalia examination
- Readiness for Enhanced Health Management: Requests information on ways to prevent sexually transmitted diseases (STDs) or infections (STIs)
- Readiness for Enhanced Health Management: Requests information on ways to prevent yeast infections.
- Readiness for Enhanced Health Management: Requests information on birth control
- Readiness for Enhanced Health Management: Requests information on cessation of menses and hormone-replacement therapy
- Readiness for Enhanced Health Management: Requests information on purpose and need for colorectal examination

Risk Diagnoses

- Risk for Infection related to unprotected sexual intercourse
- Risk for Disturbed Body Image related to perceived effects on feminine role and sexuality
- Risk for Ineffective Health Maintenance related to lack of knowledge of need for recommended colorectal examination
- Risk for Impaired Skin Integrity in rectal area related to chronic irritation secondary to diarrhea
- Risk-Prone Behavior related to sexual encounters with multiple partners
- Risk-Prone Behavior related to having unprotected intercourse with more than one partner

Actual Diagnoses

- Fear of ovarian cancer related to high incidence of risk factors
- Ineffective Sexuality Pattern related to decreased libido
- Ineffective Health Management related to lack of knowledge of external genitalia self-examination
- Acute Pain: Dysuria related to infection
- Anticipatory Grieving related to impending loss of reproductive organs secondary to gynecologic surgery
- Ineffective Sexuality Pattern related to perceptions of effects of surgery on sexual functioning and attractiveness
- Acute Pain related to surgical incision
- Acute Pain: Dyspareunia (painful intercourse) related to inadequate vaginal lubrication
- Acute Pain: Rectal related to unknown cause
- Diarrhea related to chronic inflammatory bowel disease
- Ineffective Sexuality Patterns related to feelings of loss of femininity/masculinity and sexual attractiveness secondary to chronic diarrhea or pain
- Situational Low Self-Esteem related to loss of control over bowel elimination
- Bowel Incontinence related to chronic diarrhea
- Constipation related to low intake of high fiber foods

Selected Collaborative Problems

After grouping the data, certain collaborative problems may become apparent. Remember that collaborative problems differ from nursing diagnoses in that they cannot be prevented by nursing interventions. However, these physiologic complications of medical conditions can be detected and monitored by the nurse. In addition, the nurse can use physician- and nurse-prescribed interventions to minimize the complications posed by these problems. The nurse may also have to refer the client in such situations for further treatment of the problem. Following is a list of collaborative problems that may be identified when assessing the female genitalia. These problems are worded as Risk for Complications (RC), followed by the problem:

- RC: Gonorrhea
- RC: Syphilis
- RC: *Chlamydia*
- RC: Infertility
- RC: Pregnancy
- RC: Urinary incontinence
- RC: Ovarian nodule
- RC: Abnormal Pap smear result
- RC: Vaginal bleeding
- RC: Fistula
- RC: Fissure
- RC: Hemorrhoids
- RC: Rectal bleeding
- RC: Rectal abscess

Medical Problems

After grouping the data, the client's signs and symptoms may clearly require referral to a primary care provider for medical diagnosis (e.g., uterine fibroids) and treatment.

CASE STUDY

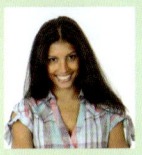

After collecting and analyzing the data for Melinda Carlisle, the nurse determines that the following conclusions are appropriate:
- Acute pain: genitalia and perianal area r/t ulcerations and vesicles from probable STI
- Situation Low Self-Esteem r/t perceived lack of assertiveness in protecting self
- Risk for Ineffective Sexuality Pattern r/t change in sexual behavior and values conflict

The nurse should refer the client to a physician for diagnosis and treatment of her genital lesions. To view an algorithm depicting the process of diagnostic reasoning for this case, go to thePoint.

Interdisciplinary Verbal Communication of Assessment Findings Using SBAR

SITUATION: MC, a 22-year-old female college student, comes into the college clinic reporting having no energy, a headache, and a 100.6°F temperature. Has had lots of vaginal and rectal pain (8 on scale of 10) and itching, burning with urination, and painful defecation. Burning radiates up back, hurts to sit, and has cramps above pubic area. Also broke out with genital lesions a few days after having sexual relations 10 days ago ("first and only") with a new partner. Does not use any protection or birth control and refuses to do so. Has a great deal of itching and pain in the vaginal area and says that "urinating and having a bowel movement hurts a lot." Pain prevents her from doing any ADLs and going to class. Took an OTC pain pill that helped somewhat.

BACKGROUND: Has regular menstrual cycle every 28 days with last one 2 weeks ago (beginning the 10th and ending the 13th). Has bloating and mild cramping with period. Urine burns her genital and anal area. Immunizations up to date, including vaccination for HPV. Has had one sexual encounter; reports attempt at anal intercourse that was not successful. States "I have always been healthy—I don't know why I behaved so stupidly and put my health at risk." Denies performance of monthly vulvar self-examination. Aware of toxic shock syndrome; wears tampons only during heavy flow days, changing every few hours. Has never had a Pap test.

ASSESSMENT: Normal hair distribution of the mons pubis, with lesions present as vesicles. Ulcerations noted as well. Labia majora with mild erythema and vesicular lesions along with mild excoriation. Labia minora dark pink, moist, and free of lesions or excoriation. Vesicles and ulcerations extend into the perianal area. Visual inspection of the anus reveals multiple vesicular lesions noted around the anal opening. Upon palpation of the inguinal area and external genitalia, no masses or edema were noted to the inguinal lymph nodes bilaterally. Mild edema noted to the labia majora. Labia minora free from edema and discharge. Bartholin glands soft, nontender, and free from discharge. No discharge from urethral opening. Routine Pap smear performed. Vaginal walls smooth and pink. Cervix slightly anterior, pink, smooth in appearance, slit-like os, without lesions or discharge present.

RECOMMENDATION: Client has Acute Pain: genitalia and perianal area r/t ulcerations and vesicles from probable STI, Situation Low Self-Esteem r/t perceived lack of assertiveness in protecting self and is at Risk for Ineffective Sexuality Pattern r/t change in sexual behavior and values conflict. The client needs to be seen by their primary care provider for further evaluation, diagnosis, and treatment of her genital lesions.

ABNORMAL FINDINGS 27-1 — Abnormalities of the External Genitalia and Vaginal Opening

When assessing the female genitalia, the nurse will see various abnormal lesions on the external genitalia as well as abnormal bulging in the vaginal opening. Some common findings follow.

SYPHILITIC CHANCRE

Syphilitic chancres often first appear on the perianal area as silvery white papules that become superficial red ulcers. Syphilitic chancres are painless. They are sexually transmitted and usually develop at the site of initial contact with the infecting organism.

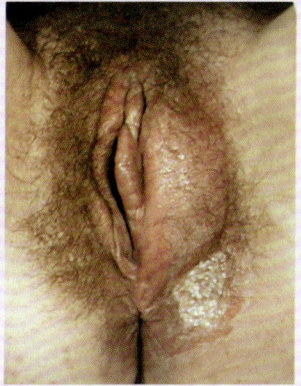

Chancre typical of syphilis. (Courtesy of Upjohn Co.)

Continued on following page

666 UNIT 3 Nursing Assessment of Physical Systems

ABNORMAL FINDINGS 27-1 · Abnormalities of the External Genitalia and Vaginal Opening (Continued)

GENITAL WARTS

Genital warts, caused by the human papilloma virus (HPV), are moist, fleshy lesions on the labia and within the vestibule. They are painless and believed to be sexually transmitted.

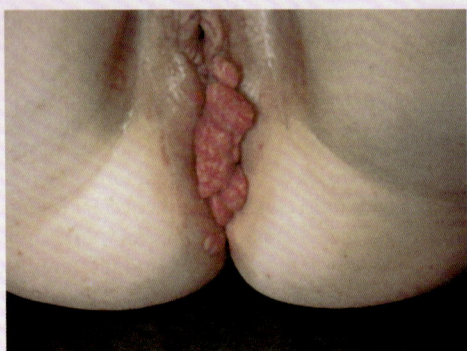

Genital warts. (Courtesy Reed & Carnrick Pharmaceuticals.)

GENITAL HERPES SIMPLEX

The initial outbreak of herpes may have many small, painful ulcers with erythematous base. Recurrent herpes lesions are usually not as extensive.

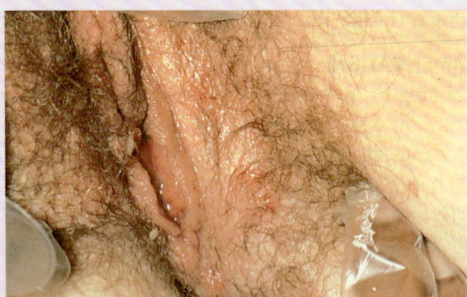

Small, painful, red-based, ulcer-like lesions of herpes simplex virus, type 2. (© 1992 Science Photo Library/CMSP.)

CYSTOCELE

A cystocele is a bulging in the anterior vaginal wall caused by thickening of the pelvic musculature. As a result, the bladder, covered by vaginal mucosa, prolapses into the vagina.

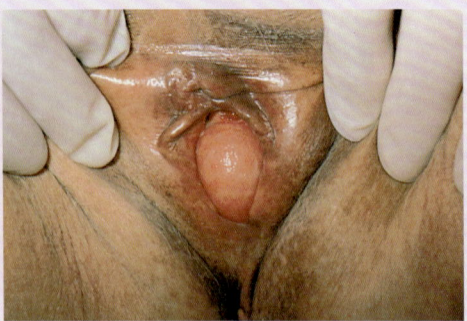

Cystocele. (© 1995 Science Photo Library/CMSP.)

RECTOCELE

A rectocele is a bulging in the posterior vaginal wall caused by weakening of the pelvic musculature. Part of the rectum covered by the vaginal mucosa protrudes into the vagina.

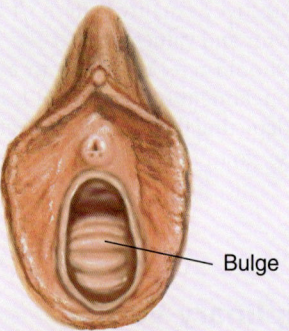

Rectocele.

UTERINE PROLAPSE

Uterine prolapse occurs when the uterus protrudes into the vagina. It is graded according to how far it protrudes into the vagina. In first-degree prolapse, the cervix is seen at the vaginal opening; in second-degree prolapse the uterus bulges outside of vaginal openings; in third-degree prolapse, the uterus bulges completely out of the vagina.

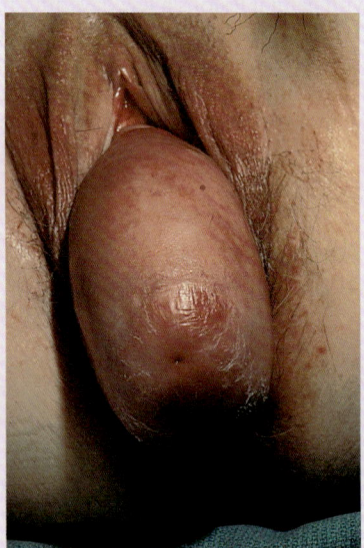

Prolapsed uterus. (© 1991, Michael English, MD/CMSP.).

ABNORMAL FINDINGS 27-2 Abnormalities of the Cervix

CYANOSIS OF THE CERVIX
The cervix normally appears bluish in the client who is in her first trimester of pregnancy. However, if the client is not pregnant, a bluish color to the cervix indicates venous congestion or a diminished oxygen supply to the tissues.

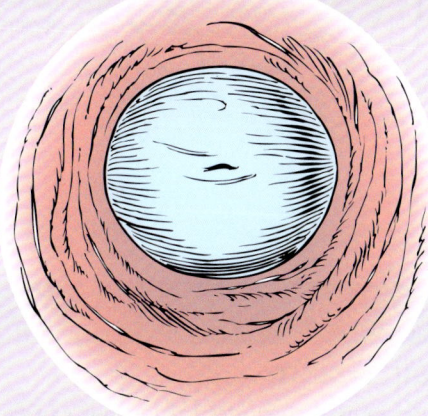

CANCER OF THE CERVIX
A hardened ulcer is usually the first indication of cervical cancer, but it may not be visible on the ectocervix. In later stages, the lesion may develop into a large cauliflower-like growth. A Pap smear is essential for diagnosis.

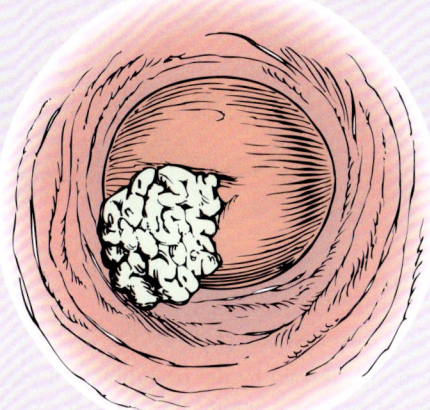

MUCOPURULENT CERVICITIS
This condition produces a mucopurulent yellowish discharge from the external os. It usually indicates infection with *Chlamydia* or gonorrhea. However, these STIs may also occur with no visible signs, although the discharge may change the cervical pH (3.8–4.2).

CERVICAL POLYP
A polyp typically develops in the endocervical canal and may protrude visibly at the cervical os. It is soft, red, and rather fragile. Cervical polyps are benign.

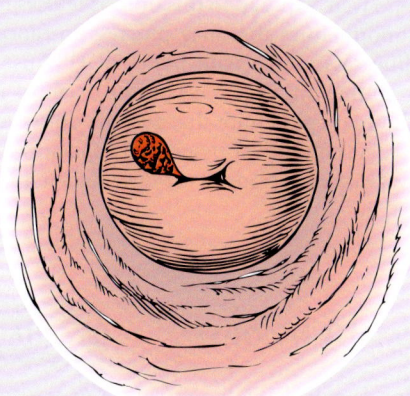

CERVICAL EROSION
This condition differs from cervical eversion in that normal tissue around the external os is inflamed and eroded, appearing reddened and rough. Erosion usually occurs with mucopurulent cervical discharge.

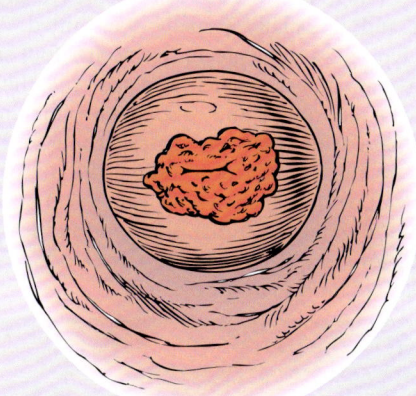

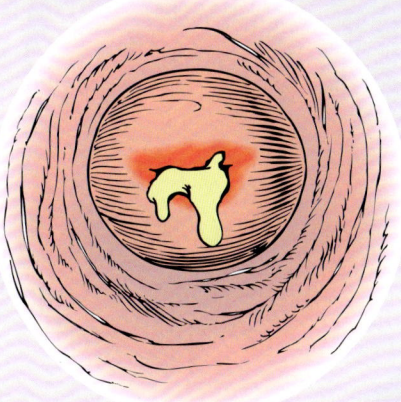

Continued on following page

ABNORMAL FINDINGS 27-2 Abnormalities of the Cervix (Continued)

MALFORMATIONS FROM EXPOSURE TO DIETHYLSTILBESTROL (DES)

DES, a drug used more than 50 years ago to prevent spontaneous abortion and premature labor, was learned to be teratogenic (capable of causing malformations in the fetus). Women who were exposed to this drug as fetuses may have cervical abnormalities that may progress to cancer. Some abnormalities associated with maternal DES use include columnar epithelium that covers most or all of the ectocervix; columnar epithelium that extends onto the vaginal wall; a circular column of tissue that separates the cervix from the vaginal wall; transverse ridge; and enlarged upper ectocervical lip.

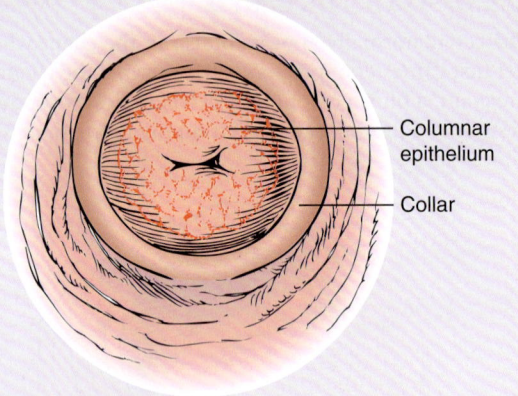

ABNORMAL FINDINGS 27-3 Vaginitis

In assessing female genitalia, the nurse may suspect vaginal infection from signs such as redness or lack of color, unusual discharge and secretions, reported itching, and other typical symptoms of the kinds of vaginitis discussed here.

TRICHOMONAS VAGINITIS (TRICHOMONIASIS)

This type of vaginal infection is caused by a protozoan organism and is usually sexually transmitted. The discharge is typically yellow-green, frothy, and foul smelling. The labia may appear swollen and red, and the vaginal walls may be red, rough, and covered with small red spots (or petechiae). This infection causes itching and urinary frequency in the client. Upon testing, the pH of vaginal secretion will be greater than 4.5 (usually 7.0 or more). If a sample of vaginal secretions is stirred into a potassium hydroxide solution (KOH prep), a foul odor (typically known as a "+" amine) may be noted.

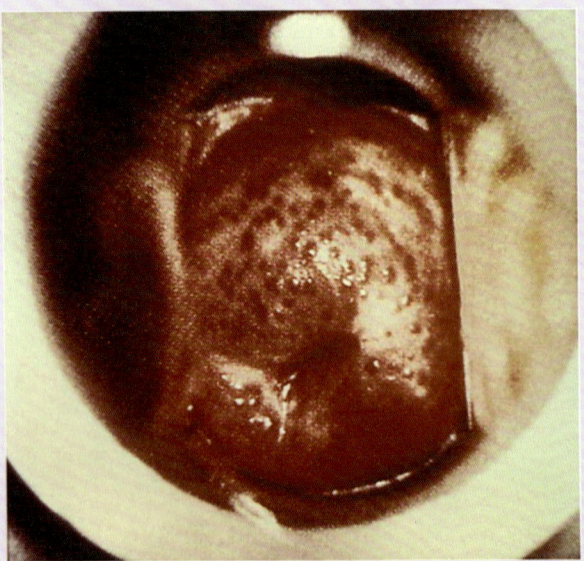

ATROPHIC VAGINITIS

Atrophic vaginitis occurs after menopause when estrogen production is low. The discharge produced may be blood-tinged and is usually minimal. The labia and vaginal mucosa appear atrophic. The vaginal mucosa is typically pale, dry, and contains areas of abrasion that bleed easily. Atrophic vaginitis causes itching, burning, dryness, and painful urination.

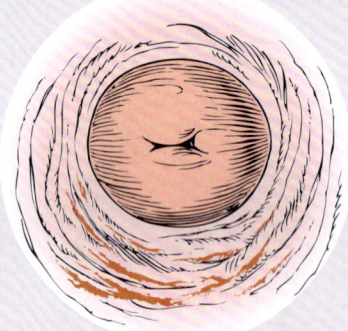

CANDIDAL VAGINITIS (MONILIASIS)

This infection is caused by the overgrowth of yeast in the vagina. It causes a thick, white, cheesy discharge. The labia may be inflamed and swollen. The vaginal mucosa may be reddened and typically contains patches of the discharge. This infection causes intense itching and discomfort.

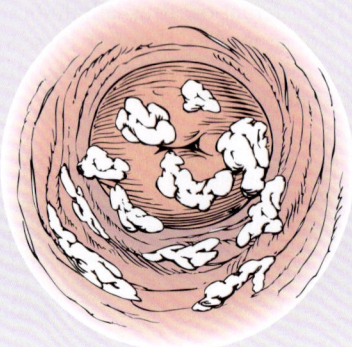

BACTERIAL VAGINOSIS

The cause of bacterial vaginosis is unknown (possibly anaerobic bacteria), but it is thought to be sexually transmitted. The discharge is thin and gray-white, has a positive amine (fishy smell), and coats the vaginal walls and ectocervix. The labia and vaginal walls usually appear normal and pH is greater than 4.5 (5.5–6.0).

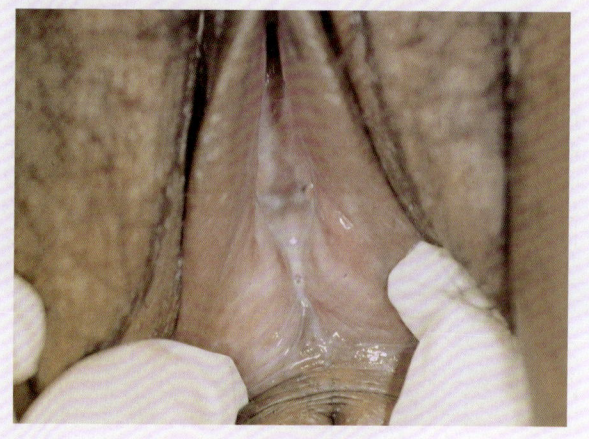

Photo credits: Trichomoniasis, *from the Centers for Disease Control and Prevention Public Health Image Library;* Bacterial vaginosis, *from Sweet, R. L., & Gibbs, R. S. [2005]. Atlas of infectious diseases of the female genital tract. Philadelphia, PA: Lippincott Williams & Wilkins.*

ABNORMAL FINDINGS 27-4 Uterine Enlargement

NORMAL ENLARGEMENT: PREGNANCY
The only uterine enlargement that is normal results from pregnancy and fetal growth. In such cases, the isthmus feels soft (Hegar sign) on palpation, and the fundus and isthmus are compressible at between 10 and 12 weeks of pregnancy.

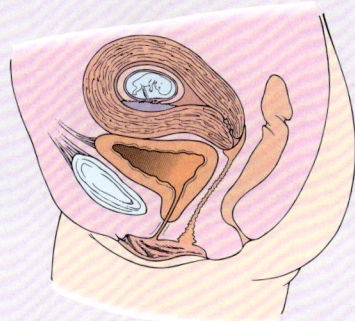

UTERINE CANCER (CANCER OF THE ENDOMETRIUM)
The uterus may be enlarged with a malignant mass. Irregular bleeding, bleeding between periods, or postmenopausal bleeding may be the first sign of a problem.

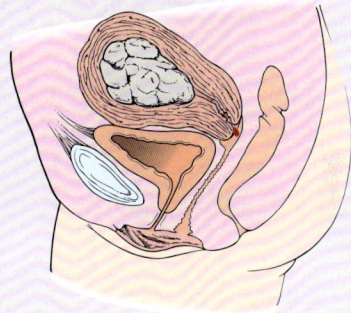

UTERINE FIBROIDS (MYOMAS)
Uterine fibroid tumors are common and benign. They are irregular, firm nodules that are continuous with the uterine surface. They may occur as one or many and may grow quite large. The uterus will be irregularly enlarged, firm, and mobile.

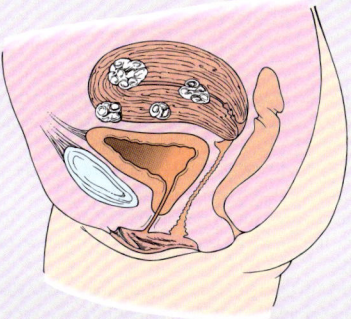

ENDOMETRIOSIS
In endometriosis, the uterus is fixed and tender. Growths of endometrial tissue are usually present throughout the pelvic area and may be felt as firm, nodular masses. Pelvic pain and irregular bleeding are common.

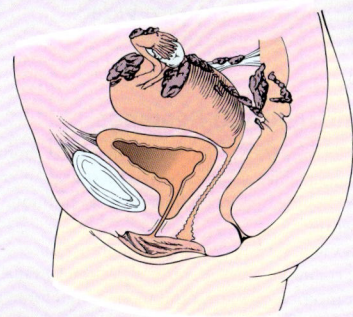

ABNORMAL FINDINGS 27-5 — Adnexal Masses

PELVIC INFLAMMATORY DISEASE (PID)
PID is typically caused by infection of the fallopian tubes (salpingitis) or fallopian tubes and ovaries (salpingo-oophoritis) with an STI (i.e., gonorrhea, *Chlamydia*). It causes extremely tender and painful bilateral adnexal masses (positive Chandelier sign).

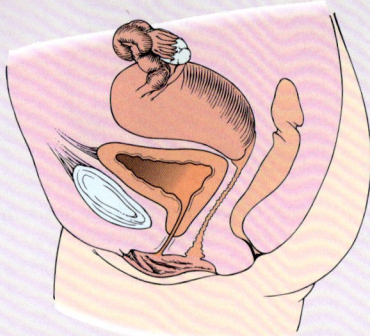

OVARIAN CANCER
Masses that are cancerous are usually solid, irregular, nontender, and fixed.

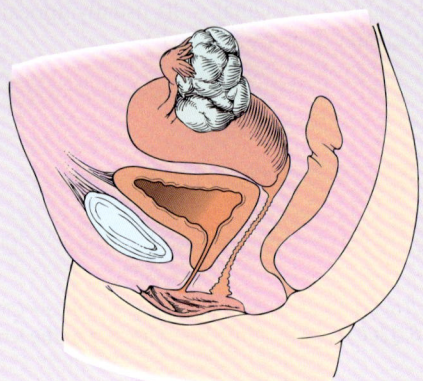

OVARIAN CYST
Ovarian cysts are benign masses on the ovary. They are usually smooth, mobile, round, compressible, and nontender.

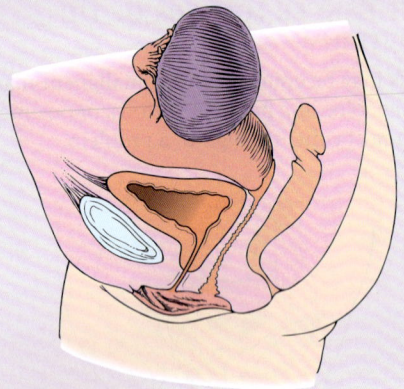

ECTOPIC PREGNANCY
Ectopic pregnancy occurs when a fertilized egg attaches to the fallopian tube and begins developing instead of continuing its journey to the uterus for development. A solid, mobile, tender, and unilateral adnexal mass may be palpated if tenderness allows. The cervix and uterus will be softened, and movement of these structures will cause pain.

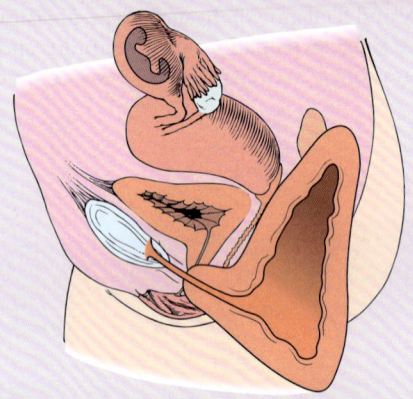

Want to know more?
A wide variety of resources to enhance your learning and understanding of this book are available on thePoint. Visit thePoint to access:
- NCLEX-Style Student Review Questions
- Watch and Learn Videos
- Concepts in Action Animations
- And more!

References and Selected Readings

American Cancer Society (ACS). (2015). Menopausal hormone therapy and cancer risk. Available at http://www.cancer.org/cancer/cancercauses/othercarcinogens/medicaltreatments/menopausal-hormone-replacement-therapy-and-cancer-risk

American Cancer Society (ACS). (2016a). American Cancer Society recommendations for colorectal cancer early detection. Available at http://www.cancer.org/cancer/colonandrectumcancer/moreinformation/colonandrectumcancerearlydetection/colorectal-cancer-early-detection-acs-recommendations

American Cancer Society (ACS). (2016b). Colorectal cancer risk factors. Available at http://www.cancer.org/cancer/colonandrectumcancer/detailedguide/colorectal-cancer-risk-factors

American Cancer Society (ACS). (2017a). Cervical cancer. Available at https://www.cancer.org/cancer/cervical-cancer.html

American Cancer Society (ACS). (2017b). Key statistics for colorectal cancer. Available at https://www.cancer.org/cancer/colon-rectal-cancer/about/key-statistics.html

American Congress of Obstetricians and Gynecologists (ACOG). (2015). Human papillomavirus vaccination. Available at http://www.acog.org/Resources-And-

Publications/Committee-Opinions/Committee-on-Adolescent-Health-Care/Human-Papillomavirus-Vaccination

American Congress of Obstetricians and Gynecologists. (2016). Pap smear (Pap test): Resource overview. Available at http://www.acog.org/Womens-Health/Pap-Smear-Pap-Test

Association of Professors of Gynecology and Obstetrics (APGO). (2008). Cervical cytology, wet prep and cervical culture collection. Available at http://apgo.org/binary/UMEC%20-%20CSC%20Cervical%20Cytology%20Final.pdf

Castleman, M. (2015). Pubic shaving: Which women, and why? Available at https://www.psychologytoday.com/blog/all-about-sex/201509/pubic-shaving-which-women-and-why

Centers for Disease Control and Prevention (CDC). (2015). HIV testing in clinical settings. Available at http://www.cdc.gov/hiv/testing/clinical/

Crooks, R., & Baur, K. (2017). *Our sexuality*. Boston, MA: Cengage Learning.

Gallup. (2015). American greatly overestimate percent gay, lesbian in U.S. Available at http://www.gallup.com/poll/183383/americans-greatly-overestimate-percent-gay-lesbian.aspx

Gay Lesbian Medical Association (GLMA). (2006). Guidelines for care of lesbian, gay, bisexual, and transgender patients. Available at http://www.qahc.org.au/files/shared/docs/GLMA_guide.pdf

Healthy People 2020. (2016). Immunization and infectious diseases. Available at https://www.healthypeople.gov/2020/topics-objectives/topic/immunization-and-infectious-diseases/objectives

Healthy People 2020. (2014/16). Cancer. Available at http://www.healthypeople.gov/2020/topics-objectives/topic/cancer

Johns Hopkins Medicine. (n.d.). Pap test. Available at http://www.hopkinsmedicine.org/healthlibrary/test_procedures/gynecology/pap_test_procedure_92,p07783/

Klatt, K. (2015). Revisiting fiber and colorectal cancer. Available at https://www.nutrition.org/asn-blog/2015/05/revisiting-fiber-and-colorectal-cancer/

Lab Tests Online. (2012). Pap smear. Available at http://labtestsonline.org/understanding/analytes/pap/tab/sample

Mayo Clinic. (2013a). Hemorrhoids. Available at http://www.mayoclinic.org/diseases-conditions/hemorrhoids/basics/definition/con-20029852

Mayo Clinic. (2013b). Vaginal atrophy. Available at http://www.mayoclinic.org/diseases-conditions/vaginal-atrophy/basics/definition/con-20025768

Mitchell, M., Bisch, S., Arntfield, S., et al. (2015). A confirmed case of toxic shock syndrome associated with use of a menstrual cup. *Canadian Journal of Infectious Diseases and Medical Microbiology, 26*(4), 218–220. Available at http://www.ncbi.nlm.nih.gov/pmc/articles/PMC4556184/

National Cancer Institute. (2009). Calcium and cancer prevention. Available at https://www.cancer.gov/about-cancer/causes-prevention/risk/diet/calcium-fact-sheet#q5

Neinstein, L. (2013). Adolescent health curriculum: Menarche. Available at http://www.usc.edu/student-affairs/Health_Center/adolhealth/content/b3menses.html

Paoletti, J. (2010). Why a woman without a uterus needs progesterone. Available at http://www.healthwatchersnews.com/2010/10/why-a-woman-without-a-uterus-needs-progesterone/

Puscheck, E. E., & Lucidi, R. S. (2012). Infertility. Available at http://emedicine.medscape.com/article/274143-overview

Rice, S. C. (2015). Postmenopausal atrophic vaginitis. Available at http://www.healthline.com/health/atrophic-vaginitis#Overview1

Thornton, S. (2015). Hemorrhoids. Available at http://emedicine.medscape.com/article/775407-overview#a7

Turner, N., & Lupton, J. (2011). Dietary fiber. *Advances in Nutrition, 2*, 151–152.

U.S. Department of Health and Human Services, Office on Women's Health. (2015). Douching fact sheet. Available at http://womenshealth.gov/publications/our-publications/fact-sheet/douching.html

U.S. Preventive Services Task Force (USPSTF). (2012). Screening for cervical cancer. Available at http://www.uspreventiveservicestaskforce.org/uspstf/uspscerv.htme.

U.S. Preventive Services Task Force (ISPSTF). (2016). Colorectal cancer: Screening. Available at http://www.uspreventiveservicestaskforce.org/Page/Document/UpdateSummaryFinal/colorectal-cancer-screening2

Velez, M., Alvarado, B., Lord, C., & Zunzunegui, M. (2010). Life course socioeconomic adversity and age at natural menopause in women from Latin America and the Caribbean. Menopause, 17(3), 552–559.

World Health Organization (WHO). (2015). HPV and cancer. Available at http://www.cancer.gov/about-cancer/causes-prevention/risk/infectious-agents/hpv-fact-sheet#q2

World Health Organization (WHO). (2016a). Cancer mortality and morbidity. Available at http://www.who.int/gho/ncd/mortality_morbidity/cancer_text/en/

World Health Organization (WHO). (2016b). Classification of female genital mutilation. Available at http://www.who.int/reproductivehealth/topics/fgm/overview/en/

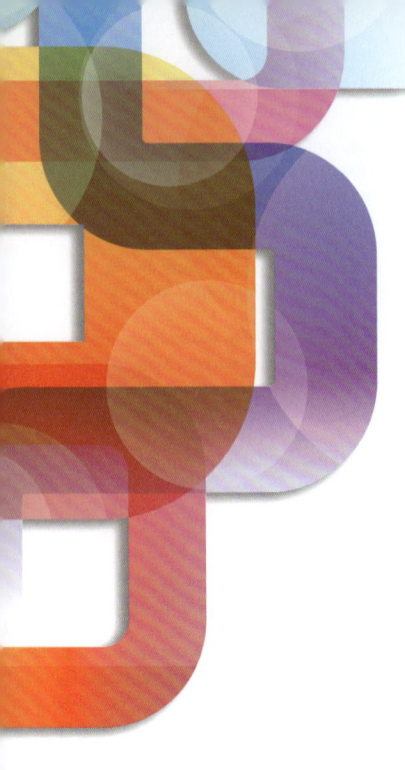

28 PULLING IT ALL TOGETHER: INTEGRATED HEAD-TO-TOE ASSESSMENT

Learning Objectives

1. Explain how to prepare yourself and the client for a complete head-to-toe integrated physical assessment.
2. Describe the purpose of all the equipment needed for a total head-to-toe physical assessment.
3. Explain how specific parts of the physical examination can be integrated into assessment of other body systems.
4. Correctly perform an integrated, head-to-toe physical assessment.
5. Differentiate between normal and abnormal findings identified during the head-to-toe assessment.
6. Analyze the data from a comprehensive nursing interview and head-to-toe integrated physical assessment to formulate valid nursing diagnoses, collaborative problems, and/or referrals.
7. Differentiate between the skills needed to complete an integrated head-to-toe routine screening versus those needed for a focused or specialty assessment of a specific body system.
8. Document and verbally report accurate assessment findings of an integrated head-to-toe physical assessment.

CASE STUDY

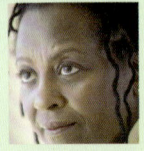

Susan Lewis presents today for a checkup. She reports that she has not had a checkup in 8 years. Ms. Lewis has type 2 diabetes and feels as though it is under control. She states that she has been having burning, numbness, and tingling in her feet for the past couple of months.

Now that you have learned how to discretely assess each body system you may be wondering how you will be able to put all these pieces together to perform a comprehensive head-to-toe assessment. While focused body systems assessments are useful when a client seeks care for a particular health concern, comprehensive assessments are completed in such instances as the client's first visit to a health care provider, to obtain an overall impression and baseline data. For practical reasons, a head-to-toe approach is more convenient for performing a comprehensive assessment, which integrates the assessment of all body systems. This approach conserves time and energy for both the client and nurse.

When using a head-to-toe approach, some body systems may be assessed in combination. For example, when performing an eye assessment you will also be performing part of the neurologic examination for cranial nerves II, III, IV, and VI, which affect vision and eye movements. When you assess the legs you will be assessing the parts of the skin (color and condition of skin on legs), peripheral vascular system (pulses, color, edema, lesions of legs), musculoskeletal system (movement, strength, and tone of legs), and neurologic system (ankle and patellar reflexes, clonus).

There is more than one correct way to integrate the entire health history and physical examination. However, it is important to develop a consistent and logical routine to avoid omitting significant data collection from your assessment. Integrating all these skills together takes time and practice. The more you practice, the faster you will perform the assessment. Performing a complete interview and total physical examination may take up to 2 hours for the novice and only 30 minutes for the skilled practitioner. Do not get discouraged; no one becomes an expert without practice. Develop a routine that is comfortable for you and the client.

It is wise to break up the assessment into segments to allow both you and the client short rest periods. The client's physical and mental statuses will determine how much of the total examination you may perform at one time. For example, if the client is having excruciating hip pain, an extensive assessment would need to wait until the client is more comfortable. If the

28 Pulling It All Together: Integrated Head-To-Toe Assessment   673

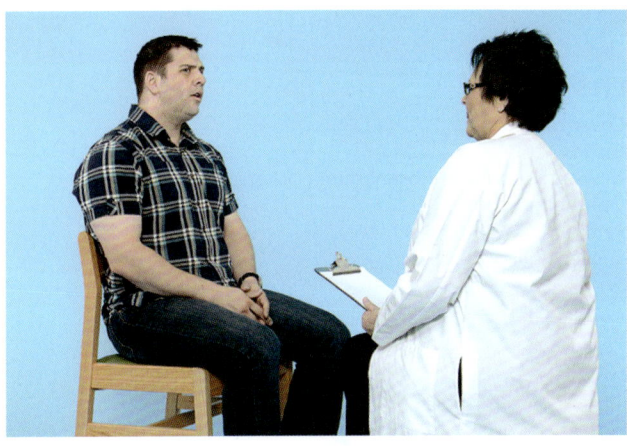

FIGURE 28-1 Nurse sitting in chair talking to client who is still in street clothes, prior to changing into a gown.

client is confused, you will need to gather data from relatives or friends and proceed in a manner that does not agitate the client.

> **CLINICAL TIP**
> Before performing a complete assessment, read your state's Nurse Practice Act to determine your legal scope of practice (what you can legally assess and diagnose).

COMPREHENSIVE HEALTH ASSESSMENT

Preparing the Client

Discuss the purpose and importance of the health history and physical assessment with your client (Fig. 28-1). For example, when you introduce yourself to your client you may want to say "Hello, my name is _____. I am the registered nurse who will be helping to take care of you today. I need to ask you questions and perform a physical examination to determine how you are doing to better plan your nursing care." Then obtain your client's permission to ask personal questions and to perform the various physical assessments (e.g., breast, thorax, genitourinary examination). Explain your respect for the client's privacy and confidentiality. Respect your client's right to refuse any part of the assessment. Explain that the client will need to change into a gown for the examination.

Equipment

Box 28-1 lists the equipment needed for a comprehensive assessment covering all body systems. However, the nurse rarely performs a total eye and ear examination, and does not normally perform genital and rectal examinations. The client often sees specialists for these examinations. The nurse, however, may perform these examinations when needed. Therefore, your equipment needs will be determined by the areas being assessed. In addition, modifications may be necessary when performing an assessment in a client's home. For example, you may use the client's bath scale in place of a platform scale.

Collecting Data

Remember to document all your subjective and objective findings, nursing diagnoses, collaborative problems, and referrals.

Collecting Subjective Data: The Comprehensive Nursing Health History

While taking the nursing health history and performing the general survey and mental status examination, make sure that the client is comfortable with seating and room temperature. See Chapter 2 for an in-depth review of the following components of a comprehensive health history:
- Biographical data
- Reasons for seeking health care
- History of present health concern using COLDSPA to explore concerns
- Personal health history
- Family health history
- Review of body systems (ROS) for current health problems
- Lifestyle and health practices profile
- Developmental level

See Appendix A for a comprehensive Nursing Health History Guide.

General Routine Screening versus Focused Specialty Assessment

The purpose of this chapter is to explain how to complete an integrated head-to-toe examination of all body systems. Depending on the specialty area and need for a more focused or total examination, the nurse will have to determine what parts of the total examination are necessary, as explained in all the prior body system chapters. See the Abbreviated Head-to-toe Physical Assessment located at the end of this chapter that may be used as needed when time and/or the situation does not allow for a total head-to-toe examination.

BOX 28-1 EQUIPMENT FOR A HEAD-TO-TOE EXAMINATION

GENERAL SURVEY

Assessment documentation forms
Balance beam scale with height attachment
Flexible tape measure
Skin-fold calipers
Stethoscope and sphygmomanometer
Thermometers
Watch with second hand

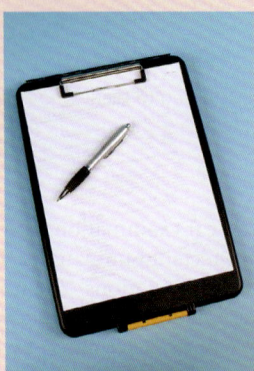
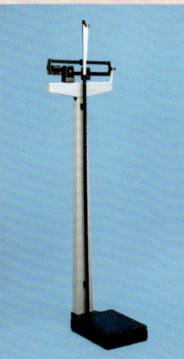
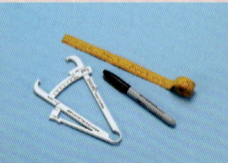
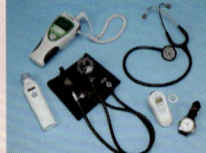

SKIN, HAIR, NAILS

Gloves
Mirror
Magnifying glass
Penlight
Ruler with centimeter markings
Skin marking pen

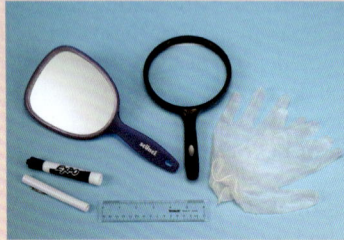

HEAD AND NECK

Stethoscope
Small cup of water for client to drink

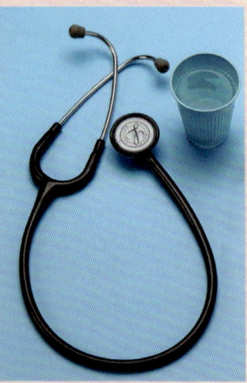

EYES

Cover card
Gloves
Newspaper print or Rosenbaum pocket screener
Ophthalmoscope
Penlight
Snellen chart

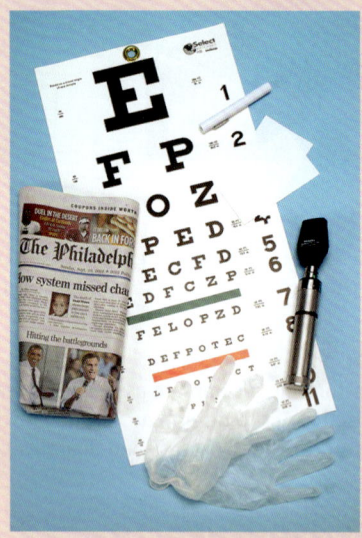

EARS

Otoscope
Tuning fork
Watch with second hand

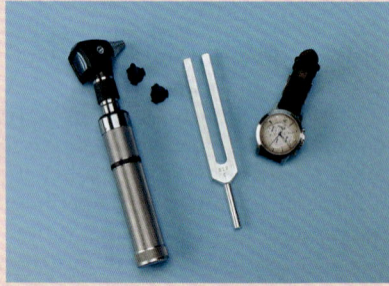

MOUTH, THROAT, NOSE, AND SINUSES

4 × 4-in gauze pad
Penlight
Short, wide-tipped speculum attached to the head of an otoscope or nasal speculum with penlight
Tongue depressor

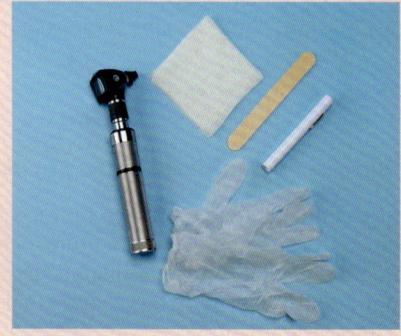

THORAX AND LUNGS
Client gown and draping sheet
Gloves and mask (for nurse if client is actively coughing)
Metric ruler
Skin marking pen
Stethoscope (diaphragm)

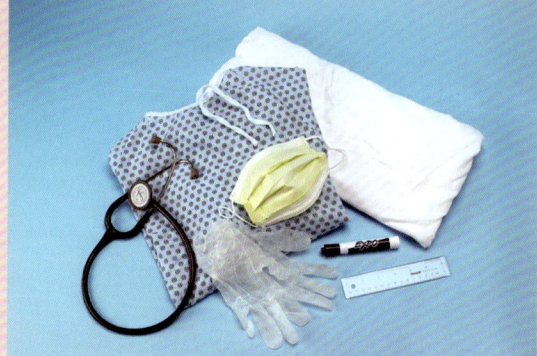

BREASTS
Client gown
Gloves for nurse
Small pillow
Metric ruler
Breast self-examination teaching pamphlet

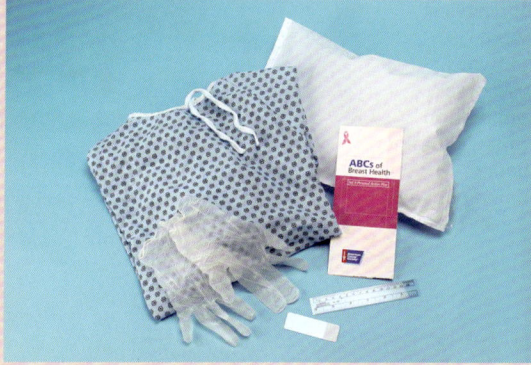

HEART AND NECK VESSELS
Client draping sheet
Metric rulers (two)
Penlight
Small pillow
Stethoscope
Watch with second hand

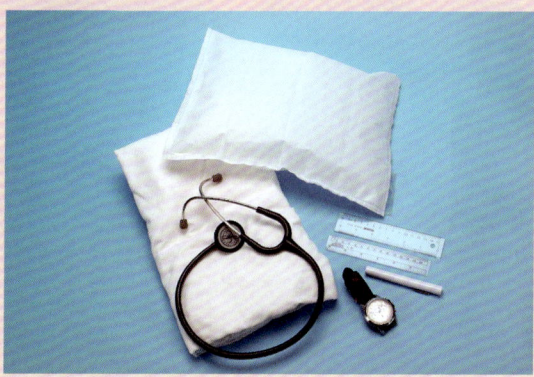

PERIPHERAL VASCULAR
Client gown
Doppler ultrasound device and conductivity gel
Flexible metric tape measure
Gauze or tissue
Skin marking pen
Sphygmomanometer
Stethoscope
Tourniquet
Watch with second hand

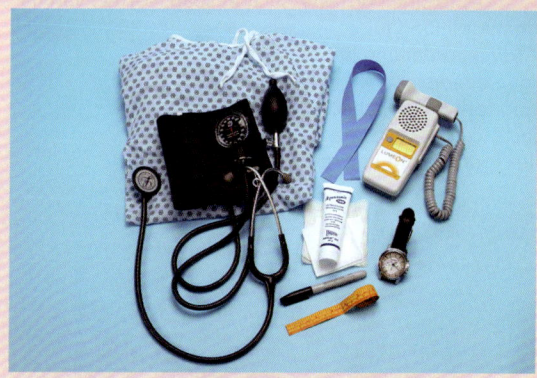

ABDOMEN
Client drape
Metric ruler
Skin marking pen
Small pillows
Stethoscope

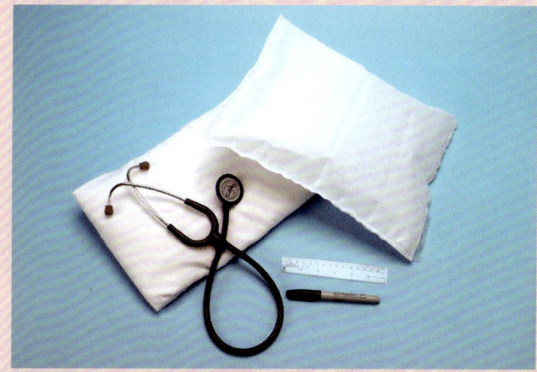

MUSCULOSKELETAL
Flexible metric tape measure
Goniometer

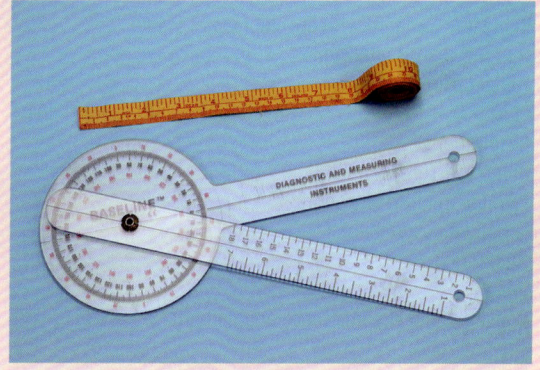

Continued on following page

BOX 28-1 EQUIPMENT FOR A HEAD-TO-TOE EXAMINATION (Continued)

NEUROLOGIC
Newsprint to read
Ophthalmoscope
Penlight
Snellen chart
Cotton-tipped applicators
Flexible metric tape measure
Sterile cotton ball and paper clip
Substances to smell or taste, such as soap, coffee, vanilla, salt, sugar, or lemon juice
Test tubes containing hot and cold water
Tongue depressor
Tuning fork (low-pitched)
Objects to feel, such as a quarter or key
Reflex (percussion) hammer

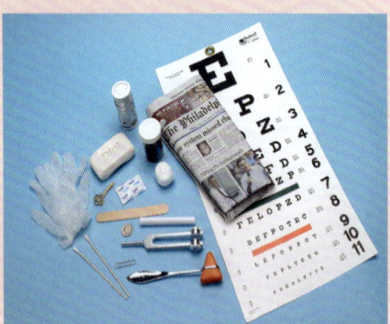

MALE GENITALIA AND RECTUM
Gloves
Water-soluble lubricant
Flashlight
Specimen card

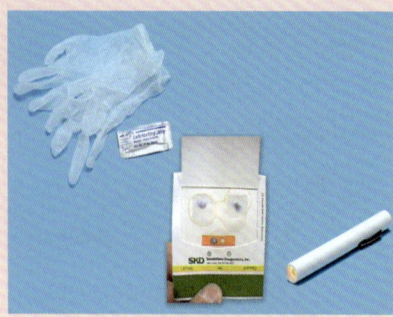

FEMALE GENITALIA AND RECTUM
Gloves (non-sterile)
Light
Hand-held mirror
Vaginal speculum
Water-soluble lubricant
Bifid spatula, endocervical broom
Large swabs for vaginal examination
Specimen container
pH paper
Feminine napkins

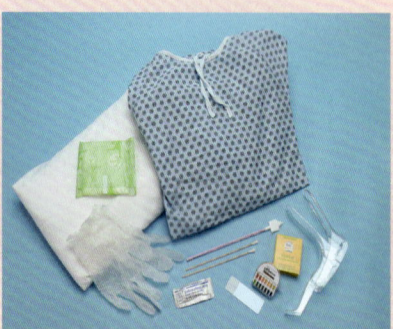

 Collecting Objective Data: Physical Assessment

GENERAL SURVEY

- Observe appearance, including:
  - Overall physical and sexual development
  - Apparent age compared with stated age
  - Overall skin coloring
  - Dress, grooming, and hygiene
  - Body build as well as muscle mass and fat distribution
  - Behavior (compare with developmental stage)
- Assess the client's vital signs:
  - Temperature
  - Pulse
  - Respirations
  - Blood pressure (Fig. 28-2)
  - Pain (as the fifth vital sign)
- Take body measurements:
  - Height (Fig. 28-3)
  - Weight
  - Waist and hip circumference and midarm circumference
  - Triceps skin-fold thickness (TSF)
- Calculate ideal body weight, body mass index (BMI), waist-to-hip ratio, mid-arm muscle area, and circumference.

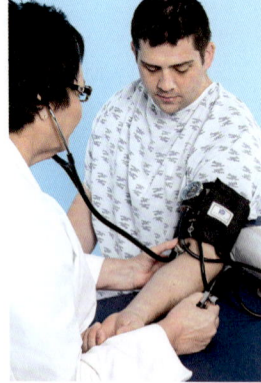

FIGURE 28-2 Assessing blood pressure.

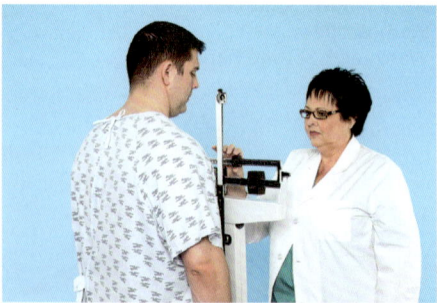

FIGURE 28-3 Measuring height.

MENTAL STATUS EXAMINATION

- In addition to data collected about the client's appearance during the general survey, observe:
  - Level of consciousness
  - Posture and body movements
  - Facial expressions
  - Speech
  - Mood, feelings, and expressions
  - Thought processes and perceptions
- Assess the client's cognitive abilities. The SLUMS (St. Louis University Mental Status) tool may be used (see Assessment Tool 6-3, in Chapter 6). If not the following need to be assessed:
  - Orientation to person, time, and place
  - Concentration, ability to focus and follow directions
  - Recent memory
  - Remote memory
  - Recall of unrelated information in 5-, 10-, and 30-minute periods
  - Abstract reasoning (e.g., explain "A stitch in time saves nine")
  - Judgment (what one would do in case of…)
  - Visual perceptual and constructional ability (draw a clock or shape of square, etc.)

SKIN

- As you perform each part of the head-to-toe assessment, assess the skin for color variations, texture, temperature, turgor, edema, and lesions (Fig. 28-4).
- As you assess the skin, teach the client how to examine their own skin to note any warning signs of skin cancer. This is a good time to teach preventative measures (e.g., sunscreen, sunglasses, hat protection, etc).

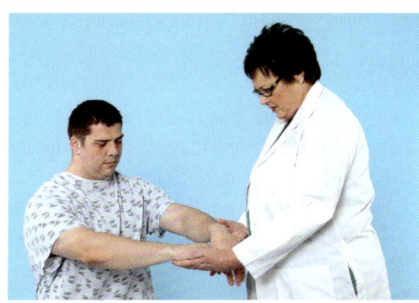

FIGURE 28-4 Assessing the skin.

HEAD AND FACE

- Inspect and palpate the head for size, shape, and configuration (Fig. 28-5).
- Note consistency, distribution, and color of hair.
- Observe the face for symmetry, facial features, expressions, and skin condition.
- Check the function of CN VII: Have the client smile, frown, show teeth, blow out cheeks, raise eyebrows, and tightly close eyes.
- Evaluate the function of CN V: Using the two ends of a paper clip opened to 5 mm, touch forehead, cheeks, and chin to see if the client can identify whether being touched by one or both ends simultaneously.
- Palpate the temporal arteries for elasticity and tenderness.
- As the client opens and closes the mouth, palpate the temporomandibular joint for tenderness, swelling, and crepitation (Fig. 28-6).

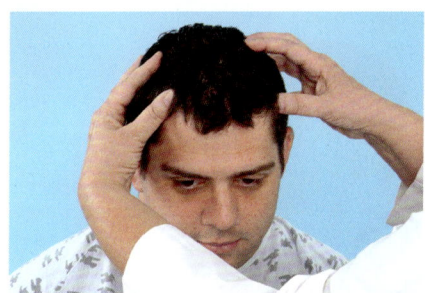

FIGURE 28-5 Inspecting the head.

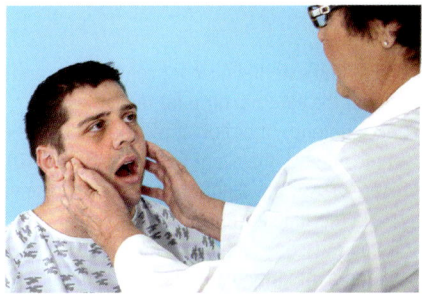

FIGURE 28-6 Palpating the temperomandibular joint.

Continued on following page

EYES

- Determine function:
  - Test vision using Snellen chart.
  - Test visual fields.
  - Assess corneal light reflex.
  - Perform cover–uncover tests if corneal light reflex test is abnormal.
- Inspect the external eye:
  - Position and alignment of the eyeball in eye socket
  - Bulbar conjunctiva and sclera
  - Palpebral conjunctiva
  - Area over lacrimal ducts
  - Cornea, lens, iris, and pupil
- Test pupillary reaction to light (Fig. 28-7).
- Test accommodation of the pupils.
- Assess corneal reflex (CN VII—facial).
- Use the ophthalmoscope to inspect*:
  - Optic disc for shape, color, size, and physiologic cup
  - Retinal vessels for color and diameter and arteriovenous (AV) crossings
  - Retinal background for color and lesions
  - Fovea centralis (sharpest area of vision) and macula
  - Anterior chamber for clarity

*These findings are RARELY visible by the novice unless the client's eye is dilated. However one may attempt to view these findings.

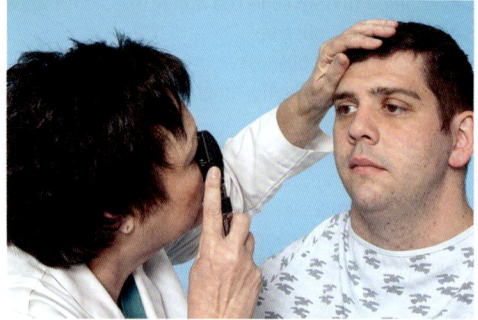

FIGURE 28-7 Testing papillary reaction to light.

EARS

- Inspect the auricle, tragus, and lobule for shape, position, lesions, discolorations, and discharge.
- Palpate the auricle and mastoid process for tenderness (Fig. 28-8).
- Use the otoscope (Fig. 28-9) to inspect:
  - External auditory canal for color and cerumen (ear wax)
  - Tympanic membrane for color, shape, consistency, and landmarks
- Test hearing
  - Whisper test
  - Weber test to assess bone conduction
  - Rinne test to compare bone conduction and air conduction

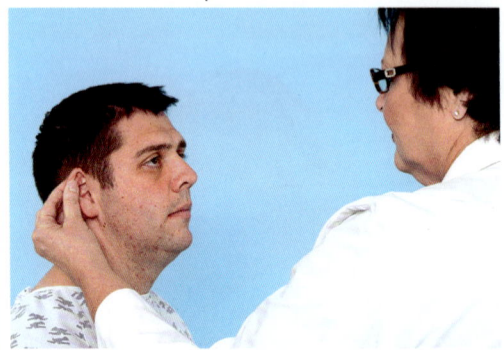

FIGURE 28-8 Palpating the auricle and mastoid process.

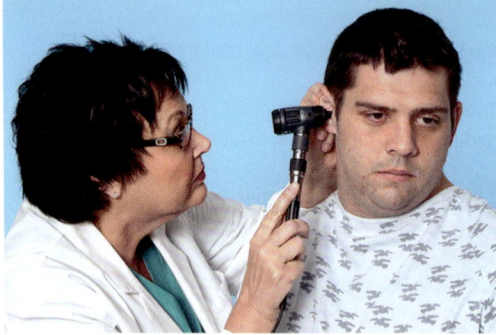

FIGURE 28-9 Using the otoscope to inspect the ear.

NOSE AND SINUSES

- Inspect the external nose for color, shape, and consistency. Palpate the external nose for tenderness.
- Check patency of airflow through the nostrils (occlude one nostril at a time and ask the client to exhale; Fig. 28-10).
- Test CN I. Ask the client to close eyes and smell for soap, coffee, or vanilla (occlude each nostril).
- Use an otoscope with a short, wide speculum to inspect the internal nose for color and integrity of nasal mucosa, nasal septum, and inferior and middle turbinates.
- Transilluminate the maxillary sinuses with a penlight to check for fluid or pus.

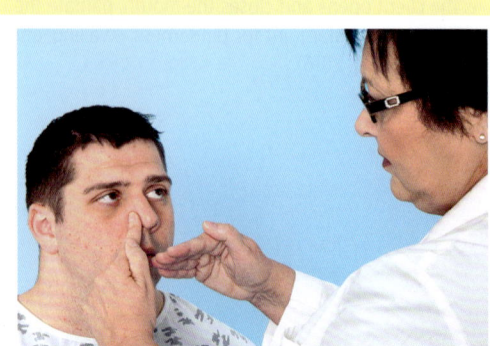

FIGURE 28-10 Checking airflow through the nostrils.

MOUTH AND THROAT

Put on gloves. Use a tongue depressor and penlight as needed.
- Inspect the lips for consistency, color, and lesions.
- Inspect the teeth for number and condition.
- Check the gums and buccal mucosa for color, consistency, and lesions.
- Inspect the hard (anterior) and soft (posterior) palates for color and integrity.
- Ask the client to say "aah" and observe the rise of uvula.
- Test CN X: Touch the soft palate to assess for gag reflex.
- Inspect the tonsils for color, size, lesions, and exudates.
- Inspect the tongue for color, moisture, size, and texture. Inspect the ventral surface of the tongue for frenulum, color, lesions, and Wharton ducts.
- Palpate the tongue for lesions (Fig. 28-11).
- Test CN IX and CN X: Assess the tongue strength by asking the client to press tongue against tongue blade.
- Assess CN VII and CN IX: Have the client close eyes. Check taste by placing salt, sugar, and/or lemon on the tongue.

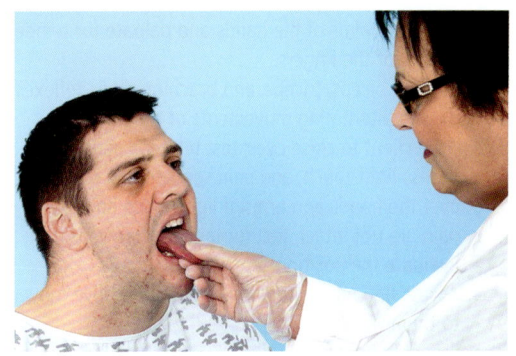

FIGURE 28-11 Palpating the tongue for lesions.

NECK

- Inspect the neck for lesions, masses, swelling, and symmetry.
- Test range of motion (ROM).
- Palpate the preauricular, postauricular, occipital, tonsillar, submandibular, submental, superficial, deep cervical chain, posterior cervical, and supraclavicular lymph nodes (Fig. 28-12).
- Palpate the trachea.
- Auscultate an enlarged thyroid for bruits. (If a bruit is present do not proceed to palpate.)
- Palpate the thyroid gland for size, irregularity, and masses (Fig. 28-13).
- Auscultate the carotid arteries for bruits. (If a bruit is present do not proceed to palpate.) Palpate the carotid arteries.

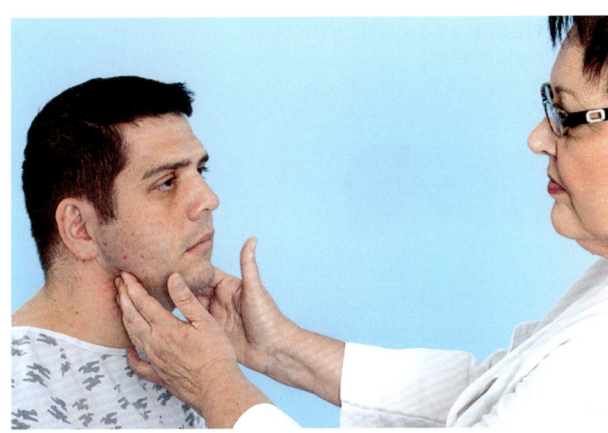

FIGURE 28-12 Palpating the lymph nodes.

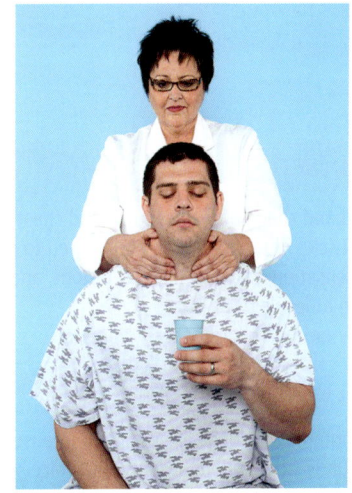

FIGURE 28-13 Palpating the thyroid gland.

ARMS, HANDS, AND FINGERS

- Inspect the upper extremities for overall skin coloration, texture, moisture, masses, and lesions.
- Test the function of CN XI spinal by shoulder shrug and turning head against resistance.
- Palpate the shoulders and arms for tenderness, swelling, and temperature (Fig. 28-14).
- Assess the epitrochlear lymph nodes.
- Test ROM of the shoulders and elbows.
- Palpate the brachial pulse.
- Palpate the ulnar and radial pulses.
- Test ROM of the wrist.

Continued on following page

ARMS, HANDS, AND FINGERS (Continued)

- Inspect the palms of the hands and palpate for temperature.
- Test ROM of the fingers.
- Assess the biceps, triceps, and brachioradialis reflexes (Fig. 28-15).
- Test rapid alternating movements of the hands.
- Ask the client to close eyes; test bilateral sensation:
  - Assess light touch, and pain sensation in scattered locations over the hands and arms. If light touch and pain are not intact, test for temperature sensation.
  - Evaluate the position sense of the fingers.
  - Assess fine motor function (rapid alternative movements, finger to thumb).
  - Test stereognosis.
  - Assess graphesthesia by writing a number in the palm of the client's hand.

Ask the client to continue sitting with arms at sides and stand behind the client. Untie the gown to expose the posterior chest.

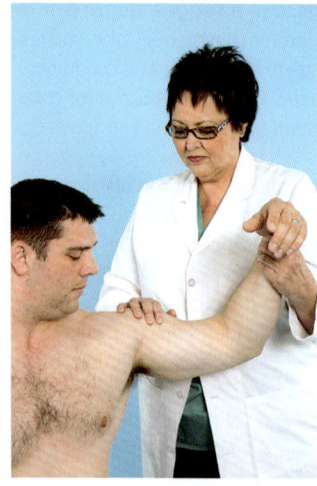

FIGURE 28-14 Palpating the shoulders and arms.

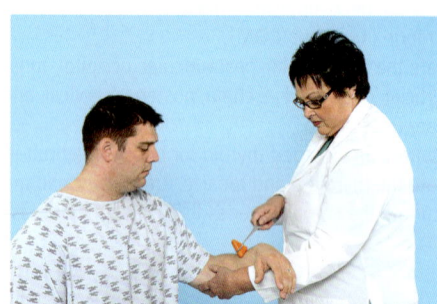

FIGURE 28-15 Testing the biceps, triceps, and brachioradialis reflexes.

POSTERIOR AND LATERAL CHEST

- Inspect the configuration and shape of the scapulae and chest wall.
- Note use of accessory muscles when breathing and related to posture.
- Palpate for tenderness, sensation, crepitus, masses, lesions, and fremitus.
- Evaluate chest expansion at levels T9 or T10.
- Percuss for tone at posterior intercostal spaces, comparing bilaterally (Fig. 28-16).
- Determine diaphragmatic excursion.

If client has respiratory symptoms and lungs are not clear to auscultation, then:
- Auscultate for breath sounds, adventitious sounds, and voice sounds (bronchophony, egophony, and whispered pectoriloquy, respectively) (Fig. 28-17).
- Test for two-point discrimination on the client's back.
- Ask the client to lean forward and exhale; use the bell of the stethoscope to listen over the apex and left sternal border of the heart.

Move to the front of the client and expose the anterior chest. Be sensitive to the client's modesty concerns.

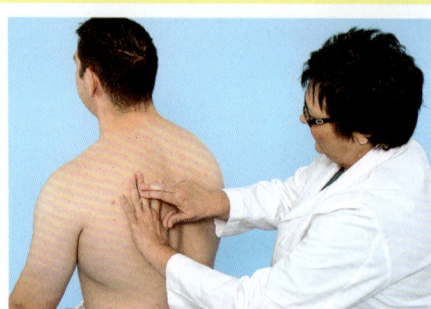

FIGURE 28-16 Percussing the posterior intercostal spaces.

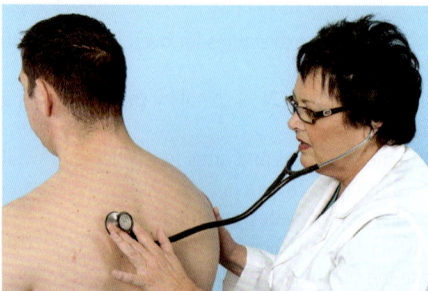

FIGURE 28-17 Auscultating the posterior chest.

ANTERIOR CHEST

- Inspect the anteroposterior diameter of the chest, slope of ribs, and color of chest.
- Note the quality and pattern of respirations (rate, rhythm, and depth).
- Observe intercostal spaces for bulging or retractions and use of accessory muscles.
- Palpate for tenderness, sensation, masses, lesions, fremitus, and anterior chest expansion.
- Percuss for tone at apices above the clavicles, then at the intercostal spaces, comparing bilaterally.
- Auscultate for anterior breath sounds, adventitious sounds, and voice sounds (Fig. 28-18).
- Pinch skin over the sternum to assess mobility (ease to pinch) and turgor (return to original shape).

Ask the client to fold the gown to the waist and sit with arms hanging freely.

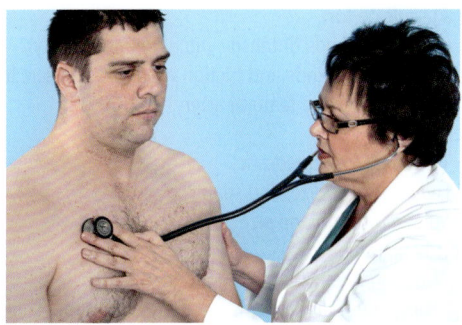

FIGURE 28-18 Auscultating the anterior chest.

BREASTS

FEMALE BREASTS

Inspect size, symmetry, color, texture, superficial venous pattern, areolas, and nipples of both breasts.

- Inspect for retractions and dimpling of the nipples: Have the client raise her arms overhead, press her hands on her hips, press her hands together in front of her, and lean forward.

Ask the client to lie down in the supine position and raise the gown over her upper chest to expose the breasts.

- Palpate each breast, tail of Spence, areola, and nipples for discharge (Fig. 28-19).
- Palpate the axillae for rashes or infection, and the anterior, central, and posterior lymph nodes.
- Teach breast self-examination if the client is interested and expresses a desire to learn.

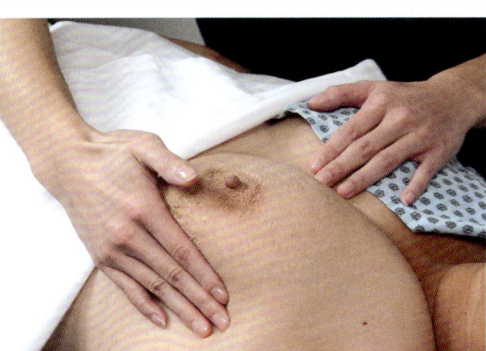

FIGURE 28-19 Palpating the breasts for discharge.

MALE BREASTS

- Inspect for swelling, nodules, and ulcerations.
- Palpate the breast tissue and axillae.

HEART

- Inspect and palpate for apical impulse.
- Palpate the apex, left sternal border, and base of the heart for any abnormal pulsations.
- Auscultate (Fig. 28-20) over the aortic area, pulmonic area, Erb point, tricuspid area, and the mitral area (apex) for:
  - Heart rate and rhythm, using diaphragm of stethoscope. If irregular, auscultate for a pulse rate deficit.
  - S_1 and S_2, using diaphragm of stethoscope
  - Extra heart sounds, S_3 and S_4, using diaphragm and bell of stethoscope
  - Murmurs, using bell and diaphragm of the stethoscope
- Ask the client to lie on left side; use bell of stethoscope to auscultate apex of the heart.

Lower the head of the examination table.

If the client is female, cover her chest with the gown and arrange draping to expose the abdomen. For male clients, arrange draping to expose the abdomen.

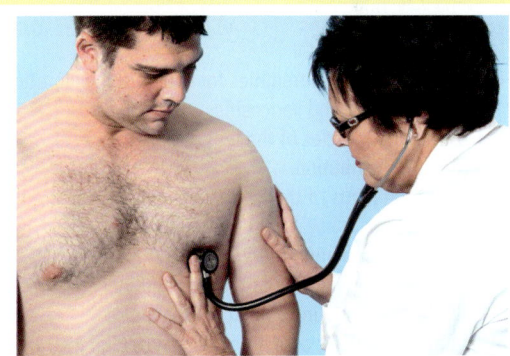

FIGURE 28-20 Auscultating the heart.

ABDOMEN

- Inspect for:
  - Overall skin color: Vascularity, striae, lesions, and rashes
  - Location, contour, and color of the umbilicus
  - Symmetry and contour of the abdomen (Fig. 28-21)
  - Aortic pulsations or peristaltic waves

Continued on following page

ABDOMEN (Continued)

- Auscultate for:
  - Bowel sounds (intensity, pitch, and frequency)
  - Vascular sounds and friction rubs (over spleen, liver, aorta, iliac artery, umbilicus, and femoral artery) (Fig. 28-22)
- Percuss for:
  - Tone over four quadrants
  - Liver location, size, and span
  - Spleen location and size
- Lightly palpate:
  - Abdominal reflex
  - Four quadrants to identify tenderness and muscular resistance
- Deeply palpate:
  - Four quadrants for masses (Fig. 28-23)
  - Aorta
  - Liver, spleen, and kidneys for enlargement or irregularities

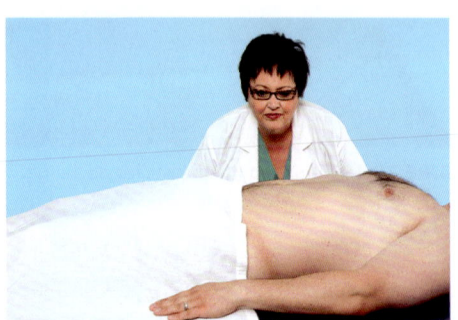

FIGURE 28-21 Inspecting the abdomen.

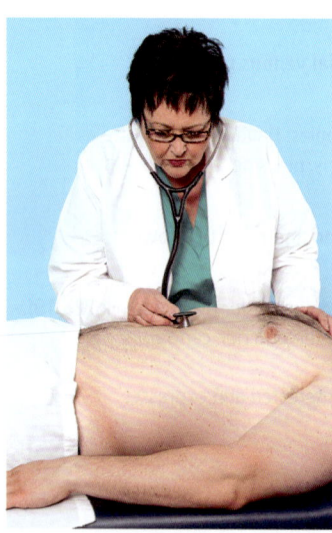

FIGURE 28-22 Auscultating the abdomen.

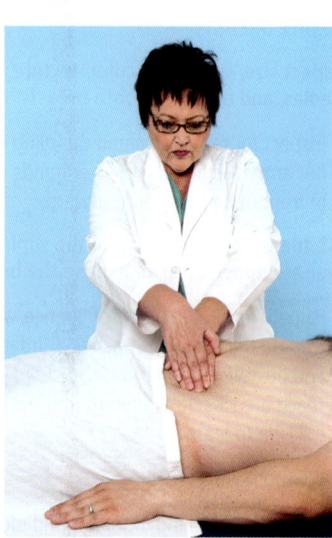

FIGURE 28-23 Palpating the abdomen.

Replace the gown and position draping so that the lower extremities are exposed.

LEGS, FEET, AND TOES

- Inspect the lower extremities for overall skin coloration, texture, moisture, masses, lesions, and varicosities.
- Observe the muscles of the legs and feet.
- Note hair distribution.
- Palpate the joints of the hips and test ROM. Palpate the femoral pulse.
- Palpate for:
  - Edema, skin temperature
  - Muscle size and tone of the legs and feet
- Palpate the knees, including popliteal pulse.
- Palpate the ankles; assess dorsalis-pedis (Fig. 28-24) and posterior-tibial pulses bilaterally. Test ROM.
- Assess capillary refill.
- Test:
  - Sensation to dull and sharp sensations
  - Two-point discrimination (on thighs)
  - Position sense of toes (Fig. 28-25)
  - Vibratory sensation on bony surface (joint) of great toe
  - Perform heel to shin test (fine motor function)

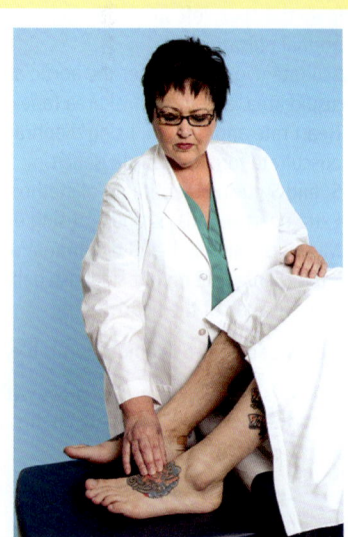

FIGURE 28-24 Assessing dorsalis-pedis pulse.

LEGS, FEET, AND TOES (Continued)

Assist the client to sit on the side of the examination table.

- Assess the patellar, Achilles, and plantar reflexes (Fig. 28-26).
- As warranted, perform special tests:
  - Position change for arterial insufficiency
  - Manual compression test
  - Trendelenburg test
  - Bulge knee test
  - Ballottement test
  - McMurray test

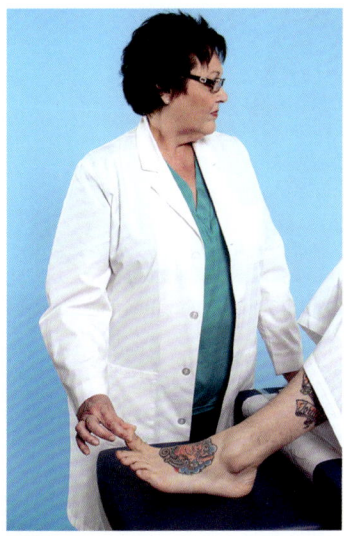
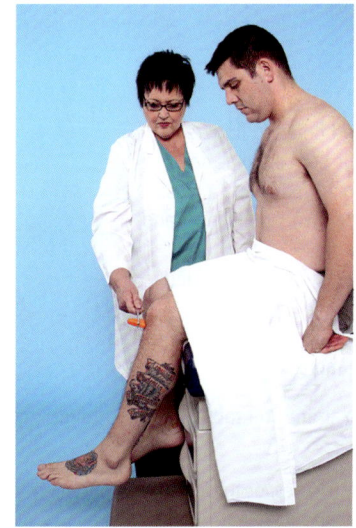

FIGURE 28-25 Testing position sense.　　**FIGURE 28-26** Testing the patellar reflex.

Secure the gown and assist the client to standing position. Assist the client to walk.

MUSCULOSKELETAL AND NEUROLOGIC SYSTEMS

Note that most areas of the musculoskeletal and neurologic systems have been integrated and already assessed throughout the examination up to this point. However, the following areas of these two major body systems need to be completed now.

- Observe spinal curvatures and check for scoliosis.
- Observe gait including base of support, weight-bearing stability, foot position, stride, arm swing, and posture.
- Observe the client as you ask the client to:
  - Walk in a heel-to-toe fashion (tandem walk) (Fig. 28-27)
  - Hop on one leg, then the other leg
  - Perform finger-to-nose test
  - Perform Romberg test—stand close to client as you check this (Fig. 28-28)

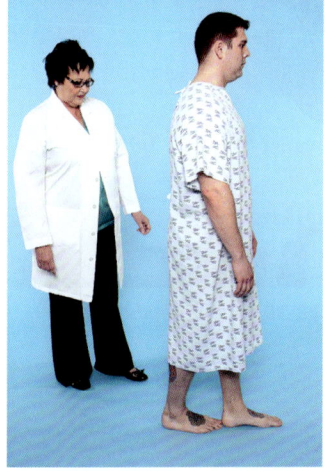
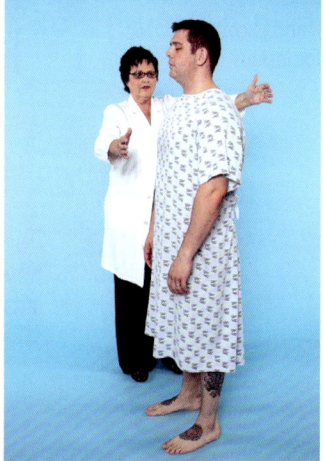

FIGURE 28-27 Tandem walk.　　**FIGURE 28-28** Romberg test.

Perform the male and female genitalia examination last, moving from the less-private to more-private examination for client comfort.

Continued on following page

GENITALIA

MALE GENITALIA AND RECTUM

Sit on a stool. Have the client stand and face you with gown raised (Fig. 28-29). Apply gloves.

- Inspect the penis, including:
  - Base of penis and pubic hair for excoriation, erythema, and infestation
  - Skin and shaft of penis for rashes, lesions, lumps, hardened or tender areas
  - Color, location, and integrity of foreskin in uncircumcised men
  - Glans for size, shape, lesions or redness, and location of urinary meatus
- Palpate for urethral discharge by gently squeezing glans.
- Inspect the scrotum, including:
  - Size, shape, and position
  - Scrotal skin for color, integrity, lesions, or rashes
  - Posterior skin (by lifting scrotal sac)
- Palpate both testis and epididymis between the thumb and first two fingers for size, shape, nodules, and tenderness. Palpate the spermatic cord and vas deferens.
- Transilluminate the scrotal contents for red glow, swelling, or masses. If a mass is found during inspection and palpation, have the client lie down, and inspect and palpate for scrotal hernia.
- As the client bears down, inspect for bulges in inguinal and femoral areas and palpate for femoral hernias.
- While the client shifts weight to each corresponding side, palpate for inguinal hernia.
- Teach testicular self-examination to adolescent and adult men.

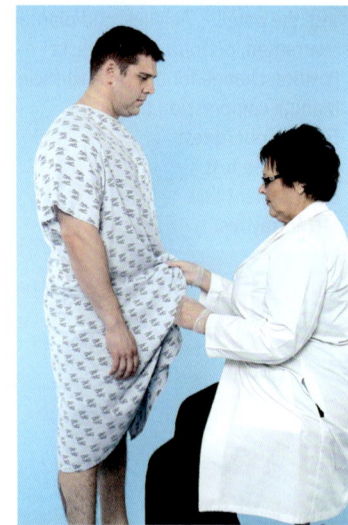

FIGURE 28-29 Inspecting the male genitalia.

Ask the client to remain standing and to bend over the examination table. Change gloves.

- Inspect:
  - Perianal area for lumps, ulcers, lesions, rashes, redness, fissures, or thickening of epithelium
  - Sacrococcygeal area for swelling, redness, dimpling, or hair
- While the client bears down or performs the Valsalva maneuver, inspect for bulges or lesions.
- Apply lubrication and use finger to palpate:
  - Anus
  - External sphincter for tenderness, nodules, and hardness
  - Rectum for tenderness, irregularities, nodules, and hardness
  - Peritoneal cavity
  - Prostate for size, shape, tenderness, and consistency
- Inspect stool for color and test feces for occult blood.

FEMALE GENITALIA

Have the female client assume the lithotomy position. (Fig. 28-30) Apply gloves. Apply lubricant as appropriate.

- Inspect:
  - Distribution of pubic hair
  - Mons pubis, labia majora, and perineum for lesions, swelling, and excoriations
  - Labia minora, clitoris, urethral meatus, and vaginal opening for lesions, swelling, or discharge
- Palpate:
  - Bartholin glands, urethra, and Skene glands
  - Vaginal opening and vaginal musculature
- Insert speculum and inspect:
  - Cervix for lesions and discharge
  - Vagina for color, consistency, and discharge
- Obtain cytologic smears and cultures.
- Perform bimanual examination; palpate:
  - Cervix for contour, consistency, mobility, and tenderness
  - Uterus for size, position, shape, and consistency
  - Ovaries for size and shape

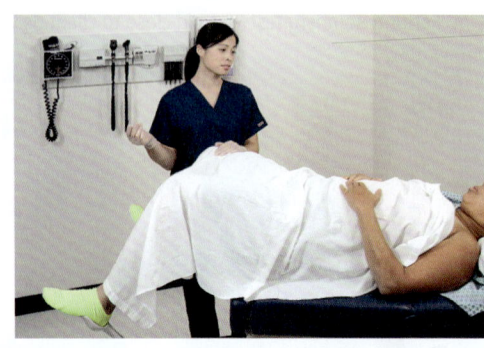

FIGURE 28-30 Lithotomy position.

Discard gloves and apply clean gloves and lubricant.

- Perform the rectovaginal examination; palpate rectovaginal septum for tenderness, consistency, and mobility.

See Appendix B for a comprehensive Physical Assessment Guide.

 Visit thePoint to watch the accompanying video for this chapter illustrating a head-to-toe physical examination, focusing on those assessment techniques most commonly used by the nurse. In the video, a student nurse performs the examination, demonstrating integration of the body systems and correct assessment technique.

Sample Documentation of a Comprehensive Adult Nursing Health History and Physical Assessment

CASE STUDY

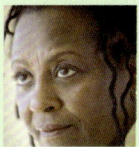

Remember Susan Lewis from the chapter opener case study? The following is a sample documentation of a comprehensive nursing health history and physical assessment performed on this client.

Biographical Data
Client's Name (use initials): S. L.
Data provided by: Client
Age and Place of Birth: 65 years old; St. Louis, Missouri
Gender: Female
Marital Status: Married
Nationality, Culture, Ethnicity: African American
Religion/Spiritual Practices: Baptist
Who Lives With Client: Husband
Significant Others: Husband, two daughters, one son
Education Level: College degree
Occupation (active/laid off/retired): Retired elementary school teacher
Primary language (written/spoken): English
Secondary language: None
Reasons for Seeking Health Care Provider: Client states: "The main reason I am here today is to get a checkup. I haven't had one in 8 years. I probably should have had one sooner because I have type 2 diabetes. I think I have it under control, but I want to make sure. Another reason I am here is because I have started to have some numbness, burning, and tingling in my feet. It is starting to really bother me, and I thought I should have it examined."
History of Present Health Concern: Client states that pain started 2 months ago, and has been getting progressively worse. She reports constant numbness, burning, or tingling in bilateral feet. At time when the feet are burning or tingling at night (about once a week), she says she is unable to sleep. Says that pain is worse when not wearing shoes and walking on a firm surface. Pain started gradually—client cannot think of any event that may have caused it. Client expressed that she thought it was arthritis and that it just happens when "you get old."

Client states that the pain is aggravated by tight shoes, temperature extremes, and extended periods of walking. She rates the pain in these situations as 5–6 on a scale of 0–10. She also notes that the pain is always present at a level of 2–3 on a scale of 0–10. The client reports that she has tried taking ibuprofen 400 mg when the pain started; however, this did not relieve the pain. She reports that the only time the discomfort decreases is when she is non–weight-bearing. Client says she is concerned about the pain getting progressively worse and the impact it may have on her life. Client denies any edema, discoloration, lesions, or changes in temperature of bilateral feet. Client denies any calf pain or cramping with ambulation.

Past Health History: Denies birth problems. Reports having usual childhood illnesses; none requiring hospitalization. Allergies: Denies allergies to medications, environment, food, or insects. Reports the following: type 2 diabetes mellitus, obesity.

Past Surgical History: Reports appendectomy at age 18 and cholecystectomy at age 56. Developed urinary tract infection (UTI) at age 57, at which time she sought medical advice and was diagnosed with type 2 diabetes. She received diabetes education with nutritional medical therapy at the time of her diagnosis.

Family Health History: Mother: History of diabetes and hypertension; deceased at age 72 due to stroke. Father: Deceased at age 63 due to complications of COPD. Maternal grandmother: Deceased, age unknown, during childbirth. Maternal grandfather: Deceased age 56 due to a mining accident. Paternal grandmother: Deceased, cause and age unknown. Paternal grandfather: Deceased, cause and age unknown.

Review of Body Systems for Current Health Problems
Skin, Hair, Nails: Describes skin and scalp as dry. Applies lotion to skin daily. Denies easy bruising, pruritus, or nonhealing sores. Describes nails as hard and brittle. Reports that hair is fine and soft. Reports washing hair weekly. Denies intolerance to heat or cold.
Head and Neck: Denies neck stiffness, swelling, difficulty swallowing, sore throat, or enlarged lymph nodes. "I get a headache about one to two times a month, but I just put a cool washcloth on my head and lie down for a bit—it usually goes away without having to take medicine."
Eyes: Has worn glasses "all my life." Cannot recall age at which they were prescribed. Reports change from bifocals to trifocals at age 60. Complains of blurred vision without glasses. Denies diplopia, itching, excessive tearing, discharge, redness, or trauma to eyes. Has yearly dilated eye examination.
Ears: Believes she is "a little slow to grasp, and I think it may be because of my hearing." Does not wear hearing aid. Cannot recall last hearing test. Denies tinnitus, pain, discharge, or trauma to ears. Does not ask for questions to be repeated.
Mouth, Throat, Nose, and Sinuses: Wears dentures. Last dental examination 3 years ago. Denies problems with proper fit, eating, chewing, swallowing, sore throat, sore tongue. Reports development of a "canker sore" if she eats strawberries. Denies difficulty with smell, pain, postnasal drip, sneezing, or frequent nosebleeds. Denies difficulty tasting foods.
Breasts: Denies pain, lumps, dimpling, retraction, discharge.
Thorax and Lungs: Denies dyspnea, orthopnea, cough, wheezing, or sputum production. Cannot remember when last chest x-ray was performed.

Heart and Neck Vessels: Denies palpitations, chest pain or pressure, and fatigue. Last EKG was 8 years ago.

Peripheral Vascular: See History of Present Health Concern. Denies claudication, cramping, skin lesions, or edema of legs and feet.

Abdomen: Denies nausea, vomiting, abdominal pain, flatulence, constipation, diarrhea, hematemesis, hematochezia, and tenesmus.

Musculoskeletal: Denies stiffness, joint pain, or swelling with activity. Reports lower back pain when carrying large amounts of food or when carrying large trays of food when she volunteers as a cook at church social functions once monthly. Improves after rest and use of ice pack to lower back.

Neurologic: Denies difficulty with speech. Denies difficulty formulating ideas or expressing feelings. States that she has a gradual loss of memory over past 5 to 6 years. Believes long-term memory is better than short-term memory. Reports that she must make a list to remember items when she does grocery shopping. Reports that she learns best by writing information down and then reviewing it. Makes major decisions jointly with husband after prayer.

Genitourinary: Reports voiding four to five times per day, clear yellow urine. Denies dysuria, hematuria, polyuria, hesitancy, incontinence, or nocturia. Menarche: approximately 12 years. Menopause: age 50 years. States "going through my change of life wasn't difficult for me physically or emotionally." Described menstrual period as regular, lasting 4 days with moderate flow. Denies postmenopausal spotting at this time. Client is gravida 3, para 3. No complications with pregnancy or childbirth. Has never used any form of contraception. Client states she is sexually active—"My husband and I have good relations." Denies pain, discomfort, or postcoital bleeding. Denies history of any sexually transmitted diseases. Denies vaginal itching, odor, or discharge. Last Pap smear: negative, 4 years ago.

Anus/Rectum: Soft, formed, medium brown BM every other day. Denies mucoid stools, melena, or hematochezia. Denies rectal bleeding, change in color, consistency, or habits.

Lifestyle and Health Practices: A typical day for client is to arise at 6:00 AM, eat breakfast, and perform light housekeeping. Client goes to community center in late morning to eat lunch, quilt, and visit. Goes home around 2:00 PM. Used to walk about four blocks with a friend every day, however, has not done this in the past 6 months. Cleans own house throughout the week, must space activities according to level of discomfort (includes dusting, vacuuming, washing). Relaxes with sewing crafts and visits with husband in the evening. Attends church-related activities mid-week and on Sunday. Bedtime is approximately 10:00 PM.

Nutrition Habits and Weight Management: Client states she is on a reduced carbohydrate/concentrated sweet diet that has approximately 1,600 calories/day intake. 24-hour diet recall: Breakfast—2 pieces whole-wheat toast, one boiled egg, 8-oz orange juice, and 2 cups decaffeinated coffee; lunch—tuna on salad with lettuce, tomatoes, and broccoli, an apple, and 8-oz skim milk; afternoon snack—Snickers candy bar, small bag plain potato chips; dinner—small serving of broiled meat, 1 cup green beans, half of cup mashed potatoes, slice of peach pie, and 8-oz glass of skim milk. Tries not to snack but admits that it is difficult not to. Drinks two 8-oz glasses of water a day. Drinks decaffeinated coffee—no tea or colas. Voices no food dislikes or intolerances.

Client expresses desire to maintain current weight. Weight tends to fluctuate ±5 lb/month—"I've always had to watch what I eat because I gain so easily."

Medication/Substance Use: No prescribed medications. Takes the following OTC medications: ibuprofen 200 mg 2 every 8 hours as needed; multivitamin l qd for past 4 years. Denies use of alcohol, tobacco, and illicit drugs.

Activity Level/Exercise-Fitness Plan: Retired elementary school teacher. Volunteers to cook for church social functions. Client expresses satisfaction with activity. However, she is concerned that she may not be able to maintain her current level of activity if the problems with her feet continue to progress.

Sleep/Rest: Goes to bed at 10:00 PM. Denies difficulty falling asleep, remaining asleep, or early morning awakening. Feels well rested when she arises at 6:00 AM. Denies use of sleep medications. Enjoys reading her Bible each evening before bed.

Self-Concept, Self-Esteem, Body Image: Describes self as normal person. Talkative, outgoing, and likes to be around people, but hates noisy environments. Happy with the person she has become and states, "I can definitely live with myself." States a weakness is that she worries about "little things" more now than she used to and tends to be irritated more easily. Client states she is capable of self-management of diabetes. Client rates own health as an 8 on a scale of 1 (worst) to 10 (best). She rates her health 5 years ago as a 10 and predicts that 5 years in the future her health will be a 6. Sees health deterioration as normal aging process and states, "I feel really good when I look at a lot of people my age with all their problems and the medicine they take."

Self-Care Responsibilities: Client seeks health care only in emergencies. Last medical examination was 8 years ago. Preventive health practices: wears seatbelt, tests smoke alarm every 6 months, has a carbon monoxide detector in home. Denies presence of firearms in the home. Handrails are present in bathtub. Denies presence of throw rugs in the home. Denies use of cell phone or texting use while driving.

Social Relationships: Describes relationship with other members of the church and community groups as friendly and "family-like." Has casual relationship with neighbors.

Family Relationships: Client has been married 55 years. Describes marital relationship as the best part of her life right now. Two daughters live in Texas with their husbands and children. Her son and his wife and baby boy live in Minnesota. All the children and their families come home once a year, and the client and her husband visit each family once a year. She expresses desire to visit her children and grandchildren more often and states, "I wish my babies lived nearby. I love being a grandma and miss them so much." Communicates with each of them several times a month by phone. Client was the fourth of five children in her family. Had a happy childhood, describes family as close and loving—"my daddy was very strict though."

Education and Work: Client went to college to be a teacher. Taught elementary school for 30 years. After her children were grown, she would work during the summer as a caterer—"I love to cook." Is retired now but still volunteers to cook for church social functions.

> ***Stress Level and Coping Styles:*** Shares confidences with husband and with a few close friends. Most stressful time in life was losing two brothers and a sister, all in the same year. States that with support of husband, children, and church, she handled it "better than most people would have." States that she prays and eats when under stress. Cannot identify any major stresses that have occurred in the last year.
>
> ***Environmental Hazards:*** Is not aware of any environmental hazards in area where she lives.
>
> ***Developmental Level—Integrity Versus Despair:*** Describes childhood as a very happy time for her. Becomes excited and smiles as she relates stories of her childhood on the farm. States that she was an average child and ran and played like all the others. Companions were brothers and sisters. Has been married for 55 years. Describes relationship with husband as close and sharing. Taught elementary school for 30 years and catered in the summer for several years. Lived in a large house until 1976. Currently lives in small, two-bedroom bungalow. Active in church and society. Volunteers at church functions. States that she enjoys being retired and lives a "comfortable" life. Does not voice financial concerns. Has begun to write a will and distribute personal heirlooms to children and grandchildren. States that she is not afraid of death and wishes to have the "business part taken care of" in order to enjoy the rest of her life with her husband.

Physical Assessment

General Survey

Ht: 5 ft 4 in; Wt: 185 lb; BMI: 31.75, Pulse: 71; Resp: 16; B/P: R arm—146/88, L arm—152/90; Temp: 98.6. Client alert and cooperative. Speech clear, without slur or stutter. Expresses ideas and feelings clearly and concisely. Makes and maintains eye contact and conversation. Follows verbal cues. Sitting on table with arms crossed and shoulder slightly slouched forward. Dress is clean and appropriate for season.

Skin, Hair, Nails

Skin: Dark brown, warm, and dry to touch. Turgor intact, with immediate recoil of skin over clavicle. Dark brown macules scattered over dorsal surfaces bilateral hands. No excoriations. Appendectomy scar right lower quadrant of abdomen is thin and well healed.

Hair: Black with scattered gray streaks, short, and curly. No scalp lesions or flaking.

Nails: Fingernails well manicured and immobile. Immediate capillary refill. No clubbing or Beau lines.

Head and Neck

Head symmetrically round, hard, and smooth, without lesions or bumps. Face is oval, smooth, and symmetric. Bilateral temporal arteries are smooth and elastic. Bilateral temporomandibular joints with full ROM and no tenderness. Neck symmetric, without bulging masses. C7 is visible and palpable. Full and controlled ROM of neck. Thyroid gland is nonvisible and nonpalpable. Trachea is midline. No lymphadenopathy noted.

Eyes

Visual acuity 20/20 corrected. Visual fields full by confrontation. Corneal light reflex with symmetric reflexion. EOMs smooth and intact. No ptosis. No redness, discharge of lid margins. Eyes symmetrical. Eyebrows sparse, with equal distribution. Conjunctiva and sclera moist and smooth. Sclera white, without increased vascularity or lesions noted. Lacrimal apparatus nonedematous and without drainage. Iris uniformly dark brown. Pupils 5 to 3 mm, equal, round, and reactive to light and accommodation. Pupils converge evenly. Funduscopic examination: Red reflex present bilaterally. No other structures visualized to examiner.

Ears

Bilateral auricles without deformity, lumps, or lesions. Mastoid processes nontender. Bilateral auditory canals contain scant amount of dark brown cerumen. Tympanic membranes pearly gray and transparent, with no bulging or retraction. Light reflex at 5:00 on the right TM and at 7:00 on the left TM. Bony structures of TM visible bilaterally. Whisper test: Unable to identify two-syllable word whispered at distance of 3 ft. Weber test: No lateralization of sound to either ear. Rinne test: AC is greater than BC in both ears.

Mouth, Throat, Nose, and Sinuses

Lips pink, smooth, and moist; no lesions or ulcerations. Buccal mucosa pink and moist, with patchy areas of dark pigment on ventral surface of tongue, gums, and floor of mouth. No ulcers or nodules. Gums pink and moist, without inflammation, bleeding, or discoloration. Hard and soft palates smooth, without lesions or masses. Tongue midline when protruded, no lesions, or masses. Uvula midline and elevates on phonation. Tonsils present, without exudate, edema, ulcers, or enlargement. Nose: External structure without deformity, asymmetry, or inflammation. Nares patent. Turbinates and middle meatus pale pink, without swelling, exudate, lesions, or bleeding. Nasal septum midline without bleeding, perforation, or deviation. Frontal and maxillary sinuses nontender.

Thorax and Lung

Respirations even, unlabored, and regular. No use of accessory muscles and no nasal flaring. Skin dark brown, without tenderness, lesion, or masses. Thorax expands symmetrically without retractions or bulging. Slope of ribs = 40 degrees. Bilateral tactile fremitus decreases below T5 posteriorly, and 4th ICS anteriorly. Percussion resonant throughout. Diaphragmatic excursion: 4 cm and equal bilaterally. Vesicular breath sounds heard in all lung fields. No adventitious sounds. No whispered pectoriloquy, bronchophony, or egophony noted.

Breasts

Breasts pendulous and symmetric. Skin dark brown, with black/brown areola. No dimpling or retraction noted bilaterally. Free movement in all positions. Nipples inverted bilaterally. No discharge expressed. No masses, thickening, tenderness, or lymphadenopathy noted.

Heart and Neck Vessels

Carotid pulses 2+ bilaterally. No carotid bruits or jugular vein distension. No precordial pulsations, heaves, lifts or vibrations visible. PMI palpable at 5th ICS, LMCL. Heart regular rate and rhythm with S_1 and S_2. No S_3 or S_4. No murmurs, gallops, rubs, splitting, clicks, or snaps.

Peripheral Vascular

Upper extremities: Equal in size and symmetric. Skin dark brown; warm and dry to touch, without edema, bruising, or lesions. Radial and brachial pulses 2+ and equal bilaterally. Allen's test: radial and ulnar arteries intact bilaterally. Epitrochlear nodes nonpalpable.

Lower extremities: Symmetric in size and shape. Skin intact, dark brown; warm and dry to touch, without edema, bruising, lesions, or increased vascularity. No inguinal lymphadenopathy. Femoral pulses 2+ and equal bilaterally, without bruits. Dorsalis pedal and posterior tibial pulses 1+ and equal bilaterally. Capillary refill <2 seconds. Position's change test is negative for arterial insufficiency.

Abdomen

Abdomen rounded and symmetric, without masses, lesions, pulsations, or peristaltic waves. Abdomen free of hair, bruising, or increased vasculature. Umbilicus in midline, without herniation, swelling, or discoloration. Bowel sounds low pitched and gurgling at 22/min. Aortic, renal, and iliac arteries without bruits. No venous hums or friction rubs over liver or spleen. Abdomen tympanic. Liver span is 8 cm in R MCL. Area of dullness over spleen at 9th ICS in left postaxillary line. No tenderness or masses noted with light or deep palpation. Liver and spleen nonpalpable.

Musculoskeletal

Posture erect. Gait steady, smooth, and coordinated with even base. Full, smooth ROM of cervical and lumbar spine. Paravertebral muscles equal in size and strength. Upper extremities and lower extremities symmetric, without lesions, nodules, deformities, or swelling. Full ROM against gravity and with resistance.

Neurologic

Mental Status Examination: Facial expressions symmetric and correlate with mood and topic discussed. Speech clear and appropriate. Follows through with train of thought. Carefully chooses words to convey feelings and ideas. Oriented to person, place, time, and events. Remains attentive and able to focus on examination during entire interaction. Short- and long-term memories intact. Vocabulary suitable to educational level.

Cranial Nerve Examination: CN I: Correctly identifies scents. CN II: 20/20 corrected vision. CN III, IV, and VI: EOMs intact. PERRLA. Lid covers 2 mm of iris; bilateral eye movement, bilateral pupil response. CN V: Identifies light touch to forehead, cheek, and chin. Bilateral corneal reflex intact. Masseter muscles contract equally and bilaterally. CN VII: Identifies sugar and salt on anterior 2/3 of tongue. Smiles, frowns, shows teeth, blows out cheeks, and raises eyebrows as instructed. CN VIII: Unable to hear whispered words from 3 ft; Weber test: equal lateralization; Rinne test: AC > BC. CN IX and X: Gag reflex intact. Client identifies sugar and salt on posterior of tongue. Uvula in midline and elevates on phonation. CN XI: Shrugs shoulders and moves head to right and left against resistance. CN XII: Tongue midline when protruded, without fasciculations. (One may also document cranial nerves I to XII intact.)

Motor and Cerebellar Examination: Muscle tone intact, with no atrophy, tremors, or weakness. No fasciculations, tics, or tremors. Muscle strength 5/5 upper and lower extremities. Gait and tandem walk intact. Romberg test negative. Alternates finger to nose with eyes closed. Rapidly opposes fingers to thumb bilaterally without difficulty. Alternates pronation and supination of hands rapidly without difficulty. Heel to shin intact bilaterally.

Sensory Status Examination: Superficial light and sharp sensation intact. Position sense of fingers intact bilaterally. Stereognosis and graphesthesia intact. Upper extremity vibratory sensation and two-point discrimination intact. Lower extremity vibratory sensation from mid-calf to ankle decreased bilaterally. Unable to distinguish vibratory sensation or proprioception of either great toe. Monofilament test reveals inability to perceive pressure of the great toe, third and fifth toe/digits bilaterally (Boulton et al., 2008).

Genitalia

Labia pink with decreased elasticity and vaginal secretions. No bulging of vaginal wall, discharge, or lesions. Skene gland not visible.

Anus/Rectum

Anal opening is hairless, moist, and closed tightly. Perianal area is without redness, lumps, lesions, or rash. No bulging or lesions with Valsalva maneuver.

Client's Strengths

- Positive attitude and outlook on life
- Motivation to maintain her health
- Strong support systems; husband and spiritual beliefs

Nursing Diagnoses

- Acute Pain in lower extremities/feet
- Impaired Physical Mobility related to decreased sensation lower extremities/feet and discomfort
- Risk for Impaired Skin Integrity related to decreased peripheral sensation
- Risk for Injury related to decreased peripheral sensation
- Risk for Ineffective Health Maintenance related to lack of knowledge concerning importance of regular medical checkups, that is, no Pap smear, and no follow-up for diabetes
- Knowledge Deficit: Signs and symptoms and treatment of hyperglycemia/hypoglycemia
- Knowledge Deficit: Self-care behaviors regarding diabetes management: Blood glucose monitoring, yearly dilated eye examination, and yearly lipid panel

Collaborative Problems

- RC: Peripheral neuropathy
- RC: Hyperglycemia, hypoglycemia

The following is a brief "Head-to-Toe Physical Assessment Guide" that may be used to establish the client's physical status. This type of assessment is frequently used by nurses at the beginning of a hospital shift when the nurse has multiple clients to whom she will provide nursing care. Often, a total physical examination is done upon admission to the hospital by the physician or nurse practitioner. Therefore, this shorter format is more practical for ongoing client assessments.

ABBREVIATED HEAD-TO-TOE PHYSICAL ASSESSMENT GUIDE

Assessment Procedure	Normal Findings	Abnormal Findings
GENERAL SURVEY		
Assess Level of Consciousness (LOC).	Awake, alert, and oriented to person, place, and time.	If altered LOC, consider the Glasgow Coma Scale.
Assess speech.	Speech clear. Makes and maintains conversation appropriately.	
Assess comfort level.	Denies pain/discomfort.	If the patient reports pain: rate the pain using the 0–10 pain scale, intervene to provide comfort measures, and evaluate the effectiveness of such interventions.
Assess skin color, temperature, moisture, turgor.	Skin: pink, warm, and dry. Immediate recoil noted at the clavicle.	Pale, pallor → anemia Erythema → infection Warmth → infection Increased tenting → dehydration
EYES		
Assess pupils.	Pupils equal, round, react to light and accommodation (PERRLA).	Pupils unequal or nonreactive to light.
CHEST		
Assess breath sounds.	Lungs: clear to auscultation (CTA) anterior and posterior (A and P), bilaterally. Respiratory rate = 18, no reports of dyspnea	Note any wheezes or crackles and identify their location (anterior or posterior, upper or lower lobes, right or left).
Assess heart sounds. Note if rhythm is irregular.	Heart: S_1 and S_2 present, regular rate (82) and rhythm. No S_3 or S_4 appreciated. No murmur, rub, or gallop (MRG).	Heart sounds irregular or irregularly irregular. Murmurs, rub, or gallop present.
ABDOMEN		
Assess contour and firmness.	Nondistended, soft, and nontender.	Distended and firm, visible palpations.
Assess bowel sounds.	Active bowel sounds noted in all 4 quadrants (+ABS × 4Q). Normal bowel sounds = 5–35/min.	Absence of bowel sounds in one or more quadrants. One must listen for 5 minutes to document absent bowel sounds.
EXTREMITIES		
Assess mobility of extremities, strength of extremities, and peripheral pulses.	Able to actively move all extremities. Equal strength, 5/5. Radial, dorsalis pedis and posterior tibia pulses 2+. No peripheral edema.	Unable to actively or passively move one or more extremities. Decreased or absent pulses, edema of one of more extremities.
OTHER		
Note any wounds or lesions.	Describe: size, shape, location, color, characteristics of any drainage, type of dressing.	
Note any drains: Jackson–Pratt, Foley catheter, Hemovac, nasogastric tube, etc.	Describe insertion site; color, consistency, and/or odor of any drainage.	

Continued on following page

ABBREVIATED HEAD-TO-TOE PHYSICAL ASSESSMENT GUIDE (Continued)

Assessment Procedure	Normal Findings	Abnormal Findings
Note any venous access devices.	Describe the location, appearance, type and size of device, type of intravenous fluids and rate of infusion, and infusion device(s).	
Note any other therapies: oxygen, telemetry, CPAP/BiPap (for sleep apnea), insulin pump, sequential compression device, external ice/heat device, continuous passive motion device, traction, TENS (transcutaneous electrical nerve stimulation) unit, etc.	Describe the presence of correct functioning of any of these devices.	

Interdisciplinary Verbal Communication of Assessment Findings Using SBAR

SITUATION: SL, a retired school teacher, requests an examination, as she has not had a physical examination in 8 years. She has type 2 diabetes but feels it is under "control." However, she has been having constant numbness, burning, and tingling in both feet for the last 2 months, which has been getting progressively worse. Aggravated by tight shoes, temperature extremes, and extended periods of walking. Rates pain in these situations as 5–6 on a scale of 0–10. Pain is worse without shoes and walking on a firm surface. But pain is always present at a level of 2–3 on a scale of 0–10. Ibuprofen does not relieve the pain. Pain decreases only when she is non–weight-bearing. Interferes with her sleep. She thinks it may be arthritis but is concerned as she has not been to a primary care provider for so long.

BACKGROUND: Developed urinary tract infection at age 57, at which time she was diagnosed with type 2 diabetes and received diabetes education with nutritional medical therapy. Mother died from stroke at age 72 with history of diabetes and hypertension. Skin and scalp dry. Nails hard and brittle. Has worn glasses all her life, changing from bifocals to trifocals at age 60. Has blurred vision without glasses. States "I think I am a little slow to grasp because of my hearing." Does not wear hearing aid. Follows reduced carbohydrate diet for main meals but eats Snickers candy bar and small bag potato chips for snacks. Takes no prescribed medications. Takes the ibuprofen 200 mg 2 every 8 hours as needed; multivitamin l qd for past 4 years. Retired elementary school teacher. Volunteers to cook for church social functions. Sees health deterioration as normal aging process and seeks health care only in emergencies. Married 55 years with two daughters and one son who are married, have children and live far away. Describes childhood as a very happy time. Has begun to write a will and distribute personal heirlooms to children and grandchildren. States that she is not afraid of death and wishes to have the "business part taken care of" in order to enjoy the rest of her life with her husband.

ASSESSMENT: Ht: 5 ft 4 in; Wt: 185 lb; BMI: 31.75; Pulse: 71; Resp: 16; B/P: R arm—146/88, L arm—152/90; Temp: 98.6. Lower extremity vibratory sensation from mid-calf to ankle decreased bilaterally. Unable to distinguish vibratory sensation or proprioception of either great toe. Monofilament test reveals inability to perceive pressure at any point bilaterally. Rest of physical assessment reveals normal findings.

RECOMMENDATION: Mrs. Lewis has acute pain in lower extremities/feet with impaired physical mobility related to decreased sensation in lower extremities/feet with discomfort. She is at risk for Impaired Skin Integrity related to decreased peripheral sensation and risk for Injury related to decreased peripheral sensation. She also has ineffective health maintenance related to lack of knowledge concerning importance of regular medical checkups, Pap smears, and follow-up for diabetes. She lacks knowledge regarding the signs and symptoms and treatment of hyperglycemia/hypoglycemia and self-care regarding diabetes management for blood glucose monitoring, yearly dilated eye examination, and yearly lipid panel. She is at risk for peripheral neuropathy, hyperglycemia, and hypoglycemia. She needs to be seen by her primary care provider for further evaluation and treatment of her diabetes.

Want to know more?

A wide variety of resources to enhance your learning and understanding of this book are available on **thePoint**. Visit thePoint to access:

NCLEX-Style Student Review Questions
Watch and Learn Videos
Concept in Action Animations
And more!

Reference and Selected Reading

Boulton, A. J., Armstrong, D. G., Albert, S. F., Frykberg, R. G., Hellman, R., Kirkman, M. S., et al; American Diabetes Association; American Association of Clinical Endocrinologists. (2008). Comprehensive foot examination and risk assessment: A report of the task force of the foot care interest group of the American Diabetes Association, with endorsement by the American Association of Clinical Endocrinologists. *Diabetes Care*, 31(8), 1679–1685.

UNIT 4

Nursing Assessment of Special Groups

29 ASSESSING CHILDBEARING WOMEN

Learning Objectives

1. Describe the physiologic and anatomical changes that occur during pregnancy.
2. Discuss risk factors associated with complications that may occur during pregnancy across the cultures and ways to reduce one's risks.
3. Interview a client for an accurate nursing history of the pregnant client.
4. Perform a physical assessment of the pregnant client using the correct techniques.
5. Differentiate between normal and abnormal findings identified during pregnancy.
6. Analyze the data from the interview and physical assessment of the pregnant client to formulate valid nursing diagnoses, collaborative problems, and/or referrals.
7. Differentiate between general routine screening versus skills needed for focused or specialty assessment of the pregnant client.
8. Document and verbally report accurate assessment findings of the pregnant client.

CASE STUDY

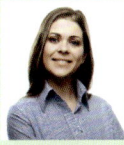

Mrs. Mary Farrow is a 29-year-old Caucasian woman, gravida 3, para 2, who presents to the clinic today for her initial prenatal examination. She states that her last menstrual period (LMP) was on September 15, approximately 16 weeks ago. Because she was so sick and unable to get transportation to the clinic, she did not come in for prenatal care earlier in this pregnancy. She reports that she has had severe nausea with vomiting for the past 8 weeks of this pregnancy.

STRUCTURE AND FUNCTION

Healthy People 2020 (2016) notes that improving the well-being of mothers, infants, and children is an important public health goal for the United States, as their well-being determines the health of the next generation and can help predict future public health challenges for families, communities, and the health care system. Additionally, pregnancy can provide an opportunity to identify existing health risks in women and thereby prevent future health problems for the women and their children.

The body experiences physiologic and anatomic changes during pregnancy. Most of these changes are influenced by the hormones of pregnancy, primarily estrogen and progesterone.

Normal physiologic and anatomic changes during pregnancy are discussed in this chapter.

Skin, Hair, and Nails

During pregnancy, integumentary system changes occur primarily because of hormonal influences. Many of these skin, hair, and nail changes fade or completely resolve after the end of the gestation. As the pregnancy progresses, the breasts and abdomen enlarge and striae gravidarum, or stretch marks—pinkish-red streaks with slight depressions in the skin—begin to appear over the abdomen, breasts, thighs, and buttocks. These marks usually fade to a white or silvery color, but they typically never completely resolve after the pregnancy.

Hyperpigmentation also results from hormonal influences (e.g., estrogen, progesterone, and melanocyte-stimulating hormone). It is most noted on the abdomen (linea nigra, a dark line extending from the umbilicus to the mons pubis) and face (chloasma, a darkening of the skin on the face, known as the facial "mask of pregnancy"). When not pregnant, women taking oral contraceptives may also experience chloasma because of the hormones in the medication.

Other skin changes during pregnancy include darkening of the areolae and nipples, axillae, umbilicus, and perineum. Scars and moles may also darken from the influence of melanocyte-stimulating hormone. Vascular changes, such as spider nevi (tiny red angiomas occurring on the face, neck, chest, arms, and legs), may occur because of elevated estrogen levels. Palmar erythema (a pinkish color on the palms of the hands) may also be noted. Pruritic urticarial papules and plaques of pregnancy (PUPPP) is a skin disorder seen during the third trimester of pregnancy, characterized by erythematous papules, plaques, and urticarial lesions. The rash begins on the abdomen and may soon spread to the thighs, buttocks, and arms. The intense itching and rash usually resolve within weeks of delivery. Acne vulgaris is an unpredictable response during pregnancy. Acne may worsen or improve. It consists of erythema, pustules, comedones, and/or cysts that appear on the face, back, neck, or chest. The activity of the eccrine sweat glands and the excretion rate of sebum onto the skin increase in normal pregnancy, whereas the activity of the apocrine sweat glands appears to decrease. The changes that occur in the endocrine system help to maintain optimal maternal and fetal health. Estrogen is primarily responsible for the changes that occur to the pituitary, thyroid, parathyroid, and adrenal glands. The increased production of hormones—especially triiodothyronine (T_3) and thyroxine (T_4)—increases the basal metabolic rate, cardiac output, vasodilation, heart rate, and heat intolerance. The basal metabolic rate increases up to 30% in a term pregnancy.

Growth of hair and nails also tends to increase during pregnancy. Some women note excessive oiliness or dryness of the scalp and a softening and thinning of the nails by the 6th week of gestation. Pregnancy hormones increase the growing phases of the hair follicle and decrease the resting phase of the hair follicle. During the postpartum period, hormone withdrawal increases the resting phase of the hair follicle and transient hair loss is noticed, commonly peaking at 3 to 4 months postpartum. This loss is normally resolved within 9 months to 1 year of delivery.

Hirsutism of the face, abdomen, and back may also be experienced during the second and third trimesters of pregnancy. Hormonal changes (androgens) cause this hair growth, which may improve after delivery.

Ears and Hearing

Pregnant women may report a decrease in hearing, a sense of fullness in the ears, or earaches because of the increased vascularity of the tympanic membrane and blockage of the eustachian tubes.

Mouth, Throat, Nose, and Sinus

Some women may note changes in their gums during pregnancy. Gingival bleeding when brushing teeth and hypertrophy are common. Occasionally epulis develop, which are small, irritating nodules of the gums. These nodules usually resolve on their own. Occasionally, the lesion may need to be surgically excised if the nodule bleeds excessively.

Vocal changes may be noted due to edema of the larynx. Nasal "stuffiness" and epistaxis are also common during pregnancy because of estrogen-induced edema and vascular congestion of the nasal mucosa and sinuses.

Thorax and Lungs

As the pregnancy progresses, progesterone influences relaxation of the ligaments and joints. This relaxation allows the rib cage to flare, thus increasing the anteroposterior and transverse diameters. This accommodation is necessary as the pregnancy progresses and the enlarging uterus pushes up on the diaphragm. The client's respiratory pattern changes from abdominal to costal. Shortness of breath is a common complaint during the last trimester. The client may be more aware of her breathing pattern and of deep respirations and more frequent sighing. Oxygen requirements increase during pregnancy because of the additional cellular growth of the body and the fetus. Pulmonary requirements increase, with the tidal volume increasing by 30% to 40%. All of these changes are normal and are to be expected during the last trimester.

Breasts

Soon after conception, the surge of estrogen and progesterone begins, causing notable changes in the mammary glands (Fig. 29-1). Breast changes noted by many women include:
- Tingling sensations and tenderness
- Enlargement of breast and nipple
- Hyperpigmentation of areola and nipple
- Enlargement of Montgomery tubercles
- Prominence of superficial veins
- Development of striae
- Expression of colostrum in the second and third trimesters

Heart

Significant cardiovascular changes occur during pregnancy. One of the most dynamic changes is the increase in cardiac output and maternal blood volume by approximately 40% to 50%. Because the heart is required to pump much harder, it actually increases in size. Its position is rotated up and to the left approximately 1 to 1.5 cm. The heart rate may increase by 10 to 15 beats/min and systolic murmurs may be heard.

Peripheral Vascular System

With the dynamic increase in maternal blood volume, a physiologic anemia (pseudoanemia) commonly develops. This

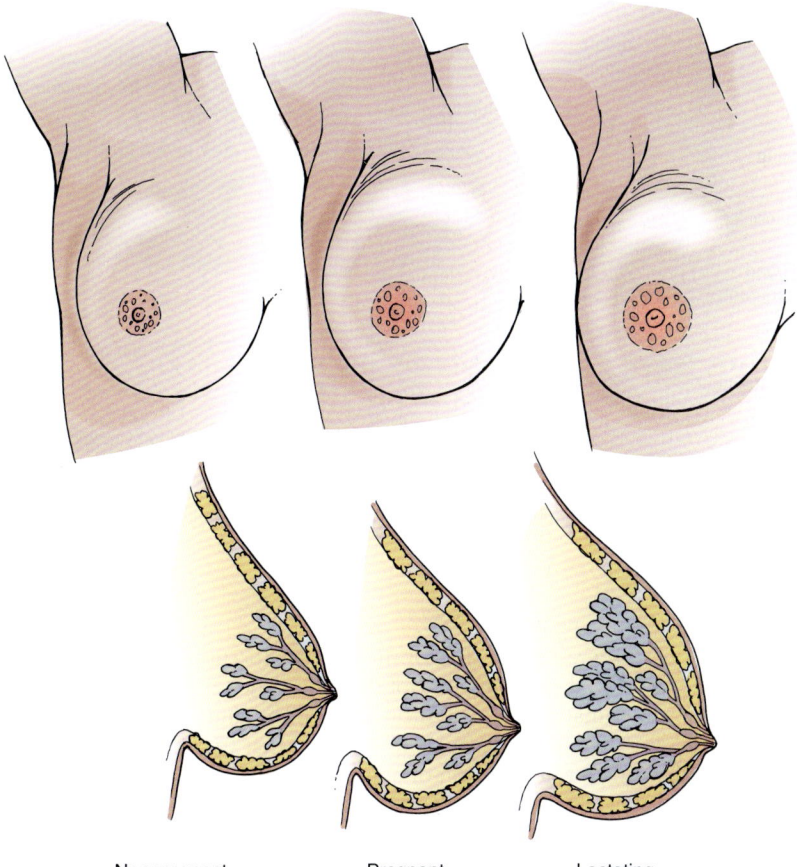

FIGURE 29-1 Breast changes during pregnancy.   Nonpregnant   Pregnant   Lactating

anemia results primarily from the disproportionate increase in blood volume compared with the increased red blood cell (RBC) production. Plasma volume increases 40% to 50% and RBC volume increases 18% to 30% by 30 to 34 weeks' gestation.

As plasma blood volume increases, the blood vessels must accommodate for this volume: progesterone acts on the vessels to make them relax and dilate. Clients often complain of feeling dizzy and lightheaded beginning with the second trimester. These effects peak at approximately 32 to 34 weeks. As the pregnancy progresses, the arterial blood pressure stabilizes and symptoms begin to resolve. Prepregnancy values return in the third trimester.

Other changes that occur during pregnancy include dependent edema and varicosities. Two thirds of all pregnant women have swelling of the lower extremities in the third trimester. Swelling is usually noted late in the day after standing for long periods. Fluid retention is caused by the increased hormones of pregnancy, increased hydrophilicity of the intracellular connective tissue, and increased venous pressure in the lower extremities. As the expanding uterus applies pressure on the femoral venous area, femoral venous pressure increases. This uterine pressure restricts venous blood flow return, causing stagnation of the blood in the lower extremities and resulting in dependent edema. Varicose veins in the lower extremities, vulva, and rectum are also common during pregnancy. Pregnant women are also more prone to development of thrombophlebitis because of the hypercoagulable state of pregnancy. Women who are placed on bedrest during pregnancy are at a very high risk for development of thrombophlebitis.

Abdomen

During pregnancy, the abdominal muscles stretch as the uterus enlarges. These muscles, known as the rectus abdominis muscles, may stretch to the point that permanent separation occurs. This condition is known as *diastasis recti abdominis*. Four paired ligaments (broad ligaments, uterosacral ligaments, cardinal ligaments, round ligaments) support the uterus and keep it in position in the pelvic cavity (Fig. 29-2). As the uterus enlarges, the client may complain of lower pelvic discomfort, which quite commonly results from stretching the ligaments, especially the round ligaments.

In the abdomen, the expanding uterus exerts pressure on the bladder, kidney, and ureters (especially on the right side), predisposing the client to kidney infection. Urinary frequency is a common complaint in the first and third trimesters. The applied pressure on the kidneys and ureters causes decreased flow and stagnation of the urine. As a result, physiologic hydronephrosis and hydroureter occur. During the second trimester, bladder pressure subsides and urinary frequency is relieved by the uterus enlarging and being lifted out of the pelvic area.

The enlarging uterus also applies pressure and displaces the small intestine. This pressure, along with the secretion of progesterone, decreases gastric motility. Gastric tone is decreased and the smooth muscles relax, decreasing emptying time of the stomach. Constipation results from these physiologic events. Heartburn, which may also result, may also be related to decreased gastrointestinal motility and displacement of the stomach. This causes reflux of stomach acid into the esophagus. Progesterone secretion also relaxes the smooth muscles

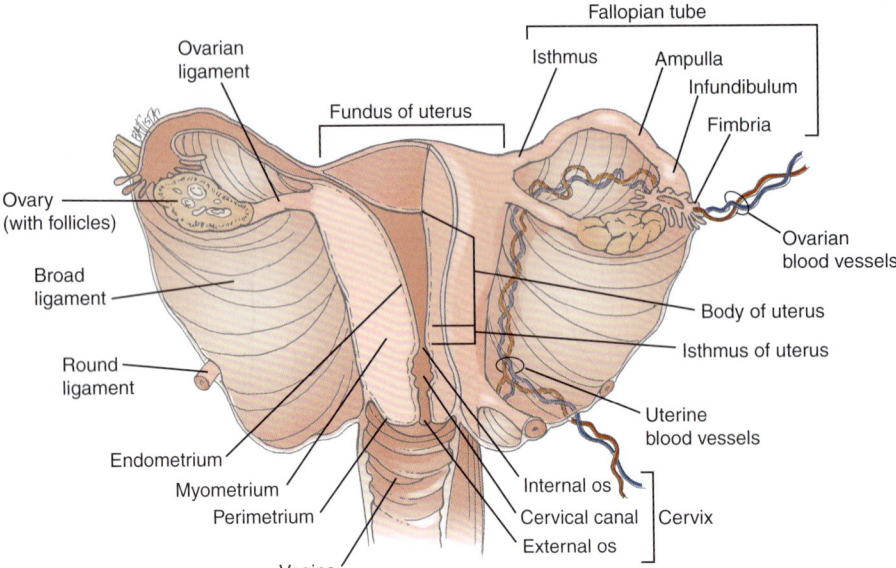

FIGURE 29-2 Anterior cross-section of the female reproductive structures.

of the gallbladder; as a result, gallstone formation may occur because of the prolonged emptying time of the gallbladder.

Other gastrointestinal symptoms include ptyalism and pica. Ptyalism, excessive salivation may occur in the first trimester. Pica, a craving for or ingestion of nonnutritional substances such as dirt or clay, is seen in all socioeconomic classes and cultures. Pica can be a major concern if the craving interferes with proper nutrition during pregnancy.

Carbohydrate metabolism is also altered during pregnancy. Glucose use increases, leading to decreased maternal glucose levels. The rise in serum levels of estrogen, progesterone, and other hormones stimulates beta-cell hypertrophy and hyperplasia, and insulin secretion increases. Glycogen is stored and gluconeogenesis is reduced. In addition, the mother's body tissues develop an increased sensitivity to insulin, thus decreasing the mother's need. As a result, maternal hypoglycemia leads to hypoinsulinemia and increased rates of ketosis. Some well-controlled insulin-dependent diabetic clients have frequent episodes of hypoglycemia in the first trimester. This buildup of insulin ensures an adequate supply of glucose, because the glucose is preferentially shunted to the fetus.

In contrast, during the second half of pregnancy, tissue sensitivity to insulin progressively decreases, producing hyperglycemia and hyperinsulinemia. Insulin resistance becomes maximal in the latter half of the pregnancy (and this is when gestational diabetes is more likely to occur) (UCSF Medical Center, 2016).

Genitalia

Before conception, the uterus is a small, pear-shaped organ that weighs approximately 44 g. Its cavity can hold approximately 10 mL of fluid. Pregnancy changes this organ, giving it the capacity to weigh approximately 1,000 g and potentially hold approximately 5 L of amniotic fluid. This dynamic change is mainly due to the hypertrophy of pre-existing myometrial cells and the hyperplasia of new cells. Estrogen and the growing fetus are primarily responsible for this growth. Once conception occurs, the uterus prepares itself for the pregnancy: ovulation ceases, the uterine endometrium thickens, and the number and size of uterine blood vessels increase.

With fetal growth, the uterus continues to expand throughout the pregnancy. At approximately 10 to 12 weeks' gestation, the uterus should be palpated at the top of the symphysis pubis. At 16 weeks' gestation, the top of the uterus, known as the fundus, should reach halfway between the symphysis pubis and the umbilicus. At 20 weeks' gestation, the fundus should be at the level of the umbilicus. For the rest of the pregnancy, the uterus grows approximately 1 cm/wk; the fundal height should equal the number of weeks pregnant (e.g., at 25 weeks' gestation, the fundal height should measure 25 cm). This formula is known as McDonald's rule. It can be calculated by taking the fundal height in centimeters and multiplying it by 8/7. With a full-term pregnancy, the fundus should reach the xiphoid process. The fundal height measurement may drop in the last few weeks of the pregnancy if the fetal head is engaged and descended in the maternal pelvis. This occurrence is known as *lightening*.

Near-term gestation, the uterine wall begins thinning out to approximately 5 mm or less. Fetal parts are easily palpated on the external abdomen in the term pregnancy. Braxton Hicks contractions (painless, irregular contractions of the uterus) may occur sporadically in the third trimester. These contractions are normal as long as no cervical change is noted.

Normal changes in the cervix, vagina, and vulva also occur during pregnancy. Cervical softening (Goodell sign), bluish discoloration (Chadwick sign), and hypertrophy of the glands in the cervical canal all occur. With these glands secreting more mucus, there is an increase in vaginal discharge, which is acidic. The mucus collects in the cervix to form the mucous plug. This plug seals the endocervical canal and prevents bacteria from ascending into the uterus, thus preventing infection. The vaginal smooth muscle and connective tissue soften and expand to prepare for the passage of the fetus through the birth canal.

Anus and Rectum

Constipation is a common problem during pregnancy. Progesterone decreases intestinal motility, allowing more time for nutrients to be absorbed for the mother and fetus. This also increases the absorption time for water into the circulation, taking fluid from the large intestine and contributing to hardening of the stool and decreasing the frequency of bowel movements. Iron supplementation can also contribute to constipation for those women who take additional iron. As a result, hemorrhoids (varicose veins in the rectum) may develop because of the pressure on the venous structures from straining to have a bowel movement. Vascular congestion of the pelvis also contributes to hemorrhoid development.

Musculoskeletal System

Anatomic changes of the musculoskeletal system during pregnancy result from fetal growth, hormonal influences, and maternal weight gain. As the pregnancy progresses, uterine growth pulls the pelvis forward, which causes the spine to curve forward, creating a gradual lordosis (Fig. 29-3). The enlarging breasts cause the shoulders to droop forward. The pregnant client typically finds herself pulling her shoulders back and straightening her head and neck to accommodate for this weight. Progesterone and relaxin (nonsteroidal hormone) induce relaxation of the pelvic joints and ligaments. The symphysis pubis, sacroiliac and sacrococcygeal joints become more flexible during pregnancy. This flexibility allows the pelvic outlet diameter to increase slightly, which reduces the risk of trauma during childbirth. After the postpartum period, the pelvic diameter will generally remain larger than the size before childbirth.

Relaxin contributes to changing the client's gait during pregnancy. The pregnant woman's gait is often described as "waddling." Gait changes are also attributed to weight gain in the uterus, fetus, and breasts. At approximately 24 weeks' gestation, the woman's center of gravity and stance change, causing her to lean back slightly to balance herself. Backaches are common during pregnancy. Along with these changes, the woman may also see an increase in shoe size, especially in width.

Neurologic System

Most neurologic changes that occur during pregnancy are discomforting to the client. Common neurologic complaints include:
- Pain or tingling feeling in the thigh: Caused by pressure on the lateral femoral cutaneous nerve
- Carpal tunnel syndrome: Pressure on the median nerve below the carpal ligament of the wrist causes a tingling sensation in the hand. Because fluid retention occurs during pregnancy, swollen tissues compress the median nerve in the wrist and produce the tingling sensations. Pain can be reproduced by performing Tinel sign and Phalen test. Up and down movement of the wrist aggravates this condition.
- Leg cramps: Caused by inadequate calcium intake.
- Dizziness and lightheadedness: In early pregnancy, the client may experience dizziness because of blood pressure slightly decreasing as a result of vasodilation and decreased vascular resistance. In later pregnancy, the client in the supine position may experience dizziness caused by the heavy uterus compressing the vena cava and aorta. This compression reduces cardiac return, cardiac output, and blood pressure. This is known as *supine hypotensive syndrome.*

CLINICAL TIP
Exposure to mosquito bites in geographical areas where Zika, dengue, or chikungunya virus are known to exist requires a more in-depth assessment. Several systems can be affected by these viruses. The serious risk to pregnant women and their fetuses due to Zika virus is just being ascertained. See Evidence-Based Health Promotion and Disease Prevention 29-1 for further details.

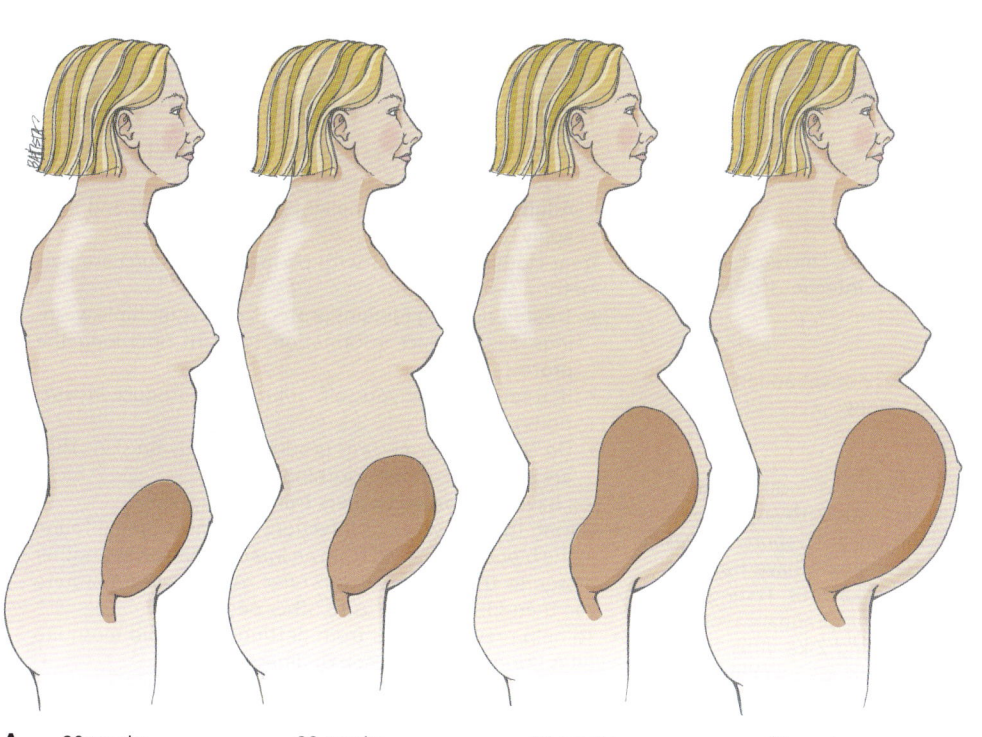
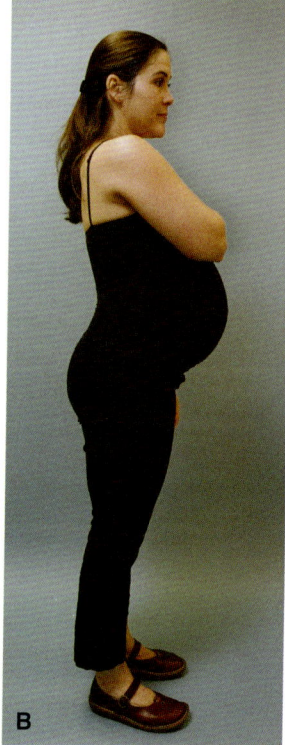

A 20 weeks   28 weeks   36 weeks   40 weeks

FIGURE 29-3 A. Postural changes during pregnancy. B. Lordosis in pregnant client.

29-1 EVIDENCE-BASED HEALTH PROMOTION AND DISEASE PREVENTION: ZIKA VIRUS INFECTION

Zika virus was first identified in Uganda in 1947 in monkeys, and in humans in 1952 in both Uganda and Tanzania (WHO, 2016). The virus has been known to circulate in Africa, Asia, the Pacific, and the Americas. In response to the recent epidemic of Zika virus infections in the Americas, by February of 2016 the CDC (2016) activated the highest level of its Emergency Operations Center and the WHO (2016) declared a Public Health Emergency of International Concern. The urgent response to the Zika virus is due to the number of cases reported, especially in Brazil and northern parts of South America, and to increased reports of birth defects (microcephaly) and Guillain–Barré syndrome in areas affected by Zika. Prior to February of 2016, there were cases in the United States, but only in persons who had travelled to Zika-infested areas and not from person-to-person transmission. However, as the disease has spread up through Central America and cases have been identified in Florida, U.S. citizens have been put on alert.

The CDC (2016) explains that the Zika virus is transmitted to people primarily through the bite of an infected *Aedes* species mosquito (*A. aegypti* and *A. albopictus*). These are the same mosquitoes that spread the dengue and chikungunya viruses. These mosquitoes typically lay eggs in standing water, such as buckets, dishes, bowls, and flower pots. They are aggressive daytime biters, but can bite at night as well. The mosquitoes become infected by biting an infected person and then spread the disease by biting another person. The virus has been shown to spread through sexual contact and blood transfusions as well. It was believed that there is no transmission of the virus via breast-feeding. However, there is evidence that the virus is transmitted across the placental barrier to the unborn infant, as it has been found in the amniotic fluid in studies of fetuses with microcephaly in mothers infected with the virus (Calvet et al., 2016).

People with the Zika virus usually have symptoms that can include mild fever, skin rashes, conjunctivitis, muscle and joint pain, malaise, or headache (WHO, 2016). These symptoms normally last for 2 to 7 days. There is no specific treatment or vaccine currently available.

HEALTHY PEOPLE 2020 GOAL

Overview
Healthy People 2020 includes the topic area of Immunization and Infectious Diseases.

Goal
The goal for this topic is general and states: "Increase immunization rates and reduce preventable infectious diseases" (Healthy People 2020, 2016).

Objectives
Unfortunately, Healthy People 2020 has not yet added objectives for prevention of Zika virus infections.

SCREENING

The CDC (2016) has updated guidelines that include a new recommendation to offer serologic testing to asymptomatic pregnant women (women who do not report clinical illness consistent with Zika virus disease) who have traveled to areas with ongoing transmission of Zika virus. Testing can be offered between 2 and 12 weeks after pregnant women return from travel to areas with ongoing Zika virus transmission. The updated guidelines also include recommendations for health care providers caring for women who reside in areas with ongoing transmission of Zika virus, including recommendations for screening, testing; and management of pregnant women and recommendations for counseling women of reproductive age (15–44 years).

RISK ASSESSMENT

Because Zika virus infection is preventable, knowing risks and practicing risk-reducing behaviors will help to stem the epidemic of this infection.

Risks include:
- Being bitten by mosquitoes that carry Zika virus (which also spread dengue and chikungunya infections)
- Development of microcephaly in fetuses of pregnant women who have Zika virus

CLIENT EDUCATION

Teach Clients (CDC, 2016)
When traveling to countries where Zika virus or other viruses spread by mosquitoes are found, remember that they bite mostly in daytime but also at night, and take the following steps:
- Wear long-sleeved shirts and long pants.
- Stay in places with air conditioning or that use window and door screens to keep mosquitoes outside.
- Sleep under a mosquito bed net if you are overseas or outside and are not able to protect yourself from mosquito bites.
- Use Environmental Protection Agency (EPA)-registered insect repellents. When used as directed, EPA-registered insect repellents are proven safe and effective, even for pregnant and breast-feeding women.
  - Always follow the product label instructions
  - Reapply insect repellent as directed.
  - Do not spray repellent on the skin under clothing.
  - If you are also using sunscreen, apply sunscreen before applying insect repellent.
- If you have a baby or child:
  - Do not use insect repellent on babies younger than 2 months of age.
  - Dress your child in clothing that covers arms and legs, or
  - Cover crib, stroller, and baby carrier with mosquito netting.
  - Do not apply insect repellent onto a child's hands, eyes, mouth, and cut or irritated skin.
  - Adults: Spray insect repellent onto your hands and then apply to a child's face.
- Treat clothing and gear with permethrin or purchase permethrin-treated items.
  - Treated clothing remains protective after multiple washings. See product information to learn how long the protection will last.
  - If treating items yourself, follow the product instructions carefully.
  - Do NOT use permethrin products directly on skin. They are intended to treat clothing.

If you have Zika, protect others from getting sick
- During the first week of infection, Zika virus can be found in the blood and passed from an infected person to another mosquito through mosquito bites. An infected mosquito can then spread the virus to other people.
- To help prevent others from getting sick, avoid mosquito bites during the first week of illness.

Prevent mosquitos from hatching in the environment
- Take care to empty standing water from all sources such as flower pots, bowls, buckets, or other areas of standing water.

HEALTH ASSESSMENT

Collecting Subjective Data: The Nursing Health History
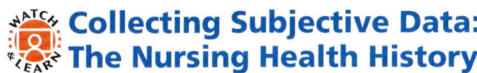

A complete health history is necessary to provide high-quality care for the pregnant client. If the examiner does not have access to a recent complete health history for the pregnant client, a complete health history should be performed before focusing on particular questions associated with the pregnancy, which are discussed in this section. The first prenatal visit focuses on collection of baseline data about the client and her partner, and identification of risk factors.

Biographical Data

Biographical data should be included in the health history. This information may include the client's name, birth date, address, and phone number. Obtaining the client's educational level, occupation, and work status helps the staff to speak to the client at the appropriate level for understanding. The health history should also include the client's significant other with phone number and contact information in case of emergency.

History of Present Health Concern

QUESTION	RATIONALE
What was your normal weight before pregnancy? Has your weight changed since a year ago? How much weight have you gained since your last menstrual period?	Optimal weight gain during pregnancy depends on the client's height and weight. Recommended weight gain in pregnancy is as follows: Underweight client, 28–40 lb; normal weight client, 25–35 lb; overweight client, 15–25 lb; obese client 11–20 lb (American College of Obstetricians and Gynecologists [ACOG], 2013). Low pregnant weight and inadequate weight gain during pregnancy contribute to intrauterine growth retardation and low birth weight. Figure 29-4 shows typical distribution of weight gain in pregnancy.
Have you had a fever or chills, except with a cold, since your last menstrual period?	Fetal exposure to cytomegalovirus has been associated with intrauterine growth retardation, developmental delay, hearing impairment, and mental retardation (Pereira et al., 2014). Newest research indicates that Zika virus is likely associated with microcephaly of the fetus (and cases of Guillain–Barré in the mothers) (Calvet et al., 2016; CDC, 2016).

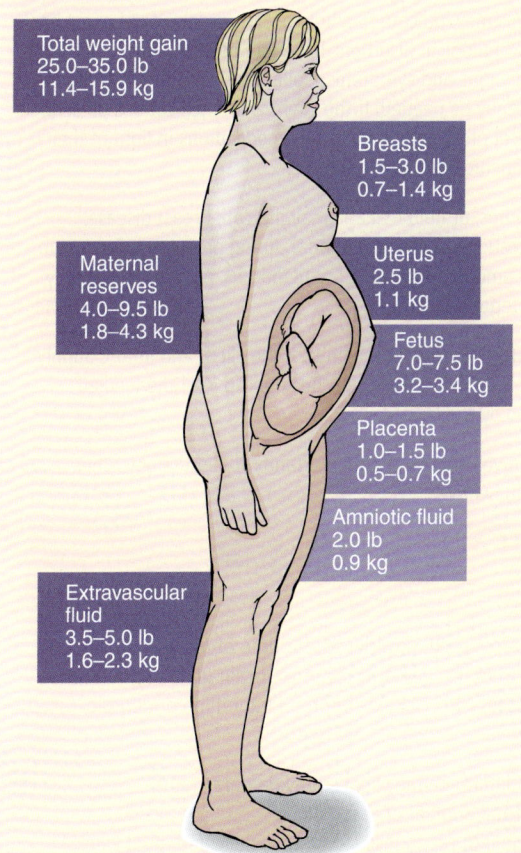

FIGURE 29-4 Distribution of weight gain during pregnancy.

Continued on following page

History of Present Health Concern (Continued)

QUESTION	RATIONALE
Is your nose often stuffed up when you don't have a cold? Have you experienced more frequent nosebleeds while pregnant?	Nasal "stuffiness" and nose bleeds (epistaxis) are common during pregnancy due to estrogen-induced edema and vascular congestion of the nasal mucosa and sinuses.
Do you have any trouble with your throat? Do you have a cough that hasn't gone away or do you have frequent chest infections?	Persistent cough and frequent chest infections may indicate pneumonia or tuberculosis.
Do you have nausea or vomiting that doesn't go away? Is your thirst greater than normal?	If proper hydration and nutrition are not maintained, the client may be at risk for hyperemesis gravidarum, cholecystitis, or cholelithiasis.
Do you ever have bloody stools? Do you have any change in bowel habits? Do you have difficulty when trying to have a bowel movement?	Changes in stool appearance and bowel habits may indicate constipation or hemorrhoids.
Do you experience a burning sensation while urinating?	Pregnant women may have asymptomatic bacteriuria. Urinary tract infections (UTIs) need to be diagnosed and treated with antibiotics. Untreated UTIs predispose the client to complications such as preterm labor, pyelonephritis, and sepsis.
Do you have vaginal bleeding, leakage of fluid, or vaginal discharge?	Vaginal bleeding may indicate placenta previa. Leakage of fluid may indicate membrane rupture. Vaginal discharge may indicate vaginal infections (e.g., bacterial vaginosis, trichomoniasis, gonorrhea, chlamydia). Untreated infections can predispose the client to preterm labor or fetal infections.
Have you lost interest in eating? Do you have trouble falling asleep or staying asleep? Do you ever feel depressed or feel like crying for no reason? Are problems at home or work bothering you? Have you ever thought of suicide? Have you ever had professional counseling (psychiatric/psychological)?	These symptoms may indicate psychological disorders. If the client has a history of psychological disorders, be aware of these and continually monitor her for signs and symptoms. Collaboration with a psychologist or psychiatrist may be needed. If the client is on medications prescribed for psychological problems, evaluate the medications in light of their possible teratogenic effects on the fetus.
Have you noticed breast pain, lumps, or fluid leakage?	Breast pain, lumps, or fluid leakage may indicate breast disease. Colostrum secretion, however, is normal during pregnancy. Colostrum varies in color among individuals. Erythematous, painful breasts may indicate a bacterial infection.
Have you thought about breast-feeding or bottle-feeding your infant?	Discuss advantages of breast-feeding for the client and infant. Supply educational resources for the client. Be supportive of the feeding method chosen by the client.
Are there any problems or concerns you may have that we haven't discussed yet?	This question gives the client an opportunity to discuss any other concerns she may have.

Personal Health History

QUESTION	RATIONALE
Will you be 35 years or older at the time the baby is born? Are you and the baby's father related to each other (e.g., cousins or other relations)?	Women who are age 35 or older at the time of delivery should be offered genetic counseling and testing. Obtain genetic information so you can assess fetal risk of abnormal karyotype or genetic disorders.

List the number of times you have been pregnant, beginning with the first pregnancy.	This data will determine the client's gravida/para status.
	• Gravida—total number of pregnancies
	• Para—number of pregnancies that have delivered at 20 weeks' gestation or greater
	  • *Term Gestation*—delivery of pregnancy 38–42 weeks
	  • *Preterm Gestation*—delivery of pregnancy after 20 weeks and before the start of 38 weeks' gestation
	  • **Abortion**—termination of pregnancy (spontaneous [miscarriage] or induced prior to the 20th week of gestation)
	  • **Living**—number of living children

QUESTION	RATIONALE
	Example: G $_\#$P $_{T\ Pt\ Ab\ L}$ G $_4$P $_{2\ 1\ 1\ 3}$ This represents a client who has been pregnant 4 times: 2 term deliveries, 1 preterm delivery, 1 spontaneous abortion, and 3 children living.
Describe your previous pregnancies including child's name, birth date, birth weight, sex, gestational age, type of delivery (if cesarean section, discuss reason). Did you experience any complications (e.g., pregnancy-induced hypertension, diabetes, bleeding, depression) during any of these pregnancies?	History of previous pregnancies helps identify clients at risk for complications during current pregnancy (e.g., preterm labor, gestational diabetes).
Describe any neonatal complications such as birth defects, jaundice, infection, or any problems within the first 2 weeks of life.	Previous neonatal complications may be hereditary and may recur in future births. Knowledge of such complications helps in detecting abnormalities early.
Describe any perinatal or neonatal losses, including when the loss occurred and the reason for the loss, if known. Have you ever had a child die in the first year of life?	Death of a child in the first year of life may indicate a risk for fetal cardiac disease or other diseases. This information is necessary for assessing fetal risk for birth defects.
Discuss previous abortions (spontaneous or elective), including procedures required and gestational age of fetus. Have you had two or more pregnancies that ended in miscarriage? Have you had a Rhogam injection after a spontaneous or elective abortion?	Previous history of abortions helps to identify women who have had habitual abortions and who may need medical treatment to maintain the pregnancy. Such medical complications that put the client at risk for habitual abortions include incompetent cervix and systemic lupus erythematosus. In the case of an Rh-negative mother carrying an Rh-positive fetus, blood cells of the fetus may get into the mother's blood. The mother's body then produces antibodies, which in a subsequent pregnancy may cross the placenta and destroy red blood cells of an Rh-positive fetus. RhoGAM protects the mother from the Rh-positive blood cells to prevent the antigen/antibody reaction (American College of Nurse Midwives, 2013).
Have you ever had a hydatidiform mole (molar pregnancy)?	Molar pregnancies occur in 1 of every 700–1,000 pregnancies in the United States and Europe. Incidence increases with the woman's age and particularly after age 45 or under 16; in multiple pregnancy or previous molar pregnancy; with Asian origin; or with late-onset menarche after 12 years of age, light menstruation, or use of oral contraceptive pills (Gestational trophoblastic disease, 2013). Recurrence of the hydatidiform mole is seen in approximately 1–2% of cases. Due to prompt diagnosis, mortality rates have been reduced to practically zero. Nearly 20% of complete moles progress to gestational trophoblastic tumors (Moore, 2015).
Have you ever had a tubal (ectopic) pregnancy (pregnancy outside of the uterus)?	Ectopic pregnancy occurs in 1 in every 50 pregnancies in the United States (American Pregnancy Association, 2017). A history of damage to the Fallopian tubes, including previous ectopic pregnancy, increases the risk of having a second ectopic pregnancy (Sivalingam et al., 2011).
Do you have regular periods? When was the first day of your last menstrual period? Was this period longer, shorter, or normal? Have you had any bleeding or spotting since your last period? Are your periods usually regular or irregular?	Menstrual history helps to determine expected date of confinement (EDC).
Describe the most recent form of birth control used. If you've used birth control pills in the past, when did you take the last pill?	Intrauterine devices in place at the time of conception place the client at risk for an ectopic pregnancy. Birth control pills should be discontinued when pregnancy is confirmed.

Continued on following page

Personal Health History (Continued)

QUESTION	RATIONALE
Have you had any difficulty in getting pregnant for more than 1 year?	Inability to conceive after trying for more than 1 year may signal reproductive complications such as infertility.
Have you ever had any type of reproductive surgery? Have you ever had an abnormal Pap smear? Have you ever had any treatment performed on your cervix for abnormal Pap smear results? When was your last Pap test, and what were the results?	Reproductive surgery and instrumentation to the cervix place the client at risk for complications during pregnancy. Conization of the cervix places the client at risk for an incompetent cervix during pregnancy.
Do you have a history of any type of sexually transmitted infection (STI) such as a chlamydial infection, gonorrhea, herpes, genital warts, or syphilis? If so, describe when it occurred and the treatment. Does your partner have a history of STI? If so, when was he treated?	Early identification and treatment of STIs prevent intrauterine complications from long-term exposure to infections.
Do you have a history of any vaginal infections such as bacterial vaginosis, yeast infection, or others? If so, when did the last infection occur and what was the treatment?	Vaginal infections need treatment. During pregnancy, medications for bacterial vaginosis, including nonteratogenic medications such as clindamycin (Cleocin 2%) or metronidazole intravaginal cream or oral tablets, may be recommended; recommended medications for yeast infections often are over the counter. Treatment for trichomoniasis is usually a single dose of metronidazole by mouth (avoid drinking alcohol for 24 hours after taking this drug because it causes nausea and vomiting); sexual partners must be treated to prevent the infection from recurring (ACOG, 2011).
Do you know your blood type and Rh factor? If you are Rh negative, do you know the Rh factor of your partner?	Rh-negative mothers should receive Rho immunoglobulin at 28 weeks' gestation and with antepartum testing (chorionic villi sampling, amniocentesis) if the partner's blood type is unknown to prevent isoimmunization.
Have you ever received a blood transfusion for any reason? If so, explain reason and provide date.	Infections (hepatitis, human immunodeficiency virus [HIV]) and antibodies can be received from contaminated blood during blood transfusions, which can be detrimental to the mother and fetus. Foreign antibodies can be life threatening for the fetus. Positive antibody screens need to be followed up to identify the antibody detected in the blood. Besides Rh antibody, other antibodies include Kell, Duffy, and Lewis. Titers should be followed to prevent fetal complications.
Do you have a history of any major medical problem (e.g., heart trouble, rheumatic fever, hypertension, diabetes, lung problems, tuberculosis, asthma, trouble with nerves and/or depression, kidney disease, cancer, convulsions or epilepsy, abnormality of female organs [uterus, cervix], thyroid problems, or hearing loss in infancy)?	Identification of any medical problem is important during pregnancy because the body undergoes so many physiologic changes. Certain medical conditions put the mother at high risk for maternal or fetal complications. Postpartum depression occurs after childbirth. Women who are most at risk have had previous depression (whether associated with previous childbirth or not), bipolar disorder, family member diagnosed with depression or other mental condition, stressful life event during or shortly after pregnancy and giving birth, complicated pregnancy or delivery, ambivalence about pregnancy, lack of emotional support, or alcohol or drug abuse (National Institute of Mental Health [NIMH], n.d.).
Do you have diabetes?	Preconceptual maternal hemoglobin A1c levels should not exceed 6.9% when conception occurs. Studies show that women with hemoglobin A1c levels that exceed 6.9% have an increased risk of fetuses with congenital malformations. When the A1c level reaches 10.4%, the rate significantly increased. (Jensen et al., 2009).

QUESTION	RATIONALE
Have you had twins or multiple gestation?	Early identification of multiple gestation is important. Refer clients with multiple gestation to an obstetrician for continued care. Multiple gestation places the client in the high-risk category during pregnancy.
Do you have a history of medication, food, or other allergies? If so, list the allergies and describe the reactions.	Identification of medication allergies is necessary to prevent complications.
Have you ever been hospitalized or had surgery (not including hospitalizations or surgery related to pregnancy)? If so, discuss the reason for the hospitalization or surgery, the date, and if the problem is resolved today.	Previous hospitalizations or surgeries must be noted to assess for potential medical complications during the pregnancy.
Are you currently taking any medications (either prescription or nonprescription) or have you taken any since you have become pregnant? If so, list the medication, the amount taken, the date you started taking it, and the reason for taking it.	Some medications are teratogenic to the fetus during pregnancy. All medications taken since the LMP need to be discussed with the practitioner.
Are your immunizations up to date? Have you received the influenza immunization this year?	Assessment for immunity for rubella and hepatitis B is performed at the initial obstetric visit along with the other prenatal labs. CDC recommends influenza vaccination for women who are pregnant during the influenza season (CDC, 2015b).

Family History

QUESTION	RATIONALE
Do you have a child with a birth defect? Do you have any type of birth defect or inherited disease such as cleft lip or cleft palate, clubfoot, hemophilia, mental retardation, or any others? Are there any members in your family with a birth defect, inherited disease, blood disorder, mental retardation, or any other problems? What is your ethnic or racial group: Jewish, Black/African, Asian, Mediterranean (e.g., Greek, Italian), French Canadian?	There is a genetic risk factor for Down syndrome, spina bifida, brain defects, chromosome problems, anencephaly, heart defects, muscular dystrophy, cystic fibrosis, hemophilia, thalassemia, sickle cell disease, and other inherited diseases. Cystic fibrosis screening should be offered to all clients during preconceptual counseling. Identification of signs and symptoms of birth defects and inherited disorders is important to assist in early interventions and treatment. **CULTURAL CONSIDERATIONS** Certain inherited disorders occur more often in particular ethnic groups such as Tay–Sachs disease in Ashkenazi Jews, Eastern Europeans, and certain French Canadians and Louisiana Cajuns (NINDS, 2016).
Has anyone in your family (grandparents, parents, siblings, children) had rheumatic fever or heart trouble before age 50 years?	Cardiovascular disease or heart defects may be inherited.
Has anyone in your family had lung problems, diabetes, tuberculosis, or asthma?	Pulmonary or endocrine disorders may be familial.
Has anyone in your family been diagnosed with any type of cancer? If so, what kind?	There is a genetic component associated with certain types of cancer.

Lifestyle and Health Practices

QUESTION	RATIONALE
Since the start of this pregnancy, have you had drinks containing alcohol?	Any oral alcohol intake puts the fetus at risk for fetal alcohol spectrum disorders (FASDs). Studies do not indicate a safe level of alcohol intake in pregnancy. Fetal alcohol spectrum disorders (FASDs) are a group of conditions that can occur in a person whose mother drank alcohol during pregnancy. Alcohol passes from the mother's blood through the umbilical cord to the fetus. The CDC (2015a) describes three types of FASDs: Fetal alcohol syndrome (FAS); Alcohol-related Neurodevelopment

Continued on following page

Lifestyle and Health Practices (Continued)

QUESTION	RATIONALE
	Disorder (ARND); and Alcohol-related Birth Defects (ARBD). Signs and symptoms of FASDs are: • Abnormal facial features, such as a smooth ridge between the nose and upper lip (this ridge is called the philtrum) • Small head size • Shorter-than-average height • Low body weight • Poor coordination • Hyperactive behavior • Difficulty with attention • Poor memory • Difficulty in school (especially with math) • Learning disabilities • Speech and language delays • Intellectual disability or low IQ • Poor reasoning and judgment skills • Sleep and sucking problems as a baby • Vision or hearing problems • Problems with the heart, kidneys, or bones
Do you smoke? If so, how much do you smoke per day? Pregnant women are half as likely as nonpregnant women to be smokers. An estimated 20.4% of women smokers continue smoking throughout their pregnancies. Variations in effectiveness of smoking cessation programs leads to between 29% and 85% of women who get a planned intervention relapsing after delivery (Fang et al., 2004).	Maternal cigarette smoking correlates with an increased incidence of perinatal mortality, preterm delivery, premature rupture of membranes, abruptio placentae, stillbirth, and bleeding during pregnancy. Smoking is also associated with decreased fetal size, low birth weight, intrauterine death, or sudden infant death syndrome (SIDS) after birth (March of Dimes, 2015), attention-deficit hyperactivity disorder (ADHD), and behavioral and learning disorders in school (CDC, 2014).
Have you used cocaine, marijuana, speed, or any street drug during this pregnancy?	Women who use cocaine, methamphetamine, or other illicit drugs during pregnancy have a higher rate of spontaneous abortions and abruptio placentae. Infants exposed to illicit drugs in utero are shown to have an increase in fetal growth issues, congenital anomalies, withdrawal, and neurobehavioral problems (such as impaired orientation and autonomic regulation) and abnormalities of muscle tone, low levels of arousal, irritability and lability of mood, decreased behavioral and autonomic regulation, and poor alertness and orientation (American Academy of Pediatrics, 2013).
Does anyone in your family consider your social habits to be a problem? Do your social habits interfere with your daily living? If so, please explain.	Women who abuse substances (e.g., alcohol, cocaine, marijuana) do not always consider their habits to be a problem. They also tend to underestimate the amount of substances used. Family members or friends may give a truer estimate of the substances abused. These habits need to be known to assist the client during pregnancy and to alert neonatal personnel after delivery to prepare for potential neonatal complications.
What is a normal daily intake of food for you? Are you on any special diet? Do you have any diet intolerances or restrictions? If so, what are they? Can you write down or tell me what you ate and drank in the last 24 hours?	Maternal nutrition has a direct relationship to maternal–fetal well-being. Daily maternal caloric intake, as reflected by weight gain, has a direct relationship to birth weight. The caloric content required to supply daily energy needs and to achieve appropriate weight gain can be estimated by multiplying the client's optimal body weight (in kilograms) by 35 kcal and adding 300 kcal to the total.
Do you eat lunchmeats or unpasteurized milk products?	Unpasteurized milk products and all deli meats should be avoided or cooked well. Undercooked meats and unpasteurized milk products or soft cheeses can cause an infection called listeriosis. Maternal infection may have few symptoms or may lead to life-threatening complications, such as septicemia or meningitis; if spread to the fetus, it may cause miscarriage in early pregnancy; or if spread to the fetus later in pregnancy, it may cause premature birth, stillbirth, or a potentially fatal infection even after birth (Mayo Clinic, 2014).

QUESTION	RATIONALE
Do you currently take any vitamin supplements? If so, what are they?	The client's balanced diet should provide an appropriate supply of vitamins required for pregnancy. Routine multivitamin supplementation is recommended for most clients who do not obtain sufficient resources from diet alone. The diet selection should be from protein-rich foods, whole-grain breads and cereals, dairy products, and fruits and vegetables. Of the minerals, iron supplementation is recommended to maintain body stores and minimize the occurrence of iron-deficiency anemia. All women of childbearing age are advised to consume 400 µg of folic acid daily to help prevent neural tube defects in the fetus. This can be achieved by eating fruits, vegetables, and fortified cereals, and/or a folic acid supplement. Women who have previously had newborns born with spinal cord defects can decrease the risk of neural tube defects in future pregnancies by supplementing the diet with folic acid 2–3 months prior to conceiving.
Activity and Exercise	
Do you exercise daily? If so, what do you do and for how long?	Daily exercise is highly recommended as long as it is tolerated well by the pregnant client. Women who are in good physical condition tend to have shorter, less difficult labors compared with women who are not physically fit.
	Regular and routine exercise may be continued as long as tolerated. Caution women not to start *new* forms of exercise during pregnancy.
Have your normal daily activities or exercise ever had a negative impact on your previous pregnancies? If so, please discuss.	Pregnant clients at high risk may be prescribed bed rest during the pregnancy to maintain a healthy pregnancy.
Do you perform any type of heavy labor (lifting >20 lb) while working or while at home? If so, please describe.	Lifting heavy weights during pregnancy has been questioned in recent years but the amount of weight and the fitness of the mother affect the overall daily amount of weight safely lifted. Lifting weights of 20 kg or more 10 times a day has been shown to be associated with preterm labor (Runge et al. 2013).
Are you easily fatigued? Do you require more sleep than 8 hours/day? Do you get fatigued with your daily routine of work/family life? Do you get fatigued by performing daily household chores, such as cleaning, running errands, etc.? If so, please describe. What are your normal sleeping patterns?	Fatigue is the most difficult symptom for many women during pregnancy, especially during the first trimester, and many also have difficulty sleeping at night, which increases the fatigue (Women's Healthcare Topics, 2012). Sleep restores the body and assists with the energy level of the client.
Do you frequently have rest periods? If so, for how long?	Pregnancy places a tremendous amount of stress on the body due to the physiologic changes that occur. Encourage rest periods.
Toxic Exposure	
Have you or your partner ever worked around chemicals or radiation? If so, please explain. Are you exposed to an excessive amount of tobacco smoke daily?	Assessment of toxic exposure can identify potential teratogens to the fetus.
Do you have a cat? If so, are you exposed to cat litter or cat feces?	Education regarding proper handling of cat litter is needed because of risk of infection (toxoplasmosis). Advise clients to have other family members change cat litter. Encourage the client to wash hands well after petting cats and to wear gloves when planting in outdoor soil if cats are present in the neighborhood.
Role and Relationships	
What is your occupation? What are your typical daily activities? Who do you interact with each day? Do you find work, activities, and the people you encounter in them supportive or stressful?	Roles and relationships outside the family may be supportive or stressful. Interpersonal support or conflict has a significant effect on depressive symptoms during pregnancy (Nelson, 2012).

Continued on following page

Lifestyle and Health Practices (Continued)

QUESTION	RATIONALE
Role and Relationships (Continued)	
Discuss your feelings about this pregnancy. Is the father of the baby involved with the pregnancy? How does your partner feel about the pregnancy? To what degree do you feel that the father of the baby will be involved with the pregnancy (e.g., not involved, interested and supportive, full caretaker of the pregnancy)?	These questions identify psychosocial issues for the client. Assess social support systems for the family.
What type of support systems do you have at home? Who is your primary support person? List the people living with you including their names, ages, relationship to you, and any health problems that they may have. Are they aware of your pregnancy?	Assessment of social structures and supportive influences is required to determine potential client needs. If additional needs are noted, contact social services for assistance.
How have you introduced this pregnancy to any siblings? What are their reactions regarding this pregnancy? Do you plan to involve the siblings in any type of education program to enhance the attachment process for the newborn?	Sibling rivalry can interfere with the bonding process between siblings. Education and preparation for the new family member (the newborn) can alleviate potential problems with sibling rivalry. Encourage siblings to attend sibling class offered at your institution.
Has anyone close to you ever threatened to hurt you? Has anyone ever hit, kicked, choked, or physically hurt you? Has anyone ever forced you to have sex?	Lack of recognition of domestic violence is one of the primary barriers to recognizing domestic violence for women. Universal screening for domestic violence is recommended for all women (see Chapter 10 for screening tools).
What is your partner's highest level of education? What is your partner's occupation or major activity? Does your partner consume alcohol? If yes, how much alcohol does your partner use daily? List type and amount. Does your partner smoke? If yes, how often does your partner smoke? List amount and frequency. Does your partner use illicit drugs? If yes, how often does your partner use illicit drugs? List drug type, amount, and frequency.	Exploration of the partner's social or cultural habits may identify needs of the family unit.

CASE STUDY

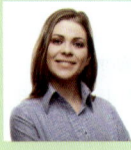

The nurse interviews Mrs. Farrow using specific probing questions. The client reports being very nauseated, with vomiting from week 4 of this 12-week pregnancy. She says that she has lost weight because she has trouble eating and keeping food down. The nurse explores Mrs. Farrow's report of nausea and vomiting using the COLDSPA mnemonic.

Mnemonic	Question	Data Provided
Character	Describe the sign or symptom (feeling, appearance, sound, smell, or taste if applicable).	Client says she feels awful with this pregnancy. She is very nauseated, fatigued, and has trouble keeping food down (she reports vomiting about 2 times daily). She has had no transportation to get to clinic for prenatal care over the past 12 weeks.
Onset	When did it begin?	The nausea and fatigue began during the 4th week of pregnancy and haven't gone away.
Location	Where is it? Does it radiate?	Client reports an overall feeling of exhaustion.
Duration	How long does it last? Does it recur?	Client reports that she has had severe nausea and fatigue with vomiting every day for the past 8 weeks.
Severity	How bad is it? How much does it bother you?	During the client's first pregnancy, she recalls being quite sick throughout the pregnancy (though not quite as bad as this time). She gained 20 lb and her son weighed 6 lb 2 oz at birth. The client's last pregnancy was normal and uneventful; she gained 30 lb and her son weighed 7 lb 6 oz at birth. She tries to eat healthily, but says she often feels too sick to eat. She tries to keep down the free fast food that her husband brings home from work every night. She denies nausea at this time but describes a level of 8 (0–10) nausea when she is around food and 10 after she has eaten, at which time she often vomits.

Mnemonic	Question	Data Provided
Pattern	What makes it better or worse?	Client states that if she is able to stay in bed and eat something before getting up, the nausea and vomiting are to a level of about 6 (scale 1–10 worse). Client reports that certain smells and being extra tired make the nausea and vomiting worse.
Associated factors/ How it **A**ffects the client	What other symptoms occur with it? How does it affect you?	Client describes excessive fatigue, with no time to rest since she is caring for two small children. She also reports financial concerns; her husband works at a fast-food chain and is looking for a better paying job. The nausea, vomiting, and fatigue add to the stress, which works in a circle, as stress makes the nausea and vomiting increase to a level of 9–10 if she is also around food.

After exploring Mrs. Farrow's reports of nausea and vomiting using COLDSPA, the nurse continues with the client history.

Mrs. Farrow is a 29-year-old woman G3 P2; LMP 16 weeks ago. She explains that she couldn't come for prenatal care until now because she was so sick, had no childcare, and no transportation. Her husband finally took off work to stay with the kids and asked a friend to drive his wife to the doctor because he is concerned. "I do know how important early prenatal care is, but I just couldn't get here." She reports a weight gain of 20 and 30 lb with previous two pregnancies. Mrs. Farrow lives with her husband and two sons in a two-bedroom trailer on land owned by her in-laws. She states that her in-laws are very supportive and help out during tough times by not charging rent. Her husband works full time at a fast-food chain restaurant but is looking for a job that pays more money. It is often hard for them to meet their financial responsibilities; however, they believe it is important for her to stay home with the children, so she does not contribute financially. She reports that, in general, she encourages healthful practices for herself and family, but because her husband gets a discount on food and soda from his workplace, they don't eat as well as she knows they should. "When I am not having this nausea and vomiting, I am eating less so I don't gain so much weight this time." MF says she is not on any prescribed medications. She is taking some prenatal vitamin capsules that she got from her local pharmacy. She occasionally takes allergy tabs for hay fever symptoms. Denies medication, food, insect, or other allergies except occasional hay fever. Denies use of herbal medicines or alternative therapies.

Mrs. Farrow's past medical history is unremarkable; her two pregnancies were term gestations and deliveries were vaginal. However, during the last pregnancy, she was diagnosed with pregnancy-induced hypertension and gestational diabetes, and labor was induced at 38 weeks' gestation.

Parents both alive and well, but live in another state. Mother was very sick while pregnant with MF and one other of three siblings. Father has mild hypertension and mild obesity. No other health problems described in family.

Mrs. Farrow does not work outside the home. Sleeps only 6 to 7 hours per night, but tries to get 7 to 8 hours per night. Exercise is keeping up with her two boys each day and housework. When feeling able, she walks her boys to a park 4 blocks from residence. Her 24-hour diet recall: Breakfast—a roll with black tea; lunch—a few crackers and cheese; dinner—a burger and fries.

Collecting Objective Data: Physical Examination

Preparing the Client

The nurse needs to provide a warm and comfortable environment for the physical assessment. After meeting the client, the nurse should quickly explain the sequence of events for the visit. Note that a full head-to-toe examination will be performed, including a pelvic examination. Pelvic cultures obtained with this examination include a Pap smear and gonorrhea and chlamydia cultures. Explain that after the examination is complete, the client will go to the laboratory for initial prenatal blood tests including complete blood count, blood type and screen, Rh status, rubella titer, serologic test for syphilis, hepatitis B surface antigen, and sickle cell anemia screen (for clients of African ancestry). Universal screening for HIV is recommended.

The first procedure involves obtaining a clean-catch, midstream urine specimen. After the client has voided, instruct her to undress. Provide adequate gowns and cover-up drapes to ensure privacy.

Equipment

- Adequate room lighting
- Ophthalmoscope
- Otoscope
- Stethoscope
- Sphygmomanometer
- Speculum
- Light for pelvic examination
- Tape measure
- Fetal Doppler ultrasound device
- Disposable gloves
- Lubricant
- Slides
- KOH (potassium hydroxide)
- Normal saline solution
- Thin prep Pap smear test

Physical Assessment

Remember these key points during the examination:
- Obtain an accurate and complete prenatal history.
- Understand and recognize cardiovascular changes of pregnancy.
- Recognize skin changes.
- Identify common complaints of pregnancy and explain what causes them.
- Correctly measure growth of uterus during pregnancy.
- Demonstrate the four Leopold maneuvers and explain their significance.

General Routine Screening versus Focused Specialty Assessment of the Pregnant Woman

Assessment of the pregnant woman is a specialty assessment. Performing a head-to-toe assessment requires experience and familiarity with changes that naturally occur in pregnancy and indicators of abnormal changes. Palpation of fetal movements, uterine contractions, fetal positioning, and fetal heart rate/rhythm, and pelvic examination of the uterus and pelvic adequacy for vaginal delivery require skill and experience for assessment of all pregnant clients.

ASSESSMENT PROCEDURE	NORMAL FINDINGS	ABNORMAL FINDINGS
General Survey: Vital Signs, Height, and Weight		
Measure blood pressure (BP). Have the client sit on the examination table.	BP range: systolic 90–134 mmHg and diastolic 60–89 mmHg. BP decreases during the second trimester because of the relaxation effect on the blood vessels. By 32–34 weeks, the client's BP should be back to normal.	Elevated BP at 9–11 weeks may be indicative of chronic hypertension, hydatidiform mole pregnancy or thyroid storm. After 20 weeks, increased BP (>140/90) may be associated with pregnancy-induced hypertension. Decreased blood pressure may indicate supine hypotensive syndrome.
Measure pulse rate.	60–90 beats/min; may increase 10–15 beats/min higher than prepregnancy levels.	Irregularities in heart rhythm, chest pain, dyspnea, and edema may indicate cardiac disease.
Take the client's temperature.	97–98.6°F.	An elevated temperature (above 100°F) may indicate infection.
Measure height and weight (Fig. 29-5).	Establish a baseline height and weight. The client with normal prepregnancy weight should gain 2–4 lb in the first trimester and approximately 11–12 lb in both the second and third trimesters for a total weight gain between 25 and 35 lb.	A sudden gain exceeding 5 lb a week may be associated with pregnancy-induced hypertension and fluid retention. Weight gain <2 lb a month may indicate insufficient nourishment.
		Guidelines for weight gain during pregnancy for singleton pregnancy:
		Low BMI (<18.5 kg/m^2): 28–40 lb; normal BMI (18.5–24.9 kg/m^2): 25–35 lb; high BMI: >25.0–29.9 kg/m^2): 15–25 lb; obese (>30.0 kg/m^2): >11–20 lb

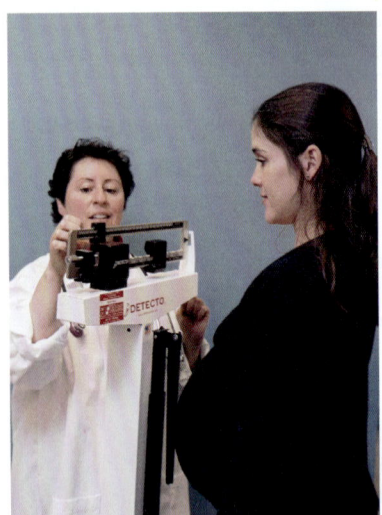

FIGURE 29-5 Weighing the pregnant client.

Observe behavior.	*First trimester:* Tired, ambivalent. *Second trimester:* Introspective, energetic. *Third trimester:* Restless, preparing for baby, labile moods (father may also experience these same behaviors).	Denial of pregnancy, withdrawal, depression, or psychosis may be seen in the client with psychological problems.
Skin, Hair, and Nails		
Inspect the skin. Note hyperpigmented areas associated with pregnancy.	Linea nigra, striae, gravidarum, chloasma, and spider nevi may be present.	Pale skin suggests anemia. Yellow discoloration suggests jaundice.

ASSESSMENT PROCEDURE	NORMAL FINDINGS	ABNORMAL FINDINGS
Observe skin for vascular markings associated with pregnancy.	Angiomas and palmar erythema are common.	
Inspect the hair and nails.	Hair and nails tend to increase in growth; softening and thinning are common.	

Head and Neck

INSPECTION AND PALPATION

Inspect and palpate the neck. Assess the anterior and posterior cervical chain lymph nodes. Also palpate the thyroid gland.	Smooth, nontender, small cervical nodes may be palpable. Slight enlargement of the thyroid may be noted during pregnancy.	Hard, tender, fixed, or prominent nodes may indicate infection or cancer. Marked enlargement of the thyroid gland indicates thyroid disease. Benign and malignant nodules as well as tenderness are noted in thyroiditis.

Eyes

INSPECTION

Inspect eyes. Examine cornea, lens, iris, and pupil. Use an ophthalmoscope to examine the fundus of the eye.	Pupils are equal and round, reactive to light, and accommodate.	Narrowing of the arterioles or AV nicking may indicate hypertension.

Ears

INSPECTION

Inspect the ears.	Tympanic membranes clear: landmarks visible.	Tympanic membrane red and bulging with pus indicates infection.

Mouth, Throat, and Nose

INSPECTION

Inspect the mouth. Pay particular attention to the teeth and the gingival tissues, which may normally appear swollen and slightly reddened.	Hypertrophy of gingival tissue is common. Bleeding may occur due to brushing teeth or dental examinations.	Epulis nodules may be present (Fig. 29-6). These may represent benign changes of the gum that may spontaneously resolve after the pregnancy.
Inspect the throat.	Throat pink, no redness or exudate.	Throat red, exudate present, tonsillary hypertrophy indicate infection.
Inspect the nose.	Nasal mucosal swelling and redness may result from increased estrogen production. Epistaxis is a common variation because of the increased vascular supply to the nares during pregnancy.	Abnormal findings are the same as those for nonpregnant clients.

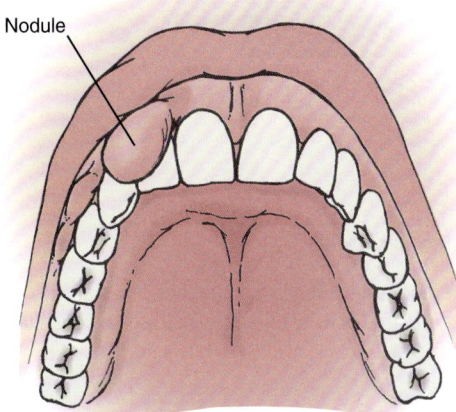

FIGURE 29-6 Epulis.

Continued on following page

708 UNIT 4 Nursing Assessment of Special Groups

ASSESSMENT PROCEDURE	NORMAL FINDINGS	ABNORMAL FINDINGS
Thorax and Lungs		
Inspect, palpate, percuss, and auscultate the chest.	Normal findings include increased anteroposterior diameter, thoracic breathing, slight hyperventilation; shortness of breath in late pregnancy. Lung sounds are clear to auscultation bilaterally.	Dyspnea, rales, rhonchi, wheezes, rubs, absence of breath sounds, and unequal breath sounds are signs of respiratory distress. Clients with a history of asthma have increased risk of perinatal morbidity/mortality, and increased risk of pregnancy-induced hypertension, preterm labor, and low birth weight (Little et al., 2012).
Breasts		
INSPECTION AND PALPATION		
Inspect and palpate the breasts and nipples for symmetry and color (Fig. 29-7).	Venous congestion is noted with prominence of veins. Montgomery tubercles are prominent. Breast size is increased and nodular. Breasts are more sensitive to touch. Colostrum is excreted, especially in the third trimester. Hyperpigmentation of nipples and areolae is evident (Fig. 29-8).	Nipple inversion could be problematic for breastfeeding. Inverted nipples should be identified in the beginning of the third trimester. Breast shields can be inserted in the bra to train the nipple to turn outward. Localized redness, pain, and warmth could indicate mastitis. Bloody discharge of the nipple and retraction of the skin could indicate breast cancer.

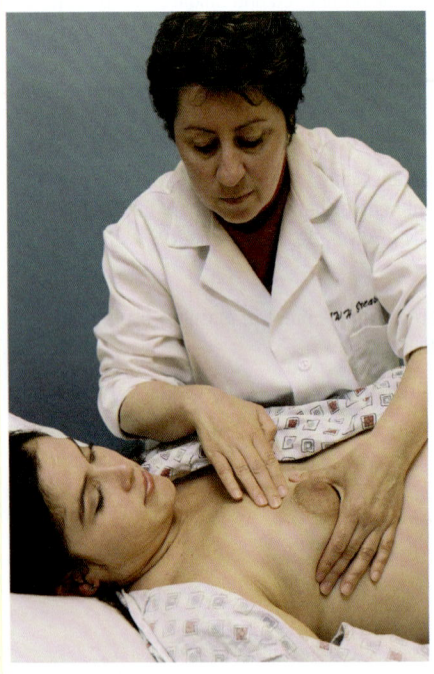

FIGURE 29-7 Palpating the breasts.

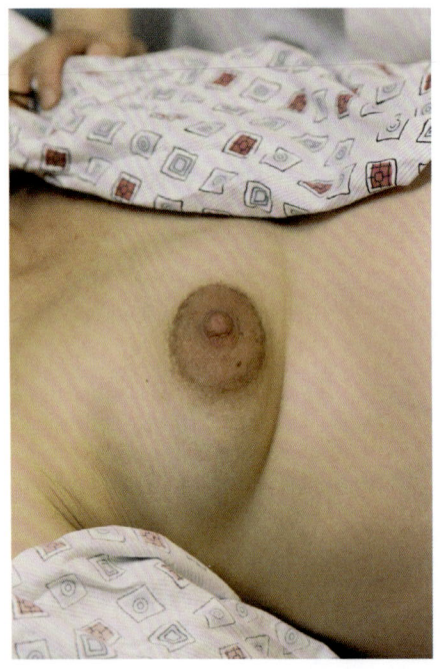

FIGURE 29-8 Hyperpigmentation of the nipples and areolae.

Heart		
AUSCULTATION		
Auscultate the heart.	Normal sinus rhythm. Soft systolic murmurs are audible during pregnancy secondary to the increased blood volume.	Irregular rhythm. Progressive dyspnea, palpitations, and markedly decreased activity tolerance indicate cardiovascular disease.

ASSESSMENT PROCEDURE	NORMAL FINDINGS	ABNORMAL FINDINGS
Peripheral Vascular		
INSPECTION AND PERCUSSION		
Inspect face and extremities. Note color and edema.	During the third trimester, dependent edema is normal. Varicose veins may also appear.	Abnormal findings include calf pain, generalized edema, and diminished pedal pulses. These findings may indicate thrombophlebitis. Facial edema may indicate pregnancy-induced hypertension with elevated blood pressure and weight gain.
Percuss deep tendon reflexes.	Normal reflexes 1–2+. Clonus is absent.	Reflexes 3–4+ and positive clonus require evaluation for pregnancy-induced hypertension.
Abdomen		
INSPECTION		
Inspect the abdomen. For this part of the examination, ask the client to recline with a pillow under her head and her knees flexed. Note striae, scars, and the shape and size of the abdomen.	Striae and linea-nigra are normal. The size of the abdomen may indicate gestational age. The shape of the uterus may suggest fetal presentation and position in later pregnancy.	Scars indicate previous surgery; be careful to note cesarean section scars and location. A transverse lie may be suspected by abdominal palpation, noting enlargement of the width of the uterus.
Palpation		
Palpate the abdomen. Note organs and any masses.	The uterus is palpable beginning at 10–12 weeks' gestation.	Abnormal masses palpable in the abdomen may indicate uterine fibroids or hepatosplenomegaly.
Palpate for fetal movement after 24 weeks.	Fetal movement should be felt by the mother by approximately 18–20 weeks.	If fetal movement is not felt, the EDC may be wrong or possibly intrauterine fetal demise may have occurred.
Palpate for uterine contractions (Fig. 29-9). Note intensity, duration, and frequency of contractions.	The uterus contracts and feels firm to the examiner.	Regular contractions before 37 completed weeks' gestation may suggest preterm labor. Braxton Hick contractions are irregular contractions that may occur anytime during the pregnancy and do not cause cervical dilation or changes in the cervix.
Palpate the abdomen. Notice the difference between the uterus at rest and during a contraction.	Intensity of contractions may be mild, moderate, or firm to palpation.	Regular contractions prior to 37 weeks' gestation suggest premature labor.

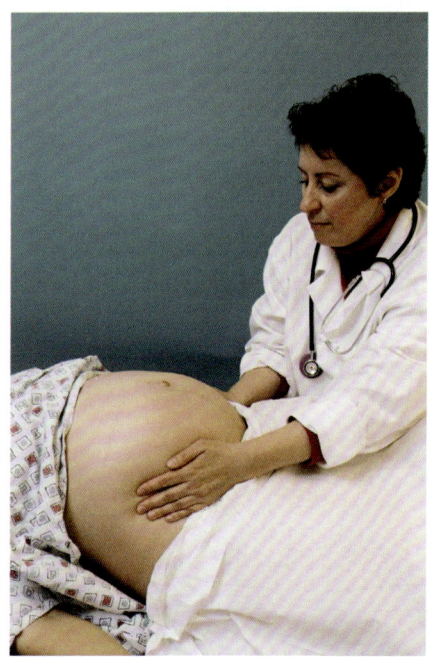

FIGURE 29-9 Palpating for uterine contractions.

Continued on following page

ASSESSMENT PROCEDURE	NORMAL FINDINGS	ABNORMAL FINDINGS

Palpation (Continued)

Time the length of the contraction from the beginning to the end. Also note the frequency of the contractions, timing from the beginning of one contraction until the beginning of the next (Fig. 29-10). The frequency of contractions is timed from the start of one contraction to the start of the next contraction. This allows the nurse to see the pattern of occurrence. Timing from the end of one contraction to the beginning of another would tell the amount of time between the contractions but that would not allow the nurse to see the pattern of occurrence.	Contraction may last 40–60 seconds and occur every 5–6 minutes.	Contractions lasting too long or occurring too frequently cause fetal distress.

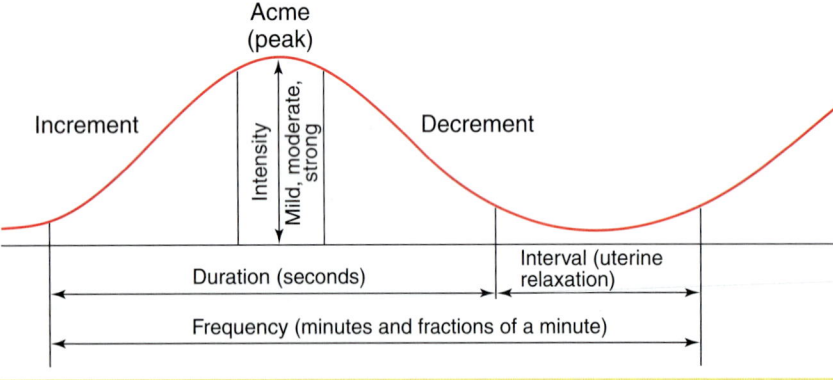

FIGURE 29-10 Contraction cycle.

Fundal Height

Measure fundal height. Do this by placing one hand on each side of the abdomen and walk hands up the sides of the uterus until you feel the uterus curve; hands should meet. Take a tape measure and place the zero point on the symphysis pubis and measure to the top of the fundus (Fig. 29-11).	Uterine size should approximately equal the number of weeks of gestation (e.g., the uterus at 28 weeks' gestation should measure approximately 28 cm) (Fig. 29-12). Measurements may vary by about 2 cm and examiners' techniques may vary, but measurements should be about the same.	Measurements beyond 4 cm of gestational age need to be further evaluated. Measurements greater than expected may indicate a multiple gestation, polyhydramnios (excess of amniotic fluid), fetal anomalies, or macrosomia (great increase in size similar to obesity). Measurements smaller than expected may indicate intrauterine growth retardation.

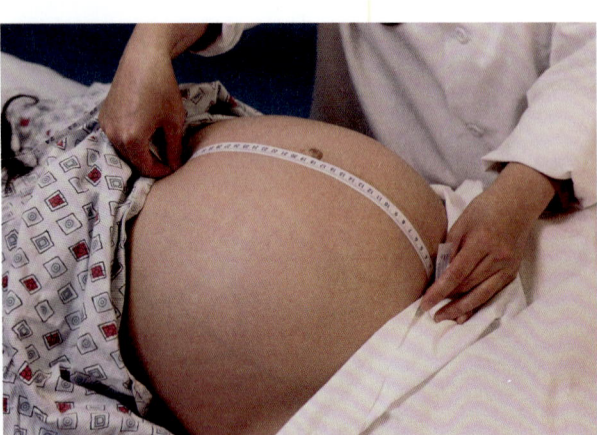

FIGURE 29-11 Measuring the fundal height.

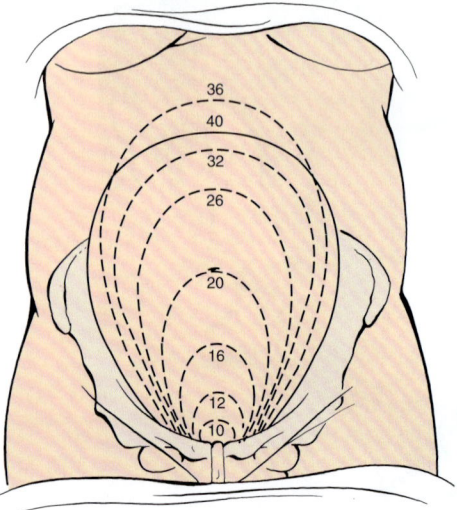

FIGURE 29-12 Approximate height of fundus at various weeks of gestation.

ASSESSMENT PROCEDURE	NORMAL FINDINGS	ABNORMAL FINDINGS
Fetal Position		
Using Leopold maneuvers, palpate the fundus, lateral aspects of the abdomen, and the lower pelvic area. Leopold maneuvers assist in determining the fetal lie (where the fetus is lying in relation to the mother's back), presentation (the presenting part of the fetus into the maternal pelvis), size, and position (the fetal presentation in relation to the maternal pelvis).	A longitudinal lie, in which the fetal spine axis is parallel to the maternal spine axis, is the expected finding. The presentation may be cephalic, breech, or shoulder. The size of the fetus may be estimated by measuring fundal height and by palpation. Fetal positions include right occiput anterior (ROA), left occiput posterior (LOP), left sacrum anterior (LSA), and so on. (Refer to a textbook on obstetrics for further detail.)	Oblique or transverse lie needs to be noted. If vaginal delivery is expected, external version can be performed to rotate the fetus to the longitudinal lie. Breech or shoulder presentations can complicate delivery if it is expected to be vaginal.
For the first maneuver, face the client's head. Place your hands on the fundal area, expecting to palpate a soft, irregular mass in the upper quadrant of the maternal abdomen (Fig. 29-13).	The soft mass is the fetal buttocks. The fetal head feels round and hard.	
For the second maneuver, move your hands to the lateral sides of the abdomen (Fig. 29-14).	On one side of the abdomen, you will palpate round nodules; these are the fists and feet of the fetus. Kicking and movement are expected to be felt. The other side of the abdomen feels smooth; this is the fetus's back.	

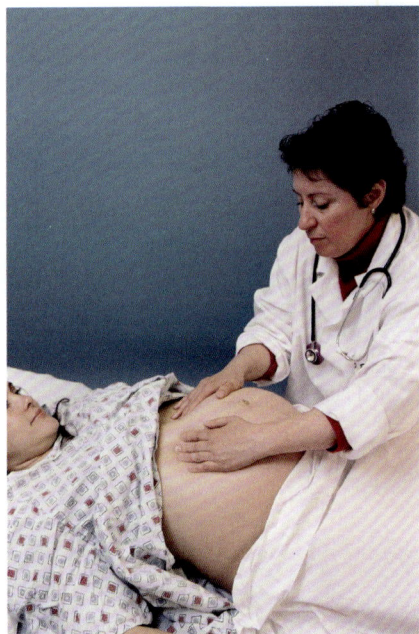

FIGURE 29-13 Leopold maneuver: first maneuver.

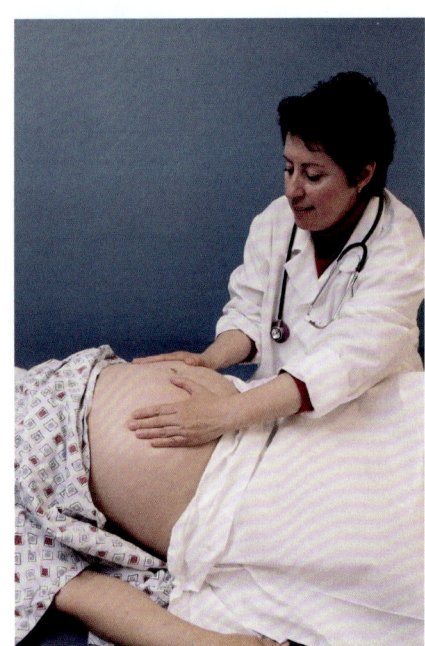

FIGURE 29-14 Leopold maneuver: second maneuver.

For the third maneuver, move your hands down to the lower pelvic area and palpate the area just above the symphysis pubis to determine the presenting part. Grasp the presenting part with the thumb and third finger (Fig. 29-15).	The unengaged head is round, firm, and ballotable, whereas the buttocks are soft and irregular.	Soft, presenting part at the symphysis pubis indicates breech presentation.

Continued on following page

712 UNIT 4 Nursing Assessment of Special Groups

ASSESSMENT PROCEDURE	NORMAL FINDINGS	ABNORMAL FINDINGS
Fetal Position (Continued)		
For the fourth maneuver, face the client's feet, place your hands on the abdomen, and point your fingers toward the mother's feet. Then try to move your hands toward each other while applying downward pressure (Fig. 29-16).	If the hands move together easily, the fetal head has not descended into the maternal pelvic inlet. If the hands do not move together and stop to resistance met, the fetal head is engaged into the pelvic inlet.	

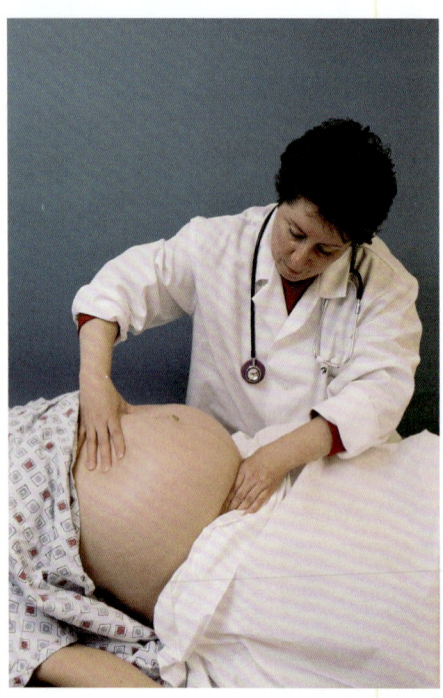

FIGURE 29-15 Leopold maneuver: third maneuver.

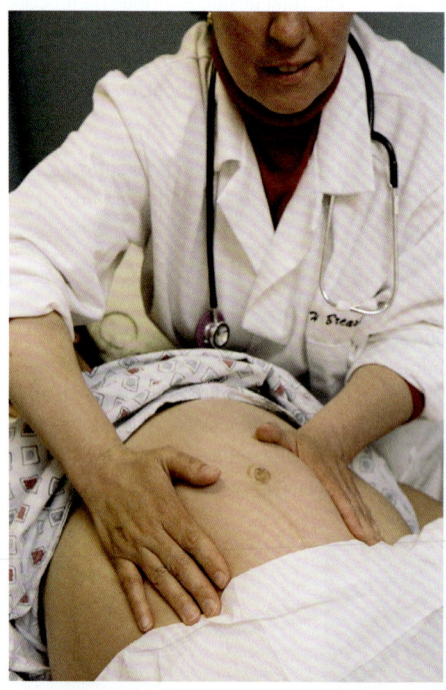

FIGURE 29-16 Leopold maneuver: fourth maneuver.

Fetal Heart		
Determine the location, rate, and rhythm of the fetal heart. Auscultate the fetal heart rate in the woman's left lower abdominal quadrant when the fetal back is positioned on maternal left, vertex position (Fig. 29-17). In breech presentations, fetal heart rate is heard in the upper quadrant of the maternal abdomen. Other locations for auscultating fetal heart rate (when the fetal back is positioned differently) are illustrated in Box 29-1. 🎯 **CLINICAL TIP** After assessing the fetal position, you can auscultate fetal heart tones best through the back of the fetus. A fetal Doppler ultrasound device can be used after 10–12 weeks' gestation to hear the fetal heartbeat. A fetoscope may also be used to hear the heartbeat after 18 weeks' gestation.	Fetal heart rate ranges from 120 to 160 beats/min. During the third trimester, the fetal heart rate should accelerate with fetal movement.	Inability to auscultate fetal heart tones with a fetal Doppler at 12 weeks may indicate a retroverted uterus, uncertain dates, fetal demise, or false pregnancy. Fetal heart rate decelerations could indicate poor placental perfusion.

ASSESSMENT PROCEDURE	NORMAL FINDINGS	ABNORMAL FINDINGS

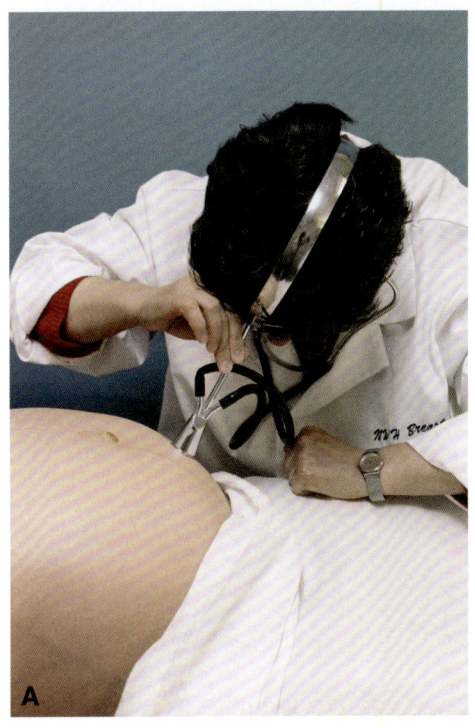 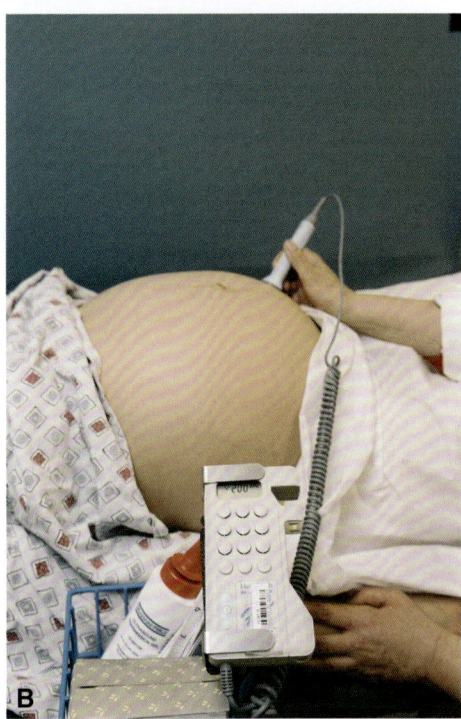

FIGURE 29-17 Auscultating the fetal heart rate with a fetoscope (**A**) and a Doppler ultrasound device (**B**).

Genitalia

EXTERNAL GENITALIA

Inspect the external genitalia. Note hair distribution, color of skin, varicosities, and scars.	Normal findings include enlarged labia and clitoris, parous relaxation of the introitus, and scars from an episiotomy or perineal lacerations (in multiparous women).	Labial varicosities, which can be painful. Evidence of female genital cutting (Box 29-2).
Palpate Bartholin and Skene glands.	There should be no discomfort or discharge with examination.	Discomfort and discharge noted with palpation may indicate infection.
Inspect vaginal opening for cystocele or rectocele.	No cystocele or rectocele.	Cystocele or rectocele may be more pronounced because of the muscle relaxation of pregnancy.

Internal Genitalia

Inspect internal genitalia (refer to gynecologic examination in textbook). Insert speculum into the vagina. Visualize the cervix, noting position and color. Obtain Pap smear and cultures if indicated. Withdraw speculum.	Cervix should look pink, smooth, and healthy. With pregnancy, the cervix may appear bluish (Chadwick sign). In multiparous women, the cervical opening has a slit-like appearance known as "fish mouth." A small amount of whitish vaginal discharge (leukorrhea) is normal.	Gonorrhea infection may present with thick, purulent vaginal discharge. A thick, white, cheesy discharge presents with a yeast infection. Grayish-white vaginal discharge, positive "whiff test" (fishy odor), and clue cells positive on microscopic wet prep (epithelial cells that have been invaded by disease-causing bacteria) are evidence of bacterial vaginosis.
Perform pelvic examination. Put on gloves lubricated with water or KY jelly, gently insert fingers into the vagina, and palpate the cervix. Estimate the length of the cervix by palpating the lateral surface of the cervix from the cervical tip to the lateral fornix.	The cervix may be palpated in the posterior vaginal vault. It should be long, thick, and closed. Cervical length should be approximately 2.3–3 cm. Positive Hegar sign (softening of the lower uterine segment) should be present (Fig. 29-18).	An effaced opened cervix may indicate an incompetent cervix if gestation is not at term, or preterm labor (Fig. 29-19).

Continued on following page

714 UNIT 4 Nursing Assessment of Special Groups

| ASSESSMENT PROCEDURE | NORMAL FINDINGS | ABNORMAL FINDINGS |

Internal Genitalia (Continued)

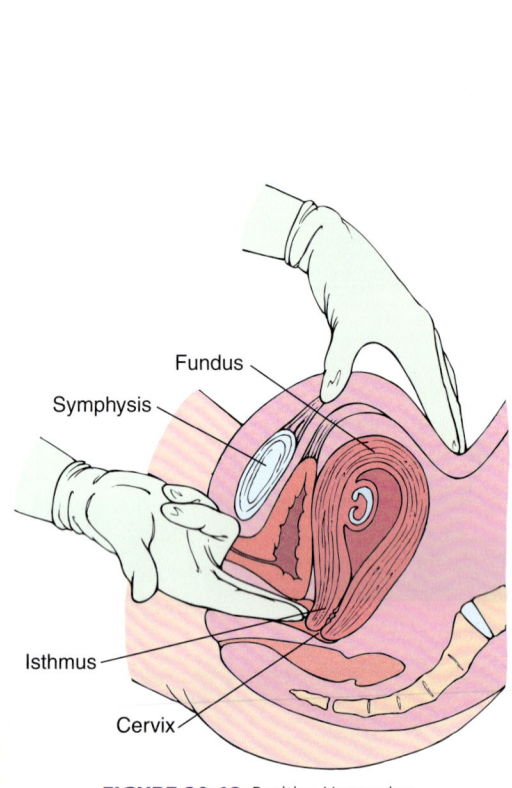

FIGURE 29-18 Positive Hegar sign.

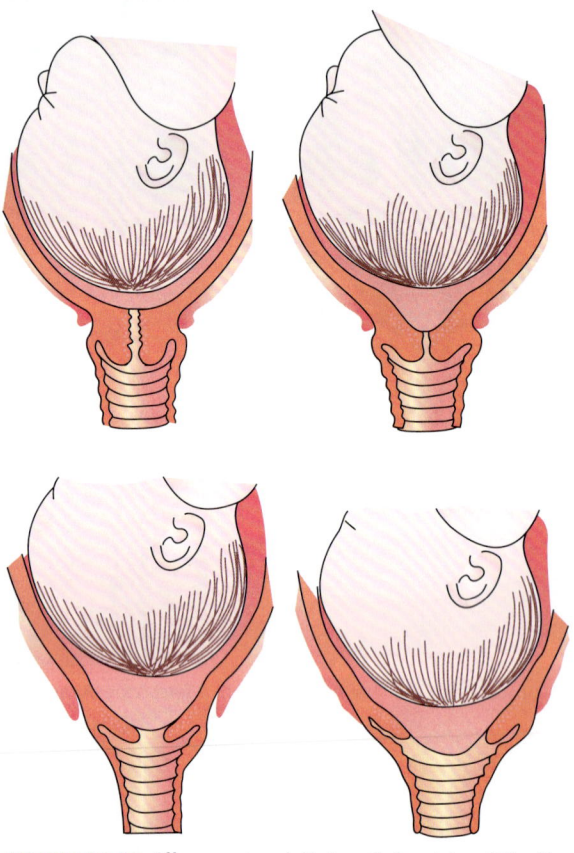

FIGURE 29-19 Effacement and dilation. Before labor, 0% effacement (*top left*). Early effacement, 30% (*top right*). Complete effacement, 100% (*bottom left*). Complete effacement and dilation (*bottom right*).

Feel for uterus. While leaving the fingers in the vagina, place the other hand on the abdomen and gently press down toward the internal hand until you feel the uterus between the two hands.

Palpate the left and right adnexa.

The uterus should feel about the size of an orange at 10 weeks (palpable at the suprapubic bone) and about the size of a grapefruit at 12 weeks.

No masses should be palpable. Discomfort with examination is due to stretching of the round ligaments throughout the pregnancy.

If uterine size is not consistent with dates, consider wrong dates, uterine fibroids, or multiple gestation.

Adnexal masses may indicate ectopic pregnancy (Fig. 29-20).

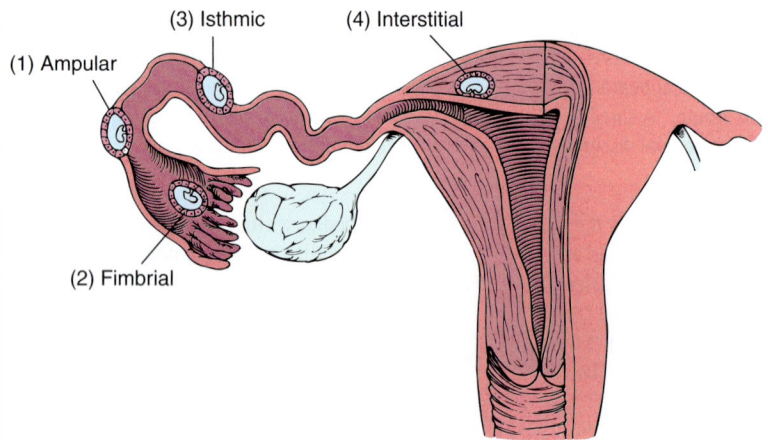

FIGURE 29-20 Sites of ectopic pregnancy.

ASSESSMENT PROCEDURE	NORMAL FINDINGS	ABNORMAL FINDINGS
Anus and Rectum		
Inspect the anus and rectum. Note color, varicosities, lesions, tears, or discharge.	Mucosa should be pink and intact. No masses, varicosities, lesions, tears, or discharge present. Hemorrhoids or varicose veins may be present. Hemorrhoids usually get bigger and more uncomfortable during pregnancy. Bleeding and infection may occur.	Masses may indicate cancer.
MUSCULOSKELETAL		
Determine pelvic adequacy for a vaginal delivery by estimating the angle of the subpubic arch. Place hands as shown in Figure 29-21, noting angle between thumb and first finger. **Determine the height and inclination of the symphysis pubis** (Fig. 29-22).	The subpubic arch should be greater than 90 degrees.	A narrow pubic arch displaces the presenting part posteriorly and impedes the fetus from passing under the pubic arch.

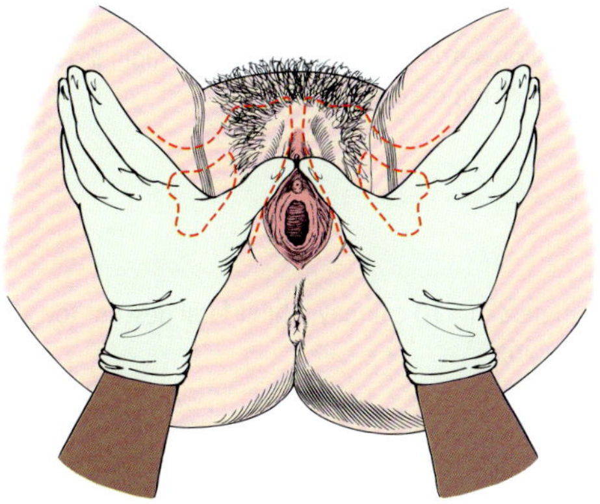

FIGURE 29-21 Estimating the angle of the subpubic arch.

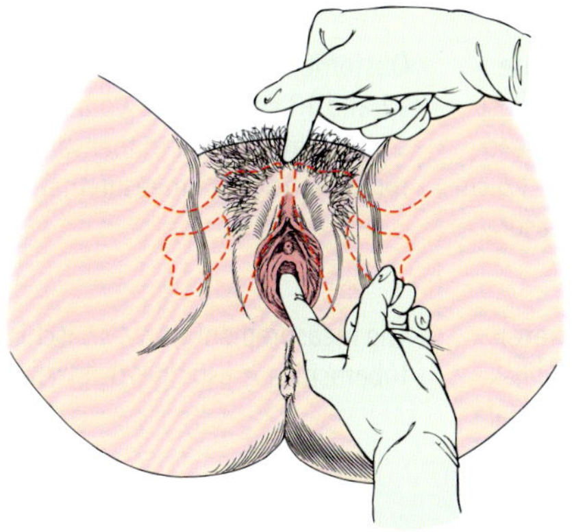

FIGURE 29-22 Determining the height and incline of the symphysis pubis.

Palpate the lateral walls of the pelvis.	Lateral walls should be straight or divergent.	Lateral walls that narrow as they approach the vagina may be problematic with vaginal delivery. Problems that may occur are shoulder dystocia, problems getting the fetus to drop into the pelvis, as well as increasing the risk of cesarean delivery.
Palpate the ischial spines. Sweep the finger posteriorly from one spine over to the other spine.	Ischial spines are small, not prominent. Interspinous diameter is at least 10.5 cm (Fig. 29-23).	Prominent spines. Interspinous diameter <10.5 cm may interfere with delivery.
Examine the sacrum and coccyx. Sweep fingers down the sacrum. Gently press back on the coccyx to determine mobility.	Gynecoid pelvis is most common. Mobile coccyx increases ease of delivery by expansion, enlarging the area in the pelvis.	Anthropoid or platypelloid pelvis with an immobile coccyx may interfere with vaginal birth. This type of pelvis may increase the risk of cesarean delivery.
Measure the diagonal conjugate. The diagonal conjugate measures the anteroposterior diameter of the pelvic inlet through which the fetal head passes first. Measure the diagonal conjugate by pressing internal hand into the sacral promontory and up; mark the spot on your hand directly below the symphysis pubis (Fig. 29-24).	Pelvic adequacy is expected if diagonal conjugate measures 12.5 cm or greater. If the middle finger cannot reach the sacral promontory, space is considered adequate.	A diagonal conjugate measuring <12.5 cm may impede vaginal delivery process.

Continued on following page

716 UNIT 4 Nursing Assessment of Special Groups

ASSESSMENT PROCEDURE	NORMAL FINDINGS	ABNORMAL FINDINGS

Anus and Rectum (Continued)

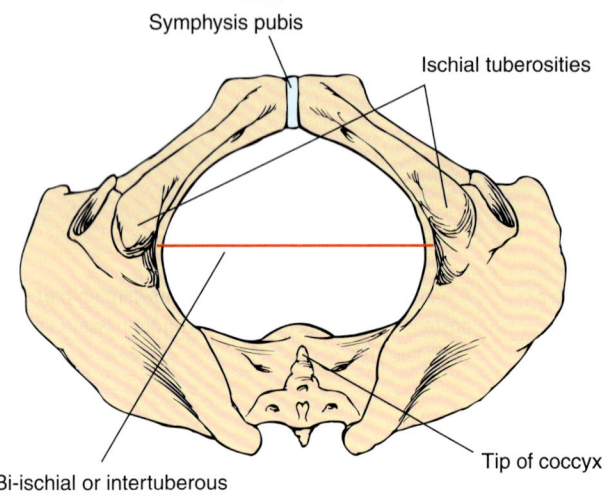

FIGURE 29-23 Ischial spines.

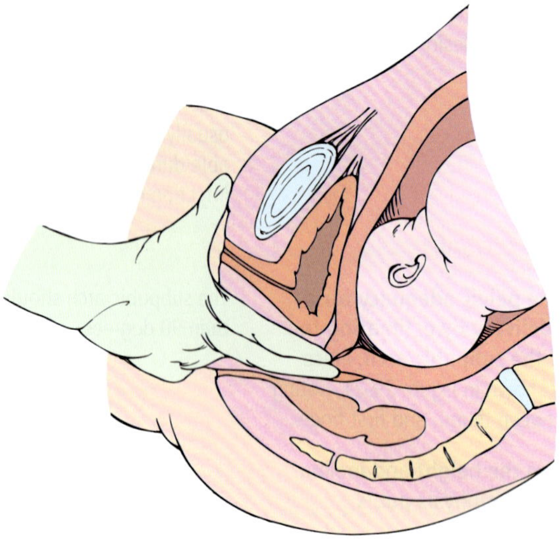

FIGURE 29-24 Measuring the diagonal conjugate.

Calculate the obstetric conjugate. The obstetric conjugate is the smallest opening through which the fetal head must pass. To calculate it, subtract 1.5 cm from the diagonal conjugate measurement (Fig. 29-25).	Obstetric conjugate is normally between 12 and 13 cm in adult women. Ultrasound may be used to measure this area for more accurate measurement.	A small obstetric conjugate may make vaginal delivery difficult or impossible.
Measure the transverse diameter of the pelvic outlet. To do this, make a fist and place it between the ischial tuberosities (Fig. 29-26).	The measurement between ischial tuberosities is usually 10–11 cm.	Diameters of <10 cm may inhibit fetal descent toward the vagina.

◎ **CLINICAL TIP**
Know the measurement of your own hand to estimate the measurement of the transverse diameter at pelvic outlet.

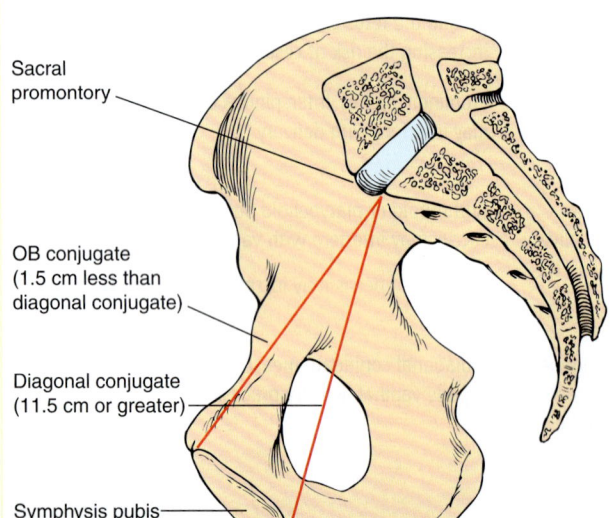

FIGURE 29-25 Pelvic structure: Obstetric (OB) conjugate, diagonal conjugate.

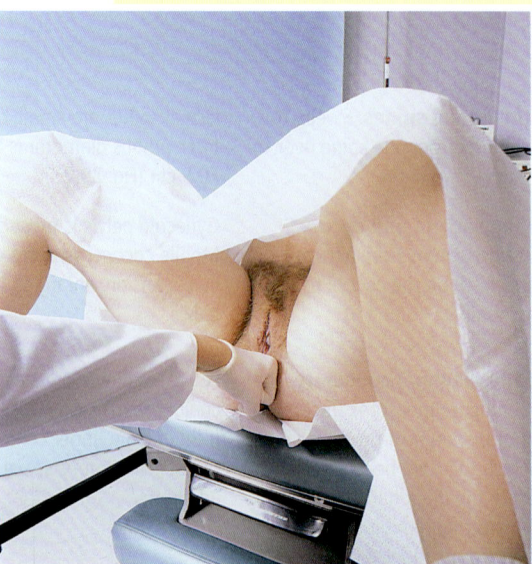

FIGURE 29-26 Using the fist to measure the pelvic outlet.

BOX 29-1 WHERE TO AUSCULTATE FETAL HEART RATE

These illustrations represent the best locations for auscultating the fetal heart rate: Left occiput anterior (LOA), right occiput anterior (ROA), left occiput posterior (LOP), right occiput posterior (ROP), left sacrum anterior (LSA), and right sacrum posterior (RSP).

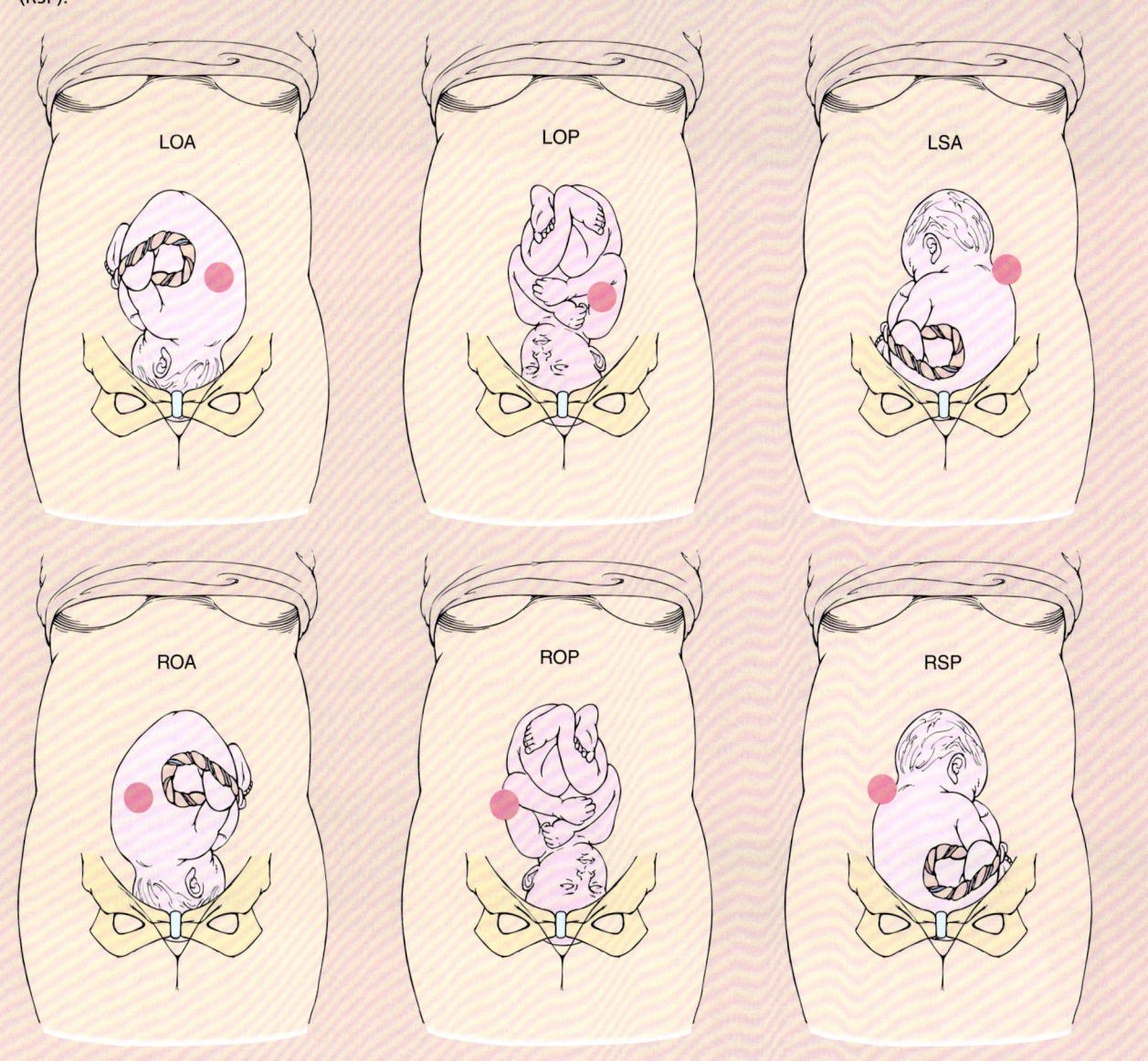

BOX 29-2 FEMALE GENITAL CUTTING (FGC)

Female genital cutting (FGC, also called female genital mutilation or female circumcision) includes piercing, cutting, removing, or sewing closed all or part of a woman's or a girl's external genitals (infibulation) for no medical reason (Womenshealth.gov, 2015). Approximately 513,000 women or girls have experienced or are at risk for experiencing this genital mutilation. Complications of pregnancy are rare, but complications of delivery include prolonged labor; excessive bleeding after the birth; higher risk for episiotomy; higher risk for cesarean section. Risks to the infant include low birth weight (less than 5 ½ lb); breathing problems; stillbirth; or early death after birth. The practice is culturally evident in many countries, especially those in northern and eastern Africa and the Middle East.

In the United States, FGC is against the law, and it is a crime to perform FGC on a girl younger than 18 or to take or attempt to take a girl out of the United States for FGC. Girls and women who have experienced FGC are not at fault and have not broken any U.S. laws.

Some women or their husbands ask for or demand reinfibulation after delivery when defibulation was necessary with the delivery. Ethical issues abound. Performing reinfibulation is discouraged, as there is no medical benefit, but if a patient insists upon the procedure and the provider is agreeable, a repair may legally be performed. The provider who agrees to do this is protected under the Federal Prohibition of Female Genital Mutilation Act of 1996, under which the initial mutilation is prohibited but not the repair (Lee & Strong, 2015).

CASE STUDY

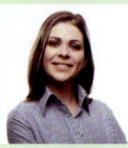

The chapter case study is now used to demonstrate a physical assessment of Mrs. Farrow. Your physical assessment reveals a blood pressure of 100/60 right arm, sitting: pulse rate 86, regular and strong; respirations 18, regular and moderately shallow; temperature 36.7°C. Her apical beat is also 86 and strong; heart sounds: S_1 and S_2 with no murmurs or clicks. Skin is warm and dry, slightly pale with light pink nail beds, pale palpebral conjunctiva, and oral mucous membranes. Abdomen moderately rounded with striae; fundal height 20 cm; fetal heart rate 158 per Doppler, right lower quadrant. Current weight 136 lb at 5 ft 9 in tall, 4 lb less than her stated usual weight. Lab values show hemoglobin (Hgb) 10.2 g/dL; hematocrit (Hct) 29.9%; RBC count $3.20 \times 10{-6}/\mu L$. Her sodium (Na) level is 129 and her potassium (K) level is 3.1. The remainder of the blood values is within normal limits. Urinalysis results are negative for protein and glucose.

Validating and Documenting Findings

Validate the assessment data that you have collected about the childbearing woman (by asking additional questions, verifying data with another health care professional, or comparing objective with subjective findings). If there are discrepancies between the objective and subjective data or if abnormal findings are inconsistent with other data, validate your data. This is necessary to verify that the data are reliable and accurate. Document the assessment data following the health care facility or agency policy.

CASE STUDY

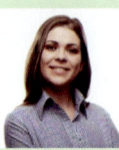

Think back to the case study. The nurse completed the following documentation of her assessment of Mrs. Farrow.

Biographical Data: MF, 29 years old, Caucasian, is a stay at home mother, married, living with husband and two sons in two-bedroom trailer. Husband works at a fast-food chain. Alert and oriented, and answers questions appropriately.

History of Present Health Concern: LMP September 15 (12 weeks ago), Gr3 P2, on first visit for prenatal care due to being very sick with this pregnancy and limited financial and transportation resources. Pregnancy affected by severe nausea, fatigue, and vomiting for last 8 weeks. Husband brings home free fast food, so nutrition not as she would like.

Personal Health History: Two past deliveries of healthy babies weighing 6 lb 2 oz and 7 lb 6 oz, but first pregnancy complicated with mild hyperemesis gravidarum throughout the pregnancy. She gained 20 lb with her first pregnancy and 30 lb with her second pregnancy. She gained 30 lb during the second pregnancy and was diagnosed with pregnancy-induced hypertension and mild gestational diabetes; labor was induced at 38 weeks' gestation. MF is not on any prescribed medications. She is taking some prenatal vitamin capsules that she got from her local pharmacy. She occasionally takes allergy tabs for symptoms of hay fever. Denies medication, food, insect, or other allergies except for occasional hay fever. Denies use of herbal medicines or alternative therapies. No other health issues described.

Family History: Parents both alive and well, but live in another state. Mother was very sick while pregnant with MF and one other of three siblings. Father has mild hypertension and mild obesity. No other health problems described in family.

Lifestyle and Health Practices: States she knows good nutrition and hydration and exercise criteria, but does not follow them due to being so sick with this pregnancy, two small children at home, financial limitations, and husband bringing home free fast food. Knows she should have come to prenatal visit much earlier, but physical, transportation, and financial issues made it difficult. Sleeps only 6–7 hours per night, but tries to get 7–8 hours per night. Exercise is keeping up with her two boys each day and housework. When feeling able, she walks her boys to a park 4 blocks from residence.

24-hour diet recall: Breakfast—a roll with black tea; lunch—a few crackers and cheese; dinner—a burger and fries.

Physical Examination Findings: Blood pressure 100/60 right arm, sitting: pulse rate 86, regular and strong; respirations 18, regular and moderately shallow; temperature 36.7°C. Apical beat also 86 and strong; heart sounds: S_1 and S_2 with no murmurs or clicks. Skin is warm and dry, slightly pale, with light pink nail beds, pale palpebral conjunctiva and oral mucous membranes. Abdomen moderately rounded with striae; fundal height 20 cm; fetal heart rate 158 per Doppler, right lower quadrant. Current weight 136 lb at 5 ft 9 in tall, 4 lb less than her stated usual weight. Lab values show hemoglobin (Hgb) 10.2 g/dL; hematocrit (Hct) 29.9%; RBC count $3.20 \times 10{-6}/\mu L$. Her sodium (Na) level is 129 and her potassium (K) level is 3.1. The remainder of the blood values is within normal limits. Urinalysis results are negative for protein and glucose.

ANALYSIS OF DATA: DIAGNOSTIC REASONING

After collecting assessment data, you will need to analyze it using diagnostic reasoning skills. The following lists some possible conclusions that may be drawn after assessment of a childbearing woman.

Selected Nursing Diagnoses

After collecting subjective and objective data pertaining to the assessment of the childbearing woman, you will need to identify abnormalities and cluster the data to reveal any significant patterns or abnormalities. These data will then be used to make clinical judgments (nursing diagnoses: health promotion, risk, or actual) about the status of the client's pregnancy. Following is a listing of selected nursing diagnoses that you may identify when analyzing data for this part of the assessment.

Health Promotion Diagnoses

- Readiness for Enhanced Health Management
- Readiness for Enhanced Childbearing Process

Risk Diagnoses

- Risk for Ineffective Childbearing Process (related to placenta placement with bleeding; premature contractions; preeclampsia)
- Risk for Deficient Fluid Volume (related to excessive nausea/vomiting)
- Risk for Injury (maternal; related to elevated arterial pressure)
- Risk for Injury (fetal; related to decreased placental perfusion due to blood loss)
- Risk for Infection (related to having cats in the household, i.e., toxoplasmosis).
- Risk for Constipation (related to decreased appetite/fiber and fluid intake).
- Risk for Unstable Blood Glucose Level (related to high carbohydrate intake and gestational diabetes)
- Risk for Stress Urinary Incontinence (related to enlarging pregnant uterus)

Actual Diagnoses

- Ineffective Childbearing Process (related to cephalopelvic disproportion and insufficiently strong contractions)
- Sleep Deprivation (related to fatigue and effects of pregnancy)
- Fatigue (related to effects of pregnancy and lack of sufficient sleep)
- Interrupted Family Coping (related to required bedrest to prevent premature labor)
- Nausea (related to hormonal effects of pregnancy)
- Electrolyte Imbalance (Hyponatremia/Hypokalemia): Less Than Body Requirements, related to vomiting, inadequate dietary intake
- Anemia (related to excessive nausea/vomiting)
- Anxiety (related to fear of loss of pregnancy)
- Imbalanced Nutrition related to lack of knowledge of proper nutrition during pregnancy

Selected Collaborative Problems

After grouping the data, certain collaborative problems may emerge. Remember that collaborative problems differ from nursing diagnoses in that they cannot be prevented with nursing interventions. However, these physiologic complications of medical conditions can be detected and monitored by the nurse. In addition, the nurse can use physician- and nurse-prescribed interventions to minimize the complications of these problems. The nurse may also have to refer the client in such situations for further treatment of the problem. Following is a list of collaborative problems that may be identified when assessing the childbearing woman. These problems are worded as Risk for Complications (RC) followed by the problem.

- RC: Anemia
- RC: Pregnancy-induced hypertension
- RC: Preeclampsia
- RC: Hyperemesis gravidarum
- RC: Gestational diabetes
- RC: Placenta previa
- RC: Spontaneous abortion

Medical Problems

After grouping the data, it may become apparent that the client has signs and symptoms that may require medical diagnosis and treatment. Referral to a primary care provider is necessary.

CASE STUDY

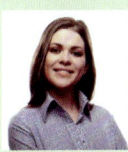

After collecting and analyzing the data for Mrs. Farrow, the nurse determines that the following conclusions are appropriate:

Nursing Diagnoses

- Risk for Ineffective Health Maintenance r/t inadequate financial resources
- Risk for Disabled Family Coping r/t inadequate resources and coming birth of third child
- Imbalanced Nutrition r/t to prolonged nausea and vomiting

Potential Collaborative Problems

- RC: Hyperemesis gravidarum
- RC: Fetal compromise
- RC: Anemia
- RC: Electrolyte imbalance

Refer the client to a nutritionist for dietary consult and to a social worker for evaluation/assistance with financial resources.

To view an algorithm depicting the process of diagnostic reasoning for this case, go to thePoint.

Interdisciplinary Verbal Communication of Assessment Findings Using SBAR

SITUATION: MF, a 29-year-old Caucasian woman, G3 P2 (term and vaginal), came to clinic for initial prenatal examination. Her LMP was 12 weeks ago. She did seek earlier prenatal care because of severe nausea with vomiting for the past 8 weeks and was unable to get child care or transportation to clinic.

BACKGROUND: Husband took off work to care for kids as he is concerned about his wife. Gained 20 and 30 lb with previous two pregnancies. Lives with husband and two sons in a two-bedroom trailer on land owned by in-laws, who are very supportive and help out during tough times by not charging rent. Husband works full time at fast-food chain. It is often hard for them to meet their financial responsibilities; however, they believe it is important for her to stay home with the children, so she does not contribute financially. Encourages healthy eating but husband gets food and soda discounts from workplace so they don't eat as well as she knows they should. Takes some prenatal vitamins and for allergy tabs for hay fever as needed. During last pregnancy diagnosed with pregnancy-induced hypertension, gestational diabetes, and induced at 38 weeks' gestation. Mother also very sick during two pregnancies. Father has mild hypertension and mild obesity. Sleeps 6 to 7 hours per night, but tries to get 7 to 8 hours. Exercises by keeping up with two boys, walking 4 blocks to park, and housework. 24-hour diet recall: Breakfast—a roll with black tea; lunch—a few crackers and cheese; dinner—a burger and fries.

ASSESSMENT: Blood pressure 100/60 right arm, sitting: pulse rate 86, regular and strong; respirations 18, regular and moderately shallow; temperature 36.7°C. Apical beat also 86 and strong; heart sounds: S_1 and S_2 with no murmurs or clicks. Skin is warm and dry, slightly pale, with light pink nail beds, pale palpebral conjunctiva and oral mucous membranes. Abdomen moderately rounded with striae; fundal height 20 cm; fetal heart rate 158 per Doppler, right lower quadrant. Current weight 136 lb at 5 ft 9 in tall, 4 lb less than her stated usual weight. Lab values show hemoglobin (Hgb) 10.2 g/dL; hematocrit (Hct) 29.9%; RBC count $3.20 \times 10-6/\mu L$. Her sodium (Na) level is 129 and her potassium (K) level is 3.1.

RECOMMENDATION: MF is at Risk for Ineffective Health Maintenance r/t inadequate financial resources; Risk for Disabled Family Coping r/t inadequate resources and coming birth of third child, and Imbalanced Nutrition r/t to prolonged nausea and vomiting. She needs to be observed for signs of Hyperemesis Gravidarum, Fetal Compromise, Anemia, and/or Electrolyte Imbalance. She should be referred to a nutritionist for dietary consult and to a social worker for evaluation/assistance with financial resources.

Want to know more?

A wide variety of resources to enhance your learning and understanding of this book are available on **thePoint**. Visit thePoint to access:

NCLEX-Style Student Review Questions	Concept in Action Animations
Watch and Learn Videos	And more!

Unfolding Patient Stories: Edith Jacobson • Part 2

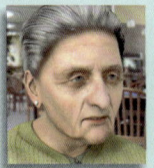

Recall from Chapter 6 Edith Jacobson, an 85-year-old female who fell at home and is hospitalized for hip surgery. Why is it important for the nurse to screen Edith for common problems associated with older adults? What syndromes are assessed with the SPICES risk screening tool for older adults? What nursing assessments are done to identify each problem, and how can the findings benefit the nursing plan of care?

Care for Edith and other patients in a realistic virtual environment: **vSim** *for Nursing* (thepoint.lww.com/vSimHealthAssessment). Practice documenting these patients' care in DocuCare (thepoint.lww.com/DocuCareEHR).

Unfolding Patient Stories: Kim Johnson • Part 2

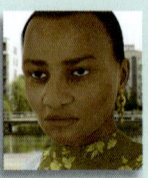

Recall from Chapter 14 Kim Johnson, a 26-year-old police officer who uses a wheelchair because of paraplegia from a complete spinal cord injury. Upon discharge from the rehabilitation center, she would like to return to her apartment (shared with a friend) that is located near her parents. Describe the community assessment the nurse would perform to evaluate the adequacy of available resources necessary for Kim's health needs, independence, and safety.

Care for Kim and other patients in a realistic virtual environment: **vSim** *for Nursing* (thepoint.lww.com/vSimHealthAssessment). Practice documenting these patients' care in DocuCare (thepoint.lww.com/DocuCareEHR).

References and Selected Readings

American Academy of Pediatrics. (2013). Prenatal substance abuse: Short- and long-term effects on the exposed fetus. Available at http://pediatrics.aappublications.org/content/pediatrics/131/3/e1009.full.pdf

American College of Nurse Midwives. (2013). RH-negative blood type and pregnancy. *Journal of Midwifery and Women's Health*, 58(6), 725–726. Available at http://onlinelibrary.wiley.com/doi/10.1111/jmwh.12140/pdf

American College of Obstetricians and Gynecologists (ACOG). (2011). *Vaginitis*. Available at http://www.acog.org/Patients/FAQs/Vaginitis#is

American College of Obstetricians and Gynecologists (ACOG). (2013). Weight gain during pregnancy: ACOG committee opinion. Available at http://www.acog.org/Resources-And-Publications/Committee-Opinions/Committee-on-Obstetric-Practice/Weight-Gain-During-Pregnancy

American Pregnancy Association. (2017). Ectopic pregnancy. Available at http://americanpregnancy.org/pregnancy-complications/ectopic-pregnancy/

Calvet, G., Aguiar, R. S., Melo, A. S., et al. (2016, February 17). Detection and sequencing of Zika virus from amniotic fluid of fetuses with microcephaly in Brazil: A case study. Available at http://www.thelancet.com/journals/laninf/article/PIIS1473-3099(16)00095-5/abstract

Centers for Disease Control and Prevention (CDC). (2014). Smoking in pregnancy: A possible risk for ADHD. Available at http://www.cdc.gov/features/smoking-adhd/

Centers for Disease Control and Prevention (CDC). (2015a). Facts about FASDs. Available at http://www.cdc.gov/ncbddd/fasd/facts.html

Centers for Disease Control and Prevention (CDC). (2015b). Pregnant women & influenza (flu). Available at http://www.cdc.gov/flu/protect/vaccine/pregnant.htm

Centers for Disease Control and Prevention (CDC). (2016). Zika virus. Available at http://www.cdc.gov/zika/index.html

Fang, W. L., Goldstein, A., Butzen, A., et al. (2004). Smoking cessation in pregnancy: A review of postpartum relapse prevention strategies. *Journal of the American Board of Family Practice, 17*, 264–275.

Gestational trophoblastic disease. (2013). Available at http://patient.info/doctor/gestational-trophoblastic-disease

Healthy People 2020. (2016). Maternal, infant, and child health. Available at https://www.healthypeople.gov/2020/topics-objectives/topic/maternal-infant-and-child-health

Institute of Medicine (IOM). (2009). Weight gain during pregnancy: Reexamining the guidelines. Available at http://www.nationalacademies.org/hmd/~/media/Files/Report%20Files/2009/Weight-Gain-During-Pregnancy-Reexamining-the-Guidelines/Report%20Brief%20-%20Weight%20Gain%20During%20Pregnancy.pdf

Jensen, D. M., Korsholm, L., Ovesen, P., et al. (2009). Peri-conceptional A1C and risk of serious adverse pregnancy outcome in 933 women with type 1 diabetes. *Diabetes Care, 32*(6), 1046–1048.

Lee, M. J., & Strong, N. (2015). Female genital mutilation: What ob/gyns need to know. Available at http://contemporaryobgyn.modernmedicine.com/contemporary-obgyn/news/female-genital-mutilation-what-obgyns-need-know-0?page=0%2C3

Little, M., Sinert, R. H., Sayah, A. J., et al. (2012). Asthma in Pregnancy. Medscape (updated March 8, 2012). Available at http://emedicine.medscape.com/article/796274-overview#showall.

March of Dimes. (2015). Smoking during pregnancy. Available at http://www.marchofdimes.org/pregnancy/smoking-during-pregnancy.aspx#

Mayo Clinic. (2014). Listeria infection. Available at http://www.mayoclinic.org/diseases-conditions/listeria-infection/basics/definition/con-20031039

Moore, L. (2015). Hydatidiform mole. Available at http://emedicine.medscape.com/article/254657-overview

National Institute of Mental Health (NIMH). (n.d.). Postpartum depression facts. Available at http://www.nimh.nih.gov/health/publications/postpartum-depression-facts/index.shtml#pub7

National Institute of Neurological Disorders and Stroke (NINDS). (2016). NINDS Tay-Sachs information page. Available at http://www.ninds.nih.gov/disorders/taysachs/taysachs.htm

Nelson, M. (2012). Ask the doctor: Stress in pregnancy. Available at http://www.chambanamoms.com/2012/01/27/ask-the-doctor-stress-in-pregnancy/

Pereira, L., Petitt, M., Fong, A., et al. (2014). Intrauterine growth restriction caused by underlying congenital cytomegalovirus infection. *Journal of Infectious Diseases, 209*(10), 1573–1584.

Runge, S. B., Pedersen, J. K., Svendsen, S. W., et al. (2013). Occupational lifting of heavy loads and preterm birth: A study within the Danish national birth cohort. *Occupational Environmental Medicine, 70*(11), 782–788. Available at http://www.medscape.com/viewarticle/813592

Sivalingam, V. N., Duncan, W. C., Kirk, E., et al. (2011). Diagnosis and management of ectopic pregnancy. *Journal of Family Planning and Reproductive Health Care, 37*(4), 231–240.

UCSF Medical Center. (2016). Diabetes in pregnancy. Available at https://www.ucsfhealth.org/education/diabetes_in_pregnancy/

Women's Healthcare Topics. (2012). Fatigue in pregnancy. Available at http://www.womenshealthcaretopics.com/preg_fatigue_during.htm

Womenshealth.gov. (2015). Female genital cutting. Available at http://womenshealth.gov/publications/our-publications/fact-sheet/female-genital-cutting.html

World Health Organization (WHO). (2016). Zika virus. Available at http://www.who.int/mediacentre/factsheets/zika/en/

30 ASSESSING NEWBORNS AND INFANTS

Learning Objectives

1. Describe the physical, motor, sensory perceptual, moral, psychosocial, and psychosexual development patterns seen in a newborn.
2. Complete a newborn history by interviewing parents about their newborn's prenatal development and by reviewing prenatal/delivery records.
3. Perform an initial physical assessment of the newborn using the correct techniques.
4. Perform subsequent follow-up physical assessments of the newborn using the correct techniques.
5. Differentiate between normal and abnormal assessment findings seen in the initial and subsequent assessments of the newborn.
6. Analyze the data from the interview and initial and subsequent physical assessments of the newborn to formulate valid nursing diagnoses, collaborative problems, and/or referrals.
7. Differentiate between general routine screening versus skills needed for focused or specialty assessment of the newborn.
8. Document and verbally report accurate assessment findings of the newborn.

CASE STUDY

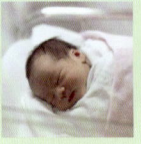

Kaitlin is a 4-day-old female infant brought into the clinic today by her mother for evaluation of jaundice. Her mother states that she is concerned about the yellowing of her skin because she feels like it is not improving over the last 2 days. She states that her daughter's skin started to turn yellow on the day she was discharged from the hospital.

Her mother is a 28-year-old gravida 1, para 1, with an unremarkable medical history. Her pregnancy was uneventful. She delivered at term, 39 weeks' gestation, via vaginal delivery with forceps. Kaitlin weighed 8 lb 10 oz and was appropriate for gestational age (AGA).

Kaitlin is a healthy term infant, with molding of the head and a cephalohematoma noted on her right anterior scalp. Mother states this has been gradually improving since delivery.

Kaitlin has been breastfeeding every 3–4 hours since birth. She was discharged to home from the hospital at approximately 36 hours of age and has been wetting approximately 8–10 diapers a day and stooling 2–3 times a day.

GROWTH AND DEVELOPMENT

A newborn, or neonate, is the term used to describe a child from birth to 28 days old. An infant refers to a child between the ages of 28 days and 1 year.

 ### Physical Development

Skin, Hair, and Nails

At birth, the newborn's skin is smooth and thin. It may appear ruddy because of visible blood circulation through the newborn's thin layer of subcutaneous fat. This thin layer of fat, combined with the skin's inability to contract and shiver, results in ineffective temperature regulation. The skin may appear mottled on the trunk, arms, or legs. The dermis and epidermis are thin and loosely bound together. This increases the skin's susceptibility to infection and irritation and creates a poor barrier, resulting in fluid loss. When the newborn's body temperature drops, the hands and/or feet may appear blue (acrocyanosis). Vernix caseosa may be visible on the skin. It appears as a thick, cheesy, white substance on the skin and is especially prevalent in skin folds. This is normal and usually absorbs into the skin.

After birth, the newborn's sebaceous glands are active because of high levels of maternal androgen. Milia develop when these glands become plugged. Eccrine glands function at birth, creating palmar sweating, which is helpful when

722

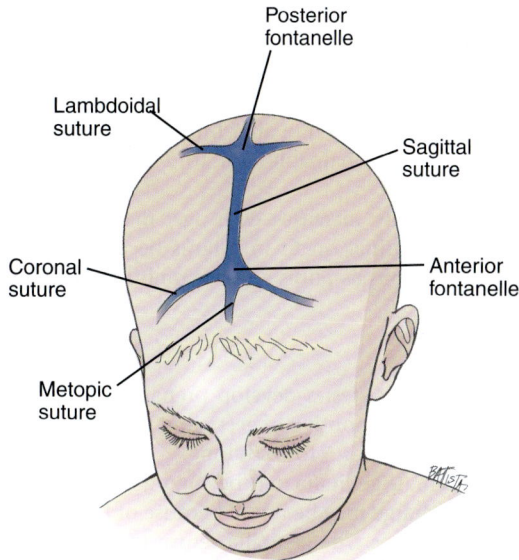

FIGURE 30-1 The infant head.

assessing pain. Apocrine glands stay small and nonfunctional until puberty.

The fine, downy hairs called *lanugo*, which appear on the newborn's body, shoulders, and/or back at birth, develop in the fetus at 3 months gestation and disappear within the first 2 weeks of life. Scalp hair-follicle growth phases occur concurrently at birth but are disrupted during early infancy. This may result in overgrowth or alopecia (hair loss).

Nails are usually present at birth. Missing or short nails usually signify prematurity, and long nails usually signify postmaturity. Nails are usually pink, convex, and smooth throughout childhood and adolescence.

Head and Neck

Head growth predominates during the fetal period. At birth, the head circumference is greater (by 2 cm) than that of the chest. The cranial bones are soft and separated by the coronal, lambdoid, and sagittal sutures, which intersect at the anterior and posterior fontanelle (Fig. 30-1). Ossification begins in infancy and continues into adulthood.

The newborn's skull is typically asymmetric (plagiocephaly) because of molding that occurs as the newborn passes through the birth canal. The skull molds easily during birth, allowing for overlapping of the cranial bones.

The posterior fontanelle usually measures 1 to 2 cm at birth and usually closes at 2 months. The anterior fontanelle usually measures 4 to 6 cm at birth and closes between 12 and 18 months.

CLINICAL TIP
A full anterior fontanelle may be palpable when the newborn cries.

Visible pulsations may also appear, representing the peripheral pulse. The sutures and fontanelles allow the skull to expand to accommodate brain growth. Brain growth is reflected by head circumference (occipital—frontal circumference), which increases six times as much during the first year as it does the second. Half of postnatal brain growth is achieved within the first year of life.

The neck is usually short during infancy (lengthening at about age 3 or 4 years). Lymphoid tissue is well developed at birth and reaches adult size by age 6 years.

Eyes

Eye structure and function are not fully developed at birth. The iris shows little pigment, and the pupils are small. The macula, which is absent at birth, develops at 4 months and is mature by 8 months. Pupillary reflex is poor at birth and improves at 5 months of age. The sclerae are clear. Small subconjunctival hemorrhages are normal after birth. Peripheral vision is developed, but central vision is not. The newborn is farsighted and has a visual acuity of 20/200. At 4 months, an infant can fixate on a singular object with both eyes simultaneously (binocularity). Tearing and voluntary control over eye muscles begin at 2 to 3 months. These functions are better developed by 9 months. Newborns cannot distinguish between colors; this ability develops by 8 months.

Ears

The inner ear develops during the first trimester of gestation. Therefore, maternal problems during this time, such as rubella, may impair hearing. Newborns can hear loud sounds at 90 decibels and react with the startle reflex. They respond to low-frequency sounds, such as a heartbeat or a lullaby, by decreasing crying and motor movement. They react to high-frequency sounds with an alerting reaction. In infants, the external auditory canal curves upward and is short and straight. Therefore, the pinna must be pulled down and back to perform the otoscopic examination. The eustachian tube is wider, shorter, and more horizontal, increasing the possibility of infection rising from the pharynx. If there is an anatomical anomaly of the ear, the neonate should be examined for renal anomalies as well, as the ears and kidneys develop at the same embryologic stage (Rashad & El-Fiky, 2007).

Mouth, Throat, Nose, and Sinus

Saliva is minimal at birth but drooling is evident by 3 months because of the increased secretion of saliva. Drooling persists for a few months until the infant learns to swallow the saliva. Drooling does not signify tooth eruption. The development of both temporary (deciduous) and permanent teeth begins in utero. Deciduous tooth eruption takes place between the ages of 6 and 24 months.

The tonsils and adenoids are small in relation to body size and hard to see at birth. The pharynx is best seen when the newborn is crying.

Newborns are obligatory nose breathers and, therefore, have significant distress when their nasal passages are obstructed. The maxillary and ethmoid sinuses begin to develop the 10th week and are present at birth. However, they are small and cannot be examined until they further develop.

Thorax and Lungs

At term gestation, the fetal lungs should be developed and the alveoli should be collapsed. The placenta performs gas exchange. Immediately after birth, the lungs aerate; blood flows through them more vigorously, causing greater expansion and relaxation of the pulmonary arteries. The decrease in pulmonary pressure closes the foramen ovale, increasing oxygen tension and closing the ductus arteriosus. The lungs continue to develop after birth, and new alveoli form until about 8 years of age.

Breasts

Ventral epidermal ridges (milk lines), which run from the axilla to the medial thigh, are present during gestation. True breasts develop along the thoracic ridge; the other breasts along the milk line atrophy. Occasionally a supernumerary nipple persists along the ridge track. At birth, lactiferous ducts are present in the nipple but there are no alveoli. Although the newborn's breasts may be temporarily enlarged from the effects of maternal estrogen, they are usually flat and remain so until puberty.

Heart

Because oxygenation takes place in the placenta in fetal circulation, the lungs are bypassed and arterial blood is returned to the right side of the heart. Blood is shunted through the foramen ovale and ductus arteriosus into the left side of the heart and out the aorta. At birth, lung aeration causes circulatory changes. The foramen ovale closes within the first hour because of the newly created low pressure in the right side of the heart, and the ductus arteriosus closes about 10 to 15 hours after birth.

When listening to the heart in the infant, systolic murmurs may be audible due to the transition from intrauterine to extrauterine life. This murmur generally resolves within 24 to 48 hours after birth. The pulse rate is usually between 120 and 160 beats/min. The rate decreases as the child ages, having a normal heart rate of 120 to 160 at birth and declining to approximately 120s at 6 months of age and down to 110s from 6 months to 1 year old. The heart should be auscultated at approximately the 4th intercostal margin to the left of the mid-clavicular line. The heart lies more horizontal in the chest and may seem enlarged with percussion. Heart sounds are also more audible in the newborn secondary to the thin subcutaneous layer of skin on the newborn.

Peripheral Vascular System

The skin should appear pink and well perfused. The hands and feet may appear blue at times (acrocyanosis), which is normal, especially when the newborn is cold. With warming, skin color should return to pink. If the infant does not respond with warming techniques (placing newborn under radiant heater or adding a layer of blankets), consider a congenital heart defect in the newborn.

Pulses should be audible at the 4th intercostal space. Pulses should be felt in extremities, assessing the radial, brachial, and femoral pulses bilaterally. Weakness or absence of femoral pulses may indicate coarctation of the aorta. Bounding pulses can be seen with patent ductus arteriosus.

Abdomen

The umbilical cord is prominent in the newborn and contains two arteries and one vein. The umbilicus consists of two parts: the amniotic portion and the cutaneous portion. The amniotic portion is covered with a gel-like substance and dries up and falls off within 2 weeks of birth. The cutaneous portion is covered with skin and draws back to become flush with the abdominal wall.

The abdomen of infants is cylindrical. Peristaltic waves may be visible in infants up to 3 months of age and may be indicative of a disease or disorder such as pyloric stenosis (Mayo Clinic, 2012).

The newborn's liver is palpable at 0.5 to 2.5 cm below the right costal margin, thereby occupying proportionately more space than at any other time after birth. In infants and small children, the liver is palpable at 1 to 2 cm below the right costal margin.

Bladder capacity increases with age; the bladder is considered an abdominal organ in infants because it is located between the symphysis pubis and the umbilicus (higher than in adults).

Genitalia

In male infants, the testes develop prenatally and drop into the scrotum during month 8 of gestation. Each testis measures about 1 cm wide and 1.5 to 2 cm long.

At birth, female genitalia may be engorged. Vaginal mucoid or bloody discharge may be noted because of the influence of maternal hormones. The genitalia return to normal size in a few weeks and remain small until puberty.

Anus, Rectum, and Prostate

Meconium is passed during the first 24 hours of life, signifying anal patency. Stools are passed by reflex, and anal sphincter control is not reached until 1.5 to 2 years of age after the nerves supplying the area have become fully myelinated. Meconium not passed within 24 hours of birth could signify a problem. In boys, the prostate gland is underdeveloped and not palpable.

Musculoskeletal System

At birth, the newborn should have full range of motion (ROM) of all extremities. Many newborns have feet that may appear deformed in position due to the intrauterine position of extremities. The feet should turn to the normal position with ease by the examiner.

The hips should also be checked for dislocation and ease of movement by performing the Ortolani test and Barlow sign.

The newborn vertebral column differs in contour from the normal adult vertebral column. The spine has a single C-shaped curve at birth. By 3 to 4 months, the anterior curve in the cervical region develops from the infant raising its head when prone.

Neurologic System

The neurologic system is not fully developed at birth. Motor control is maintained by the spinal cord and medulla, and most actions in the newborn are primitive reflexes. As myelinization develops and the number of brain neurons grows rapidly, from the 30th week of gestation through the first year of life, voluntary control and advanced cerebral functions appear and the more primitive reflexes diminish or disappear. The nervous system grows rapidly during fetal and early postnatal life, reaching 25% of adult capacity at birth, 50% by age 1 year, 80% by age 3, and 90% by age 7.

Newborns have rudimentary sensation. Any stimulus must be strong to cause a reaction, and the response is not localized. A strong stimulus causes a vigorous response of crying with whole-body movements. As myelinization develops, stimulus localization becomes possible and the child responds in a more localized manner. Motor control develops in a head-to-neck to trunk-to-extremities sequence.

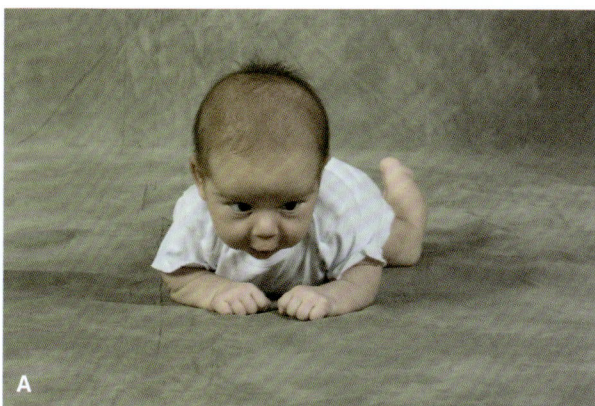
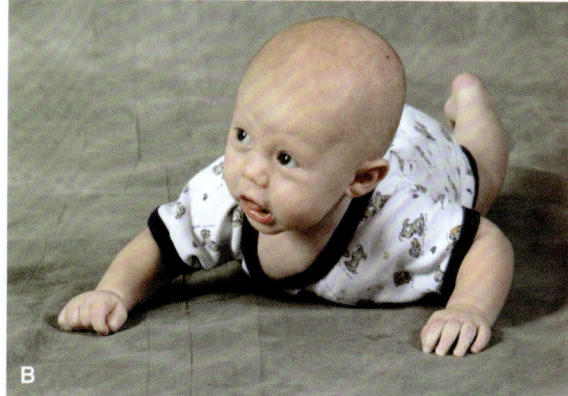
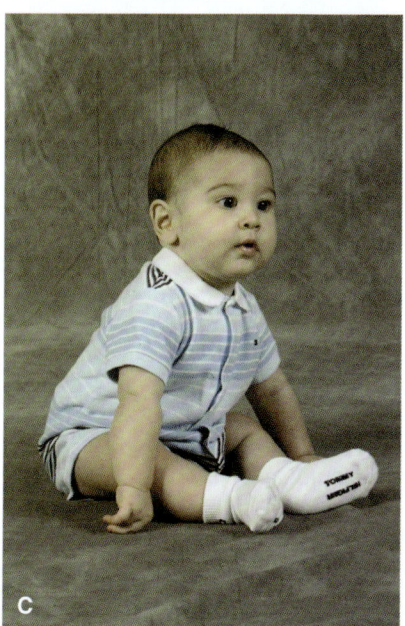
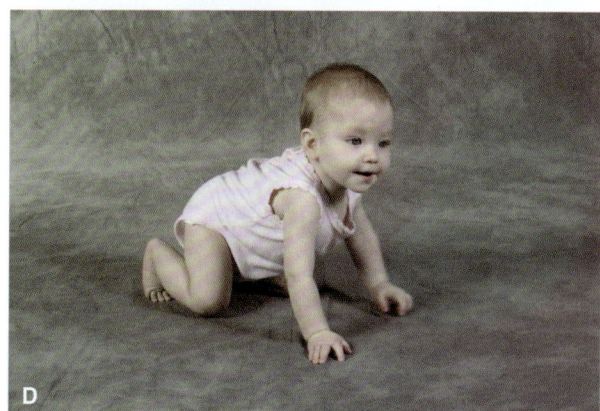
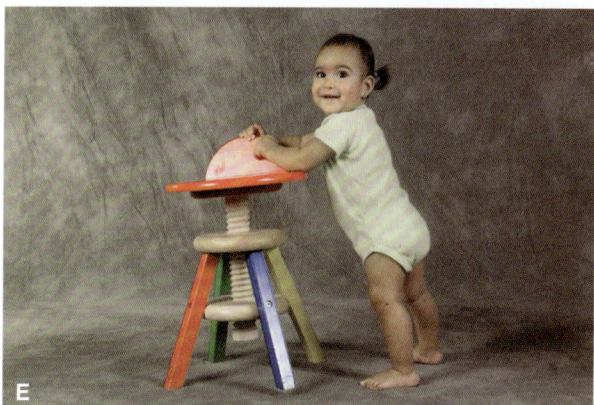

FIGURE 30-2 Growth and development of the infant. **A.** At 4 weeks, this infant turns the head when lying in a prone position. **B.** At 12 weeks, this infant pushes up from a prone position. **C.** At 21 weeks, this infant sits up but tilts forward for balance. **D.** At 30 weeks, this infant is crawling around and on the go. **E.** At 43 weeks, this infant is getting ready to walk.

Motor Development

Gross Motor

Newborns can turn their heads from side to side when prone unless they are lying on a soft surface. This inability to turn their head while lying on a soft surface makes suffocation a real concern. By 3 to 4 months, there is almost no head lag and the infant may push up to prone position. Infants roll from front to back at 5 months and sit unsupported by 6 to 7 months. They pull to stand by 9 months, cruise by 10 months, and walk when hand held by 12 months. Figure 30-2 displays gross motor development of the infant.

Fine Motor

The grasp reflex is present at birth and strengthens at 1 month. This reflex fades at 3 months, at which time an infant can actively hold a rattle. Five-month-old infants can grasp voluntarily, and 7-month-old infants can hand-to-hand transfer. The pincer grasp develops by 9 months, and 12-month-old infants will attempt to build a two-block tower (Fig. 30-3).

Sensory Perception Development

Visual

The newborn's visual impressions are unfocused, and the ability to distinguish between colors is not developed until approximately 8 months of age. Therefore, stimuli should be bright, simple, moving, and, preferably black and white (e.g., a mobile that consists of black-and-white circles and cubes).

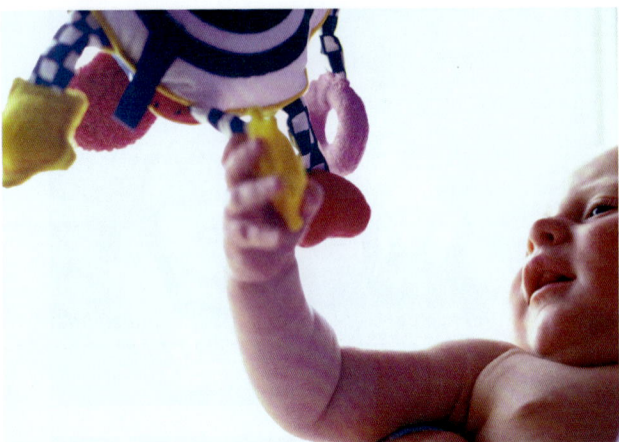

FIGURE 30-3 Development of the pincer grasp. (Used with permission from T. Kyle & S. Carman, *Essentials of pediatric nursing* (2nd ed.). Philadelphia, PA: Lippincott Williams & Wilkins, p. 77.)

Auditory

Newborns can distinguish sounds and turn toward voices and other noises. They may be very familiar with their mother's voice, and other sounds gradually gain significance when associated with pleasure. Infants normally attend to the human voice. Therefore, question parents as to whether their child turns his or her head toward the spoken voice or loud noises.

Olfactory

Smell is fully developed at birth, and newborns can differentiate the smell of their mother's milk and parents' body odors.

Tactile

Touch is well developed at birth, especially the lips and tongue. Touch should be used frequently because infants enjoy rocking, warmth, and cuddling.

Cognitive and Language Development (Piaget) (see Chapter 7 for in-depth discussion and references)

The sensorimotor stage, from birth to around 18 months, involves the development of intellect and knowledge of the environment gained through the senses. During this stage, development progresses from reflexive activity to purposeful acts. At the completion of this stage, the infant achieves a sense of object permanence (retains a mental image of an absent object; sees self as separate from others). An emerging sense of body image parallels sensorimotor development.

Crying is the first means of communication, and parents can usually differentiate cries. Cooing begins by 1 to 2 months, laughing and babbling by 3 to 4 months, and consonant sounds by 3 to 4 months. The infant begins to imitate sounds by 6 months. Combined syllables ("mama") are vocalized by 8 months, and the infant understands "no-no" by 9 months. "Mama" and "dada" are said with meaning by 10 months, and the infant says a total of 2 to 4 words with meaning by 12 months.

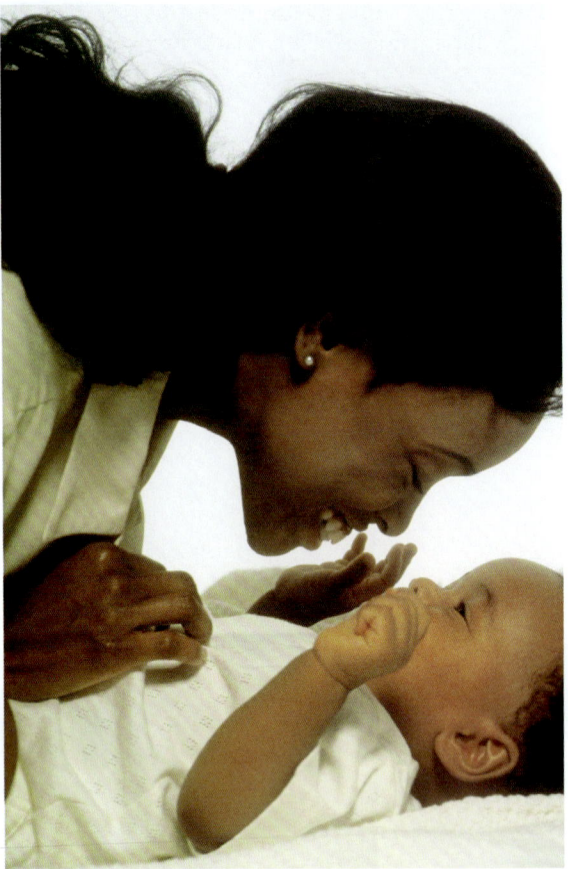

FIGURE 30-4 The infant–caregiver relationship fosters trust.

Moral Development (Kohlberg) (see Chapter 7 for in-depth discussion and references)

Although Kohlberg's theory of moral development begins with toddlerhood, infants cannot be overlooked. Child moral development begins with the value and belief system of the parents and the infant's own development of trust. Parental discipline patterns may start with the young infant in the form of interventions for crying behaviors. Stern discipline and withholding love and affection may affect infant moral development. Love and affection are the building blocks of an infant's developing sense of trust (Fig. 30-4).

Psychosocial Development (Erikson) (for more comprehensive discussions and references, see Chapter 7)

The crisis faced by an infant (birth to 1 year) is termed *trust versus mistrust*. In this stage, the infant's significant other is the "caretaking" person. Developing a sense of trust in caregivers and the environment is a central focus for an infant. This sense of trust forms the foundation for all future psychosocial tasks. The quality of the caregiver–child relationship is a crucial factor in the infant's development of trust. An infant who receives attentive care learns that life is predictable and that his or her needs will be met promptly; this fosters trust. In contrast, an infant experiencing consistently delayed needs gratification develops a sense of uncertainty, leading to mistrust of caregivers and the environment. An infant commonly seeks comfort from a security blanket or other object such as a favorite stuffed animal.

Psychosexual Development (Freud) (see Chapter 7 for in-depth discussion and references)

In the *oral stage* of development, from birth to 18 months, the erogenous zone is the mouth, and sexual activity takes the form of sucking, swallowing, chewing, and biting. In this stage, the infant meets the world by crying, tasting, eating, and early vocalization; biting, to gain a sense of having a hold on and having greater control of the environment; and grasping and touching, to explore texture variations in the environment.

Normal Infant Nutritional Requirements

Breast milk is the most desirable complete food for the first 6 months of a child's life. However, commercially prepared, iron-fortified formula is an acceptable alternative. Formula intake varies per infant. Most infants take 100-cal/kg body weight/day. This amount of formula should be offered to the infant every 3 to 4 hours, approximately four to six times a day.

Solids are not recommended before 4 months of age due to the presence of the protrusion or sucking reflexes and the immaturity of the gastrointestinal tract and the immune system. Key behaviors that indicate the infant is ready before introducing solid foods are: Baby is able to hold the head in an upright position, able to sit without support, is mouthing hands or toys, appears interested in what the parent is eating (Mayo Clinic, 2016). For most infants, it does not matter what the first solid foods are, but Mayo Clinic provides some guidelines to consider. First, start simple with single-ingredient foods that contain no salt or sugar. Offer the chosen food for 3 to 5 days to see if diarrhea occurs. If tolerated well, another simple food can be added. Next begin adding fruits and vegetables one at a time. By 8 to 10 months, finely chopped finger foods can be added. Essential ingredients that must be added by 4 months are iron and zinc, which are found in pureed meats and single-grain iron-fortified cereal (cultural variation using beans and lentils is also acceptable) (see Mayo Clinic, 2016, for further details). Verify with a health care provider the recommended iron supplementation for the infant. This is based on prematurity, term, and whether the infant is breastfed or formula-fed (with variations depending on the formula).

For exclusively breastfed infants, the American Academy of Pediatrics (AAP) recommended in 2008 a daily intake of vitamin D of 400 IU/day for all infants and children beginning in the first few days of life (reported and supported by Centers for Disease Control and Prevention [CDC], 2015). Human milk typically contains a vitamin D concentration of 25 IU per liter or less. Therefore, a supplement of 400 IU per day of vitamin D meets the requirement for all breastfed infants.

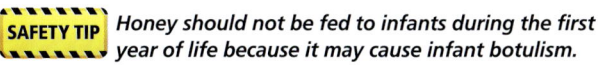 *Honey should not be fed to infants during the first year of life because it may cause infant botulism.*

Normal Infant Sleep Requirements and Patterns

Sleep patterns vary among infants. During the first month, most infants sleep when not eating. By 3 to 4 months, most infants sleep 9 to 11 hours at night. By 12 months, most infants take morning and afternoon naps. Bedtime rituals should begin in infancy to prepare the infant for sleep and prevent future sleep problems.

SAFETY TIP *Because of the possibility of SIDS (sudden infant death syndrome), caution parents to place their young infants to sleep in the supine or side-lying position.*

HEALTH ASSESSMENT

Collecting Subjective Data: The Nursing Health History for the Infant

[Note that the initial assessment of a neonate takes place at birth and does not include subjective data. The neonate assessment is placed after this section on collecting subjective data to provide consistency for the physical assessment of both the neonate and the infant.]

Interviewing Parents

The initial assessment of the newborn occurs immediately after delivery. Therefore, parent interviewing is not performed. However, the nurse needs to get a complete history of the mother before and during pregnancy. Delivery record information is also imperative for the initial newborn assessment. This information is usually obtained from the maternal hospital chart.

For subsequent infant assessments, the nurse interviews the parent(s).

Use a friendly, nonjudgmental approach when interviewing the family. Portray proficiency and competence when talking with the parents. Explain the purpose of the interview and clarify any misunderstandings during this time. Explain the importance of getting accurate information about the infant to ensure that the correct diagnosis and treatment are provided for the infant. Realize that common behaviors of the family may not be portrayed at this setting. The unfamiliar setting and concerns for the infant, especially if the infant is ill, may cause the parents to be very nervous and anxious during the interview. Providing a safe, relaxed environment will help the parents to be calm and be able to answer questions accurately.

Cultural variations may also exist with the family. The nurse should provide a nonjudgmental environment, using active listening skills and providing empathy as appropriate.

Be aware of barriers to effective nurse–parent communication. These include time constraints, frequent interruptions, lack of privacy, and language differences as well as provider callousness and cultural insensitivity. Make every effort to prevent these barriers. Providing enough time for the interview, keeping interruptions to a minimum, maintaining client privacy, and using interpreters when language barriers exist will help with obtaining accurate information regarding the infant's history.

Biographical Data

QUESTION	RATIONALE
What is the infant's name? Nickname? What are the parents' or caregivers' names?	Knowing personal information about the infant and caregivers helps to establish rapport with the infant and family.
Who is the infant's primary health care provider, and when was the infant's last well-child care appointment?	This determines the infant's access to health care. It tells the nurse where to find the client's previous medical information/record.
Where does the infant live? (address)	In addition, assess the family's living conditions.
Do the parents and infant live in the same residence? Are the infant's parents married, single, divorced, LGBTQ (lesbian, gay, bisexual, transgender, queer, and/or questioning)? Who else lives in this residence? What are the parents' ages?	This indicates the availability of potential caregivers and support people for the infant. It also helps to define familial relationships.
What is the infant's age? What is the infant's date of birth?	This provides a reference for assessing the infant's developmental level.
Is the infant adopted, foster, or natural?	Certain health problems run in families. It is helpful to know the infant's genetic relationship with the parents.
What is the infant's ethnic origin? Religion?	This information helps the nurse to examine special needs and beliefs that may affect the infant's or family's health care.
What do the infant's parents do for a living?	This provides insight into the economic status of the family.

History of Present Health Concern

Elicit the reason for seeking care and ask questions about the infant's current health status.

QUESTION	RATIONALE
Describe the infant's general state of health. Does the infant have a chronic illness (cystic fibrosis, Down syndrome, sickle cell, congenital heart disease, PKU, G6PD, etc.)?	Obtaining baseline information about the infant helps to identify important areas of assessment.

Personal Health History

QUESTION	RATIONALE
Ask about the mother's pregnancy: Was the pregnancy planned? How did you feel when you found out you were pregnant?	The caregiver's answer may provide insight into her feelings about the infant. Negative feelings about the pregnancy may or may not lead to difficulty attaching emotionally to the newborn and affect the psychological and behavioral functioning of the infant (The Royal College of Midwives, 2012).
When did you first receive prenatal care? How was your general health during pregnancy?	Prenatal information helps to identify potential health problems for the infant.
Did you have any problems with your pregnancy?	Reviewing the prenatal history will help the nurse to assess for possible complications for the infant after delivery. An example would include a mother who develops gestational diabetes during pregnancy. Infants born to mothers with gestational diabetes are at higher risk for having unstable blood glucose levels after delivery.
Did you have any accidents during this pregnancy?	Prenatal trauma (motor vehicle accidents, domestic violence) can increase the risk of complications for the fetus/newborn.
Did you take any medications during pregnancy?	Certain medications should not be taken during pregnancy and may be teratogenic (harmful to the infant).
Did you use any tobacco, alcohol, or drugs during this pregnancy?	Smoking, alcohol, and drug use may cause complications or anomalies in the fetus.

QUESTION	RATIONALE
Ask about delivery of the newborn: Do you have information on the duration of labor, PROM, GBS status, Rhogam, late decellerations, artificial ROM, induction, meconium, shoulder dystocia, LGA, hip dysplasia, etc?	Delivery details and complications are pertinent for assessing fetal injury and potential risk for infection.
Where was the infant born (hospital, home, with or without a midwife or other care provider)? What type of delivery did you have? Any anesthesia? Type? Complications?	Information regarding the delivery of the infant provides information relative to the initial newborn assessment/evaluation and follow-up that might be needed. Infants born via cesarean section are at higher risk for having respiratory problems.
Were there any problems during the delivery? Did you have any vaginal infections at time of delivery?	Complications at delivery may predispose the infant to complications after birth. Long labors, prolonged rupture of membranes, and undiagnosed vaginal infections predispose the infant to sepsis.
What was the infant's Apgar score at 1 and 5 minutes?	Knowing the Apgar score helps to identify the infant's respiratory/cardiac status immediately after delivery and prepare for potential respiratory/cardiac complications after birth.
What were the infant's weight, length, and head circumference? Did the infant have any problems after birth (e.g., feeding, jaundice)?	Documentation of the infant's weight, length, and head circumference are documented at birth. These components are monitored to assess for adequate nutrition and growth at regular intervals. Documentation of problems following delivery should be reassessed to verify that the condition has resolved for normal growth and development.
Ask about past illnesses or injuries: Has the infant ever been hospitalized? Has the infant ever had any major illnesses?	Previous illnesses and hospitalizations may affect the present examination.
What immunizations has the infant received thus far? Has your infant had any reactions to immunizations?	This helps identify risk for infection and/or potential reactions to immunizations.
Does the infant have any allergies? If so, what is the specific allergen? How does the infant react to it?	This identifies allergens and helps the nurse plan to prevent exposure.
What prescriptions, over-the-counter medications, devices, treatments, and home or folk remedies is the infant taking? Please provide the name of the drug, dosage, frequency, and reason it is administered.	It is always important to know what treatments or medications are being used for an infant. If there are potential side effects or adverse effects associated with the medication or practice, these can be explored with the parents.

Family History

QUESTION	RATIONALE
Please list any chronic health conditions in the family.	Certain conditions tend to run in families and increase the infant's risk for such conditions.
Genogram: two generations.	This helps to identify risk factors.
Does the infant have family members with communicable diseases?	This also helps to identify risk factors.

Lifestyle and Health Practices

QUESTION	RATIONALE
Is the infant being breast or bottle fed? What foods and fluids does the infant eat or drink?	Feeding patterns help the nurse to assess nutrition and gastrointestinal function.
What are the infant's sleep patterns?	Sleep patterns vary, according to the infant's age.
In what position does the infant sleep?	Due to the risk of sudden infant death syndrome (SIDS), it is recommended to lay the infant in the supine or side-lying position.

Continued on following page

Review of Systems

QUESTION	RATIONALE
Skin, Hair, Nails	
Has your infant had any changes in hair texture?	Changes may indicate an underlying problem. However, hair at birth may be lost as the female hormones transmitted via the placenta are reduced.
Does your infant exhibit scaling on the scalp?	Cradle cap is a common problem.
Has your infant been exposed to any contagious disease such as measles, chickenpox, lice, ringworm, scabies, and the like?	This helps to identify risks for health problems.
Has your infant ever had any rashes or sores? Does your infant have diaper rash? If so, how is this being treated?	Diaper rash is a common finding in infants. Knowing the treatment can help with assessment of safe versus unsafe approaches.
Has your infant had any excessive bruising or burns?	This helps to assess for child abuse. Excessive bruising or burns suggest abuse.
Does your infant have any birthmarks?	Birthmarks are normal findings. Mongolian spots may be confused with birthmarks by parents or caregivers, or with abuse if the caregiver is not familiar with these as normal variations.
Head and Neck	
Has your infant ever had a head injury?	Head injuries may cause neurologic problems.
Did the fontanelles close on schedule? Does the infant have head control? If so, at what age did this occur?	These questions assess normal growth and development.
Eyes and Vision	
Does your infant have any unusual eye movements? Does your infant excessively cross eyes?	This helps to determine eye and vision development.
Does your infant blink when necessary?	Absent blinking is abnormal in newborns. If the newborn does not blink when shown a bright light by 2–4 weeks, then the newborn should be referred for evaluation by a health care provider for newborns (On Track, n.d.).
Is your infant able to focus on moving objects?	By 1 month, the infant should be able to follow a moving object or light.
Does the infant's pupil appear cloudy?	Cloudiness of the eyeball may indicate the presence of cataracts.
Ears and Hearing	
Does your infant turn his/her head to the human voice? (Infants should respond to the human voice.) Does the infant respond to loud noise?	Infants who do not respond to the human voice or loud voices may have a hearing loss.
Has your infant had frequent ear infections? Tubes in ears?	Frequent otitis media is a risk factor for hearing loss.
Does anyone in the infant's home smoke?	Smoking increases the risk of otitis media.
Mouth, Throat, Nose, and Sinuses	
Does your infant have any teeth?	No teeth by age one is a variation of normal.
Does your infant attend day care?	Attending day care increases risk of upper respiratory infections (through exposure to other children).
Thorax and Lungs	
Has your infant ever had cough, wheezing, shortness of breath, grunting, nasal flaring, chest retractions during the day, at night or during feedings? If so, when does it occur? Has your infant had frequent or severe colds?	Positive answers to any of these questions may indicate respiratory disorders.

QUESTION	RATIONALE
Heart and Neck Vessels	
Does your infant become fatigued or short of breath during feedings?	Infants who fatigue easily with feedings may have a congenital heart defect or disorder, cystic fibrosis, or Down syndrome.
Peripheral Vascular System	
Does your infant ever experience bluing of the extremities? Does your infant ever experience bluing of the skin, lips, and/or nail beds?	Acrocyanosis, blue discoloration of the extremities, is a common, benign finding in newborns (especially after delivery) and resolves with increasing body temperature.
	Cyanosis, bluing of the skin, lips, and/or nail beds (especially after crying or eating), is an abnormal finding. Cyanosis may be seen in newborns with cardiac defects.
Abdomen	
Are you breast- or bottle-feeding? What foods does the infant eat? Do you prop the infant's bottle? Do you put the infant to bed with a bottle?	Feeding patterns help the nurse to assess nutrition and gastrointestinal function. Infants should not have bottles propped or be put to bed with a bottle.
Has your infant ever had any vomiting?	Excessive vomiting may indicate neurologic disorder.
Has your infant exhibited symptoms of abdominal pain (drawing knees to chest, excessive, inconsolable crying, cries when eating, or cries excessively when having a bowel movement/urination)? Please describe.	Exhibiting symptoms of pain may indicate problems with gastrointestinal system.
Genitalia	
How often does your infant urinate? How many wet diapers do you change per day?	The caregiver's answer helps the nurse to assess the genitourinary system.
Is the infant prone to frequent diaper rash?	Diaper rash (irritant contact dermatitis) is common in infants.
What do you do to reduce the rash if present?	Knowing the approach the caregiver takes to diaper rash helps to evaluate the efficacy and safety of the approach.
Anus and Rectum	
How often does your infant have bowel movements? What does it look like?	These questions help to assess gastrointestinal function.
Is there any history of bleeding, constipation, diarrhea, or hemorrhoids?	Constipation and diarrhea may occur due to diet. Evaluate the infant's dietary intake and teach the caregiver any necessary changes to control the problem. Other causes for constipation and diarrhea may be infection, obstruction, or other abnormalities of the gastrointestinal tract. Bleeding and hemorrhoids are not normal in the infant. This may indicate a problem with the gastrointestinal tract.
Musculoskeletal System	
Has your infant ever had limited range of motion (ROM), joint pain, stiffness, paralysis?	These questions assess musculoskeletal development.
Has your infant ever had any fractures? Have you noticed any bone deformities?	Frequent fractures may indicate child abuse or osteomalacia.
Neurologic System	
Has your infant ever had a seizure?	Seizures indicate a neurologic or other systemic disorder.
Has your infant ever experienced any problems with motor coordination?	If the infant is not meeting developmental landmarks, it may indicate an underlying problem.

CASE STUDY

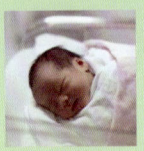

The nurse interviews Kaitlin's mother using specific probing questions. Kaitlin's mother reports her concern about the increasing yellowing of Kaitlin's skin over the last 2 days since discharge at 36 hours from birth. The nurse explores the mother's concerns regarding Kaitlin's health using the COLDSPA mnemonic.

Mnemonic	Question	Data Provided
Character	Describe the sign or symptom (feeling, appearance, sound, smell, or taste if applicable). Describe the color of the skin.	"Faint, yellow discoloration of her skin."
Onset	When did it begin?	"Two days ago, when we were discharged from the hospital."
Location	Where is it? Does it radiate? Does it occur anywhere else?	"Feet, legs, abdomen and chest."
Duration	How long does it last? Does it recur?	"Yellow discoloration is constant and progressing up her body."
Severity	How bad is it? Or How much does it bother you?	"I am very concerned about her color because this same thing happened to my sister's son and he ended up in the hospital."
Pattern	What makes it better or worse?	"Nothing changes the color. It seems to be getting more yellow each day."
Associated factors/How it Affects the client	What other symptoms occur with it? How does it affect you?	"I am worried about the color because I was told it would improve after 2–3 days. It seems to be getting worse instead of better."

After investigating the mother's reports of Kaitlin's jaundice, the nurse continues with the health history. Kaitlin's mother is a 28-year-old, gravida 1, para 1, with an unremarkable medical history. She and her husband had been trying to conceive for approximately 6 months, so they were thrilled to find out they were expecting a baby. She began her prenatal care at approximately 6 weeks' gestation. She had a healthy pregnancy.

Initially she experienced some nausea and vomiting, but this resolved after 6 weeks into the pregnancy. The only medications taken during her pregnancy were prenatal vitamins and an occasional Tylenol for headaches. No tobacco or alcohol was consumed during the pregnancy.

Kaitlin was delivered at term, 39 weeks' gestation, via vaginal forceps delivery. Kaitlin weighed 8 lb 10 oz, was 21 in long, and was AGA. Her Apgar scores were 9 and 9. She was a healthy newborn baby. However, the day of discharge her skin began to turn slightly yellow. The only other feature that is remarkable is the cephalohematoma on the right side of her scalp that is still resolving.

Family history is remarkable for her maternal side of the family and includes hypertension, glaucoma, hypothyroidism, and stroke. Paternal family history is positive for hypertension, early myocardial infarction of grandfather (at 50 years old), glaucoma, and kidney stones. All close family relatives are alive and well, with no one having any communicable diseases at this time.

The review of systems for Kaitlin is positive for her skin color turning yellow on the 2nd day of life, sclerae still white. She has a cephalohematoma on the right side of her scalp, approximately 2 cm in diameter, which her mother says is getting smaller. She has not been taken out of the house since she has been home; therefore, there is not any known exposure to communicable disease or other infections.

She startles easily by jerking her body and blinking when she hears a loud noise. She is breastfeeding every 3–4 hours and having approximately 8–10 wet/stool diapers a day. When not eating, she is usually sleeping. Kaitlin moves all extremities well and expresses a lusty cry when she is hungry. She is easily consoled when held and fed. Her motor skills are appropriate for a 4-day-old infant.

Collecting Objective Data: Physical Examination

The purpose of the newborn/infant examination is to identify normal physiologic and developmental changes of the newborn/infant. Performing a head-to-toe physical examination of the infant can accomplish this. Early detection of changes or problems in the newborn/infant is important for early diagnosis and treatment.

Preparing the Infant and Caregiver

Make sure that the caregiver understands the examination process. The infant should be fully unclothed, lying in a basinet or tabletop and never left unattended. A blanket will be used to cover the infant to prevent cooling. Explain to the caregiver that each body system will be uncovered as examined to prevent cooling of the infant. A complete head-to-toe examination will be performed.

For the complete infant physical assessment, advise the caregiver that the heart, lungs, and abdomen will be auscultated/percussed. Skin will be evaluated for color, birthmarks, and rash. Head, weight, and length will be measured for growth. The eyes, ears, nose, throat, and genitalia will also be inspected. Reflexes will be evaluated by performing appropriate tests. Explain that the Denver Development Examination will be performed to assess normal developmental milestones. Encourage the caregiver to ask questions during the examination.

Equipment

- Denver Development Kit
- Measuring tape
- Ophthalmoscope
- Otoscope
- Scale
- Stethoscope
- Thermometer

Physical Assessment

At birth, the newborn will undergo an *initial physical assessment*. This special assessment is performed to evaluate:

- Apgar score
- Vital signs
- Measurements
- Gestational age
- Newborn reflexes

These assessments are performed in order to evaluate the newborn's transition from intrauterine to extrauterine life and to detect any health concerns that may require prompt intervention. The initial assessment is performed immediately after birth, while the infant is supine and under a radiant warmer.

Subsequent physical assessments of the infant are performed using the following guide. Physical assessment of the infant is a complete head-to-toe examination that also includes developmental screening.

General Routine Screening versus Focused Specialty Assessment of the Newborn

General Routine Screening
- Test distant visual acuity.
- Test near visual acuity.
- Test visual fields for gross peripheral vision.
- Inspect the eyelids and eyelashes.
- Observe the position and alignment of the eyeball in the eye socket.
- Inspect the bulbar conjunctiva and sclera.
- Inspect the lacrimal apparatus.
- Inspect the iris and pupil.
- Test pupillary reaction to light.

Focused Specialty Assessment
- Perform corneal light reflex test.
- Perform cover test.
- Perform the cardinal fields of gaze test.
- Inspect the palpebral conjunctiva.
- Palpate the lacrimal apparatus.
- Inspect the cornea and lens.
- Test accommodation of pupils.
- Use opthalmoscope to inspect the optic disc, retinal vessels and background, fovea and macula, and anterior chamber.

INITIAL NEWBORN ASSESSMENT

Assessment Procedure	Normal Findings	Abnormal Findings
APGAR SCORE		
Assign Apgar scores at 1 and at 5 minutes after delivery. The Apgar score is an assessment of the infant's ability to adapt to extrauterine life. Assess the following:	The score is 8–10. See Table 30-1 for Apgar scoring.	A score of less than 8 may indicate poor transition from intrauterine to extrauterine life.
Auscultate apical pulse.	The pulse is greater than 100 bpm.	Pulse is less than 100 bpm, indicating bradycardia. Absent heartbeat indicates fetal demise.

TABLE 30-1 Apgar Scoring

	Scores 0	Scores 1	Scores 2
Heart rate	Absent	<100 bpm	>100 bpm
Respiratory rate	Absent	Slow, irregular	Good, lusty cry
Reflex irritability	No response	Grimace, some motion	Cry, cough
Muscle tone	Flaccid, limp	Flexion of extremities	Active flexion
Color	Cyanotic, pale	Pink body, acrocyanosis	Pink body, pink extremities

Inspect chest and abdomen for respiratory effort.	The newborn is crying.	The newborn has absent, slow, or irregular respirations.

Continued on following page

INITIAL NEWBORN ASSESSMENT (Continued)

Assessment Procedure	Normal Findings	Abnormal Findings
Stroke back or soles of feet.	Crying	Delayed neurologic function may be seen in grimace, no response.
Inspect muscle tone by extending legs and arms. Observe degree of flexion and resistance in extremities.	The extremities are flexed, and you note active movement.	Delayed neurologic function may be seen in grimace or no response.
Inspect body and extremities for skin color.	The full body should be pink, but acrocyanosis is common in newborns whether preterm or full term.	The newborn is cyanotic, pale.

VITAL SIGNS

Monitor axillary temperature (Fig. 30-5).	Temperature is 97.5–99°F (36.4–37.2°C).	A temperature of less than 97.5°F (36.4°C) indicates hypothermia, which may suggest sepsis. A temperature of greater than 99°F (37.2°C) indicates hyperthermia, which may indicate infection or improper monitoring of temperature probe.

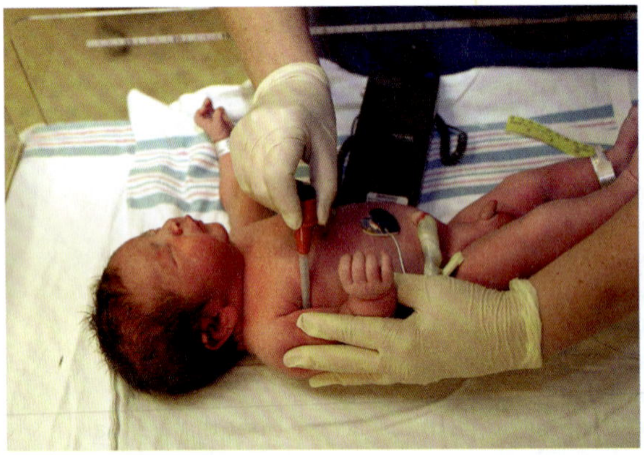

FIGURE 30-5 Measuring the newborn's axillary temperature.

Inspect and auscultate lung sounds.	Breathing is easy and nonlabored. The lungs are clear bilaterally.	Abnormal findings include labored breathing, nasal flaring, rhonchi, rales, retractions, or grunting.
Monitor respiratory rate.	Rate is 30–53 breaths/min (PedsCases, 2016).	A rate less than 30 or greater than 60 breaths/min is seen with respiratory distress.
Auscultate apical pulse.	Pulse is regular and within a range of 120–140 beats/min while at rest. The rate may rise to 180 beats/min when crying or fall to 100 beats/min when sleeping.	An irregular pulse or a rate above 180 beats/min while crying or below 100 beats/min while sleeping may indicate cardiac abnormalities.

MEASUREMENTS

Weigh the newborn using a newborn scale (Fig. 30-6). The child should be unclothed.	The newborn weighs between 2,500 and 4,000 g.	Weight is less than 2,500 g or greater than 4,000 g.
Measure length (Fig. 30-7).	The newborn is 44–55 cm.	Length is less than 44 or greater than 55 cm.

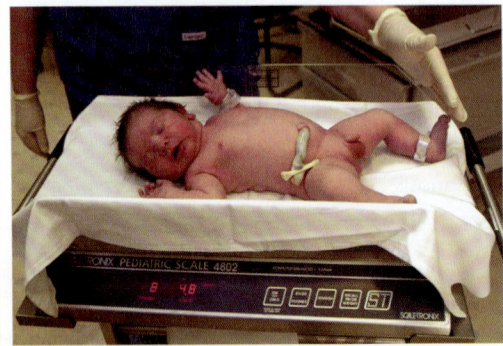

FIGURE 30-6 Weighing the newborn.

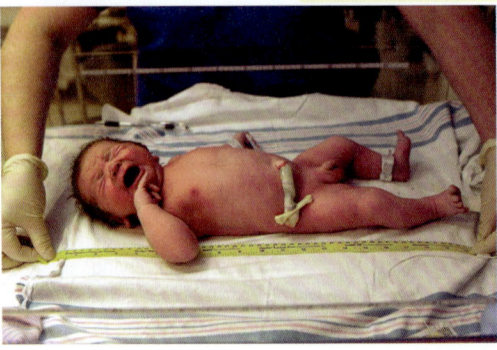

FIGURE 30-7 Measuring the length of the newborn.

Assessment Procedure	Normal Findings	Abnormal Findings
Measure head circumference (Fig. 30-8). (See instructions under Subsequent Assessment.)	Circumference is 33–35.5 cm.	Circumference is less than 33 cm or greater than 35.5 cm. This may indicate microcephaly, improper brain growth, premature closing of the sutures, intrauterine infection, or chromosomal defect.

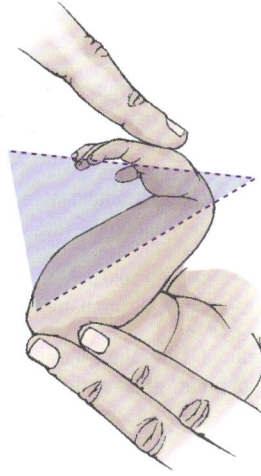

FIGURE 30-8 Measuring the circumference of an infant's head (© B. Proud).

Assessment Procedure	Normal Findings	Abnormal Findings
Measure chest circumference. Place tape measure at nipple line and wrap around infant.	Circumference is 30–33 cm (1–2 cm less than head).	Circumference is less than 29 cm or greater than 34 cm.

GESTATIONAL AGE

Assess gestational age within 4 hours after birth to identify any potential age-related problems that may occur within the next few hours. This examination requires assessing the newborn's neuromuscular and physical maturity. Use the Ballard Scale to rate.

Assessment Procedure	Normal Findings	Abnormal Findings
To assess neuromuscular maturity (with the newborn in supine position):		
Inspect posture (with the newborn undisturbed).	Arms and legs are flexed.	In premature children, the newborn's arms and legs may be limp and extend away from the body.
Assess for square window sign. Bend the wrist toward the ventral forearm until resistance is met. Measure angle.	Angle is 0–30 degrees (Fig. 30-9A).	Premature newborns may have a square window measurement of less than 30 degrees (Fig. 30-9B).

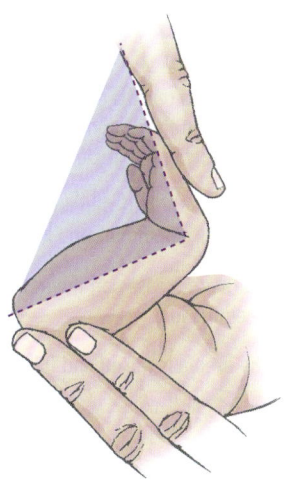

A B

FIGURE 30-9 Square window sign: (A) term infant; (B) preterm infant.

Continued on following page

INITIAL NEWBORN ASSESSMENT (Continued)

Assessment Procedure	Normal Findings	Abnormal Findings
Test arm recoil. Bilaterally flex elbows up.	Elbow angle is less than 90 degrees and the arm rapidly recoils to a flexed state.	In premature children, elbow angle may be greater than 110 degrees and delayed recoil may be seen.
Assess popliteal angle. Flex the thigh on top of the abdomen; push behind the ankle and extend the lower leg up towards the head until resistance is met. Measure the angle behind the knee.	The angle should be less than 100 degrees.	Premature children may have a popliteal angle of greater than 100 degrees.
Assess for Scarf sign. Lift the arm across the chest toward the opposite shoulder until resistance is met; note location of the elbow in relation to midline of the chest.	Elbow position is less than midline of the chest (Fig. 30-10A).	In premature children, elbow position is at midline of the chest or greater (toward opposite shoulder; Fig. 30-10B).

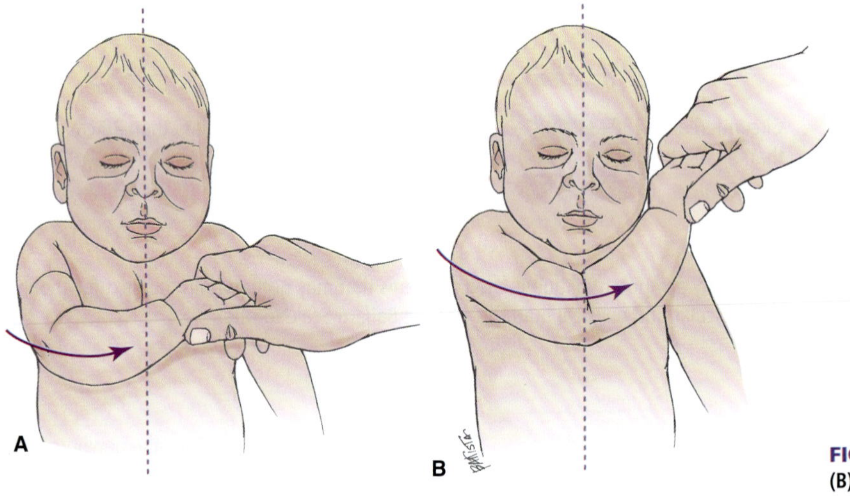

FIGURE 30-10 Scarf sign: **(A)** term infant; **(B)** preterm infant.

Assessment Procedure	Normal Findings	Abnormal Findings
Perform heel-to-ear test. Keeping buttocks flat on the bed, pull leg toward the ear on the same side of the body; inspect popliteal angle and proximity of the heel to the ear.	Popliteal angle is less than 90 degrees; the heel is distal from the ear.	In premature infants, popliteal angle may be greater than 90 degrees, and the heel may be proximal to the ear.

To assess for physical maturity:

Assessment Procedure	Normal Findings	Abnormal Findings
Inspect the skin.	Inspection reveals parchment, few or no vessels on the abdomen, and crackling, especially in the ankle area.	Inspection reveals translucent, visible veins; rash; leathery, wrinkled skin that is seen in most postmature children.
Inspect for lanugo.	Normally there is thinning and balding on the back, shoulders, and knees.	In premature children, abundant amounts of fine hair may be seen on the face.
Inspect the plantar surface of the feet for creases.	There are creases on the anterior two thirds or entire sole.	Transverse crease on sole only, no creases, or fewer creases indicate prematurity.
Inspect and palpate breast bud tissue with the middle finger and forefinger; measure bud in millimeters.	The areola is raised and full.	In premature infants, there may be an absence of breast tissue and a bud less than 3 mm.
Observe ear cartilage in the upper pinna for curving. Fold the pinna down toward the side of the head and release; note recoil of the ear.	Normally you find a well-curved pinna, well-formed cartilage, and instant recoil.	With prematurity, you may find a slightly curved pinna and slow recoil.

Assessment Procedure	Normal Findings	Abnormal Findings
Inspect the genitals. *Male:* Assess scrotum for rugae and palpate position of testes. *Female:* Inspect labia majora, labia minora, and clitoris. **Determine score rating:** Use Figure 30-11. Mark the boxes that most closely represent each observation.	*Male:* There are deep rugae; testes are positioned down in scrotal sac. *Female:* The labia majora covers the labia minora and clitoris. Score totals 35–45.	*Male:* There is decreased presence of rugae; testes are positioned in upper inguinal canal. *Female:* In prematurity, the labia majora and labia minora are equally prominent and the clitoris is prominent. Score totals less than 35 or greater than 45.

NEUROMUSCULAR MATURITY

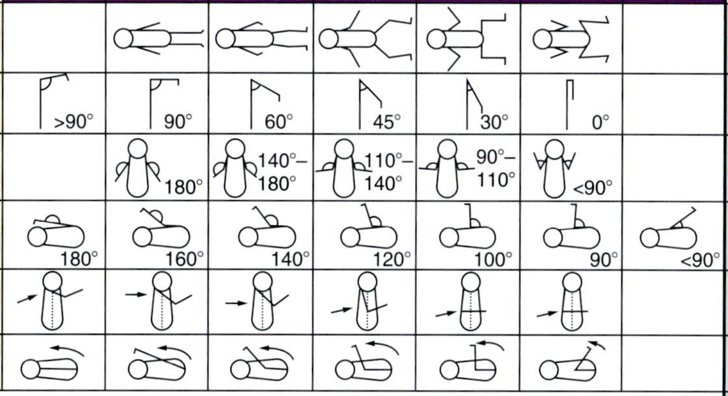

NEUROMUSCULAR MATURITY SIGN	SCORE −1	0	1	2	3	4	5	RECORD SCORE HERE
POSTURE								
SQUARE WINDOW (Wrist)	>90°	90°	60°	45°	30°	0°		
ARM RECOIL		180°	140°–180°	110°–140°	90°–110°	<90°		
POPLITEAL ANGLE	180°	160°	140°	120°	100°	90°	<90°	
SCARF SIGN								
HEEL TO EAR								
						TOTAL NEUROMUSCULAR MATURITY SCORE		

PHYSICAL MATURITY

PHYSICAL MATURITY SIGN	SCORE −1	0	1	2	3	4	5	RECORD SCORE HERE
SKIN	sticky, friable, transparent	gelatinous, red, translucent	smooth, pink, visible veins	superficial peeling and/or rash, few veins	cracking pale areas, rare veins	parchment, deep cracking, no vessels	leathery, cracked, wrinkled	
LANUGO	none	sparse	abundant	thinning	bald areas	mostly bald		
PLANTAR SURFACE	heel-toe 40–50 mm:−1 <40 mm:−2	>50 mm no crease	faint red marks	anterior transverse crease only	creases ant. 2/3	creases over entire sole		
BREAST	imperceptible	barely perceptible	flat areola no bud	stippled areola 1–2 mm bud	raised areola 3–4 mm bud	full areola 5–10 mm bud		
EYE-EAR	lids fused loosely: −1 tightly: −2	lids open pinna flat stays folded	sl. curved pinna; soft; slow recoil	well-curved pinna; soft but ready recoil	formed and firm instant recoil	thick cartilage, ear stiff		
GENITALS (Male)	scrotum flat, smooth	scrotum empty, faint rugae	testes in upper canal, rare rugae	testes descending, few rugae	testes down, good rugae	testes pendulous, deep rugae		
GENITALS (Female)	clitoris prominent and labia flat	prominent clitoris and small labia minora	prominent clitoris and enlarging minora	majora and minora equally prominent	majora large, minora small	majora cover clitoris and minora		
						TOTAL PHYSICAL MATURITY SCORE		

SCORE
Neuromuscular ____
Physical ____
Total ____

MATURITY RATING

Score	Weeks
−10	20
−5	22
0	24
5	26
10	28
15	30
20	32
25	34
30	36
35	38
40	40
45	42
50	44

GESTATIONAL AGE (weeks)
By dates ____
By ultrasound ____
By exam ____

FIGURE 30-11 New Ballard scale. Used to rate neuromuscular and physical maturity of gestational age.

NEWBORN REFLEXES

Assessment Procedure	Normal Findings	Abnormal Findings
Assess newborn reflexes. See Box 30-1 for techniques.	See Box 30-1.	See Box 30-1.

SUBSEQUENT INFANT PHYSICAL ASSESSMENT

Assessment Procedure	Normal Findings	Abnormal Findings
GENERAL APPEARANCE AND BEHAVIOR		
Observe general appearance. Observe hygiene. Note interaction with parents and yourself (and siblings if present). Note also facies (facial expressions) and posture.	Child appears stated age; is clean, has no unusual body odor, and clothing is in good condition and appropriate for climate. Child is alert, active, responds appropriately to stress of the situation. Child is appropriately interactive for age, seeks comfort from parent; appears happy. Newborn's arms and legs are in flexed position.	Note any facies that indicate acute illness, respiratory distress. Flaccidity or rigidity in newborn may be from neurologic damage, sepsis, or pain. Poor hygiene and clothes may indicate neglect, poverty. Infant does not appear stated age (mental retardation, abuse, neglect).
DEVELOPMENTAL ASSESSMENT		
Screen for cognitive, language, social, and gross and fine motor developmental delays in the beginning of the physical assessment in infants. Growth and development of the newborn/infant may be assessed using the Denver Developmental Screening Test (DDST; Assessment Tool 30-1). This test is used to guide the nurse to the appropriate developmental milestones for the child's gross motor, language, fine motor, and personal social development.	Infant meets normal parameters for age (see information contained in subjective data section) Gross and fine motor skills should be appropriate for the child's developmental age. Head control should be acquired by 4 months of age. Hand preference is developed during the preschool years.	Infant lags in earlier stages. Gross and fine motor skills that are inappropriate for developmental age and lack of head control by age 6 months may indicate cerebral palsy. Hand preference that is not developed during preschool years may indicate paresis on opposite side.
VITAL SIGNS		
Assess temperature. Use rectal, axillary, skin, or tympanic route when assessing the temperature of an infant. **The rectal temperature is most accurate.** To take a rectal temperature in a newborn, lay the child supine and lift lower legs up into the air, bending the legs at the hips. Insert lubricated rectal thermometer no more than 2 cm into rectum. Temperature registers in 3–5 minutes on a rectal thermometer. **Axillary and/or tympanic temperature may also be used.** For axillary temperature, place the thermometer under axilla, holding arm close to chest for approximately 3–5 minutes. For tympanic temperature, use digital tympanic thermometer as directed in manufacturer's instructions.	Temperature is 99.4°F (because of excess heat production).	Temperature may be altered by exercise, stress, crying, environment, diurnal variation (highest between 4 and 6 PM). Both hyperthermic and hypothermic conditions are noted in infants.
Note apical pulse rate. Count the pulse for a full minute (Fig. 30-12).	Awake and resting rates vary with the age of the child. For a newborn to 1-month-old child, it should be 120–160 beats/min. When crying, the heart rate may increase up to 180 beats/min. Rate decreases gradually with age. At 6 months to 1 year, rate is approximately 110 beats/min.	Pulse may be altered by medications, activity, and pain as well as pathologic conditions. Bradycardia (<100 beats/min) in an infant is usually an ominous finding. Tachycardia may also indicate cardiac/respiratory problems or sepsis.

Assessment Procedure	Normal Findings	Abnormal Findings

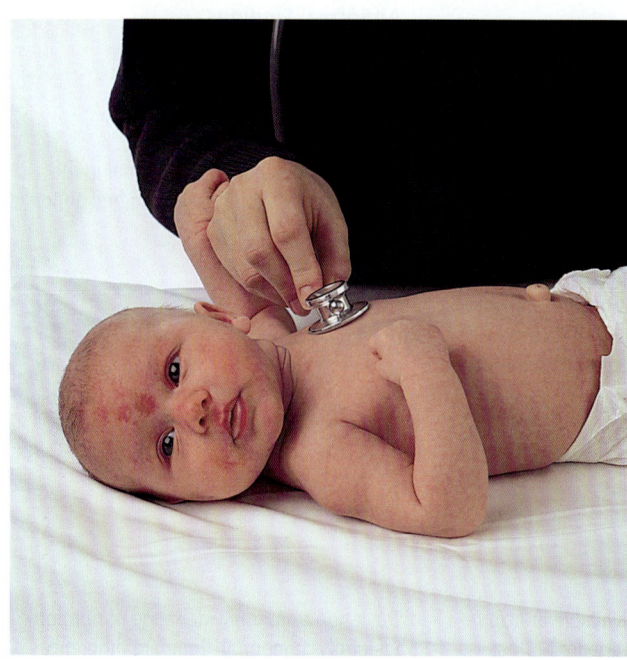

FIGURE 30-12 Auscultating apical pulse rate in the infant (© B. Proud).

Assess respiratory rate and character. Measure respiratory rate and character in infants by observing abdominal movements.

Neonates: Rate is 30–60 breaths/min.

Breathing is unlabored; lung sounds clear. Newborns are obligatory nose breathers.

Respiratory rate and character may be altered by medications, positioning, fever, and activity, as well as pathologic conditions. Retractions, see-saw respirations, apnea greater than 15 seconds, grunting, nasal flaring, stridor, rale, tachypnea greater than 60 breaths/min should be further evaluated for respiratory distress.

Evaluate infant blood pressure, if necessary.

Normal findings are specific to age and size and are included in Chapter 31.

◎ CLINICAL TIP
If the blood pressure reading is too high for age, the cuff may be too small; it should cover two thirds of the infant's upper arm. If the blood pressure reading is too low for age, the cuff may be too large. Chapter 8 explains how to take a blood pressure reading.

Evaluate newborn blood pressure: A Doppler stethoscope should be used or an electronic Dinamap machine may be used to record blood pressure readings in the newborn.

◎ CLINICAL TIP
Make sure the newborn or infant is not crying during the measurement, as this can elevate blood pressure.

Continued on following page

SUBSEQUENT INFANT PHYSICAL ASSESSMENT (Continued)

Assessment Procedure	Normal Findings	Abnormal Findings
MEASUREMENTS		

Measure length.

Determine height by measuring the recumbent length. Fully extend the body, holding the head in midline and gently grasping the knees, pushing them downward until the legs are fully extended and touching the table (Fig. 30-13).

If using a measuring board, place the head at the top of the board and the heels firmly at the bottom. Without a board, use paper under the infant and mark the paper at the top of the head and bottom of the heels. Then measure the distance between the two points. Plot height measurement on an age- and gender-appropriate growth chart.

For normal findings see the growth charts available at http://www.cdc.gov/growth-charts.

CULTURAL CONSIDERATIONS
Asian and African American newborns are smaller than Caucasian newborns. Asian children are smaller at all ages.

Significant deviation from normal in the growth charts would be considered abnormal.

Measure weight. Measure weight on an appropriately sized beam scale with nondetectable weights. Weigh an infant lying or sitting on a scale that measures to the nearest 0.5 oz or 10 g (Fig. 30-14). Weigh an infant naked. Plot weight measurement on age- and gender-appropriate growth chart.

See the growth charts available at http://www.cdc.gov/growthcharts for normal findings.

Deviation from the wide range of normal weights is abnormal. Compare differences by referencing the growth charts available at http://www.cdc.gov/growthcharts.

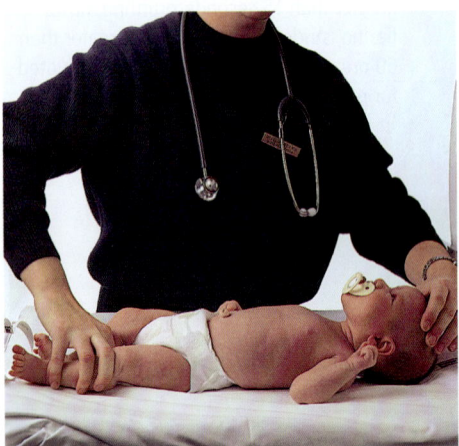

FIGURE 30-13 Positioning for measuring an infant.

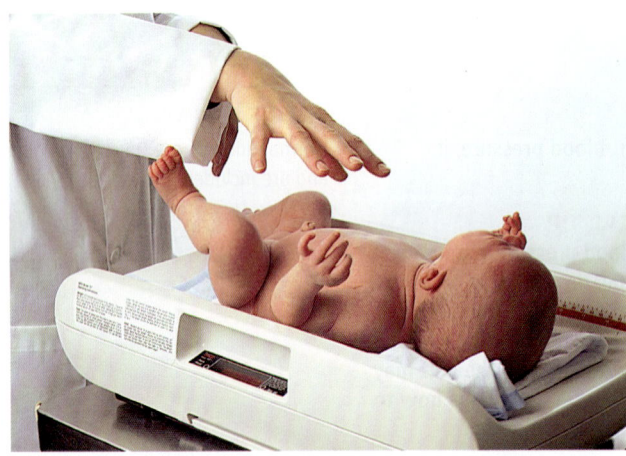

FIGURE 30-14 Weighing an infant (© B. Proud).

Determine head/chest circumference. Measure head circumference (HC) or occipital frontal circumference (OFC) at every physical examination for infants and toddlers younger than 2 years and older children when conditions warrant.

HC (OFC) measurement should fall between the 5th and 95th percentiles and should be comparable to the child's height and weight percentiles.

Abnormal circumference of head includes less than 29 cm and greater than 34 cm. HC (OFC) not within the normal percentiles may indicate pathology. Those greater than 95% may indicate macrocephaly. Those under the 5th percentile may indicate microcephaly.

If necessary, determine chest circumference by measuring the chest at the nipple line. Plot the measurements for both the head and chest on standardized growth charts specific for gender from birth to 36 months.

Chest circumference is not normally measured after the newborn period but continues to increase in size.

Assessment Procedure	Normal Findings	Abnormal Findings
SKIN, HAIR, AND NAILS		
Assess for skin color, odor, and lesions.	Newborn skin color ranges from pale white with pink, yellow, brown, or olive tones to dark brown or black. Acrocyanosis (sluggish perfusion of peripheral circulation) may be present. Mottling (general red/white discoloration of the skin) may be noted when chilled. No strong odor should be evident, and the skin should be lesion free. 🌐 **CULTURAL CONSIDERATIONS** Bruising or burning may also be from cultural practices such as cupping or coining. Petechiae or bruising may be noted on the presenting part (head, buttocks, face chest) in newborns due to rapid pressure and release with delivery. Common newborn skin variations include: • Physiologic jaundice • Birthmarks • Milia (Fig. 30-15A) • Erythema toxicum (Fig. 30-15B) • Telangiectatic nevi (stork bites) (Fig. 30-15C). • Café au lait spots <1.5 cm (Fig. 30-15D) • Benign hemangioma • Port-wine stain (nevus flammeus): flat macule, reddish/purple in color noted at birth, which is caused from capillary dilation on the surface of the skin. These usually do *not* fade over time (Fig. 30-15E). Strawberry mark: raised reddish papule, usually 2–3 cm in diameter, that does not blanch with pressure (Fig. 30-15F). These are caused from capillaries compressed together and usually fade by 5–7 years of age. • Another common variation is harlequin sign (one side of the body turns red; the other side is pale). There is a distinct color line separation at midline. The cause is unknown. 🌐 **CULTURAL CONSIDERATIONS** Dark-skinned newborns have lighter skin color than their parents. Their color darkens with age. Bluish pigmented areas called Mongolian spots (Fig. 30-15G) may be noted on the sacral areas or upper buttocks of Asian, African American, Native American, and Mexican American infants.	Yellow skin may indicate jaundice or passage of meconium in utero secondary to fetal distress. Jaundice within 24 hours after birth is pathologic and may indicate hemolytic disease of the newborn. Blue skin suggests cyanosis, pallor suggests anemia, and redness suggests fever, irritation. Ecchymoses in various stages or in unusual locations or circular burn areas suggest child abuse. Petechiae, lesions, or rashes may indicate blood disorders or neurologic disorders. Abnormal skin lesions include: Café au lait spots: if there are 6 or more hyperpigmented macules, greater than 1.5 cm in diameter, it may indicate neurofibromatosis, an inherited neurocutaneous disease.
Palpate for texture, temperature, moisture, turgor, and edema.	Skin is soft, warm, and slightly moist. Vernix caseosa (cheesy, white substance that is found on the skin, especially in skin folds) is a common finding; it eventually absorbs into the skin. Skin turgor should have quick recoil. Edema may be present around the eyes and genitalia of the newborn.	Pallor, ruddy complexion, and jaundice should be further evaluated for cardiac anomalies and blood disorders.

Continued on following page

SUBSEQUENT INFANT PHYSICAL ASSESSMENT (Continued)

Assessment Procedure	Normal Findings	Abnormal Findings

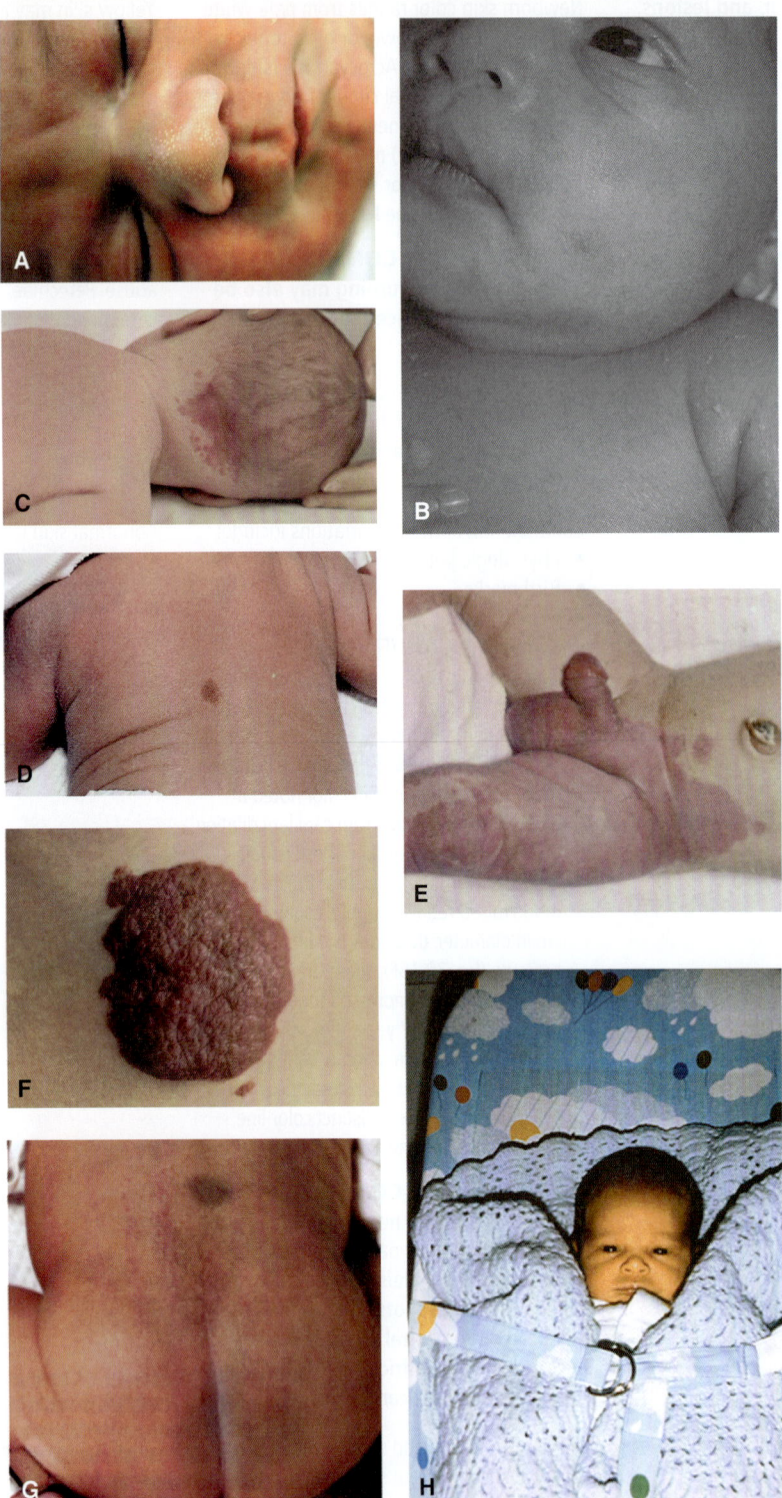

FIGURE 30-15 A. Milia. B. Erythema toxicum neonatorum. C. Telangiectatic nevi. D. Café-au-lait spot. E. Port-wine stain (nevus flammeus). F. Strawberry hemangioma. G. Mongolian spots. H. Jaundice in newborn.

Assessment Procedure	Normal Findings	Abnormal Findings
Inspect and palpate hair. Observe for distribution, characteristics, and presence of any unusual hair on body.	Hair is normally lustrous, silky, strong, and elastic. Lanugo—fine, downy hair that covers parts of the body, such as the shoulders, back, and sacral area—may be seen in the newborn or young infant. **CULTURAL CONSIDERATIONS** African American children usually have hair that is curlier and coarser than Caucasian children.	Dirty, matted hair may indicate neglect. Tufts of hair over spine may indicate spina bifida occulta.
Inspect and palpate nails. Note color, texture, shape, and condition of nails.	**CULTURAL CONSIDERATIONS** Dark-skinned children have deeper nail pigment. Nails extend to end of fingers or beyond and are well formed.	Blue nailbeds indicate cyanosis. Yellow nailbeds indicate jaundice. Blue-black nailbeds suggest a nailbed hemorrhage.

HEAD, NECK, AND CERVICAL LYMPH NODES

Inspect and palpate the head. Note shape and symmetry. In newborns, inspect and palpate the condition of fontanelles and sutures (Fig. 30-16).	Head is normocephalic and symmetric. In newborns, the head may be oddly shaped from molding (overriding of the sutures) during vaginal birth. The diamond-shaped anterior fontanelle measures about 4–5 cm at its widest part; it usually closes by 12–18 months. The triangular posterior fontanelle measures about 0.5–1 cm at its widest part and should close at 2 months of age.	A very large head is found with hydrocephalus. An oddly shaped head is found with premature closure of sutures (possibly genetic). One-sided flattening of the head suggests prolonged positioning on one side. A third fontanelle between the anterior and posterior fontanelle is seen with Down syndrome. Premature closure of sutures (craniosynostosis) may result in caput succedaneum (edema from trauma), which crosses the suture line, and cephalohematoma (bleeding into the periosteal space), which does not extend across the suture line (Fig. 30-17). Craniotabes may result from osteoporosis of the outer skull bone. Palpating too firmly with the thumb or forefinger over the temporoparietal area will leave an indentation of the bone. Bulging fontanelle indicates increased cranial pressure. Microcephaly is seen with infants who have been exposed to congenital infections.

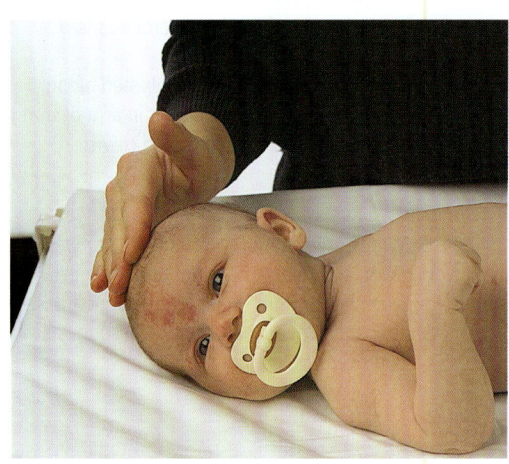

FIGURE 30-16 Palpating the anterior fontanelle (© B. Proud).

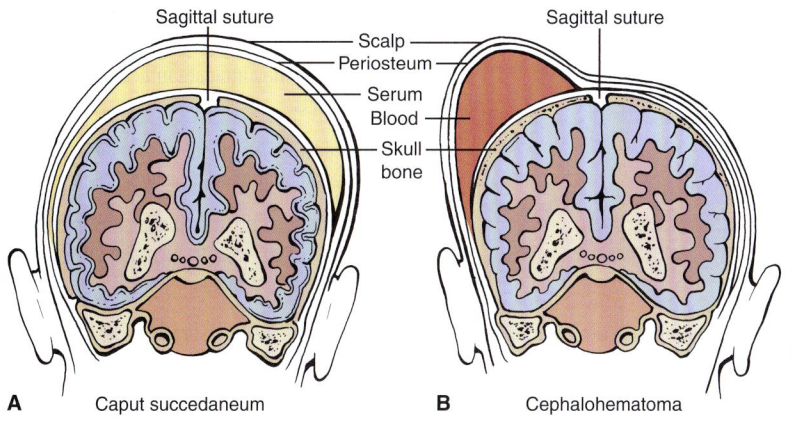

FIGURE 30-17 Premature suture closure may result in caput succedaneum (**A**) and cephalohematoma (**B**).

Continued on following page

SUBSEQUENT INFANT PHYSICAL ASSESSMENT (Continued)

Assessment Procedure	Normal Findings	Abnormal Findings
Test head control, head posture, and ROM.	Full ROM—up, down, and sideways—is normal. Infants should have head control by 4 months of age.	Hyperextension is seen with opisthotonos or significant meningeal irritation. Limited range of motion may indicate torticollis (wry neck).
Inspect and palpate the face. Note appearance, symmetry, and movement. Palpate the parotid glands for swelling.	Face is normally proportionate and symmetric. Movements are equal bilaterally. Parotid glands are normal size.	Unusual proportions (short palpebral fissures, thin lips, and wide and flat philtrum, which is the groove above the upper lip) may be hereditary or they may indicate specific syndromes such as Down syndrome and fetal alcohol syndrome. Unequal movement may indicate facial nerve paralysis. Abnormal facies may indicate chromosomal anomaly.
Inspect and palpate the neck. Palpate the thyroid gland and trachea. Also inspect and palpate the cervical lymph nodes for swelling, mobility, temperature, and tenderness. ◎ **CLINICAL TIP** The thyroid is very difficult to palpate in an infant because of the short, thick neck.	The neck is usually short with skin folds between the head and shoulder during infancy. The isthmus is the only portion of the thyroid that should be palpable. The trachea is midline. Lymph nodes are usually nonpalpable in infants. Clavicles are symmetrical and intact.	Implications of some abnormal findings include the following: • Short, webbed neck suggests anomalies or syndromes such as Down syndrome. • Distended neck veins may indicate difficulty breathing. • Enlarged thyroid or palpable masses suggest a pathologic process. • Shift in tracheal position from midline suggests a serious lung problem (e.g., foreign body or tumor). • Crepitus when clavicle palpated along with decreased movement in arm of that side may indicate fractured clavicle.

EYES

Assessment Procedure	Normal Findings	Abnormal Findings
Inspect the external eye. Note the position, slant, and epicanthal folds of the external eye.	Inner canthus distance approximately 2.5 cm, horizontal slant, no epicanthal folds. Outer canthus aligns with tips of the pinnas. 🌐 **CULTURAL CONSIDERATIONS** Epicanthal folds (excess of skin extending from roof of nose that partially or completely covers the inner canthus) are normal findings in Asian children, whose eyes also slant upward.	Wide-set position (hypertelorism), upward slant, and thick epicanthal folds suggest Down syndrome. "Sun-setting" appearance (upper lid covers part of the iris) suggests hydrocephalus.
Observe eyelid placement, swelling, discharge, and lesions. Inspect the lacrimal duct.	Eyelids have transient edema, absence of tears.	Eyelid inflammation may result from infection. Swelling, erythema, or purulent discharge may indicate infection or blocked tear ducts. Purulent discharge seen with sexually transmitted infections (gonorrhea, chlamydia). Lacrimal duct obstruction is common in the newborn and leads to increased discharge from the affected eye.
Inspect the sclera and conjunctiva for color, discharge, lesions, redness, and lacerations.	Sclera and conjunctiva are clear and free of discharge, lesions, redness, or lacerations. Small subconjunctival hemorrhages may be seen in newborns.	Yellow sclera suggests jaundice; blue sclera may indicate osteogenesis imperfecta ("brittle bone disease").

Assessment Procedure	Normal Findings	Abnormal Findings
Observe the iris and the pupils.	Typically, the iris is blue in light-skinned infants and brown in dark-skinned infants; permanent color develops within 9 months. Brushfield spots (white flecks on the periphery of the iris) may be normal in some infants. Pupils are equal, round, and reactive to light and accommodation (PERRLA).	Brushfield spots may indicate Down syndrome. Sluggish pupils indicate a neurologic problem. Miosis (constriction) indicates iritis or narcotic use or abuse. Mydriasis (pupillary dilation) indicates emotional factors (fear), trauma, or use of certain drug.
Inspect the eyebrows and eyelashes.	Eyebrows should be symmetric in shape and movement. They should not meet midline. Eyelashes should be evenly distributed and curled outward.	Sparseness of eyebrows or lashes could indicate skin disease.
Perform visual acuity tests. Assess visual acuity by observing infant's ability to gaze at an object.	Visual acuity is difficult to test in infants; test by observing the infant's ability to fix on and follow objects. Normal visual acuity is as follows: • Birth: 20/100 to 20/400 • 1 year: 20/200 By 4 weeks of age, the infant should be able to fixate on objects. By 6–8 weeks, eyes should follow a moving object. By 3 months, the infant is able to follow and reach for an object.	Children with a one-line difference between eyes should be referred for ophthalmology examination.
Perform extraocular muscle tests. Hirschberg test: Shine light directly at the cornea while the infant looks straight ahead.	In the Hirschberg test, the light reflects symmetrically in the center of both pupils. Light causes pupils to vasoconstrict bilaterally and blink reflex occurs. Blink reflex also occurs as an object is brought towards the eyes. By 10 days of age, when turning the head, the infant's eyes should follow the position of the head.	Unequal alignment of light on the pupils in the Hirschberg test signals strabismus. Doll's eye reflex is an abnormal reflex that occurs when the eyes do not follow or adjust to movement of the head.
Perform ophthalmoscopic examination. The procedure is the same as for adults. Distraction is preferred over the use of restraint, which is likely to result in crying and closed eyes. Careful ophthalmoscopic examination of newborns is difficult without the use of mydriatic medications.	Red reflex is present. This reflex rules out most serious defects of the cornea, aqueous chamber, lens, and vitreous humor. When visualized, the optic disc appears similar to an adult's. A newborn's optic discs are pale; peripheral vessels are not well developed.	Absence of the red reflex indicates cataracts. Papilledema is unusual in children of this age owing to the ability of the fontanelles and sutures to open during increased intracranial pressure. Disc blurring and hemorrhages should be reported immediately. Abnormal findings include congenital defects, such as cataracts.
EARS		
Inspect external ears. Note placement, discharge, or lesions of the ears.	Top of pinna should cross the eye-occiput line and be within a 10-degree angle of a perpendicular line drawn from the eye-occiput line to the lobe. No unusual structure or markings should appear on the pinna.	Low-set ears with an alignment greater than a 10-degree angle (Fig. 30-18) suggest retardation or congenital syndromes. Abnormal shape may suggest renal disease process, which may be hereditary. Preauricular skin tags or sinuses suggest other anomalies of the ears or renal system.

Continued on following page

SUBSEQUENT INFANT PHYSICAL ASSESSMENT (Continued)

Assessment Procedure	Normal Findings	Abnormal Findings
Inspect internal ear. The internal ear examination requires an otoscope. The nurse should always hold the otoscope in a manner that allows for rapid removal if the child moves. Have the caregiver hold and restrain the child. Because an infant's external canal is short and straight, pull the pinna down and back (Fig. 30-19).	No excessive cerumen, discharge, lesions, excoriations, or foreign body in external canal. Amniotic fluid/vernix may be present in canal of the ear of the newborn. Tympanic membrane is pearly gray to light pink, with normal landmarks. Tympanic membranes redden bilaterally when child is crying or febrile.	Presence of foreign bodies or cerumen impaction. Purulent discharge may indicate otitis externa or presence of foreign body. Purulent, serous discharge suggests otitis media. Bloody discharge suggests trauma, and clear discharge may indicate cerebrospinal fluid leak. Perforated tympanic membrane may also be noted.

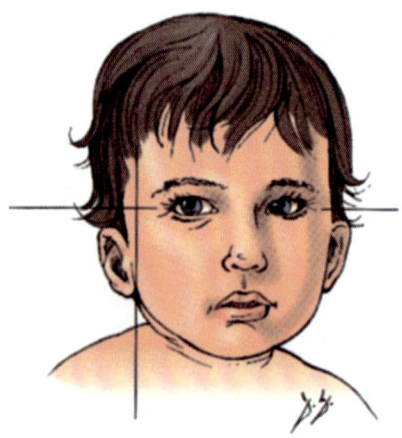

FIGURE 30-18 Low-set ears with alignment greater than 10-degree angle.

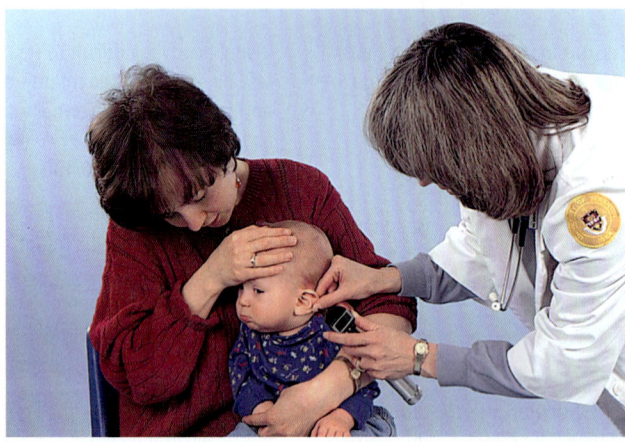

FIGURE 30-19 To examine the ears of an infant, restrain the child and pull the pinna down and back (© B. Proud).

Assess the mobility of the tympanic membrane by pneumatic otoscopy. This consists of creating pressure against the tympanic membrane using air. To do this, create a seal in the external canal and direct a puff of air against the tympanic membrane. Create the seal by using the largest speculum that will comfortably insert into the ear canal. Cover the tip with rubber for a better and more comfortable seal. Attach a pneumatic bulb to the otoscope and squeeze the bulb lightly to direct air against the tympanic membrane.	Tympanic membrane is mobile; moves inward with positive pressure (squeeze of bulb) and outward with negative pressure (release of bulb).	Immobility indicates fluid behind tympanic membrane.
Hearing acuity. In the infant, test hearing acuity by noting the reaction to noise. Stand approximately 12 in from the infant and create a loud noise (e.g., clap hands, shake/squeeze a noisy toy). Routine newborn hearing screening is performed in most newborn nurseries 24–48 hours after birth or prior to discharge.	A newborn will exhibit the startle (Moro) reflex and blink eyes (acoustic blink reflex) in response to noise. Older infant will turn head.	Absence of reactions to noise may indicate a hearing deficit. Audiometry results outside normal range suggest hearing deficit.

MOUTH, THROAT, NOSE, AND SINUSES

Inspect mouth and throat. Note the condition of the lips, palates, tongue, and buccal mucosa.	Epstein's pearls—small, yellow-white retention cysts on the hard palate and gums—are common in newborns and usually disappear in the first weeks of life. In infants, a sucking tubercle (pad) from the friction of sucking may be evident in the middle of the upper lip.	White discharge noted on the tongue or buccal mucosa is thrush. Cleft lip and/or palate are congenital abnormalities.

Assessment Procedure	Normal Findings	Abnormal Findings
Observe the condition of the gums. When teeth appear, count teeth and note location.	Gums appear pink and moist. Teeth may begin erupting at 4–6 months. Teeth develop in sequential order. By 10 months, most infants have two upper and two lower central incisors.	Abnormal findings include lesion and edema.
Note the condition of the throat and tonsils. Also observe the insertion and ending point of the frenulum.	Tonsils are not visible in newborns. As the infant gets older, it is possible but still difficult to see tonsils.	Extension of the frenulum to the tip of tongue may interfere with extension of the tongue, which causes speech difficulties.
Inspect nose and sinuses. To inspect the nose and sinuses, avoid using the nasal speculum in infants and young children. Instead, push up the tip of the nose and shine the light into each nostril. Observe the structure and patency of the nares, discharge, tenderness, and any color or swelling of the turbinates. ◎ **CLINICAL TIP** **Infants are obligatory nose breathers.** Consequently, obstructed nasal passages may precipitate serious health conditions, making it very important to assess the patency of the nares in the newborn. If, after suctioning fluid and mucus from the nares, you suspect obstruction, insert a small-lumen catheter into each nostril to assess patency.	Nose is midline in face, septum is straight, and nares are patent. No discharge or tenderness is present. Turbinates are pink and free of edema. Milia are small, white papules found on the nose, forehead, and chin. They develop from retention of sebum in sebaceous pores. They usually resolve spontaneously within a few weeks.	Choanal atresia is blockage of the posterior nares in the newborn. If the blockage is bilateral, the newborn is at risk for acute respiratory distress. Immediate referral is necessary. Deviated septum may be congenital or caused by injury. Foul discharge from one nostril may indicate a foreign body.
THORAX		
Inspect the shape of the thorax.	Infant's thorax is smooth, rounded, and symmetric.	Abnormal shapes of the thorax include pectus excavatum and pectus carinatum.
Observe respiratory effort, keeping in mind that newborns and young infants are obligatory nose breathers.	Respirations should be unlabored and regular in all ages except for immediate newborn period, when respirations are irregular (see "Vital Signs" section). Some newborns, especially the premature, have periodic irregular breathing, sometimes with apnea (episodes when breathing stops) lasting a few seconds. This is a normal finding if bradycardia does not accompany irregular breathing.	Retractions (suprasternal, sternal, substernal, intercostal) and grunting suggest increased inspiratory effort, which may be due to airway obstruction. Periods of apnea that last longer than 15 seconds and are accompanied by bradycardia may be a sign of a cardiovascular or central nervous system (CNS) disease. Nasal flaring, tachypnea, and seesaw movement of the chest indicate respiratory distress.
Percuss the chest. During percussion of the lungs, note tone elicited.	Hyperresonance is the normal tone elicited in infants because of thinness of the chest wall.	A dull tone may indicate a mass, fluid, or consolidation.
Auscultate for breath sounds and adventitious sounds. If a newborn's lung sounds seem noisy, auscultate the upper nostrils.	Breath sounds may seem louder and harsher in young children because of their thin chest walls. No adventitious sounds should be heard, although transmitted upper airway sounds may be heard on auscultation of thorax.	Diminished breath sounds suggest respiratory disorders such as pneumonia or atelectasis. Stridor (inspiratory wheeze) is a high-pitched, piercing sound that indicates a narrowing of the upper tracheobronchial tree. Expiratory wheezes indicate narrowing in the lower tracheobronchial tree. Rhonchi and rales (crackles) may indicate a number of respiratory diseases such as pneumonia, bronchitis, or bronchiolitis.

Continued on following page

SUBSEQUENT INFANT PHYSICAL ASSESSMENT (Continued)

Assessment Procedure	Normal Findings	Abnormal Findings

BREASTS

Inspect and palpate breasts. Note shape, symmetry, color, tenderness, discharge, lesions, and masses.

Newborns may have enlarged and engorged breasts with a white liquid discharge resulting from the influence of maternal hormones (Fig. 30-20). This condition resolves spontaneously within days.

A palpable mass of the breast is abnormal. The newborn or infant may have extra nipples noted on the chest or abdomen, called *supernumerary nipples*.

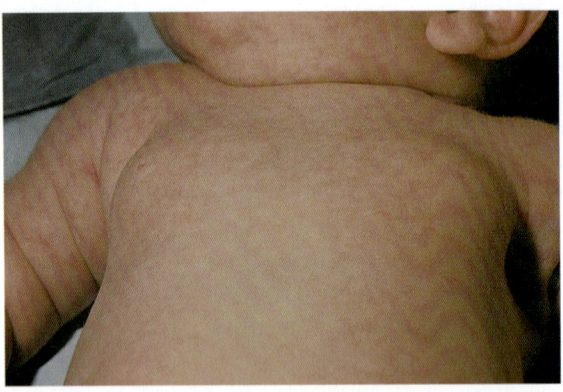

FIGURE 30-20 The enlarged breasts of this newborn are normal, resulting from the influence of maternal hormones (© 1994 Science Photo Library/CMSP).

HEART

Inspect and palpate the precordium. Note lifts, heaves, apical impulse (Fig. 30-21).

The apical pulse is at the 4th intercostal space (ICS) until the age of 7 years, when it drops to the 5th. It is to the left of the midclavicular line (MCL) until age 4.

A systolic heave may indicate right ventricular enlargement. Apical impulse that is not in proper location for age may indicate cardiomyopathy, pneumothorax, or diaphragmatic hernia.

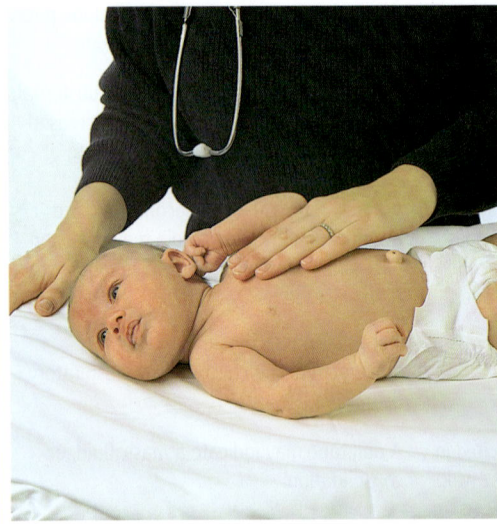

FIGURE 30-21 Palpate the infant's chest for lifts and heaves (© B. Proud).

Auscultate heart sounds. Listen to the heart. Note rate and rhythm of apical impulse, S_1, S_2, extra heart sounds, and murmurs. Keep in mind that sinus arrhythmia is normal in infants. Heart sounds are louder, higher pitched, and of shorter duration in infants. A split S_2 at the apex occurs normally in some infants and S_3 is a normal heart sound in some children. A venous hum also may be normally heard in children.

Normal heart rates are cited in the previous "Vital Signs" section. Innocent murmurs, which are common throughout childhood, are classified as systolic; short duration; no transmission to other areas; grade III or less; loudest in pulmonic area (base of heart); low-pitched, musical, or groaning quality that varies in intensity in relation to position, respiration, activity, fever, and anemia. No other associated signs of heart disease should be found.

Murmurs that do not fit the criteria for innocent murmurs may indicate a disease or disorder. Extra heart sounds and variations in pulse rate and rhythm also suggest pathologic processes.

Assessment Procedure	Normal Findings	Abnormal Findings
ABDOMEN		
Inspect the shape of the abdomen.	In infants, the abdomen is prominent in supine position.	A scaphoid (boat-shaped; i.e., sunken with prominent rib cage) abdomen may result from malnutrition or dehydration. Distended abdomen may indicate pyloric stenosis.
Inspect umbilicus. Note color, discharge, evident herniation of the umbilicus.	Umbilicus is pink, with no discharge, odor, redness, or herniation. Cord should demonstrate three vessels (two arteries and one vein). Remnant of cord should appear dried 24–48 hours after birth.	Inflammation, discharge, and redness of umbilicus suggest infection. Diastasis recti (separation of the abdominal muscles) is seen as a midline protrusion from the xiphoid to the umbilicus or pubis symphysis. This condition is secondary to immature musculature of abdominal muscles and usually has little significance. As the muscles strengthen, the separation resolves on its own. A bulge at the umbilicus suggests an umbilical hernia (Fig. 30-22), which may be seen in newborns; many disappear by the age of 1 year. **CULTURAL CONSIDERATIONS** Umbilical hernias are seen more frequently in African American children. Abnormal insertion of cord, discolored cord, or two-vessel cord could indicate genetic abnormalities; however, these are also seen in newborns without abnormalities.

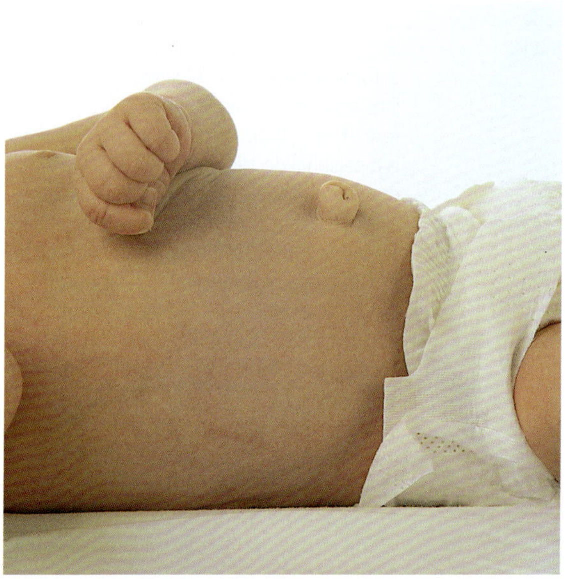

FIGURE 30-22 Umbilical hernia.

Assessment Procedure	Normal Findings	Abnormal Findings
Auscultate bowel sounds. Follow auscultation guidelines for adult clients provided in Chapter 23.	Normal bowel sounds occur every 10–30 seconds. They sound like clicks, gurgles, or growls.	Marked peristaltic waves almost always indicate a pathologic process such as pyloric stenosis.
Palpate for masses and tenderness. Palpate abdomen for softness or hardness.	Abdomen is soft to palpation and without masses or tenderness.	A rigid abdomen is almost always an emergent problem. Masses or tenderness warrants further investigation. Hirschsprung disease could also be considered, especially with a rigid abdomen. The most common finding is failure to have a bowel movement within 48 hours after birth.
Palpate liver. Palpate the liver the same as you would for adults (see Chapter 23).	Liver is usually palpable 1–2 cm below the right costal margin in young children. The liver is hard to palpate in the newborn.	An enlarged liver with a firm edge that is palpated more than 2 cm below the right costal margin usually indicates a pathologic process.
Palpate spleen. Palpate the spleen the same as you would for adults.	Spleen tip may be palpable during inspiration. The spleen is difficult to palpate in the newborn.	Enlarged spleen is usually indicative of a pathologic process.
Palpate kidneys. Palpate the kidneys the same as you would for adults.	The tip of the right kidney may be palpable during inspiration.	Enlarged kidneys are usually indicative of a pathologic process.
Palpate bladder. Palpate the bladder the same as you would for adults.	Bladder may be slightly palpable in infants and small children.	An enlarged bladder is usually due to urinary retention but may be due to a mass.

Continued on following page

SUBSEQUENT INFANT PHYSICAL ASSESSMENT (Continued)

Assessment Procedure	Normal Findings	Abnormal Findings
MALE GENITALIA		
Inspect penis and urinary meatus. Inspect the genitalia, observing size for age and any lesions. 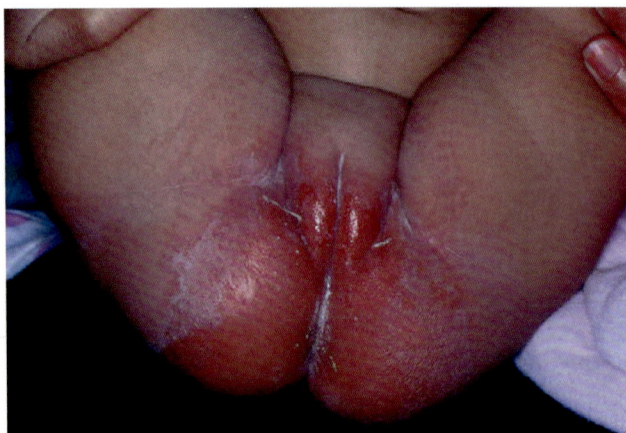 **FIGURE 30-23** Diaper rash, a common finding in infants.	Penis is normal size for age, and no lesions are seen. Diaper rash, however, is a common finding in infants (Fig. 30-23). The foreskin is retractable in uncircumcised child. Urinary meatus is at tip of glans penis and has no discharge or redness. Penis may appear small in large for gestational age (LGA) boys because of overlapping skin folds. For circumcised boys, the site is dry with minimal swelling and drainage.	An unretractable foreskin in a child older than 3 months suggests phimosis. Paraphimosis is indicated when the foreskin is tightened around the glans penis in a retracted position. Hypospadias (urinary meatus on the ventral surface of glans) and epispadias (urinary meatus on dorsal surface of glans) are congenital disorders (see Chapter 26). Circumcision has become a topic of discussion due to increased anti-circumcision activism (Strobbe, 2014). Strobbe quotes findings and conclusions by the CDC and other researchers about circumcision: Circumcision is a personal decision often based on cultural or religious beliefs. Studies in Africa have suggested that circumcision may reduce the spread of HIV-AIDS; the benefits of circumcision have become even more clear over the last 10 years of studies in Africa. Acceptance of circumcision has swung widely in the United States from about 25% of males in 1900, to a high of 64.9% in 1981, and back down to about 58% in 2010. Stobbe lists the reasons for the CDC's conclusion, based on strong evidence, that male circumcision can: • Cut a man's risk by 50–60% of becoming infected with HIV from an infected female partner • Reduce the risk by 30% of becoming infected with genital herpes or human papilloma virus • Lower the risk of UTI in infancy and of cancer of the penis in adulthood However, research evidence does not show that circumcision can stop the spread of AIDS to women or to a same sex partner. The final conclusion is that the decision to circumcise or not is personal, even in light of the evidence.
Inspect and palpate scrotum and testes. To rule out cryptorchidism, it is important to palpate for testes in the scrotum in infants. 🎯 **CLINICAL TIP** When palpating the testicles in the infant, you must keep the cremasteric reflex in mind. This reflex pulls the testicles up into the inguinal canal and abdomen, and is elicited in response to touch, cold, or emotional factors.	Scrotum is free of lesions. Testes are palpable in scrotum, with the left testicle usually lower than the right. Testes are equal in size, smooth, mobile, and free of masses. If a testicle is missing from the scrotal sac but the scrotal sac appears well developed, suspect physiologic cryptorchidism. The testis has originally descended into the scrotum but has moved back up into the inguinal canal because of the cremasteric reflex and the small size of the testis. You should be able to milk the testis down into the scrotum from the inguinal canal. This normal condition subsides at puberty.	Absent testicle(s) and atrophic scrotum suggest true cryptorchidism (undescended testicles). This suggests that the testicle(s) never descended. This condition occurs more frequently in preterm than term infants because testes descend at 8 months of gestation. It can lead to testicular atrophy and infertility, and increases the risk for testicular cancer. Hydroceles are common in infants. They are a collection of fluid along the spermatic cord within the scrotum that can be transilluminated (see Chapter 26, Abnormal Findings 26-2). They usually resolve spontaneously.

Assessment Procedure	Normal Findings	Abnormal Findings
Inspect and palpate inguinal area for hernias. Observe for any bulge in the inguinal area. Using your pinky finger, palpate up the inguinal canal to the external inguinal ring if a hernia is suspected.	No inguinal hernias are present.	A scrotal hernia is usually caused by an indirect inguinal hernia that has descended into the scrotum. It can usually be pushed back into the inguinal canal. This mass will not transilluminate. A bulge in the inguinal area or palpation of a mass in the inguinal canal suggests an inguinal hernia. Indirect inguinal hernias occur most frequently in children (see Chapter 26).
FEMALE GENITALIA		
Inspect external genitalia. Note labia majora, labia minora, vaginal orifice, urinary meatus, and clitoris.	Labia majora and minora are pink and moist. Newborn's genitalia may appear prominent because of influence of maternal hormones. Bruises and swelling may be caused by breech vaginal delivery. Pseudomenstruation (blood-tinged discharge), smegma (cheesy white discharge) of the sebaceous gland. Reddish, orange, pink-tinged urine, or stains on diaper may also be normal due to uric acid crystals.	Enlarged clitoris in newborn combined with fusion of the posterior labia majora suggests ambiguous genitalia.
ANUS AND RECTUM		
Inspect the anus. The anus should be inspected in infants. Spread the buttocks with gloved hands; note patency of anal opening, presence of any lesions and fissures, and condition and color of perianal skin.	The anal opening should be visible and moist. Perianal skin should be smooth and free of lesions. Perianal skin tags may be noted. Meconium is passed within 24–48 hours after birth.	Imperforate anus (no anal opening) should be referred. Pustules may indicate secondary infection of diaper rash. No passage of meconium stool could indicate no patency of anus or cystic fibrosis.
MUSCULOSKELETAL		
Assess arms, hands, feet, and legs. Note symmetry, shape, movement, and positioning of the feet and legs. Perform neurovascular assessment. **CLINICAL TIP** If the client is a newborn, keep in mind that the feet may retain their intrauterine position and appear deformed (positioned outward or inward from normal right angle to the leg). This is normal if the foot easily returns to its normal position with manipulation (either scratch along the lateral edge of the affected foot or gently push the forefoot into its normal position).	Feet and legs are symmetric in size, shape, and movement. Extremities should be warm and mobile, with adequate capillary refill. All pulses (radial, brachial, femoral, popliteal, pedal) should be strong and equal bilaterally. There is an inward (pointing toward center of the body) positioning of the forefoot with the heel in normal straight position; it resolves spontaneously. Tibial torsion, also common in infants and toddlers, consists of twisting of the tibia inward or outward on its long axis, and is usually caused by intrauterine positioning; this typically corrects itself by the time the child is 2 years old.	Short, broad extremities, hyperextensible joints, and palmar simian crease may indicate Down syndrome. Polydactyly (extra digits) and syndactyly (webbing) are sometimes found in children with mental retardation. Absent femoral pulses may indicate coarctation of the aorta. Neurovascular deficit in children is usually secondary to trauma (e.g., fracture). Fixed-position (true) deformities do not return to normal position with manipulation. Metatarsus varus is inversion (a turning inward that elevates the medial margin) and adduction of the forefoot. Talipes varus is adduction of the forefoot and inversion of the entire foot. Talipes equinovarus (clubfoot) is indicated if foot is fixed in the following position: adduction of forefoot, inversion of entire foot, and equinus (pointing downward) position of entire foot.
Assess for congenital hip dysplasia. Assessing for hip dysplasia is an important aspect of the physical examination for infants. The assessment should be performed at each visit until the child is about 1 year old. (Several tests are described below.)	Equal gluteal folds and full hip abduction are normal findings.	Unequal gluteal folds and limited hip abduction are signs of congenital hip dysplasia.

Continued on following page

SUBSEQUENT INFANT PHYSICAL ASSESSMENT (Continued)

Assessment Procedure	Normal Findings	Abnormal Findings
Begin by assessing the symmetry of the gluteal folds. Also assess hip abduction using the maneuvers below.		
Perform Ortolani maneuver to test for congenital hip dysplasia (Fig. 30-24). With the infant supine, flex infant's knees while holding your thumbs on midthigh and your fingers over the greater trochanters; abduct the legs, moving the knees outward and down toward the table.	Negative Ortolani sign is normal.	Positive Ortolani sign: A click heard along with feeling the head of the femur slip in or out of the hip.

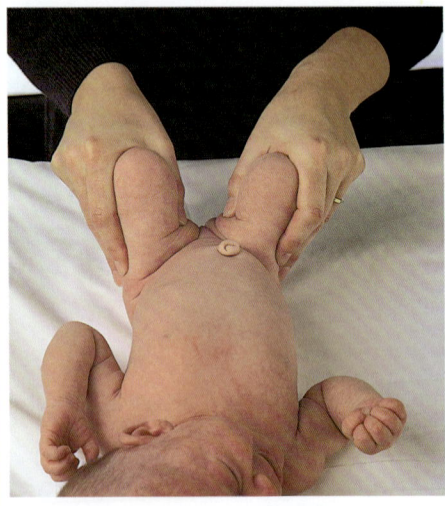

FIGURE 30-24 Performing the Ortolani maneuver.

Perform Barlow maneuvers (Fig. 30-25). With the infant supine, flex the infant's knees while holding your thumbs on midthigh and your fingers over the greater trochanters; adduct legs until thumbs touch.	Negative Barlow sign is normal.	Positive Barlow sign: A feeling of the head of the femur slipping out of the hip socket (acetabulum).
Assess spinal alignment. Observe spine and posture.	In newborns, the spine is flexible, with convex dorsal and sacral curves. In infants younger than 3 months, the spine is rounded (Fig. 30-26).	In newborns, flaccid or rigid posture is considered abnormal. In older infants and children, abnormal posture suggests neuromuscular disorders such as cerebral palsy.

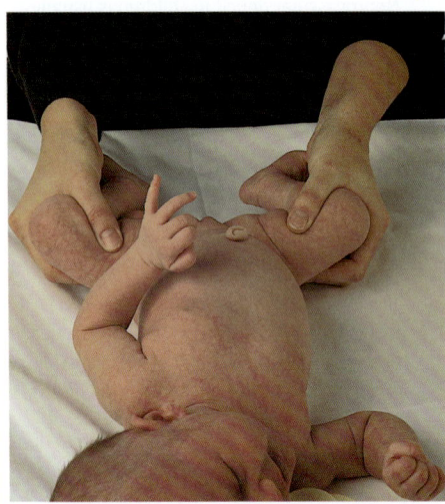

FIGURE 30-25 Performing the Barlow maneuver.

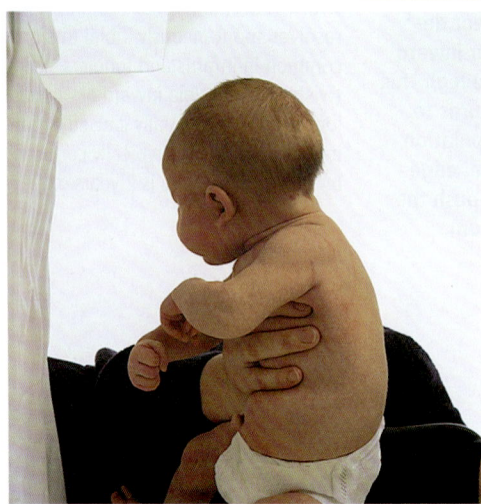

FIGURE 30-26 The spine is rounded in infants under 3 months old.

Assessment Procedure	Normal Findings	Abnormal Findings
Assess joints. Note ROM, swelling, redness, and tenderness.	Full ROM and no swelling, redness, or tenderness.	Limited ROM, swelling, redness, and tenderness indicate problems ranging from mild injuries to serious disorders.
Assess muscles. Note size and strength. (e.g., Can the infant bear weight on the legs?)	Muscle size and strength should be adequate for the particular age and should be equal bilaterally.	Inadequate muscle size and strength for the particular age indicate neuromuscular disorders such as muscular dystrophy.
NEUROLOGIC SYSTEM		
Assess the newborn's and infant's cry, responsiveness, and adaptation.	The newborn's and infant's cries are lusty and strong; responds appropriately to stimuli and quiets to soothing when held in the *en face* position (Fig. 30-27).	Inappropriate response to stimuli suggests CNS disorders or problems. An inability to quiet to soothing and gaze aversion is seen in "cocaine babies." Infantile reflexes present when inappropriate, absent, or asymmetric may indicate a CNS problem.

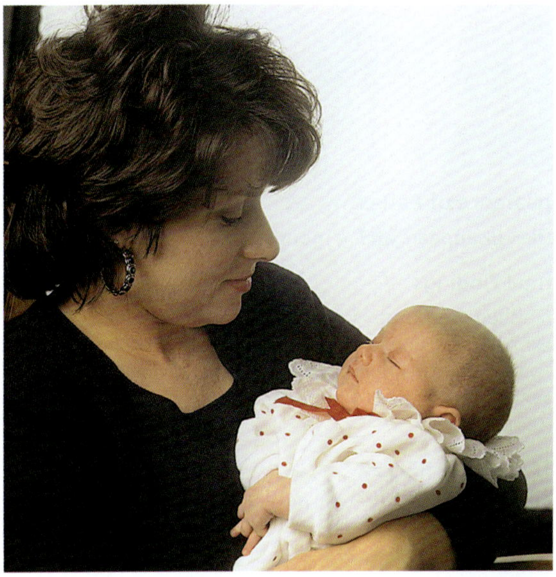

FIGURE 30-27 The newborn quiets to soothing when held *en face*.

Test deep tendon and superficial reflexes.	Infantile reflexes are present when appropriate, and are symmetric. The Babinski response is normal in children younger than 2 years (this response usually disappears between 2 and 24 months), and triceps reflex is absent until age 6. Ankle clonus (rapid, rhythmic plantar flexion) in response to eliciting ankle reflex is common in newborns.	Absence or marked intensity of these reflexes, asymmetry, and presence of Babinski response after age 2 years may demonstrate pathology.
Test motor function. See Developmental Assessment section in the beginning of the subsequent infant physical assessment.		

BOX 30-1 NEWBORN REFLEXES: DIFFERENTIATING NORMAL AND ABNORMAL FINDINGS

The reflexes illustrated and described are the most commonly tested newborn reflexes. These reflexes are present in all normal newborns, and most disappear within a few months after birth. Therefore, absence of a reflex at birth or persistence of a reflex past a certain age may indicate a problem with central nervous system function.

ROOTING REFLEX

To elicit the rooting reflex, touch the newborn's upper or lower lip or cheek with a gloved finger or sterile nipple. The newborn will move the head toward the stimulated area and open the mouth.

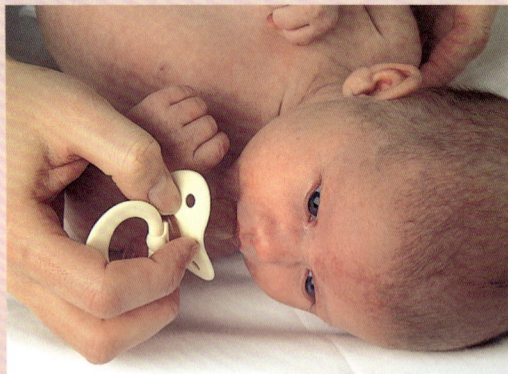

Disappearance of Reflex
The rooting reflex disappears by 3–4 months.

Abnormal Findings
Absence of a rooting indicates serious CNS disease.

SUCKING REFLEX

Place a gloved finger or nipple in the newborn's mouth, and note the strength of the sucking response. (A diminished response is normal in a recently fed newborn.)

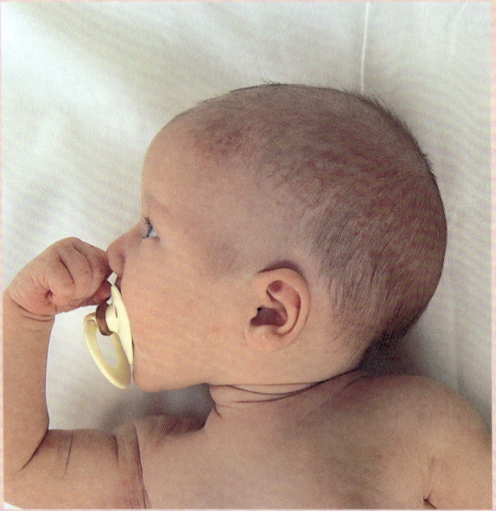

Disappearance of Reflex
This reflex disappears at 10–12 months.

Abnormal Findings
A weak or absent sucking reflex may indicate a neurologic disorder, prematurity, or CNS depression caused by maternal drug use or medication during pregnancy.

PALMAR GRASP REFLEX

Press your fingers against the palmar surface of the newborn's hand from the ulnar side. The grasp should be strong—you may even be able to pull the newborn to a sitting position.

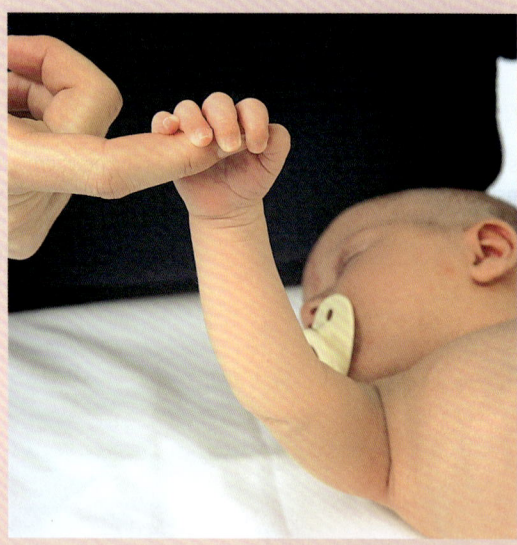

Disappearance of Reflex
This reflex disappears at 3–4 months.

Abnormal Findings
A diminished response usually indicates prematurity; no response suggests neurologic deficit; asymmetric grasp suggests fracture of the humerus or peripheral nerve damage. If this reflex persists past 4 months, cerebral dysfunction may be present.

PLANTAR GRASP REFLEX

Touch the ball of the newborn's foot. The toes should curl downward tightly.

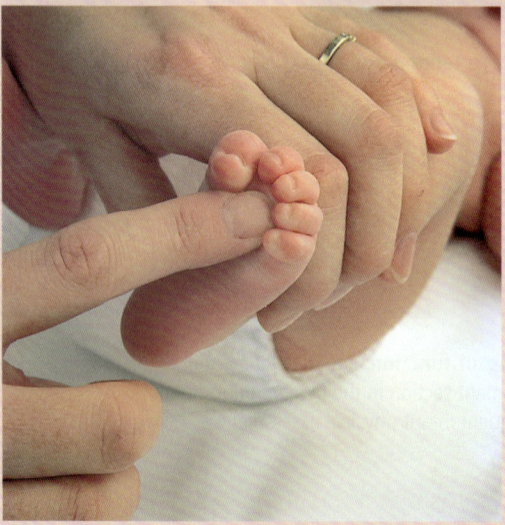

Disappearance of Reflex
This reflex disappears at 8–10 months.

Abnormal Findings
A diminished response usually indicates prematurity; no response suggests neurologic deficit.

TONIC NECK REFLEX

The newborn should be supine. Turn the head to one side, with newborn's jaw at the shoulder. The tonic neck reflex is present when the arm and leg on the side to which the head is turned extend and the opposite arm and leg flex. This reflex usually does not appear until 2 months of age.

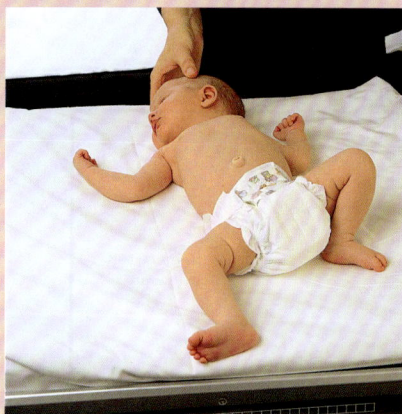

Disappearance of Reflex

This reflex disappears by 4–6 months. The reflex may not occur every time that the examiner tries to elicit it, in which case, repeat stimulus of turning head to one side to re-elicit the response.

Abnormal Findings

If this reflex persists until later in infancy, brain damage is usually present.

MORO (OR STARTLE) REFLEX

The Moro reflex is a response to sudden stimulation or an abrupt change in position. This reflex can be elicited by using either one of the following two methods:

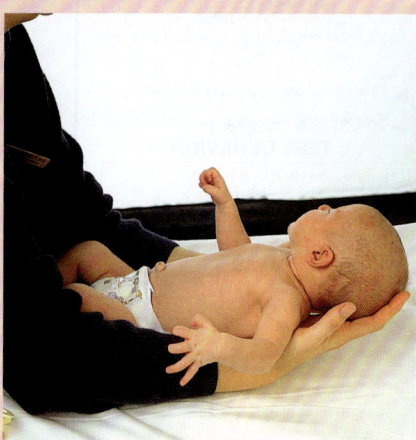

1. Hold the infant with the head supported and rapidly lower the whole body a few inches.
2. Place the infant in the supine position on a flat, soft surface. Hit the surface with your hand or startle the infant in some way.

The reflex is manifested by the infant slightly flexing and abducting the legs, laterally extending and abducting the arms, forming a "C" with thumb and forefinger, and fanning the other fingers. This is immediately followed by anterior flexion and adduction of the arms. All movements should be symmetric.

Disappearance of Reflex

This reflex disappears by 3 months.

Abnormal Findings

An asymmetric response suggests injury of the part that responds more slowly. Absence of a response suggests CNS injury. If the reflex was elicited at birth and disappears later, cerebral edema or intracranial hemorrhage is suspected. Persistence of the response after 4 months suggests CNS injury.

BABINSKI REFLEX

Hold the newborn's foot and stroke up the lateral edge and across the ball. A positive Babinski reflex is fanning of the toes. Many normal newborns will not exhibit a positive Babinski reflex; instead, they will exhibit the normal adult response, which is flexion of the toes. Response should always be symmetric bilaterally.

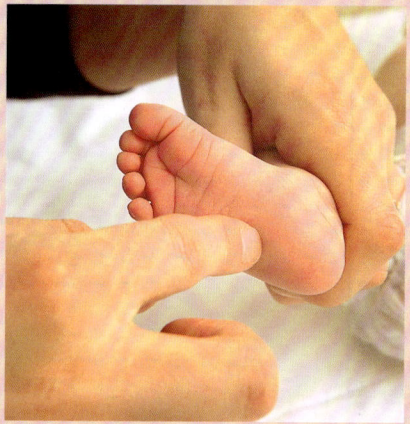

Disappearance of Reflex

This reflex disappears within 2 years.

Abnormal Findings

A positive response after 2 years suggests pyramidal tract disease.

STEPPING REFLEX

Hold the newborn upright from behind, provide support under the arms, and let the newborn's feet touch a surface. The reflex response is manifested by the newborn stepping with one foot and then the other in a walking motion.

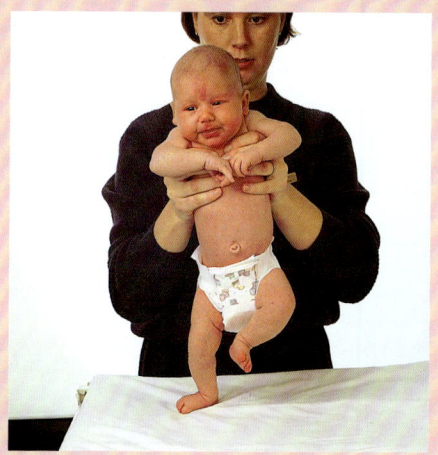

Disappearance of Reflex

This reflex usually disappears within 2 months.

Abnormal Findings

An asymmetric response may indicate injury of the leg, CNS damage, or peripheral nerve injury.

ASSESSMENT TOOL 30-1 Using the Denver Developmental Screening Test

The following is an example of the Denver Developmental Screening Test (DDST), which assesses a child's gross motor, language, fine motor, and personal social development according to the child's age. Testing kits, test forms, and reference manuals (which must be used to ensure accuracy in administering the test) may be ordered from Denver Developmental Materials Inc. (Denverii.com) (DenverDevelopmentalMaterials@gmail.com).

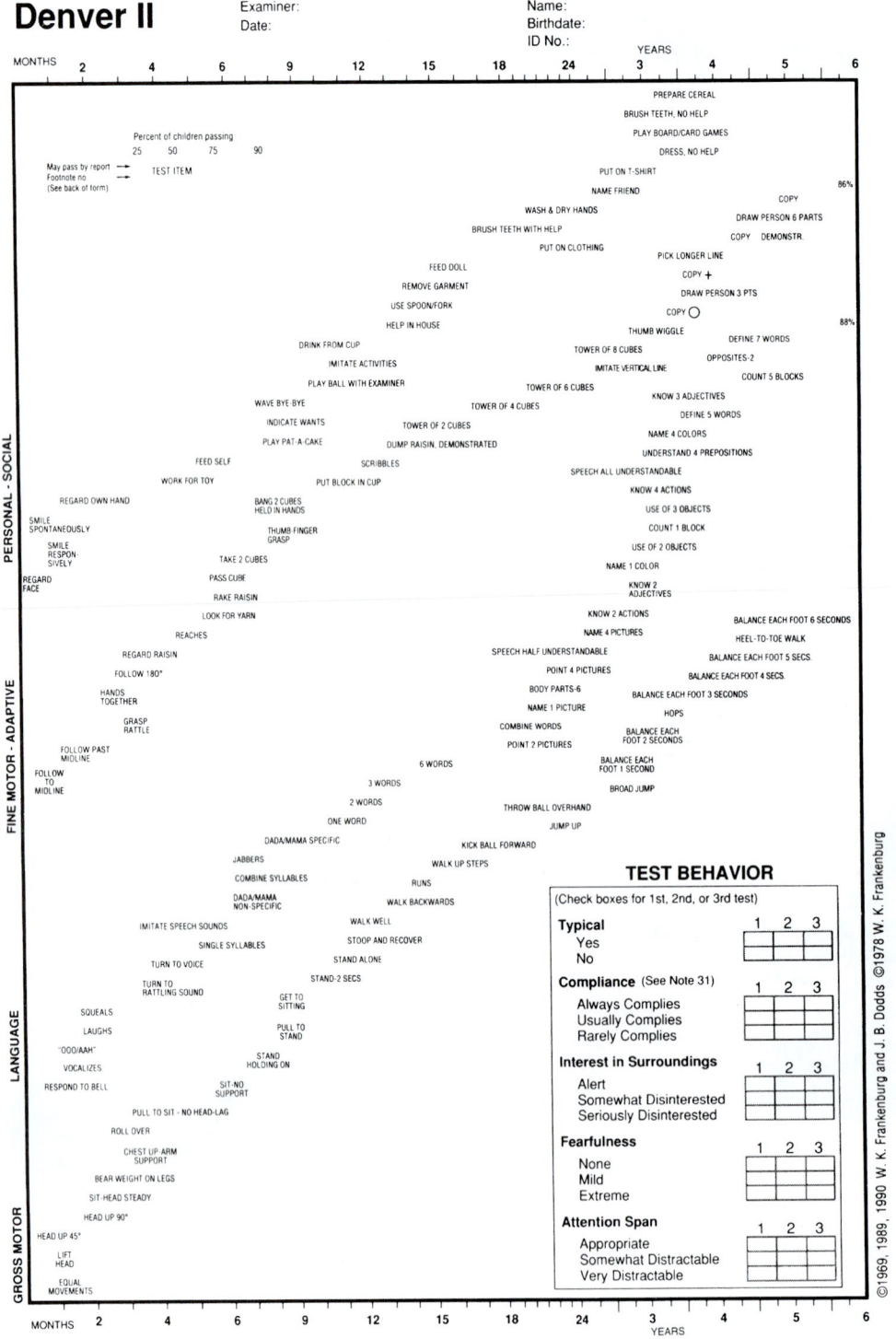

Testing kits, test forms, and reference manuals (which must be used to ensure accuracy in administration of the test) for the DDST may be ordered from Denver Developmental Materials Incorporated, P.O. Box 6919, Denver, CO 80206-0919. (Reprinted with permission from William K. Frankenburg, M.D.)

ASSESSMENT TOOL 30-1 Using the Denver Developmental Screening Test (Continued)

DIRECTIONS FOR ADMINISTRATION

1. Try to get child to smile by smiling, talking or waving. Do not touch him/her.
2. Child must stare at hand several seconds.
3. Parent may help guide toothbrush and put toothpaste on brush.
4. Child does not have to be able to tie shoes or button/zip in the back.
5. Move yarn slowly in an arc from one side to the other, about 8 in above child's face.
6. Pass if child grasps rattle when it is touched to the backs or tips of fingers.
7. Pass if child tries to see where yarn went. Yarn should be dropped quickly where it is out of sight from tester's hand without arm movement.
8. Child must transfer cube from hand to hand without help of body, mouth, or table.
9. Pass if child picks up raisin with any part of thumb and finger.
10. Line can vary only 30 degrees or less from tester's line.
11. Make a fist with thumb pointing upward and wiggle only the thumb. Pass if child imitates and does not move any fingers other than the thumb.

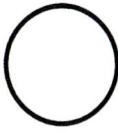 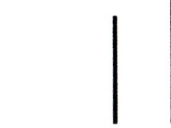 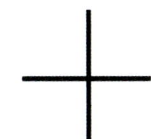 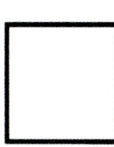

12. Pass any enclosed form. Fail continuous round motions.
13. Which line is longer? (Not bigger.) Turn paper upside down and repeat. (pass 3 of 3 or 5 of 6)
14. Pass any lines crossing near midpoint.
15. Have child copy first. If failed, demonstrate.

When giving items 12, 14, and 15, do not name the forms. Do not demonstrate 12 and 14.

16. When scoring, each pair (2 arms, 2 legs, etc.) counts as one part.
17. Place one cube in cup and shake gently near child's ear, but out of sight. Repeat for other ear.
18. Point to picture and have child name it. (No credit is given for sounds only.) If less than 4 pictures are named correctly, have child point to picture as each is named by tester.

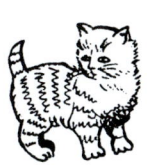 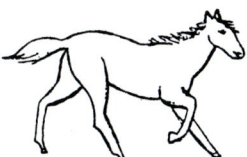 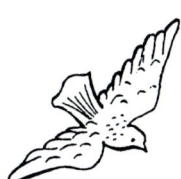 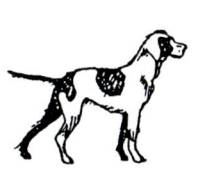 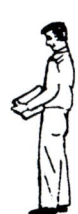

19. Using doll, tell child: Show me the nose, eyes, ears, mouth, hands, feet, tummy, hair. Pass 6 of 8.
20. Using pictures, ask child: Which one flies?… says meow?… talks?… barks?… gallops? Pass 2 of 5, 4 of 5.
21. Ask child: What do you do when you are cold?… tired?… hungry? Pass 2 of 3, 3 of 3.
22. Ask child: What do you do with a cup? What is a chair used for? What is a pencil used for? Action words must be included in answers.
23. Pass if child correctly places and says how many blocks are on paper. (1, 5).
24. Tell child: Put block on table; under table; in front of me, behind me. Pass 4 of 4. (Do not help child by pointing, moving head or eyes.)
25. Ask child: What is a ball?… lake?… desk?… house?… banana?… curtain?… fence?… ceiling? Pass if defined in terms of use, shape, what it is made of, or general category (such as banana is fruit, not just yellow). Pass 5 of 8, 7 of 8.
26. Ask child: If a horse is big, a mouse is__? If fire is hot, ice is__? If the sun shines during the day, the moon shines during the__? Pass 2 of 3.
27. Child may use wall or rail only, not person. May not crawl.
28. Child must throw ball overhand 3 ft to within arm's reach of tester.
29. Child must perform standing broad jump over width of test sheet (8 1/2 in).
30. Tell child to walk forward, ⚬⚬⚬⚬→ heel within 1 in of toe. Tester may demonstrate. Child must walk 4 consecutive steps.
31. In the second year, half of normal children are noncompliant.

OBSERVATIONS:

Concept Mastery Alert

A rigid abdomen in an infant is an emergency situation because it signifies peritoneal irritation from either blood or infection. A palpable mass would be cause for concern and would require referral, but it is not an emergency situation.

CASE STUDY

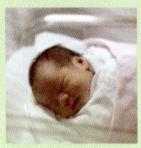

The chapter case study is now used to demonstrate the physical examination performed on Kaitlin when she was brought into the office for evaluation of jaundice. Performing a physical examination on a 4-day-old infant is best done when the infant is in a quiet and alert state.

At birth, her Apgar scores were 9 at 1 minute and 9 at 5 minutes.

For the physical examination, Kaitlin is placed on her back in the basinet, undressed except for her diaper, and a newborn blanket is draped over her to keep her warm. While she is quiet, her heart and lungs are auscultated with the stethoscope, with a heart rate of 150 beats/min, regular and without murmur. Her respiratory rate is 46 breaths/min, clear to auscultation, with regular and unlabored respirations. She is moving all extremities well, with arms and legs tucked close to the body. When touched on her arms or legs, she exerts resistance with movement and during examination begins to cry. Her hips are negative for Ortolani and Barlow maneuvers. Gluteal folds are symmetrical. Her skin is pink, with light-yellow discoloration on her feet, legs, and abdomen up to the nipple line on her chest. She has small amount of milia on her nose and a birthmark on her right elbow, tan macule with smooth borders, measuring 2 mm × 2 mm.

Vital signs are all within normal range.

Kaitlin is weighed and measured; she is 8 lb 5 oz, 21 in long. The circumference of her head and chest are 34 and 32 cm, respectively. She is AGA.

Her head is still slightly molded; her anterior and posterior fontanelles are smooth, flat, and appropriate for size. She has a 2-cm firm, palpable nodule on the right side of her scalp. She does not exhibit any signs of pain with palpation.

Her neck is full without masses, with full range of motion.

Eyes are clear; sclerae are white without jaundice.

Her face is symmetrical when smiling and crying. No edema of eyes or face. Ears are placed symmetrical, with the pinna equal to the eye-occipital line.

Ears are pink; tympanic membrane pink with landmarks visible. Mouth is pink, with pink gums, good suck reflex. Anterior/posterior palates are intact. Nose is clear, with patent nares. Neck is smooth; no palpable masses, no lymphadenopathy present. Clavicles are symmetrical. Chest expands equally with each respiration.

Lungs are clear to auscultation bilaterally. Heart with normal sinus rhythm, without murmur. All pulses (radial, brachial, femoral, popliteal, pedal) are palpable bilaterally. Nipple line symmetrical, with no palpable mass.

Abdomen is soft, nondistended, with active bowel sounds all quadrants. No palpable masses. Cord is drying, no drainage or erythema noted. Female genitalia with labia majora covering labia minora. No discharge or edema noted. Anus is pink and mother states that she has had several stools since delivery. Spine is closed, with normal curvature of the spine.

Validating and Documenting Findings

Validate the assessment data you have collected (by asking additional questions, verifying data with another health care professional, or comparing objective with subjective findings). This is necessary to verify that the data are reliable and accurate. Document the assessment data following the health care facility or agency policy.

CASE STUDY

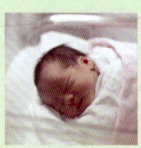

The nurse documents the following subjective and objective assessment findings of Kaitlin's infant examination.

Biographical data: Kaitlin is a 4-day-old infant being evaluated for jaundice. Her mother brings her into the office today and Kaitlin is calm, alert, and cooperative during the examination.

Reason for Seeking Care: "My daughter has been jaundiced for the past several days and I can't tell if it is getting worse or better."

The chapter case study is now used to demonstrate the physical examination performed on Kaitlin when she was brought into the office for evaluation of jaundice. Performing a physical examination on a 4-day-old infant is best done when the infant is in a quiet and alert state.

History of Present Health Concern: Mother states that Kaitlin's skin color has been yellow since discharge from the hospital. She is breastfeeding approximately every 2–3 hours each day. She is wetting approximately 8–10 diapers a day, with having at least two bowel movements daily.

Personal Health History: At birth, her Apgar scores were 9 at 1 minute and 9 at 5 minutes. Mother has not weighed infant since discharge from the hospital, but appears to be gaining weight and growing per mother. Her medical history is unremarkable. She is sleeping, eating, voiding, and having regular bowel habits. She has some colic in the early evening but is easy to console. No current medications. No known allergies. Mother states that at nighttime she will occasionally sleep longer and she is allowing her to do this, but not missing too many feedings. Mother also states that with the frequent feedings, mother has started to note some tenderness with her nipples, but is already improving.

Family History: Unremarkable for liver or pancreatic cancer.

Lifestyle and Health Practices: She is an infant, therefore she does not have any exposure to alcohol or tobacco. No exposure to alcohol or tobacco use in the household.

Physical Examination Findings: For the physical examination, Kaitlin is placed on her back in the basinet, undressed except for her diaper, and a newborn blanket is draped over her to keep her warm. While she is quiet, her heart and lungs are auscultated with the stethoscope, with a heart rate of 150 beats/min, regular and without murmur. Her respiratory rate is 46 breaths/min, clear to auscultation, with regular and unlabored respirations. She is moving all extremities well, with arms and legs tucked close to the body. When touched on her arms or legs, she exerts resistance with movement, and during examination begins to cry. Her hips are negative for Ortolani and Barlow maneuvers. Gluteal folds are symmetrical. Her skin is pink, with light yellow discoloration on her feet, legs, and abdomen up to the nipple line on her chest. She has small amount of milia on her nose and a birthmark on her right elbow, tan macule with smooth borders, measuring 2 mm × 2 mm.

Vital signs are all within normal range.

Kaitlin is weighed and measured; she is 8 lb 5 oz, 21 in long. The circumference of her head and chest are 34 and 32 cm, respectively. She is AGA.

Her head is still slightly molded; her anterior and posterior fontanelles are smooth, flat, and appropriate for size. She has a 2-cm, firm nodule on right side of her scalp.

Her neck is full without masses, with full range of motion.

Eyes are clear, sclerae are white without jaundice.

Her face is symmetrical when smiling and crying. No edema of eyes or face. Ears are placed symmetrical with the pinna equal to the eye-occipital line.

Ears are pink, tympanic membrane pink with landmarks visible. Mouth is pink, with pink gums, good suck reflex. Anterior/posterior palates are intact. Nose is clear, with patent nares. Neck is smooth; no palpable masses, no lymphadenopathy present. Clavicles are symmetrical. Chest expands equally with each respiration.

Lungs are clear to auscultation bilaterally. Heart with normal sinus rhythm, without murmur. All pulses (radial, brachial, femoral, popliteal, pedal) are palpable bilaterally. Nipple line symmetrical, with no palpable mass.

Abdomen is soft, nondistended, with active bowel sounds all quadrants. No palpable masses. Cord is drying; no drainage or erythema noted. Female genitalia with labia majora covering labia minora. No discharge or edema noted. Anus is pink and mother states that she has had several stools since delivery. Spine is closed, with normal curvature of the spine.

ANALYSIS OF DATA: DIAGNOSTIC REASONING

After collecting assessment data, analyze the data using diagnostic reasoning skills. Following are some possible conclusions that may be drawn after assessment of the newborn and infant.

Selected Nursing Diagnoses

Health Promotion Diagnoses

- Readiness for Enhanced Breastfeeding
- Readiness for Enhanced Parenting

Risk Diagnoses

- Risk for Impaired Skin Integrity related to allowing wet diaper to remain on baby for more than an hour at a time
- Risk for Ineffective Infant Feeding Pattern related to mother's lack of sleep and omitting feeding times during night
- Risk for Ineffective Breastfeeding related to fear of breastfeeding with sore nipples
- Risk for Disturbed Maternal-Fetal Dyad related to comorbidity in pregnancy

Actual Diagnoses

- Deficient Knowledge (family) regarding condition, treatment, prognosis of infant related to unfamiliar diagnosis of jaundice

Selected Collaborative Problems

After grouping the data, it may become apparent that certain collaborative problems emerge. Remember that collaborative problems differ from nursing diagnoses in that they cannot be prevented with nursing interventions alone. However, these physiologic complications of medical conditions can be detected and monitored by the nurse. In addition, the nurse can use physician- and nurse-prescribed interventions to minimize the complications of these problems. The nurse may also have to refer the client in such situations for further treatment of the problem. Following is a list of collaborative problems seen more frequently in the newborn or infant. However, other collaborative problems seen in the adult are also seen in pediatric clients. These problems are worded as Risk for Complications (RC) followed by the problem.

- RC: Hypoglycemia
- RC: Thrush
- RC: Subconjunctival hemorrhage
- RC: Hip displacement
- RC: Failure to thrive
- RC: Kernicterus
- RC: Skin rash

Medical Problems

After grouping the data, the client's signs and symptoms may clearly require medical diagnosis and treatment. Referral to a primary care provider is necessary.

CASE STUDY

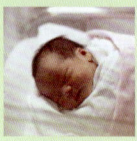

After collecting and analyzing the data for Kaitlin, the nurse determines that the following conclusions are appropriate:

Nursing Diagnoses
- Risk for Injury r/t side effects of phototherapy treatment
- Readiness for Enhanced Knowledge (how to recognize worsening jaundice in newborn)

Potential Collaborative Problems
- RC: Neonatal jaundice

To view an algorithm depicting the process of diagnostic reasoning for this case, go to **thePoint**.

Interdisciplinary Verbal Communication of Assessment Findings Using SBAR

SITUATION: Kaitlin, a 4-day-old female, is brought to clinic by mother for the faint yellowing discoloration of her skin on her feet, legs, abdomen, and chest that has not improved over last 2 days since she was discharged from hospital. Yellow discoloration is progressing up her body.

BACKGROUND: Mother is 28-year-old gravida 1, para 1 who had an uneventful pregnancy with a vaginal term delivery (39 weeks' gestation). Kaitlin weighed 8 lb 10 oz (AGA). Breastfeeding every 3–4 hours since birth. Wets 8–10 diapers a day and has stools 2–3 times a day. Apgar scores were 9 at 1 minute and 9 at 5 minutes. Has some colic in the early evening but easy to console.

ASSESSMENT: 8 lb 5 oz, 21 in long. Head and chest circumference: 34 and 32 cm, respectively. Heart rate 150 beats/min, regular without murmur; respiratory rate 46 breaths/min, clear to auscultation, with regular and unlabored respirations. Skin is pink, with light yellow discoloration on her feet, legs, and abdomen up to the nipple line on her chest. Has small amount of milia on nose and a birthmark on her right elbow, tan macule with smooth borders, measuring 2 mm × 2 mm. She has molding of the head with a cephalohematoma on right anterior scalp, that "has been gradually improving since delivery." She has a 2-cm, firm nodule on right side of her scalp. Sclerae white without jaundice.

RECOMMENDATION: Kaitlin is at risk for injury r/t side effects of phototherapy treatment. Her mother is ready for enhanced knowledge (how to recognize worsening jaundice in newborn). She needs to be further evaluated for neonatal jaundice.

Want to know more?

A wide variety of resources to enhance your learning and understanding of this book are available on **thePoint**. Visit thePoint to access:

- NCLEX-Style Student Review Questions
- Watch and Learn Videos
- Concept in Action Animations
- And more!

References and Selected Readings

Apgar, V. (1953, July, August). A proposal for a new method of evaluation of the newborn infant. *Current Researchers in Anesthesia and Analgesia.* Available at http://profiles.nlm.nih.gov/ps/access/CPBBKG.pdf

Ballard, J. L., Khoury, J. C., Wedig, K., Want, L., Eilers-Walsman, B. L., & Lipp, R. (1991). New Ballard score: Expanded to include extremely premature infants. *Journal of Pediatrics, 19*(3), 417–423.

Centers for Disease Control and Prevention (CDC). (2015). Vitamin D supplementation. Available at https://www.cdc.gov/breastfeeding/recommendations/vitamin_d.htm

Mayo Clinic. (2012). Pyloric stenosis. Available at http://www.mayoclinic.org/diseases-conditions/pyloric-stenosis/symptoms-causes/dxc-20163857

Mayo Clinic. (2016). Solid foods: How to get your baby started. Available at http://www.mayoclinic.org/healthy-lifestyle/infant-and-toddler-health/in-depth/healthy-baby/art-20046200

On Track. (n.d.). Children's development: Infants (0–14 months): Signs of atypical development in infants. Available at http://www.beststart.org/OnTrack_English/3-infant.html

PedsCases. (2016). Pediatric vital signs reference chart. Available at http://www.pedscases.com/pediatric-vital-signs-reference-chart

Rashad, M., & El-Fiky, S. (2007). Prevalence of renal anomalies in children with auricular malformations among attendance of Genetics Clinic in Ain Shams University. *Egyptian Journal of Medical Human Genetics. 8*(2). Available at http://www.ajol.info/index.php/ejhg/article/view/42618

Strobbe, M. (2014, December 2). CDC: Circumcision outweighs risks. Available at https://www.yahoo.com/news/cdc-circumcision-benefits-outweigh-risks-134651002.html?ref=gs

The Royal College of Midwives. (2012). Maternal emotional wellbeing and infant development. Available at https://www.rcm.org.uk/sites/default/files/Emotional%20Wellbeing_Guide_WEB.pdf

31 ASSESSING CHILDREN AND ADOLESCENTS

Learning Objectives

1. Describe the physical, motor, cognitive, language, psychosocial, psychosexual, and moral growth and development of children and adolescents.
2. Interview children, adolescents, and their parents or caregivers as appropriate for an accurate nursing history.
3. Perform a physical assessment of children and adolescents using the correct techniques.
4. Differentiate between normal and abnormal findings of children and adolescents.
5. Describe the findings frequently seen with assessing children and adolescents.
6. Analyze the data from the interview and physical assessment of children and adolescents to formulate valid nursing diagnoses, collaborative problems, and/or referrals.
7. Communicate interview and assessment findings through clear concise documentation and verbal reports.

CASE STUDY

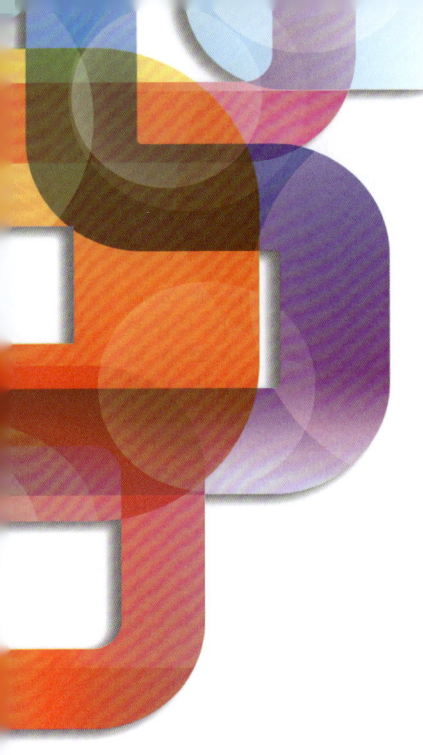

Carsen is a 13-year-old boy who presents with his mother for a well-child visit. Current health and illness status: Has been well since last health care visit at age 12 years; currently complaining of right ear pain, runny nose, and cough. No other health concerns or medications.

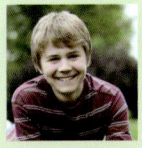

GROWTH AND DEVELOPMENT

Physical Development

Skin, Hair, and Nails

During early childhood, the skin develops a tighter bond with the dermis, making it more resistant to infection, irritation, and fluid loss. Skin color appears pink and evenly distributed and may include normal variations such as freckles. The texture is smooth because the skin has not had years of exposure to the environment and because the hair is less coarse than in adulthood. The sebaceous glands and eccrine glands are minimally active, with the eccrine glands producing little sweat.

During the toddler years, scalp hair grows coarser, thicker, and darker, and usually loses curliness. Fine hair becomes visible on the distal portions of the upper and lower extremities.

As the child ages, skin structure and function remain stable until puberty, when adrenarche (adrenocortical maturation) signals the onset of increased sebum production from the sebaceous glands, a process that continues until late adolescence. Sebum is involved in the development of acne. The apocrine glands also respond more to emotional stimulation and heat, with the end result being body odor.

Head and Neck

During infancy, body growth predominates and the head grows proportionately to body size, reaching 90% of its full adult size by age 6 years. Facial bone growth is variable, especially for the nasal and jaw bones. During the toddler years, the nasal bridge is low and the mandible and maxilla are small, making the face seem small compared with the whole skull. During the school-age years, the face grows proportionately faster than the rest of the cranium, and secondary teeth appear too large for the face. In adolescence, the nose and thyroid cartilage enlarge in boys. Lymph tissue is well developed at birth and continues to grow rapidly until age 10 or 11 years, exceeding adult size before puberty, after which the tissue atrophies and stabilizes to adult dimensions by the end of adolescence.

Eyes

During childhood, the eyes are less spherical than adult eyes. In addition, children remain farsighted until age 6 or 7 years, when they achieve a visual acuity of 20/20.

Ears

As the child grows, the inner ear matures. In older children, the eustachian tube lengthens but it may become occluded from growth of lymphatic tissue, specifically the adenoids. The canal shortens and straightens as the child ages, and the pinna can be pulled up and back as in the adult.

Mouth, Nose, Throat, and Sinuses

Children have 20 deciduous teeth, which are lost between the ages of 6 and 12 years. Permanent teeth begin forming in the

761

jaw by age 6 months and begin to replace temporary teeth at age 6 years, usually starting with the central incisors. Permanent teeth appear earlier in African Americans than in Caucasians and in girls before boys.

Nasal cartilage grows during adolescence with the secondary sex characteristics. Growth starts at age 12 or 13 years and reaches full size by 16 years in girls and 18 years in boys. The maxillary and ethmoid sinuses are present at birth, but they are small and cannot be examined until they develop, when the child is much older. The frontal sinuses develop around ages 7 to 8 years, and the sphenoid sinuses develop after puberty.

The tonsils and adenoids rapidly grow, reaching maximum development by ages 10 to 12 years. At this point, they may be about twice their adult size. However, as with other lymphoid tissue, tonsils and adenoids atrophy to stable adult dimensions by the end of adolescence.

Thorax and Lungs

The lungs continue to develop after birth, and new alveoli form until about 8 years of age. Thus, in a child with pulmonary damage or disease at birth, pulmonary tissue may regenerate and the lungs can eventually attain normal respiratory function. The child will have 300 million alveoli by adolescence.

The chest wall is thin, with very little musculature. The ribs are soft and pliable, with the xiphoid process movable. The airways of children are also smaller and narrower than in adults; therefore, children are at risk for airway obstruction from edema and infections in the lungs. A child's respiratory rate is much faster than an adult's rate: children younger than 7 years tend to be abdominal breathers. In children between 8 and 10 years of age, respiratory rates lower and breathing becomes thoracic, like adults' breathing.

Breasts

In girls, breast growth is stimulated by estrogen at the onset of puberty. Between 8 and 13 years of age, thelarche (breast development) may occur; breasts continue to develop in stages (Table 31-1). Breasts enlarge primarily as a result of fat deposits. However, the duct system also grows and branches, and masses of small cells develop at the duct endings. These masses are potential alveoli. Tenderness and asymmetric development are common, and anticipatory guidance and reassurance are needed. Gynecomastia, enlargement of breast tissue in boys, may be noted in some male adolescents. This is related to pubertal changes and is usually temporary. However, use of marijuana and anabolic steroids are two of several external causes of gynecomastia.

Heart

In children, the heart is positioned more horizontally in the chest. The apical impulse is felt at the 4th intercostal space left of the mid-clavicular line in young children. By the time the child is 7 years old, the apical pulse reaches the 5th intercostal space and the mid-clavicular line. Heart sounds are louder, higher pitched, and of shorter duration in children. Physiologic splitting of the second sound, which widens with inspiration, may be heard in the second left intercostal space. A third heart sound (S_3) may be heard at the apex and is present in one third of all children.

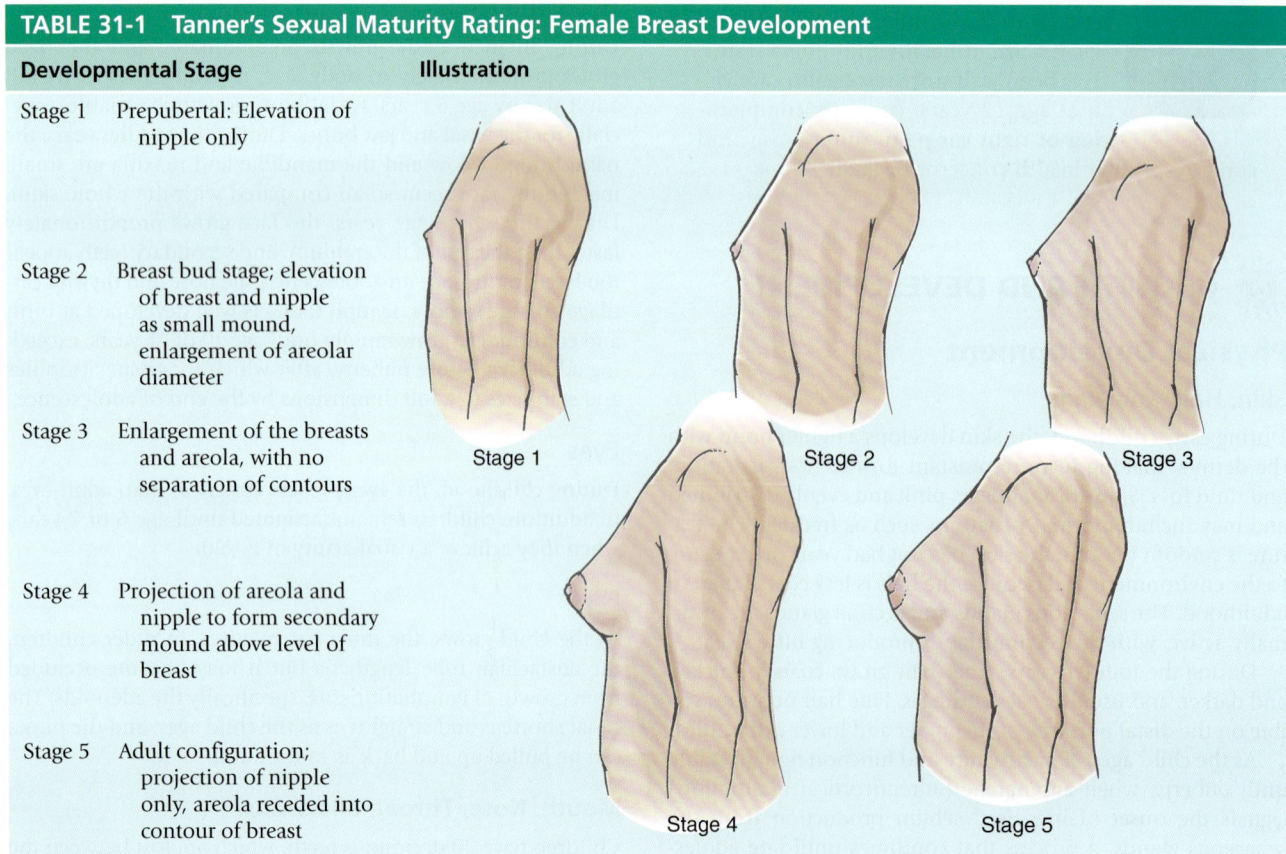

TABLE 31-1 Tanner's Sexual Maturity Rating: Female Breast Development

Developmental Stage		Illustration
Stage 1	Prepubertal: Elevation of nipple only	
Stage 2	Breast bud stage; elevation of breast and nipple as small mound, enlargement of areolar diameter	
Stage 3	Enlargement of the breasts and areola, with no separation of contours	
Stage 4	Projection of areola and nipple to form secondary mound above level of breast	
Stage 5	Adult configuration; projection of nipple only, areola receded into contour of breast	

Tanner, J. M. (1962). *Growth at adolescence* (2nd ed.). Oxford: Blackwell Scientific Publications.

Sinus arrhythmia is normal and reaches its greatest degree during adolescence. Some children may have physiologic murmurs that do not indicate disease. The heart rate decreases as the child gets older, usually dropping to about 85 beats/min by 8 years of age. Athletic adolescents may have even lower heart rates.

Abdomen

The abdomen of small children is cylindrical, prominent in the standing position, and flat when supine. The abdomen of toddlers appears prominent and gives the child what is popularly called a pot-belly appearance. The contours of the abdomen change to adult shapes during adolescence. Peristaltic waves may be visible in thin children; they may also be indicative of a disease or disorder.

The tip of the right kidney may be felt in young children, especially during inspiration.

In small children, the liver is palpable at 1 to 2 cm below the right costal margin. The spleen may be palpable below the left costal margin at 1 to 2 cm. Often, in older children these structures are not palpable.

Genitalia

Male genitalia generally develop over a 2- to 5-year period, beginning from preadolescence to adulthood. In the adolescent male, enlargement of the testes is an early sign of puberty, occurring between the ages of 9.5 and 13.5 years. Pubic hair signifies the onset of puberty in boys. Pubic hair development and penile enlargement are concurrent with testicular growth (Table 31-2). Axillary hair development occurs late in puberty. It follows definitive penile and testicular enlargement in boys. Facial hair in boys also develops at this time. The onset of spontaneous nocturnal emission of seminal fluid is a sign of puberty similar to menarche in females. During puberty, the prostate gland grows rapidly to twice its prepubertal size under the influence of androgens.

In female adolescents, puberty is the time that estrogen stimulates the development of the reproductive tract and secondary sex characteristics. The external genitalia increase in size and sensitivity, whereas the internal reproductive organs increase in weight and mass. Pubic hair begins growing early in puberty (2 to 6 months after thelarche) and follows a distinct

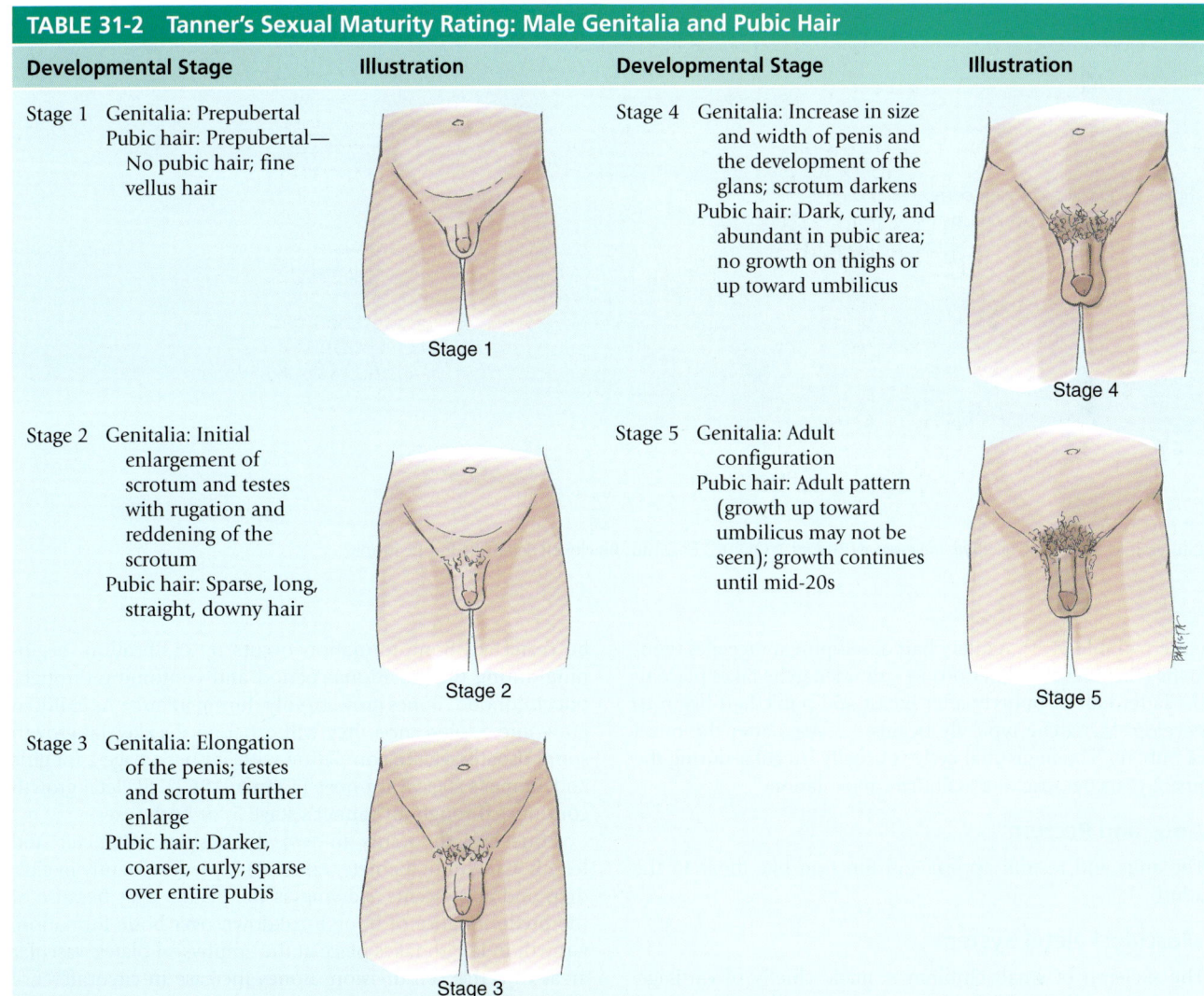

TABLE 31-2 Tanner's Sexual Maturity Rating: Male Genitalia and Pubic Hair

Developmental Stage	Illustration	Developmental Stage	Illustration
Stage 1 — Genitalia: Prepubertal; Pubic hair: Prepubertal—No pubic hair; fine vellus hair	Stage 1	Stage 4 — Genitalia: Increase in size and width of penis and the development of the glans; scrotum darkens. Pubic hair: Dark, curly, and abundant in pubic area; no growth on thighs or up toward umbilicus	Stage 4
Stage 2 — Genitalia: Initial enlargement of scrotum and testes with rugation and reddening of the scrotum. Pubic hair: Sparse, long, straight, downy hair	Stage 2	Stage 5 — Genitalia: Adult configuration. Pubic hair: Adult pattern (growth up toward umbilicus may not be seen); growth continues until mid-20s	Stage 5
Stage 3 — Genitalia: Elongation of the penis; testes and scrotum further enlarge. Pubic hair: Darker, coarser, curly; sparse over entire pubis	Stage 3		

Tanner, J. M. (1962). *Growth at adolescence* (2nd ed.). Oxford, England: Blackwell Scientific Publications.

TABLE 31-3 Tanner's Sexual Maturity Rating: Female Pubic Hair

Developmental Stage	Illustration	Developmental Stage	Illustration
Stage 1 Prepubertal: No pubic hair; fine vellus hair		Stage 4 Dark, curly, and abundant on mons pubis; no growth on medial thighs	
Stage 2 Sparse, long, straight, downy hair		Stage 5 Adult pattern of inverse triangle; growth on medial thighs	
Stage 3 Darker, coarser, curly; sparse over mons pubis			

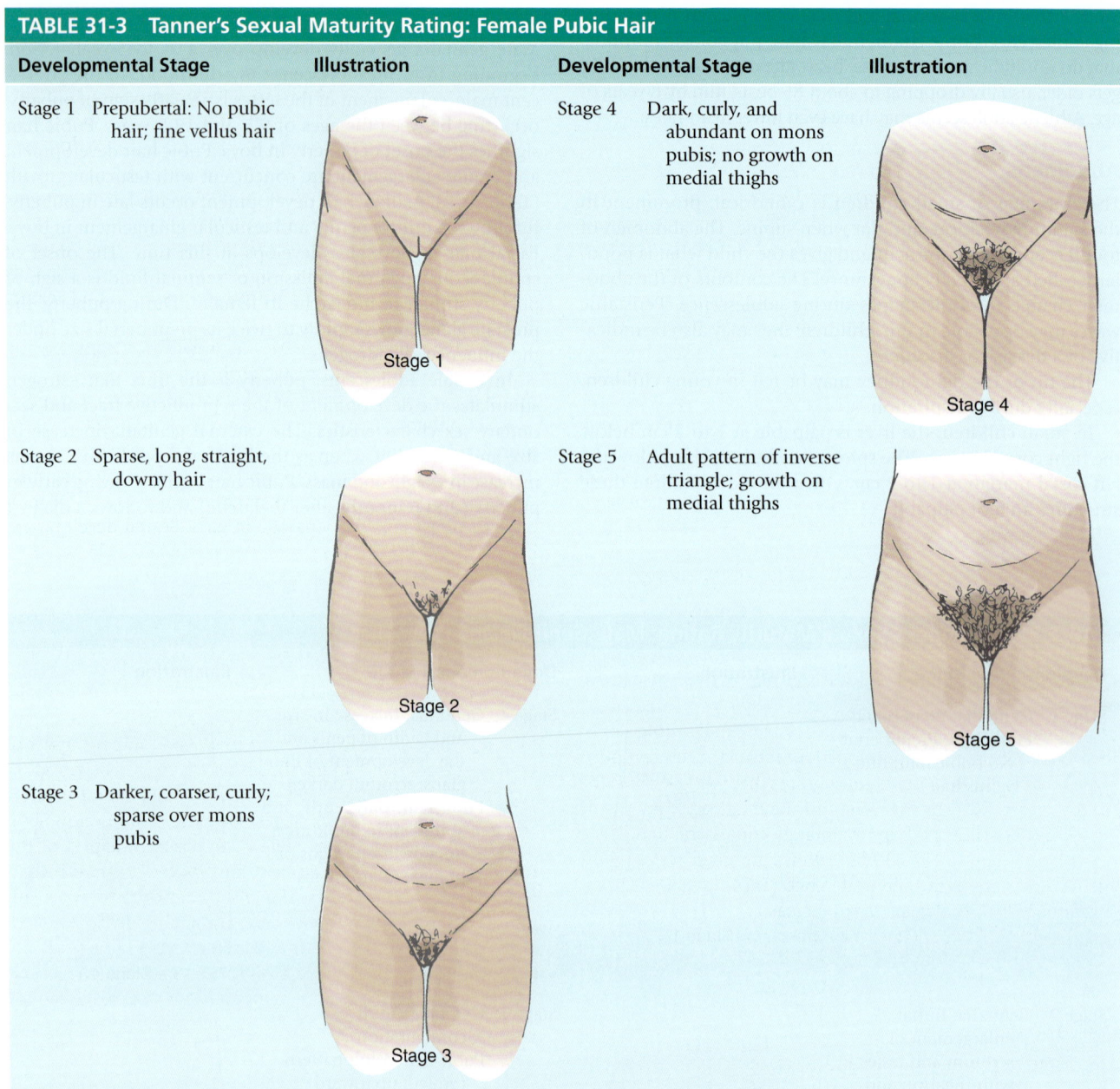

Tanner, J. M. (1962). *Growth at adolescence* (2nd ed.). Oxford, England: Blackwell Scientific Publications.

pattern (Table 31-3). Axillary hair development precedes menarche (first menstrual period) in girls. Menarche takes place in the latter half of puberty after breast and pubic hair begin to develop. Menarche typically begins 2.5 years after the onset of puberty. The menstrual cycle is usually irregular during the first 2 years because of physiologic anovulation.

Anus and Rectum
The anus and rectum appear and function like those in the adult.

Musculoskeletal System
The skeleton of small children is made chiefly of cartilage, accounting for the relative softness and malleability of the bones and the relative ease with which certain deformities can be corrected. Bone formation occurs by ossification, beginning during the gestational period and continuing throughout childhood. Bones grow rapidly during infancy. As children grow into adolescence, they will experience a skeletal growth spurt, usually seen in correlation with Tanner's stage 2 for girls and Tanner's stage 3 for boys (Tanner, 1962). Skeletal growth continues throughout Tanner's stage 5 for both sexes.

Bone growth occurs in two dimensions: diameter and length. Growth in diameter takes place predominantly in children and adolescents, slowing as the person ages because of the predominance of bone breakdown over bone formation. Growth in length takes place at the epiphyseal plates, vascular areas of active cell division. Bones increase in circumference and length under the influence of hormones, primarily pituitary growth hormone and thyroid hormone.

Muscle growth is related to growth of the underlying bone. Individual fibers, ligaments, and tendons grow throughout childhood. Bone and muscle development is influenced by use of the extremities. If extremities are not used, minimal growth of the muscle will occur. Walking and weight-bearing activities stimulate bone and muscle growth.

The anterior curve in the lumbar region of the vertebral column develops between the ages of 12 and 18 months, when the toddler starts to stand erect and walk.

Muscle growth contributes significantly to weight gain in the child. Individual fibers grow throughout childhood, and growth is considerable during the adolescent growth spurt, which usually peaks at 12 years in girls and 14 years in boys.

Neurologic System

Motor control develops in a head-to-neck to trunk-to-extremities sequence. Development takes place in an orderly progression, but each child develops at his or her own pace. The norms demonstrate wide variation among individuals as well as within a single individual under different circumstances.

Growth Patterns

Pediatric growth charts are available at http://www.cdc.gov/growthcharts.

Toddlers

Height and weight increase in a step-like rather than linear fashion, reflecting the growth spurts and lags characteristic of toddlerhood. The toddler's characteristic protruding abdomen results from underdeveloped abdominal muscles. Bow-leggedness typically persists through toddlerhood because the leg muscles must bear the weight of the relatively large trunk. The height at age 2 years approximately equals one half of the child's adult height. The child's birth weight quadruples by the age of 2.5 years. Head circumference (HC) equals chest circumference by 1 to 2 years. Total increase in HC in the second year of life is 2.5 cm; the rate then increases slowly at 0.5 in per year until the age of 5 years. Primary dentition (20 deciduous teeth) is completed by the age of 2.5 years.

Preschoolers

Preschoolers are generally slender, graceful, and agile. The average 4-year-old is 101.25 cm tall and weighs 16.8 kg (37 lb).

School-Age Children

During the school-age period, girls often grow faster than boys, often surpassing boys in height and weight. During preadolescence extending from about ages 10 to 13, children commonly experience rapid and uneven growth compared with age mates. The average 6-year-old child is 112.5 cm tall and weighs 21 kg (46 lb), whereas the average 12-year-old child is 147.5 cm tall and weighs 40 kg (88 lb). Beginning around age 6, permanent teeth erupt and deciduous teeth are gradually lost. Caries, malocclusion, and periodontal disease become evident.

Adolescents

From 20% to 25% of adult height is achieved in adolescence. Girls grow 5 to 20 cm until about age 16 or 17. Boys grow 10 to 30 cm until about 18 or 20 years of age. From 30% to 50% of adult weight is achieved during adolescence (http://www.cdc.gov/growthcharts). Adolescence encompasses puberty—the period during which primary and secondary sex characteristics begin to develop and reach maturity. In girls, puberty begins between the ages of 8 and 14 years, and is completed within 3 years. In boys, puberty begins between the ages of 9 and 16 years, and is completed by age 18 or 19 years. During adolescence, hormonal influence causes important developmental changes.

Body mass reaches adult size, sebaceous glands become active, and eccrine sweat glands become fully functional. Apocrine sweat glands develop, and hair grows in the axillae, areola of the breast, and genital and anal regions. Body hair assumes characteristic distribution patterns and texture changes (see Tables 31-1, 31-2, and 31-3).

During puberty, girls experience growth in height, weight, breast development, and pelvic girth with expansion of uterine tissue. Menarche typically occurs about 2.5 years after onset of puberty. Boys experience increases in height, weight, muscle mass, and penis and testicle size. Facial and body hair growth and voice deepening also occur. The onset of spontaneous nocturnal emissions of seminal fluid is an overt sign of puberty, analogous to menarche in girls. Sexual development is evaluated by noting the specific stages that take place in boys and girls.

Motor Development

Nurses must possess baseline knowledge of the fundamental principles of motor development, sensory perception, cognitive and language development, moral development, psychosocial development and psychosexual development as well as strategies for assessment and client teaching. Several theories exist regarding the various stages and phases of development. It is suggested that nurses review the basic principles of the major theorists, such as Erikson and Piaget, to refresh their frames of reference. Information about these theorists is readily accessible in any basic or developmental psychology text. The Denver Developmental Screening Test is also available for guidance when assessing the child's motor, language, and social development at each particular age (see Chapter 30, Assessment Tool 30-1).

Toddlers

Motor development should be evaluated at well-child visits. Using the Denver Developmental Tool can assist the nurse in noting the developmental milestones of the child at the particular age.

The major gross motor skill is locomotion. At 15 months, toddlers walk without help (Fig. 31-1). At 18 months, they walk upstairs with one hand held. At 24 months, toddlers walk up and down stairs one step at a time. At 30 months, they jump with both feet.

Fifteen-month-old toddlers can build a two-block tower and scribble spontaneously. At 18 months, they can build a three- to four-block tower. Toddlers at 24 months imitate a vertical stroke; at 30 months, they build an eight-block tower and copy a cross.

Sample questions for toddlerhood include:
- When did your child first walk?
- Can your toddler walk up and down steps?
- Can your toddler jump with both feet?
- Does your toddler spontaneously scribble?

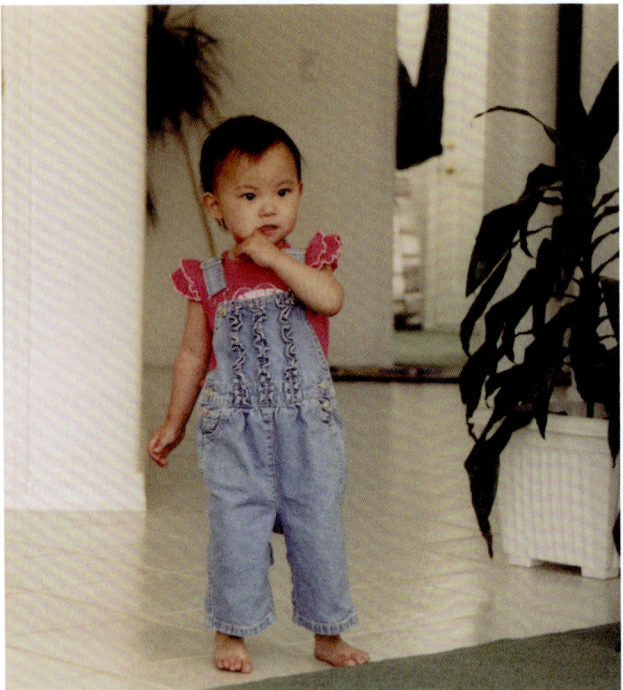

FIGURE 31-1 The toddler is proud of her ability to stand and walk without help.

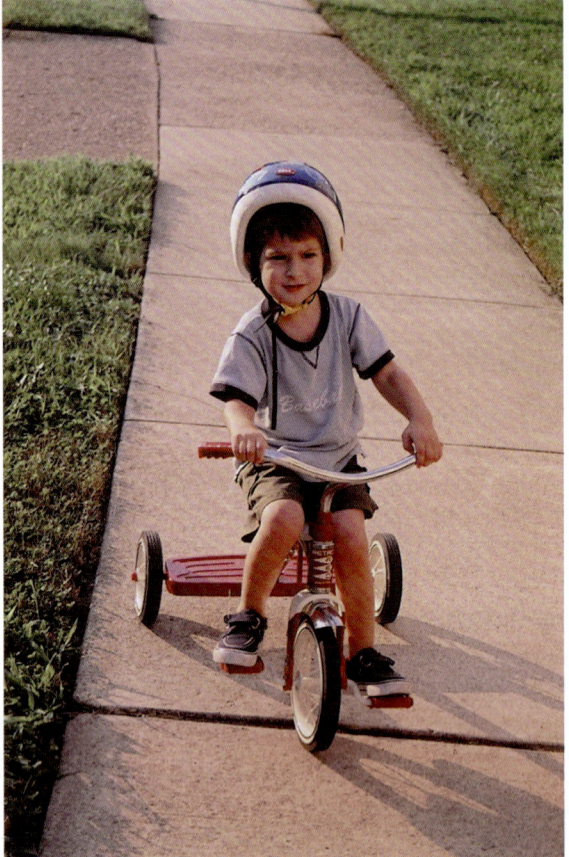

FIGURE 31-2 This preschooler enjoys riding a tricycle.

Preschoolers

At 3 years old, children can ride a tricycle (Fig. 31-2), go upstairs using alternate feet, stand on one foot for a few seconds, and broad jump. Four-year-old children can skip, hop on one foot, catch a ball, and go downstairs using alternate feet. At 5 years, children can skip on alternate feet, throw and catch a ball, jump rope, and balance on alternate feet with eyes closed.

Three-year-old children can build a tower of up to 10 blocks, build three-block bridges, copy a circle, and imitate a cross. At 4 years old, children can lace shoes, copy a square shape, trace a diamond shape, and add three parts to a stick figure. Five-year-old children can tie shoelaces, use scissors well, copy diamond and triangle shapes, add seven to nine parts to a stick figure, and print a few letters and numbers and their first name.

Sample questions for preschoolers include:
- Can your preschooler run, hop, and skip?
- Can your preschooler lace shoes?
- Can your preschooler write his or her first name?

School-Age Children

Skills acquired during the school years include bicycling, rollerskating, rollerblading, and skateboarding. Running and jumping improve progressively, and swimming is added to the child's repertoire.

Printing skills develop in the early school years; script skills in later years. School-age children also develop greater dexterity and competence for crafts (Fig. 31-3), video games, and computers.

Sample questions for school-age children include:
- Can your school-age child ride a bicycle?
- Can your school-age child write script?

Adolescents

Gross motor skills have reached adult levels, and fine motor skills continue to be refined.

Sample questions for the adolescent include:
- Does your adolescent have a job, hobby, or interest that involves hand skills? If so, how is his or her performance?
- Does your adolescent participate in sports?

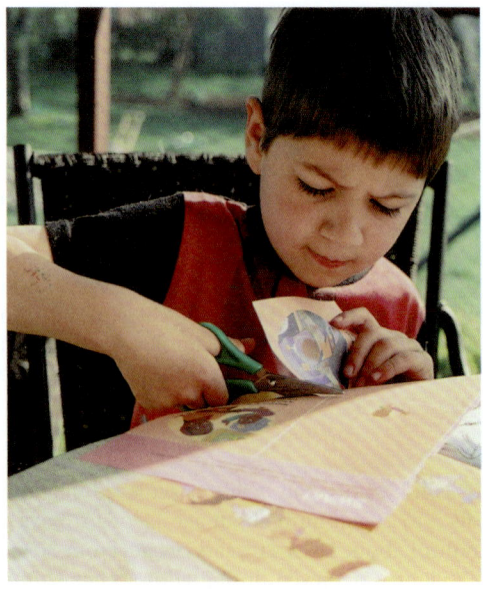

FIGURE 31-3 This 6-year-old enjoys cutting shapes with safety scissors.

Sensory Perception

Toddlers

Toddlers' visual acuity and depth perception improve, and they are able to recall visual images. Toddlers begin learning the ability to listen and comprehend. As every parent knows, listening is different from hearing. This ability includes attending to what is heard, discriminating sound qualities, creating cognitive associations with previous learning, and remembering. The olfactory and gustatory senses are influenced by voluntary control, and are associated with other sensory and motor areas. Therefore, toddlers refuse to eat anything that looks unpleasant to them. Children also begin to learn conditioned reactions to odors at this age.

Preschoolers

Color and depth perception become fully developed. Preschoolers may be aware of visual difficulties. Hearing reaches its maximum level and listening further develops. Preschoolers usually enjoy vision and hearing testing.

School-Age Children

Visual capacity reaches adult level (20/20) by age 6 or 7 years. Hearing acuity is almost complete.

Adolescents

All senses have reached their mature capacity by adolescence.
Sample questions to assess for vision problems include:
- Does your child frequently rub the eyes?
- Does your child become irritable with close work?
- Does your child blink repeatedly?
- Does your child ever appear cross-eyed?
- Does your child strain to see distant objects or sit close to the TV?
- Does your child reverse letters or numbers?
- Does your child ever complain of headache?

Sample questions to assess for hearing deficits include:
- Does your child respond to verbal commands? (Remember that we can only test hearing, not listening.)
- Does your child sit too close to the TV?
- Does your adolescent blast the stereo? (This may not indicate a hearing deficit, as it is typical behavior; however, it can lead to hearing deficit.)
- Does your child have any speech difficulties?

Sample questions to assess sense of smell and taste include:
- Does your child ever complain of having difficulty with his sense of smell?
- Does your child experience difficulty with taste?

Cognitive and Language Development

Toddlers

The sensorimotor phase (between ages 12 and 24 months) involves two substages in toddlerhood: tertiary circular reactions (ages 12 to 18 months) involving trial-and-error experimentation and relentless exploration and mental combinations (ages 18 to 24 months) during which the toddler begins to devise new means for accomplishing tasks through mental calculations. Toddlers go through a preconceptual substage of the preoperational phase typical of preschoolers. During this time, the child uses representational thought to recall the past, represent the present, and anticipate the future. As toddlers get older, they begin to enter the preoperational phase. This phase is described in the following section on preschoolers.

At 15 months, toddlers use expressive jargon. At 2 years, they say 300 words and use 2- to 3-word phrases and pronouns. At 2.5 years, toddlers give their first and last names and use plurals.

Sample nursing history questions for toddlers include:
- Can your toddler name some body parts?
- Can your toddler state first and last name?
- Does your toddler imitate adults?
- Does your toddler put two words together to form a sentence? (e.g., "me go")?

Preschoolers

This stage of preoperational thought (ages 2 to 7 years) consists of two phases. In the preconceptual phase, extending from ages 2 to 4, the child forms concepts that are not as complete or logical as an adult's; makes simple classifications; associates one event with a simultaneous one (transductive reasoning); and exhibits egocentric thinking.

In the intuitive phase extending from ages 4 to 7, the child becomes capable of classifying, quantifying, and relating objects but remains unaware of the principles behind these operations; exhibits intuitive thought processes (is aware that something is right but cannot say why); is unable to see viewpoint of others; and uses many words appropriately but without a real knowledge of their meaning. Preschoolers exhibit magical thinking and believe that thoughts are all powerful. They may feel guilty and responsible for bad thoughts, which, at times, may coincide with the occurrence of a wished event (e.g., wishing a sibling was dead and the sibling suddenly needs to be hospitalized).

Three-year-old children can say 900 words, 3- to 4-word sentences, and can talk incessantly. Four-year-old children can say 1,500 words, tell exaggerated stories, and sing simple songs. This is also the peak age for "why" questions. Five-year-old children can say 2,100 words, and know four or more colors, the names of the days of the week, and the months.

Sample questions for preschoolers include:
- Does your preschooler tell fantasy stories or have an imaginary friend?
- Does your preschooler have an invisible friend?
- Can your preschooler make simple classifications (e.g., dogs and cats)?
- Is your preschooler "chatty"? Does your preschooler frequently ask "why?"
- Can your preschooler name at least four colors?

School-Age Children

A child aged 7 to 11 years is in the stage of concrete operations marked by inductive reasoning, logical operations, and reversible concrete thought. Specific characteristics of this stage include movement from egocentric to objective thinking: seeing another's point of view; seeking validation and asking questions; focusing on immediate physical reality with inability to transcend the here and now; difficulty dealing with remote, future, or hypothetical matters; development of various mental classifying and ordering activities; and development of the principle of conservation of volume, weight, mass, and numbers. Typical activities of a child at this stage may include collecting and sorting objects (e.g., baseball cards, dolls, marbles); ordering items according to size, shape, weight, and other criteria; and considering options and variables when problem solving. Electronic games (X-Box, PlayStation) are popular with this age group.

Children develop formal adult articulation patterns by the ages of 7 to 9 years. They learn that words can be arranged in terms of structure. The ability to read is one of the most significant skills learned during these years (Fig. 31-4).

Sample questions for school-age children include:
- Can your school-age child see another's point of view?
- Does your school-age child collect things (e.g., baseball cards, dolls)?
- Does your school-age child try to solve problems?
- How well does your school-age child do in school? (Also ask school-age child and compare the answers.)
- How well does your school-age child read?

Adolescents

In the development of formal operations, which commonly occurs from the ages of 11 to 15 years, the adolescent develops abstract reasoning. This period consists of three substages:
- Substage 1: The adolescent sees relationships involving the inverse of the reciprocal.
- Substage 2: The adolescent develops the ability to order triads of propositions or relationships.
- Substage 3: The adolescent develops the capacity for true formal thought.

In true formal thought, the adolescent thinks beyond the present and forms theories about everything, delighting especially in considerations of "that which is not." However, adolescents in this age group do not have futuristic thoughts. They do not relate current events "here and now" to long-term results (2 years from now). An example of this includes teenagers who are sexually active and who may not consider the consequences of sexual activity (pregnancy and parenthood).

Sample nursing history questions for adolescents include:
- Do you consider your adolescent to be a problem solver?
- How well does your adolescent do in school? (Also ask the adolescent and compare the responses.)

Moral Development (Kohlberg)

(see Chapter 7 for in-depth discussion and references)

Toddler

A toddler is typically at the first substage of the preconventional stage involving punishment and obedience orientation in which he or she makes judgments on the basis of avoiding punishment or obtaining a reward. Discipline patterns affect a toddler's moral development. For example, physical punishment and withholding privileges tend to give the toddler a negative view of morals; withholding love and affection as punishment leads to feelings of guilt in the toddler. Appropriate disciplinary actions include providing simple explanations about why certain behaviors are unacceptable, praising appropriate behavior, and using distraction when the toddler is headed for danger.

Preschooler

A preschooler is in the preconventional stage of moral development, which extends to 10 years. In this phase, conscience emerges, and the emphasis is on external control. The child's moral standards are those of others, and he or she observes them either to avoid punishment or reap rewards.

School-Age Child

A child at the conventional level of the role conformity stage (generally ages 10 to 13 years) has an increased desire to please others. The child observes and, to some extent, externalizes the standards of others. The child wants to be considered "good" by those people whose opinion matters to the child.

Adolescent

Development of the postconventional level of morality occurs at about age 13, marked by the development of an individual conscience and a defined set of moral values. For the first time, the adolescent can acknowledge a conflict between two socially accepted standards and try to decide between them. Control of conduct is now internal, both in standards observed and in reasoning about right or wrong.

Sample nursing history questions for toddlerhood through adolescence include:
- Does your child understand the difference between right and wrong?
- Do you discuss family values with your child?
- Do you have family rules? How are they implemented?
- How are disciplinary measures handled?
- Has your child ever had any problems with lying, cheating, or stealing?
- Has your child ever required disciplinary action at school?
- Has your child ever violated the law?

For a more in-depth discussion of Kohlberg, see Chapter 7.

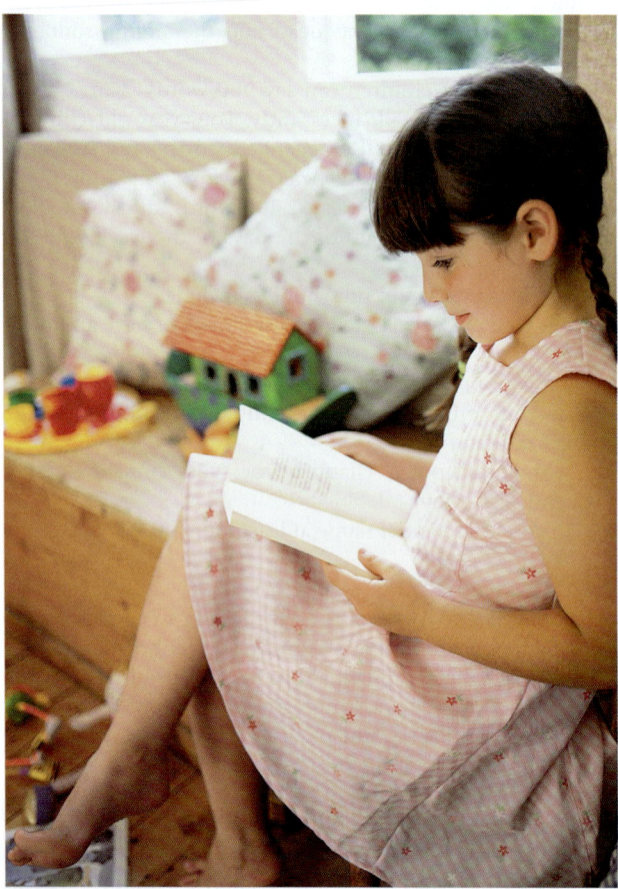

FIGURE 31-4 Reading is a milestone achievement for a school-age child.

Psychosocial Development (Erikson)

(see Chapter 7 for in-depth discussion and references)

Toddler

Erikson terms the psychosocial crises facing a child between ages 1 and 3 years *autonomy versus shame and doubt*. The psychosocial theme is "to hold on; to let go." The toddler has developed a sense of trust and is ready to give up dependence to assert a budding sense of control, independence, and autonomy (Fig. 31-5). The toddler begins to master the following:
- Individuation—differentiation of self from others
- Separation from parent(s)
- Control over bodily functions
- Communication with words
- Acquisition of socially acceptable behavior
- Egocentric interactions with others

The toddler has learned that his or her parents are predictable and reliable. The toddler begins to learn that his or her own behavior has a predictable, reliable effect on others. The toddler learns to wait longer for needs gratification. The toddler often uses "no" even when meaning "yes." This is done to assert independence (negativistic behavior). A sense of shame and doubt can develop if the toddler is kept dependent when capable of using newly acquired skills or if made to feel inadequate when attempting new skills. A toddler often continues to seek a familiar security object, such as a blanket, during times of stress.

Sample questions for the toddler include:
- Does your toddler try to do things for himself or herself (e.g., feed, dress)?
- Does your toddler have temper tantrums? How are they handled?
- Does your toddler frequently use the word "no"?
- At what age was your toddler completely toilet trained?
- Does your toddler actively explore the environment?

Preschooler

Between the ages of 3 and 6 years, a child faces a psychosocial crisis that Erikson terms *initiative versus guilt*. The child's significant other is the family. At this age, the child has normally mastered a sense of autonomy and moves on to master a sense of initiative. A preschooler is an energetic, enthusiastic, and intrusive learner with an active imagination. Conscience (an inner voice that warns and threatens) begins to develop. The child explores the physical world with all senses and powers. Development of a sense of guilt occurs when the child is made to feel that his or her imagination and activities are unacceptable. Guilt, anxiety, and fear result when the child's thoughts and activities clash with parental expectations. A preschooler begins to use simple reasoning and can tolerate longer periods of delayed gratification.

Sample questions for the preschooler include:
- Does your preschooler have an active imagination?
- Does your preschooler imitate adult activities?
- Does your preschooler engage in fantasy play?
- Does your preschooler frequently ask questions?
- Does your preschooler enjoy new activities?

School-Age Child

Erikson terms the psychosocial crisis faced by a child aged 6 to 12 years *industry versus inferiority*. During this period, the child's radius of significant others expands to include school and instructive adults. A school-age child normally has mastered the first three developmental tasks—trust, autonomy, and initiative—and now focuses on mastering industry. A child's sense of industry grows out of a desire for real achievement. The child engages in tasks and activities that he or she can carry through to completion. The child learns rules and how to compete with others, and to cooperate to achieve goals. Social relationships with others become increasingly important sources of support. The child can develop a sense of inferiority stemming from unrealistic expectations or a sense of failing to meet standards set for him or her by others. The child's self-esteem sags because of feelings of inadequacy.

Sample questions for the school-age child include:
- What are your school-age child's interests/hobbies?
- Does your school-age child interact well with teachers, peers?
- Does your school-age child enjoy accomplishments?
- Does your school-age child shame self for failures?
- What is your school-age child's favorite activity?

Adolescent

Erikson terms the psychosocial crisis faced by adolescents (aged 13 to 18 years) *identity versus role diffusion*. For an adolescent, the radius of significant others is the peer group. To adolescents, development of who they are and where they are going becomes a central focus. Adolescents continue to redefine their self-concept and the roles that they can play with certainty. As rapid physical changes occur, adolescents must reintegrate previous trust in their body, themselves, and how they appear to others. The inability to develop a sense of who one is and what one can become results in role diffusion and inability to solve core conflicts.

Sample questions for adolescents include:
- Does your adolescent have a peer group?
- Does your adolescent have a best friend?
- Does your adolescent exhibit rebellious behavior at home?
- How does your adolescent see self as fitting in with peers?
- What does your adolescent want to do with his or her life?

Psychosexual Development (Freud)

(see Chapter 7 for in-depth discussion and references)

It is suggested that children of all ages be questioned about sexual abuse. This may be elicited by asking, "Has anyone ever touched you where or when you did not want to be touched?"

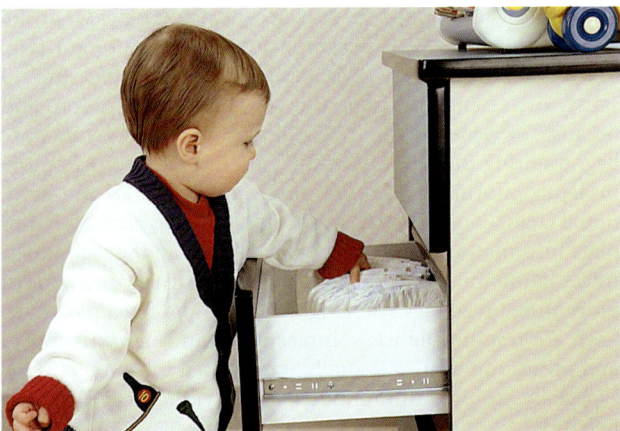

FIGURE 31-5 Toddlers love to assert their sense of control, independence, and autonomy.

Toddler

In the *anal stage*, typically extending from ages 8 months to 4 years, the erogenous zone is the anus and buttocks, and sexual activity centers on the expulsion and retention of body waste. In this stage, the child's focus shifts from the mouth to the anal area with emphasis on bowel control as he or she gains neuromuscular control over the anal sphincter. Toddlers experience both satisfaction and frustration as they gain control over withholding and expelling, containing and releasing. The conflict between "holding on" and "letting go" gradually resolves as bowel training progresses; resolution occurs once control is firmly established. Toilet training is a major task of toddlerhood (Fig. 31-6). Readiness is not usual until 18 to 24 months of age. Bowel training occurs before bladder; night bladder training usually does not occur until 3 to 5 years of age. Masturbation can occur from body exploration. Toddlers learn words associated with anatomy and elimination and can distinguish the sexes.

Sample questions for the toddler include:
- Does your toddler have any problems with toilet training?
- Does your toddler masturbate?

Preschooler

In the *phallic stage*, extending from about 3 to 7 years of age, the child's pleasure centers on the genitalia and masturbation. Many preschoolers masturbate for physiologic pleasure. The Oedipal stage occurs, marked by jealousy and rivalry toward the same-sex parent and love of the opposite-sex parent. The Oedipal stage typically resolves in the late preschool period with a strong identification with the same-sex parent. Sexual identity is developed during this time. Modesty may become a concern, and the preschooler may have fears of castration. Because preschoolers are keen observers but poor interpreters, the child may recognize but not understand sexual activity. Before answering a child's questions about sex, parents should clarify what the child is really asking and what the child already thinks about the specific subject. Questions about sex should be answered simply and honestly, providing only the information that the child requests; additional details can come later.

Sample questions for the preschooler include:
- Does your preschooler masturbate?
- Does your preschooler know what sex he or she is?
- Has your preschooler asked questions about sex, childbirth, and the like?

School-Age Child

The *latency period*, extending from about 5 to 12 years, represents a stage of relative sexual indifference before puberty and adolescence. During this period, development of self-esteem is closely linked with a developing sense of industry in gaining a concept of one's value and worth. Preadolescence begins near the end of the school-age years and discrepancies in growth and maturation between the sexes become apparent. School-age children have acquired much of their knowledge of and many of their attitudes toward sex at a very early age. During the school-age years, the child refines this knowledge and these attitudes. Questions about sex require honest answers based on the child's level of understanding.

Sample questions for the school-age child include:
- Does your school-age child interact with same-sex peers?
- What has your school-age child been told about puberty and sex?

Adolescent

In the *genital stage*, which extends from about ages 12 to 20 years, an adolescent focuses on the genitals as an erogenous zone and engages in masturbation and sexual relations with others. During this period of renewed sexual drive, adolescents experience conflict between their own needs for sexual satisfaction and society's expectations for control of sexual expression. Core concerns of adolescents include body image development and acceptance by the opposite sex. Relationships with the opposite sex are important (Fig. 31-7). Adolescents engage in sexual activity for pleasure, to satisfy drives and curiosity, as a conquest, for affection, and because of peer pressure. Teaching about sexual function, begun during the school years, should expand to cover more in-depth information on the physical, hormonal, and emotional changes of puberty. An adolescent needs accurate, complete information on sexuality and cultural and moral values. Information must include how pregnancy occurs; methods of preventing pregnancy stressing that male and female partners both are responsible for contraception; and transmission of and protection against sexually transmitted infections (STIs), especially acquired immunodeficiency syndrome (AIDS) and hepatitis.

A full, confidential sexual/sexuality history should be obtained from adolescents. This history includes questioning

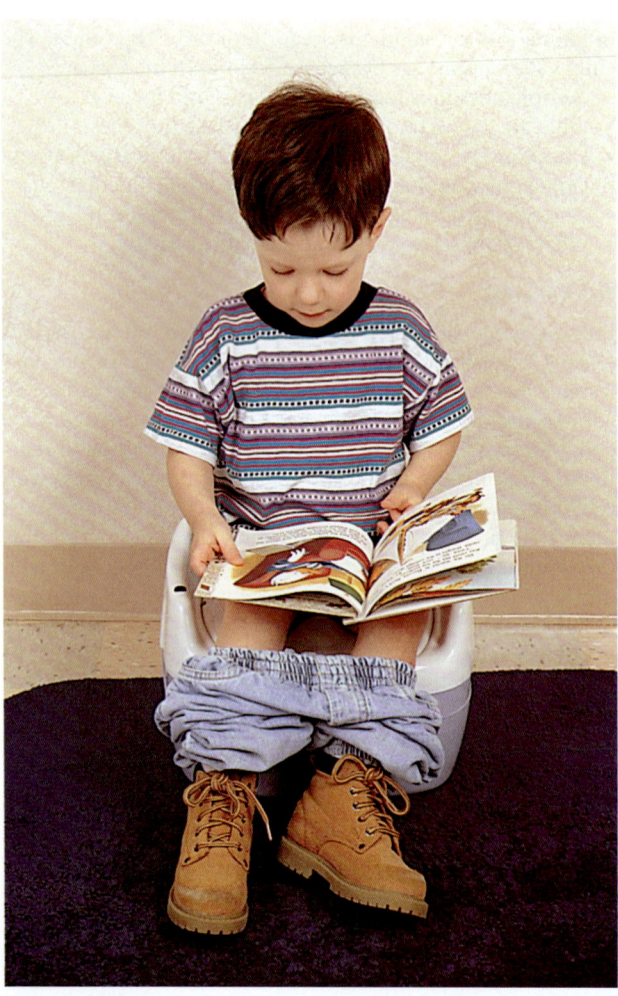

FIGURE 31-6 Toilet training is a major task of toddlerhood.

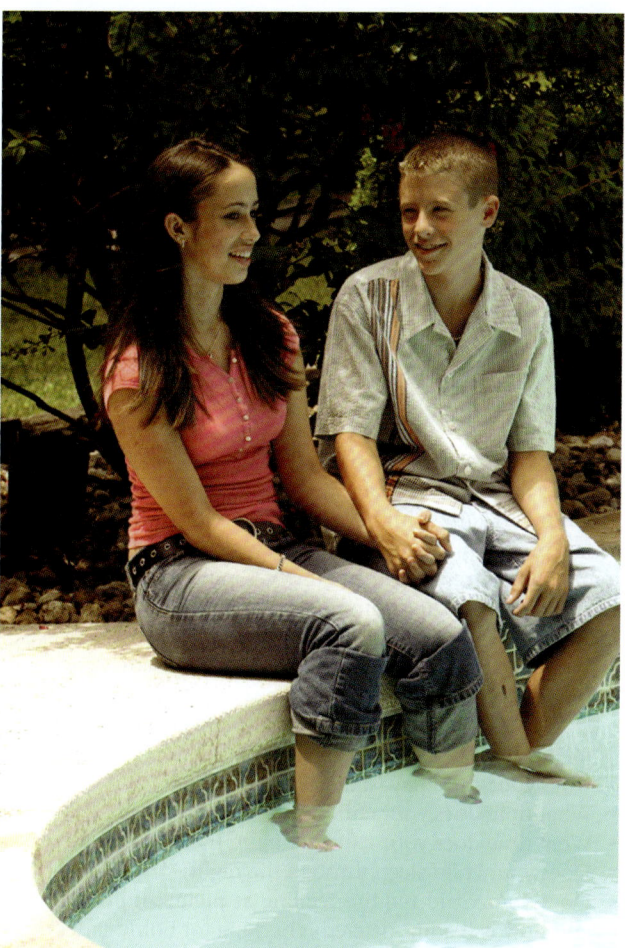

FIGURE 31-7 During adolescence, relationships with the opposite sex are important stepping stones to adulthood.

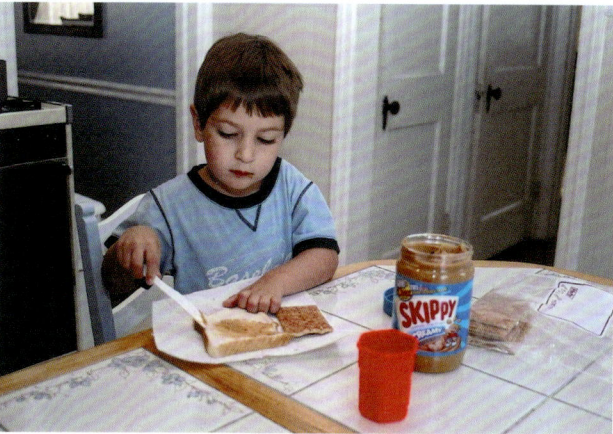

FIGURE 31-8 This toddler enjoys helping prepare his lunch.

previously noted in the reproductive review of systems as well as:
- What is your sexual preference?
- How do you feel about becoming a man/woman?

Normal Nutritional Requirements

Proper nutrition is necessary for childhood growth and development. Food and feeding are important parts of growing up, with needs and desires changing as the child grows (Fig. 31-8). Guidelines about nutritional requirements for each age group are provided by the U.S. Department of Health and Human Services and the U.S. Department of Agriculture. See the entire table at the following website: http://health.gov/dietaryguidelines/2015/guidelines/.

Attention has been drawn to the higher incidence of obesity in children. According to the CDC (2017), approximately 17% of children and adolescents aged 2 to 19 years old are obese. Obesity among children and adolescents has tripled since 1980, a difference having been noted in the prevalence of obesity between racial and ethnic disparities.

The CDC reports that in 2007 to 2008, Hispanic boys ages 2 to19 years old were more likely to be obese than non-Hispanic white males. Non-Hispanic black girls were more likely to be obese than non-Hispanic white girls.

Although obesity in preschool children aged 2 to 5 years remains high, it has decreased significantly from 13.9% in 2003–2004 to 8.4% in 2011–2012 (CDC, 2015). General overviews for each phase of nutrition follow.

Toddlers

Growth rate slows dramatically during the toddler years, thus decreasing the need for calories, protein, and fluid. Starting at about 12 months, most toddlers are eating the same foods as the rest of the family. At 18 months, many toddlers experience physiologic anorexia and become picky eaters. They experience food jags, eating large amounts one day and very little the next. They like to feed themselves and prefer small portions of appetizing foods. Frequent, nutritious snacks can replace a meal. Food should not be used as a reward or a punishment. Milk should be limited to no more than 1 quart per day to ensure intake and absorption of iron-enriched foods to prevent anemia. Recommendations for screening for anemia should be based on age, sex, and risk of anemia.

Preschoolers

Requirements are similar to those of the toddler. Three- and 4-year-old children may still be unable to sit with family during meals. Four-year-old children are picky eaters. Five-year-old children are influenced by food habits of others. A 5-year-old child tends to be focused on the "social" aspects of eating: table conversation, manners, willingness to try new foods, and help with meal preparation and cleanup.

School-Age Children

A school-age child's daily caloric requirements diminish in relation to body size. Caregivers should continue to stress the need for a balanced diet from the food pyramid because resources are being stored for the increased growth needs of adolescence. Children are exposed to broader eating experiences in the school lunchroom; they may still be a picky eaters but should be more willing to try new foods. Children may trade, sell, or throw away home-packed school lunches. At home, the child should eat what the family eats; the patterns that develop then stay with the child into adulthood.

Adolescents

An adolescent's daily intake should be balanced among the foods in the pyramid; average daily caloric intake requirements vary with sex and age. Adolescents typically eat whatever they have at break activities; readily available nutritious snacks provide good insurance for a balanced diet. Milk (calcium) and protein are needed in quantity to aid in bone and muscle growth. Maintaining adequate quality and quantity of daily intake may be difficult because of factors such as busy schedule, influence of peers, and easy availability of fast foods. Family eating patterns established during the school years continue to influence an adolescent's food selection. Female adolescents are very prone to negative dieting behaviors. Common dietary deficiencies include iron, folate, and zinc.

Nursing History Questions Related to Nutrition

Sample nursing history questions for toddlerhood to adolescence include:

- What does your child eat in a typical day?
- Is your child on any special type of diet? If so, what for?
- What types of food does your child like/dislike most?
- Does your child have any feeding problems?
- Is your child allergic to any foods? If so, how does your child react to those foods?
- Does your child take any vitamin or mineral supplements?
- How much fluid does your child drink per day?
- Is your water fluorinated? If not, does your child take supplements?
- Has your child had any recent weight gain or loss?

These questions should be also asked directly of adolescents when parents are not present:

- Does your child have any concerns with body image?
- Has your child been on any self-imposed diet?
- How often does your child weigh himself or herself?
- Has your child ever used any of the following methods for weight loss: self-induced vomiting? Laxatives? Diuretics? Excessive exercise? Fasting?

Normal Activity and Exercise

Activity and exercise are important components of a child's life and, therefore, should be assessed when a complete subjective examination is being performed. Play, activity, and exercise patterns can give the nurse valuable clues about the overall health of a child. Box 31-1 describes play characteristics across childhood. This assessment also allows the examiner to provide health promotion teaching.

Sample nursing history questions for toddlerhood to adolescence include:

- What is your child's activity like during a typical 24-hour day (including activities of daily living [ADLs], play, and school)?
- What are your child's favorite activities and toys?
- How many hours of television or video games does your child watch or play per day? What are his or her favorite programs/movies? Do you discuss TV shows/movies with your child?
- Are there any restrictions on TV watching (content, hours, relationship to chores/homework)?
- What chores does your child do at home? (school-age child/adolescent)
- Does the older child/adolescent work outside the home? What does he or she do?
- How many hours does he or she work during the school year?
- Does the work interfere with school or social life?
- Why does your child work?
- Does your child have any problems that restrict physical activity?
- Does your child require any special devices to manage with ADLs/play?
- At what age did your child first walk?
- Can your child keep up with his or her peers?
- Does your child have any hobbies/interests (ages 6 and older)?
- What sports does your child participate in?

Normal Sleep Requirements and Patterns

Sleep is an integral part of health assessment. Lack of sleep can affect all areas of health including cognitive, physical, and emotional health. Children require varying amounts of sleep based primarily on their age. They also have varying sleep habits that correlate with their developmental status. Sample nursing history questions for toddlerhood to adolescence include:

- Where does your child sleep; what type of bed?
- With whom does your child sleep?
- Does your child use a sleep aid (blanket, toy, night light, medication, beverage)?
- Does your child have a bedtime ritual?
- What time does your child go to bed at night?
- What time does your child get up in the morning?
- Does your child sleep through the night?
- Does your child require feeding at night, and, if so, what and how is it administered (checking for bottle caries)?
- What is your child's nap schedule, and how long does your child sleep for naps?
- Is your child's sleep restful or restless; any snoring or breathing problems?
- Does your child sleepwalk or sleeptalk?
- Does your child have nightmares or night terrors?
- If your child has sleep problems, what do you do?
- Does your child or adolescent sleep with any light on in the room (even a dim one)?
- Does your child or adolescent use a cell phone, computer, or tablet within 4 hours of bedtime? (see Ford, 2016 for effect on sleep)

Toddlers

Total sleep requirements decrease during the second year and average about 12 hours per day. Most toddlers nap once a day until the end of the second or third year. Sleep problems are common and may be due to fears of separation. Bedtime rituals and transitional objects, such as a blanket or stuffed toy, are helpful.

Preschoolers

The average preschooler sleeps 11 to 13 hours per day. Preschoolers typically need an afternoon nap until age 5, when most begin kindergarten. Bedtime rituals persist and sleep problems are common. These include nightmares, night terrors, difficulty settling in after a busy day, and stretching bedtime rituals to delay sleep. Continuing reassuring bedtime rituals with relaxation time before bedtime should help the child settle in. The daytime nap may be eliminated if it seems

| BOX 31-1 | CHARACTERISTICS OF PLAY AMONG CHILDREN |

TODDLERS
Toddlers engage in parallel play—they play alongside, not with, others. Imitation is one of the most common forms of play and locomotion skills can be enhanced with push–pull toys. Toddlers change toys frequently because of short attention spans.

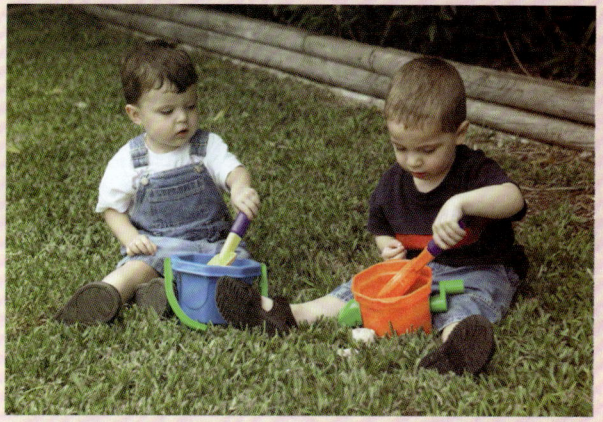

PRESCHOOLERS
Typical preschool play is associative—interactive and cooperative with sharing. Preschoolers need contact with age mates. Activities, such as jumping, running and climbing, promote growth and motor skills. Preschoolers are at a typical age for imaginary playmates. Imitative, imaginative, and dramatic play are important. TV and video games should only be a part of the child's play and parents should monitor content and amount of time spent in use. Associative play materials include dress-up clothes and dolls, housekeeping toys, play tents, puppets, and doctor and nurse kits. Curious and active preschoolers need adult supervision, especially near bodies of water and gym sets.

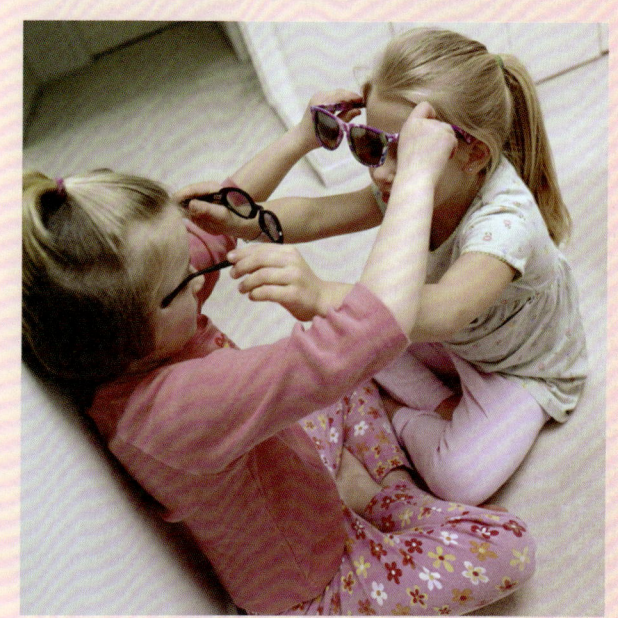

SCHOOL-AGE CHILDREN
Play becomes more competitive and complex during the school-age period. Characteristic activities include joining team sports, secret clubs, and "gangs"; scouting or like activities; working complex puzzles, collecting, playing quiet board games; reading; and hero worshiping. Rules and rituals are important aspects of play and games.

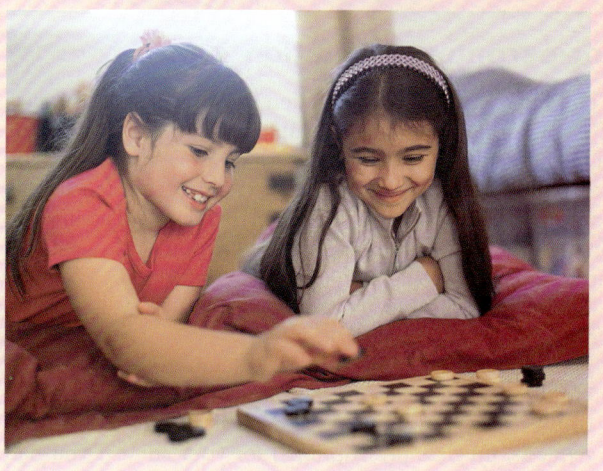

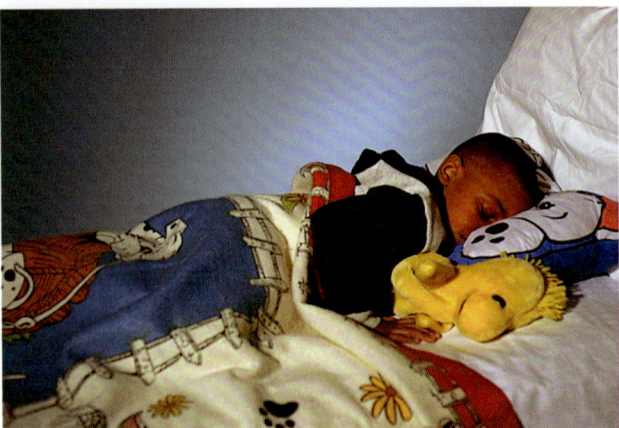

FIGURE 31-9 A security object, such as a favorite toy, can help a preschooler to sleep (© B. Proud).

to interfere with nighttime sleep. For many preschoolers, a security object and night light continue to help relieve anxiety/fears at bedtime (Fig. 31-9).

School-Age Children

School-age children's individual sleep requirements vary but typically range from 8 to 9.5 hours per night. Because the growth rate has slowed, children actually need less sleep at this age than during adolescence. The child's bedtime can be later than during the preschool period but should be firmly established and adhered to on school nights. Reading before bedtime may facilitate sleep and set up a positive bedtime pattern. Children may be unaware of fatigue and, if allowed to remain up, will be tired the next day.

Adolescents

During adolescence, rapid growth, overexertion in activities, excessive use of blue-light-emitting devices (cell phone, TV, tablet, computer, and LED lights), and a tendency to stay up late commonly interfere with sleep and rest requirements (Ford, 2016). In an attempt to "catch up" on missed sleep, many adolescents sleep late at every opportunity. Each adolescent is unique in the number of sleep hours required to stay healthy and rested.

Socioeconomic Situation

A family's socioeconomic situation greatly affects all aspects of a child's life including development, nutrition, and overall health and functioning. Low socioeconomic status has the greatest adverse effect on health, and many children in this country live below the poverty level. Therefore, it is critical to obtain this assessment to initiate intervention strategies at the earliest opportunity.

Sample nursing history questions for infancy to adolescence include:
- Does your child have health care insurance?
- Would you seek more medical assistance (e.g., in the way of preventive screenings, checkups, sick visits, medication requests, eyeglass prescriptions) for your child if you had the money to do so?
- Do you have any financial difficulties with which you need assistance?
- How would you describe your family's living conditions?

Relationship and Role Development

The development of relationships and a role within groups is a crucial aspect of childhood. The ability of children to establish high-quality relationships and form specific roles in the early years significantly determines their ability to form high-quality relationships and roles in adulthood.

Culture is an important factor in a person's relationship and role development. Things to consider include whether the child's culture/ethnicity is a minority within the major cultural group; the traditional role of children in the particular child's culture; and whether there is male or female dominance in the particular culture. Another major influence on the child's development of relationships and roles is the structure of the family. Various family structures include two-parent families, single-parent families, blended families, homosexual parent families, families with an adopted child, or families with a foster child.

Early intervention in and early prevention of poor relationships between children and their caregivers, siblings, peers, and influential adults outside the immediate family are vital. Therefore, assessment of this aspect of a child's life is extremely important. It is important to ask the parent or caregiver as well as the child questions because they may have differing views concerning the nature of the child's relationships.

Sample nursing history questions for toddlerhood to adolescence (*specifically geared to parent or caregiver*) include:
- What is your family structure?
- With what culture or ethnic group does your family identify?
- How would you describe your family support system?
- Who is your child's primary caretaker (especially for smaller children, not in school)?
- What is your child's role in the family?
- What are the family occupations and schedules?
- How much time do you spend with your children and what activities do you participate in when you are together?
- Have there been any changes in the family lately—divorce, birth, deaths, moves?
- How does your child get along with parents, siblings, extended family, teachers, and peers?
- Discuss your child's circle of friends.
- What disciplinary measures do you use?

Sample nursing history questions for toddlerhood to adolescence (*specifically geared to child and/or adolescent*) include:
- How do you get along with your parents? brothers? sisters?
- What activities does the family do together?
- What chores do you do around the house?
- What would you consider your role in the family?
- What are the names of your family members and friends?
- Do you have a best friend?
- What do you like best about family/friends?
- What do you dislike about family/friends?
- What do you do/share with your friends?
- Do your parents know your friends? Do they like them?
- Do you get along with the other kids at school?
- Do you get along with your teacher(s)?

Self-Esteem and Self-Concept Development

Childhood is the time when individuals develop the self-esteem and self-concept that shapes them in adult life (Table 31-4). Therefore, an assessment of this nature is

TABLE 31-4 Self-Concept Development

Developmental Stage	Self-Concept
Toddler/Preschoolers	Greater sense of independence.
School-agers	More aware of differences, norms, and morals; sensitive to social pressures.
Adolescents	Self-concept crystallizes in later adolescence when child focuses on physical and emotional changes and peer acceptance.

crucial to provide health promotion teaching, prevent future problems, and intervene with current problems. This is a good time to ask questions regarding the child's values and beliefs because these areas tend to influence significantly a person's self-concept. This assessment requires that the same questions be asked of both the parent and child, because their opinions may be significantly different. Reassure the parent and child that all answers discussed will be kept confidential.

Sample nursing history questions for toddler to adolescence include (also ask these questions directly to the child; these questions are given in italics):

- How would you describe your child? *How would you describe yourself?*
- What does your child do best? *What do you do best?*
- In what areas does your child need improvement? *In what areas do you think you need improvement?*
- Is your child ever overly concerned about his or her weight? *Do you like your present weight? What would you like to weigh?*
- Are culture and religion important factors in your home? *Are culture and religion important to you?*
- In what religion is the child being reared? *What religion are you?*
- How does your child define right and wrong? *How would you decide if something were right or wrong?*
- What are your family values? *What values are important to you?*
- What are your child's goals in life? *What are your goals in life?*

Coping and Stress Management

Childhood is full of stressors and fears, including the developmental crises of transition to each life stage and common

TABLE 31-5 Stressors in Children

Group	Stressors
Young children	Change in daily structure New sibling Separation
Older children	Starting school Long vacations Moving Change in family structure (remarriage) Christmas
Adolescents	Pregnancy Peer loss Breakup with boy/girlfriend
All children	Parental loss (divorce, death, jail)

TABLE 31-6 Common Childhood Fears

Developmental Stage	Fear Factors
Infants	Loud noises; falling and sudden movements in the environment; stranger anxiety begins around age 6 months
Toddlers	Loss of parents—separation anxiety; stranger anxiety; loud noises; going to sleep; large animals; certain people (doctor, Santa Claus); certain places (doctor's office); large objects or machines
Preschoolers	The dark; being left alone, especially at bedtime; animals (particularly large dogs); ghosts and other supernatural beings; body mutilation; pain; objects and people associated with painful experiences
School-agers	Failure at school; bullies; intimidating teachers; supernatural beings; storms; staying alone; scary things in TV and movies; consequences related to unattractive appearance; death
Adolescents	Relationships with people of the opposite sex; homosexual tendencies; ability to assume adult roles; drugs; AIDS; divorce; gossip; public speaking; plane and car crashes; death

childhood fears such as the dark and being left alone (Tables 31-5 and 31-6). The ways in which children cope with stress and fear can affect their development and how they will handle subsequent life events. Coping mechanisms vary depending on developmental level, resources, situation, style, and previous experience with stressful events (Table 31-7). The ability

TABLE 31-7 Coping Mechanisms in Children

Developmental Stage	Coping Mechanisms
Infants	Restlessness; rocking; playing with toys; crying; thumb sucking; sleeping
Toddlers/Preschoolers	Asking questions; wanting order; holding favorite toy; learning by trial and error; tantrums; aggression; thumb sucking; withdrawal; regression
School-agers	Trying problem solving; communicating; fantasizing; acting out situations; quiet; denial; regression; reaction formation
Adolescents	Problem solving; philosophical discussions; conforming with peers; asserting control; acting out; using drugs/alcohol; denial; projection; rationalization; intellectualization

of a child to cope is often influenced by individual temperament. Temperament involves the child's style of emotional and behavioral responses across situations. Temperament is biologic in origin; however, it is influenced by environmental characteristics and patterned by the society. This is significant because short- and long-term psychosocial adjustments are shaped by the goodness of fit between the child's temperament and the social environment.

Sample nursing history questions for infancy to adolescence include (*questions asked of a child appear in italics*):

- What does your child do when he or she gets angry or frustrated? *What do you do when you get angry or frustrated?*
- What does your child do when he or she gets tired? *What do you do when you get tired?*
- When your child has a tantrum, how do you handle it?
- What things make your child scared? *What things scare you?*
- What does he or she do when scared? *What do you do when you're scared?*
- What kinds of things does your child worry about? *What kinds of things do you worry about?*
- When your child has a problem, what does he or she do? *When you have a problem, what do you do?*
- Have there been any big problems or changes in your family lately? *Have there been any big problems or changes in your family lately?*
- Is there a problem with alcohol or drugs? *Do you use tobacco, alcohol, or drugs?*
- Has your child ever run away from home? *Have you ever run away from home?*
- How does your child react when needs are not met immediately, and what do you do about it? *What do you do when you are sad? What do you do when you are angry?*
- Is your child "accident prone," and why do you think he or she is? *Did you ever think about hurting yourself? Did you ever think about killing yourself?* (Box 31-2)

HEALTH ASSESSMENT

Collecting Subjective Data: The Nursing Health History

The complete pediatric nursing history is one of the most crucial components of child health care. Many of the materials and questions are unique to this population. The nursing history interview usually provides an opportunity to observe the caregiver–child or parent–child interaction and to participate in early detection of health problems and prevention of future difficulties.

Nurses must have the communication skills needed to elicit data about the child and family within a framework that incorporates biographic data, current health status, past history, family history, a review of each body system, knowledge of growth and development, and lifestyle and health practices–related information. It is important to keep in mind that data collected in one category may have relevance to another category. For example, data collected about the condition of the child's skin, hair, and nails may indicate a problem in the area of nutrition.

Because infants and children are uniquely different from adults, a separate subjective assessment that focuses on questions suited for this population is vital. Subjective assessment of children encompasses interviewing and compiling a complete nursing history. General interviewing techniques used for the adult are used in the pediatric setting. However, in pediatrics, someone other than the client, usually the parent, gives the history. Thus, the interview becomes the onset of a relational triad between the nurse, the child or adolescent, and the parents. Nurses establish a comfortable, yet professional, rapport that forms the foundation for the ongoing therapeutic relationship. Nurses accomplish this by developing communication and interviewing skills that incorporate the needs of

---

BOX 31-2   SUICIDE ASSESSMENT: RISKS AND SIGNS

Suicide is a leading killer of young people, particularly teenagers. The nurse can be instrumental in detecting signs of impending suicide and, possibly, intervening to prevent it. During the nursing assessment, asking the following questions may help uncover a young client's suicidal thoughts:

- Have you ever thought of hurting or killing yourself ? (Hurting is different from killing.)
- (If the answer is "yes," ask:) When did you think of killing yourself? How did you plan to do it?
- Did you ever try to kill yourself before? Did you receive any help after the incident?
- Do you believe that there are other options besides suicide to resolve problems?

Children and adolescents who verbalize planned, lethal means to commit suicide, and who feel that they do not have any other options, are at extremely high risk of carrying out their plan—especially if they have attempted suicide in the past. Some risk factors and warning signs of potential suicide include the following:

RISK FACTORS

- Previous attempt
- Suicide of family member or close friend
- History of abuse, neglect, or psychiatric hospitalization
- Persistent depression
- Mental disorder (e.g., voices tell child to kill self)
- Substance abuse
- Difficult home situation
- Incarceration
- Few social opportunities; isolation
- Firearms in the home

WARNING SIGNS

- Seems preoccupied with death themes, as in books, music, art, films, or TV shows
- Gives away valued possessions
- Talks about death, especially own
- Acts recklessly or adopts antisocial behavior
- Experiences rapid change in school performance
- Has episode of sudden cheerfulness after being depressed
- Exhibits dramatic change in everyday behaviors, such as sleeping and eating
- Smokes continuously (chain smoking)
- Expresses sense of worthlessness or hopelessness

both the parent and child or adolescent, treating both as equal partners.

Interviewing

Interviewing Parents

The parental interview entails more than just fact gathering. The tone of future contacts is established as parents begin to develop a trusting relationship with the nurse (Fig. 31-10). Parents expect health professionals to be sources of information and education, and they assess professional competence during the initial contact. Therefore, it is important that the nurse use a friendly, nonjudgmental approach while demonstrating proficiency as a practitioner. Rarely is the interview just data gathering; it is also a forum for rapport building, explaining, and health teaching.

Introductory Stage

As with all clients, the nurse–parent relationship begins with the introduction, when nurses explain their roles and the purpose of the interview. Clarification and consistency are crucial from the start because parents may be anxious about the child's condition or uncomfortable about their roles, especially if the setting is a hospital. Anxiety may be overt or masked, even demonstrated by negative behaviors such as hostility.

Cultural variations may also affect parental reactions and response. Active listening facilitates the use of leads and better enables nurses to keep the interview focused on specific concerns. It also allows nurses to uncover clues that further the interview, to seek validation of perceptions and responses that may have alternate meanings, and to provide reassurance for both the expressed and hidden concerns that parents may be experiencing.

Encouraging Talk

By encouraging parents to talk, you can identify information that affects all aspects of a child's life. Some parents take the lead without prompting (e.g., "He's been pulling up his legs like he's in pain"). Others offer vague concerns (e.g., "…she's just not acting right") and need more direction. However, all have significant information about their child. You can further encourage verbalization through communication techniques such as open-ended questioning ("How does Sarah behave when she isn't acting just right?") and focus directing ("When does Darryl have the pain?"). Communication skills allow nurses to elicit information in all patient groups, even in the most difficult situations.

The atmosphere should create an exchange of information rather than one directed solely by the nurse. Use problem solving, collaboration, and anticipatory guidance. For example, ask the parent, "What do you see as the problem?" Once the problem is identified, lead the parent through the problem-solving process to arrive at a solution. Parents should also be asked what they found to be effective or ineffective in managing their child's problems. Anticipatory guidance promotes an exchange because parents can better participate in discussions of their child's future developmental trends.

Be aware of the barriers to effective nurse–parent communication. These include time constraints, frequent interruptions, lack of privacy, and language differences as well as provider callousness and cultural insensitivity. Make every effort possible to avoid these barriers. Allow adequate time and privacy for every interview and keep interruptions at a minimum. Interpreters can assist when language differences are present.

Always display a warm, professional manner when interacting with clients and families, and be sensitive to cultural differences displayed in values, beliefs, and customs.

Interviewing Children and Adolescents

As noted earlier, the child or adolescent and parent are treated as equal partners in the health care triad. Include the child in the introductory stage of the interview and observe for signs of readiness to evaluate the level of participation. Readiness evaluation includes questioning the parents about how the child copes with stressful situations and what the child has been told about this particular health encounter.

Communication Techniques

Direct communication—such as open-ended and closed-ended questions, age-appropriate humor, and dialogue strategies—is usually more beneficial when used with indirect communication techniques including sentence completion, mutual storytelling, and using drawings, play (the universal language of children), and magic.

Play as Communication

Talk to the child at eye level (be aware of cultural variations in eye contact) and actively engage children through play and verbalization. Play is one of the most valuable communication techniques when working with children; it allows for the discovery of important clues to children's development and illness behaviors. Rushing creates anxiety; therefore, take time to listen and to allow children to feel comfortable. Privacy and confidentiality are important in pediatric nursing, especially when assessing the adolescent. Children or adolescents may be anxious, fearful, or embarrassed. Respect their emotions.

Explain the interview process and assessment procedures in clear and honest terms. State directions in a positive manner, and offer choices only when available and appropriate. Use honest praise to reinforce positive behaviors; gratuitous praise is quickly recognized by children and may decrease the child's trust in the nurse.

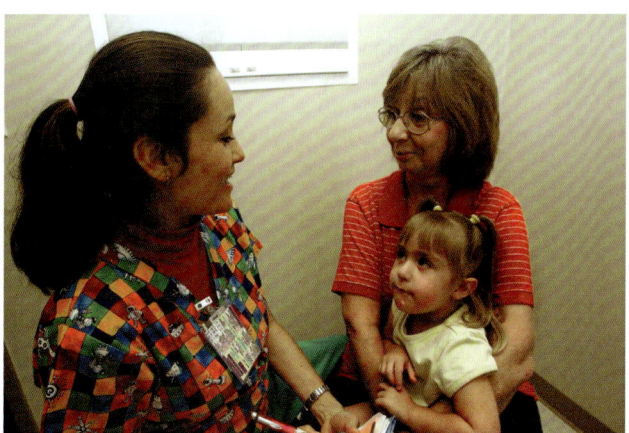

FIGURE 31-10 Developing a trusting relationship with the parent(s) is an essential aspect of the interview process.

BOX 31-3 AGE-SPECIFIC INTERVIEW TECHNIQUES

Each child responds differently during the assessment interview according to developmental status, severity and perception of illness, experience with health care, intrusiveness of procedures, and the child's own uniqueness. The following are some guidelines for adapting the interview techniques to the child's status.

TODDLERS: SENSORIMOTOR TO PREOPERATIONAL STAGES

Trial-and-error experimentation and relentless exploration are typical in the early toddler stage; later, the toddler uses representational thought in intellectual development. Children under 5 years of age are egocentric. A toddler's attention span ranges between 5 and 10 minutes.

- Encourage parental presence.
- Provide careful and simple explanations just before procedure.
- Use play as a communication technique.
- Tell child it is okay to cry.
- Encourage expression through toys.
- Use simple terminology; child's receptive language is more advanced than his or her expressive language.
- Allow child to be close to parent—be alert for separation anxiety.

Acknowledge child's favorite toy or a unique characteristic about the child.

PRESCHOOLERS: PREOPERATIONAL STAGE

Preschoolers progress from making simple classifications and associating one event with a simultaneous one to classifying and quantifying and exhibiting intuitive thought processes. A preschooler's attention span ranges between 10 and 15 minutes. Preschoolers use magical thinking.

- Explain why things are as they are, simply.
- Validate child's perceptions.
- Avoid threatening words.
- Use simple visual aids.
- Involve child in teaching by allowing child to do something (e.g., handling equipment).
- Allow child to ask questions.
- Use child's toys for expression; use miniature equipment on toys.
- Avoid using words that have double meaning.
- Explain sensations that the child will experience.
- Answer "why" questions with simple explanations.
- Be direct and concrete; do not use analogies, abstractions, or words with more than one meaning. Avoid slang (such as "laugh your head off"—preschoolers interpret literally).
- Ask simple questions.
- Allow child to manipulate equipment.

Use the child's active imagination—use toys, puppets, and play.

SCHOOL-AGE CHILDREN: OPERATIONAL STAGE

Egocentric thinking progresses to objective thinking in school-age children who begin using inductive reasoning, logical operations, and reversible concrete thought. A school-age child's attention span ranges between 30 and 45 minutes. Use books and other visual aids to advance the assessment interview.

- Remember to remain concrete (i.e., avoid abstractions).
- Use group discussion to educate children among their peers; also use games.
- Provide health teaching; perform demonstrations.
- Give more responsibility to child.
- School-age children like explanations and need assistance in vocalizing their needs.

Allow children to engage in discussions.

ADOLESCENTS: FORMAL OPERATIONS STAGE

Abstract thought develops, as does thinking beyond the present and forming theories about everything.

- Give adolescents control whenever possible.
- Use scientific explanations and make expectations clear.
- Explore expected parental level of involvement before initiating it.
- Involve adolescents in planning.
- Clearly explain how body will be affected.
- Anticipate feelings of anger and grief.
- Use peers with common situation to help with teaching.
- Encourage expression of ideas and feelings.
- Maintain confidentiality; facilitate trust.
- Give adolescents your undivided attention.
- Make expectations clear.
- Ask to speak to adolescent alone.
- Encourage open and honest communication.
- Be nonjudgmental; respect views, differences, and feelings.

Ask open-ended questions.

Touch

Touch is a powerful communication tool. However, the child may find touch intrusive if the nurse has not yet begun to formulate a relationship with the child. Cultural taboos may also prohibit touch. Therefore, it is prudent to communicate with the child at a "safe distance" until the relationship begins to form.

Developmental Considerations

It is important to be familiar with developmentally oriented approaches to interviewing children. Box 31-3 presents specific developmentally oriented approaches that may be used in interviewing children and adolescents.

These approaches are important to know because barriers can exist when communicating with children. For example, some nurses overestimate the understanding abilities of young children and underestimate those of older children and adolescents. This creates frustration for all involved. Be habitually aware of children's cognitive status when interacting with them. Another barrier develops when the child is excluded altogether. Children and adolescents can be eager participants and should be treated as such.

Finally, although many children are eager participants, others need encouragement, especially toddlers and preschoolers who may react with crying and lack of cooperation.

Avoid power struggles and instead rely on empathy, developmental strategies, parental assistance, and a good sense of humor.

Adolescent Concerns

Adolescents are neither children nor adults. Therefore, treat them accordingly. Privacy is essential, as are respect and confidentiality. General health issues may or may not be discussed with the parent present. However, sensitive issues, such as sex, sexuality, drugs, and alcohol, are best handled without parental presence. Trust and genuineness are important; do not "talk down" to adolescents or mimic their language style. The approach should be as a professional, not as a peer, parent, or big sister or brother (Fig. 31-11). Use open-ended and specific questions to avoid "yes/no" answers; use silence sparingly because it may be viewed as threatening to this age group. Be aware of your own nonverbal and facial expressions. Approach delicate issues with sensitivity and a nonjudgmental, matter-of-fact manner to keep them from appearing to be focal points. History taking provides an excellent opportunity for health teaching with adolescents, who are eager to learn about their ever-changing bodies. Encourage the adolescent to ask questions and then answer any questions throughout the history.

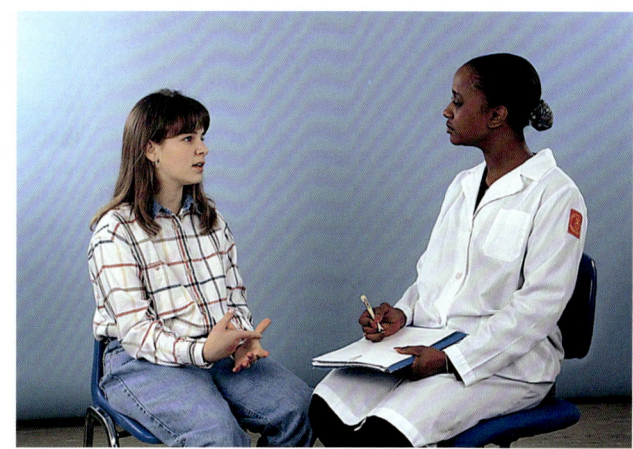

FIGURE 31-11 Handle sensitive issues with adolescents by establishing trust and genuineness (© B. Proud).

Biographic Data

QUESTION	RATIONALE
What is the child's name? Nickname? What are the parents' or caregivers' names?	Knowing personal information about the child and caregivers helps to establish rapport with child and family.
Who is the child's primary health care provider, and when was the child's last well-child care appointment? (Guidelines for primary health care provider visits, developed by the Committee on Practice and Ambulatory Medicine and the American Academy of Pediatrics [AAP], can be found in table format on thePoint.)	This determines the child's access to health care. It tells the nurse where to find the client's previous medical information/record.
Where does the child live? (Address) Do the parents and child live in the same residence? Who else lives in this residence? Are the child's parents married, single, divorced, homosexual? What are the parents' ages?	This provides insight into living conditions and family dynamics, which contribute to the child's health.
What is the child's age? What is the child's date of birth?	This provides a reference for assessing the child's developmental level.
Is the child adopted, foster, natural?	Certain health problems run in families. It is helpful to know the child's genetic relationship with the parents.
What is the child's ethnic origin? Religion?	This information helps the nurse to examine special needs and beliefs that may affect the client or family's health care.
What do the child's parents do for a living?	This provides insight into the economic status of the family.

History of Present Health Concern

The purpose of asking about the child's current health status is to determine why the child was brought in for an examination. For some examinations, the child and parents may have no symptoms to report. In this case, the parent and child should be asked to describe the general state of the child's health (see Personal Health History section).

QUESTION	RATIONALE
If there is a perceived problem with the child's health or if the child or parent notices symptoms, the same focus questions that are asked for each body system for the adult client are used for the child (e.g., location, intensity, duration). However, for the child, it is important to ask both the parent and the child (if possible) to get the most accurate information. When asking the child about symptoms, the following techniques are usually helpful: • Ask the child to point with one finger to where the pain or symptom is located.	Conflicting information may clue the nurse in to other areas that may need to be assessed.

Continued on following page

History of Present Health Concern (Continued)

QUESTION	RATIONALE
• Use a pain scale developed for children such as the FACES Pain Rating Scale characters ranging from a happy face signifying no pain to a tearful face signifying the worst pain); the Oucher scale (six photographs of children's faces ranging from "no hurt" to "biggest hurt you could ever have"—also comes with scale from 0 to 100); or a numeric scale (straight line with numbers from 0 to 10 representing no pain to worst pain). Figure 31-12 illustrates the FACES and numeric pain-rating scales.	

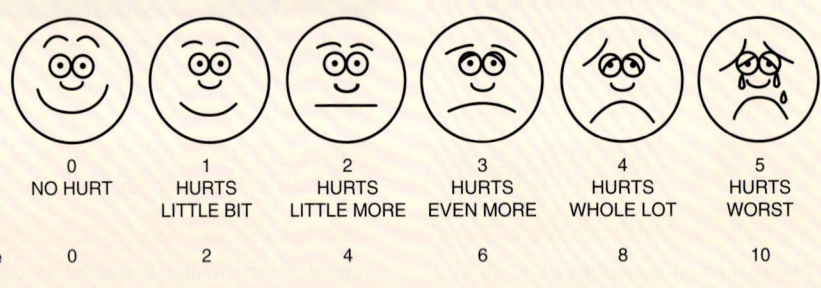

Explain to the person that each face is for a person who feels happy because he has no pain (hurt) or sad because he has some or a lot of pain. Face 0 is very happy because he doesn't hurt at all. Face 1 hurts just a little bit. Face 2 hurts a little more. Face 3 hurts even more. Face 4 hurts a whole lot. Face 5 hurts as much as you can imagine, although you don't have to be crying to feel this bad. Ask the person to choose the face that best describes how he is feeling.

Rating scale is recommended for persons age 3 years and older.

Brief word instructions: Point to each face using the words to describe the pain intensity. Ask the child to choose face that best describes own pain and record the appropriate number.

FIGURE 31-12 Pain rating scales: Numerical scale and FACES pain rating scale. (Used with permission from Hockenberry, M. J., & Wilson D. (2009). *Wong's essentials of pediatric nursing* (8th ed.). St. Louis, MO: Mosby–Elsevier.)

Personal Health History

Personal history is important information to collect when assessing children. Certain problems and conditions can be associated with a difficult birth experience, whether the child was immunized, genetic conditions acquired from parents, and the like. Obviously, most of this information must come from the birth parent. If the child is a foster child or adopted, some of the information may be obtained from hospital records.

QUESTION	RATIONALE
Was this child's pregnancy planned? How did you feel when you found out you were pregnant?	The caregiver's answer may provide insight into her feelings about the child.
When did you first receive prenatal care? How was your general health during pregnancy?	Prenatal information helps to identify potential health problems for the child.
Did you have any problems with your pregnancy?	It is important to identify problems during pregnancy to help to identify potential complications for the child.
Did you have any accidents during this pregnancy?	Trauma or domestic violence that involved any type of physical trauma to the abdomen should be identified for possible complications for the infant/child.
Did you take any medications during pregnancy?	Certain medications should not be taken during pregnancy and may be harmful to the child.
Did you use any tobacco, alcohol, or drugs during this pregnancy?	Smoking, alcohol, and drug use may cause complications or anomalies with the fetus.

QUESTION	RATIONALE
Ask about delivery of the child or adolescent: • Where was the child or adolescent born? • What type of delivery did you have? • Were there any problems during the delivery? Did you have any vaginal infections at time of delivery? • What was the child's or adolescent's Apgar score? • What were the child's or adolescent's weight, height, and head circumference? Did the child or adolescent have any problems after birth (e.g., feeding, jaundice)?	Delivery details and complications are pertinent for assessing fetal injury and potential risk for infection.
Ask about past illnesses or injuries: • Has the child or adolescent ever been hospitalized? • Has the child or adolescent ever had any major illnesses? • Has the child or adolescent ever experienced any major injuries?	Previous illnesses and hospitalizations may affect the present examination.
Ask the parent, and child or adolescent, if possible, to describe the child's or adolescent's general state of health and compare it with how it was 1 and 5 years ago (if age appropriate).	Obtaining baseline information about the client helps to identify important areas of assessment. **CLINICAL TIP** If the answer is "good," ask what "good" means to them. "Good" could mean "only one cold this year" for a generally healthy child or "only two hospitalizations this year" for a child with a chronic illness such as cystic fibrosis.
Does the child have a chronic illness?	Chronic illnesses may explain or affect assessment findings. Chronic illness, such as asthma, or disability, such as cerebral palsy, must be established early in the history to allow for better assessment and teaching strategies.
Does the child have any allergies? If so, what is the specific allergen? How does the child react to it? **CLINICAL TIP** Some parents consider medication side effects to be allergic responses (e.g., diarrhea that is common after antibiotic use) and need information to differentiate side effects from actual allergies.	Allergies are very common during childhood. Nurses need to ask what the specific allergen is and how the child reacts to it.
What prescriptions; over-the-counter medications, devices, and treatments; and home or folk remedies is the child taking? Please provide the name of the drug, dosage, frequency, and reason it is administered.	It is always important to know what medications a client is taking, especially young clients. The child may be taking a combination of medications that are incompatible or a folk remedy that is harmful (e.g., azarcon, used in Mexico for digestive problems, contains lead). **CULTURAL CONSIDERATIONS** Greta and azarcon (also known as alarcon, coral, luiga, marialuisa, or rueda) are Hispanic traditional medicines taken for upset stomach (empacho), constipation, diarrhea, and vomiting, and are also used on teething babies. They are fine orange powders with lead content as high as 90% (CDC, 2013).
What immunizations has the child or adolescent received thus far? Has your child or adolescent had any reactions to immunizations? (See Tables of immunization recommendations by pediatric age group on thePoint.)	This helps to identify risk for infection and/or potential reactions to immunizations.

Family History

The questions asked about family history for the child and adolescent are basically the same types of questions that are asked of the adult client (e.g., whether certain diseases/conditions run in the family, the age and cause of death for blood relatives, and family members with communicable diseases). This is an area of the subjective assessment in which the nurse focuses primarily on the parent for the necessary information. An exception might be if the child is older or is an adolescent and knows a great deal about his or her family history. As with the past history information, if the child or adolescent is adopted or a foster child, family history information may not be known. An important reason for collecting these data is to implement preventive teaching at a young age. Word the following sample questions to address either the parent or the child/adolescent as appropriate.

Continued on following page

Family History (Continued)

QUESTION	RATIONALE
Do certain diseases/conditions run in the family?	Certain conditions tend to run in families and increase the client's risk for such conditions.
Please list the ages and causes of death for blood relatives.	This helps to identify risk factors.
Does the child or adolescent have family members with communicable diseases?	This also helps to identify risk factors.

Lifestyle and Health Practices

QUESTION	RATIONALE
What activities are you involved with at school, or after school activities? Are you involved in sports at school or city league sports, such as baseball, basketball, and the like?	Involvement in activities, such as sports or clubs at school or in afterschool programs, provides the examiner with knowledge regarding the child's or teen's exercise habits and social, academic, musical and artistic interests.
Do you use tobacco or alcohol products?	Smoking and alcohol use increase the risk of cancer and lung disease. Asking the child or teen about use of these products will help to identify underage use of products, in which case counseling is suggested.
What is your typical diet during the day? How many meals do you eat per day? Do you start the day out by eating breakfast? During the school year, do you usually eat school-prepared meals? What snacks are consumed? What fluids are consumed? Are caffeinated beverages consumed?	Assessment of dietary habits is important to identify the child's nutritional habits. Adequate nutrition is imperative during the childhood years for proper growth and development. The nurse can determine if counseling regarding nutritional habits for the child and/or parent is needed.
Are you sexually active?	Identifying sexual activity in the adolescent is important to establish and determine the need for counseling for sexual activity.
Do you spend much time using a cell phone, computer, or tablet, or watching LED television?	Blue light or blue/violet light from these sources penetrates deeply into the retina and has been shown to interfere with melatonin production and reduce REM sleep, which can affect behavior and produce a sense of tiredness throughout the day (Ford, 2016).

Review of Systems

It is essential that pertinent subjective data be collected for each body system. Many of the questions for each body system asked of the adult are asked of the parent, child, or adolescent. The additional nursing history questions listed in the following sections for each system are of special concern for children and adolescents.

QUESTION	RATIONALE
Skin, Hair, Nails	
Has your child or adolescent had any changes in hair texture?	Changes may indicate an underlying problem.
Does your child or adolescent complain of scalp itching?	Itching may indicate lice, seborrhea, allergies, or ringworm.
Have you noticed any changes in your child's or adolescent's nails? Color? Cracking? Shape? Lines?	Changes may indicate an underlying problem.
Has your child or adolescent been exposed to any contagious disease such as measles, chickenpox, lice, ringworm, scabies, and the like?	These communicable diseases are common in childhood.
Has your child or adolescent ever had any rashes or sores? Acne?	Rashes may represent a number of diseases/disorders. Acne is a common problem for adolescents. They often have a hard time talking about it, but they want treatment.
Has your child or adolescent had any excessive bruising or burns?	This helps to assess for child abuse. Excessive bruising or burns suggest abuse.

QUESTION	RATIONALE
Does your child or adolescent use any cosmetics? Have tattoos? Have any pierced body parts?	This provides insight into personal habits.
Does your child or adolescent have any birthmarks?	This helps to identify any lesions and lets the examiner know to assess areas for changes.

Head and Neck

Has your child or adolescent ever had a head injury?	Head injuries may cause neurologic problems.
Does your child or adolescent experience headaches? How frequently?	Many neurologic disorders cause headaches.
Has your child or adolescent ever had swollen neck glands for any significant length of time?	This may indicate an underlying disorder.
Has your child or adolescent ever experienced any neck stiffness?	Stiffness may indicate disorders such as meningitis.

Eyes

Does your child or adolescent excessively cross eyes?	Eye crossing may indicate visual or neurologic problems.
Does your child or adolescent frequently rub the eyes or blink repeatedly?	This could indicate visual problems.
Does your child or adolescent strain/squint to see distant objects?	These suggest visual problems.
Has your child's or adolescent's vision been tested?	Children require regular vision screening.
Does your child or adolescent wear glasses or contact lenses? Are they worn when needed? Do the glasses or contact lenses help your child or adolescent to see better?	This helps to gauge usage and if the prescription needs to be reassessed.

Ears

Does your child or adolescent appear to be paying attention when you speak?	Children/adolescents should respond. A child or adolescent who often appears to not be paying attention may have a hearing deficit or neurologic disorder.
Does your child speak? At what age did talking start?	It is important to assess developmental milestones.
Does your child or adolescent listen to loud music?	This is common behavior among adolescents and usually does not indicate hearing deficit. However, it can lead to a hearing deficit. Preventative education may be needed.
Does your child or adolescent use a hearing aid? If so, has it improved the child's ability to interact and understand others?	This helps to evaluate the effectiveness of the hearing aid.
Has your child or adolescent had frequent ear infections? Tubes in ears?	Frequent ear infections may contribute to hearing loss.
How frequently does your child or adolescent have hearing tested?	Screening for hearing deficits should be done regularly.

Mouth, Throat, Nose, and Sinuses

Has your child or adolescent ever had any difficulty swallowing or chewing?	Difficulty may indicate a mechanical/neurologic disorder.
Has your child or adolescent ever had strep throat, tonsillitis, pharyngitis, or any other mouth or throat infections? Does your child or adolescent get frequent oral lesions?	Past infections may affect current condition.
When did your child's teeth erupt? When did your child lose baby teeth? When did adult teeth erupt?	See Chapter 30 for a schedule for teeth eruption.
Does your child or adolescent have any dental problems? Does your child or adolescent visit the dentist regularly? Wear any dental appliances?	Children/adolescents should visit the dentist twice a year. If child/adolescent has frequent dental problems, provide education about dental care and preventive care.

Continued on following page

Review of Systems (Continued)

QUESTION	RATIONALE
Mouth, Throat, Nose, and Sinuses (Continued)	
Does your child or adolescent experience nosebleeds?	Nosebleeds may occur with allergies, trauma, nose-picking, or foreign bodies.
Does your child or adolescent have any sinus problems?	Sinus pain may indicate allergies or infection.
Thorax and Lungs	
Has your child or adolescent ever had cough, wheezing, shortness of breath, nocturnal dyspnea? If so, when does it occur?	Many respiratory problems, such as asthma and bronchitis, are frequently seen in children. They may affect current health status.
Has your child or adolescent received the influenza and pneumonia vaccines?	American Academy of Pediatrics (AAP, 2015) recommends that children and adolescents who are 6 months old and older, including all children and adolescents, receive influenza immunization annually. According to the CDC (2016), pneumococcal conjugate vaccine (PVC13) should be administered to all children under 5 years old and to those 6 and older if certain risk factors are present (see CDC, 2016).
Does your child or adolescent smoke? When did your child or adolescent start smoking? How much does he or she smoke? **CLINICAL TIP** Ask adolescents and older school-age children about smoking, including smokeless tobacco, in private.	Smoking increases the risk for many diseases, including lung cancer. Provide appropriate client teaching.
Is your child or adolescent exposed to secondhand smoke?	Respiratory infections are more common in children exposed to secondhand smoke.
Breasts and Lymphatics	
Has your daughter started developing breasts (thelarche)? If so, when did development start?	This helps to determine the child's/adolescent's sexual development stage.
Have you noticed any abnormal breast development in your son or young daughter?	Gynecomastia is enlargement of breast tissue in males. It is a normal finding during puberty. See Tanner's Sexual Maturity Rating (Table 31-1) for growth and development of breast tissue for girls.
Heart and Neck Vessels	
Has your child or adolescent ever experienced chest pain, heart murmurs, congenital heart disease, or hypertension?	All of these symptoms indicate possible cardiac problems.
Has your child or adolescent ever complained of fatigue? Does your child or adolescent have difficulty keeping up with peers when running or exercising?	Fatigue may result from decreased cardiac output. Heart problems may impede the child's or adolescent's ability to perform physical activities.
Has your child or adolescent ever fainted?	Children or adolescents who faint should be screened for cardiac problems.
Has your child or adolescent ever turned "blue" during activity?	This may suggest cardiac arrhythmia.
Do you believe that your child or adolescent is meeting the normal growth requirements for his or her age?	Children or adolescents with congenital heart disease may grow and develop more slowly than other children.
Peripheral Vascular System	
Does your child or adolescent ever experience bluing of the extremities? Do your child's or adolescent's hands and/or feet get unusually cold?	Cyanosis and/or coldness in the extremities suggests vascular problems.
Has your child or adolescent ever had problems with blood clots?	A history of blood clots increases the risk of recurrence.

QUESTION	RATIONALE
Abdomen	
Has your child or adolescent ever had any excessive vomiting? Abdominal pain? Please describe.	Excessive vomiting may be associated with gastrointestinal problems. Abdominal pain may accompany many disorders/problems.
Does your child or adolescent have any digestive problems (e.g., irritable bowel, constipation)?	Bowel problems should be explored further.
Has your child or adolescent ever experienced any trauma to the abdomen?	Trauma may result in injuries or contribute to disorders.
Does your child or adolescent have any hernias?	
Genitalia and Sexuality	
How often does your child urinate? How many wet diapers do you change per day?	This helps to determine nutritional habits, e.g., is the child receiving enough fluids?
At what age was your child toilet (bladder) trained? Night?	This helps to determine whether and when the child reaches developmental milestones.
Does your child ever wet his or her pants?	If there is a history of enuresis, obtain routine that family follows to deal with problem.
Is there any history of frequency, burning, pain during urination?	These genitourinary problems should be further explored.
Do you have any concerns about your child or adolescent related to masturbation, asking/answering questions about sex, not respecting others' privacy, or wanting too much privacy?	This helps to assess the child's or adolescent's sexual development.
Has anyone ever touched your child or adolescent in a way that made him or her feel uncomfortable? (Make sure to ask the parent *and* child or adolescent this question.)	It is important to screen for sexual abuse.
Has the child or adolescent started puberty, thelarche, menarche? See Tables 31-1, 31-2, and 31-3 for Tanner's stages of sexual development.	
Has your child or adolescent started having wet dreams (nocturnal emissions)?	Pubescent clients should be reassured that nocturnal emissions are normal.
Who is/are the source(s) of sex/AIDS education? (Questions to the adolescent about sexuality and reproductive issues should be asked privately at each office visit. Interactive counseling directed at the adolescent's risks and goals between the provider and adolescent should be tailored to risk–reduction practices.)	This helps to determine the child's need for sexual education.
Do you know how to perform breast self-examination or testicular self-examination?	Breast and testicular self-examinations are important screening tools that the nurse should teach adolescents.
Ask about menstruation: • How old were you when you started menstruating? • When was your last menstrual period (LMP)? • What is your menstrual cycle schedule? Has it always been this way? • What is your bleeding like? Light, moderate, heavy? • Do you experience any cramps? Tell me about them. • Do you experience any other physical or emotional discomfort associated with menstruation? • Do you use tampons? How frequently do you change them?	This assesses the client's development and gynecologic needs.
Assess sexual history: • What was your age at first intercourse?	A careful sexual history should be taken for all sexually active clients.

Continued on following page

Review of Systems (Continued)

QUESTION	RATIONALE
Genitalia and Sexuality (Continued)	
For adolescent or parent: Have you received information regarding the human papillomavirus vaccine that can reduce the incidence of cervical, vulvar, vaginal, and anal cancer? Have you received the vaccine?	HPV is associated with cervical, vulvar, and vaginal cancer in females, penile cancer in males, and anal and oropharyngeal cancer in both females and males. HPV vaccine is recommended for routine vaccination at age 11 or 12 years, for females aged 13 through 26 years and males aged 13 through 21 years not vaccinated previously. Vaccination is also recommended through age 26 years for men who have sex with men and for immunocompromised persons (including those with HIV infection) if not vaccinated previously. There are three approved vaccines for preventing human papilloma virus (HPV). The vaccine comes in 2-valent, 9-valent, and 14-valent forms (CDC, MMWR, 2015).
Have you ever had a Pap smear? Do you experience any discomfort/pain with intercourse?	NOTE: There is much controversy over pelvic examinations, when they should begin, when they should no longer be done, and how extensive the examination should be (bimanual palpation or not). ACOG (2016) continues to recommend beginning pelvic examinations at age 21 but ACOG is reviewing the new USPSTF (2016a) recommendation that there is insufficient evidence to determine the benefits or harms of performing pelvic screening exams in asymptomatic, nonpregnant adult women. (This does not apply to pelvic examinations performed for the purposes of screening for specific disorders for which the USPSTF has already issued a recommendation, i.e., cervical cancer, gonorrhea, and Chlamydia.) The USPSTF (2016b) recommends that all women aged 25 or less who are sexually active be screened for STIs.
How many sexual partners do you have/have you had?	
What type of contraception do you use and how do you use it? Do you use condoms? How do you use them?	Contraceptive education (preventive education) should be provided, along with stressing the importance of abstinence.
Have you ever had a sexually transmitted infection?	STIs can have long-term health effects and may indicate unprotected sexual activity.
Were you ever pregnant? What was the result of that pregnancy?	Pregnancy, spontaneous abortion, or elective abortion may affect the adolescent's reproductive health and may indicate unprotected sexual activity.
Have you had or considered having a gynecologic examination?	This examination should be performed for all sexually active adolescent girls, and is suggested as a routine examination for those older than 21 years of age (USPSTF, 2016a).
Anus and Rectum	
How often does your child or adolescent have a bowel movement? What does it look like?	This helps to assess the child's/adolescent's nutritional intake and gastrointestinal function.
At what age was your child toilet trained (bowel)?	This helps to determine whether and when the child reaches developmental milestones.
Does your child ever soil his or her pants?	With a history of encopresis, obtain the routine that the family follows to deal with the problem.
Is there any history of bleeding, constipation, diarrhea, rectal itching, or hemorrhoids?	Constipation may cause rectal bleeding and/or pain. Rectal bleeding needs further investigation if not controlled with treatment for constipation. Child abuse (sodomy) should also be suspected. Rectal itching may be a sign of pinworms or infection.
	Hemorrhoids are very unusual in children, unless they are chronically constipated. Hemorrhoids may indicate an intra-abdominal mass.

QUESTION	RATIONALE
Musculoskeletal System	
Has your child or adolescent ever had limited range of motion, joint pain, stiffness, paralysis? Have you noticed any bone deformity?	A positive history of any of these requires further investigation.
Has your child or adolescent ever had any fractures?	Frequent fractures may suggest a disorder of the musculoskeletal system or child abuse.
Has your child or adolescent ever used any corrective devices (orthopedic shoes, scoliosis brace)?	This should be noted as it may affect/explain findings during the physical examination.
Describe your child's or adolescent's posture.	Children, especially females, should be screened for scoliosis.
Is your child or adolescent involved in any sports? What type of protective gear does your child or adolescent use?	Provide appropriate client teaching about safety and protective gear as needed.
Neurologic System	
Does your child or adolescent have any learning disabilities? Does your child or adolescent have any attention problems at home or at school?	Learning disabilities may hinder a child's performance at school and/or indicate a neurologic disorder.
Has your child or adolescent ever experienced any problems with memory?	Memory problems may indicate neurologic disorders.
Has your child or adolescent ever had a seizure?	Seizures may indicate a neurologic or cardiovascular disorder.
Has your child or adolescent ever had a head injury?	Head trauma may cause intracranial bleeding or other injuries.
Has your child or adolescent ever experienced any problems with motor coordination?	Uncoordinated movements or difficulty with coordination may indicate neurologic disorders.

CASE STUDY

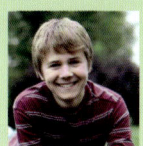

The nurse interviews Carsen using specific probing questions, using the COLDSPA mnemonic as a guide.

Mnemonic	Question	Data Provided
Character	Describe the sign or symptom (feeling, appearance, sound, smell, or taste if applicable).	"My ear hurts."
Onset	When did it begin?	"Yesterday."
Location	Where is it? Does it radiate? Does it occur anywhere else?	"Inside my right ear and down to my jaw."
Duration	How long does it last? Does it recur?	"It hurts all the time."
Severity	How bad is it? or How much does it bother you?	"Really bad." Client gives the pain a rating of 8 on a scale of 1–10.
Pattern	What makes it better or worse?	"Tylenol and heat made it a little better."
Associated factors/ How it **A**ffects the client	What other symptoms occur with it? How does it affect you?	"My head hurts and my nose is stuffy. I keep coughing. I can't sleep and I can't think in school either because I feel bad all over."

The nurse continues with the health history. Carsen is a 13-year-old boy who presents with his mother for a well-child visit. He tells the nurse that he has been healthy until yesterday when he developed pain in his right ear, along with a runny nose and cough. He has experienced a low-grade fever and is not sleeping during the nighttime. He has a headache and finds it difficult to concentrate at school. He denies use of tobacco products or alcohol.

Family history is remarkable for his grandparents having heart disease and glaucoma. Mother and father are both healthy. He has one older sister, who is alive and well. No current exposure to communicable diseases.

The review of systems for Carsen is positive for having right ear pain, runny nose, and cough. He has had a low-grade fever, up to 100.0°F.

BOX 31-4 HEALTHY PEOPLE 2020 OBJECTIVES FOR EARLY AND MIDDLE CHILDHOOD

Healthy People 2020 (HealthyPeople.gov, 2014a; 2014b) has newly developed goals and objectives for the topics Early and Middle Childhood, and Adolescent Health.

EARLY AND MIDDLE CHILDHOOD

The goal for early and middle childhood is to document and track population-based measures of health and well-being for early and middle childhood populations over time in the United States.

The following objectives were developed for childhood:
1. (Developmental) Increase the proportion of children who are ready for school in all five domains of healthy development: physical development, social-emotional development, approaches to learning, language, and cognitive development.
2. Increase the proportion of parents who use positive parenting and communicate with their doctors or other health care professionals about positive parenting.
3. (Developmental) Reduce the proportion of children who have poor quality of sleep.
4. Increase the proportion of elementary, middle, and senior high schools that require school health education.
5. (Developmental) Increase the proportion of children with ADHD who receive recommended treatment.

Immunization-related objectives include:
1. Reduce, eliminate, or maintain elimination of cases of vaccine-preventable diseases.
2. Reduce early-onset group B streptococcal disease.
3. Reduce meningococcal disease.
4. Reduce invasive pneumococcal infections.
5. Achieve and maintain effective vaccination coverage levels for universally recommended vaccines among young children.
6. Increase the proportion of children aged 19–35 months who receive the recommended doses of DTaP, polio, MMR, Hib, hepatitis B, varicella, and PCV vaccines. Decrease the proportion of children in the United States who receive zero doses of recommended vaccines by 19–35 months.
7. Maintain vaccination coverage levels for children in kindergarten.
8. Increase routine vaccination coverage levels for adolescents.
9. Increase the proportion of children and adults who are vaccinated annually against seasonal influenza.
10. Increase the scientific knowledge of vaccine safety and adverse events.
11. Increase the proportion of providers who have had vaccination coverage levels among children in their practice population measured within the past year.
12. Increase the proportion of children under 6 years of age whose immunization records are in fully operational, population-based immunization information systems.
13. Increase the number of states collecting kindergarten vaccination coverage data according to CBC minimum standards.
14. Increase the number of states that have 80% of adolescents with two or more age-appropriate immunizations recorded in immunization information systems (adolescents aged 11–18 years).
15. Reduce hepatitis A infections.
16. Reduce chronic hepatitis B infections in infants and young children (perinatal infections).
17. Reduce hepatitis B infections.

ADOLESCENT HEALTH

The Healthy People 2020 (2014a) goal for Adolescent Health is to improve the healthy development, health, safety, and well-being of adolescents (ages 10–19) and young adults (ages 20–24). The following objectives have been developed for adolescents:
1. Increase the proportion of adolescents who have had a wellness checkup in the past 12 months.
2. Increase the proportion of adolescents who participate in extracurricular and/or out-of-school activities.
3. Increase the proportion of adolescents who are connected to a parent or other positive adult caregiver.
4. Increase the proportion of adolescents who transition to self-sufficiency from foster care.
5. Increase educational achievement of adolescents and young adults.
6. Increase the proportion of schools with a school breakfast program.
7. Reduce the proportion of adolescents who have been offered, sold, or given an illegal drug on school property.
8. Increase the proportion of adolescents whose parents consider them to be safe at school.
9. Increase the proportion of middle and high schools that prohibit harassment based on a student's sexual orientation or gender identity.
10. Reduce the proportion of public schools with a serious violent incident.
11. Reduce adolescent and young adult perpetration of, and victimization by, crimes.

Adapted from HealthyPeople.gov. (2014a). Adolescent health (available at https://www.healthypeople.gov/2020/topics-objectives/topic/Adolescent-Health) and HealthyPeople.gov. (2014b). Early and middle childhood (available at http://www.healthypeople.gov/2020/topicsobjectives2020/overview.aspx?topicid=10).

BOX 31-5 DEVELOPMENTAL APPROACHES TO THE PHYSICAL ASSESSMENT

Children in each age group respond differently to the hands-on physical assessment; however, the following guidelines should be kept in mind:

TODDLERS
Allow toddler to sit on parent's lap; enlist parent's aid; use play; praise cooperation.

PRESCHOOLERS
Use story telling; use doll and puppet play; give choices when able.

SCHOOL-AGERS
Maintain privacy; use gown; explain procedures and equipment; teach about their bodies.

ADOLESCENTS
Ensure privacy and confidentiality; provide option of having parent present or not; emphasize normality; provide health teaching.

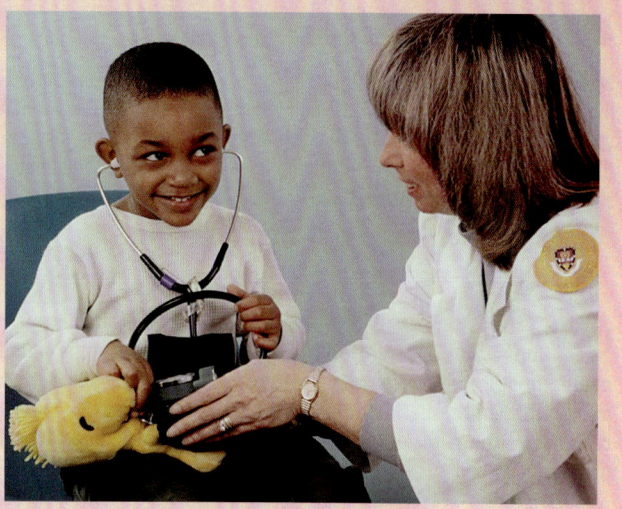

Puppet or doll play is a great way to prepare a preschooler for physical examination (© B. Proud).

Collecting Objective Data: Physical Examination

Preparing the Client

In most cases, physical assessment involves a head-to-toe examination that encompasses each body system. When examining children, alter the sequence to accommodate the child's developmental needs. Complete less threatening and least intrusive procedures, such as general inspection and heart and lung auscultation, first to secure the child's trust. Explain what you will be doing and what the child can expect to feel; allow the child to manipulate the equipment before it is used. Try to perform examination in a comfortable, nonthreatening area. The temperature should be warm, the room well lit, and all threatening instruments out of the child's view. The room should contain age-appropriate diversions such as toys and cartoons for younger children and posters for adolescents. If the child is uncooperative, first assess the reason (usually fear) then intervene appropriately. If still unsuccessful, involve parents, use a firm approach, and complete the examination as quickly but completely as possible. Involve the child in the physical examination at all times unless it is stressful for him or her.

Equipment
- Denver Developmental Kit
- Ophthalmoscope
- Otoscope with nasal speculum
- Scale/stadiometer
- Snellen Eye Chart
- Stethoscope

Physical Assessment

Key points to keep in mind during the physical assessment include:
- Recognize how techniques and demeanor for interviewing and examining children differ among the age groups and from those used for interviewing and examining adults. Box 31-5 gives developmental approaches to the physical examination.
- Evaluate growth and development patterns according to the different pediatric age groups and across body systems.
- Recognize children who are difficult to examine because of anxiety or fear.
- Develop forms of age-appropriate "play" to distract less cooperative children, so physical examination can be completed.

Focused Specialty Assessment of the Child or Adolescent

Assessment of children and adolescents is a focused specialty area for nurses. Development of these skills requires knowledge and experience with pediatric clients. The nurse learns to vary her approach and interaction as appropriate with the age of the child or adolescent and availability of the parent or care giver. The extent of each assessment depends on the child or adolescent's presenting problem, setting, equipment availability and scope of assessment experience of the nurse or pediatric nurse practitioner. For example, the Denver Developmental Screening Test requires special testing equipment and knowledge and experience with using this tool.

ASSESSMENT PROCEDURE	NORMAL FINDINGS	ABNORMAL FINDINGS
General Appearance and Behavior		
Note overall appearance. Observe hygiene, interaction with parents and with you (and siblings if present). Note also facies (facial expressions), posture, nutritional status, speech, attention span, and level of cooperation.	Child appears stated age, is clean, appears well nourished, and has no unusual body odor. Clothing is in good condition and appropriate for climate.	Lack of eye contact indicates many things including anxiety or significant psychosocial problems. **CULTURAL CONSIDERATIONS** Lack of eye contact is normal for certain cultural groups such as Asians and Native Americans.
CLINICAL TIP Behavioral observation is one of the most important assessments to make with children and adolescents because alterations usually signify health problems.	Child is alert, active, responds appropriately to stress of the situation, and maintains eye contact. Child is appropriately interactive for age, seeks comfort from parent; appears happy or appropriately anxious because of examination. Child is attentive and speech is appropriate for age, follows age-appropriate commands, and is reasonably cooperative. Toddler is lordotic when standing; preschooler is slightly bowlegged; older child demonstrates straight and well-balanced posture.	Deviations from normal that can be discerned from a child's appearance or behavior follow. Certain facies may indicate fear, anxiety, anger, allergies, acute illness, pain, mental deficiency, or respiratory distress. A child's posture or movement may indicate pain, low self-esteem, rejection, depression, hostility, or aggression. Hygiene gives insight into neglect, poverty, mental illness or retardation, knowledge deficit regarding hygiene (e.g., teen parent). Abnormal behavior may suggest neurologic problems (head trauma, cranial lesions), metabolic problems (diabetic ketoacidosis), psychiatric disorders, or psychosocial problems. Abnormal development (child does not appear stated age) may indicate mental retardation, abuse, neglect, or psychiatric disorders.
Developmental Assessment		
Screen for cognitive, language, social, and gross and fine motor developmental delays in the beginning of the physical assessment for preschoolers. Use a standardized assessment tool such as Draw a Person, Revised Prescreening Developmental Questionnaire, or the Denver Developmental Screening Test II (DDST). In Chapter 30, Assessment Tool 30-1 presents the DDST II and directions for its use.	Child meets normal parameters for age. See information contained in the Growth and Development section.	Child lags in earlier stages.
Vital Signs		
Assess temperature. Use rectal, axillary, skin, or tympanic route when assessing temperature. For children older than 4 years of age, the oral route can be used in addition to the other routes (see Chapter 8 for techniques for taking temperature). **SAFETY TIP** *Use of the rectal route is rare these days, and should only be used when absolutely necessary because of increased discomfort in older children. Rectal temperatures are also contraindicated in certain circumstances, such as the immunosuppressed child as well as the child who has diarrhea, a bleeding disorder, a perforated anus, or a history of rectal surgery.*	Temperature is 98.6°F.	Temperature may be altered by exercise, stress, crying, environment, diurnal variation (highest between 4 PM and 6 PM). Both hyperthermic and hypothermic conditions are noted in children.

ASSESSMENT PROCEDURE	NORMAL FINDINGS	ABNORMAL FINDINGS
Assess pulse rate. Count the pulse for a full minute. Children younger than 2 years old should have apical pulse measured. Radial pulses may be taken in children over 2 years old (Fig. 31-13).	Awake and resting rates vary with the age of the child: • 3 months–2 years: 80–150 • 2–10 years: 70–110 • 10 years–adult: 55–90 🎯 **CLINICAL TIP** Athletic adolescents tend to have lower pulse rates.	Pulse may be altered by apprehension or anxiety, medications, activity, and pain, as well as pathologic conditions.
Assess respiratory rate. Monitor respirations in children older than 1 year the same as for adults.	Normal ranges are as follows: **Respiratory Rates in Children** | Age	Normal Respiratory Rate
---	---
Infants (<1 year)	30–53
Toddler (1–2 years)	22–37
Preschool (3–5 years)	20–28
School-age (6–11 years)	18–25
Adolescent (12–15 years)	12–20 | (From PedsCases, 2016, Pediatric vital signs reference chart. Available at http://www.pedscases.com/pediatric-vital-signs-reference-chart)	Respiratory rate and character may be altered by medications, positioning, fever, activity, and anxiety or fear as well as pathologic conditions.

Evaluate blood pressure. Blood pressure should be measured annually in children 3 years and older, and in all ages when conditions warrant it. The appropriate cuff width is 50–75% of the upper arm (Fig. 31-14). The length should encircle the circumference without overlapping. A small diaphragm should be used for the stethoscope. If for some reason the arm cannot be used, a measurement can be taken on the thigh. If children younger than 3 years old require a blood pressure reading, a Doppler stethoscope should be used.	Normal ranges are as follows:
	• Systolic
	  • 1–7 years = age in years + 90
	  • 7–18 years = (2 × age in years) + 90
	• Diastolic
	  • 1–6 years = 53–66
	  • 6–18 years = age in years + 52
		Systolic and diastolic BP above 95th percentiles for age and sex after three readings is considered high blood pressure.
		
		🎯 **CLINICAL TIP**
		If the blood pressure reading is too high for age, the cuff may be too small; it should cover two thirds of the child's upper arm. If the blood pressure reading is too low for age, the cuff may be too large. Chapter 8 explains how to take a blood pressure reading.

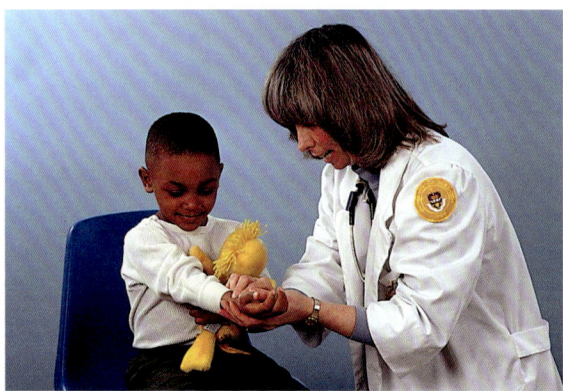

FIGURE 31-13 Measuring radial pulse in a child over 2 years (© B. Proud).

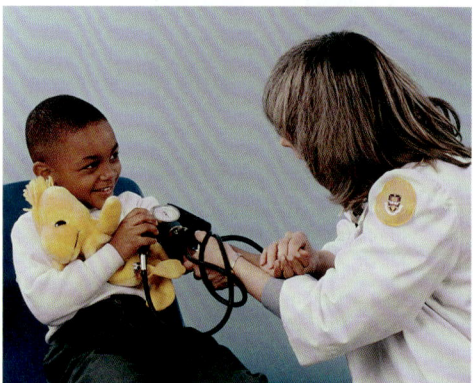

FIGURE 31-14 Measuring the child's blood pressure requires a cuff that is appropriately sized (© B. Proud).

Measurements

Measure height. In a child younger than 2 years, determine height by measuring the recumbent length. Fully extend the body, holding the head in midline and gently grasping the knees and pushing them	See the growth charts available at http://www.cdc.gov/growthcharts for normal findings. **CULTURAL CONSIDERATIONS** Asian children are smaller at all ages.	Significant deviation from normal in the growth charts would be considered abnormal.

Continued on following page

ASSESSMENT PROCEDURE	NORMAL FINDINGS	ABNORMAL FINDINGS
Measurements (Continued)		
downward until the legs are fully extended and touching the table. If using a measuring board, place the head at the top of the board and the heels firmly at the bottom. Without a board, use paper under the child and mark the paper at the top of the head and bottom of the heels. Then measure the distance between the two points. Determine an older child's height by having the shoeless child stand as straight as possible with head midline and vision line parallel between the ceiling and floor (Fig. 31-15). The child's back, buttocks, and back of heels should be against the wall; measure height with a stadiometer. Plot height measurement on an age- and gender-appropriate growth chart (birth to 36 months and 2–20 years).		

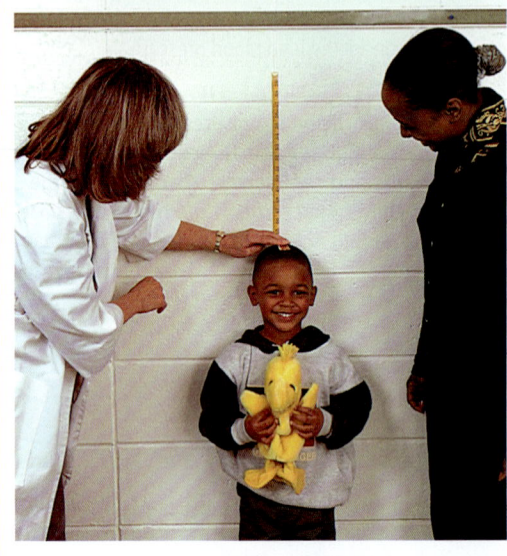

FIGURE 31-15 Measuring the height of a preschooler (© B. Proud).

Measure weight on an appropriately sized beam scale with nondetectable weights. Weigh a small child lying or sitting on a scale that measures to the nearest 0.5 oz or 10 g. Weigh an older child standing on a scale that measures to the nearest 0.25 lb or 100 g. Weigh an older child in underpants or light gown to respect modesty. Plot weight measurement on age- and gender-appropriate growth chart (birth to 36 months and 2–20 years).	For normal findings see growth charts available at http://www.cdc.gov/growthcharts.	Deviation from the wide range of normal weights is abnormal. See the growth charts available at http://www.cdc.gov/growth-charts and compare differences.
Measure head circumference (HC) or occipital frontal circumference (OFC) at every physical examination for toddlers younger than 2 years and older children when conditions warrant. Plot the measurement on standardized growth charts specific for gender.	HC (OFC) measurement should fall between the 5th and 95th percentiles, and should be comparable to the child's height and weight percentiles.	HC (OFC) not within the normal percentiles may indicate pathology. Those greater than 95% may indicate macrocephaly. Those under the 5th percentile may indicate microcephaly. Increased HC (OFC) in children older than 3 years may indicate separation of cranial sutures due to increased intracranial pressure.

ASSESSMENT PROCEDURE	NORMAL FINDINGS	ABNORMAL FINDINGS
Skin, Hair, and Nails		
INSPECTION AND PALPATION		
Observe skin color, odor, and lesions.	Skin color ranges from pale white with pink, yellow, brown, or olive tones to dark brown or black. No strong odor should be evident, and the skin should be lesion free. Normal skin variations (Box 31-6) include: • Port-wine stains • Hemangiomas • Café-au-lait spots (normal in small numbers)	Yellow skin may indicate jaundice or intake of too many yellow vegetables, especially noticeable in infants (sclera remain white if associated with eating vegetables). Blue skin suggests cyanosis; pallor suggests anemia; and redness suggests fever, irritation, or allergies. Body piercing may be cultural or a fad, but excessive piercing may indicate underlying self-abusive tendencies. If tattoos appear to be "homemade," consider the possibility of contamination with hepatitis B virus or HIV from infected needles. Urine odor suggests incontinence, dirty diaper, or uremia. Salty sweat may indicate cystic fibrosis (a parent may report that the child's skin tastes salty when the parent kisses the child). Ecchymoses in various stages or in unusual locations or circular burn areas suggest child abuse. **CULTURAL CONSIDERATIONS** Bruising or burning may also be from cultural practices such as cupping or coining. Petechiae, lesions, or rashes may indicate serious disorders. More than six café-au-lait spots may indicate neurovascular disease.
Palpate for texture, temperature, moisture, turgor, and edema.	Skin should be soft, warm, and slightly moist, with good turgor and without edema.	Excessive dryness suggests poor nutrition, excessive bathing, or an endocrine disorder. Flaking or scaling suggests eczema or fungal infections. Poor skin turgor indicates dehydration or malnutrition; edema suggests renal or cardiac disorders; periorbital edema may indicate pathology but may also be due to recent crying, sleeping, or allergies. Russell sign (abrasion or scarring on joints of the index and middle finger) suggests self-induced vomiting. Bite marks may indicate child abuse or self-abusive behavior (psychiatric disorders, mental retardation).
Inspect and palpate hair. Observe for distribution, characteristics, infestation, and presence of any unusual hair on body.	Hair is normally lustrous, silky, strong, and elastic. Fine, downy hair covers the body. Adolescents may display a variety of hairstyles and hair colors to assert independence and group conformity. **CULTURAL CONSIDERATIONS** African American children usually have hair that is curlier and coarser than Caucasian children.	Dirty, matted hair may indicate neglect. Dull, dry, brittle hair may indicate poor nutrition, hypothyroidism, excessive use of chemical hair products (teens). Grayish or brown oval bodies suggest ticks or lice. Balding (alopecia) suggests neglect, trichotillomania (hair pulling), skin diseases, or chemotherapy.

Continued on following page

ASSESSMENT PROCEDURE	NORMAL FINDINGS	ABNORMAL FINDINGS
Skin, Hair, and Nails (Continued)		
		Tufts of hair over the spine may indicate spina bifida occulta.
		Coarse body hair in a prepubertal child or older girl may be due to an endocrine disorder.
		Pubic hair growth in a child younger than 8 years may indicate precocious adrenarche or precocious puberty.
Inspect and palpate nails. Note color, texture, shape, and condition of nails.	Nails should be clean and groomed. Pink undertones should be seen. Adolescents may color or pierce nails. 🌐 **CULTURAL CONSIDERATIONS** Dark-skinned children have deeper nail pigment.	Blue nailbeds indicate cyanosis. Yellow nailbeds suggest jaundice. Blue-black nailbeds are found with nailbed hemorrhage. White color suggests fungal infection. Scaly lesions also indicate fungal infections, especially in adolescents who use artificial nails.
		Short, ragged nails are common with nail biting; dirty, uncut nails suggest poor hygiene. Concave shape, "spoon nails" (koilonychia) indicate iron-deficiency anemia. Clubbing indicates chronic cyanosis.
		Macerated thumb tip is found with thumb sucking.
		Inflammation at the nail base indicates paronychia.
Head, Neck, and Cervical Lymph Nodes		
INSPECTION AND PALPATION		
Inspect and palpate the head. Note shape and symmetry.	Head is normocephalic and symmetric.	Very large head is hydrocephalus. Oddly shaped head suggests premature closure of sutures (possibly genetic).
		Presence of a third fontanelle located between the anterior and posterior fontanelle indicates Down syndrome.
		Craniotabes—from osteoporosis of the outer skull bone. Palpating too firmly with the thumb or forefinger over the temporoparietal area will leave an indentation of the bone.
Test head control, head posture, and range of motion (ROM).	Full ROM—up, down, and sideways—is normal.	Hyperextension suggests opisthotonos or significant meningeal irritation.
		Limited ROM suggests torticollis (wry neck).
Inspect and palpate the face. Note appearance, symmetry, and movement (have child make faces). Palpate the parotid glands for swelling.	Face is normally proportionate and symmetric. Movements are equal bilaterally. Parotid glands are normal size. 🎯 **CLINICAL TIP** Some adolescents may appear to have unusual skin tones or markings from applying makeup as a form of self-expression.	Unusual proportions (short palpebral fissures, thin lips, and wide and flat philtrum, which is the groove above the upper lip) may be hereditary or may indicate specific syndromes, such as Down syndrome (Fig. 31-16) and fetal alcohol syndrome. Other findings may indicate the following: • Unequal movement—facial nerve paralysis • Enlarged parotid gland—mumps or bulimia • Abnormal facies—chromosomal anomaly • Crease across nose, shiners (dark circles under eyes), and mouth agape—allergies (allergic facies)

ASSESSMENT PROCEDURE	NORMAL FINDINGS	ABNORMAL FINDINGS
Inspect and palpate the neck. Palpate the thyroid gland and the trachea. Also inspect and palpate the cervical lymph nodes for swelling, mobility, temperature, and tenderness (Fig. 31-17).	The isthmus is the only portion of the thyroid that should be palpable. The trachea is midline. Lymph nodes are usually nonpalpable in adolescents. "Shotty" lymph nodes (small, nontender, mobile) are commonly palpated in children between the ages of 3 and 12 years.	Implications of some abnormal findings include the following: • Short, webbed neck—anomalies or syndromes • Distended neck veins—difficulty breathing • Enlarged thyroid or palpable masses—pathologic processes • Shift in tracheal position from midline—serious lung problem (e.g., foreign body or tumor) • Enlarged, firm lymph nodes—Hodgkin disease or HIV infection • Enlarged, warm, and tender lymph nodes—lymphadenitis or infection in the head and neck area that is drained by the affected node

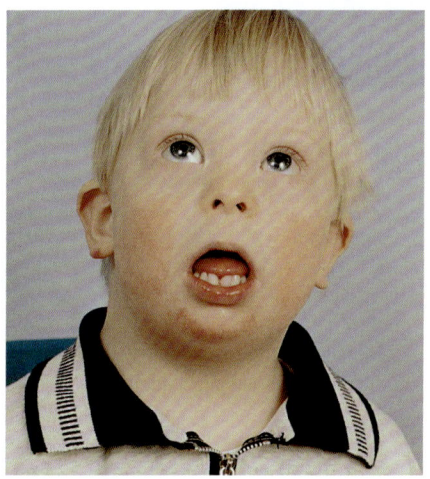

FIGURE 31-16 Down syndrome results from a genetic abnormality (© B. Proud).

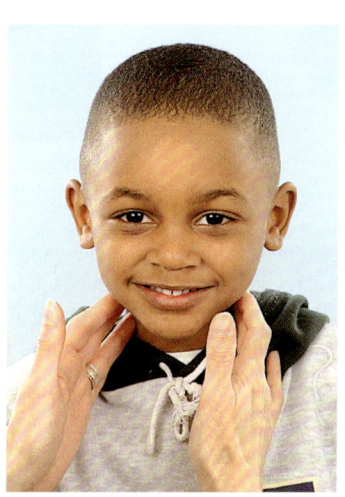

FIGURE 31-17 Palpating the cervical lymph nodes (© B. Proud).

Mouth, Throat, and Sinuses

INSPECTION

ASSESSMENT PROCEDURE	NORMAL FINDINGS	ABNORMAL FINDINGS
Note the condition of the lips, palates, tongue, and buccal mucosa (Fig. 31-18).	Lips, tongue, and buccal mucosa appear pink and moist. No lesions are present.	Dry lips may indicate mouth breathing or dehydration. Stomatitis suggests infection or immunodeficiency. Koplik spots (tiny, white spots on red bases) on the buccal mucosa may be a prodromal sign of measles. Cleft lip and/or palate are congenital abnormalities (Fig. 31-19).
Observe the condition of the teeth and gums.	Deciduous teeth begin to develop between 4 and 6 months; all 20 erupt by 36 months; teeth begin to fall out around 6 years, when permanent tooth eruption begins and progresses until all 32 have erupted.	Dental caries may herald "bottle caries syndrome." Enamel erosion may indicate bulimia.
Note the condition of the throat and tonsils. Also observe the insertion and ending point of the frenulum.	Tonsils are easily seen by age 6, when they increase to adult dimensions. They reach maximum size (about twice adult size) between the ages of 10 and 12 years. Atrophy to stable adult dimensions usually occurs by the end of adolescence.	Tonsillar or pharyngeal inflammation suggests infection. Extension of the frenulum to the tip of the tongue may interfere with extension of the tongue, which causes speech difficulties.

Continued on following page

796   UNIT 4   Nursing Assessment of Special Groups

ASSESSMENT PROCEDURE	NORMAL FINDINGS	ABNORMAL FINDINGS

Mouth, Throat, and Sinuses (Continued)

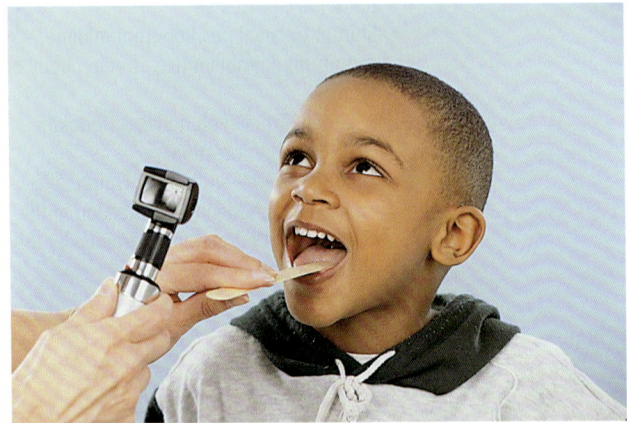

FIGURE 31-18 Inspecting the mouth (© B. Proud).

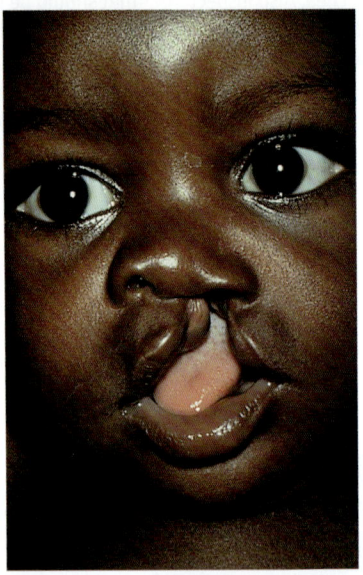

FIGURE 31-19 Cleft lip (© 1991 National Medical Slide Bank/CMSP).

Inspect nose and sinuses. To inspect the nose and sinuses, avoid using the nasal speculum in young children. Instead, push up the tip of the nose and shine the light into each nostril. Observe the structure and patency of the nares, discharge, tenderness, and any color or swelling of the turbinates.	Nose is midline in face, septum is straight, and nares are patent. No discharge or tenderness is present. Turbinates are pink and free of edema.	Deviated septum may be congenital or caused by injury. Foul discharge from one nostril may indicate a foreign body. Pale, boggy nasal mucosa with or without possible polyps suggests allergic rhinitis. Nasal polyps are also seen in children with cystic fibrosis.

PALPATION

Palpate the sinuses in older children if sinusitis is suspected. The sinuses of young children are not palpable.	No tenderness palpated over sinuses.	Tender sinuses suggest sinusitis.

Eyes

INSPECTION

Inspect the external eye. Note the position, slant, and epicanthal folds of the external eye.	Inner canthus distance approximately 2.5 cm, horizontal slant, noepicanthal folds. Outer canthus aligns with tips of the pinnas (Fig. 31-20).	Wide-set position (hypertelorism), upward slant, and thick epicanthal folds suggest Down syndrome. "Sun-setting" appearance (upper lid covers part of the iris) suggests hydrocephalus.

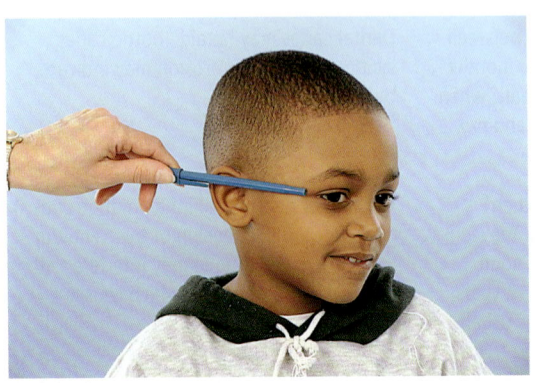

FIGURE 31-20 Outer canthus is in alignment with the tip of the pinna (© B. Proud).

ASSESSMENT PROCEDURE	NORMAL FINDINGS	ABNORMAL FINDINGS
	CULTURAL CONSIDERATIONS Epicanthal folds (excess of skin extending from roof of nose that partially or completely covers the inner canthus) are normal findings in Asian children, whose eyes also slant upward.	
Observe eyelid placement, swelling, discharge, and lesions.	No swelling, discharge, or lesions of eyelids.	Eyelid inflammation may result from blepharitis, hordeolum, or dacryocystitis (inflammation or blockage of lacrimal sac or duct.) Ptosis (drooping eyelids) suggests oculomotor nerve palsy, congenital syndrome, or a familial trait. A painful, edematous, erythematous area on the eyelid may be a hordeolum (stye). A nodular, nontender lesion on the eyelid may be a chalazion (cyst). Swelling, erythema, or purulent discharge may indicate infection or blocked tear ducts. Sunken area around eyelids may indicate dehydration. Periorbital edema suggests fluid retention.
Inspect the sclera and conjunctiva for color, discharge, lesions, redness, and lacerations.	Sclera and conjunctiva are clear and free of discharge, lesions, redness, or lacerations.	Yellow sclera suggests jaundice, blue sclera may indicate osteogenesis imperfecta ("brittle bone disease"), and redness may indicate conjunctivitis.
Observe the iris and pupils.	Pupils are equal, round, and reactive to light and accommodation (PERRLA).	Brushfield spots may indicate Down syndrome. Sluggish pupils indicate a neurologic problem. Miosis (constriction) indicates iritis or narcotic use or abuse. Mydriasis (pupillary dilation) indicates emotional factors (fear), trauma, or drug use.
Finally, inspect the eyebrows and eyelashes.	Eyebrows should be symmetric in shape and movement. They should not meet midline. Eyelashes should be evenly distributed and curled outward.	Sparseness of eyebrows or lashes could indicate skin disease or deliberate pulling out of hairs (usually due to anxiety or habit). Corneal abrasions are common during childhood and may not be easily visible to the naked eye.
Perform visual acuity tests. Use the following diagnostic tools to perform visual acuity testing: • Snellen letter chart • Snellen symbol chart (E chart; used for preschoolers) • Blackbird Preschool Vision Screening Test (uses modified E that resembles a bird and a story to engage children's attention) • Faye symbol chart (uses pictures) **CLINICAL TIP** Fatigue, anxiety, hunger, and distractions interfere with vision testing. Testing should precede procedures that create discomfort.	Normal visual acuity is as follows: • 1 year: 20/200 • 2 years: 20/70 • 5 years: 20/30 • 6 years and up: 20/20 Children should be able to differentiate colors by age 5.	Children with a one-line difference between eyes should be referred. Children should also be referred for abnormal visual acuity or inability to distinguish colors. Visual impairment can indicate congenital defects (cataracts), malignant tumors, chronic disease (diabetes), drug use, trauma, enzyme deficiencies, or refractive errors (myopia, hyperopia, astigmatism).
Perform extraocular muscle tests.	In the cover test, the eyes remain focused.	Eye movement is present during the cover test; this may indicate strabismus.

Continued on following page

ASSESSMENT PROCEDURE	NORMAL FINDINGS	ABNORMAL FINDINGS
Eyes (Continued)		
Cover test: Have the child cover one eye and look at an interesting object (Fig. 31-21). Observe the uncovered eye for any movement. When the child is focused on the object, remove the cover and observe that eye for movement. **Hirschberg test:** Shine light directly at the cornea while the child looks straight ahead. 🎯 **CLINICAL TIP** Use a toy, a puppet, and the parent to focus the child's eyes. Older children, including adolescents, focus better if they are given something to focus on instead of being told to "look straight ahead."	In the Hirschberg test, the light reflects symmetrically in the center of both pupils.	Unequal alignment of light on the pupils in the Hirschberg test signals strabismus.

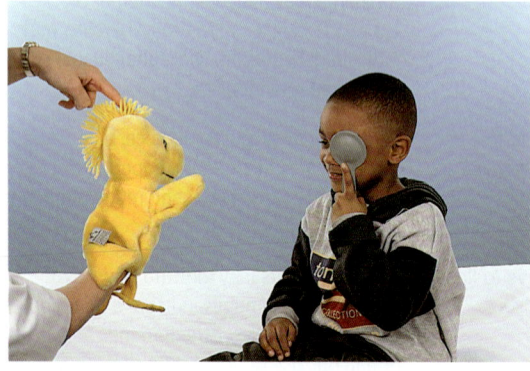

FIGURE 31-21 Performing the cover test (© B. Proud).

Inspect the internal eye. Perform ophthalmoscopic examination. The procedure is the same as for adults. Distraction is preferred over the use of restraint, which is likely to result in crying and closed eyes.	Red reflex is present. This reflex rules out most serious defects of the cornea, aqueous chamber, lens, and vitreous humor. When visualized, the optic disc appears similar to an adult's.	Absence of the red reflex indicates cataracts. Papilledema is unusual in children under 3 years of age owing to the ability of the fontanelles and sutures to open during increased intracranial pressure. Report disc blurring and hemorrhages immediately.
Ears		
Inspect external ears. Note placement, discharge, or lesions of the ears.	The top of the pinna should cross the eye-occiput line and be within a 10-degree angle of a perpendicular line drawn from the eye-	Low-set ears with an alignment greater than a 10-degree angle suggest mental retardation or congenital syndromes (Fig. 31-22).

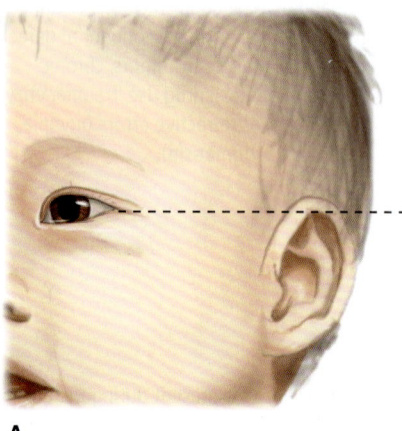 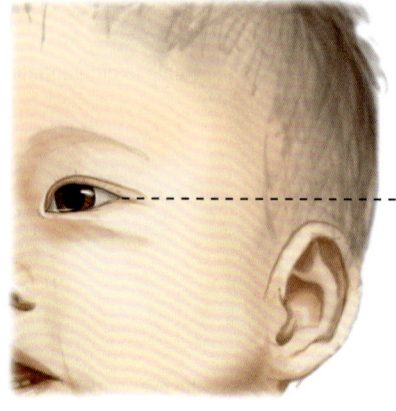

A **B**

FIGURE 31-22 **A.** Top of pinna above eye-occiput line. **B.** Pinna below eye-occiput line.

ASSESSMENT PROCEDURE	NORMAL FINDINGS	ABNORMAL FINDINGS
	occiput line to the lobe. No unusual structure or markings should appear on the pinna.	Abnormal shape may suggest renal disease process, which may be hereditary. Preauricular skin tags or sinuses suggest other anomalies of ears or the renal system.
Inspect internal ear. The internal ear examination requires using an otoscope and, for toddlers, restraint by (1) having a parent hold the seated child in the lap while holding the child's hands with one hand and the child's head sideways against chest or (2) laying the child supine, with the parent holding the child's arms up over the head. Then the nurse can gently but firmly hold child's head to the side. Regardless of technique used, the nurse should always hold the otoscope in a manner that allows for rapid removal if the child moves. Unlike an infant's external canal, which is short and straight, an older child's canal shortens and becomes less straight, like the adult's. Gently pull the pinna up and back, as you would for an adult.	No excessive cerumen, discharge, lesions, excoriations, or foreign body are in external canal. Tympanic membrane is pearly gray to light pink, with normal landmarks. Tympanic membranes redden bilaterally when child is crying or febrile.	Presence of foreign bodies or cerumen impaction (Fig. 31-23). Purulent discharge may indicate otitis externa or presence of foreign body. Purulent, serous discharge suggests otitis media. Bloody discharge suggests trauma, and clear discharge may indicate cerebrospinal fluid leak. Perforated tympanic membrane may also be noted.

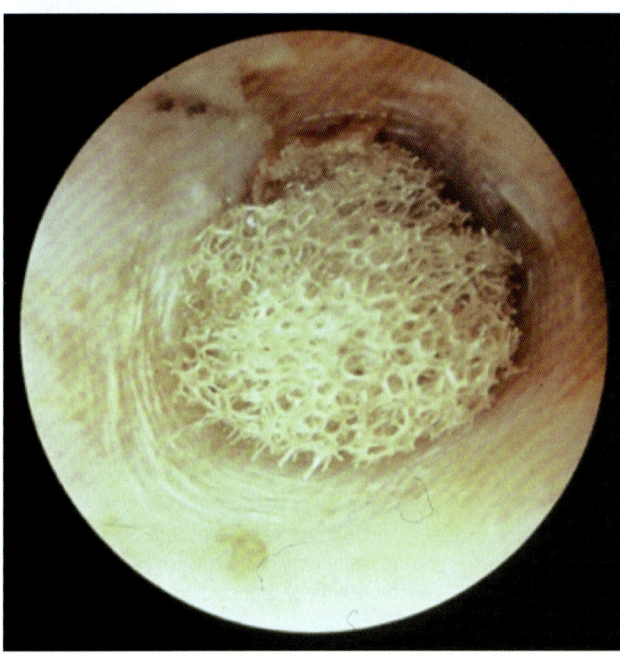

FIGURE 31-23 Presence of foreign body or cerumen impaction.

Assess the mobility of the tympanic membrane by pneumatic otoscopy. This consists of creating pressure against the tympanic membrane using air. To do this, you need to create a seal in the external canal and direct a puff of air against the tympanic membrane. Create the seal by using the largest speculum that will comfortably insert into the ear canal. Cover the tip with rubber for a better and more comfortable seal. Attach a pneumatic bulb to the otoscope and squeeze the bulb lightly to direct air against the tympanic membrane.	Tympanic membrane is mobile; moves inward with positive pressure (squeeze of bulb) and outward with negative pressure (release of bulb).	Immobility suggests chronic (serous) otitis media; decreased mobility may occur with acute otitis media.

Continued on following page

ASSESSMENT PROCEDURE	NORMAL FINDINGS	ABNORMAL FINDINGS
Ears (Continued)		
Test hearing acuity. Test acuity initially by whispering questions from a distance of approximately 8 ft. If hearing deficit is suspected, complete audiometric testing should be performed. Audiometry measures the threshold of hearing for frequencies and loudness. In addition, all children should have audiometric testing performed before entering school.	Answers whispered questions. Audiometry results are within normal ranges.	Failure to respond to whispered questions may indicate hearing deficit. Audiometry results outside normal range suggest hearing deficit.
Thorax and Lungs		
INSPECTION		
Inspect the shape of the thorax.	By age 5–6 years, the thoracic diameter reaches the adult 1:2 or 5:7 ratio (anteroposterior to transverse).	Abnormal shapes of the thorax include pectus excavatum and pectus carinatum.
Children under 7 years old are abdominal breathers.	Respirations should be unlabored and regular in all ages. Respirations should be: 2–10 years: 20–28 breaths/min 10–18 years: 12–20 breaths/min	Retractions (suprasternal, sternal, substernal, intercostal) and grunting suggest increased inspiratory effort, which may be due to asthma, atelectasis, pneumonia, or airway obstruction. Periods of apnea that last longer than 20 seconds and are accompanied by bradycardia may be a sign of a cardiovascular or central nervous system (CNS) disease.
PERCUSSION AND AUSCULTATION		
Percuss and auscultate the lungs. During percussion of the lungs, note tone elicited.	Hyperresonance is the normal tone elicited in young children because of thinness of the chest wall. This diminishes as the child ages and the chest wall develops.	A dull tone may indicate a mass, fluid, or consolidation.
Auscultate for breath sounds and adventitious sounds. If a toddler's lung sounds seem noisy, auscultate the upper nostrils. Toddlers with an upper respiratory infection may transmit noisy breathing from the upper nostrils to the upper lobes of the lungs. Encourage deep breathing in children; try one of the following techniques: blow out light on otoscope (Fig. 31-24), blow cotton ball in air, blow pinwheel, "race" paper off table.	Breath sounds may seem louder and harsher in young children because of their thin chest wall. No adventitious sounds should be heard, although transmitted upper airway sounds may be heard on auscultation of thorax.	Diminished breath sounds suggest respiratory disorders such as pneumonia or atelectasis. Stridor (inspiratory wheeze) is a high-pitched, piercing sound that indicates a narrowing of the upper tracheobronchial tree. Expiratory wheezes indicate narrowing in the lower tracheobronchial tree. Rhonchi and rales (crackles) may indicate a number of respiratory diseases such as pneumonia, bronchitis, or bronchiolitis.

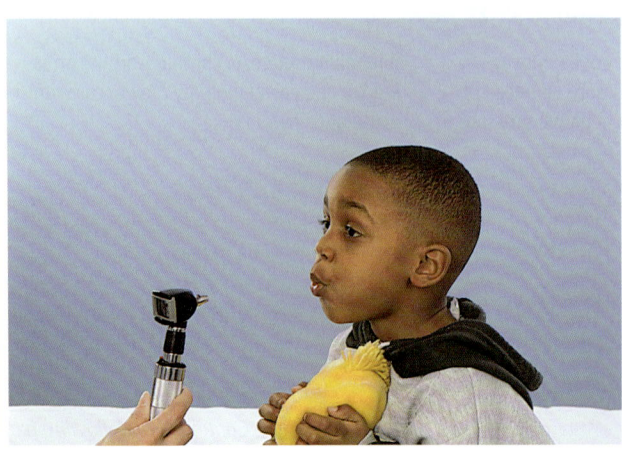

FIGURE 31-24 To encourage deep breathing, ask a child to blow out the light on an otoscope or a penlight (© B. Proud).

ASSESSMENT PROCEDURE	NORMAL FINDINGS	ABNORMAL FINDINGS
Breasts		
Inspect and palpate breasts. Note shape, symmetry, color, tenderness, discharge, lesions, and masses.	Breasts are flat and symmetric in prepubertal children. Obese children may appear to have breast tissue.	Redness, edema, and tenderness indicate mastitis. Enlargement in adolescent boys suggests gynecomastia. Masses in the adolescent female breast usually indicate cysts or trauma.
Assess stage of breast/sexual development of girl client. Teach breast self-examination to adolescents.	See Tanner's sexual maturity rating in Table 31-1.	Breast development before age 8 may indicate precocious puberty or thelarche. Lack of breast development after age 13 may indicate delayed puberty and/or a pathologic process.
Heart		
INSPECTION AND PALPATION		
Inspect and palpate the precordium. Note lifts and heaves. Palpate apical impulse (Fig. 31-25).	The apical pulse is at the 4th intercostal space (ICS) until the age of 7 years, when it drops to the 5th. It is to the left of the mid-clavicular line (MCL) until age 4 years, at the MCL between the ages of 4 and 6 years, and to the right at age 7 years.	A systolic heave may indicate right ventricular enlargement. Apical impulse that is not in proper location for age may indicate cardiomyopathy, pneumothorax, or diaphragmatic hernia.

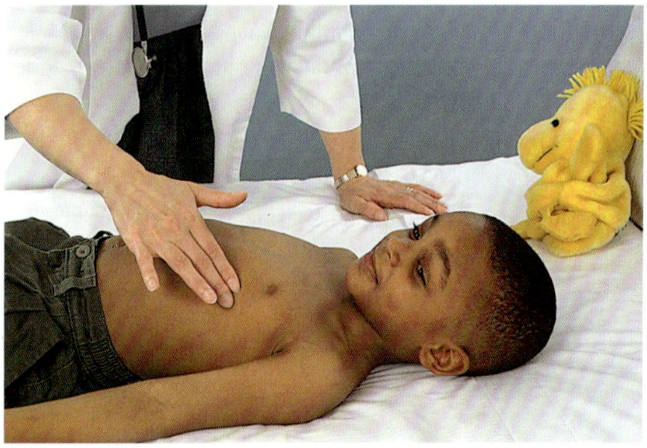

FIGURE 31-25 To palpate a preschooler's apical pulse, place your hand at the 4th intercostal space to the left of the mid-clavicular line (© B. Proud).

AUSCULTATION		
Auscultate heart sounds. Listen to the heart. Note rate and rhythm of apical impulse, S_1, S_2, extra heart sounds, and murmurs. ⊙ **CLINICAL TIP** Keep in mind that sinus arrhythmia is normal in young children. Heart sounds are louder, higher pitched, and of shorter duration in children. A split S_2 at the apex occurs normally in some children, and S_3 is a normal heart sound in some children. A venous hum also may be normally heard in children.	Normal heart rates are cited in the "Vital Signs" section earlier. Innocent murmurs, which are common throughout childhood, are classified as systolic; short duration; no transmission to other areas; grade III or less; loudest in pulmonic area (base of heart); low-pitched, musical, or groaning quality that varies in intensity in relation to position, respiration, activity, fever, and anemia. No other associated signs of heart disease.	Murmurs that do not fit the criteria for innocent murmurs may indicate a disease or disorder. Extra heart sounds and variations in pulse rate and rhythm also suggest pathologic processes.
Abdomen		
INSPECTION		
Inspect the shape of the abdomen.	In children up to 4 years of age, the abdomen is prominent in standing and supine positions. After 4 years of age, the abdomen appears slightly prominent when standing, but flat when supine until puberty.	A scaphoid (boat-shaped; i.e., sunken with prominent rib cage) abdomen may result from malnutrition or dehydration.

Continued on following page

ASSESSMENT PROCEDURE	NORMAL FINDINGS	ABNORMAL FINDINGS
Abdomen (Continued)		
Inspect umbilicus. Note color, discharge, evident herniation of the umbilicus.	Umbilicus is pink, no discharge, odor, redness, or herniation.	Inflammation, discharge, and redness of umbilicus suggest infection. Diastasis recti (separation of the abdominal muscles) is seen as midline protrusion from the xiphoid to the umbilicus or pubis symphysis. This condition is secondary to immature musculature of abdominal muscles and usually has little significance. As the muscles strengthen, the separation resolves on its own. A bulge at the umbilicus suggests an umbilical hernia, which may be seen in newborns; many disappear by the age of 1 year, and most by 4 or 5 years of age. **CULTURAL CONSIDERATIONS** Umbilical hernias are seen more frequently in African American children.
AUSCULTATION		
Auscultate bowel sounds. Follow auscultation guidelines for adult clients provided in Chapter 23.	Normal bowel sounds occur every 10–30 seconds. They sound like clicks, gurgles, or growls.	Marked peristaltic waves almost always indicate a pathologic process such as pyloric stenosis.
PALPATION		
Palpate for masses and tenderness. Palpate abdomen for softness or hardness. **CLINICAL TIP** To decrease ticklishness, have the child help by placing his or her hand under yours, using age-appropriate distraction techniques, and maintaining conversation focused on something other than the examination (Fig. 31-26).	Abdomen is soft to palpation and without masses or tenderness.	A rigid abdomen is almost always an emergent problem. Masses or tenderness warrants further investigation.

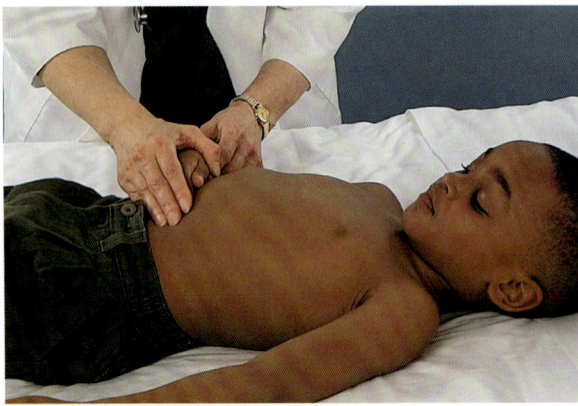

FIGURE 31-26 Let a child help palpate his or her abdomen to decrease ticklishness (© B. Proud).

Palpate liver. Palpate the liver the same as you would for adults (see Chapter 23).	Liver is usually palpable 1–2 cm below the right costal margin in young children.	An enlarged liver with a firm edge that is palpated more than 2 cm below the right costal margin usually indicates a pathologic process.

ASSESSMENT PROCEDURE	NORMAL FINDINGS	ABNORMAL FINDINGS
Palpate spleen. Palpate the spleen the same as you would for adults.	Spleen tip may be palpable during inspiration.	Enlarged spleen is usually indicative of a pathologic process.
Palpate kidneys. Palpate the kidneys the same as you would for adults.	The tip of the right kidney may be palpable during inspiration.	Enlarged kidneys are usually indicative of a pathologic process.
Palpate bladder. Palpate the bladder the same as you would for adults.	Bladder may be slightly palpable in small children.	An enlarged bladder is usually due to urinary retention but may be due to a mass.
Male Genitalia		
Inspect penis and urinary meatus. Inspect the genitalia, observing size for age and any lesions. ⊙ **CLINICAL TIP** Use distraction or teaching (such as testicular self-examination) when examining the genitalia in older children and adolescents to decrease embarrassment.	Penis is normal size for age, and no lesions are seen. The foreskin is retractable in uncircumcised child. Urinary meatus is at the tip of the glans penis and has no discharge or redness. Penis may appear small in obese boys because of overlapping skin folds.	An unretractable foreskin in a child older than 3 months suggests phimosis. Paraphimosis is indicated when the foreskin is tightened around the glans penis in a retracted position. Hypospadias, urinary meatus on the ventral surface of the glans, and epispadias, urinary meatus on the dorsal surface of the glans, are congenital disorders (see Abnormal Findings 26-1). Discharge, redness, or lacerations may indicate abuse in young children but may occur from infections or a foreign body. Discharge in adolescents may be due to STI, infection, or irritation.
Inspect and palpate scrotum and testes. To rule out cryptorchidism, it is important to palpate for testes in the scrotum in young boys. ⊙ **CLINICAL TIP** When palpating the testicles of a young boy, you must keep the cremasteric reflex in mind. This reflex pulls the testicles up into the inguinal canal and abdomen and is elicited in response to touch, cold, or emotional factors. Have young boys sit with knees flexed and abducted. This lessens the cremasteric reflex and enables you to examine the testicles.	Scrotum is free of lesions. Testes are palpable in the scrotum, with the left testicle usually lower than the right. Testes are equal in size, smooth, mobile, and free of masses. If a testicle is missing from the scrotal sac but the scrotal sac appears well developed, suspect physiologic cryptorchidism. The testis has originally descended into the scrotum but has moved back up into the inguinal canal because of the cremasteric reflex and the small size of the testis. You should be able to milk the testis down into the scrotum from the inguinal canal. This normal condition subsides at puberty.	Absent testicle(s) and atrophic scrotum suggest true cryptorchidism (undescended testicles; see Chapter 26). This suggests that the testicle(s) never descended. This condition occurs more frequently in preterm than term infants because testes descend at 8 months of gestation. It can lead to testicular atrophy and infertility, and increases the risk for testicular cancer. Hydroceles are common in infants. They are fluid-filled masses that can be transilluminated (see Abnormal Findings 26-2). They usually resolve spontaneously. A scrotal hernia is usually caused by an indirect inguinal hernia that has descended into the scrotum. It can usually be pushed back into the inguinal canal. This mass will not transilluminate. A painless nodule on the testis may indicate testicular cancer, which appears most frequently in males aged 15–34 years; therefore, testicular self-examination (TSE) should be taught to all boys 14 years old and older.
Inspect and palpate inguinal area for hernias. Observe for any bulge in the inguinal area. Ask the child to bear down or try to lift something heavy to elicit a possible hernia. Using your pinky finger, palpate up the inguinal canal to the external inguinal ring if a hernia is suspected.	No inguinal hernias are present.	A bulge in the inguinal area or palpation of a mass in the inguinal canal suggests an inguinal hernia. Indirect inguinal hernias occur most frequently in children (see Chapter 26).
Assess sexual development. Note public hair pattern, and size and development of penis and scrotum.	See Tanner's Sexual Maturity Ratings in Table 31-2.	Pubic hair growth, enlargement of the penis to adolescent or adult size, and enlarged testes in a boy less than 8 years of age suggest precocious puberty.

Continued on following page

ASSESSMENT PROCEDURE	NORMAL FINDINGS	ABNORMAL FINDINGS
Female Genitalia		
Inspect external genitalia. Note labia majora, labia minora, vaginal orifice, urinary meatus, and clitoris. ◎ **CLINICAL TIP** Have female children assist with genitalia examination by using their hands to spread the labia. This helps to decrease any stress and embarrassment.	Labia majora and minora are pink and moist. Young girls have flattened majora, thin minora, small clitoris, and thin hymen. Starting at school age, the labia become fuller and the hymen thickens. This progresses until puberty, when the genitalia develop adult characteristics. No discharge from vagina or meatus; no redness or edema present normally.	Partial or complete labia minora adhesions are sometimes seen in girls younger than 4 years of age. Referral is necessary to disintegrate the thin, membranous adhesion. An imperforate hymen (no central orifice) is sometimes seen and is not significant unless it persists until puberty and causes problems with menstruation. Discharge from vagina or urinary meatus, redness, edema, or lacerations may suggest abuse in the young child. However, infections or a foreign body in the vagina may cause these symptoms. Discharge in adolescents suggests STI, infection, or irritation.
Inspect internal genitalia. An internal genitalia examination is not routinely performed in the child although it may be called for if infection, bleeding, a foreign body, disease, or sexual abuse is suspected. A pediatric specialist should perform the examination. An internal genital examination consisting of both the speculum and bimanual examinations is recommended for all sexually active adolescents. An internal examination may be indicated in the adolescent who has discharge or suspects an STI. The procedure is the same as for the adult. Time and care must be taken for adequate teaching and reassurance.	See Chapter 27 for normal findings.	See Chapter 27 for abnormal findings.
Assess sexual development. Note pubic hair pattern.	See Tanner's Sexual Maturity Ratings in Table 31-3 for normal findings.	Growth of pubic hair in young girls (<8 years of age) suggests precocious puberty. Unusual pubic hair distribution in pubertal girls may indicate a disorder. For example, a male pattern of hair growth may suggest polycystic ovary disease.
Anus and Rectum		
INSPECTION AND PALPATION		
Inspect the anus. The anus should be inspected in children and adolescents. Perform quickly at the end of the genitalia examination to limit embarrassment in the older child and adolescent. Spread the buttocks with gloved hands, and note patency of anal opening, presence of any lesions and fissures, and condition and color of perianal skin.	The anal opening should be visible, moist, and hairless. No hemorrhoids or lesions. Perianal skin should be smooth and free of lesions. Perianal skin tags may be noted.	Imperforate anus (no anal opening) should be referred. Hemorrhoids are unusual in children and could be due to chronic constipation, but may be caused by sexual abuse or abdominal pressure from lesion. Bleeding and pain often indicate tears or fissures in the anus, which often cause constipation because of pain of passing stool. Pustules may indicate secondary infection of diaper rash. A dark ring around the anus may indicate heavy-metal poisoning. Lacerations, purulent discharge, or extreme apprehension during examination may indicate physical or sexual abuse.
Palpate rectum. This internal examination is not routinely performed in children or adolescents. However, it should be performed	Prostate gland is nonpalpable in young boys. Bimanual rectoabdominal examination in girls may reveal small midline mass (cervix).	If other masses are palpated, they are considered abnormal; no other structures are palpable until adolescence.

ASSESSMENT PROCEDURE	NORMAL FINDINGS	ABNORMAL FINDINGS
if symptoms suggest a problem. The child should be in a supine position with the legs flexed. Provide reassurance throughout the examination. If the child is old enough, ask the child to bear down. This helps to relax the sphincter. Slowly insert a gloved, lubricated finger (the pinky finger may be used for comfort, but the index finger is more sensitive) into the anal opening, aiming the finger toward the umbilicus.		

Musculoskeletal

INSPECTION

Assess feet and legs. Note symmetry, shape, movement, and positioning of the feet and legs. Perform neurovascular assessment.	Feet and legs are symmetric in size, shape, movement, and positioning (Fig. 31-27). Extremities should be warm and mobile, with adequate capillary refill. All pulses (radial, brachial, femoral, popliteal, pedal) should be strong and equal bilaterally. A common finding in children (up to 2 or 3 years old) is metatarsus adductus deformity. This is an inward positioning of the forefoot with the heel in normal straight position, which resolves spontaneously. Tibial torsion, also common in infants and toddlers, consists of twisting of the tibia inward or outward on its long axis, is usually caused by intrauterine positioning, and typically corrects itself by the time the child is 2 years old.	Short, broad extremities, hyperextensible joints, and palmar simian crease may indicate Down syndrome. Polydactyly (extra digits) and syndactyly (webbing) are sometimes found in children with mental retardation.

Fixed-position (true) deformities do not return to normal position with manipulation. Metatarsus varus is inversion (a turning inward that elevates the medial margin) and adduction of the forefoot.

Talipes varus is adduction of the forefoot and inversion of the entire foot.

Talipes equinovarus (clubfoot) is indicated if foot is fixed in the following position: adduction of the forefoot, inversion of the entire foot, and equinus (pointing downward) position of the entire foot (Fig. 31-28).

Neurovascular deficit in children is usually secondary to trauma (e.g., fracture). |

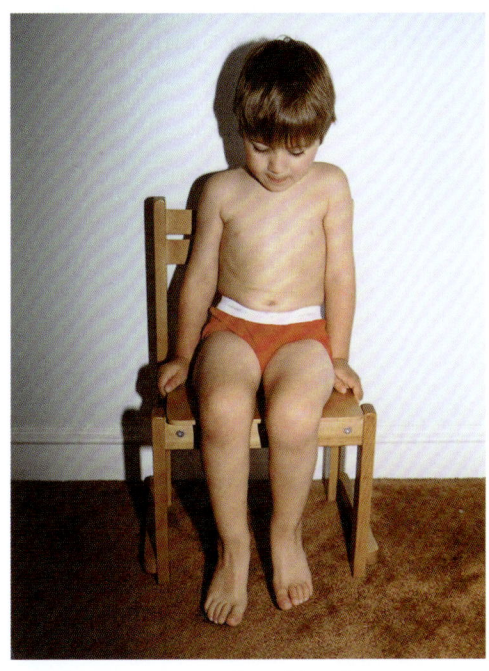

FIGURE 31-27 Normally positioned feet and legs.

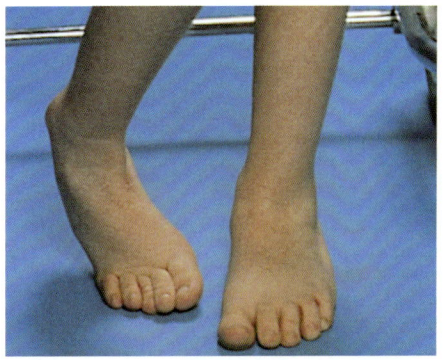

FIGURE 31-28 Talipesequinovarus, also called clubfoot (© 1995 Science Photo Library/CMSP).

Continued on following page

ASSESSMENT PROCEDURE	NORMAL FINDINGS	ABNORMAL FINDINGS
Musculoskeletal (Continued)		
Assess spinal alignment. Observe spine and posture. Assess for scoliosis (Fig. 31-29).	By 12–18 months, the lumbar curve develops. Toddlers display lordotic posture. Findings in older children and adolescents are similar to those in adults.	Kyphosis may result from poor posture or from pathologic conditions. Scoliosis usually is idiopathic and is more common in adolescent girls. Abnormal posture suggests neuromuscular disorders such as cerebral palsy (Fig. 31-30). Extremities that are asymmetric in size, shape, and movement indicate scoliosis or hip disease.
Assess gait. Observe gait initially when the child enters the examination room. This enables you to observe the child when he or she is unaware of being observed and gait	Toddlers have a wide-based gait and are usually bow-legged (genu varum). Children aged 2–7 are usually knock-kneed (genu valgum; see Fig. 31-31). Gait in older children is the same as in adults.	"Toeing in" or "toeing out" indicates problems such as tibial torsion or clubfoot. Limping may indicate congenital hip dysplasia (toddlers); synovitis (preschoolers); Legg–Calvé–Perthes disease (school-age children);

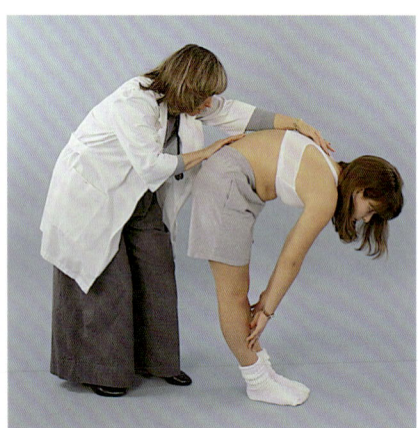

FIGURE 31-29 Assessing spinal curvature for scoliosis (© B. Proud).

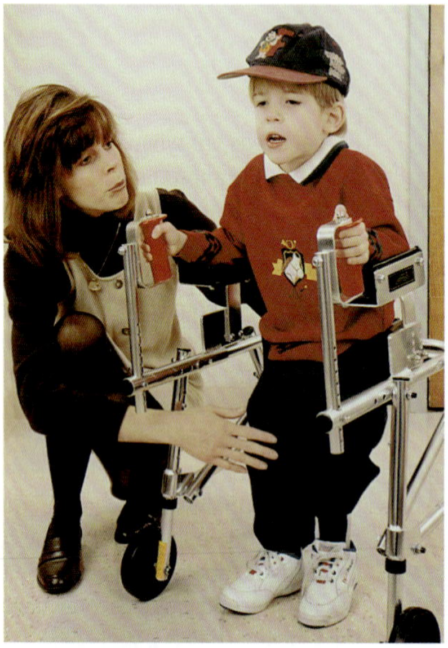

FIGURE 31-30 Neuromuscular weakness is a hallmark of cerebral palsy.

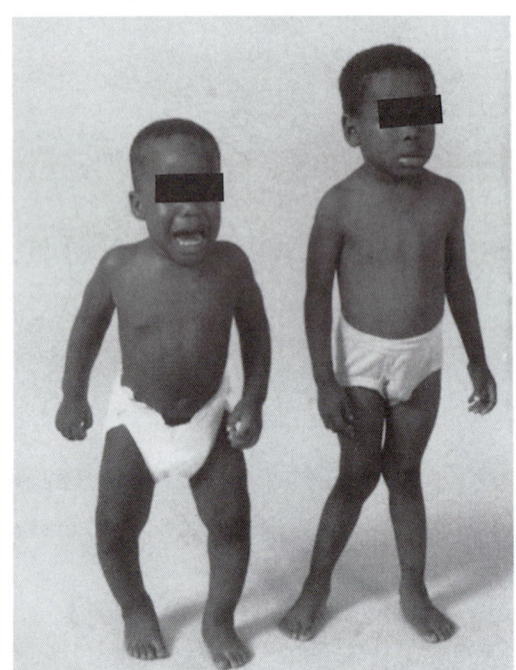

FIGURE 31-31 (A) Genu varum (bow legs); (B) genu valgum (knock knees)

ASSESSMENT PROCEDURE	NORMAL FINDINGS	ABNORMAL FINDINGS
is most natural. Later, have the child walk to and from the parent (the child should be barefoot), and observe gait.		slipped capital femoral epiphysis, scoliosis (adolescents). When a child is wearing shoes, limping usually suggests poorly fitting shoes or presence of a pebble. Many abnormal gaits are noted in cerebral palsy.
Assess joints. Note ROM, swelling, redness, and tenderness.	Full ROM and no swelling, redness, or tenderness.	Limited ROM, swelling, redness, and tenderness indicate problems ranging from mild injuries to serious disorders, such as rheumatoid arthritis.
Assess muscles. Note size and strength.	Muscle size and strength should be adequate for the particular age and should be equal bilaterally.	Inadequate muscle size and strength for the particular age indicate neuromuscular disorders such as muscular dystrophy.

Neurologic

INSPECTION

Much of the neurologic examination of children older than age 2 years is performed in much the same way as for adults.

> **CLINICAL TIP**
> As with adults, integrate the neurologic assessment into the overall assessment, observing the child first in the natural state, then purposefully. Playing games such as "Simon Says" can help elicit responses from young children.

Test cerebral function. Assess level of consciousness, behavior, adaptation, and speech.	The child should be alert and active, respond appropriately, and relate well to the parent and the nurse. Increased independence will be demonstrated with age. By the age of 3 years, speech should be easily understood.	Abnormal findings include altered level of consciousness and inappropriate responses. Maladaptation is displayed by an inability to relate well to parent and nurse, lack of independence with age, inappropriate responses to commands, hyperactivity, and poor attention span. Although physiologic disfluency is normal in preschoolers, unintelligible speech by age 3 years, prolonged stuttering, slurring, and lisping indicate speech disorders or neurologic problems. Slurring may also be indicative of substance abuse, drug toxicity, or conditions such as diabetic ketoacidosis.
Test cranial nerve function. Test cranial nerve function in young people the same way as for adults when possible.	Normal findings are the same as for adults.	Alterations in cranial nerve function demonstrate problem or pathologic process.
Test deep tendon and superficial reflexes. Test deep tendon and superficial reflexes in young people the same way as for adults.	Normal findings are the same as for adults, except that the Babinski response is normal in children younger than 2 years (this response usually disappears between 2 and 24 months), and triceps reflex is absent until age 6.	Absence or marked intensity of these reflexes, asymmetry, and presence of Babinski response after age 2 years may demonstrate pathology. Sustained (continuous) ankle clonus is abnormal and suggests CNS disease.

Continued on following page

UNIT 4 Nursing Assessment of Special Groups

ASSESSMENT PROCEDURE	NORMAL FINDINGS	ABNORMAL FINDINGS
Neurologic (Continued)		
Test balance and coordination. Balance and coordination in a child are tested in much the same way as for an adult. Have the child hop, skip, and jump, when appropriate for developmental age.	School-age children and adolescents should be able to perform most balance and coordination tests.	Abnormal findings include unstable gait, lack of coordination of movements, and a positive Romberg test. These may indicate a number of problems, including CNS disease and neuromuscular disorders.
Test sensory function. Same as for adults, when possible.	Sensitivity to touch and discrimination should be present. The thresholds of touch, pain, and temperature are higher in older children.	Absent or decreased sensitivity to touch and two-point discrimination may indicate paresthesia.
Test motor function. Tests for motor function in children are similar to tests for adults. Also watch for hand preference.	Gross and fine motor skills should be appropriate for the child's developmental age. Hand preference is developed during the preschool years.	Gross and fine motor skills that are inappropriate for developmental age and lack of head control by age 6 months may indicate cerebral palsy. Hand preference that is not developed during preschool years may indicate paresis on the opposite side.
Observe for "soft signs." Soft signs of neurologic problems are controversial, because these signs do not always indicate a pathologic process.	Soft signs disappear with age.	Soft signs include but are not limited to: • Short attention span • Poor coordination of position • Hypoactivity • Impulsiveness • Labile emotions • Distractibility • No demonstration of handedness • Language and articulation problems • Learning problems

---

BOX 31-6   COMMON SKIN VARIATIONS IN CHILDREN AND ADOLESCENTS

PORT-WINE STAIN

This birthmark consisting of capillaries is dark red or bluish and darkens with exertion or temperature exposure. It appears as a large, irregular, macular patch on the scalp or face. Unlike a hemangioma, this birthmark does not fade with time.

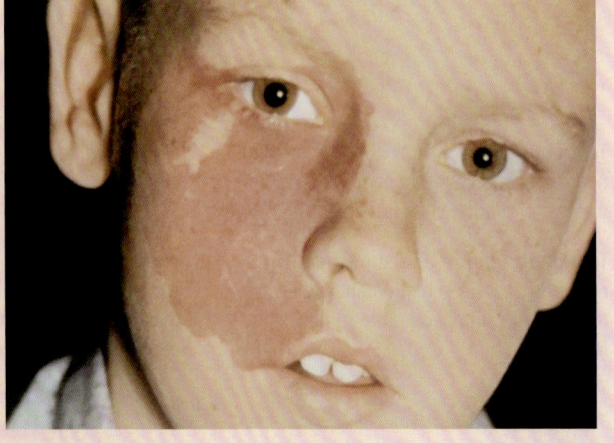

HEMANGIOMA

This skin variation is caused by an increased amount of blood vessels in the dermis. A series of photographs of children with hemangiomas are presented demonstrating variations in morphology: **(A)** Example of a child with an isolated focal hemangioma; **(B)** example of a child with multiple cutaneous hemangiomas; **(C)** example of a child with a facial segmental hemangioma occupying the periorbital, temporal, cheek, and chin areas of the face. Segmental hemangiomas are prone to ulceration as can be seen in this child around the left nasolabial crease.

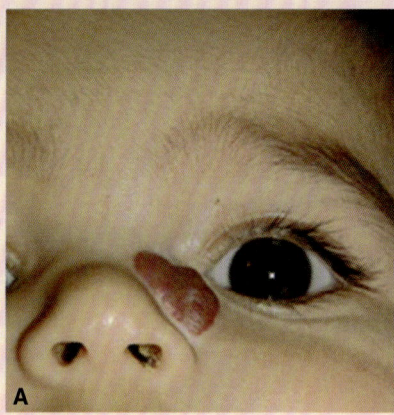
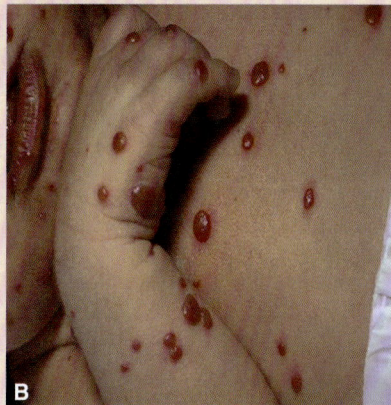
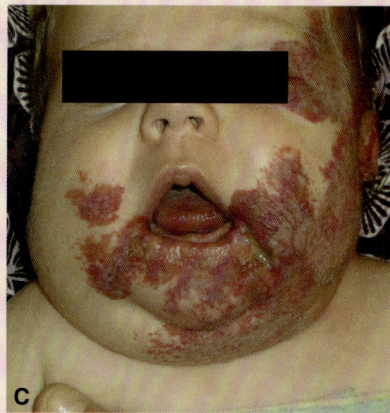

CAFÉ-AU-LAIT SPOT

This birthmark is a light brown, round or oval patch. If there are more than six separate, large (>1.5 cm) patches, an inherited neurocutaneous disease may be present.

BODY PIERCING AND TATTOOS IN ADOLESCENTS

Adolescents express their identity in different ways. Body piercing and tattoos make a strong statement.

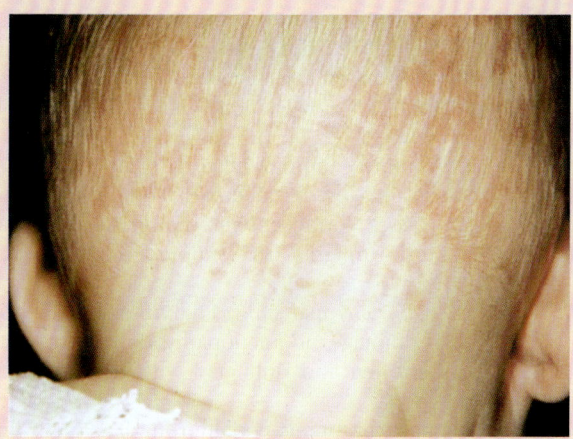
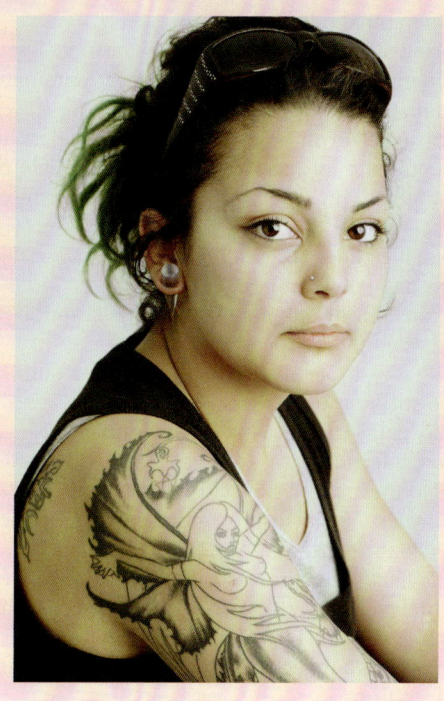

Validating and Documenting Findings

Validate findings by asking additional questions, verifying data with another health care professional, or comparing objective with subjective findings. Documentation for children and adolescents is the same as that for adults. Nurses document what they observed, palpated, percussed, and auscultated. Descriptions should be objective, accurate, and concise, yet comprehensive. Avoid terms such as *good*, *poor*, and *normal*. Phrases and standardized abbreviations are preferable to full sentences, and a sequential manner should be followed.

CASE STUDY

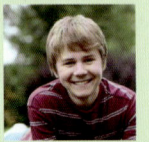

The nurse documents the following subjective and objective assessment findings of Carsen's examination.

Subjective Data

Carsen, 13 years old, is brought into the office with his mother for well-child care.

Current Health and Illness Status: Has been well since last health care visit at age 12 years old; reports right ear pain for past 3 days, no other health concerns or medications.

Past Health History: Birth FTNSVD (full-term, normal, spontaneous delivery), BW (birth weight) 7 lb; no problems. Otitis media at age 6 months. Allergies (and reaction to same): None. Immunization status: UTD (up to date).

Growth and Developmental Milestones: Has grown 1 in in height in 1 year.

Body Mass Index is 25.

He is a concrete thinker and problem solver and reports straight As in school. Socializes with friend his own age. Coordination is improving with the sports he plays, such as basketball and track.

Physical Examination Findings: Well adolescent, with history of occasional ear infections in past.

Integument: No lesions, bruising.

Head: No trauma, headaches.

Eyes: Visual acuity, no problems by history; last eye examination: has not had formal eye examination; no drainage, infections.

Ears: Hearing acuity, no problems by history; last hearing examination 2 years ago; no drainage. Right tympanic membrane red and bulging. Left tympanic membrane dull.

Nose: No bleeding, congestion, mild clear nasal discharge, nasal membranes gray.

Mouth: No lesions, soreness; no tooth eruption, last dental examination 6 months ago.

Throat: No sore throats, hoarseness, difficulty swallowing.

Neck: No stiffness, tenderness.

Chest: No pain, cough, wheezing, shortness of breath, asthma, infections.

Breasts: No thelarche, lesions, discharge.

Cardiovascular: No history of murmurs, exercise tolerance, dizziness, palpitations, congenital defects.

Gastrointestinal: Appetite excellent; bowel habits (one soft, brown BM/day); no food intolerances, nausea, vomiting, pain, history of parasites.

Genitourinary: No urgency, frequency, discharge, urinary tract infections.

Gynecologic: N/A.

Musculoskeletal: No pain, swelling, fractures, mobility problems.

Neurologic: No tremors, unusual movements, seizures.

Lymphatic: No pain, swelling or tenderness, enlargement of spleen or liver.

Endocrine/metabolic: Growth patterns follow 75th percentile; no polyuria, polydipsia, polyphagia.

Psychiatric History: Unremarkable. No developmental disorder.

Family History: Diabetes (maternal grandmother); hypertension (paternal grandfather).

Nutritional History: Eats three meals a day with snacks of healthy foods during the day. Has had increased appetite with growth spurt. No problems with feeding self. Takes multivitamin daily.

Sleep History: Bedtime is 10:00 PM, awakens at 7 AM. No sleeping disorders.

Psychosocial History: Lives with mother, father, and older sister. Mother is 42 years old, father is 43 years old, sister is 17 years old. Mother works outside the home and is vice president at a local bank; mother completed graduate school. Father is employed full time as a chemical engineer and completed his Masters in Science degree.

Cultural background is Italian/Irish; religion, Catholic.

No financial difficulties. Attends school during the day and plays sports in the evenings. Likes to play basketball and football. No history of domestic violence; no guns in household.

Objective Data

General Appearance: alert, active, well-developed, well-nourished 13-year-old male, in no acute distress.

Developmental Assessment: Cognitive: Concrete thinker, Active in school groups, such as the scholar bowl.

Emotional: Self-identity versus role confusion experiments under safe environment.

Social Development: Expresses more tolerance and appreciation in self and of others.

Vital Signs: BP 90/50; P 100; T 100.4 F. Wt: 150 lb, Ht: 5 ft 8 in

Skin: Pink, moist, appropriate turgor, face T-zone are with open and closed comedones, nails pink and hard.

Head and neck: Normocephalic, hair clean, no scalp lesions or birthmarks, neck supple, no lymph nodes palpable.

Mouth, throat, nose, and sinus: Pharynx red with thick purulent drainage, no adenopathy, nares patent, turbinates swollen and dull gray with thick purulent discharge.

Eyes: Sclerae clear, pupils equally round, react to light and accommodation (PERRLA).

Ears: External ear canals free of cerumen impaction, foreign body, discharge. Right tympanic membrane red and bulging. Left tympanic membrane gray with dull landmarks.

Heart/lungs: Normal sinus rhythm, no murmurs. Rate 90 beats/min. Lungs clear to auscultation bilaterally. Hyperresonance percussed over lung fields.

Thorax: Round and symmetric.

Abdomen: Soft, no masses or organomegaly.

Genitalia and rectum: Tanner's stage 2, no discharge or lesions. Penis circumcised.

Spine: Straight, no tufts or dimples.

Musculoskeletal: Adequate muscle strength and tone, range of motion within normal.

Neurologic: Cranial nerves II to XII intact, deep tendon reflexes 2+, negative Babinski reflex, sensitive to touch.

Coordination: Gross and fine motor movement appropriate for age.

ANALYSIS OF DATA: DIAGNOSTIC REASONING

After collecting subjective and objective data pertaining to children and adolescents, identify abnormal findings and client's strengths. Then cluster the data to reveal any significant patterns or abnormalities. These data may then be used to make clinical judgments about the status of the child or adolescent.

Selected Nursing Diagnoses

Following is a listing of selected nursing diagnoses (health promotion, risk, or actual) that you may identify when analyzing the cue clusters.

Health Promotion Diagnoses

- Readiness for Enhanced Health Management during the growing years

Risk Diagnoses

- Risk for Obesity related to lack of knowledge of how to eat nutritious diet as normal adolescent
- Risk for Deficient Fluid Volume related to decreased fluid and food intake × 2 days and increased metabolic needs associated with elevated temperature
- Risk for Injury to teeth related to developmental age and sports activities
- Risk for Injury related to attempts to insert foreign objects (Q-Tips) into ear

Actual Diagnoses

- Impaired Skin Integrity: Acne related to endocrine changes
- Acute pain related to red, bulging tympanic membrane

Concept Mastery Alert

Acne consists of pustules and macules on the face. It is usually found in adolescence when hormone changes are occurring. Therefore, an appropriate nursing diagnosis would be Impaired Skin Integrity.

Selected Collaborative Problems

After grouping the data, certain collaborative problems may become apparent. Remember that collaborative problems differ from nursing diagnoses in that they cannot be prevented with nursing interventions alone. However, these physiologic complications of medical conditions can be detected and monitored by the nurse. In addition, the nurse can use physician- and nurse-prescribed interventions to minimize the complications of these problems. The nurse may also have to refer the client in such situations for further treatment of the problem. Following is a list of collaborative problems seen more frequently in the pediatric client. However, other collaborative problems seen in the adult are also seen in pediatric clients. These problems are worded as Risk for Complications (RC), followed by the problem:

- RC: Altered skin integrity
- RC: Upper respiratory infection
- RC: Hearing impairment
- RC: Systemic infection

Medical Problems

After grouping the data, the client's signs and symptoms may clearly require medical diagnosis and treatment. Referral to a primary care provider is necessary.

CASE STUDY

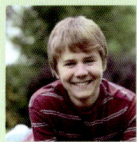

After collecting and analyzing the data for Carsen, the nurse determines that the following conclusions are appropriate:
- Acute pain r/t red, bulging tympanic membrane
- Risk for Deficient Fluid Volume r/t decreased fluid and food intake × 2 days and increased metabolic needs associated with elevated temperature

Potential collaborative problems include the following:
- RC: Ear infection
- RC: Hearing impairment
- RC: Systemic infection
- RC: Permanent scarring

To view an algorithm depicting the process of diagnostic reasoning for this case, go to thePoint.

Interdisciplinary Verbal Communication of Assessment Findings Using SBAR

SITUATION: Carsen, a 13-year-old boy, came in with his mother for a well-child visit. Current health and illness status: Reports right internal constant ear pain (8 on a scale of 1–10) that radiates down to jaw. Pain relieved to a 4 with Tylenol. Clear runny nasal discharge with thick yellow mucous; stuffy nose, and nonproductive cough. Has had low-grade fever up to 100.0°F for last 3 days. Experiencing insomnia and difficulty concentrating at school due to coughing, head hurting, and feeling "bad all over."

BACKGROUND: Has been well since last health care visit at age 12 years until yesterday. Family history is remarkable for his grandparents having heart disease and glaucoma. Mother and father are both healthy. He has one older sister, who is well. No current exposure to communicable diseases. Otitis media at age 6 months. Immunizations up to date.

ASSESSMENT: Alert, active, well-developed, well-nourished 13-year-old male, in no acute distress. BP 90/50; P 100; T 100.4 F. Wt: 150 lb, Ht: 5 ft 8 in. Pharynx red with thick, purulent drainage, no adenopathy, nares patent, turbinates swollen and dull gray, with thick purulent discharge. External ear canals free of cerumen impaction, foreign body, and discharge. Right tympanic membrane red and bulging. Left tympanic membrane gray with dull landmarks.

RECOMMENDATION: Carsen has acute right ear pain r/t red, bulging tympanic membrane. He is at risk for a deficient fluid volume r/t decreased fluid and food intake × 2 days and increased metabolic needs associated with elevated temperature. He needs to be seen by his primary care provider for further assessment and treatment of right ear pain and infection to prevent future tympanic membrane scarring, hearing impairment, and development of a systemic infection.

Want to know more?

A wide variety of resources to enhance your learning and understanding of this book are available on thePoint. Visit thePoint to access:

NCLEX-Style Student Review Questions

Watch and Learn Videos

Concept in Action Animations

And more!

References and Selected Readings

American Academy of Pediatrics (AAP). (2015). Recommendations for prevention and control of influenza in children, 2015-2016. Available at http://pediatrics.aappublications.org/content/early/2015/09/01/peds.2015-2920

American College of Obstetricians and Gynecologists (ACOG). (2016). ACOG statement on USPSTF draft recommendations on pelvic exams. Available at http://www.acog.org/About-ACOG/News-Room/Statements/2016/ACOG-Statement-on-USPSTF-Draft-Recommendations-on-Pelvic-Exams

Centers for Disease Control and Prevention (CDC). (2013). Folk medicine. Available at http://www.cdc.gov/nceh/lead/tips/folkmedicine.htm

Centers for Disease Control and Prevention (CDC). (2015). Childhood obesity facts: Prevention of childhood obesity in the United States, 2011-2012. Available at http://www.cdc.gov/obesity/data/childhood.html

Centers for Disease Control and Prevention (CDC), Morbidity and Mortality Weekly Report (MMWR). (2015, March 27). Use of 9-Valent Human Papillomavirus (HPV) Vaccine: Updated HP vaccination recommendations of the Advisory Committee on Immunization Practices. *Morbidity and Mortality Weekly Report (MMWR), 64*(11), 300-304. Available at http://www.cdc.gov/mmwr/preview/mmwrhtml/mm6411a3.htm

Centers for Disease Control and Prevention (CDC). (2016). Pneumococcal vaccine. Available at http://www.cdc.gov/vaccines/vpd-vac/pneumo/default.htm?s_cid=cs_797

Centers for Disease Control and Prevention (CDC). (2017). Childhood obesity facts. Available at https://www.cdc.gov/obesity/data/childhood.html

Ford, H. (2016). Seeing blue: The impact of excessive blue light exposure. *Review of Optometry*. Available at https://www.reviewofoptometry.com/article/seeing-blue-the-impact-of-excessive-blue-light-exposure

HealthyPeople.gov. (2014a). Adolescent health. Available at https://www.healthypeople.gov/2020/topics-objectives/topic/Adolescent-Health

HealthyPeople.gov. (2014b). Early and middle childhood. Available at https://www.healthypeople.gov/2020/topics-objectives/topic/early-and-middle-childhood

Tanner, J. (1962). *Growth at adolescence* (2nd ed.). Oxford, England: Blackwell Scientific.

U.S. Preventive Services Task Force (USPSTF). (2016a). Draft recommendation statement: Gynecological conditions: Periodic screening with the pelvic examination. Available at https://www.uspreventiveservicestaskforce.org/Page/Document/draft-recommendation-statement157/gynecological-conditions-screening-with-the-pelvic-examination

U.S. Preventive Services Task Force (USPSTF). (2016b). USPSTF recommendations for STI screening. Available at https://www.uspreventiveservicestaskforce.org/Page/Name/uspstf-recommendations-for-sti-screening

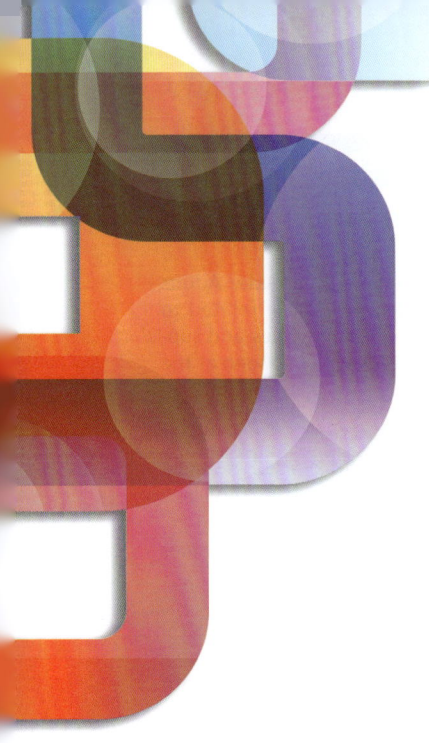

32 ASSESSING OLDER ADULTS

Learning Objectives

1. Describe the common structural and the functional changes of all body systems often seen as one ages.
2. Differentiate between common variations and the atypical presentation of disease and illness (known as geriatric syndromes) seen in the older adult.
3. Interview the older adult for an accurate nursing history of the genitalia, anus, and rectum.
4. Perform a physical assessment of the older adult using the correct techniques.
5. Analyze the data from the interview and physical assessment of the older adult to formulate valid nursing diagnoses, collaborative problems, and/or referrals.
6. Differentiate between general routine screening versus skills needed for focused or specialty assessment of the older adult.
7. Document and verbally report accurate assessment findings of the older adult.

CASE STUDY

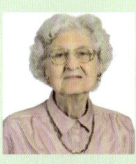

Mrs. Doris Miller, an 82-year-old Caucasian widow, is being seen for home health care. Mrs. Miller fell in her home 3 weeks ago and was hospitalized for repair and pinning of a fractured right femur. She is now living with her daughter, Delores Ralston, who reports that Mrs. Miller can put just enough weight on her right leg to use a walker, but needs assistance with bathing, cooking, and dressing. She says that her mother is not eating very well and seems to be choking easily, especially when she is drinking, and that she complains frequently of a "dry mouth." Mrs. Miller's case will be followed throughout the chapter, describing modifications in the approach, assessment and analysis of data needed by the nurse when assessing an older adult.

CHALLENGES TO HEALTH ASSESSMENT OF THE OLDER ADULT

Common physical findings in older adult clients have been identified throughout the preceding body system chapters. It is not, however, the physiologic changes of aging alone that warrant a special approach to assessment of the older client. Many older adults are healthy, active, and independent despite these normal physical changes in their bodies. It is, rather, that advancing age has a tendency to place a person at greater risk for chronic illness and disability. The term *frail elderly* describes the vulnerability of the "old-old" (generally mid-eighties, nineties, and centenarians) to be in poorer health, to have more chronic disabilities, and to function less independently. It is the frail elderly that are the focus of this chapter (see the Evidence-Based Health Promotion and Disease Prevention 32-1: Older Adults).

Loss of Physiologic Reserve

Some type of disability (e.g., difficulty in hearing, vision, cognition, ambulation, self-care, or independent living) was reported by 36% of people age 65 and over in 2012, and many with more severe disabilities need assistance to meet daily needs (Administration on Aging [AOA], 2014). The AOA surveys are mostly of uninstitutionalized adults, but also report that about 1.3 million older adults are in nursing homes (almost half are age 85 and over).

Greco et al. (2014) note that most definitions of frailty in the elderly describe a syndrome marked by loss of function, strength, and physiologic reserve, which leaves them susceptible to sickness and death. Additional aspects of frailty include cognitive impairment, depression, and decline in mobility, strength, endurance, nutrition, and physical activity. Weakness and fatigue are central to almost all definitions of frailty. Charansonney (2011) defined the loss of physiologic reserve of aging and frailty as the aging body's inability to make an appropriate adaptation to environmental challenges. Sarcopenia (skeletal muscle mass decrease) and sarcopenic obesity (muscle mass decrease with excessive body fat), common in aging, are related to functional impairments in older adults (Batsis et al., 2015).

DNA damage occurs throughout the body, again causing changes in cells, enzymes, ion, and nutrient production and much more, including decreases in metabolism (National Institute on Aging, 2015). For instance, by the age of 70, the metabolism has lost 85% of its original function. This decrease

32-1 EVIDENCE-BASED HEALTH PROMOTION AND DISEASE PREVENTION: OLDER ADULTS

According to Healthy People 2020 (2017), older adults are among the fastest growing age. In 2014, 14.5% (46.3 million) of the U.S. population was aged 65 or older and is projected to reach 23.5% (98 million) by 2060. These older adults are at high risk for developing chronic illnesses and related disabilities. Aging adults experience higher risk of chronic disease. In 2012, 60% of older adults managed two or more chronic conditions, including: heart disease, cancer, chronic bronchitis or emphysema, stroke, diabetes mellitus, and Alzheimer's disease.

The Healthy People 2020 (2017) objectives for older adults are many and varied, but are designed to promote healthy outcomes for this population. Many factors affect the health, function, and quality of life of older adults. Preventive health services are valuable for maintaining the quality of life and wellness of older adults. The Patient Protection and Affordable Care Act of 2010 includes provisions related to relevant Medicare services. However, preventive services are underused, especially among certain racial and ethnic groups.

The ability to complete basic daily activities may decrease if illness, chronic disease, or injury limits physical or mental abilities of older adults. These limitations make it hard for older adults to remain at home. Early prevention and physical activity can help prevent such declines. However, Healthy People 2020 reports that less than 60% of older adults engage in enough physical activity, and fewer do strength training. Minority populations often have lower rates of physical activity.

Most older adults want to remain in their communities as long as possible, but often there is not enough support available to help them. States that invest in such services show lower rates of growth in long-term care expenditures.

Healthy People 2020 (2017) reported that each year, one out of three older adults falls. Falls often cause severe disability among survivors, with injuries leading to fear of falling, sedentary behavior, impaired function, and a lower quality of life. Falls are the leading cause of death due to unintentional injury among older adults; deaths and injuries can be prevented by addressing risk factors.

An additional stress is that of caregivers. Caregivers for older adults living at home are typically unpaid family members; increased caregiver stress often results in unnecessary nursing home placement.

Elder abuse is another related concern. Healthy People 2020 reported that 1–2 million older adults in the United States are injured or mistreated by a loved one or a caregiver. A measure of elder abuse has been added to encourage data collection on this issue.

Behaviors such as participation in physical activity, self-management of chronic diseases, or use of preventive health services can improve health outcomes. Housing and transportation services affect the ability of older adults to access care. People from minority populations tend to be in poorer health and use health care less often than people from nonminority populations. The quality of health and social services available to older adults and their caregivers affects their ability to manage chronic conditions and long-term care needs effectively.

HEALTHY PEOPLE 2020 (2017) GOAL

Improve the health, function, and quality of life of older adults.

HEALTHY PEOPLE 2020 (2017) OBJECTIVES FOR OLDER ADULTS

The Healthy People objectives for the new topic Older Adults include a variety of objectives, divided into those related to prevention and those related to long-term services and supports. The details of these many objectives may be seen at the Healthy People 2020 website.

PREVENTION

OA-1: Use of Welcome to Medicare benefit
OA-2: Older adults up to date on clinical preventive services

OA-4: Receipt of diabetes self-management benefits by older adults
OA-5: Reduce functional limitations in older adults
OA-6: Increase proportion of older adults with reduced physical or cognitive function who engage in leisure-time activities
OA-7: Increase the proportion of health care work force with geriatric certification

LONG-TERM SERVICES AND SUPPORTS

OA-8: Need for long-term services and support

OA-10: Reduce rate of pressure ulcer hospitalizations
OA-11: Reduce emergency department visits due to falls among older adults
OA-12: Increase data collection and publication of information on elder abuse, neglect, and exploitation

SCREENING

Screening of older adults focuses on functional status, home safety including fall risk, abuse risk, physical activity level, social support, use of federal and specific disease-related services, and all areas that support healthy function, quality of life, and continued health of older adults. The U.S. Preventive Services Task Force (USPSTF, 2014) has a work group focused entirely on the complex topics associated with screening of older adults. The scope of topics and related recommendations focused on older adults is long—only the list of topics under review or already developed is included here. For details, see the USPSTF website. USPSTF topics that focus on older adults and are currently under review include:

- Falls Prevention in Older Adults
- Hearing Loss in Older Adults
- Vitamin D for Osteoporosis Prevention
- Multivitamins for Cardiovascular Disease and Cancer Prevention
- Dementia Screening

The following topics either include specific recommendations for adults ages 65 years and older or target preventive services primarily provided to older adults, diseases that carry a higher burden for older adults, or diseases that generally occur in older adults.

- Abdominal Aortic Aneurysm Screening
- Breast Cancer Screening
- Carotid Artery Stenosis Screening
- Cervical Cancer Screening
- Colorectal Cancer Screening
- Coronary Heart Disease Screening
- Dementia Screening
- Hormone Replacement Therapy
- Immunizations, Adult
- Osteoporosis Screening

- Ovarian Cancer Screening
- Peripheral Arterial Disease Screening
- Prostate Cancer Screening
- Thyroid Disease Screening
- Vision Screening in Older Adults

RISK ASSESSMENT

For the older adult, risks exist in the areas noted by Healthy People 2020 (2017): functional status, home safety including fall risk, abuse risk, physical activity level, social support, use of federal and specific disease-related services, and all areas that support healthy function, quality of life, and continued health of older adults, taking into consideration geriatric syndromes as well. Because of the complexity, a full assessment as described in this chapter and use of recommended tools to determine risks in each area are needed to assess risks.

CLIENT EDUCATION

As noted earlier, the complexity of assessing and teaching older adults and family members devoted to caring for older adults makes a specific client education topic list too long to include here.

---

in metabolism leads to less toleration to cold, weight gain, and a decreased efficiency in the body's use of glucose. Cellular aging affects organ function. For instance, by the age of 85, lung capacity has decreased by 50%; muscle strength by 45%; and kidney function by 30%. In the presence of these normal changes of aging, the physiologic reserve is reduced and the body is less able to resist illness.

Atypical Presentation of Illness

When the physiology of advanced age is combined with comorbidity, assessment is complicated. In fact, the signs and symptoms of illness often present differently in the oldest-old. Adverse events (AE) or adverse drug effects (ADE) in this population often include falls, confusion, incontinence, generalized weakness, and lethargy. These responses are associated with the most common geriatric syndromes, which are conditions with potential multiple causes found in the elderly. The most common conditions identified as geriatric syndromes are pressure ulcers, incontinence, falls, functional decline, and delirium; and associated factors, sometimes classified as separate geriatric syndromes, include malnutrition, eating and feeding problems, sleeping problems, dizziness and syncope, and self-neglect (Brown-O'Hara, 2013).

Knowing the older person's usual daily patterns and functional level is the best baseline against which to compare assessment data. For example, new-onset incontinence for the 92-year-old resident of an assisted living facility who still drives her own car should not be viewed as a normal consequence of aging. The incontinence could be the result of an infection or worsening heart failure. A more subtle presentation of these same problems could be signaled by complete incontinence in a 92-year-old man with severe cognitive impairment who until very recently had only occasional incontinence. Clearly, the key to recognizing pathology and illness in the very old is in knowing the person's baseline functional status and recognizing a deviation from it.

Symptoms of disease and disability in the very old frequently manifest as incontinence, falls, weakness and lethargy, confusion, changes in sleep or level of alertness, and loss of appetite or weight loss. Not only do these syndromes describe the common and most recognizable ways in which disease often presents itself in the frail elderly, they also describe the consequences of physiologic stress. For example, incontinence and confusion are often signs of infection in the frail older adult. The incontinence and confusion can easily lead to a fall when the older person attempts to walk to the bathroom, but on the way experiences lightheadedness caused by dehydration and postural hypotension. The fall may result in a hip fracture and immobility, which may lead to a pressure ulcer, urinary tract infection (UTI), and delirium. This type of cascade of unfortunate events often leads a frail but independent older adult living at home to disability and dependence.

Risk screening tools, such as SPICES (Box 32-1), may be used to monitor the population of high-risk frail older adults for some of the more common nonspecific indicators of disease. Because the oldest-old have the highest prevalence of chronic illness and comorbidity, one disease may mask the symptoms of another. For example, the fatigue and dyspnea of severe congestive heart failure may mask the anemia caused by a duodenal ulcer. A severe illness is more likely to affect multiple organ systems as the body's reserves and ability to respond to physiologic stress are impaired. For instance, pneumonia will typically precipitate congestive heart failure.

To complicate the assessment process even more, medications often result in significant adverse effects rather than improving the symptoms in frail older adults. Often another drug is used to treat the adverse drug effect and the problems spiral into a nearly indecipherable multiplicity of symptoms. The second and expanded version of the Beers Criteria for Potentially Inappropriate Medication (PIM) Use in the Elderly (American Geriatrics Society, 2015) identifies medications noted by experts to have potential risks that outweigh their potential benefits for people older than 65 years of age, regardless of their level of frailty.

Thus, collection of subjective data from the frail older adult must take into consideration the more common ways in which diseases and disorders present in older adults. Information regarding falls, weakness, incontinence, confusion,

---

BOX 32-1 COMMON PROBLEMS IN OLDER ADULTS WARRANTING FURTHER INVESTIGATION AS IDENTIFIED BY THE ACRONYM "SPICES"

- **S**kin impairment
- **P**oor nutrition
- **I**ncontinence
- **C**ognitive impairment
- **E**vidence of falls or functional decline
- **S**leep disturbances

Adapted from Wallace, M., & Fulmer, T. (2008). Fulmer SPICES: An overall assessment tool for older adults. Available at http://www.annalsoflongtermcare.com/article/6911.

sleep difficulties, and loss of appetite is essential. Finally, the client's family, social, and economic resources and/or environment must be assessed to determine any relationship to the client's symptoms. For example, isolation, physical barriers, or neglect may precipitate physiologic and functional decline.

Collecting Subjective Data: The Nursing Health History

Adapting Interview Techniques

In today's youth-oriented culture, it is not uncommon to think of physical frailty as a serious problem. If older people experience some degree of declining health, fear of increasing dependency may be paramount in their minds. Many older adult clients approach clinicians with hesitation because they have known friends and family members who have become sicker or died as a result of intervention. They may also be reluctant to admit health problems because they fear being admitted to a hospital or nursing home. It is essential that the nurse adapt routine interviewing techniques to always stress the positive habits that have helped the older person to live to an advanced age. For example, it is important to look for good nutritional habits as well as to identify which foods are to be avoided, or to focus on everyday activities that keep an older person ambulatory in addition to identifying risk factors for falls. The nurse needs to acknowledge the older client's accomplishments that have made life meaningful.

Determining Functional Status

Functional assessment is an evaluation of the person's ability to carry out the basic self-care activities of daily living (ADLs), such as bathing, eating, grooming, and toileting. There are many tools available for measuring ability to perform ADLs. One commonly used tool that is thought to be the most appropriate for assessing functional status in older adults (Wallace & Shelkey, 2007) is the Katz Activities of Daily Living (Assessment Tool 32-1), which include those activities necessary for well-being as an individual in a society. These activities, known as Instrumental Activities of Daily Living (IADLs) (Assessment Tool 32-2), focus primarily on household chores (such as cooking, cleaning, laundry), mobility-related activities (such as shopping and transportation), and cognitive abilities (such as money management, using the telephone, and making decisions affecting basic safety and social needs). Functional ability is determined by the dynamic interplay of the frail elder's physiologic status; emotional and cognitive statuses; and the physical, interpersonal, and social environments. A major purpose of assessing the frail older adult is to correctly identify and describe the client's ability to perform ADLs.

Biographical Data

Cultural norms were not always as informal as they are today. Many older adults grew up when older people were not addressed by their first names except by those very close to them. One should always begin the interview by addressing an older person as "Mr.," "Mrs.," or "Ms.," or with an appropriate title such as "Reverend" or "Doctor." In general, younger people

---

ASSESSMENT TOOL 32-1 Katz Activities of Daily Living

ACTIVITIES	INDEPENDENCE	DEPENDENCE
Points (1 or 0)	(1 Point) NO supervision, direction or personal assistance	(0 Points) WITH supervision, direction, personal assistance, or total care
Bathing Points: _____	(1 POINT) Bathes self completely or needs help in bathing only a single part of the body such as the back, genital area, or disabled extremity.	(0 POINTS) Needs help with bathing more than one part of the body, getting in or out of the tub or shower. Requires total bathing by care giver.
Dressing Points: _____	(1 POINT) Gets clothes from closets and drawers, and puts on clothes and outer garments complete with fasteners. May have help tying shoes.	(0 POINTS) Needs help with dressing self or needs to be completely dressed.
Toileting Points: _____	(1 POINT) Goes to toilet, gets on and off, arranges clothes, cleans genital area without help.	(0 POINTS) Needs help transferring to the toilet, cleaning self or uses bedpan or commode.
Transferring Points _____	(1 POINT) Moves in and out of bed or chair unassisted. Mechanical transferring aides are acceptable.	(0 POINTS) Needs help in moving from bed to chair or requires a complete transfer.
Continence Points: _____	(1 POINT) Exercises complete self-control over urination and defecation.	(0 POINTS) Is partially or totally incontinent of bowel or bladder.
Feeding Points: _____	(1 POINT) Gets food from plate into mouth without help. Preparation of food may be done by another person.	(0 POINTS) Needs partial or total help with feeding or requires parenteral feeding.
Total Points = _____	6 = High (patient independent)	0 = Low (patient very dependent)

Adapted with permission from Gerontological Society of America. Katz, S., Down, T. D., Cash, H. R., & Grotz, R. C. (1970). Progress in the development of the index of ADL. *Gerontologist, 10,* 20–30.

ASSESSMENT TOOL 32-2 Lawton Scale for Instrumental Activities of Daily Living (IADLs)

Instructions: Start by asking the client to describe his or her functioning in each category; then complement the description with specific questions as needed.

ABILITY TO TELEPHONE
1. Operates telephone on own initiative: looks up and dials numbers, etc.
2. Answers telephone and dials a few well-known numbers.
3. Answers telephone but does not dial.
4. Does not use telephone at all.

SHOPPING
1. Takes care of all shopping needs independently.
2. Shops independently for small purchases.
3. Needs to be accompanied on any shopping trip.
4. Completely unable to shop.

FOOD PREPARATION
1. Plans, prepares, and serves adequate meals independently.
2. Prepares adequate meals if supplied with ingredients.
3. Heats and serves prepared meals, or prepares meals but does not maintain adequate diet.
4. Needs to have meals prepared and served.

HOUSEKEEPING
1. Maintains house alone or with occasional assistance (e.g., heavy work done by domestic help).
2. Performs light daily tasks such as dishwashing and bed making.
3. Performs light daily tasks but cannot maintain acceptable level of cleanliness.
4. Needs help with all home maintenance tasks.
5. Does not participate in any housekeeping tasks.

LAUNDRY
1. Does personal laundry completely.
2. Launders small items; rinses socks, stockings, and so on.
3. All laundry must be done by others.

MODE OF TRANSPORTATION
1. Travels independently on public transportation, or drives own car.
2. Arranges own travel via taxi, but does not otherwise use public transportation.
3. Travels on public transportation when assisted or accompanied by another.
4. Travel is limited to taxi, automobile, or ambulette, with assistance.
5. Does not travel at all.

RESPONSIBILITY FOR OWN MEDICATION
1. Is responsible for taking medication in correct dosages at correct time.
2. Takes responsibility if medication is prepared in advance, in separated dosages.
3. Is not capable of dispensing own medication.

ABILITY TO HANDLE FINANCES
1. Manages financial matters independently (budgets, writes checks, pays rent and bills, goes to bank); collects and keeps track of income.
2. Manages day-to-day purchases but needs help with banking, major purchases, controlled spending, and so on.
3. Incapable of handling money.

Scoring: Circle one number for each domain. Total the numbers circled. Total score can range from 8 to 28. The lower the score, the more independence. Scores are only good for individual patients. Useful to see score comparison over time.

Lawton, M. P. (1971). Functional assessment of elderly people. *Journal of the American Geriatrics Society, 9*(6), 465–481. Reprinted by permission of Blackwell Science, Inc.

---

today are more likely to feel comfortable sharing personal information with regard to finances, personal likes and dislikes, and feelings than are older adults. Many older people are also aware of their vulnerability with regard to scams and fraud. Thus, they are reluctant (for good reasons) to give out personal information. An important maxim of geriatric care is: "Collect no more information than is essential for optimal care." If the client is cognitively impaired, a trusted caregiver may need to be involved in the history. Being sensitive to the older adult's need to be respected and acknowledged is essential.

Assessing Sexuality in Older Adults

Many people believe the myth that older adults do not have sex. Studies show that this is not true for many. The release from fears of pregnancy, from interruptions by children in the home, and from work-related schedules allows more relaxed opportunities for older couples to enjoy and express their intimacy and sexuality. Brick (2015) noted that she has received questions from hundreds of persons aged 50 to 90 on the subject of sexuality in older age, and noted that the questions themselves provide powerful evidence of the poignant concerns people have about sex and intimacy in mid and later life. She emphasized that older adults deserve respect, and respect for their sexual histories and sexual journey; that sexuality is a positive, life-affirming force. She provides information for sexual education for older adults. Loss of intimacy is among the greatest losses for many older adults. Those with spouses or significant others find intimacy in many forms and not just in the act of intercourse. For many, changes in the aging body or chronic diseases make intercourse difficult. One role of the nurse may involve helping the older client to explore different expressions of intimacy if necessary.

> **CLINICAL TIP**
> Health care providers often create barriers for elderly clients' expressions of their sexuality (Muliira & Muliira, 2013).

Men's and women's aging bodies change in a number of ways. Bloom lists these changes for women: labia and tissue covering the pubic bone lose firmness; vaginal walls become less elastic and the vagina drier; the clitoris may become overly sensitive; uterine contractions with orgasm may be painful. Changes for men: the entire male sexual response tends to slow, with delays in erection, need for more manual stimulation to achieve erection, prolonging of the plateau phase between erection and ejaculation, shorter and less forceful orgasm, rapid loss of penile firmness after orgasm, and a marked increase in the time before another erection can be achieved after orgasm, even up to a week in very aged men.

Many diseases and medications can result in pain, erectile dysfunction, or embarrassment and impair sexual expression in the elderly as for other clients. The most important factors for continued sexual expression, according to Bloom, are a willing spirit and flexibility to adapt to conditions encountered with aging. A playful and fun spirit helps to overcome many obstacles.

> **CLINICAL TIP**
> STIs, including HIV/AIDS, occur in elderly as well as younger people. STI transmission among the elderly is unfortunately a common and growing problem. McDaniel (2016) reported that in 2013, *Chlamydia* infections among Americans 65 and over increased by 31% and syphilis by 52%. The Centers for Disease Control and Prevention (CDC, 2016a) reported that in 2014, people aged 50 and older accounted for 17% (7,391) of HIV diagnoses in the United States. Forty percent of people aged 55 and older were diagnosed with AIDS at the time of HIV diagnosis (i.e., diagnosed late in the course of the infection). In addition to the decrease in use of condoms after a woman completes menopause, many older adults simply do not believe themselves susceptible to AIDS. Also, there is more difficulty with diagnosis and detection of AIDS symptoms. For example, night sweats, chronic fatigue, weight loss, dementia, and swollen lymph nodes mimic other disease symptoms and the natural aging process.

History of Present Health Concern

QUESTION	RATIONALE
Mental Status	
Have you noticed any changes in your ability to concentrate or think clearly enough to keep up with your daily activities? If so, about when did this begin and describe what you have noticed? > **CLINICAL TIP** > If the older adult is too lethargic, agitated, or medically unstable to respond, appears excessively distracted, offers inconsistencies, or cannot answer specific questions or describe daily activities, then family or professional caregivers should be queried with regard to how current cognition and behavior compares with the client's prior level of function.	A common symptom of acute illness in the frail older adult is a sudden deterioration of cognition. The aging brain is more vulnerable to deficits in oxygenation and nutrition. Changes in cognition that have occurred suddenly and recently (e.g., the past few days or within the past week or two) must *always* be assumed to be the result of a disease or illness, and must be thoroughly assessed and appropriately referred for treatment. Although intellectual capacity does not diminish with advancing age, the brain does become more susceptible to injury. When such a change in cognition develops over a short time and is characterized by a change in level of alertness from extreme lethargy to agitation, it is called delirium (see Table 32-1). Delirious people may continuously shift attention from one stimulus to another, abruptly and inappropriately, making speech difficult to understand and conversation hard to follow. Disorientation is more often to time and place rather than to self, and delusions and hallucinations may occur.
Use the Saint Louis University Mental Status (SLUMS) (see Assessment Tool 6-3) and the Confusion Assessment Method (CAM) to assess mental status (see Assessment Tool 6-4).	These tools are validated and provide early warning of possible mental status deterioration. If assaults to the brain are not reversed quickly enough, irreversible brain tissue damage can ensue. Changes in cognition that have occurred suddenly and recently (e.g., the past few days or within the past week or two) must *always* be assumed to be the result of a disease or illness, and must be thoroughly assessed and appropriately referred for treatment.
Do you believe that you have more problems with memory than most? Do you believe that life is empty? Have you recently had to drop many of your activities and interests?	Depression is not more common in old age. However, symptoms of depression in older adults more commonly manifest as changes in cognition (memory deficits, paranoia, and agitation) and physical symptoms (muscle aches, joint pains, gastrointestinal [GI] disturbances, headache, and weight loss) than they do in younger adults. Depression in older adults has even been called "pseudodementia." It can also be a symptom of certain physical disorders, especially endocrine disorders such as hypothyroidism, pancreatic and adrenal disorders, and cancers of all types. Certain antihypertensives, antianxiety drugs, and hormones may also precipitate depressive symptoms.

QUESTION	RATIONALE
Open-ended questions usually yield the most beneficial information when screening for depression in older adults. However, when time is limited or whenever warning signs are noted, a screening instrument such as the short version of the Geriatric Depression Scale (Yesavage & Brink, 1983) should be used for further validation (see Box 32-2).	When more than five questions are answered as indicated on the tool, a high probability of depressive symptoms exists. The purpose of a screening tool is not to confirm a diagnosis, but rather to point out the need for a more in-depth assessment or referral.
Are you concerned about changes in your memory (see Assessment Tool 32-3)? Are you bothered by anger or inability to control your frustrations with day-by-day living?	By 85 years of age, nearly half the population will be exhibiting signs of the most common type of dementia, Alzheimer disease (AD). Dementia is a broad diagnostic category that includes multiple physical disorders characterized by alterations in memory, abstract thinking, judgment, and perception. Unlike delirium, dementias are characterized by gradual decline in cognitive function to the extent that daily functions are affected (ADLs or IADLs), usually over months or years. Although impaired memory is generally characterized as the key diagnostic criteria for AD, the earliest signs may more often be behavioral and characterized by irritability, aggression or angry outbursts, suspiciousness, or even withdrawal.
Functional Ability To Perform Activities of Daily Living	
Are you able to carry out the basic self-care activities of daily living (ADLs), such as bathing, eating, grooming, and toileting? Use the Katz Activities of Daily Living Assessment Tool 32-1, to assess the older adult's ability to achieve well-being as an individual in a society. Use the Lawton Scale for Instrumental Activities of Daily Living Assessment Tool 32-2, to assess the individual's ability to perform household chores (such as cooking, cleaning, laundry), mobility-related activities (such as shopping and transportation), and cognitive abilities (such as money management, using the telephone, and making decisions affecting basic safety and social needs).	Functional ability is determined by the dynamic interplay of the frail elder's physiologic status; emotional and cognitive statuses; and the physical, interpersonal, and social environments. A major purpose of assessing the frail older adult is to correctly identify and describe the client's ability to perform ADLs.
Falls	
Do you ever need to grab onto something because you feel like you're going to stumble or fall? Have you ever used anything to steady yourself when you're walking?	Risk factor assessment for falls is important because the fall can be a symptom of another problem needing attention. A fall can be the symptom of a treatable medical condition, the result of an adverse response to a medication, or a problem associated with chronic illness and frailty.
	The nurse must be sensitive to an older adult's fears and anxieties. Loved ones are also concerned with the safety threat imposed by falls and the possible guilt associated with not being available at the time that a fall occurs. Although the fear of falling is a realistic and common fear, the need to stay active both before and after a fall is even greater.
	Falling is not a normal part of aging. Limitations in activity are not the appropriate response to a positive fall assessment. The risk of falling can be minimized by a comprehensive assessment followed by appropriate medical, exercise, and adaptive environmental interventions.
Have you had any recent falls? What were you doing? Where did it occur? What other kinds of feelings or symptoms did you have when you fell (e.g., headache, confusion)?	The history should determine the circumstances surrounding any previous falls of the past 3 months to determine if a pattern exists. The pattern and circumstances surrounding the fall can provide valuable clues with regard to the physical, medication-related, or environmental basis for the fall. For example, falls occurring with standing up and associated with dizziness may point to orthostatic hypotension and an adverse reaction to medication. If the client reports tripping or slipping in the absence of stiffness, weakness, or other symptoms, an environmental basis such as shoes or floors with a slick surface or loose carpeting or rugs may be suspected.

Continued on following page

History of Present Health Concern (Continued)

QUESTION	RATIONALE
Falls (Continued)	
Do you ever feel lightheaded or dizzy when you get up from a chair or a bed?	Lightheadedness or dizziness can indicate postural hypotension or other vascular conditions.
Do you have any difficulty when getting up out of bed or from sitting in a chair? Does stiffness and soreness inhibit your ability to move about? Do you ever feel like your legs are going to "give way" or that they are weak? If so, describe. What is your usual daily pattern of activity? Exercise routine?	Clients may benefit from exercises to improve flexibility, fitness, and endurance and to delay functional decline. Exercises can benefit even those who have led sedentary lifestyles or who already have some functional deficits.
Do you have any discomfort in your legs with activity? Would you describe the discomfort as pain, cramping, aching, fatigue, or weakness in the calf? Do your hips, thighs, and/or buttocks hurt with ambulation? If so, how far can you walk before the pain occurs? Does the pain go away with rest?	These symptoms are commonly associated with intermittent claudication, a circulatory disorder affecting the peripheral blood vessels of the leg. Symptoms are usually bilateral and progressive.
Weakness: Fatigue and Dyspnea	
How has your energy level changed in the last few days or weeks? How does it affect your daily activities such as cooking, household chores, or activities outside the home (e.g., shopping, social, church)? When is your energy at its lowest level? When does it seem to be at its best? ⊙ **CLINICAL TIP** When an older adult complains of weakness and fatigue, anemia must always be ruled out. Anemia is always a symptom of an underlying pathology. A few common causes in older adults are GI bleeding and nutritional deficiencies (especially B_{12}, folate, and iron). Anticoagulants and nonsteroidal anti-inflammatory drugs (NSAIDs) increase the risk of GI bleeding.	Self-reported fatigue and weakness, as well as a decline in physical activity and appetite, are common elements of frailty syndrome. The progression of the weakness and how it relates to ADLs and IADLs provides clues as to possible etiologies. For example, a sudden and severe fatigue that affects self-care activities such as bathing and dressing may be more likely to have an acute cause such as infection, myocardial infarction, or a dysrhythmia such as atrial fibrillation. Diminishing energy over months or weeks is more likely to indicate a more insidious pathology such as a slow GI bleed, arthritis and pain, or even depression.
Do you ever experience shortness of breath? If so, is it related to activity? (Specific questions about endurance, stair climbing, or ADLs are necessary for quantifying the extent of the problem.) Does it occur at rest or when lying down? How many pillows do you use? Any pain with breathing?	Dyspnea is a frequently reported symptom associated with common illnesses among older adult clients, including chronic obstructive pulmonary disease (COPD), asthma, lung cancer, and heart failure. Older adults with chronic respiratory or cardiac problems who experience some constant degree of dyspnea are unlikely to seek care or note dyspnea unless there is a change in functional capabilities.
Do you seem to be breathing faster? Sweating? Do you experience anorexia (loss of appetite) or fatigue?	In the frail older adult, an increase in respirations, sweating, or overall malaise may be the only indication of a respiratory problem (American Association of Colleges of Nursing [AACN], 2012).
Do you have a recurrent cough? Does it ever have blood in it? Do you use tobacco or have you in the past?	A recurrent cough, fatigue, weight loss, shortness of breath, and productive cough (sometimes blood-tinged) are hallmarks of lung cancer, which is the second most common type of cancer in men over age 75, with incidence rising in women (CDC, MMWR, 2014).
Have you experienced weight loss or changes in your health along with a chronic cough?	Weight loss, night sweats, or changes in respiratory status, such as coughing, may be signs of tuberculosis (TB) or other medical conditions. Debilitated older adults are at increased risk of TB. In addition, glucocorticosteroid therapy and nutritional deficiencies depress the immune system, thereby exacerbating the chances of reactivating a dormant TB infection.

QUESTION	RATIONALE
Have you received the pneumococcal vaccine within the past 6 years? Do you get annual flu vaccines?	Pneumonia is the most common cause of infection-related deaths in older adults. The Pneumococcal vaccine (either PCV13 or PCV23) is recommended once a lifetime for those over age 65 and PCV23 is additionally recommended for those at risk for pneumococcal disease who are from 2 to 64 years (CDC, 2016b). Debilitated and institutionalized older adults are particularly at risk for serious influenza-related illness. There can be significant loss of fluid through sustained coughing with pneumonia.

Weakness: Nutrition and Hydration

QUESTION	RATIONALE
Have you experienced any change in your appetite (including nausea and vomiting) in the past 6 months? If yes, when did you first notice a decline in appetite? Did you have any other health problem at about this same time? Did you start taking any new medication at this time? (See Assessment Tool 32-4.)	A loss of appetite is a nearly universal cofactor of both physical and mental diseases in older adults.
Can you describe what you eat in an average day? (Compile a 24-hour food and fluid diary noting food preferences and cravings, vitamin and food supplement intake, and dietary restrictions, e.g., salt). On a day when your appetite is smaller, how would your eating habits change? A screening tool (Box 32-3) may be helpful in identifying those at risk for being malnourished.	A sudden loss of appetite is most often a symptom of disease or an adverse medication effect. Because the aged body is housing a "smaller engine," the minimum caloric intake does decrease in old age. Even healthy older adults consume only an estimated 1,200–1,600 calories per day. This has led to the general consensus that older adults need nutrient-dense foods to ingest enough essential nutrients. A 3-day food diary, with 1 day being a weekend day, is the most reliable method of obtaining a diet history. Sarcopenia (skeletal muscle mass decrease) and sarcopenic obesity (skeletal muscle mass decrease combined with excess body fat) result from decreased physical activity and decreased protein intake and are associated with functional decline (Batsis et al., 2015).
Do you limit the kind or amount of food you eat because of problems with your teeth or dentures (e.g., biting apples or chewing meat)? An oral health assessment tool (Assessment Tool 32-5) may help to detect problems.	Oral health is a vital component of good nutrition, socialization, and a positive self-concept. Untreated oral health problems are a common cause of discomfort that may interfere with chewing and digestion.
Do you ever feel like you're choking when you drink water or feel like food is catching in your throat?	Dysphagia is a frequent problem associated with neurologic conditions as well as when food is not sufficiently chewed or there is insufficient saliva to mix with food. Dysphagia increases risk of choking, aspiration, dehydration, and malnutrition. Signs and symptoms of dysphagia range from weak or hoarse voice, pocketing of food, coughing after food or fluids to drooling.
How much fluid do you think you drink each day?	Fluid intake of less than 1,500 mL daily (excluding caffeine-containing beverages) is a possible indicator of dehydration. The fluid requirement for older adults without cardiac or renal disease is approximately 30 ml/kg of body weight per day. Loss of appetite almost always coexists with inadequate hydration. Decreased thirst sensation is common with aging, and decreased mobility makes it less possible for the frail older adult to respond to an already diminished sense of thirst. Drug use may contribute to dehydration as well. For example, diuretics are widely used in treating cardiovascular and renal disease, as are fluid restrictions.

Urinary Incontinence (UI)

QUESTION	RATIONALE
Do you ever have any urine leakage or problems controlling your urine flow? (Explain to the client that many illnesses and medications can cause problems with urine control. This is not normal just because one is getting older, but it is a common problem.)	The CDC (2014, p. 5) reported that 50.9% of noninstitutionalized persons aged 65 and over reported a urinary leakage and/or accidental bowel leakage and of them, 43.8% reported a urinary leakage. The incidence of UI is higher for older adults who are institutionalized

Continued on following page

History of Present Health Concern (Continued)

QUESTION	RATIONALE
Urinary Incontinence (UI) (Continued)	
	and cognitively impaired. Incidence of new-onset incontinence among hospitalized older adults has been reported at 35–42% (Zürcher et al., 2011). Loss of bladder function or control can be an embarrassing and demeaning problem. Unfortunately, many older adults believe in error that problems with bladder control are a normal and expected part of aging. Incontinence is often associated with chronic conditions such as stroke, multiple sclerosis (MS), prostatitis, and UTI. It may also be the result of a fecal impaction, constipation, or an adverse drug effect.
(Male) Do you have difficulty starting a stream of urine? Frequency? Nighttime frequency? Dribbling? If yes, do you ever take any cold or sinus medications or medication to help you sleep?	Benign prostatic hypertrophy occurs in up to 90% of men over age 80 and is thought to be due to a decrease in testosterone and increase in estrogen within the prostate, promoting prostate cell growth (Urology Care Foundation, 2017). It may result in urinary frequency, difficulty starting a stream of urine, nocturia, and urinary retention with overflow incontinence and an increased risk of UTIs. Over-the-counter drugs with anticholinergic side effects (e.g., cold/sinus preparations and sleep medications) may contribute to urinary retention or add to obstructive symptoms.
How long has the leakage (or use client's descriptive words) been going on? Has it ever suddenly gotten worse?	Any new onset of incontinence or exacerbation may indicate an infection. In the hospitalized older adult, UTI ranks high as a suspected cause for any new onset of incontinence. UTI is the most common hospital-acquired bacterial infection. UTI must also be a concern for older adults at home or in long-term care because it is the most frequent source of bacteremia for these people. A UTI is particularly perplexing in older adults because it presents in such an atypical way (i.e., without fever, or elevation in white blood cell counts, or dysuria, or urinary frequency). Even more common symptoms of a UTI in the frail older adult may be confusion, lethargy, anorexia, and nocturia.
What activities are associated with your loss of urine control?	The client's activities during an episode of incontinence may help to determine the type of incontinence and, therefore, its treatment. See Box 32-4 for a description of the kinds of urinary incontinence.
Bowel Elimination	
Do you have any problems with bowel elimination?	As people age, GI motility decreases because of a loss of muscle tone and atrophy. Dehydration, immobility, and poor intake exacerbate the likelihood of constipation. Adequate fluid intake, dietary fiber, and moderate exercise are key factors in maintaining efficient elimination.
Have you had a change in bowel habits recently? Have you ever had blood in your stools? Have you had your stools tested for blood? What medications do you take?	The guaiac stool test to detect occult blood is a common test administered to detect abnormalities of the GI tract. Clients with a past history of polyps, adenomas, and inflammatory bowel disease (IBD) are at increased risk for colorectal cancer in old age. Warning signs include rectal bleeding, unexplained weight loss, and a change in bowel habits. NSAIDs, such as aspirin and naproxen, corticosteroids, and anticoagulants such as warfarin may promote GI bleeding.
Pain Assessment	
Do you have pain, discomfort, aching, or soreness? If so, is the discomfort worse with activity? Relieved by rest? Do you have problems with grasping, reaching, or activities that use your hands, arms, back, or legs?	Functional limitations and pain are common consequences of inflammatory joint disease in frail older adults. The combination of pain and functional impairment may predispose the client to social isolation and depression.

QUESTION	RATIONALE
Pain scales used with adults are also usually valid in evaluating pain in an elderly client, except in the more severe stages of dementia. For those with moderate levels of dementia but who are still able to verbalize, short and frequent questioning about pain using words such as "hurting," "soreness," "aching," or "uncomfortable" may be useful. For nonverbal demented individuals, behaviors such as grimacing, striking out, and moaning should be routinely evaluated to identify pain as well as to evaluate the degree to which the pain is being relieved (Box 32-5). Many of the behaviors commonly labeled as "aggressive" or "combative" are the result of untreated pain (Douzijian et al., 2002).	Molton and Terrill (2014) reported an estimated 60–75% of persons over age 65 have some level of persistent pain, which tends to limit physical activity, leading to greater pain and disability, possible weight gain, and obesity, which again contribute to further pain of weight-bearing joints. Sleep and social isolation also result.

TABLE 32-1   Comparing Delirium and Dementia

Delirium (Mayo Clinic, 2015)	Dementia (Alzheimer's Association, 2016)
Definition A serious disturbance in mental abilities that results in confused thinking and reduced awareness of your environment. The start of delirium is usually rapid—within hours or a few days.	A general term for a decline in mental ability severe enough to interfere with daily life; not a specific disease but an overall term that describes a wide range of symptoms. Two most common types are Alzheimer disease (60–80%) and vascular dementia after a stroke.

Causes, Risk Factors, Contributing Factors
 • Severe or chronic medical illness
 • Changes in metabolic balance (such as low sodium)
 • Medication
 • Infection
 • Surgery
 • Alcohol or drug withdrawal
	• Age
	 • Family history
	 • Genetics (specific genes)
	 • Combined factors including:
	   • Head trauma
	   • Brain health/heart health connection
	   • Vascular disease (diabetes, hypertension, high cholesterol)
	   • Latino or African American due to more vascular risks;
	   • Unhealthy behaviors in aging, such as: smoking, excessive alcohol intake, lack of exercise (or sedentary lifestyle), not socially connected; poor diet (especially affect heart health)

Symptoms
 Symptoms usually begin over a few hours or a few days, tend to fluctuate throughout the day, may include periods of no symptoms, tend to be worse at night when dark and things look less familiar. Primary signs and symptoms include those below:
 • Reduced awareness of the environment
   This may result in:
   • An inability to stay focused on a topic or to switch topics
   • Getting stuck on an idea rather than responding to questions or conversation
   • Being easily distracted by unimportant things
   • Being withdrawn, with little or no activity or little response to the environment
 • Poor thinking skills (cognitive impairment) This may appear as:
   • Poor memory, particularly of recent events
   • Disorientation, e.g., not knowing where you are or who you are
   • Difficulty speaking or recalling words
   • Rambling or nonsense speech
   • Trouble understanding speech
   • Difficulty reading or writing
	While symptoms of dementia can vary greatly, at least two of the following core mental functions must be significantly impaired to be considered dementia:
	 • Memory
	 • Communication and language
	 • Ability to focus and pay attention
	 • Reasoning and judgment
	 • Visual perception

Continued on following page

TABLE 32-1　Comparing Delirium and Dementia (Continued)

Delirium (Mayo Clinic, 2015)	Dementia (Alzheimer's Association, 2016)
• Behavior changes 　This may include: 　• Seeing things that don't exist (hallucinations) 　• Restlessness, agitation or combative behavior 　• Calling out, moaning or making other sounds 　• Being quiet and withdrawn—especially in older adults 　• Slowed movement or lethargy 　• Disturbed sleep habits 　• Reversal of night-day sleep-wake cycle • Emotional disturbances 　This may appear as: 　• Anxiety, fear or paranoia 　• Depression 　• Irritability or anger 　• A sense of feeling elated (euphoria) 　• Apathy 　• Rapid and unpredictable mood shifts 　• Personality changes	

Mayo Clinic. (2015). Delirium. Available at http://www.mayoclinic.org/diseases-conditions/delirium/basics/definition/con-20033982
Alzheimer's Association. (2016). What is dementia? Available at http://www.alz.org/what-is-dementia.asp
Alzheimer's Association. (2016). Alzheimer's disease: Risk factors. Available at http://www.alz.org/alzheimers_disease_causes_risk_factors.asp

BOX 32-2　SELF-ASSESSMENT: GERIATRIC DEPRESSION SCALE

Choose the best answer for how you felt over the past week.

1. Are you basically satisfied with your life?　Yes/No
2. Have you dropped many of your activities and interests?　Yes/No
3. Do you feel that your life is empty?　Yes/No
4. Do you often get bored?　Yes/No
5. Are you hopeful about the future?　Yes/No
6. Are you bothered by thoughts you can't get out of your head?　Yes/No
7. Are you in good spirits most of the time?　Yes/No
8. Are you afraid that something bad is going to happen to you?　Yes/No
9. Do you feel happy most of the time?　Yes/No
10. Do you often feel helpless?　Yes/No
11. Do you often get restless and fidgety?　Yes/No
12. Do you prefer to stay at home, rather than going out and doing new things?　Yes/No
13. Do you frequently worry about the future?　Yes/No
14. Do you feel you have more problems with memory than most?　Yes/No
15. Do you think it is wonderful to be alive now?　Yes/No
16. Do you often feel downhearted and blue?　Yes/No
17. Do you feel pretty worthless the way you are now?　Yes/No
18. Do you worry a lot about the past?　Yes/No
19. Do you find life very exciting?　Yes/No
20. Is it hard for you to get started on new projects?　Yes/No
21. Do you feel full of energy?　Yes/No
22. Do you feel that your situation is hopeless?　Yes/No
23. Do you think that most people are better off than you are?　Yes/No
24. Do you frequently get upset over little things?　Yes/No
25. Do you frequently feel like crying?　Yes/No
26. Do you have trouble concentrating?　Yes/No
27. Do you enjoy getting up in the morning?　Yes/No
28. Do you prefer to avoid social gatherings?　Yes/No
29. Is it easy for you to make decisions?　Yes/No
30. Is your mind as clear as it used to be?　Yes/No

For scoring, reverse the answers for Nos. 1, 5, 7, 9, 15, 19, 21, 27, 29, and 30, then count the total number of "yes" answers.

Scoring: 0–10 = within normal range; 11 or higher = possible indication of depression.

Brink T. L., Yesavage J. A., Lum O., Heersema P., Adey M. B., Rose T. L. (1982). Screening tests for geriatric depression. Clinical Gerontologist, *1*, 37–44.

ASSESSMENT TOOL 32-3　Short Blessed Test

Client:_____　　　DATE: _____

Age: _____

SHORT BLESSED TEST (SBT) ADMINISTRATION AND SCORING GUIDELINES[1]

A spontaneous self-correction is allowed for all responses without counting as an error.

1. What is the year? Acceptable Response: The exact year must be given. An incomplete but correct numerical response is acceptable (e.g., 01 for 2001).
2. What is the month? Acceptable Response: The exact month must be given. A correct numerical answer is acceptable (e.g., 12 for December).

ASSESSMENT TOOL 32-3 Short Blessed Test (Continued)

3. The clinician should state: "I will give you a name and address to remember for a few minutes. Listen to me say the entire name and address and then repeat it after me."

    It is important for the clinician to carefully read the phrase and give emphasis to each item of the phrase. There should be a 1-second delay between individual items.

    The trial phrase should be readministered until the subject is able to repeat the entire phrase without assistance or until a maximum of three attempts. If the subject is unable to learn the phrase after three attempts, a "C" should be recorded. This indicates that the subject could not learn the phrase in three tries.

    Whether or not the trial phrase is learned, the clinician should instruct, "Good, now remember that name and address for a few minutes."

4. "Without looking at your watch or clock, tell me about what time it is." This is scored as correct if the time given is within plus or minus 1 hour. If the subject's response is vague (e.g., almost 1 o'clock), the clinician should prompt for a more specific response.

5. Counting. The instructions should be read as written. If the subject skips a number after 20, an error should be recorded. If the subject starts counting forward during the task or forgets the task, the instructions should be repeated and one error should be recorded. The maximum number of errors is two.

6. Months. The instructions should be read as written. To get the subject started, the examiner may state: "Start with the last month of the year. The last month of the year is_____." If the subject cannot recall the last month of the year, the examiner may prompt this test with "December"; however, one error should be recorded. If the subject skips a month, an error should be recorded. If the subject starts saying the months forward upon initiation of the task, the instructions should be repeated and no error recorded. If the subject starts saying the months forward during the task or forgets the task, the instructions should be repeated and one error recorded. The maximum number of errors is two.

7. Repeat. The subject should state each item verbatim. The address number must be exact (i.e., "4200" would be considered an error for "42"). For the name of the street (i.e., Market Street), the thoroughfare term is not required to be given (i.e., leaving off "drive" or "street") or to be correct (i.e., substituting "boulevard" or "lane") for the item to be scored correct.

8. The final score is a weighted sum of individual error scores. Use the table below to calculate each weighted score and sum for the total.

FINAL SBT SCORE AND INTERPRETATION

Item #	Errors (0–5)	Weighting Factor	Final Item Score
1		× 4	
2		× 3	
3		× 3	
4		× 2	
5		× 2	
6		× 2	
			Sum Total = _____ (Range 0–28)

INTERPRETATION

A screening test in itself is insufficient to diagnose a dementing disorder. The SBT is, however, quite sensitive to early cognitive changes associated with Alzheimer disease. Scores in the impaired range (see below) indicate a need for further assessment. Scores in the "normal" range suggest that a dementing disorder is unlikely, but a very early disease process cannot be ruled out. More advanced assessment may be warranted in cases in which other objective evidence of impairment exists.

- In the original validation sample for the SBT (Katzman et al., 1983), 90% of normal scores 6 points or less. Scores of 7 or higher would indicate a need for further evaluation to rule out a dementing disorder, such as Alzheimer disease.
- Based on clinical research findings from the Memory and Aging Project,[2] the following cut points may also be considered:
  - 0–4   Normal Cognition
  - 5–9   Questionable Impairment (evaluate for early dementing disorder)
  - 10 or more Impairment Consistent with Dementia (evaluate for dementing disorder)

These guidelines and scoring rules are based on the administration experience of faculty and staff of the Memory and Aging Project, Alzheimer's Disease Research Center (ADRC), Washington University School of Medicine, St. Louis (John C. Morris, MD, Director & PI; morrisj@abraxas.wustl.edu). For more information about the ADRC, visit: http://alzheimer.wustl.edu or call 314–286–2881.

Morris, J. C., Heyman, A., Mohs, R. C., et al. (1989). The Consortium to Establish a Registry for Alzheimer's Disease (CERAD). Part I. Clinical and neuropsychological assessment of Alzheimer's disease. *Neurology,* 39(9), 1159–1165.

ASSESSMENT TOOL 32-4 Mini Nutritional Assessment (MNA-SF)

Mini Nutritional Assessment
MNA®

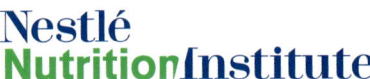

Last name: _____ First name: _____

Sex: _____ Age: _____ Weight, kg: _____ Height, cm: _____ Date: _____

Complete the screen by filling in the boxes with the appropriate numbers. Total the numbers for the final screening score.

Screening

A Has food intake declined over the past 3 months due to loss of appetite, digestive problems, chewing or swallowing difficulties?
0 = severe decrease in food intake
1 = moderate decrease in food intake
2 = no decrease in food intake ☐

B Weight loss during the last 3 months
0 = weight loss greater than 3 kg (6.6 lbs)
1 = does not know
2 = weight loss between 1 and 3 kg (2.2 and 6.6 lbs)
3 = no weight loss ☐

C Mobility
0 = bed or chair bound
1 = able to get out of bed / chair but does not go out
2 = goes out ☐

D Has suffered psychological stress or acute disease in the past 3 months?
0 = yes   2 = no ☐

E Neuropsychological problems
0 = severe dementia or depression
1 = mild dementia
2 = no psychological problems ☐

F1 Body Mass Index (BMI) (weight in kg) / (height in m^2) ☐
0 = BMI less than 19
1 = BMI 19 to less than 21
2 = BMI 21 to less than 23
3 = BMI 23 or greater ☐

IF BMI IS NOT AVAILABLE, REPLACE QUESTION F1 WITH QUESTION F2.
DO NOT ANSWER QUESTION F2 IF QUESTION F1 IS ALREADY COMPLETED.

F2 Calf circumference (CC) in cm
0 = CC less than 31
3 = CC 31 or greater ☐

Screening score
(max. 14 points) ☐☐

12-14 points: ☐ Normal nutritional status
8-11 points: ☐ At risk of malnutrition
0-7 points: ☐ Malnourished

For further information, visit: www.mna-elderly.com.
Vellas, B., Villars, H., Abellan, G., et al. (2006). Overview of the MNA®—Its History and Challenges. *Journal of Nutrition Health and Aging, 10,* 456–465.
Rubenstein, L. Z., Harker, J. O., Salva, A., Guigoz, Y., Vellas, B. (2001). Screening for Undernutrition in Geriatric Practice: Developing the Short-Form Mini Nutritional Assessment (MNA-SF). *Journals of Gerontology, 56A,* M366–M377.
Guigoz, Y. (2006). The Mini-Nutritional Assessment (MNA®) Review of the Literature—What does it tell us? *Journal of Nutrition Health and Aging, 10,* 466–487.
Kaiser, M. J., Bauer, J. M., Ramsch, C., et al. (2009). Validation of the Mini Nutritional Assessment Short-Form (MNA®-SF): A practical tool for identification of nutritional status. *Journal of Nutrition Health and Aging, 13,* 782–788.
®Société des Produits Nestlé S.A., Vevey, Switzerland, Trademark Owners.
© Nestlé, 1994, Revision 2009. N67200 12/99 10M

ASSESSMENT TOOL 32-5 The Geriatric Oral Health Assessment Index

Indicate, in the past 3 months, how often you feel the way described in each of the following statements. Circle one answer for each.

	1	2	3	4	5
1. How often did you limit the kind or amounts of food you eat because of problems with your teeth or dentures?	Always	Often	Sometimes	Seldom	Never
2. How often did you have trouble biting or chewing any kinds of food such as firm meat or apples?	Always	Often	Sometimes	Seldom	Never
3. How often were you able to swallow comfortably?[a]	Always	Often	Sometimes	Seldom	Never
4. How often have your teeth or dentures prevented you from speaking the way you wanted?	Always	Often	Sometimes	Seldom	Never
5. How often were you able to eat anything without feeling discomfort?[a]	Always	Often	Sometimes	Seldom	Never
6. How often did you limit contacts with people because of the condition of your teeth or dentures?	Always	Often	Sometimes	Seldom	Never
7. How often were you pleased or happy with the looks of your teeth and gums or dentures?[a]	Always	Often	Sometimes	Seldom	Never
8. How often did you use medication to relieve pain or discomfort from around your mouth?	Always	Often	Sometimes	Seldom	Never
9. How often were you worried or concerned about the problems with your teeth, gums, or dentures?	Always	Often	Sometimes	Seldom	Never
10. How often did you feel nervous or self-conscious because of problems with your teeth, gums, or dentures?	Always	Often	Sometimes	Seldom	Never
11. How often did you feel uncomfortable eating in front of people because of problems with your teeth or dentures?	Always	Often	Sometimes	Seldom	Never
12. How often were your teeth or gums sensitive to hot, cold, or sweets?	Always	Often	Sometimes	Seldom	Never

Total Score:_____

[a]Items 3, 5, 7 are reverse scored with a "1" for never and a "5" for always. All other items are a "1" for always.

KA Atchison and TA Dolan. Development of the Geriatric Oral Health Assessment Index. *J Dent Educ* 1990, 54, 680–687. Copyright © 1990 American Dental Education Association.

BOX 32-3 SELF-ASSESSMENT: NSI CHECKLIST TO DETERMINE YOUR NUTRITIONAL HEALTH

The warning signs of poor nutritional health are often overlooked. Use this checklist to find out if you or someone you know is at nutritional risk.

Read the statements below. Circle the number in the "yes" column for those that apply to you or someone you know. For each "yes" answer, score the number in the box. Total your nutritional score.

	YES
I have an illness or condition that made me change the kind and/or amount of food I eat.	2
I eat fewer than 2 meals per day.	3
I eat few fruits or vegetables or milk products.	2
I have 3 or more drinks of beer, liquor, or wine almost every day.	2
I have tooth or mouth problems that make it hard for me to eat.	2
I don't always have enough money to buy the food I need.	4
I eat alone most of the time.	1
I take 3 or more different prescribed or over-the-counter drugs a day.	1
Without wanting to, I have lost or gained 10 pounds in the last 6 months.	2
I am not always physically able to shop, cook, and/or feed myself.	2
TOTAL	_____

Continued on following page

BOX 32-3 SELF-ASSESSMENT: NSI CHECKLIST TO DETERMINE YOUR NUTRITIONAL HEALTH (Continued)

Total Your Nutritional Score. If it's —

0–2	Good! Recheck your nutritional score in 6 months.
3–5	You are at moderate nutritional risk. See what can be done to improve your eating habits and lifestyle. Your office on aging, senior nutrition program, senior citizens center, or health department can help. Recheck your nutritional score in 3 months.
6 or more	You are at high nutritional risk. Bring this checklist the next time you see your doctor, dietitian, or other qualified health or social service professional. Talk with them about any problems you may have. Ask for help to improve your nutritional health.

Remember that warning signs suggest risk, but do not represent a diagnosis of any condition.

These materials are developed and distributed by the Nutrition Screening Initiative, a project of:

AMERICAN ACADEMY
OF FAMILY PHYSICIANS
THE AMERICAN
DIETETIC ASSOCIATION
THE NATIONAL COUNCIL
ON THE AGING, INC.

The Nutrition Screening Initiative • 1010 Wisconsin Avenue, NW • Suite 800 • Washington, DC 20007
The Nutrition Screening Initiative is funded in part by a grant from Ross Products Division of Abbott Laboratories, Inc.

BOX 32-4 UNDERSTANDING URINARY INCONTINENCE: ASSESSMENT AND INTERVENTION

TYPES OF INCONTINENCE

The signs and symptoms associated with the involuntary loss of urine have been clustered into three categories: urge, stress, and overflow incontinence. Any one or a combination of all three types may be present in an individual. Voiding diaries are useful for determining the type of incontinence that is occurring based on the amount, timing, and associated symptoms of incontinent episodes.

Voiding Diary

Time	Drinks		Voiding	
	Kind	How much	How many times	How much
6–7 AM	coffee	2 cups	I	medium
7–8 AM	orange juice	1 glass	II	lots
8–9 AM	—	—	I	little
9–10 AM	—	—	—	—
10–11 AM	water	1 glass	I	medium

Time	Leaks/Accidents	Strength of urge	Activity at the time of leak
6–7 AM		strong	no leak
7–8 AM		strong	
8–9 AM	I		frying eggs
9–10 AM			
10–11 AM			

Urge Incontinence

Urge incontinence is the involuntary loss of urine associated with an abrupt and strong desire to void. It is frequently caused by a neurologic disorder such as a cerebrovascular accident (CVA) or multiple sclerosis (MS), which impairs the ability of the bladder or urinary sphincter to contract and relax.

Stress Incontinence

Stress incontinence is the involuntary loss of urine during coughing, sneezing, laughing, or other physical activities that increase abdominal pressure. In women, stress incontinence may result from weakened and relaxed muscles from the combined effects of aging superimposed on the effects of childbirth.

> **CLINICAL TIP**
> Atrophic vaginitis from estrogen deficiency usually results in symptoms of urge incontinence as well as stress incontinence (mixed incontinence).

Overflow Incontinence

Overflow incontinence is the involuntary loss of urine associated with overdistention of the bladder. Prostatic hypertrophy is a common cause in men; diabetic neuropathy is a common cause in both sexes.

Functional Incontinence

Functional incontinence is the inability to get to the bathroom in time or to understand the cues to void due to problems with mobility or cognition.

STEPS OF ASSESSMENT

The nursing assessment varies somewhat depending on the client's general health status and whether the problem is an acute or chronic one. In general, however, a comprehensive nursing assessment can be described as a five-step process that includes screening for an infection with urinalysis, obtaining a voiding diary, evaluating functional status, compiling a health history, and performing a physical examination. Key features within the five steps follow:

- Record all incontinent and continent episodes for 3 days in a voiding diary.
- Review medication for any newly prescribed drugs that may be triggering incontinence. Follow up with physician regarding need to discontinue therapy or change medication.
- Rule out constipation or fecal impaction as a source of urinary incontinence. If client has had no bowel movement within last 3 days or is oozing stool continuously, check for impaction by digital examination or abdominal palpation. Problem should be treated if identified.
- Assess functional status along with signs and symptoms as they relate to incontinence. Contributors to incontinence may include immobility, insufficient fluid intake, and confusion. Accompanying signs and symptoms include polyuria, nocturia, dysuria, hesitancy, poor or interrupted urine stream, straining, suprapubic or perineal pain, urgency and characteristics of incontinent episodes (precipitated by walking, coughing, getting in and out of bed, and so forth).
- Consult physician regarding physical examination and need to measure postvoid residual volume by straight catheterization (particularly if client dribbles, reports urgency, has difficulty starting stream). Components of the physical examination include direct observation of urine loss using a cough stress test; abdominal, rectal, genital, and pelvic examination; and identification of neurologic abnormalities. Abdominal and vaginal examinations are performed to detect prolapse or a palpable bladder after micturition.

INTERVENTIONS

The physician is responsible for identifying and treating the conditions causing reversible or chronic incontinence. A physical therapist may play a role in identifying specific activities that are associated with incontinent episodes. Either a nurse or physical therapist may be involved in teaching Kegel exercises to help relieve stress incontinence. When functional incontinence and urgency have been identified, the expertise of an occupational therapist in appropriate dressing and undressing and for choosing incontinence aids may be beneficial.

BOX 32-5 INDICATORS OF PAIN IN THE COGNITIVELY IMPAIRED

- Medical diagnoses known to commonly cause pain such as arthritis, osteoporosis, fractures, cancer, and history of back pain
- Pain history and use of analgesics
- Family or professional caregiver reports of possible pain
- Behavioral patterns of aggressiveness or resisting care
- Rubbing on specific areas of body
- Vocalizations, such as moaning (yelling, or increases in the loudness of existing vocalizations)

CASE STUDY

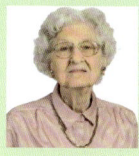

The case study introduced at the beginning of the chapter is now used to demonstrate how a nurse would use the COLDSPA mnemonic to explore Mrs. Miller's presenting concerns and continue to interview her for a health assessment, adapting the assessment for her as an older adult.

Mnemonic	Question	Data Provided
Character	Describe the sign or symptom (feeling, appearance, sound, smell, or taste if applicable). In this case, describe the pain.	Constant right leg and hip pain, rated between 5 and 7 on 10-point pain scale, all the time when awake.
Onset	When did it begin?	When I fell and broke my leg.
Location	Where is it? Does it radiate? Does it occur anywhere else?	Right leg and hip. Back becomes "achy" when sitting.

Mnemonic	Question	Data Provided
Duration	How long does it last? Does it recur?	It lasts all the time I am awake.
Severity	How bad is it? How much does it bother you?	Rates the pain as 5–7 on a 0–10 scale; rates the mental anguish as a 9–10 on a 0–10 scale.
Pattern	What makes it better or worse?	Takes two types of "medicine" for the pain. Helps to "take the edge off but only for a little while." Sitting too long or getting up out of the chair or bed makes it much worse. Bearing weight on right leg when using walker makes it "hurt real bad."
Associated factors/How it Affects the client	What other symptoms occur with it? How does it affect you?	"Achy back when I am sitting. I hate to have to get up to go to the toilet (bedside commode). I hate being so dependent on others and unable to do things for myself."

After exploring Mrs. Miller's complaints of leg pain, the nurse continues with the health history.

Mrs. Miller fell in her own home 3 weeks ago and was hospitalized for repair and pinning of a fractured right femur. She is sitting in a chair and appears to be thin, pale, and distracted as you enter the room and introduce yourself. Mrs. Miller answers some of your questions appropriately, but frequently apologizes for her appearance and defers to her daughter to answer any questions with regard to her recent fall and hospitalization. She says in a very weak, raspy voice, "I don't know how I ended up here. I don't know what I'd do without Delores, but if I could just walk and didn't hurt so bad everything would be OK … I've always been able to take care of things. This just all seems like such of a fuss over nothing." She describes pain to be especially in her right hip and leg, which increases when she sits for long periods in the same position. She rates the pain as between a 5 and a 7 on a 10-point scale. She reaches up to wipe her eyes with a tissue that she is holding in her right hand with noticeably contracted fingers with swan-neck deformities and enlarged distal, interphalangeal joints.

Delores reports that Mrs. Miller can put just enough weight on her right leg to use a walker, but needs assistance with bathing, cooking, and dressing. She says that her mother is not eating very well and seems to be choking easily, especially when she is drinking, and that she complains frequently of a "dry mouth." Bed pads are used to manage a small amount of incontinence during the night. Delores is setting the alarm for 3:00 AM to assist her mother onto a bedside commode. Mrs. Miller has a history of Parkinson's, osteoarthritis, osteoporosis, and mitral valve disease. She has fallen numerous times, but this was the first time that she broke any bones with the fall. Her current medications are Sinemet 25/250 mg every day; warfarin 5 mg every day; MS Contin 15 mg every 12 hours; morphine sulfate 10-mg oral solution (10 mg per 2.5 mL) every 8 hours prn for breakthrough pain; levothyroxine 0.05 mg every AM; Miralax every other day as needed for constipation.

Collecting Objective Data: Physical Examination

There is often a fine line between deterioration of function from aging and deterioration from disease. For this reason, it is crucial to integrate the subjective, functional, and physical assessments. The significance of a physical finding is often determined by the effect it has on the person's level of comfort and ability to function. A medical pathology should be suspected whenever any physical or functional change has occurred suddenly (days to weeks).

An efficient and effective way to determine the significance of physical findings in an older adult is to collect subjective data while you are conducting a physical examination. Because medication is often a primary method of treating disease in this country and polypharmacy is such a common occurrence in older adults, sudden changes or abnormalities noted in the physical examination must always be analyzed for the possibility of being the result of an adverse drug effect. Because many diseases have a "silent" presentation in older adults, an in-depth, comprehensive physical examination is especially important to detect and treat disease in a timely way.

Preparing the Client

It is essential that the nurse be sensitive to the client's need for privacy as well as the client's wishes for a caregiver to remain in the room during all or parts of the assessment. It is important to keep the temperature of the examination room warmer than may be comfortable for younger adults. Also, eliminate background noise as much as possible. Keep in mind that older adults with physical disabilities may need assistance with dressing and with repositioning of body parts during the examination. Allow additional time in deference to the client's need for independence as well as your need to know how much the client can do independently.

Equipment

In addition to the equipment needed for performing a complete adult physical examination, the following items will be needed for assessing the functional capacity of the frail older adult:
- Newspaper or book and lamplight for vision testing
- Lemon slice or mint for sense of smell test
- Pudding or food of pudding consistency and spoon for swallowing examination (a teacup with water to swallow may also be used)

- Food and fluid diary sheets or forms
- Nestlé MNA elderly nutritional assessment form (Assessment Tool 32-4)
- Two or three pillows for client comfort and positioning
- Straight-backed chair for "Get Up and Go" test

Physical Assessment

The nurse needs to examine his or her own attitudes or stereotypical assumptions about older adults. The examination of a frail older adult usually takes longer than that of a younger adult because of the chronic conditions, disabilities, and ensuing discomfort that many frail older adults experience. It is best to limit the length of the examination. This may mean that a complete assessment may require several sessions over a period of time. The client may feel less hurried if paperwork, such as a health questionnaire, can be completed at home either by the client alone or with the help of a caregiver. Some modifications and techniques appropriate for an examination of the frail older adult include:

- When interacting with an older adult, remember that it may be more acceptable to be more formal than informal. For example, address the client by first name only if the client specifically requests that you do so.
- Keep your voice volume down even if you anticipate that the client will have difficulty hearing. Speaking clearly and at a moderate pace is more beneficial in cases of hearing loss. Remember to face clients when speaking with them.
- Do not assume that clients cannot answer questions if they have a cognitive impairment. However, if the impairment has significantly affected function or verbal expression, give only one-step directions and avoid questions that require two responses. The cognitively impaired older adult with few remaining verbal abilities may have no or only minimal loss of the ability to comprehend nonverbal cues.
- If you need to question caregivers or collateral sources to validate or clarify information, avoid consulting them in the presence of the client.

General Routine Screening versus Focused Specialty Assessment of the Older Adult

A comprehensive assessment of the older adult requires expertise and experience. Geriatric expert nurses understand that older adults often present their illnesses in a unique manner not typically seen in younger adults. An in-depth understanding of geriatric syndromes and functional abilities is necessary to perform and complete an accurate assessment of the older adult. Thus, assessment of the older adult is considered a specialty assessment.

ASSESSMENT PROCEDURE	NORMAL FINDINGS OR VARIATIONS	ABNORMAL FINDINGS
Measure and record the client's height and weight, noting weight changes, changes in appetite, nausea and vomiting, and problems with swallowing or chewing (see Assessment Tool 32-4). **CLINICAL TIP** Suspect drug toxicity in clients taking medications such as digoxin, theophylline, quinidine, or antibiotics if client reports nausea or diarrhea.	Antral cells and intestinal villi atrophy, and gastric production of hydrochloric acid decreases with age. The ability to smell and taste decreases with age, which can also diminish appetite. Medications can also decrease sense of smell and taste in older people.	Indicators of malnutrition include poor wound healing, bruising, dental deterioration, poor appetite and fluid intake, weight loss. Client weighs less than 80% of ideal body weight. Client has had 10% loss in body weight over past 6 months or 5% loss in body weight over past month. Chronic diseases such as cancer and arthritis are associated with increases in inflammatory chemicals that can cause anorexia and fatigue. A certain degree of anorexia also always accompanies pain—especially chronic pain. (See Chapter 9 for a discussion of pain assessment.) Toxic levels of drugs must always be suspected when appetite loss is sudden and severe.
Review laboratory test values (complete blood count, and vitamin B_{12}, cholesterol, albumin, and prealbumin levels).		Hemoglobin level is lower than 12 g/dL. Hematocrit is lower than 35. Vitamin B_{12} level is lower than 100 μg/mL. Indicators of poor nutritional status include: Serum cholesterol level lower than 160 mg/dL Serum albumin level lower than 3.5 g/dL Serum prealbumin levels (used to monitor improvement of nutritional status) that do not increase 1 mg/dL/day

Continued on following page

ASSESSMENT PROCEDURE	NORMAL FINDINGS OR VARIATIONS	ABNORMAL FINDINGS
Evaluate hydration status as you would nutritional status. Because muscle mass decreases and fatty tissues increase, the elderly client is at increased risk for dehydration. Begin with accurate serial measurements of weight, careful review of laboratory test findings (serial serum sodium level, hematocrit, osmolality, BUN level, and urine-specific gravity), and a 2–3-day diary of fluid intake and output.	Normal findings include stable weight and stable mental status. **CLINICAL TIP** Increases over time in laboratory values are usually indicators of deteriorating hydration (even though values may be within normal limits).	Sudden weight loss; fever; dry, warm skin; furrowed, swollen, and red tongue; decreased urine output; lethargy; and weakness are all signs of dehydration. An acute change in mental status (particularly confusion), tachycardia, and hypotension may indicate severe dehydration, which may be precipitated by certain medications such as diuretics, laxatives, tricyclic antidepressants, or lithium.

Skin and Hair

INSPECTION AND PALPATION

Inspect and palpate skin lesions. Wear gloves when palpating lesions. Note whether lesions are flat or raised, palpable or nonpalpable. Also note color, size, and exudates, if any. 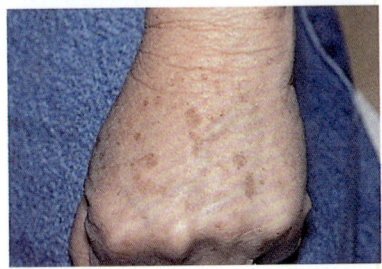 Note color, texture, integrity, and moisture of skin and sensitivity to heat or cold. **CLINICAL TIP** Room humidifiers, avoidance of harsh deodorants or soaps, and use of lanolin-containing products after bathing (while skin is still moist) may help to relieve effects of dry skin.	Despite decrease in total number of melanocytes, hyperpigmentation occurs in sun-exposed skin (neck, face, and arms). Although dermatologic lesions are common, many are benign. Benign findings include: • Venous lakes: Reddish vascular lesions on ears or other facial areas resulting from dilation of small, red blood vessels. • Skin tags: Acrochordons, flesh-colored pedunculated lesions. • Seborrheic keratoses: Tan, brown, or reddish, flat lesions commonly found on fair-skinned persons in sun-exposed areas. • Cherry angiomas: Small, round, red spots. • Senile purpura: Vivid purple patches (lesion should not blanch to touch). • Lentigines: Hyperpigmentation in sun-exposed areas appear as brown, pigmented, round or rectangular patches (Fig. 32-1). Often called "liver spots." **FIGURE 32-1** Solar lentigines are very common on aging skin. Elastic collagen is gradually replaced with more fibrous tissue and loss of subcutaneous tissue. Decreased vascularity and diminished neurologic response to temperature changes and atrophy of eccrine sweat glands increases risk of hyperthermia and hypothermia. Somewhat transparent, pale skin with an overall decrease in body hair on lower extremities. Dry skin is common. Skin may wrinkle and tent when pinched. **CLINICAL TIP** Pinching skin is not an accurate test of turgor in older adults.	The combination of environmental exposure and diminished immunity increases risk of skin cancer and cutaneous infections such as ringworm, and candidal infections of the mouth, vagina, and nail beds. This risk is increased by predisposing conditions such as diabetes mellitus, malnutrition, and steroid or antibiotic use. Abnormal findings include: • Actinic keratoses, round or irregularly shaped tan, scaly lesions that may bleed or be inflamed (premalignancy). • Waxy or raised lesions, especially on sun-exposed areas (basal cell carcinoma) • Irregularly shaped lesions or scaly, elevated lesions (squamous cell carcinoma, melanoma) • Herpes zoster vesicles (shingles) draining clear fluid or pustules atop an erythematous base following a clear, linear pattern and accompanied by pain. More than half of older adults with shingles will have neuralgia that persists after resolution of the skin lesions. • Pinpoint-sized, red-purple, nonblanchable petechiae (common sign of platelet deficiency) • Large bruises may result from anticoagulant therapy, a fall, renal or liver failure, or elder abuse. Extremely thin, fragile skin (friable skin) with excessive purpura (possibly from corticosteroid use). Dry, warm skin, furrowed tongue, and sunken eyes from dehydration (especially when the client has decreased urinary output; increased serum sodium, BUN, and creatinine levels; increased osmolality and hematocrit values; tachycardia; and mental confusion). Sudden heat or cold intolerance could be signs of thyroid dysfunction. Torn skin (possibly the result of abrasive tape used to hold bandages or tubes in place).

ASSESSMENT PROCEDURE	NORMAL FINDINGS OR VARIATIONS	ABNORMAL FINDINGS
Inspect and palpate hair and scalp.	Loss of pigmentation causes graying of scalp, axillary, and pubic hair. Mild hair growth on upper lip of women may appear as result of decreased estrogen-to-testosterone ratio. Toenails usually thicken while fingernails often become thinner. Both usually become yellowish and dull.	Patchy or asymmetric hair loss is abnormal.

Head and Neck

INSPECTION

Inspect head and neck for symmetry and movement. Observe facial expression (Fig. 32-2).	Atrophy of face and neck muscles Reduced range of motion (ROM) of head and neck. Shortening of neck due to vertebral degeneration and development of "buffalo hump" at top of cervical vertebrae.	Abnormalities include: • Asymmetry of mouth or eyes possibly from Bell's palsy or cerebrovascular accident (CVA). • Marked limitation of movement or crepitation in back of neck from cervical arthritis. • Involuntary facial or head movements from an extrapyramidal disorder such as Parkinson disease or some medications. • Reported episodic, unilateral, shock-like or burning pain of the face or continuous pain, which may be postherpetic, tic douloureux, or caused by dental caries or an abscess. ◎ **CLINICAL TIP** In cognitively impaired older adults, sleep disturbances or agitation may be the only sign of neuropathic pain.

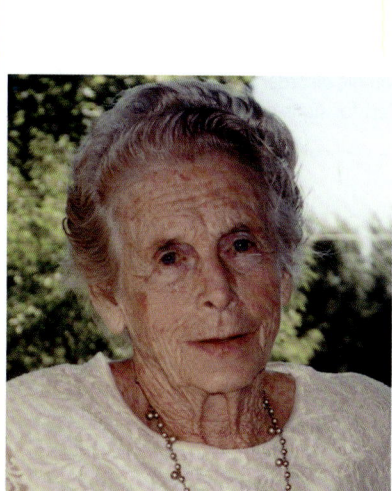

FIGURE 32-2 Observe facial expression.

Mouth and Throat

INSPECTION

Inspect the gums and buccal mucosa for color and consistency.	Slight decrease in saliva production.	Saliva-depressing medications include antihistamines, antipsychotics, and antihypertensives; any drug with anticholinergic side effects may promote dental caries and increase risk of pneumonia.
If the client is wearing dentures, inspect them for fit. Then ask the client to remove them for the rest of the oral examination.	Resorption of gum ridge commonly results in poorly fitting dentures. Tooth surfaces may be worn from prolonged use.	Loose-fitting dentures or inability to close mouth completely may also be the result of a significant weight gain or loss. Foul-smelling breath may indicate periodontal disease. Whitish or yellow-tinged patches in mouth or throat may be candidiasis from use of steroid inhalers or antibiotics.
Examine the tongue. Observe symmetry and size.	Tongue is pink and moist.	A swollen, red, and painful tongue may indicate vitamin B or riboflavin deficiency.

Continued on following page

ASSESSMENT PROCEDURE	NORMAL FINDINGS OR VARIATIONS	ABNORMAL FINDINGS
Mouth and Throat (Continued)		
Observe the client swallowing food or fluids (Fig. 32-3).	Mild decrease in swallowing ability.	Coughing, drooling, pocketing, or spitting out food after intake are all possible signs of dysphagia (difficulty swallowing). A drooping mouth, chronic congestion, or a weak or hoarse voice (especially after eating or drinking) also suggests dysphagia. If swallowing difficulties are observed, complete a nutritional assessment and refer the client for a barium swallow examination. **SAFETY TIP** Help the client who reports dysphagia to lean slightly forward with the chin tucked in toward the neck when swallowing and offer food that has a pudding-like consistency to minimize the risk of aspiration.
Test gag reflex. Depress the posterior third of the tongue, and note gag reflex.	Gag reflex may be slightly sluggish.	Absence of a gag reflex may be the result of a neurologic disorder and indicates the need to be alert for signs of aspiration pneumonia.

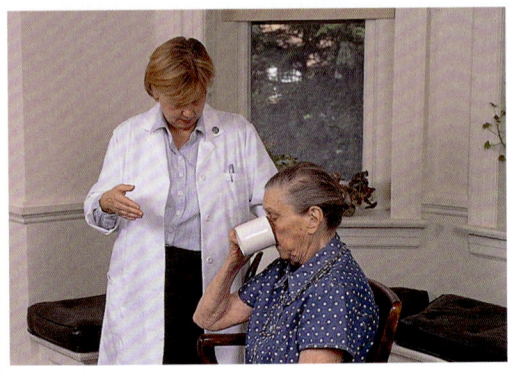

FIGURE 32-3 Assessing for swallowing problems (© B. Proud).

Nose and Sinuses

INSPECTION

Inspect the nose for color and consistency.	Nose and nasal passages are not inflamed, and skin and mucous membranes are intact. Nose may seem more prominent on face because of loss of subcutaneous fat. Nasal hairs are coarser.	Edema, redness, swelling, or clear drainage, which may indicate allergies or rhinitis. **◎ CLINICAL TIP** Relocation into a newly constructed residential or long-term care facility should be investigated as a possible cause of allergic or nonallergic rhinitis. New carpet, cabinetry of fiberboard, and paint fumes can elicit a nonallergic vasomotor response as well as an allergic one.
Evaluate the sense of smell. Have the client close the eyes and smell a common substance, such as mint, lemon, or soap (Fig. 32-4).	Slightly diminished sense of smell and ability to detect odors.	Client cannot identify strong odor. This may cause a decrease in appetite and may be a safety concern. **SAFETY TIP** Alert clients with diminished smell to the importance of smoke alarms and routine inspections of stoves and furnaces.
Test nasal patency. Ask the client to breathe while blocking one nostril at a time (Fig. 32-5).	Client breathes with reasonable ease.	Client reports feeling of inadequate breath intake, which may result from nasal polyps, a deviated septum, or allergic or infectious rhinitis or sinusitis.

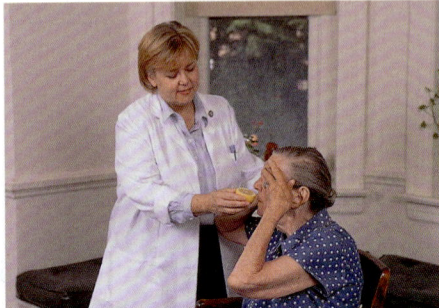

FIGURE 32-4 Assessing sense of smell (© B. Proud).

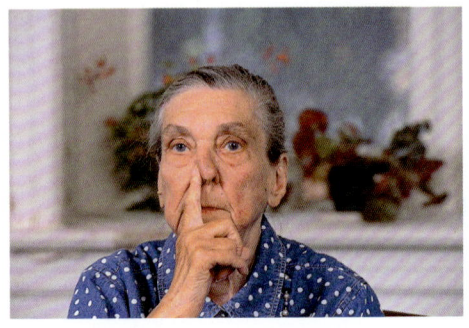

FIGURE 32-5 Testing nasal patency (© B. Proud).

ASSESSMENT PROCEDURE	NORMAL FINDINGS OR VARIATIONS	ABNORMAL FINDINGS
PALPATION		
Palpate the frontal and maxillary sinuses for consistency and to elicit possible pain. **SAFETY TIP** *Older adult clients with nasogastric feeding tubes are at increased risk for sinusitis related to the obstruction.*	No lesions or pain.	Client reports pain, congestion, and dryness; inflammation is evident. ◉ **CLINICAL TIP** Older adult clients may self-treat sinus pain and/or nasal congestion with decongestants and antihistamines, which may further dry the nasal passages and prevent normal sinus drainage. These drugs may also aggravate hypertension (in clients taking antihypertensive drugs) and exacerbate cardiac dysrhythmias. In clients taking antibiotics for sinusitis, watch for adverse effects on renal function. Because antibiotics also may kill normal bacteria, watch for signs of candidal or *Clostridium difficile* infection in the GI tract, mouth, or vagina.

Eyes and Vision

INSPECTION

ASSESSMENT PROCEDURE	NORMAL FINDINGS OR VARIATIONS	ABNORMAL FINDINGS
Inspect eyes, eyelids, eyelashes, and conjunctiva. Also observe eye and conjunctiva for dryness, redness, tearing, or increased sensitivity to light and wind.	Skin around the eyes becomes thin, and wrinkles appear normally with age. Stretched skin in eyelid may produce feeling of heaviness and a tired feeling. In lower eyelid, "bags" form. Excessive stretching of lower eyelid may cause it to droop downward, which keeps it from shutting completely and can cause dryness, redness, or sensitivity to light and wind. Eyes are described as irritated or having a "scratchy sensation."	A turning in of the lower eyelid (entropion) is more common and causes the eyelashes to touch the conjunctiva and cornea. Severe entropion may result in an ulcerous corneal infection. Abnormalities in blinking may result from Parkinson disease; dull or blank staring may be a sign of hypothyroidism.
Inspect the cornea and lens. Also ask the client when he or she last had an eye and vision examination by an optometrist or ophthalmologist. ◉ **CLINICAL TIP** To detect glaucoma, tonometry should be performed every 1–2 years on everyone older than 35 years of age. Elevated intraocular pressure indicates the need for referral to an ophthalmologist and confirmation with applanation tonometry.	An arcus senilis, a cloudy or grayish ring around the iris, and decreased pigment in iris are normal age-related changes. The lens loses elasticity, which results in decreased ability to change shape (presbyopia). A loss of transparency in the crystalline lens of the eyes is a natural part of aging process. Exposure to sunlight, smoking, and inherited tendencies increases risk. A thickening of the bulbar conjunctiva that grows over the cornea (called pterygium) may interfere with vision.	Cataracts most commonly affect people after age 55 and result in a yellowish or brownish discoloration of the lens. Common symptoms include painless blurring of vision, glare and halos around lights, poor night vision, colors that look dull or brownish. Location and extent of cloudiness determine degree to which a person's vision is affected.
Inspect the pupils. With a penlight or similar device, test pupillary reaction to light (Fig. 32-6).	Overall decrease in size of pupil and ability to dilate in dark and constrict in light may occur with advanced age. This results in poorer night vision and decreased tolerance to glare.	An irregularly shaped pupil may indicate removal of a cataract. Asymmetric pupillary reaction response may be due to a neurologic condition.
Test vision. Ask the client to read from a newspaper or magazine. Use only room lighting for the initial reading (Fig. 32-7). Use task lighting for a second reading.	Impaired near vision is indicative of presbyopia (farsightedness), a common finding in older adults. Also common are slight decreases in peripheral vision and difficulty in differentiating blues from greens.	A significant decrease in central vision, to the extent needed for ADLs, may signal a cataract in one or both eyes.

Continued on following page

836 UNIT 4 Nursing Assessment of Special Groups

ASSESSMENT PROCEDURE	NORMAL FINDINGS OR VARIATIONS	ABNORMAL FINDINGS
Eyes and Vision (Continued)		
Ask about changes in vision, trouble with night vision, or differences in vision with left versus right eye.	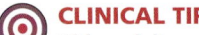 **CLINICAL TIP** Older adults generally require 2–3 times more diffuse and task lighting.	*Macular* (the *macula* is a thin membrane in the center of the retina) *degeneration* is suspected if the client has difficulty in seeing with one eye. The disorder almost always becomes bilateral. Related findings include blurry words in the center of the page or doorframes that don't appear straight. Refer the client to an ophthalmologist for evaluation (see Abnormal Findings 32-1).

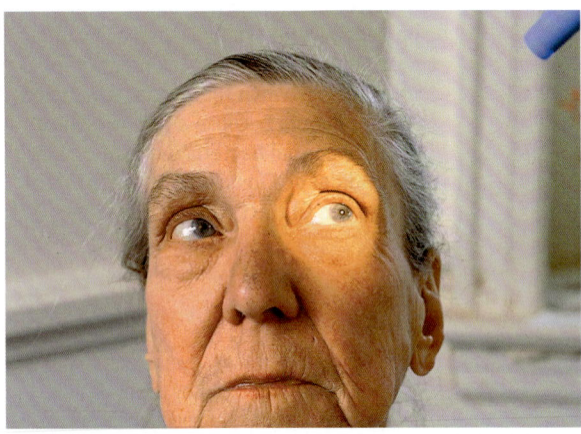

FIGURE 32-6 Testing pupillary reaction (© B. Proud).

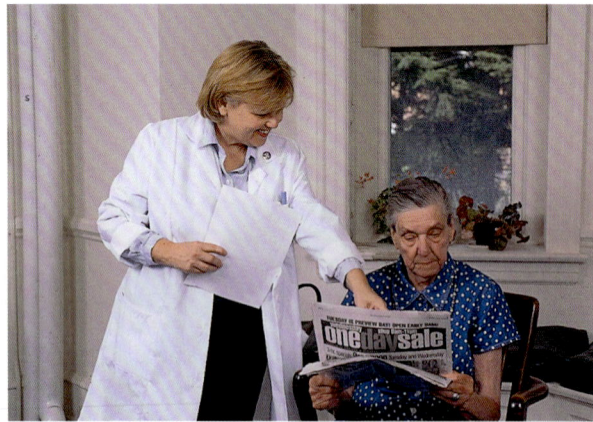

FIGURE 32-7 Reading with room lighting (© B. Proud).

Ask client about small specks or "clouds" that move across the field of vision.	With aging, tiny clumps of gel may develop within the eye. These are referred to as "floaters." They should occur occasionally and not increase significantly in frequency.	A noticeable loss of vision—including cloudiness, distortion of familiar objects, and occasionally blind spots or floaters—is a common symptom of diabetic retinopathy. New floaters, or an increase in frequency of floaters associated with flashes of light, may be a sign of retinal detachment. This requires immediate referral to prevent blindness (Abnormal Findings 32-1).
Ears and Hearing		
INSPECTION		
Inspect the external ear. Observe shape, color, and hair growth. Also look for lesions or drainage.	Hairs may become coarser and thicker in the external ear, especially in men. Earlobes may elongate and pinna increases in length and width.	Inflammation, drainage, or swelling may be from infection.
Perform an otoscopic examination to determine quantity, color, and consistency of cerumen.	Cerumen production decreases, leading to dryness and tendency toward accumulation.	Hard, dark brown cerumen signals impaction of the auditory canal, which commonly causes a conductive hearing loss.
		A darkened hole in the tympanic membrane or patches indicates perforation or scarring of the tympanic membrane.
Perform the voice–whisper test. This is a functional examination to detect obvious (conversational) hearing loss. Instruct the client to put a hand over one ear and to repeat the sentence you say.	The inability to hear high-frequency sounds (presbycusis), or to discriminate a variety of simultaneous sounds and soft consonant sounds or background noises, is due to degeneration of hair cells of inner ear.	Inability to hear the whispered sentence indicates a hearing deficiency and the need to refer the client to an audiologist for testing.

32 Assessing Older Adults   837

ASSESSMENT PROCEDURE	NORMAL FINDINGS OR VARIATIONS	ABNORMAL FINDINGS
Stand approximately 2 ft away from the client and whisper a sentence (Fig. 32-8). **CLINICAL TIP** Assess hearing acuity before as well as after the otoscopic examination if cerumen is removed during the examination. If you are facing the client, hold your hand close to your mouth so that the client cannot read your lips.		**CLINICAL TIP** Raising one's voice to someone with presbycusis usually only makes it more difficult for them to hear. Speaking more slowly will usually lower the frequency and be more therapeutic.

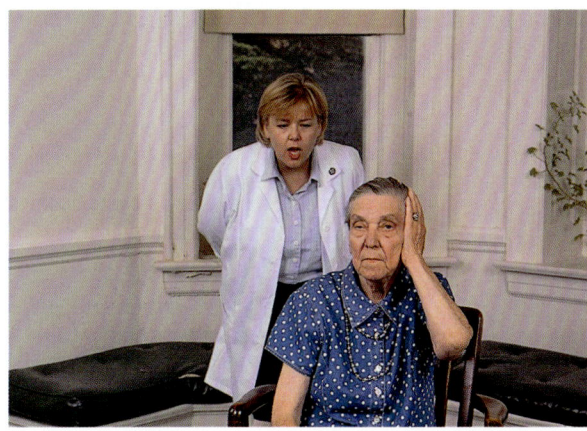

FIGURE 32-8 Assessing hearing with the voice-whisper test (© B. Proud).

Thorax and Lungs

INSPECTION

Inspect the shape of the thorax. Note respiratory rate, rhythm, and quality of breathing.	Decreased elasticity of alveoli causes lungs to recoil less during expiration. There is also loss of resilience that holds the thorax in a contracted position, loss of skeletal muscle strength in the thorax and abdomen, decreased vital capacity, increased residual volume, and slight barrel chest. Increased reliance on diaphragmatic breathing and increased work of breathing.	Williams (2009) describes the normal respiratory rate for elderly individuals living independently as 12–18 breaths/min and for those in long-term care as 16–25 breaths/min. Rates above 20–25 indicate abnormality such as infection, congestive heart failure, or other conditions. A rate less than 10 breaths/min indicates hypoventilation, which may be associated with myxedema, central nervous system depressants, or CNS disease. Significant loss of aerobic capacity and dyspnea with exertion is usually due to disease, exposure over a lifetime to pollutants, smoke, or severe or prolonged lack of exercise.

PERCUSSION

Percuss lung tones as you would in a younger adult.	Resonant, except in the presence of structural changes such as kyphosis or a slight barrel chest, when hyperresonance may occur.	Consolidation of infection will cause dullness to percussion; alveolar retention of air, as occurs in emphysema, results in hyperresonance. **SAFETY TIP** Supine positioning, shallow breathing, and poor dental hygiene increase the risk of pulmonary infection.

Continued on following page

ASSESSMENT PROCEDURE	NORMAL FINDINGS OR VARIATIONS	ABNORMAL FINDINGS
Thorax and Lungs (Continued)		
		Pneumonia is the most common cause of infection-related deaths in older adults and is called the "silent killer." It seldom presents as the classic triad of cough, fever, and pleuritic pain. Instead, subtle changes such as an increase in respiratory rate and sputum production, confusion, loss of appetite, and hypotension are more likely to be the presenting symptoms (Sapkota, 2012). The CURB-65 Score for pneumonia severity (American Academy of Family Physicians [AAFP], 2006) is recommended for any older person suspected to have pneumonia.
AUSCULTATION		
Auscultate lung sounds as you would in a younger adult.	Vesicular sounds should be heard over all areas of air exchange. However, because lung expansion may be diminished, it may be necessary to emphasize taking deep breaths with the mouth open during the examination. This may be very difficult for those with dementia.	Breath sounds may be distant over areas affected by kyphosis or the barrel chest of aging. Rales and rhonchi are heard only with diseases, such as pulmonary edema, pneumonia, or restrictive disorders. Diminished breath sounds, wheezes, crackles, rhonchi that do not clear with cough, and egophony are common signs of consolidation caused by pneumonia.
Heart and Blood Vessels		
BLOOD PRESSURE		
Measure blood pressure.	Blood pressure increases as elasticity decreases in arteries with proportionately greater increase in systolic pressure, resulting in a widening of pulse pressure.	Refer any client with blood pressure exceeding 160/90 mmHg to the health care provider for follow-up. A sudden and increasingly widened pulse pressure, especially in combination with other neurologic abnormalities and a change in mental status, is a classic sign of increased intracranial pressure (which in elderly clients may be due to a hemorrhagic stroke or hematoma).
Take blood pressure to detect actual or potential orthostatic hypotension and, therefore, the risk for falling. Measure pressure with the client in lying, sitting, and standing positions. Also measure pulse rate (Fig. 32-9A). Have the client lie down for 5 minutes; take the pulse and blood pressure; at 1 minute, take blood pressure and pulse after client is sitting and again at 1 minute after client stands (Fig. 32.9B). **SAFETY TIP** *If dizziness occurs, instruct client to sit a few minutes before attempting to stand up from a supine or reclining position.*	An older adult's baroreceptor response to positional changes is slightly less efficient. A slight decrease in blood pressure may occur.	Orthostatic hypotension occurs when blood pressure falls upon standing. The ICD-10 criteria for orthostatic hypotension are a 20-mmHg decrease in systolic pressure or a 10-mmHg decrease in diastolic pressure 3 minutes after the person has risen from supine to standing. Symptoms generally include dizziness, blurred vision, and syncope (ICD-10-CM Diagnostic Code, 2016). A serious consequence is the potential for lightheadedness and dizziness, which may precipitate hip fracture or head trauma from a fall. **CLINICAL TIP** Some sources of orthostatic hypotension include medications, such as antihypertensives, diuretics, and drugs with anticholinergic side effects (anxiolytics, antipsychotics, hypnotics, tricyclic antidepressants, and antihistamines).

ASSESSMENT PROCEDURE	NORMAL FINDINGS OR VARIATIONS	ABNORMAL FINDINGS

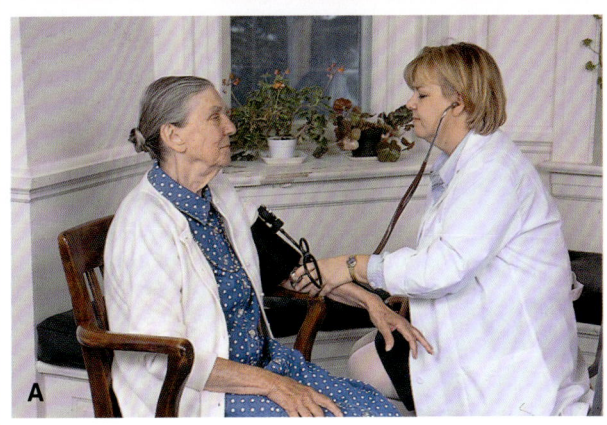 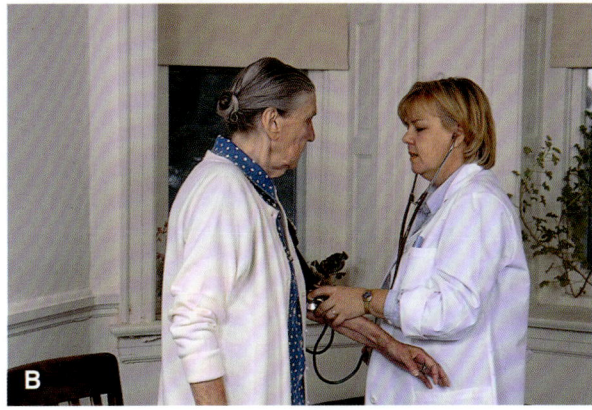

FIGURE 32-9 **A.** Assessing blood pressure (© B. Proud). **B.** Assessing blood pressure when standing.

EXERCISE TOLERANCE

Measure activity tolerance. Evaluate, either by reviewing results of stress testing or by observing the client's ability to move from a sitting to a standing position (Fig. 32-10) or to flex and extend fingers rapidly.

🎯 **CLINICAL TIP**
Poor lower body strength, especially in the ankles, may impair the ability of the frail older adult to rise from a chair to a standing position. Poor upper body strength, especially in the shoulders, may impede the ability to push up from a bed or chair or to extend and flex fingers.

The maximal heart rate with exercise is less than in a younger person. The heart rate will also take longer to return to its pre-exercise rate.

Rise in pulse rate should be no greater than 10–20 beats/min. The pulse rate should return to the baseline rate within 2 minutes.

A rise in pulse rate greater than 20 beats/min and a rate that does not return to baseline within 2 minutes is an indicator of exercise intolerance. Cardiac dysrhythmias as determined by stress testing are also indicative of exercise intolerance.

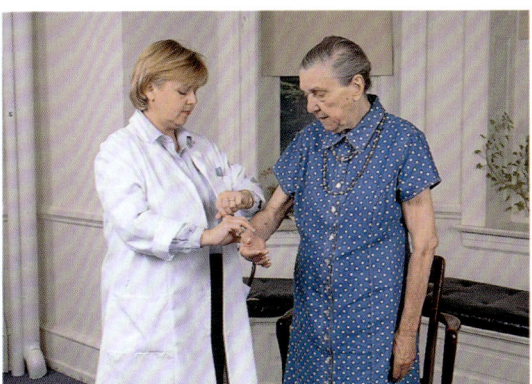

FIGURE 32-10 Assessing heart rate after the client rises from a sitting position provides clues to his or her tolerance of physical exertion (© B. Proud).

PULSES

Determine adequacy of blood flow by palpating the arterial pulses in all locations (carotid, brachial, radial, femoral, popliteal, posterior tibial, and dorsalis pedis) for strength and quality (Fig. 32-11).

Proximal pulses may be easier to palpate due to loss of supporting surrounding tissue. However, distal lower extremity pulses may be more difficult to feel or even be nonpalpable. The dorsalis pedis pulse is absent in up to 12% of the population (Judge, 2007).

Insufficient or absent pulses are a likely indication of arterial insufficiency. Partially obstructed blood flow increases the risk of ulcers and infection. Completely obstructed blood flow is a medical emergency requiring immediate intervention to prevent gangrene and possible amputation.

Continued on following page

UNIT 4 Nursing Assessment of Special Groups

ASSESSMENT PROCEDURE	NORMAL FINDINGS OR VARIATIONS	ABNORMAL FINDINGS
Heart and Blood Vessels (Continued)		
SAFETY TIP *Palpate carotid arteries gently and one side at a time to avoid stimulating vagal receptors in the neck, dislodging an existing plaque, or causing syncope or a stroke.*		**SAFETY TIP** *The absence of a pulse in a client who previously had a pulse, though weak, should be reported immediately to the primary provider. Loss of a pulse reflects loss of blood flow to an extremity and needs to be referred to the primary care provider. Color temperature, sensation, and movement of lower extremities would also need to be noted and reported to the primary care provider.*

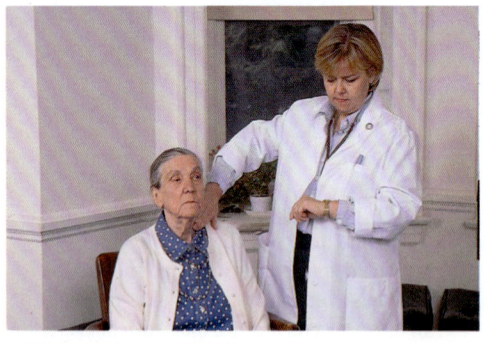

FIGURE 32-11 Palpating the carotid artery to assess blood flow (© B. Proud).

ARTERIES AND VEINS

Auscultate the carotid, abdominal, and femoral arteries (Fig. 32-12).	No unusual sound should be heard.	A bruit is abnormal; refer the client for further care because of the high risk of CVA from a carotid embolism or an abdominal or femoral aneurysm.

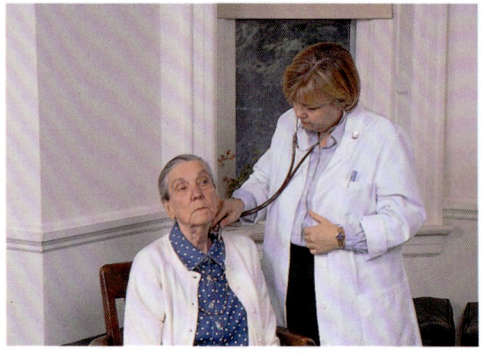

FIGURE 32-12 Use the bell of the stethoscope to listen for bruits (© B. Proud).

Evaluate arterial and venous sufficiency of extremities. Elevate the legs above the level of the heart and observe color, temperature, size of the legs, and skin integrity.	Hair loss with advanced age (cannot be used singly as an indicator of arterial insufficiency).	Leg pain associated with walking, burning or cramping, duskiness or mottling when the leg is in a dependent position; paleness with elevation; cool, thin, shiny skin; thickened, brittle nails; and diminished pulses are signs of arterial insufficiency.
Inspect and palpate veins while client is standing.	Prominent, bulging veins are common, as are spider veins. Varicose veins appear raised above the skin, often dark purple or blue, gnarled or cord-like, and are considered common unless symptoms appear. Symptoms include pain, itching, swelling, burning, leg heaviness or tiredness, skin discoloration. Symptoms typically worsen throughout the day, are partially relieved by elevation or wearing compression socks or stockings, sometimes lead to development of a clot (phlebitis) indicated by pain, heat, hardness, and discoloration (Hager, n.d.)	Unilateral warmth, tenderness, and swelling may be indications of thrombophlebitis.

ASSESSMENT PROCEDURE	NORMAL FINDINGS OR VARIATIONS	ABNORMAL FINDINGS
HEART		
Inspect and palpate the precordium.	The precordium is still, not visible, and without thrills, heaves, palpable pulsations (noted exception may be the apex of the heart if close to the surface).	Heaves are felt with an enlarged right or left ventricular aneurysm. Thrills indicate aortic, mitral, or pulmonic stenosis and regurgitation that may originate from rheumatic fever. Pulsations suggest an aortic or ventricular aneurysm, right ventricular enlargement, or mitral regurgitation.
Auscultate heart sounds.	A soft systolic murmur heard best at the base of the heart may result from calcification, stiffening, and dilation of the aortic and mitral valve. **CLINICAL TIP** The accumulation of lipofuscin, amyloid, collagen, and fats in the pacemaker cells of the heart and loss of pacemaker cells in the sinus node predispose the older adult to dysrhythmias, even in the absence of heart disease.	Abnormal heart sounds are generally considered to be disease related only if there is additional evidence of compromised cardiovascular function. However, any previously undetected extra heart sound warrants further investigation. S_3 and S_4 sounds may reflect the cardiac and fluid overloads of congestive heart failure, aortic stenosis, cardiomyopathy, or myocardial infarction. **SAFETY TIP** *Falls, dyspnea, fatigue, and palpitations are common symptoms of dysrhythmias in older adults.* If client has atrial fibrillation one may use the CHADS2-VASC scoring tool to calculate one risk for stroke at Huang, (2016).
Breasts		
INSPECTION AND PALPATION		
Inspect and palpate breast and axillae. When viewing axillae and contour of the breasts, assist a client with arthritis to raise the arms over the head. Do this gently and without force and only if it is not painful for the client. If the breasts are pendulous, assist the client to lean slightly so that the breasts hang away from the chest wall, enabling you to best observe symmetry and form. **CLINICAL TIP** A greater percentage of elderly women have had radical mastectomies. If so, inquiring about pain and swelling from lymphedema is important.	The breasts of elderly women are often described as pendulous due to the atrophy of breast tissue and supporting tissues and the forward thrust of the client brought about by kyphosis. Decreases in fat composition and increase in fibrotic tissue may make the terminal ducts feel more fibrotic and palpable as linear, spoke-like strands. The nipples may turn in slightly and the areola and any hair surrounding it may nearly disappear.	Pain upon palpation may indicate an infectious process or cancer. Breast tenderness, pain, or swelling may be side effects of hormone replacement therapy and an indication that a lower dosage is needed. Nipples that appear retracted and cannot be everted, or any retraction of only one nipple may indicate breast cancer. Male breast enlargement (gynecomastia) may result from a decrease in testosterone.
Inspect skin under breasts.	Skin intact without lesions or rashes.	Macerated skin under the breasts may result from perspiration or fungal infection (usually seen in an immunocompromised client).

Continued on following page

ASSESSMENT PROCEDURE	NORMAL FINDINGS OR VARIATIONS	ABNORMAL FINDINGS
Abdomen		
MOTILITY		
Assess GI motility and auscultate bowel sounds. Review fiber intake and laxative use. **CLINICAL TIP** Risk of constipation is increased by diminished physical activity, decreased fluid intake, decreased fiber in diet, and by ingestion of certain medications, such as iron or narcotics.	5–30 bowel sounds/min are heard. A decrease in gastric emptying time occurs with aging and may cause early satiety. Intestinal motility is generally reduced from a general loss of muscle tone.	Absence of bowel sounds and vomiting of undigested food is abnormal. Decreased motility is exacerbated by common pathologies such as Parkinson disease, stroke, and diabetes mellitus. Results in propensity for chronic constipation and diverticula. **SAFETY TIP** *If diverticula become infected, emergency treatment may be required to prevent perforation and sepsis.* Hiatal hernia that manifests by postprandial chest fullness, heartburn, or nausea.
Determine absorption or retention problems in older adult clients receiving enteral feedings. **CLINICAL TIP** An abdominal radiograph, flat plate, should be taken to check for correct placement of newly inserted nasogastric tubes.	Less than 100 mL residual is a normal finding for intermittent feedings.	More than 100 mL residual measured before a scheduled feeding is a sign of insufficient absorption and excessive retention. Abdominal distention, diarrhea, fluid overload, aspiration pneumonia, or fluid/electrolyte imbalances may indicate excessive retention although mental status changes may be the first or only sign.
Inspect and percuss the abdomen in the same manner as for younger adults. **CLINICAL TIP** The loss of abdominal musculature that occurs with aging may make it easier to palpate abdominal organs.	Liver, pancreas, and kidneys normally decrease in size, but the decrease is not generally appreciable upon physical examination. Atrophy of intestinal villi is a common aging change.	Anorexia, abdominal pain and distention, impaired protein digestion, and vitamin B_{12} malabsorption suggest inflammatory gastritis or a peptic ulcer. Abdominal distention, cramping, diarrhea, and increased flatus are signs of lactose intolerance, which may occur for the first time in old age. Bruits over aorta suggest an aneurysm. If present, do not palpate because this could rupture the aneurysm. Guarding upon palpation, rebound tenderness, or a friction rub (sounds like pieces of sandpaper rubbing together) often suggests peritonitis, which could be secondary to ruptured diverticuli, tumor, or infarct.
Palpate the bladder. (Ask client to empty bladder before the examination.) If the bladder is palpable, percuss from symphysis pubis to umbilicus. If the client is incontinent, postvoid residual content may also need to be measured.	Empty bladder is not palpable or percussible.	Full bladder sounds dull. More than 100 mL drained from bladder is considered abnormal for a postvoid residual. A distended bladder with an associated small-volume urine loss may indicate overflow incontinence (see Box 32-4).
Genitalia		
FEMALE		
Inspect external genitalia. Assist the client into the lithotomy position. Inspect the urethral meatus and vaginal opening.	Many atrophic changes begin in women at menopause. Pubic hair is usually sparse, and labia are flattened. Clitoris is decreased in size. The size of the ovaries, uterus, and cervix also decreases.	Redness or swelling from the urethral meatus indicates a possible UTI.

ASSESSMENT PROCEDURE	NORMAL FINDINGS OR VARIATIONS	ABNORMAL FINDINGS
CLINICAL TIP Arthritis may make the lithotomy position particularly uncomfortable for the older woman, necessitating changes. If the client has breathing difficulties, elevating the head to a semi-Fowler position may help.		
Ask the client to cough while in the lithotomy position.	No leakage of urine occurs.	Leakage of urine that occurs with coughing is a sign of stress incontinence and may be due to lax pelvic muscles from childbirth, surgery, obesity, cystocele, rectocele, or a prolapsed uterus.
CLINICAL TIP Incontinence is not a normal part of aging. If embarrassment or acceptance is preventing the client from acknowledging the problem, the genital examination may be a more acceptable time to introduce the topic.		**CLINICAL TIP** In noncommunicative clients, an excoriated perineum may be the result of incontinence, which warrants further investigation.
Test for prolapse. Ask the client to bear down while you observe the vaginal opening.	No prolapse is evident.	A protrusion into the vaginal opening may be a cystocele, rectocele, or uterine prolapse, which is a common sequelae of relaxed pelvic musculature in older women.
Perform a pelvic examination. Put on disposable gloves and use a small speculum if the vaginal opening has narrowed with age. Use lubrication on the speculum and hand because natural lubrication is decreased.	Vagina narrows and shortens. A loss of elastic tissue and vascularity in the vagina results in a thin, pale epithelium. Atrophic changes are intensified by infrequent intercourse. Loss of elasticity and reduced vaginal lubrication from diminishing levels of estrogen can cause dyspareunia (painful intercourse). Sexual desire and pleasure are not necessarily diminished by these structural changes, nor do women lose capacity for orgasm with age. Because the ovaries, uterus, and cervix shrink with age, the ovaries may not be palpable.	Atrophic vaginitis symptoms can mimic malignancy, vulvar dystrophies, and infections (MacBride et al., 2010).
Test pelvic muscle tone. Ask the woman to squeeze muscles while the examiner's finger is in the vagina. Assess perineal strength by turning fingers posterior to the perineum while the woman squeezes muscles in the vaginal area.	The vaginal wall should constrict around the examiner's finger, and the perineum should feel smooth.	If the client has a cystocele, the examiner's finger in the vagina will feel pressure from the anterior surface of the vagina. In clients with uterine prolapse, protrusion of the cervix is felt down through the vagina. A bulging of the posterior vaginal wall and part of the rectum may be felt with a rectocele.
MALE		
Inspect the male genital area with the client in standing position if possible.	The decline in testosterone brings about atrophic changes. Pubic hair is thinner. Scrotal skin is slightly darker than surrounding skin, and is smooth and flaccid in the older man. Penis and testicular size decrease, scrotum hangs lower.	Scrotal edema may be present with portal vein obstruction or heart failure. Lesions on the penis may be a sign of infection. Associated symptoms of infection frequently include discharge, scrotal pain, and difficulty with urination.
Observe and palpate for inguinal swelling or bulges suggestive of hernia in the same manner as for a younger male.	No swelling or bulges are present.	Masses or bulges are abnormal, and pain may be a sign of testicular torsion. A mass may be due to a hydrocele, spermatocele, or cancer.
Auscultate the scrotum if a mass is detected; otherwise, palpate the right and left testicle using the thumb and first two fingers.	No detectable sounds or masses are present.	Bowel sounds heard over the scrotum may suggest an indirect inguinal hernia. Masses are abnormal, and the client should be referred to a specialist for follow-up examination.

Continued on following page

ASSESSMENT PROCEDURE	NORMAL FINDINGS OR VARIATIONS	ABNORMAL FINDINGS
Anus, Rectum, and Prostate		
INSPECTION AND PALPATION		
Inspect the anus and rectum.	The anus is darker than the surrounding skin. Bluish, grape-like lumps at the anus are indicators of hemorrhoids.	Lesions, swelling, inflammation, and bleeding are abnormalities. If hemorrhoids account for discomfort, the degree to which bleeding, swelling, or inflammation interferes with bowel activity generally determines if treatment is warranted.
Put on gloves to palpate the anus and rectum. ◎ **CLINICAL TIP** The left side-lying position with knees tucked up toward the chest is the preferred one for comfort. Pillows may be needed for positioning and client comfort.	No masses, polyps, internal hemorrhoids, rectal prolapse, or fecal impaction palpated.	Palpation of internal masses could indicate polyps, internal hemorrhoids, rectal prolapse, cancer, or fecal impaction. Obliteration of the median sulcus is felt with prostatic hyperplasia.
Palpate the prostate in the male client.	The prostate is normally soft or rubbery-firm and smooth, and the median sulcus is palpable. Some degree of enlargement (benign prostate hypertrophy [BPH]) almost always occurs by age 85, as does a decrease in amount and viscosity of seminal fluid. Sperm count may decrease by as much as 50%. Orgasm may be briefer and time to obtain an erection may increase. These changes alone, however, do not usually result in any loss of libido or satisfaction.	A hard, asymmetrically enlarged, and nodular prostate is suggestive of malignancy (Swartz, 2014, p. 461). A tender and softer prostate is more common with prostatitis. Fever and painful urination are common with acute prostatitis. Obstructive symptoms are seen with both malignancy and infection of the prostate.
Musculoskeletal System		
INSPECTION AND PALPATION		
Observe the client's posture and balance when standing, especially the first 3–5 seconds. ◎ **CLINICAL TIP** The ability to reach for everyday items without losing balance can be assessed by asking the client to remove an object from a shelf that is high enough to require stretching or standing on the toes and to bend down to pick up a small object, such as a pen, from the floor.	Client stands reasonably straight with feet positioned fairly widely apart to form a firm base of support. This stance compensates for diminished sense of proprioception in lower extremities. Body usually bends forward as well.	A "humpback" curvature of the spine, called kyphosis, usually results from osteoporosis. The combination of osteoporosis, calcification of tendons and joints, and muscle atrophy makes it difficult for the frail older adult to extend the hips and knees fully when walking. This impairs the ability to maintain balance early enough to prevent a fall. Client cannot maintain balance without holding onto something or someone. Postural instability increases the risk of falling and immobility from the fear of falling.
Observe the client's gait by performing the timed "Get Up and Go" test (Fig. 32-13): 1. Have the client rise from a straight-backed armchair, stand momentarily, and walk about 3 m toward a wall. 2. Ask the client to turn without touching the wall and walk back to the chair, then turn around and sit down. 3. Using a watch or clock with a second hand, time how long it takes the client to complete the test.	Widening of pelvis and narrowing of shoulders. Client walks steadily without swaying, stumbling, or hesitating during the walk. The client does not appear to be at risk of falling.	Shuffling gait, characterized by smaller steps and minimal lifting of the feet, increases the risk of tripping when walking on uneven or unsteady surfaces. Abnormal findings from the timed "Get Up and Go" test include hesitancy, staggering, stumbling, and abnormal movements of the trunk and arms.

ASSESSMENT PROCEDURE	NORMAL FINDINGS OR VARIATIONS	ABNORMAL FINDINGS
4. Score performance on a 1–5 scale: • 1 = normal • 2 = very slightly abnormal • 3 = mildly abnormal • 4 = moderately abnormal • 5 = severely abnormal	Older adult clients without impairments in gait or balance can complete the test within 10 seconds.	People who take more than 30 seconds to complete the test tend to be dependent in some ADLs such as bathing, getting in and out of bed, or climbing stairs.

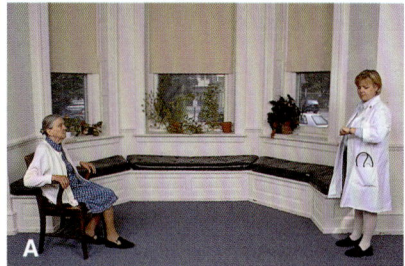 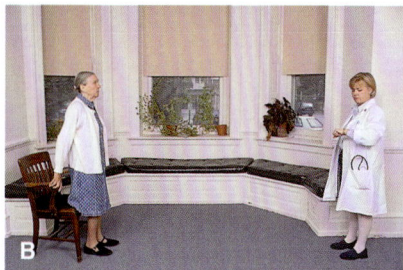 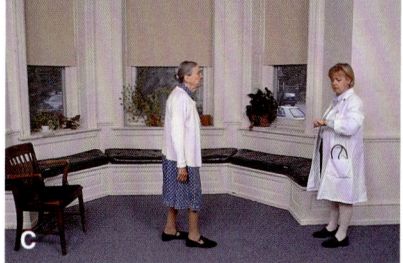
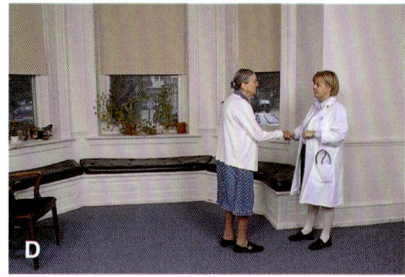 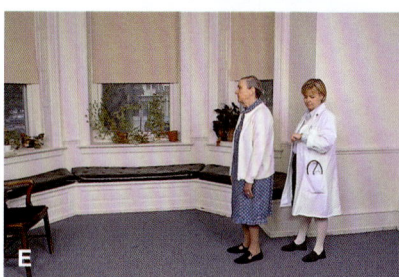 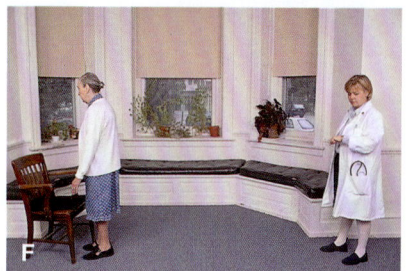
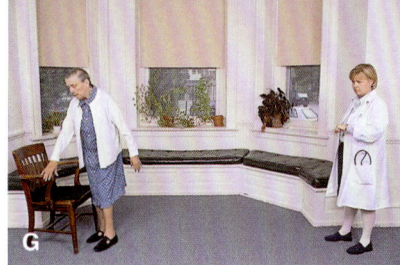 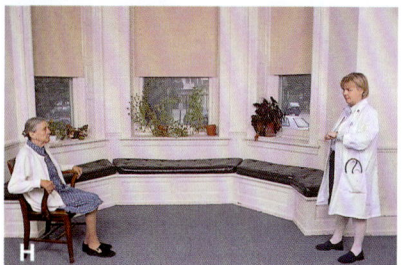

FIGURE 32-13 "Get up and go test" (© B. Proud).

Inspect the general contour of limbs, trunk, and joints. Palpate wrist and hand joints.	Enlargement of the distal, interphalangeal joints of the fingers, called Heberden nodes, are indicators of degenerative joint disease (DJD), a common age-related condition involving joints in the hips, knees, and spine as well as the fingers (Fig. 32-14).	With accumulated damage and loss of cartilage, bony overgrowths protrude from the bone into the joint capsule, causing deformities, limited mobility, and pain. Hand deformities such as ulnar deviation, swan-neck deformity, and boutonniere deformity are of concern because of the limitations they impose on activities of daily living and related pain.

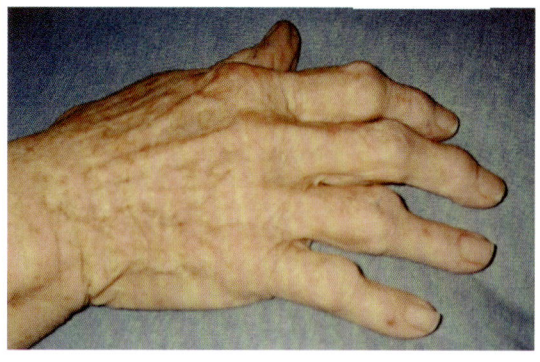

FIGURE 32-14 Degenerative joint disease.

Continued on following page

UNIT 4 Nursing Assessment of Special Groups

ASSESSMENT PROCEDURE	NORMAL FINDINGS OR VARIATIONS	ABNORMAL FINDINGS
Musculoskeletal System (Continued)		
Test ROM. Ask client to touch each finger with the thumb of the same hand, to turn wrists up toward the ceiling and down toward the floor, to push each finger against yours while you apply resistance, and to make a fist and release it (Fig. 32-15).	There is full ROM of each joint and equal bilateral resistance.	Limitations in ROM or strength may be due to DJD, rheumatoid arthritis, or a neurologic disorder, which, if unilateral, suggests CVA. Signs of pain such as grimacing, pulling back, or verbal messages are indicators of the need to do a pain assessment. Grating, popping, crepitus, and palpation of fluid are also abnormalities. Crepitus and joint pain that is worse with activity and relieved by rest in the absence of systemic symptoms is often associated with DJD.
Assess ROM and strength of shoulders and elbows (Fig. 32-16A and Fig. 32-16B).	There is full ROM of each joint and equal strength.	Tenderness, stiffness, and pain in the shoulders and elbows (and hips), which is aggravated by movement, are common signs associated with polymyalgia rheumatica (PMR).
Assess hip joint for strength and ROM in the same manner as for a younger adult.	Intact flexion, extension, and internal and external rotation.	Hip pain that is worse with weight bearing and relieved with rest may indicate DJD. There is usually also an associated crepitation and decrease in ROM.

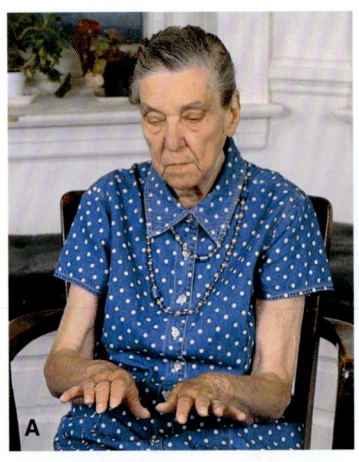
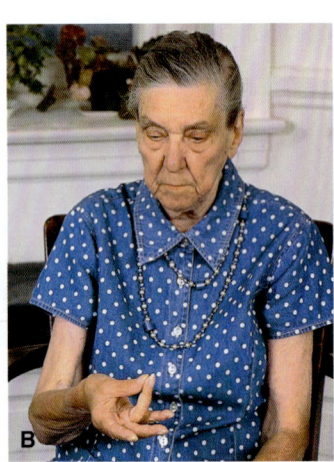
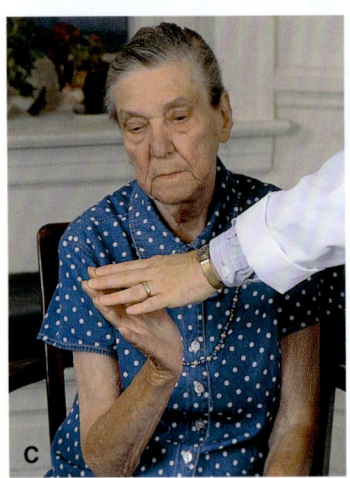
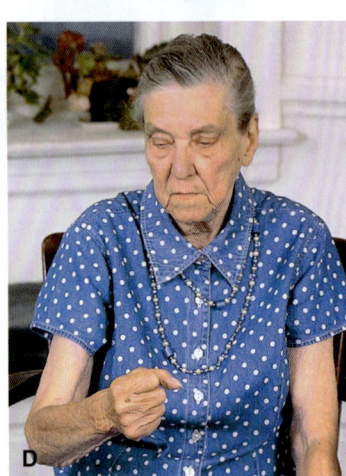

FIGURE 32-15 Testing wrist range of motion (© B. Proud).

ASSESSMENT PROCEDURE	NORMAL FINDINGS OR VARIATIONS	ABNORMAL FINDINGS

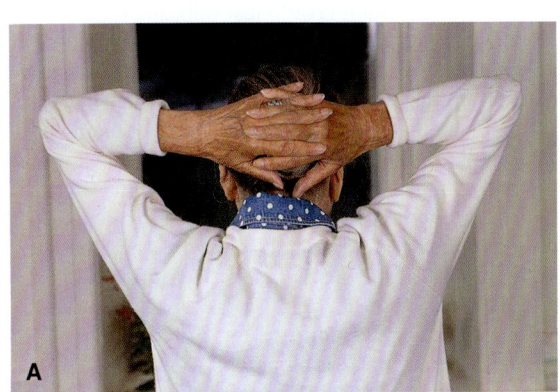 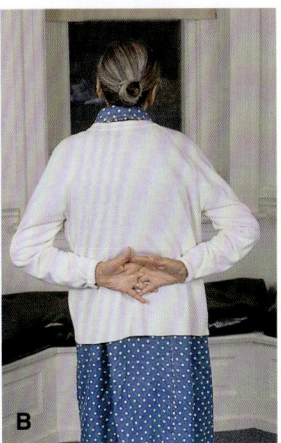

FIGURE 32-16 Testing shoulder (A) and elbow (B) range of motion (© B. Proud.)

Assessment Procedure	Normal Findings or Variations	Abnormal Findings
		Complaints of hip or thigh pain, external rotation and adduction of the affected leg, and leg shortening, and an inability to bear weight are the most common signs of a hip fracture in the elderly (Bhatti, 2015).
Inspect and palpate knees, ankles, and feet. Also assess comfort level, particularly with movement (flexion, extension, rotation).	The common problems associated with the aged foot, such as soreness and aching, are most frequently due to improperly fitting footwear.	A great toe overriding or underlying the second toe may be hallux valgus (bunion). Bunions are associated with pain and difficulty walking.
		Other abnormal findings may be enlargement of the medial portion of the first metatarsal head and inflammation of the bursae over the medial aspect of the joint.
Inspect client's muscle bulk and tone.	Atrophy of the hand muscles may occur with normal aging.	Muscle atrophy can result from rheumatoid arthritis, muscle disuse, malnutrition, motor neuron disease, or diseases of the peripheral nervous system.
		Increased resistance to passive ROM is a classic sign of Parkinson disease, especially in clients with bradykinesia. Decreased resistance may also suggest peripheral nervous system disease, cerebellar disease, or acute spinal cord injury.

Neurologic System

Assessment Procedure	Normal Findings or Variations	Abnormal Findings
Observe for tremors and involuntary movements.	Resting tremors increase in older adults. In the absence of an identifiable disease process, they are not considered pathologic.	The tremors of Parkinson's may occur when the client is at rest. They usually diminish with voluntary movement. They usually begin in the hand and may affect only one side of the body (especially early in the disease). The tremors are accompanied by muscle rigidity.

Sensory System

Assessment Procedure	Normal Findings or Variations	Abnormal Findings
Test sensation to pain, temperature, touch position and vibration as you would for a younger adult.	Touch and vibratory sensations may diminish normally with aging.	Unilateral sensory loss suggests a lesion in the spinal cord or higher pathways; a symmetric sensory loss suggests a neuropathy that may be associated with a condition such as diabetes.
Assess positional sense by using the Romberg test as presented in Chapter 25. The exceptions to the test are clients who must use assistive devices such as a walker.	There is minimal swaying, without loss of balance.	Significant swaying, with appearance of a potential fall.

CASE STUDY

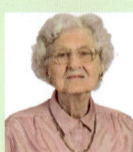

The chapter case study is now used to demonstrate a physical assessment of Mrs. Miller's post fall status.

Your physical examination reveals a resting tremor of the hands, and several large bruises on her right shoulder, upper arm, and hip. She has slight ectropion and reddened eyes. You note crepitus and a grating, popping sound bilaterally when you assist her to raise her arms as well as increased resistance and rigidity. Mrs. Miller's blood pressure is 85/45 on the right and 108/64 on the left. Her heart rate is 92 and irregularly irregular. Lung sounds are clear but only heard in the upper lobes. Her height is reported at 5 ft and her weight prior to the fall and hospitalization was 89 lb. Although her skin is pale, thin, and dry in most areas, it appears intact and well cared for. Incision line on right leg is dry, slightly red, but without swelling or drainage. However, some redness is noted on the elbows and sacrum, and the antecubital spaces are moist with some beginning maceration. Mrs. Miller has 1+ pitting pedal edema bilaterally.

Validating and Documenting Findings

The prevalence of chronic conditions in the frail elderly redefines the meaning of normalcy. The ability of the older adult to function in everyday activities, albeit with environmental and pharmacologic interventions, is a more meaningful measure of normalcy than are physical findings alone. Thus the objective and subjective data must reflect a functional and physical assessment.

CASE STUDY

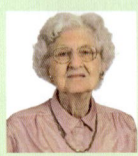

Think back to the case study. The nurse completed the following documentation of her assessment of Mrs. Doris Miller.

Biographical Data: Mrs. Doris Miller, an 82-year-old Caucasian widow. Currently lives with daughter, Delores Ralston. Sitting in chair, appears to be thin, pale, and distracted. Answers some questions appropriately, but frequently apologizes for her appearance and defers to her daughter to answer any questions with regard to her recent fall and hospitalization.

Reason for Home Health Care Visit: Fell in her own home 3 weeks ago and was hospitalized for repair and pinning of a fractured right femur.

History of Present Health Concern: Delores reports that Mrs. Miller can put just enough weight on her right leg to use a walker, but is not stable and the pain is too much to bear weight for any walking distance; needs assistance with bathing, cooking, and dressing; is not eating very well and seems to choke easily, especially when she is drinking, and that she complains frequently of a "dry mouth." Uses bed pads to manage a small amount of incontinence during the night, and daughter gets her up at 3:00 AM to bedside commode. Mrs. Miller says in a very weak, raspy voice, "I don't know how I ended up here. I don't know what I'd do without Delores but if I could just walk and didn't hurt so bad everything would be OK … I've always been able to take care of things. This just all seems like such of a fuss over nothing." She reaches up to wipe her eyes with a tissue that she is holding in her right hand with noticeably contracted fingers with swan-neck deformities and enlarged distal, interphalangeal joints.

Personal History: Past history of Parkinson's, osteoarthritis, osteoporosis, and mitral valve disease. Has had numerous falls, but this is first broken bone. Current medications: Sinemet 25/250 mg every day; warfarin 5 mg every day; MS Contin 15 mg every 12 hours; MS 10-mg oral solution (10 mg per 2.5 mL) every 8 hours prn for breakthrough pain; levothyroxine 0.05 mg every AM; Miralax every other day as needed for constipation.

Physical Examination Findings: Height 5 ft and weight prior to hospitalization 89 lb. BP 85/45 on the right and 108/64 on the left. Heart rate 92 bpm and irregularly irregular. Lung sounds are clear but only heard in the upper lobes. Skin pale, thin, and dry in most areas, and appears intact and well cared for. Several large bruises on her right shoulder, upper arm, and hip. Incision line 6 in on right leg dry, slightly red, but without swelling or drainage. However, some redness noted on elbows and sacrum, and the antecubital spaces are moist with some beginning maceration. Mrs. Miller has 1+ pitting pedal edema bilaterally. Crepitus and a grating, popping sound noted bilaterally as well as increased resistance and rigidity noted when assisted with raising arms.

ANALYSIS OF DATA: DIAGNOSTIC REASONING

After collecting subjective and objective data pertaining to the older adult, identify abnormal findings and client strengths using diagnostic reasoning. Then, cluster the data to reveal any significant patterns or abnormalities.

Selected Nursing Diagnoses

Following is a listing of selected nursing diagnoses (health promotion, risk, or actual) that you may identify when analyzing the cue clusters.

Health Promotion Diagnosis

- Readiness for Enhanced Effective Caregiving

Risk Diagnoses

- Risk for Caregiver Role Strain related to complexity of illness and lack of resources
- Risk for Ineffective Family Coping related to emotional conflicts secondary to chronic illness of parent
- Risk for Social Isolation related to inability to communicate effectively, decreased mobility, effects of chronic illness, or pain

- Risk for Imbalanced Nutrition, Less Than Body Requirements related to dysphagia or decreased desire to eat secondary to altered level of consciousness
- Risk for Constipation related to decreased physical mobility, decreased intestinal motility, lower fluid intake, reduced fiber and bulk in diet, and effects of medications
- Risks for Impaired Skin Integrity related to loss of subcutaneous tissue, immobility, malnutrition
- Risk for Ineffective Thermoregulation related to loss of subcutaneous tissue, atrophy of eccrine sweat glands, decreased functioning of sebaceous glands
- Risk for Disturbed Sensory Perception: Visual—related to dry eyes, loss of lens transparency, slow pupil constriction; Auditory—related to presbycusis
- Risk for Impaired Gas Exchange related to diminished recoil of lungs, less elastic alveoli, and loss of skeletal muscle strength
- Risk for Loneliness related to changing role and decreasing functional status

Actual Diagnoses

- Caregiver Role Strain related to severity of illness, complexity of caregiving tasks
- Diversional Activity Deficit related to impaired mobility or impaired thought processes
- Fatigue related to compromised circulatory or respiratory system and/or effects of medications
- Grieving related to debilitating effects of chronic illness
- Hopelessness related to deteriorating physical condition
- Chronic Sorrow of parent, caregiver, or individual client related to chronic physical or mental disability of client
- Ineffective Therapeutic Regimen Management related to lack of community resources
- Impaired Physical Mobility related to pain, age, pathologic changes in joints, or neuromuscular impairment
- Powerlessness related to unpredictability of complex disease processes and complex treatments
- Ineffective Protection related to decreased immunity
- Activity Intolerance related to weakness, fatigue, or pain related to joint and muscle deterioration and subsequent disuse of joints
- Ineffective Role Performance related to chronic illness
- Functional Urinary Incontinence related to immobility or dementia
- Wandering related to cognitive impairment, disorientation, and sedation
- Bathing/Hygiene Self-Care Deficit related to impaired physical or cognitive functioning
- Dressing/Grooming Self-Care Deficit related to impaired physical or cognitive functioning
- Acute Confusion related to adverse effects of medication, infection, or dehydration

Selected Collaborative Problems

Often, abnormalities identified in the nursing assessment (including functional) will require a collaborative approach. Since the geriatric syndromes (GSs) are usually caused by acute pathology, they almost always require referral and/or nurse–physician collaboration. After grouping the data, certain collaborative problems may become apparent. Remember that collaborative problems differ from nursing diagnoses in that nursing interventions cannot prevent them. However, these physiologic complications of medical conditions can be detected and monitored by the nurse. In addition, the nurse can use physician- and nurse-prescribed interventions to minimize the complications of the problems. In such situations, the nurse may also have to refer the client for further treatment of the problem. Following is a list of collaborative problems that may be identified when assessing the frail elderly client. These problems are worded as Risk for Complications (RC), followed by the problem. It is important to remember, however, that any complication in the very old is likely to manifest as any one of the following GSs.

- *Geriatric Syndromes: Falls*
  - RC: Cardiac—syncope, orthostasis, dysrhythmias
  - RC: Musculoskeletal—loss of strength, osteoporosis, osteoarthritis
  - RC: Neurologic—dizziness, poor balance and gait, intracranial hemorrhage
  - RC: Sensory—loss of vision
  - RC: Infection
- *Geriatric Syndromes: Urinary Incontinence*
  - RC: Urinary obstruction—prostatic hypertrophy
  - RC: Infection
  - RC: Constipation, fecal impaction
  - RC: Adverse medication effect
- *Geriatric Syndromes: Acute Mental Status Decline*
  - RC: Infection—pneumonia, urinary tract, sepsis
  - RC: Adverse medication effect
  - RC: Dehydration
  - RC: Cardiovascular—heart failure, cerebrovascular accident (CVA)
  - RC: Metabolic—hypothyroidism/hyperthyroidism, hypoglycemia
  - RC: Depression
- *Weakness, Fatigue, Anorexia, and Dyspnea*
  - RC: Cancer
  - RC: Pain
  - RC: Dysphagia
  - RC: Adverse medication effect
  - RC: Renal failure

Medical Problems

After grouping the data, the client's signs and symptoms may clearly require medical diagnosis and treatment. Referral to a primary care provider is necessary.

CASE STUDY

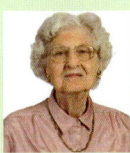

After collecting and analyzing the data for Mrs. Doris Miller, the nurse determines that the following conclusions are appropriate.

Risk Diagnoses
- Risk for Impaired Skin Integrity r/t decreased mobility; some redness on elbows, sacrum, and beginning maceration in antecubital spaces; and 1+ pitting edema bilaterally.

Actual Diagnoses
- Powerlessness r/t unpredictability of complex disease processes and treatments
- Grieving r/t debilitating effects of chronic illness and loss of independence from poststatus pain and medication effects

A collaborative problem identified is Geriatric Syndromes: Falls. (Mrs. Miller is under the care of her surgeon and other physicians. Any increase in symptoms that would indicate an increasing potential risk for falls from the interactions of her complex disease status should be reported to the appropriate health professional.)

To view an algorithm depicting the process for diagnostic reasoning in this case, go to thePoint.

Interdisciplinary Verbal Communication of Assessment Findings Using SBAR

SITUATION: DM, an 82-year-old Caucasian widow, presents with constant right leg and hip pain (5–7 on 10-point scale) when awake. Pain is increased with extended sitting and when getting out of chair or bed, and bearing weight on right leg when using walker. Pain slightly relieved when she takes MS Contin 15 mg every 12 hours; morphine sulfate 10-mg oral solution (10 mg per 2.5 mL) every 8 hours prn for breakthrough pain. Also has back aches when sitting. Client is not eating well and chokes easily when drinking. Has a frequent "dry mouth." Does not like to use bedside commode and "hates being so dependent and unable to do things." Rates mental anguish 9–10 on 10-point scale.

BACKGROUND: DM lives with daughter and is receiving home health care for bathing, cooking, and dressing, as she is recovering from repair and pinning of fractured right femur caused by fall in home 3 weeks ago. Bed pads are used to manage a small amount of incontinence during the night. Client has a history of Parkinson's, osteoarthritis, osteoporosis, and mitral valve disease. She has fallen numerous times, but this was the first time that she broke any bones. Her current medications in addition to the pain meds are Sinemet 25/250 mg every day; warfarin 5 mg every day; levothyroxine 0.05 mg every AM; Miralax every other day as needed for constipation.

ASSESSMENT: Answers some questions appropriately, but is distracted and frequently apologizes for appearance. Refers to daughter to answer questions related to recent fall and surgery. States in weak, raspy voice: "I don't know how I ended up here and I don't know what I'd do without Delores."

Height 5 ft and weight prior to hospitalization 89 lb. Pale and thin. BP 85/45 on the right and 108/64 on the left. Heart rate 92 bpm and irregularly irregular. Has slight ectropion and reddened eyes. Has contracted fingers with swan-neck deformities and enlarged distal, interphalangeal joints appear intact. Has resting tremor of the hands. Crepitus and a grating, popping sound noted bilaterally when assisted to raise her arms, as well as increased resistance and rigidity. Several large bruises on right shoulder, upper arm, and hip. Incision line 6 in on right leg dry, slightly red, but without swelling or drainage. However, some redness noted on elbows and sacrum, and antecubital spaces moist with some beginning maceration. Lung sounds clear but only heard in the upper lobes. Has 1+ pitting pedal edema bilaterally. Appears well cared for.

RECOMMENDATION: DM is at risk for Impaired Skin Integrity r/t decreased mobility; some redness on elbows, sacrum, and beginning maceration in antecubital spaces; and 1+ pitting edema bilaterally. She is experiencing Powerlessness r/t unpredictability of complex disease processes and treatments. She is also suffers from Grieving r/t debilitating effects of chronic illness and loss of independence from poststatus pain and medication effects. A plan is needed to promote her independence yet ensure safety measures. Collaborative problems include Risk for Aspiration r/t choking when swallowing liquids. She also has the Geriatric Syndrome: Falls for which she and her daughter need teaching regarding safety and fall prevention strategies. She needs to be seen by her primary care provider to be reevaluated for management of her continuous pain and swallowing difficulties.

ABNORMAL FINDINGS 32-1 Age-Related Abnormalities of the Eye

Common age-related abnormalities of the eye include glaucoma, macular degeneration, retinal detachment, and diabetic retinopathy.

GLAUCOMA

The client with glaucoma is usually symptom free. In older adults, diabetes and atherosclerosis are conditions that increase the risk of glaucoma. The disorder is caused by increased pressure that can destroy the optic nerve and cause blindness if not treated properly. An acute form of glaucoma can occur at any age and is a true medical emergency because blindness can result in a day or two without treatment. Rainbow-like halos or circles around lights, severe pain in the eyes or forehead, nausea, and blurred vision may occur with the acute form of glaucoma.

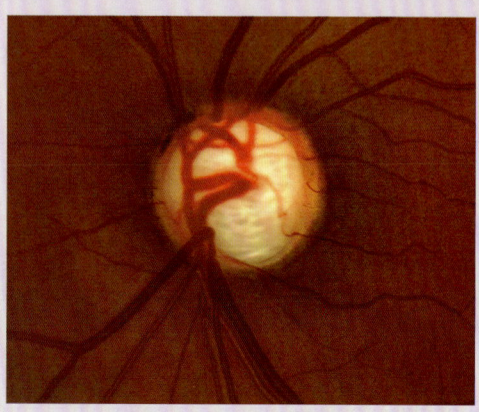

Glaucomatous cupping.

MACULAR DEGENERATION

Macular degeneration, a gradual loss of central vision, is caused by aging and thinning of the micro-thin membrane in the center of the retina called the macula. Additional risk factors include sunlight exposure, family history, and Caucasian race. Most cases begin to develop after age 50, but damage may be occurring for months to years before symptoms occur. Peripheral vision is not affected, and the condition may occur initially in only one eye. Only about 10% of all age-related macular degeneration leaks occur in the small blood vessels in the retinal pigment epithelium. This type accounts for the most serious loss of vision.

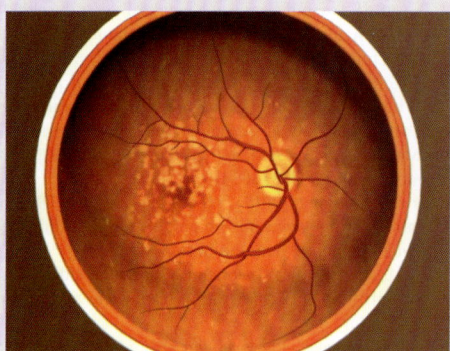

Funduscopic view of intermediate age-related macular degeneration.

RETINAL DETACHMENT

Retinal detachment occurs at a greater frequency with aging as the vitreous pulls away from its attachment to the retina at the back of the eye, causing the retina to tear in one or more places. A retinal detachment is always a serious problem. Blindness will result if the detachment is not treated.

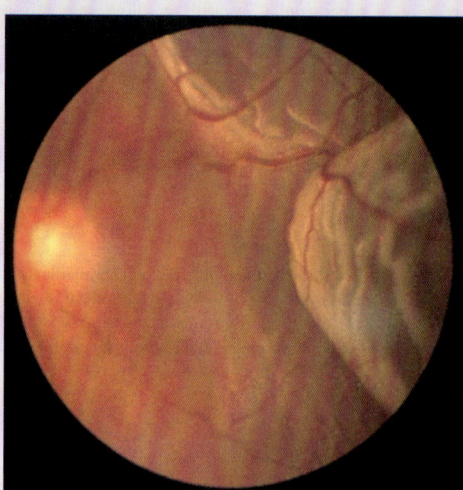

Ophthalmoscopic photograph of retinal detachment.

DIABETIC RETINOPATHY

Many older adults have diabetes, which can lead to cataracts, glaucoma, and diabetic retinopathy. Of those with diabetes mellitus, about 90% will develop diabetic retinopathy to some degree. The more serious of the two forms of the disease, proliferative diabetic retinopathy, occurs most often among those who have had diabetes for more than 25 years. People with the advanced form of the disease usually experience a noticeable loss of vision, including cloudiness, distortion of familiar objects, and, occasionally, blind spots or floaters. If not treated, diabetic retinopathy will lead to connective scar tissue, which over time can shrink, pulling on the retina and resulting in a retinal detachment. In the early stages of the milder form of the disease, background diabetic retinopathy, the person may be unaware of problems because the loss of sight is usually gradual and mainly affects peripheral vision.

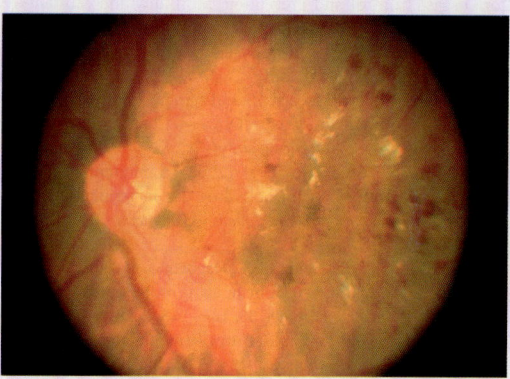

Ocular fundus of a patient with background diabetic retinopathy.

Image credits: Glaucoma, *Tasman, W., & Jaeger, E. (Eds.). (2001). The Wills Eye Hospital atlas of clinical ophthalmology (2nd ed.). Philadelphia, PA: Lippincott Williams & Wilkins;* Macular degeneration, *from the National Eye Institute, National Institutes of Health, Baltimore, MD;* Retinal detachment, *from Moore, K. L., & Dailey, A. F. (2006). Clinically oriented anatomy (5th ed., p. 967). Philadelphia, PA: Lippincott Williams & Wilkins;* Diabetic retinopathy, *from Klintworth, G. K. (2008). The eye. In R. Rubin & D. E. Strayer (Eds.)* Rubin's pathology; Clinicopathologic foundations of medicine *(5th ed., p. 1257). Philadelphia, PA: Lippincott Williams & Wilkins.*

Want to know more?

A wide variety of resources to enhance your learning and understanding of this book are available on thePoint. Visit thePoint to access:

NCLEX-Style Student Review Questions   Concept in Action Animations
Watch and Learn Videos   And more!

References and Selected Readings

Administration on Aging. (2014). A profile of older Americans: 2014. Available at http://www.aoa.gov/Aging_Statistics/Profile/2014/docs/2014-Profile.pdf

Alzheimer's Association. (2016). Alzheimer's disease: Risk factors. Available at http://www.alz.org/alzheimers_disease_causes_risk_factors.asp

American Academy of Family Physicians (AAFP). (2006). CURB-65 and CRB-65 severity scores for community-acquired pneumonia. Available at http://www.aafp.org/fpm/2006/0400/fpm20060400p41-rt2.pdf

American Association of Colleges of Nursing (AACN). (2012). Competencies to improve care of older adults. Available at http://www.aacn.nche.edu/education-resources/competencies-older-adults

American Geriatrics Society. (2015). The Beers criteria for potentially inappropriate medication (PIM) use in the elderly. Available at http://onlinelibrary.wiley.com/doi/10.1111/jgs.13702/full

Batsis, J., MacKenzie, T., Lopez-Jimenez, F., & Bartels, S. (2015). Sarcopenia, sarcopenic obesity, and functional impairments in older adults: National Health and Nutrition Examination Survey 1999–2004. *Nutrition Research, 35*(12), 1031–1039. doi: 0.1016/j.nutres.2015.09.003

Bhatti, N. (2015). Hip fracture clinical presentation. Available at http://emedicine.medscape.com/article/87043-clinical

Brick, P. (2015). Sexuality, intimacy and aging: It's time to talk! Available at http://www.asaging.org/blog/sexuality-intimacy-and-aging-it%E2%80%99s-time-talk

Brown-O'Hara, T. (2013). Geriatric syndromes and their implications for nursing. *Nursing, 43*(1), 1–3. Available at http://journals.lww.com/nursing/Fulltext/2013/01000/Geriatric_syndromes_and_their_implications_for.1.aspxdoi: 10.1097/01.NURSE.0000423097.95416.50

Centers for Disease Control and Prevention (CDC). (2014). Prevalence of incontinence among older Americans. Available at http://www.cdc.gov/nchs/data/series/sr_03/sr03_036.pdf

Centers for Disease Control and Prevention (CDC). (2016a). HIV among people aged 50 and over. Available at http://www.cdc.gov/hiv/group/age/olderamericans/

Centers for Disease Control and Prevention (CDC). (2016b). Pneumococcal vaccination. Available at http://www.cdc.gov/vaccines/vpd-vac/pneumo/default.htm?s_cid=cs_797

Centers for Disease Control and Prevention, Morbidity and Mortality Weekly Report (CDC, MMWR). (2014). Lung cancer incidence trends among men and women – United States, 2005–2009. Available at http://www.cdc.gov/mmwr/preview/mmwrhtml/mm6301a1.htm

Charansonney, O. (2011). Physical activity and aging: A life-long story. Available at http://www.discoverymedicine.com/Olivier-L-Charansonney/2011/09/09/physical-activity-and-aging-a-life-long-story/

Douzjian, M., Wilson, C., Shultz, M., et al. (2002). A program to use pain control medication to reduce psychotropic drug use in residents with difficult behavior. *Nursing home medicine: The Annals of Long-term Care*, 1–7. Available at http://www.mmhe.com

Greco, A., Paroni, G., Seripa, D., Addante, F., Dagostino, M., & Aucella, F. (2014). Frailty, disability and physical exercise in the aging process and in chronic kidney disease. *Kidney Blood Pressure Research, 39*, 164–168. doi:10.1159/000355792

Hager, E. (n.d.). Varicose veins. Available at https://vascular.org/patient-resources/vascular-conditions/varicose-veins

Healthy People 2020. (2017). Older adults. Available at https://www.healthypeople.gov/2020/topics-objectives/topic/older-adults

Huang, C. (2016). CHA_2DS_2-VASc score for atrial fibrillation stroke risk. Available at http://www.mdcalc.com/cha2ds2-vasc-score-atrial-fibrillation-stroke-risk/

ICD-10-CM Diagnostic Code. (2016). Orthostatic hypotension. Available at http://www.icd10data.com/ICD10CM/Codes/I00-I99/I95-I99/I95-/I95.1

Judge, N. (2007). Neurovascular assessment. *Nursing Standard, 21*(45), 39–44. Available at http://www.snjourney.com/ClinicalInfo/Systems/PDF/NeuroVas%20Assessment.pdf

Katzman, R., Brown, T., Fuld, P., et al. (1983). Validation of a short orientation-memory concentration test of cognitive impairment. *American Journal of Psychiatry, 140*, 734–739.

MacBride, M., Rhodes, D., & Shuster, L. (2010). Vulvovaginal atrophy. *Mayo Clinic Proceedings, 85*(1), 87–94. doi: 10.4065/mcp.2009.0413

Mayo Clinic. (2015). Delirium. Available at http://www.mayoclinic.org/diseases-conditions/delirium/basics/definition/con-20033982

McDaniel, D. (2016). Sex and seniors – a new reality for the elderly. Available at http://www.huffingtonpost.com/derrick-y-mcdaniel/sex-and-seniors-stds-a-ne_b_9619778.html

Molton, I., & Terrill, A. (2014). Overview of persistent pain in older adults. Available at http://www.apa.org/pubs/journals/releases/amp-a0035794.pdf

Muliira, J., & Mulirra, R. (2013). Sexual health for older women. *Sultan Qaboos University Medical Journal, 13*(4), 469–476. Available at http://www.ncbi.nlm.nih.gov/pmc/articles/PMC3836634/

National Institute on Aging. (2015). What happens when DNA becomes damaged. Available at https://www.nia.nih.gov/health/publication/genetics-aging-our-genes/what-happens-when-dna-becomes-damaged

Sapkota, N. (2012). Symptoms of pneumonia in the elderly often missed by caregivers. Available at http://www.prweb.com/releases/pneumonia/elderly/prweb9188784.htm

Swartz, M. (2014). *Textbook of physical diagnosis: History and examination*. Philadelphia, PA: Elsevier Task Force on Aging Research Funding (2009). Sustaining the commitment. Available at http://www.agingresearch.org

Urology Care Foundation. (2017). What is benign prostatic hypertrophy (BPH)? Available at http://urologyhealth.org/urologic-conditions/benign-prostatic-hyperplasia-(bph)

U.S. Preventive Services Task Force (USPSTF). (2014). Focus on older adults. Available at http://www.uspreventiveservicestaskforce.org/Page/Name/focus-on-older-adults

Wallace, & Shelkey, M. (2007). Katz Index of Independence in Activities of Daily Living (ADL). Available at http://consultgerirn.org/uploads/File/trythis/try_this_2.pdf

Williams, M. (2009). The basic geriatric respiratory examination. Available at http://www.medscape.com/viewarticle/712242

Yesavage, J. A., & Brink, T. L. (1983). Development and validation of a geriatric depression screening scale: A preliminary report. *Journal of Psychiatric Research, 17*, 37–49.

Zürcher, S., Saxer, S., & Schwendimann, R. (2011). Urinary incontinence in hospitalised elderly patients: Do nurses recognise and manage the problem? *Nursing Research & Practice* [Online]. Available at http://www.hindawi.com/journals/nrp/2011/671302/

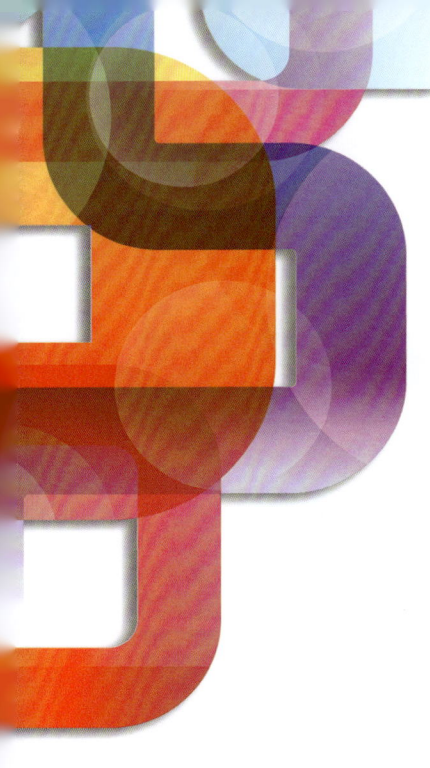

33 ASSESSING FAMILIES

Learning Objectives

1. Define family.
2. Interview and assess a family for structure, development, and function.
3. Determine a family's life cycle stage and related tasks.
4. Construct a genogram for a three-generational family.
5. Construct a family attachment diagram and ecomap.
6. Discuss theoretic concepts of family function (family systems theory, Bowen's family system theory, and communication theory)
7. Use Bowne's theory to determine the level of self-differentiation of a family and its members and to detect triangle within a family.
8. Describe the importance of effective family communication.
9. Analyze the data from the family interview and assessment to formulate valid nursing diagnoses, collaborative problems, and/or referrals.
10. Differentiate between general routine screening versus skills needed for focused or specialty assessment of the family.
11. Document and verbally report accurate family assessment findings.

CASE STUDY

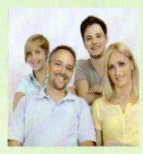

The Ross family has returned to the clinic for help in dealing with Dan's recent diagnosis and treatment of type 1 diabetes. Dan is a 17-year-old high school senior who is scheduled to leave for college in 6 months. He was diagnosed with type 1 diabetes 4 months ago. He is not following the diet–exercise–insulin protocol (prescribed 4 months ago). Dan has been seen by the physician and in the emergency department (ED) five times in the past 4 months for complications resulting from not following the protocol. The physician refers the Ross family to the nurse to help the family address the identified problem of Dan's refusal to follow the protocol. Because the diet and food preparation affect the whole family, sister Jenna attends the family session as well. The Ross family case will be discussed throughout the chapter.

CONCEPTUAL BACKGROUND

Family nursing is more than family centered care (Bell, 2013). Family nursing is about relationships. Nurses are well aware of the need for establishing a relationship with all clients, but Bell (2011; 2014) has asserted that the relationship between the nurse and the family is at a deeper level than the average nurse–client relationship and change depends on this relationship. Illness reverberates within and outside relationships, especially the effect of serious illness. As the authors say, serious illness can "strengthen, renew, and deepen relationships" or "cause relationships to become conflicted, troubled, fragmented, and broken" (p. 3). It is for this reason that Bell recommends focusing family assessment on relationships, and to include in the relationships those with the illness. The nurse must relate to the family in a way that creates a context for change.

Terms Related to Family Assessment

To assess a family, the nurse must first determine who constitutes a family. The traditional definition of family is based on relationships of blood, marriage, or adoption. This definition has evolved over the years, and a number of different groups of people living together are now considered to be families (e.g., single-parent families, extended families, communes, gay and lesbian couples, multigenerational families; Fig. 33-1). Therefore, at the beginning of the 21st century, those involved in family nursing incorporated a broader definition of family, thought to be more relevant to the times: "Family refers to two or more individuals who depend on one another for emotional, physical and economic support. The members of the family are self-defined" (Kaakinen et al., 2015, p. 5). Based on this definition, it is relatively simple for the nurse to

854   UNIT 4   Nursing Assessment of Special Groups

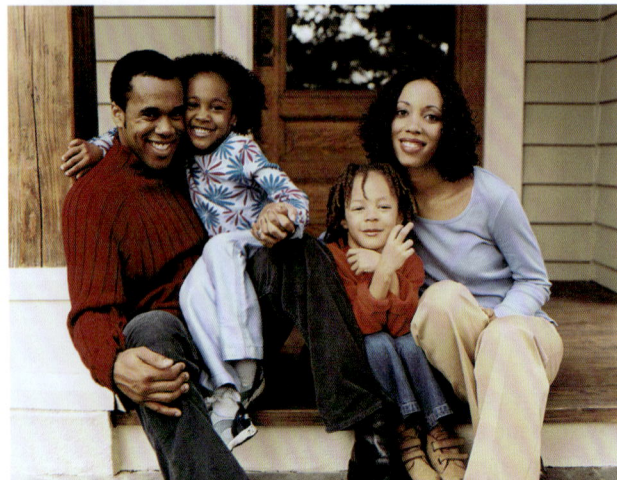
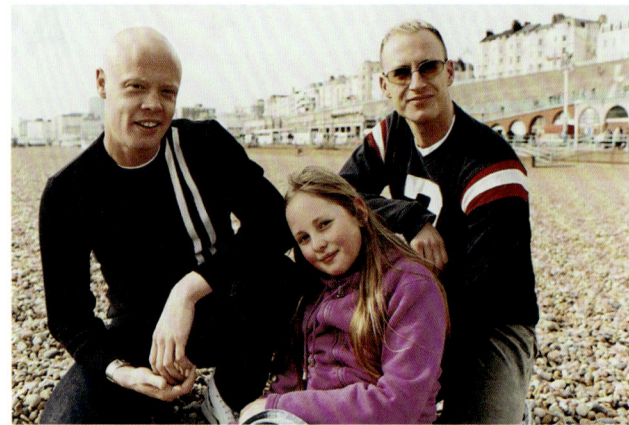
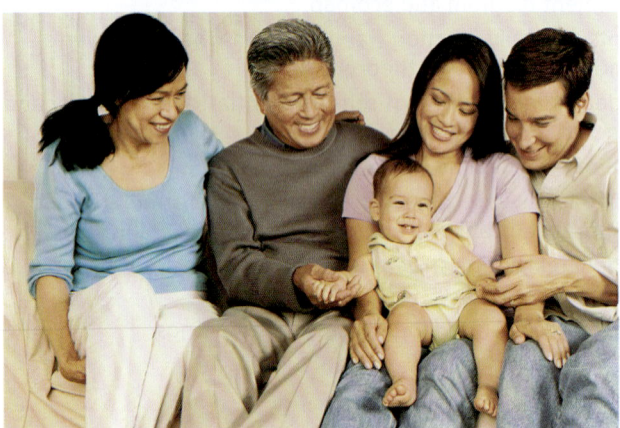
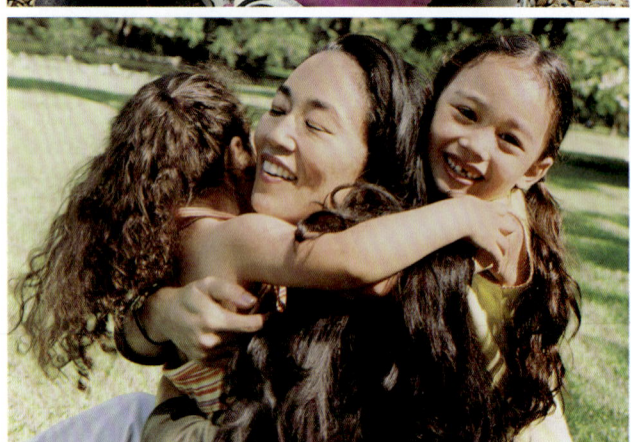

FIGURE 33-1 A few examples of many family compositions.

determine who constitutes a family: *the family is whoever they say they are.*

CLINICAL TIP
If there is disagreement within a family about who is a part of the family and who is not, the nurse should note this difference of opinion and determine that the family for the assessment consists of those people who interact the most frequently.

The Relationship Between Families and Illness

Among the many reasons for nurses to understand the concepts of family assessment, three stand out as important to a nursing assessment text:
- An ill person's family is an essential part of the context in which the illness occurs.
- The family members, the ill person, and even the illness itself interact in such a way that no one component can be separated from the rest.
- The statistics on family caregiving show that families are very much involved in providing care for an ill family member. (For an overview of the many people involved in caring for ill, chronically ill, or disabled family members in the United States, see Box 33-1.)

The dynamic interactions of the ill family member, the illness, and the other family members will become clear as the elements of family assessment are described throughout this chapter.

BOX 33-1   FAMILY CAREGIVING STATISTICS

If you're a caregiver, you are not alone. You've probably heard that before, but you may not know just how much company you have. A recent study of caregiving in the United States by the Family Caregivers Alliance (2016) reported that approximately 43.5 million caregivers have provided unpaid care to an adult or child in the past 12 months. About 65% of care recipients are female and 75% of caregivers are female. The average age of caregivers is 49.2 years and of care recipients is 69.4 years, with 47% of these being over 75 years. The number of persons cared for, their ages, and their conditions vary widely. Most caregivers (85%) provide care for relatives.

An important factor affecting the nation's economy is that the cost of this unpaid care has been estimated to be approximately $470 billion per year.

In addition to the relative cost of caregiving, there is additional cost to the caregiver due to the effect on work. Many continue to work, and many have to make adjustments relative to their work. The stresses and schedule disruptions undoubtedly affect worker productivity and health.

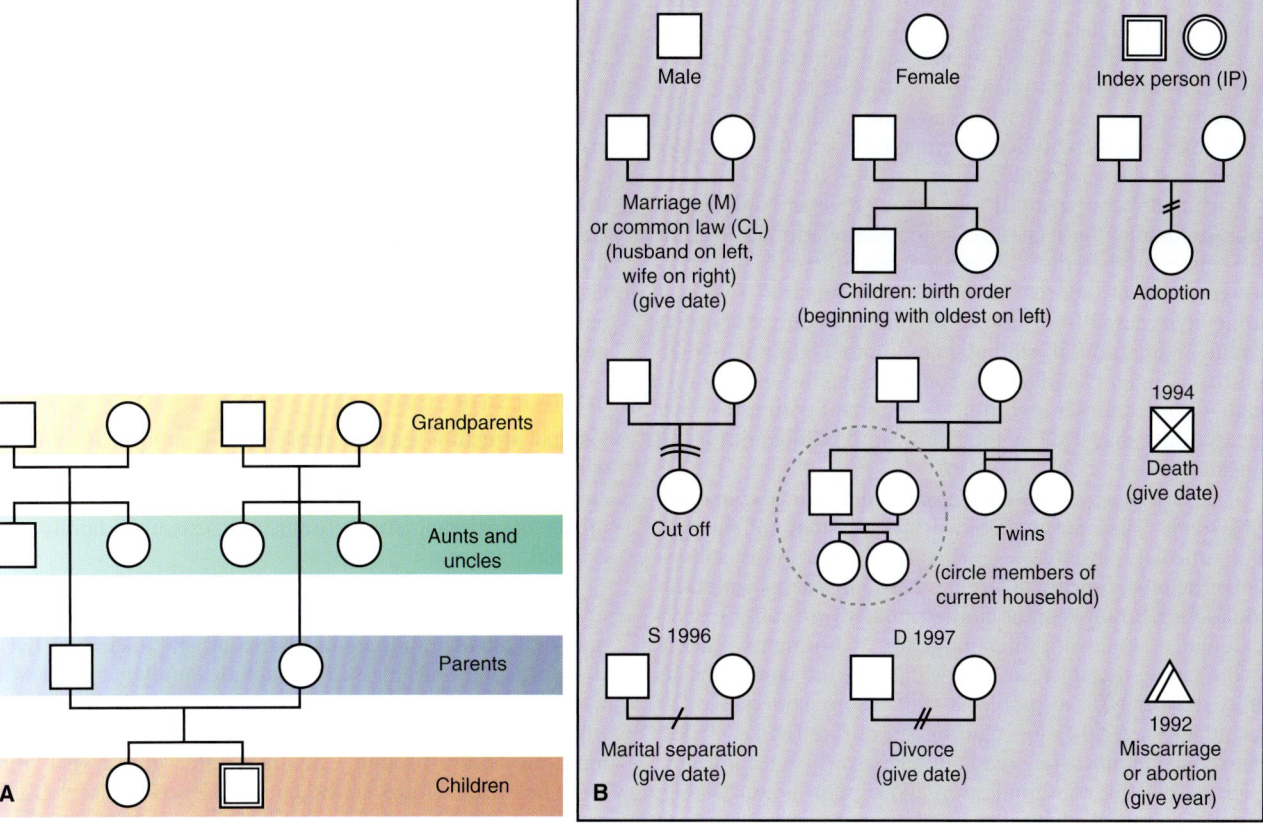

FIGURE 33-2 A. Format used for genogram. B. Symbols used in genogram.

Framework of Family Assessment

In recent years, a variety of nursing models or frameworks have been developed as tools for assessing the family. Nurses have developed these models on the basis of family theories because none of the nonnursing fields has captured the necessary elements of the nursing care of families. The framework used in this chapter for assessing the family is a modified combination of the Calgary Family Assessment Model (Wright & Leahey, 2013) and Friedman's Family Assessment Model (Friedman et al., 2003). Regardless of which model or framework you use to assess the family, there are three essential components of family assessment especially prominent in all family assessment models: structure, development, and function. Environmental components, cultural–ethnic variations, and areas of family coping, family stress, and family communication are usually incorporated into these three essential components. However, some models of family assessment may address them separately.

Family Structure

Family structure has three elements: internal structure, external structure, and context. Some theorists focus on a structural–functional framework that, when applied to family assessment, examines the interaction between the family and its internal and external environment (Friedman et al., 2003). Other theorists separate the assessment of family structure from assessment of family function within the structural component. This chapter focuses on the interaction between the family structure and its internal and external environment.

Internal Structure

The internal structure of a family refers to the ordering of relationships within the confines of that family. It consists of all the details in the family that define the structure of the family. Elements of internal structure include family composition, gender (and gender roles), rank order, subsystems, boundaries, and power structure.

Family composition can be illustrated by recording the family tree graphically as a genogram. A genogram helps the nurse to view the whole family as a unit. It shows names, relationships, and other information such as ages, marriages, divorces, adoptions, and health data. Behavior and health–illness patterns can be examined using the genogram because both of these patterns tend to repeat through the generations. Figure 33-2 illustrates the format and symbols used for a simple three-generation family genogram.

A family member's *gender* often determines his or her role and behavior in the family. Beliefs about male and female roles and behaviors vary from one family to another. Also, there may be female or male subsystems that share common interests or activities.

Rank order refers to the sibling rank of each family member. For instance, families often treat the oldest child differently from the way they treat the youngest child. The rank order and gender of each family member in relation to other siblings' rank order and gender make a difference in how the person will eventually relate to a spouse and children. For example, an older sister of a younger brother may bring certain expectations of how women relate to men into a marriage. If the older sister marries a man who is an older brother to a younger sister, there may be conflict or competition because each may expect to be the responsible leader.

Each member of a family may belong to several *subsystems*. Subsystems may be related to gender, generational position (parents, grandparents, children), shared interests or activities (e.g., music, sports, hobbies), or to function (work at home, work away from home). Examples of subsystems are parent–child, spousal, sibling, grandmother–granddaughter, mother–daughter, and father–son. Subsystems in a family relate to one another according to rules and patterns, which are often not perceived by the family until pointed out by an outsider.

Boundaries keep subsystems separate and distinct from other subsystems. They are maintained by rules that differentiate the particular subsystem's tasks from those of other subsystems. The most functional families have subsystems with clear boundaries; however, some connection between subsystems is maintained along with the boundaries. According to a theory by the family therapist Salvador Minuchin, the family and its subsystems may have problems with connectedness, so that boundaries are either too rigid or too diffuse (Kafka, 2008). Disengaged families have rigid boundaries, which leads to low levels of effective communication and support among family members. Enmeshed families have diffuse boundaries, which make it difficult for individuals to achieve individuation from the family.

Power structure relates to the influences each member has on the family processes and function. Some distribution of power is necessary to maintain order so that the family can function. There is usually a power hierarchy, with the parents having more authority than the children. In the most functional families, parents have a sense of shared power and children gain increasing power as they mature and become more responsible.

A tool to help the nurse and family examine family relationships based on structure is the Family Attachment Diagram. This is a diagram of the family members' interactions. It represents the reciprocal nature and quality of interactions. Figure 33-3 represents both a nuclear family with close and balanced relationships and a family with some conflicting, negatively attached relationships.

External Structure

External structure refers to those outside groups or things to which the family is connected. External structures may influence aspects of the internal structure of the family. Two elements of external structure include extended family and external systems.

Extended family may consist of family members not residing in the home but with whom the family interacts frequently such as grandparents or an aunt and uncle who live a short distance away. It also may include family members with whom the family interacts infrequently such as a first cousin who lives across the country and with whom the family communicates only through Christmas cards and a visit once every few years. However, the family feels confident that this cousin would be supportive in time of need. Another type of extended family is the "cut-off" family member. An example would be a brother who left home many years ago and with whom there is no contact at all. This brother may still be considered extended family.

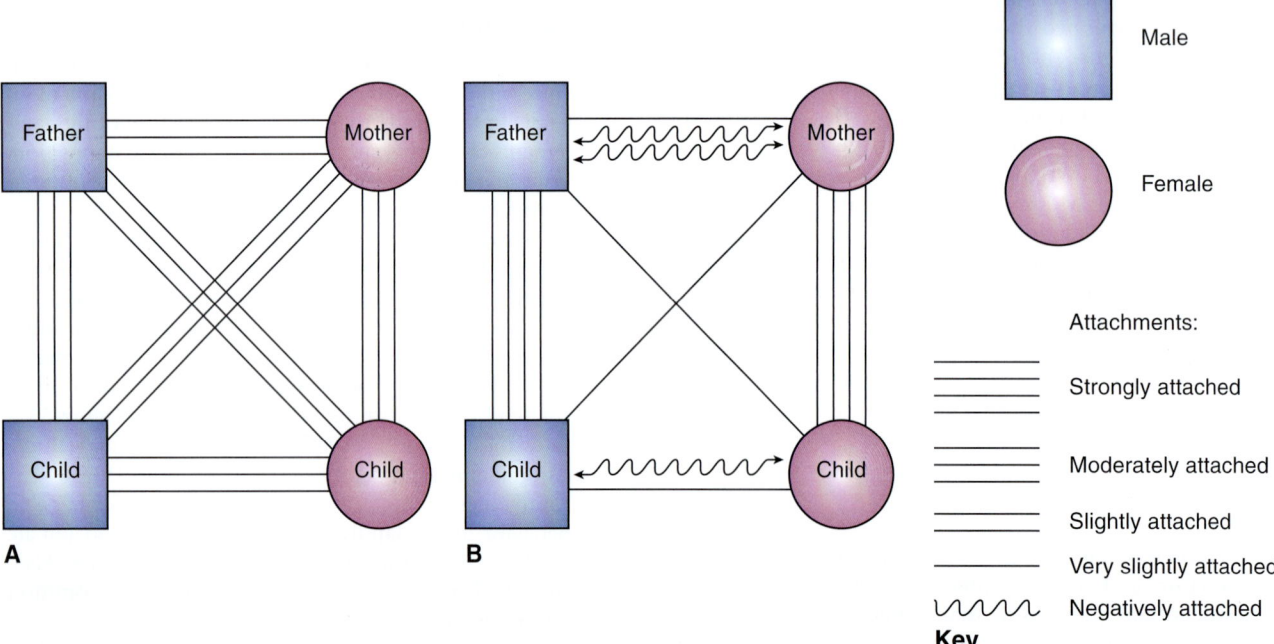

FIGURE 33-3 Family attachment diagram: nuclear family with close, balanced relationship (A); nuclear family with some conflicting, negatively attached relationships (B).

External systems are those systems that are larger than the family and with which the family interacts. These systems include institutions, agencies, and significant people outside the family. Some specific examples of external systems include a family's health center, school, jobs, volunteer agency, church, recreational organizations, friends, neighbors, coworkers, and extended family (only those with whom interaction is frequent).

An ecomap can be used to assess the family members' interactions with the systems outside the family. The diagram, illustrated in Figure 33-4, is similar to the attachment diagram and shows the positive or conflicting nature of the family's relationships with outside groups or organizations.

Context

The context of a family refers to the interrelated conditions in which the family exists: it is the family's setting. Four elements make up the context of the family structure: race or ethnicity, social class, religion, and environment.

Race or ethnicity may influence family structure and interactions. Assessment should include how much the family identifies with and adheres to traditional practices of a particular culture, whether the family's practices are similar to those of the neighborhood of residence, and whether the family has more than one ethnic or racial makeup.

The effects of *social class* and *religion* provide context for the family structure and lifestyle. A couple from different social classes or different religions may bring different expectations into the family system.

Environmental characteristics of the residence, neighborhood, and family and *neighborhood interactions* clarify the context for the family structure and interactions.

Family Development

Like individuals, families go through stages of growth and development. These stages of development are as important to the health and well-being of the family as they are to the individual. In fact, a static family structure is dysfunctional. Friedman (1998) developed theories about family life-cycle stages and associated tasks. The stages and tasks of the traditional nuclear family are presented in Box 33-2. For indepth information on nontraditional two parent families, please see McGoldrick, Preto & Carter, 2016.

Family Function

Friedman (1998) and Friedman et al. (2003) defined five basic family functions: affective, socialization and social placement, reproductive, economic, and health care. For the purposes of this chapter's approach to family assessment, however, the components of family function are organized into four areas:

- *Instrumental:* Instrumental function is the ability of the family to carry out activities of daily living (ADLs) in normal circumstances and in the presence of a family member's illness.
- *Affective and socialization:* Affective function refers to the family's response to all members' needs for support, caring, closeness, intimacy, and the balance of needs for separateness and connectedness. Socialization function refers to the family's ability to bring about healthy socialization of children.
- *Expressive:* Expressive function refers to communication patterns used within the family. Members of well-functioning families are able to express a broad range of emotions; clearly express feelings and needs; encourage feedback; listen attentively to one another; treat one another with respect; avoid displacing, distorting, or masking verbal messages; avoid negative circular communication patterns; and use encouraging versus punishment methods to influence behavior.
- *Health care:* Assessment of health care function is useful for the nurse. It refers to family members' beliefs about a health problem; its etiology, treatment, and prognosis; and the role of professionals. Whether all family members agree or some members disagree with the beliefs helps the nurse to understand the family. The family's health promotion practices are also assessed.

Concept Mastery Alert

The *affective function* refers to all family members' needs for support, caring, closeness, intimacy, and the balance of needs for separateness and connectedness. The *instrumental function* is the ability of the family to carry out activities of daily living.

Theoretical Concepts of Family Function

Some components of family function discussed previously are based on theoretical concepts found in systems theory, Bowen's family system theory, and communication theory. It is important for the nurse to have a good understanding of these concepts before performing an assessment of family function.

Systems Theory

Systems theory holds that a system is composed of subsystems interconnected to the whole system and to each other by means of an integrated and dynamic self-regulating feedback mechanism.

Wright and Leahey (2013) list the major concepts of systems theory that apply to families: A family is part of a larger suprasystem and is also composed of many subsystems (e.g., parent–child, sibling, marital); the family as a whole is greater than the sum of its parts; a change in one family member affects all family members; the family is able to create a balance between change and stability; and family members' behaviors are best understood from a view of circular rather than linear causality. For example, any behavior of family member A affects family member B, and B's behavior then affects A. Therefore, rather than an individual causing a family problem, the behavior pattern or system causes another behavior.

Bowen's Family System Theory

The family therapist Bowen (The Bowen Center, n.d.; Titelman, 2008) developed several concepts that are widely used to assess family function. Bowen views the nuclear family as part of a multigenerational extended family with patterns of

858 UNIT 4 Nursing Assessment of Special Groups

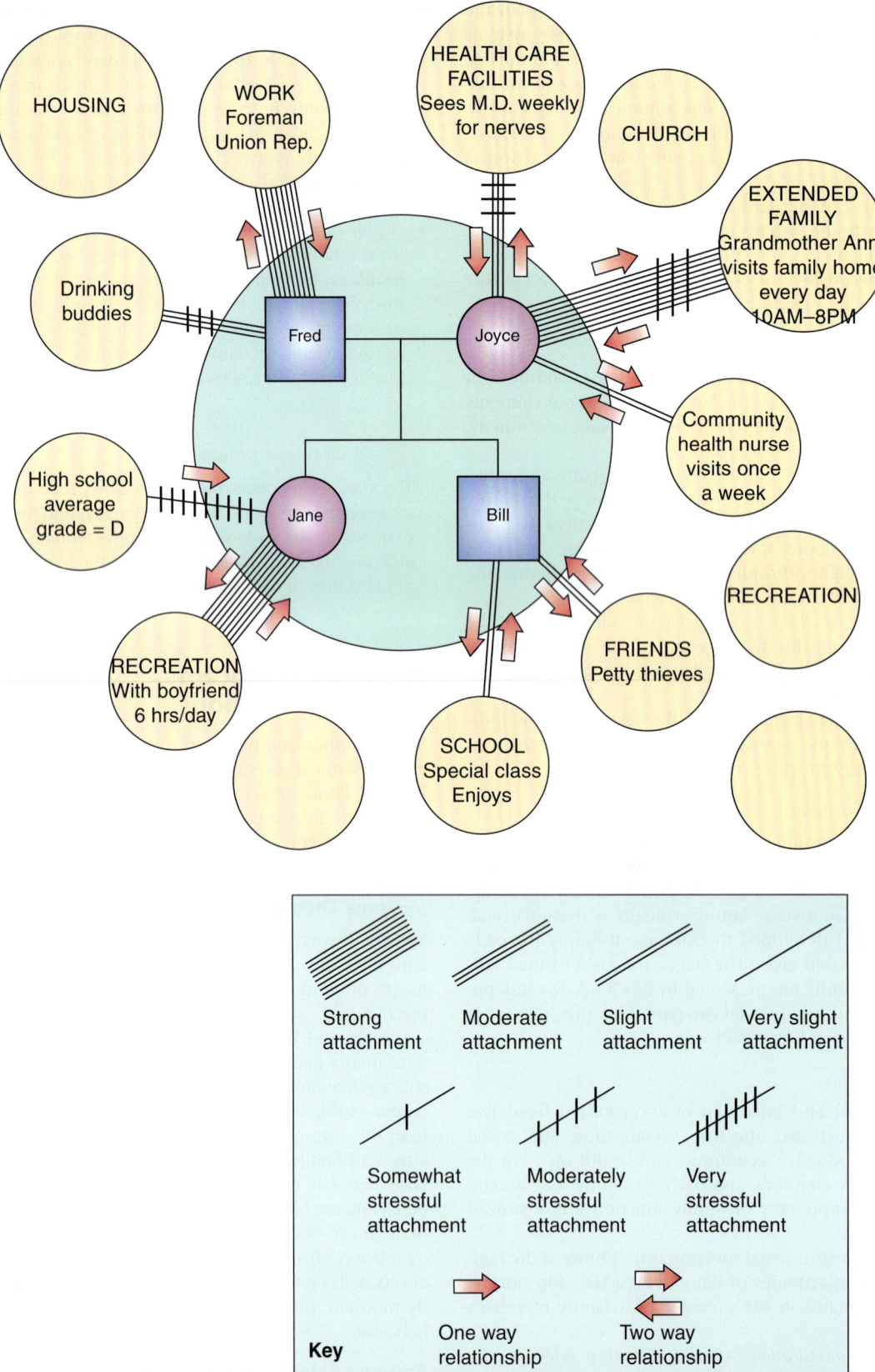

FIGURE 33-4 An ecomap is used to assess family members' interactions with systems outside the family.

BOX 33-2 FAMILY LIFE CYCLES

TWO-PARENT NUCLEAR FAMILY LIFE CYCLE
Stage I—Beginning Families (stage of marriage)
Tasks
- Establishing a mutually satisfying marriage
- Relating harmoniously to the kin network
- Planning a family (decisions about parenthood)

Stage II—Childbearing Families (oldest child is infant through 30 months)
Tasks
- Setting up the young family as a stable unit (integrating new baby into family)
- Reconciling conflicting developmental tasks and needs of various family members
- Maintaining a satisfying marital relationship
- Expanding relationships with extended family by adding parenting and grandparenting roles

Stage III—Families with Preschool Children (2.5–6 years)
Tasks
- Meeting family members' needs for adequate housing, space, privacy, and safety
- Socializing the children
- Integrating new child members while still meeting the needs of other children
- Maintaining healthy relationships within the family (marital and parent–child) and outside the family (extended family and community)

Stage IV—Families with Schoolchildren (6–13 years)
Tasks
- Socializing the children, including promoting school achievement and fostering of healthy peer relations of children
- Maintaining a satisfying marital relationship
- Meeting the physical health needs of family members

Stage V—Families with Teenagers (13–20 years)
Tasks
- Balancing of freedom with responsibility as teenagers mature and become increasingly autonomous
- Refocusing the marital relationship
- Communicating openly between parents and children

Stage VI—Launching Young Adults (from first to last child leaving home)
Tasks
- Expanding the family circle to include new family members acquired by marriage of children
- Continuing to renew and readjust in the marital relationship
- Assisting aging and ill parents of the husband or wife

Stage VII—Middle-Aged Parents (empty nest through retirement)
Tasks
- Providing a health-promoting environment
- Sustaining satisfying and meaningful relationships with aging parents and adult children
- Strengthening the marital relationship

Stage VIII—Family in Retirement and Old Age (retirement to death of both spouses)
Tasks
- Maintaining a satisfying living arrangement
- Adjusting to a reduced income
- Maintaining marital relationships
- Adjusting to loss of spouse
- Maintaining intergenerational family ties
- Continuing to make sense out of one's existence (life review and integration)

Adapted from Friedman, M., Bowden, V., & Gones, E. 2003. *Family nursing: Research, theory, and practice* (5th ed., pp. 114–131). Upper Saddle River, NJ: Prentice Hall.

---

relating that tend to repeat over generations. When the pattern continues across generations, it is called the *multigenerational transmission process*. Bowen theorizes that familial emotional and interaction patterns are reflected in eight interwoven concepts. Two of these concepts—differentiation of self and triangles—are especially important to grasp for assessment of family function.

Differentiation of Self

Differentiation of self is assessed in relation to the boundaries of the subsystems in the structure of the family. This concept is based on a balance of emotional and intellectual levels of function. The emotional level, associated with lower brain centers, relates to feelings. The intellectual level, associated with the cerebral cortex, relates to cognition. How connected these levels, or systems, are affects the person's social functioning. The greater the balance between thinking and feeling, the higher the differentiation of self and the better the person is at managing anxiety.

The Bowen Center (n.d.) provides a summary of key elements of the concept of differentiation of self. The family with highly differentiated adult members is flexible in its interactions, seeks to support all members, understands each member as unique, and encourages members to develop differently from one another. Family roles are assigned on the basis of knowledge, skill, and interest.

The family with low levels of differentiation has adult members who demonstrate impulsive actions, who have difficulty delaying gratification, who cannot analyze a situation before reacting, and who cannot maintain intimate interpersonal relationships (similar to the developmental level of a 2-year-old child). Intense, short-term relationships are the norm, and emotionally based reactions can escalate into violence. Family roles are assigned on the basis of family tradition.

A moderately differentiated person is less dominated by emotions, but personal relationships are often emotion dominated. Life is rule bound, and thinking is usually dualistic (things and people are black and white, good or bad, smart or stupid). A situation cannot be perceived from any but a personal perspective. The person tends to "fuse" or become enmeshed with another in emotional relationships, losing the

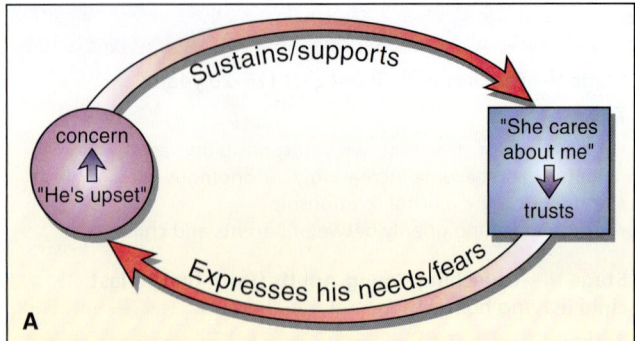 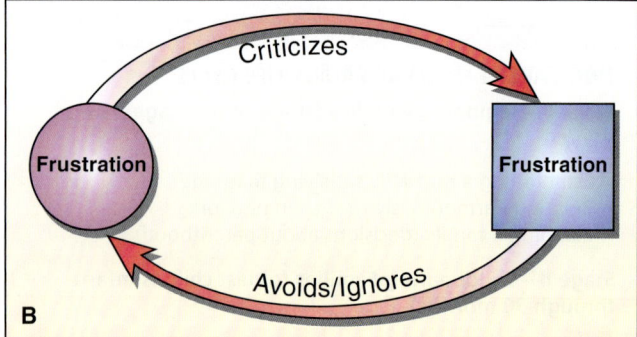

FIGURE 33-5 A. Positive circular communication. B. Negative circular communication.

self in the efforts to please the other. Families with moderately differentiated members exhibit rigid patterns of interactions that are rule bound and have defined roles and acceptable behaviors.

Triangles

Triangles are discussed in relation to subsystems of family structure. Titelman (2008) describes Bowen's triangle as a relational pattern or emotional configuration that exists among one or two family members and another person, object, or issue. Triangles exist in all families; who makes up a triangle can change depending on the situation. However, when two people avoid dealing with emotional closeness or an issue that produces anxiety, the two people may use a third person to evade the stress. For instance, a wife may pull in a child as a third person in the couple's relationship; the husband may distance himself from the conflict by deeper involvement in work. As the intensity of the relationship changes, the amount of interaction is usually balanced, so that as two members move closer, the third withdraws.

Communication Theory

Communication theory concerns the sending and receiving of both verbal and nonverbal messages. The focus is on how individuals interact with one another. According to Wright and Leahey (2013, pp. 34–36), the major concepts of communication theory applied to families are:
- All nonverbal communication is meaningful.
- All communication has two major channels for transmission (digital, or verbal, communication; and analog or analogic communication, which includes all types of nonverbal communication as well as music, poetry, and painting)
- A dyadic (two-person) relationship has varying degrees of symmetry and complementarity (both of which may be healthy depending on context).
- All communication consists of two levels: content (what is said) and relationship (of those interacting).

Circular Communication

One example of a feedback system in communications is circular communication which is a reciprocal communication between two people. Wright and Leahey (2013, p. 128) note that most relationship issues have a pattern of circular communication. One person speaks and the other person interprets what is heard, then reacts and speaks on the basis of the interpretation, creating a circular feedback loop based on the individuals' perceptions and reactions.

Circular communication can be positive or negative. An example of negative circular communication is as follows: An angry wife criticizes her husband; the husband feels angry and withdraws; the wife becomes even angrier and criticizes more; the husband becomes angrier and withdraws further. Each person sees the problem as the other's, and each person's communication influences the other person's behavior. Positive and negative circular communication patterns are illustrated in Figure 33-5.

FAMILY ASSESSMENT

Wright and Leahey (2013) assert that family knowledge can be obtained and applied even in very brief meetings with a family.

Technique

Wright and Leahey provide a guide to a 15-minute (or shorter) family interview (pp. 263–277). Key elements of the interview, which occurs only in the context of a therapeutic relationship, are manners, therapeutic conversation, family genogram (and ecomap as appropriate), therapeutic questions, and commendations. See Box 33-3 for a summary of the interview technique, which reflects successful interview techniques in any form of family nursing. Essential points follow.

Manners

The simple acts of good manners that invite a trusting relationship are:

BOX 33-3 TIPS FOR CONDUCTING THE 15-MINUTE FAMILY INTERVIEW

- Introduce yourself and use good manners in interactions.
- Seek opportunities to involve family in care delivery and decision making.
- Use active listening, create family genograms (ecomaps), and ask key therapeutic questions to help family members (and the nurse) better understand the family's needs and beliefs about themselves and the illness.
- Seek opportunities to commend individuals and the family.

- Always call the client(s) by name.
- Introduce yourself by name.
- Examine your attitude and adjust responses to convey interest and acceptance.
- Explain your role for the time you will spend with the client/family.
- Explain any procedure before entering the room with equipment to perform the procedure.
- Keep appointments and promises to return.
- Be honest.

Therapeutic Conversation

Therapeutic conversation is purposeful and time limited; however nurse–family communications are therapeutic even though the nurse may not think of them as such (Wright & Leahey, 2013, p. 266). The art of listening is paramount. The nurse *not only* makes information giving and client involvement in decision making an integral part of the care delivery process but also seeks opportunities to engage in purposeful conversations with families. Nurse–family therapeutic conversations can include such basic ideas as:

- Invitations to accompany the client to the unit, clinic, or hospital
- Inclusion of family members in health care facility admission procedures
- Encouragement to ask questions during client orientation to a health care facility
- Acknowledgment of client and family's expertise in managing health problems by asking about routines at home
- Presentation of opportunities to practice how client will handle different interactions in the future such as telling family members and others that they cannot eat certain foods
- Consultation with families and clients about their ideas for treatment and discharge (Wright & Leahey, 2013, pp. 268–274)

Family Genograms and Ecomaps

The genogram (see Fig. 33-2) acts as a continuous visual reminder to caregivers to "think family." In addition, the ecomap (see Fig. 33-4) illustrates the family's interactions with outside systems.

Commendations

Offer at least one or two commendations during each meeting with the family. The individual or family can be commended on strengths, resources, or competencies observed or reported to the nurse. Commendations are observations of behavior. Look for patterns, not one-time occurrences to commend. Examples include "Your family shows much courage in living with your wife's cancer for 5 years"; "Your son is so gentle despite feeling so ill" (Wright & Leahey, 2000, p. 282). The commendations offer family members a new view of themselves. Wright and Leahey propose that many families experiencing illness, disability, or trauma have a "commendation-deficit disorder" (p. 282). Changing the view of themselves helps the family members to look differently at the health problem and more toward solutions.

General Routine Screening versus Focused Specialty Assessment of the Family

Family assessment varies with the nurse's level of education in family nursing and with the type of family nursing care to be provided. The usual approach to family assessment taken by nurses who are not specialists in family nursing is to focus on the individual as client and the family as context for the client's illness and care. This type of family assessment focuses on determining strengths and problem areas within the family's structure and function that influence development of the illness and the family's ability to support the client.

A more advanced knowledge of family nursing is required to care for the family as client. Using this approach, the nurse views the family unit as a system and does not focus on any one family member. Instead, the nurse works at all times simultaneously with a mental picture of the family system and the individuals in the system. The nurse caring for the family system can still provide care to the individual when necessary, but the primary assessment and interventions are directed toward the family as a dynamic system. The information provided in this chapter is relevant to either approach, but omits expert family systems nursing concepts.

Assessment Procedure

To complete a family assessment of structure, function, and development, the following outline provides a pattern and suggested questions to include. As appropriate, incorporate some of the following interview components/techniques in your practice.

ASSESSMENT PROCEDURE	NORMAL FINDINGS	ABNORMAL FINDINGS
Family Structure		
INTERNAL FAMILY STRUCTURE		
Assess family composition. Use a genogram and fill in as much information as possible. Ask the following questions: • What is the family type (nuclear, three-generation, single-parent)?	Family identifies family type and members of the family. A new baby born into family or young adult moving out reflects normal life-cycle tasks. Death is also a normal part of life, but it is not often viewed as a family strength.	A new baby or a young adult moving out may cause excessive stress for family. Death of a family member often causes a variety of different reactions including denial, extreme grief, depression, guilt, and even relief.

Continued on following page

ASSESSMENT PROCEDURE	NORMAL FINDINGS	ABNORMAL FINDINGS
Family Structure (Continued)		
• Who does the family consider to be family? • Has anyone recently moved in or out? Has anyone recently died?		Serious family problems may result when family members react to, and deal with, the death differently.
Determine gender roles in the family. Gender often determines an expected family role. Ask each family member the following question: What are the expected behaviors for men in your family? For women? 🎯 **CLINICAL TIP** It is important to ask both the men and women what they perceive to be the roles of men and women in the family because they may perceive the roles differently.	Family members understand and agree on expected gender-related behaviors; expected behaviors are flexible.	Rigid, traditional gender-related behaviors reduce the family's flexibility for meeting family needs. One or more family members have different beliefs about expected behaviors for men and women, which can lead to family conflict.
Evaluate rank order. Spousal rank order often plays a significant role in family harmony. Ask spouses: What rank order did you have in your childhood family (e.g., older sister, youngest brother)? Using the family's answers and information you know concerning birth order, ask yourself: Are spouses' birth rank orders likely to be complementary or competitive?	Complementary birth order of spouses can support each spouse's interaction with the other based on past experiences with siblings (e.g., older brother marries younger sister).	Competitive birth order of spouses may result in problems. For example, if an older brother marries an older sister, both may be used to being the responsible leader.
Assess subsystems and boundaries. See "Family Function" for questions.	Family subgroups are present and appear healthy. Permeable boundaries are present.	Family subgroups are absent or appear excessively strong, excluding other family members. Rigid or diffuse boundaries are present.
Evaluate the family power structure. Ask the family to rate the structure of the family on a scale with chaos (no leader) at one end, equality in the middle, and domination by one individual at the other end. If the family is dominated by one individual, ask the clients who that person is.	A power hierarchy with parents equally in control, but tending toward egalitarian and flexible power shifts, is considered normal. This type of structure demonstrates respect for all family members and encourages family development and effective functioning.	Chaotic or authoritarian power structures tend to prevent effective family functioning and individual development.
EXTERNAL STRUCTURE		
Assess the extended family. Ask the following: "Are extended family members available to help support your immediate family?"	Extended family can provide emotional and other support to the family.	Lack of extended family or no contact with extended family results in no support for immediate family.
Assess external systems. Ask the family questions about relationships with external systems (e.g., agencies and people outside immediate family). Use an ecomap to record and view these relationships. Then ask yourself the following questions based on the ecomap: What relationship is there between the family and external systems?	Positive relationships with external systems are beneficial to the family.	Conflicting relationships with external systems add stress to the family.

ASSESSMENT PROCEDURE	NORMAL FINDINGS	ABNORMAL FINDINGS
Are external systems overinvolved or underinvolved with the family?	Balanced involvement with external systems adds to the health of the family.	Too little or too much involvement with external systems can prevent the family from effectively using resources to meet its needs. In addition, either overinvolvement or underinvolvement with external systems can add great stress to the immediate family.
Assess context. Ask questions that relate to ethnicity, social class, religion, and environment. How does the family's race or ethnicity affect the family structure and function? How does the family's race or ethnicity affect interactions with neighbors? How does the family's race or ethnicity affect interactions with external systems?	A family that has a strong ethnic identity and lives in a similar ethnic society will usually have plentiful support. Living in a safe environment and with others of similar social class may positively affect family stress levels. Having all family members of the same racial/ethnic and social class backgrounds tends to reduce family stress (Wilt, 2002).	Racial or ethnic difference from the neighborhood or larger society can produce misunderstanding and negatively affect communications and interactions. Being of a social class different from those of the surrounding society or living in an unsafe environment may increase family stress. Different racial/ethnic or social class backgrounds within the family may increase family stress.
What social class is most representative of the family? Do social class factors affect the family's ability to meet its needs?	Cultural, social, and economic factors of the family's social class support the family's ability to meet its needs.	Cultural, social, and economic resources associated with social class may be inadequate to meet family needs.
Is religion important to the family?	Religion provides the family with supportive spiritual beliefs.	Religious controversies among family members may produce family conflict.
Are environmental characteristics of the residence and neighborhood adequate to meet family needs?	The residence and neighborhood are safe, and necessary resources are available.	The residence or neighborhood is not safe. Resources are not readily available.
Family Development: Life-Cycle Stages and Tasks		
Ask the family questions about the family's life-cycle stage(s). Can the family meet the tasks of the current life-cycle stage(s) with which it is dealing?	The family has successfully met the tasks of previous life-cycle stages and can meet the tasks of its current life-cycle stage.	The family has not adequately met tasks of previous life-cycle stages and may be unable to meet tasks of the current stage.
Family Function		
Assess instrumental function. Evaluate if the family can carry out routine ADLs. Does a family member's illness affect the family's ability to carry out ADLs?	The family has successfully met routine daily living needs of all family members. The family can continue to carry out ADLs even with the added stress of an ill family member.	The family cannot carry out one or more ADLs. The added stress of caring for an ill family member prevents the family from adequately carrying out one or more ADLs.
Note affective and socialization function. Observe family interactions and ask questions to determine if family members provide mutual support and nurturance to one another.	Families that can meet psychological needs for support and nurturance of family members provide an opportunity for each individual adequately to self-differentiate and reach emotional maturity.	Families that cannot provide for psychological needs for support and nurturance make self-differentiation and emotional health of the members unlikely.
Are parenting practices appropriate for healthy socialization of the children?	Parenting practices based on respect, guidance, and encouragement (rather than punishment) promote socialization.	Parenting practices based on control, coercion, and punishment discourage socialization. Chapter 10 discusses nursing assessment of families using violence.
What function do subgroups serve within the family?	Subgroups are flexible and assist the family to meet changing needs.	Rigid subgroups do not easily change to meet individual needs.

Continued on following page

ASSESSMENT PROCEDURE	NORMAL FINDINGS	ABNORMAL FINDINGS
Family Function (Continued)		
Are there alliances that produce triangles?	Flexible alliances and triangles form to maintain family functioning.	Rigid alliances and triangles are formed to balance negative forces and stress. They are used as coping mechanisms.
What function do boundaries serve within the family?	Permeable boundaries encourage emotional development and self-differentiation of family members.	Rigid or diffuse boundaries discourage emotional development and self-differentiation.
Are family members enmeshed (overly involved with each other)? Disengaged (underinvolved with each other)?	Adequate involvement of family members without enmeshment or disengagement serves as support for family function and individual development.	Enmeshed or disengaged family members cannot adequately self-differentiate.
Evaluate expressive function. Ask the family questions and observe interactions to assess emotional communication. Do all family members express a broad range of both negative and positive emotion?	Open expression and acceptance of feelings and emotions within a family encourage positive family functioning.	Lack of acceptance of emotional expression or acceptance of emotional expression by only some family members tends to prevent effective family development and functioning.
Assess verbal communication. Are verbal messages clearly stated?	Clear verbal messages increase open communication.	Displaced, masked, or distorted messages obstruct open communication and may reflect underlying problems in family functioning.
Assess nonverbal communication. Do nonverbal communications match verbal content?	Clear and open communications have verbal and nonverbal elements that match.	Nonverbal communications that do not match verbal content suggest a lack of honesty or openness in the communication.
Assess circular communication. Is there an evident pattern of circular communication? If so, is it negative or positive?	Positive circular communication helps to build up the participants.	Negative circular communication reinforces interpersonal conflict and prevents an understanding of the intended message.
Assess the family's health care function. Ask the following questions: • What do family members believe about the etiology, treatment, prognosis of the health problem? • What do family members believe about the role of professionals, role of the family, and level of control the family has relative to the health problem? Are family members' beliefs in agreement or discord?	Agreement among family members reduces conflict.	Disagreement among family members produces conflict and draws on energy and emotional resources needed to handle the health problem.
What strengths do the family members believe they have for coping with the health problem?	If the family members perceive strengths, they will be more likely to cope effectively.	If the family members do not perceive strengths, they will have difficulty coping with the health problem.
Are the family's health promotion practices supportive of family health?	A pattern of health promotion practices provides a basis for building in health care for a particular health problem.	A family that has little practice of health promotion behaviors will have difficulty incorporating health care practices for a particular problem into its routines.
Assess for multigenerational patterns. Look back over the assessment and determine if there are any multigenerational patterns evident in any categories.	Multigenerational patterns of positive behaviors are often seen in effectively functioning families.	Multigenerational patterns of ineffective or destructive behaviors make change more difficult.

CASE STUDY

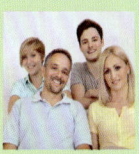

After establishing a therapeutic relationship with the Ross family, the nurse interviews the family, using therapeutic questions. The family reports family stress and conflict about Dan's (a 17-year-old high school senior) recent diagnosis of type 1 diabetes. The nurse explores this health concern using the COLDSPA mnemonic.

Mnemonic	Question	Data Provided
Character	Describe the sign or symptom (feeling, appearance, sound, smell, or taste if applicable). In this case, describe the family members' reactions to the diagnosis and treatment of Dan's diabetes.	Family conflict has developed over Dan not following the prescribed diet-exercise-insulin protocol. Repeated visits to the ED and the threats to his long-term health have exacerbated the family stress.
Onset	When did it begin?	Four months ago at diagnosis.
Location	Where is it? Does it radiate? Does it occur anywhere else?	The conflict between Dan and his parents and his sister have escalated.
Duration	How long does it last? Does it recur?	The conflicted interactions have become more frequent as the time nears for Dan to go away to university.
Severity	How bad is it? How much does it bother you?	All family members describe the conflict and its effect as very stressful, both to their interactions as a family and, for Dan, to his interactions with his peers.
Pattern	What makes it better or worse?	Mealtimes make it worse, and there is increasing family stress with repeated visits to ED.
Associated factors/How it **A**ffects the client	What other symptoms occur with it? How does it affect you?	Dan's age of 17 brings up the issues of family development states beginning to change, anticipation of Dan exiting the family when he leaves for college, as well as his developmental tasks being threatened by his inability to "be like his friends."

The nurse interviews the family about structure. The family is composed of two parents and two adolescent children (son Dan, 17 years old, and daughter Jenna, 12 years old)—a two-generation family. Family members agree on expected gender-related behaviors, which are flexible. The wife is the youngest daughter of her family, and the husband is the oldest son of his family. Subgroups and triangles between family members are flexible. The boundaries between subgroups are permeable. The nurse explores power. The two parents report that they are equally in control, but the children are consulted for decisions that affect the family. The nurse asks about extended family and support systems. Mr. Ross's mother lives in a nearby town but is not able to provide physical support to the family, although she is emotionally supportive. The family is positively involved in the local church, Dan has a group of supportive friends, and the parents enjoy being involved with the local garden club. Time spent with groups outside the family is balanced evenly with time spent with the immediate family. The nurse asks about the environment. The family lives in a safe home and in a neighborhood with people of similar ethnicity. The family's cultural, social, and economic factors support their ability to live well. The family is currently able to meet the tasks of its life-cycle stage, although the family is facing Dan's departure for college in 6 months' time. The family has met routine ADL needs of its members. The family provides the psychological needs for support and nurturance of all family members, although Dan does not feel supported and the family is conflicted on how best to support him with the new diagnosis and treatment protocol. Family members feel free to express and accept feelings and emotions openly, although Dan's increasing rebellious attitude and anger are new and are increasing family stress. Completing the Ross family assessment, the nurse asks questions about diabetes within the family and how the family has handled stressful situations in the past. The nurse asks how everyone feels about Dan's disease and treatment. Both the parents and Jenna appear tense when describing the effect of trying to deal with Dan's disease and his refusal to follow the protocol. Mr. and Mrs. Ross express frustration with inability to get Dan to follow the doctor's orders. Dan expresses frustration at having a disease and at being asked to follow a protocol that makes him different from his friends and unable to do the things that they do (e.g., partying). Dan expresses frustration at having his parents tell him what to do. Jenna expresses frustration at Dan for upsetting the family, especially at mealtime, particularly in regard to what family members eat and how they interact. When the nurse asks the family about Dan's disease and treatment, Dan and his parents describe a good understanding of the disease and reasons for the protocol. Multigenerational patterns of positive behaviors are described by this family. The nurse observes family interactions during the assessment. Negative circular communication is seen between Dan and his parents and sister.

Validating and Documenting Findings

Validate the family assessment data that you have collected (by asking additional questions, verifying data with another health care professional, or comparing objective with subjective findings). This is necessary to verify that the data are reliable and accurate. Document the assessment data following the health care facility or agency policy.

CASE STUDY

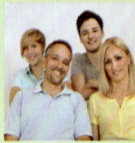

Think back to the case of the Ross family. The nurse completes the following documentation, including a genogram (Fig. 33-6).

Biographical Data: Two parents: Alan, 40; Kate, 38. Two children: Dan, 17; Jenna, 12.

Family Assessment: Members agree on expected gender roles and are flexible. Mrs. Ross is the youngest daughter of her family; Mr. Ross is the oldest son of his family. Subgroups and triangles between family members are flexible. Boundaries between subgroups are permeable.

Two parents equally in control; children consulted for decisions affecting family. Mr. Ross's mother lives close by. She cannot provide physical care, but she is emotionally supportive. Family is positively involved in the local church, Dan and Jenna each have a group of supportive friends, and the parents are involved with the local garden club.

Time spent outside the family is balanced with time spent with the family.

Live in a safe home and in a neighborhood with people of similar ethnicity. Cultural, social, and economic factors support ability to live well. Currently able to meet the tasks of its life-cycle stage, although Dan leaves for college in 6 months. Meets routine ADLs. Meets the psychological needs for support and nurturance of all family members. Dan does not feel supported and the family is conflicted on how best to support him with the new diagnosis and treatment protocol. Family members feel free to express and accept feelings and emotions openly, although Dan's increasing rebellious attitude and anger are new and are increasing family stress. Family recognizes risk to Dan's long-term health, but Dan does not believe the danger outweighs the restrictions the disease management has imposed on his life. Multigenerational patterns are positive. Negative circular communication seen between Dan and his parents and sister.

ANALYSIS OF DATA: DIAGNOSTIC REASONING

After collecting subjective and objective data pertaining to family assessment, identify abnormal findings and client strengths using diagnostic reasoning. Then, cluster the data to reveal any significant patterns or abnormalities. The following sections provide possible conclusions that the nurse may make after assessing a family.

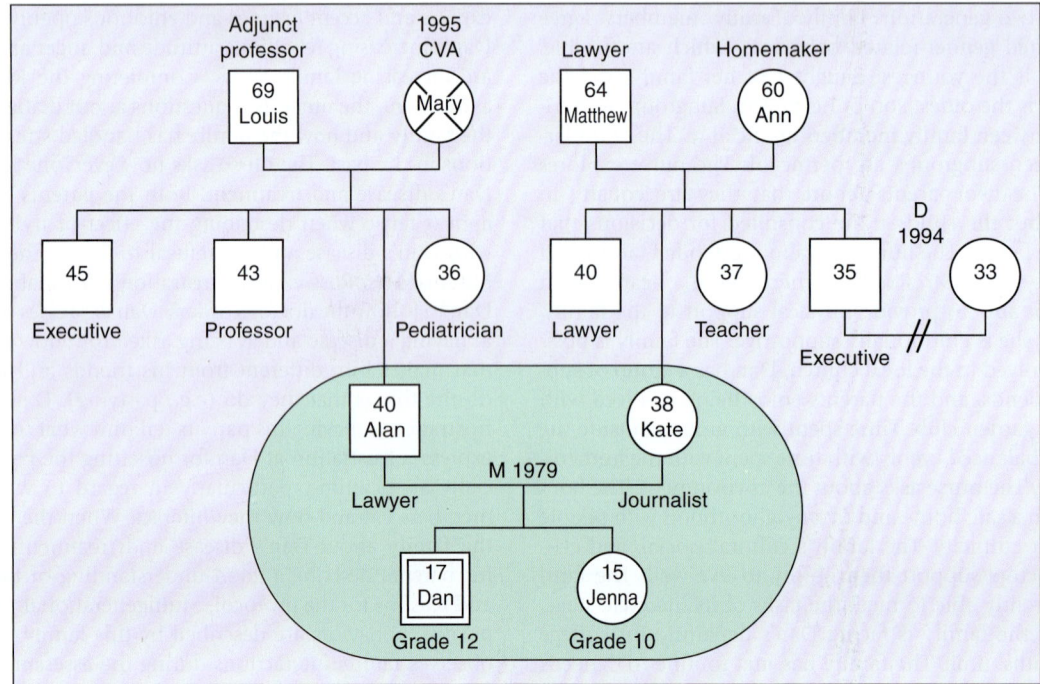

FIGURE 33-6 Genogram of the Ross family.

Selected Nursing Diagnoses

The following is a list of selected nursing diagnoses that may be identified when analyzing data from a family assessment.

Health Promotion Diagnoses
- Readiness for Enhanced Family Coping
- Readiness for Enhanced Spiritual Well-Being
- Readiness for Enhanced Parenting
- Readiness for Enhanced Home Maintenance
- Readiness for Enhanced Family Processes

Risk Diagnoses
- Risk for Caregiver Role Strain
- Risk for Impaired Parent/Infant/Child Attachment
- Risk for Impaired Parenting
- Risk for Compromised Family Coping
- Risk for Dysfunctional Family Processes
- Risk for Impaired Home Maintenance

Actual Diagnoses
- Caregiver Role Strain
- Interrupted Family Processes
- Compromised Family Coping
- Ineffective Family Coping: Disabling
- Dysfunctional Family Processes: Alcoholism
- Interrupted Family Processes
- Impaired Home Maintenance
- Ineffective Family Health Management
- Parental Role Conflict
- Impaired Parenting
- Impaired Social Interaction
- Loneliness
- Spiritual Distress
- Ineffective Role Performance

Selected Collaborative Problems

After grouping the data, certain collaborative problems may emerge. Remember that collaborative problems differ from nursing diagnoses in that they cannot be prevented by nursing interventions. However, these physiologic complications of medical conditions can be detected and monitored by the nurse. In addition, the nurse can use physician- and nurse-prescribed interventions to minimize the complications of these problems. The nurse may also have to refer the client in such situations for further treatment of the problem. Following is a list of collaborative problems that may be identified when assessing the family. These problems are worded as Risk for Complications (RC), followed by the problem.
- RC: Marital conflict
- RC: Child abuse
- RC: Spouse abuse

Medical Problems

After grouping the data, it may become apparent that the family has signs and symptoms that may require medical or mental health professional diagnosis and treatment. Referral to a primary care provider is necessary.

CASE STUDY

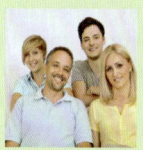

The nurse uses diagnostic reasoning to analyze the data collected on the Ross family to arrive at the following possible conclusions.

Nursing Diagnoses
- Compromised Family Coping
- Interrupted Family Processes
- Ineffective Family Health Management
- Risk for Ineffective Family Coping: Disabling
- Readiness for Enhanced Family Processes
- Readiness for Enhanced Family Coping

Potential Collaborative Problems
- RC: Depression (one or more family members)
- RC: Marital Conflict

To view an algorithm depicting the process for diagnostic reasoning in this case, go to thePoint.

Interdisciplinary Verbal Communication of Assessment Findings Using SBAR

SITUATION: The Ross family (parents: Alan, 40; Kate, 38. Two children: Dan, 17; Jenna, 12) come to clinic for help in dealing with Dan's recent diagnosis and treatment for type 1 diabetes. Dan, high school senior going to college in 6 months, was diagnosed with type 1 diabetes 4 months ago. He is not following the diet–exercise–insulin protocol. He has been seen by his physician and in the ED five times in past 4 months for DM complications from not following the protocol. Because the diet and food preparation affect the whole family, sister Jenna is also present.

BACKGROUND: Family flexible with expected behaviors and subgroups and triangles between family members. Parents make most decisions but consult children if decision affects whole family. Mr. Ross's mother provides emotional but not physical support. Family active in local church; Dan has a group of supportive friends. Time is balanced between time spent with groups outside the family and time spent with the immediate family. Family meets the tasks of its life-cycle stage. Dan does not feel supported and the family is conflicted on how best to support him with the new diagnosis and treatment protocol. Family members able to express emotions openly, although Dan's rebellious attitude and anger are new and are increasing family stress.

ASSESSMENT: Both the parents and Jenna appear tense when describing the effect of trying to deal with Dan's disease and his refusal to follow the protocol. Mr. and Mrs. Ross express frustration with inability to get Dan to follow the doctor's orders. Dan expresses frustration at having a disease and at being asked to follow a protocol that makes him different from his friends and unable to do the things that they do (e.g., partying). Dan expresses frustration at having his parents tell him what to do. Jenna expresses frustration at Dan for upsetting the family, especially at mealtime, particularly in regard to what family members eat and how they interact. When the nurse asks the family about Dan's disease and treatment, Dan and his parents describe a good understanding of the disease and reasons for the protocol. Multigenerational patterns of positive behaviors are described by this family. However, negative circular communication is seen between Dan and his parents and sister. Family recognizes risk to Dan's long-term health, but Dan does not believe the danger outweighs the restrictions the disease management has imposed on his life.

RECOMMENDATION: This family has Compromised Family Coping, Interrupted Family Processes, and Ineffective Family Health Management. They are ready for Enhanced Family Processes and Enhanced Family Coping. There is a risk for Ineffective Family Coping: Disabling, possible Depression (one or more family members), and Marital Conflict. A plan needs to be developed that is acceptable for Dan to effectively manage his own diabetes in preparation for college.

Want to know more?

A wide variety of resources to enhance your learning and understanding of this book are available on thePoint. Visit thePoint to access:

NCLEX-Style Student Review Questions
Watch and Learn Videos
Concept in Action Animations
And more!

References and Selected Readings

Bell, J. (2011). Relationships: The heart of the matter in family nursing [Editorial]. *Journal of Family Nursing, 17*(1), 3–10.

Bell, J. (2013). Family nursing is more than family centered care [Editorial]. *Journal of Family Nursing, 19*(4), 411–417. doi:10.1177/1074840713512750

Bell, J. (2014). Advanced practice competencies: Family systems nursing. Available at http://janicembell.com/2014/10/advanced-practice-competencies-family-systems-nursing/

Family Caregivers Alliance. (2016). Caregiver statistics: Demographics. Available at https://www.caregiver.org/caregiver-statistics-demographics

Friedman, M. (1998). *Family nursing: Theory and practice* (4th ed.). Norwalk, CT: Appleton & Lange.

Friedman, M., Bowden, V., & Jones, E. (Eds.). (2003). *Family nursing: Research, theory and practice* (5th ed.).Upper Saddle River, NJ: Prentice Hall.

Kaakinen, J., Coehlo, D., Steele, R., Tabacco, A., & Hanson, S. (2015). *Family health care nursing: Theory, practice, and research* (5th ed.). Philadelphia, PA: F.A. Davis.

Kafka, P. (2008). Structural family therapy: An effective approach to understanding and healing families. Available at http://pauline-kafka.suite101.com/structural-family-therapy-a61267

McGoldrick, M., Preto, N., & Carter, B. (2016). *The expanding family life cycle* (5th ed.). Boston, MA: Pearson.

The Bowen Center. (n.d.). Bowen theory. Available at http://www.thebowencenter.org/pages/theory.html

Titelman, P. (Ed.). (2008). *Triangles: Bowen family systems theory perspectives.* New York: The Haworth Press.

Wilt, J. (2002). Normal families facing unique challenges: The psychosocial functioning of multiracial couples, parents and children. *The New School Psychology Bulletin, 9*(1), 34–41. Available at http://www.thebowencenter.org/pages/theory.html

Wright, L., & Leahey, M. (2000). *Nurses and families: A guide to family assessment and intervention.* Philadelphia, PA: F. A. Davis.

Wright, L., & Leahey, M. (2013). *Nurses and families: A guide to family assessment and intervention* (6th ed.). Philadelphia, PA: F.A. Davis.

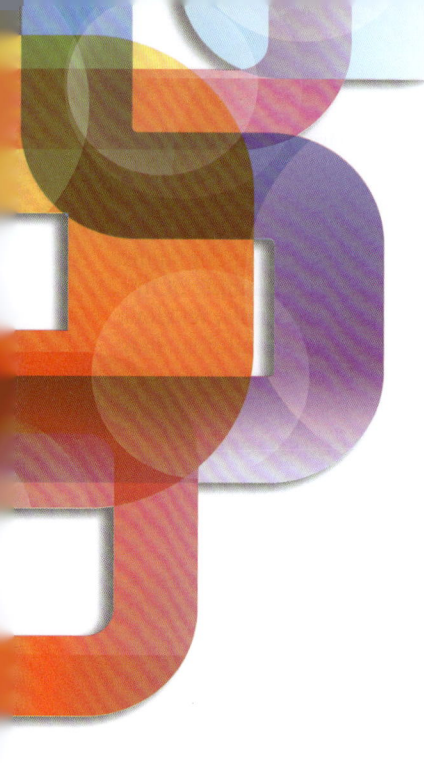

34 ASSESSING COMMUNITIES

Learning Objectives

1. Discuss various definitions of "community."
2. Explore how the history of a community affects its current health status.
3. Discuss risk factors associated with placing the community's health at risk.
4. Describe how to obtain information and effectively interview community members to obtain an accurate history of the community.
5. Complete an effective community assessment using a variety of resources to obtain necessary data.
6. Differentiate between skills needed to assess community resources needed for a client and a complete comprehensive community assessment.
7. Differentiate between normal and abnormal findings that affect the health of a community and its members.
8. Analyze the data from the interview and assessment of a community to formulate valid nursing diagnoses, collaborative problems, and/or referrals.
9. Communicate community interview and assessment findings through clear concise documentation and verbal reports.
10. Differentiate between general routine screening versus skills needed for focused or specialty assessment of a community.

CASE STUDY

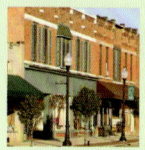

As part of a statewide public health initiative and assessment of resources, a nurse evaluates the town of Maple Grove. The small, rural Midwestern community was originally settled by Native Americans, but later was settled by German immigrants who established a lumber/logging industry. Over the years, the economic base has deteriorated and the population has decreased over the last 10 years to fewer than 2,500 people. Median household and median personal income are below the national averages, and the unemployment rate is higher than the national average. Ethnic composition is predominantly Caucasian of German descent and the predominant religion is Lutheran. Health care resources are available in the region, but only a few are located in the community itself. The nurse's assessment of Maple Grove will be discussed throughout the chapter. It is an abbreviated case study of an assessment of a small town. In actual practice, a thorough assessment of a community would require more in-depth data collection than is described in this vignette. Such assessments may be quite lengthy, which is beyond the scope of this book.

CONCEPTUAL FOUNDATIONS

The purpose of community assessment is to determine the health-related concerns of its members, regardless of the type of the community. The nurse gets to know the community, its people, its history, and its culture through the assessment process. A thorough and accurate assessment provides the foundation for diagnosis and for planning appropriate nursing interventions.

Definition of Community

A thorough assessment of a community first requires an understanding of the concept of community. *Community* may be defined several ways depending on the conceptual view of the term, but two common ways of understanding it are community of place and community of interest. A combination of place and interest are reflected in the sociologic perspective. Three definitions are offered from the field of sociology (Sociology Guide, 2011):

1. Collections of people with a "particular social structure"
2. A group with a "sense of belonging or community spirit"
3. A group for which "all the daily activities of a community, work and nonwork, take place within the geographical area, which is self contained"

Another definition of *community* that is broad enough to encompass place and interest is an "open social system

869

characterized by people in a place over time who have common goals" (Maurer & Smith, 2013, p. 341).

Classification of community, then, depends on the definition. For purposes of assessment, communities are classified according to either location or social relationship. The first classification is a geopolitical community in which people have a time-and-space relationship. Geopolitical communities may be determined by natural boundaries such as rivers, lakes, or mountain ranges. For example, the Mississippi River separates the states of Missouri and Illinois. Geopolitical boundaries also may be manmade: counties, cities, voting districts, or school districts. Another example of a geopolitical community is a census tract, which is determined by the government to organize demographic data collection.

As noted previously, communities also may be classified by relationships among a group of people. These communities are usually centered on a specific goal or function. For example, a group such as Mothers Against Drunk Driving (MADD) may center on eliciting support for a new ordinance regulating hours of bars and taverns. These types of communities can be organized to address a common interest or problem, such as a state student nurses' association or a support group for family and friends of Alzheimer's patients. Another example of this type of community is a group of people with similar religious or political beliefs. Any number of social communities may exist within the boundaries of a geopolitical community.

Models of Community Assessment

A number of different models or frameworks have been used to provide the structure for assessing both geopolitical and social communities.

The Community as Partner model provides a comprehensive guide for data collection (Fig. 34-1) (Anderson &

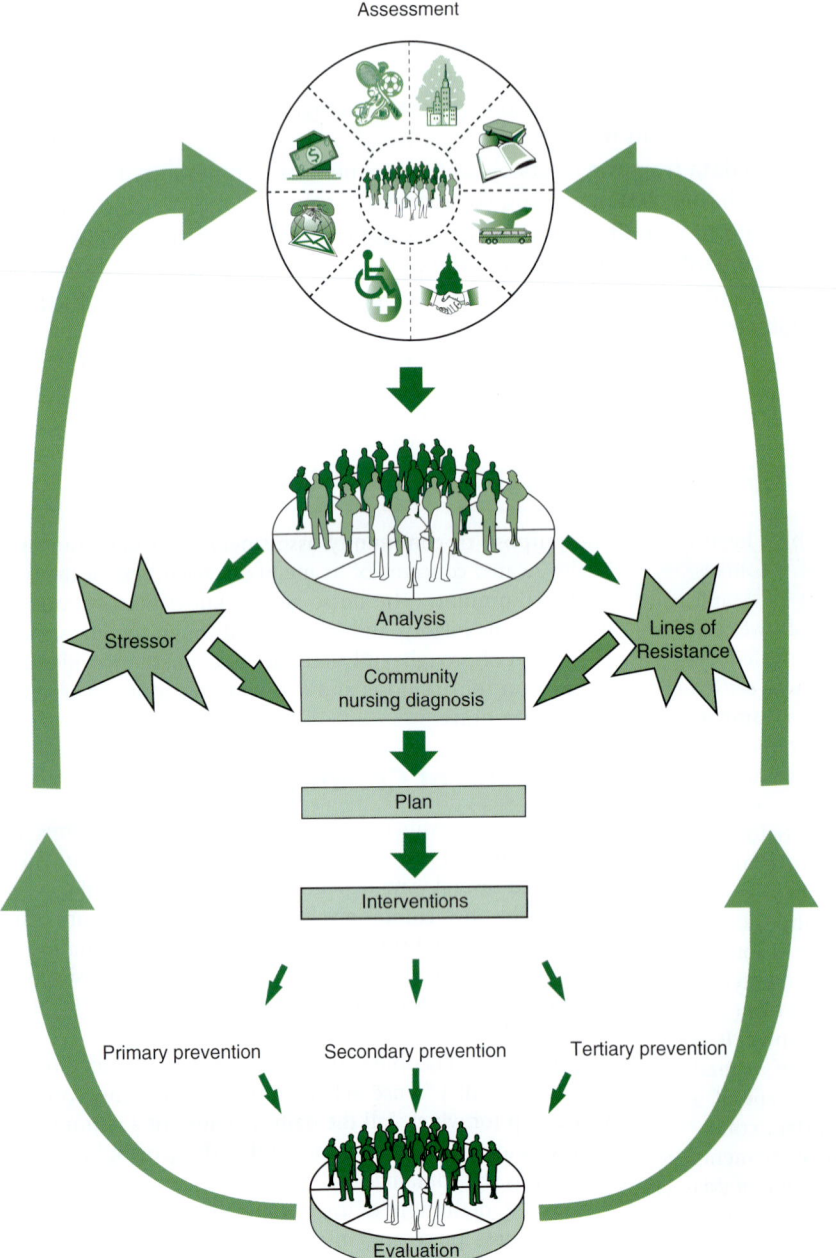

FIGURE 34-1 Community as Partner model (From Anderson, E., & McFarlane, J. (2014). *Community as Partner* (7th ed.) Philadelphia, PA: Wolters Kluwer Health.)

McFarlane, 2015). Central to the model are the people, or core, of the community. This component includes demographic information as well as information about the history, culture, values, and beliefs of the people. Also identified are eight subsystems that are affected by the people of the community and that directly contribute to the health status of the community. These include housing, fire and safety, health, education, economics, politics and government, communication, and recreation. Community assessment in this model follows Neuman's systems nursing theory model, which includes identifying stressors and lines of defense and resistance that affect, in this case, the community. The Community as Partner model has been adapted for use in this chapter.

The Centers for Disease Control and Prevention (CDC, 2016) has a specific assessment for community emergencies, but is useful for both disaster and nondisaster settings. The Community Assessment for Public Health Emergency Response (CASPER) is an epidemiologic technique designed to provide quickly and at low-cost household-based information about a community. The Casper toolkit (CDC, 2012) provides guidelines on data collection tool development, methodology, sample selection, training, data collection, analysis, and report writing.

COMMUNITY ASSESSMENT

Community assessment involves both subjective and objective data collection using a variety of methods. Subjective data collection includes perceptions of the community by the nurse as well as by members of the community. The nurse should spend time in the community to "get to know" the people and get a sense of their values and beliefs.

Through the process of participant observation, the nurse hopes to become accepted as a member of the community. This method of data collection allows the nurse to participate in the daily life of the community, make observations, and obtain information about the structures and influences that affect the community. The nurse should ask key members or leaders of the community as well as "typical" residents to provide further information and insight about the community. Objective methods of data collection include using surveys and analyzing existing data such as census information, health records, and other public documents. (See http://guides.lib.unc.edu/CommunityHealhAssessment from University of North Carolina Health Sciences Library [2015] for how to locate data and statistics for a community assessment.)

The assessment section outlines a step-by-step assessment of the community. Within each assessment topic, three aspects of community should be considered: people, environment, and health. The nursing component is inherent throughout each topic considered.

> **General Routine Screening versus Focused Specialty Assessment of Communities**
>
> All nurses need to be aware of how the community in which clients live has an influence on their holistic health status. However, nurses working in acute care would not perform a complete community assessment but would assess the community resources available to their clients. A complete community assessment would be completed by a Community, Public Health Nurse, or Advanced Practice Nurse in order to meet the needs of the clients in a specific community.

ASSESSMENT PROCEDURE	NORMAL FINDINGS	ABNORMAL FINDINGS
Community History		
Study the history of the community. Look for this information at the local library or ask local residents. Use this information to gain insights into the health practices and belief systems of community members.	The community history should include initial development, any specific ethnic groups that may have settled there, past economic trends, and past population trends.	The history of some communities may include episodes that have had a disruptive influence on the people of the community such as relocation because of repeated flooding, a history of racial or ethnic problems, or the closing of a factory.
Demographic Information		
Obtain age and gender information from census data. Age is the most important risk factor for health-related problems. Gender may be another important risk factor.	A healthy/typical community has a distribution of individuals in various age ranges: younger than 5 years, 5–19, 20–34, 35–54, 55–64, and 65+ years, as well as no significant difference between percentages of men and women.	Communities with a large percentage of elderly people or very young children generally have more health-related issues. Communities with a preponderance of women of child-bearing age may need to improve access to or expand family planning and prenatal services as well as well-baby programs.
Study census figures and state and local population reports. Use this information to learn about racial and ethnic groups that reside in the community.	Programs and special screening are congruent with the needs of the racial and ethnic groups in the community.	Special programs and screenings are not available in proportion to the racial and ethnic population.

Continued on following page

ASSESSMENT PROCEDURE	NORMAL FINDINGS	ABNORMAL FINDINGS
Demographic Information (Continued)		
Obtain vital statistics data. These data can be obtained from the National Center for Health Statistics, state and local agencies, and from hospital records. These include birth and death records as well as crude death rates (age and cause), specific death rates, and infant–maternal mortality. Morbidity (disease) data also are important indicators of the health status of the community.	Expected birth, death, and morbidity data should generally reflect overall rates for the United States. See Boxes 34-1, 34-2, and 34-3 for age-related causes of mortality.	Higher-than-expected birth, death, and morbidity rates, especially age- and cause-specific rates, may indicate a lack of services or programs in critical areas. For example, higher-than-expected teen birth rates may be related to a lack of family planning services or education; high mortality rates associated with motor vehicles, especially when alcohol is involved, indicate that alcohol awareness programs should be instituted; and greater-than-expected rates of tuberculosis or sexually transmitted infections (STIs) indicate that primary and secondary prevention efforts should be increased.
Refer to the U.S. Census Bureau for the following information: Number of people per household, their marital status, and the stability of the population.	The Census Bureau identifies three major types of households: Married couple (Fig. 34-2), female householder (no husband present), and male householder (no woman present). The nature and size of households in the United States have changed significantly in the last 50 years. Household size has decreased from 3.3–2.58 persons per household. The number of divorced people has quadrupled since 1970. According to the U.S. Census Bureau (2015a), just over 50% of adults today live with a spouse, which has decreased from 70% in 1967. The U.S. Census Bureau (2015b) reported that in 2013, there were 7 million unmarried partner households, in 2014 there were 58 million households maintained by unmarried women or men, and 34 million people lived alone. The number of female family households or sole providers (for families with children under 18 years of age) had risen from 10.8% in 1960 to 40.4% in 2011 (Wang et al., 2013). Generations United (2015) reported that by 2010, one in six Americans lived in multigenerational family households (16.1%). Americans also are a mobile population, moving for education, jobs, or retirement. A healthy community adjusts to these changes and organizes to meet the needs of the population.	**S**ingle parents (teenage mothers and fathers, in particular) are at greater risk for health problems, especially those related to role overload. This occurs because single parents often have to assume the role of the missing parent in addition to their own roles. Single mothers report a higher incidence of children's academic and behavioral problems than mothers in two-parent families. Unmarried people have a higher mortality rate than do married people. Older adults living alone also are at higher risk for health problems. In addition, some immigrant groups, such as migrant farm families, are at higher risk. Communities that do not adapt to meet the needs of the mobile population compromise the continuity and quality of care for these people.

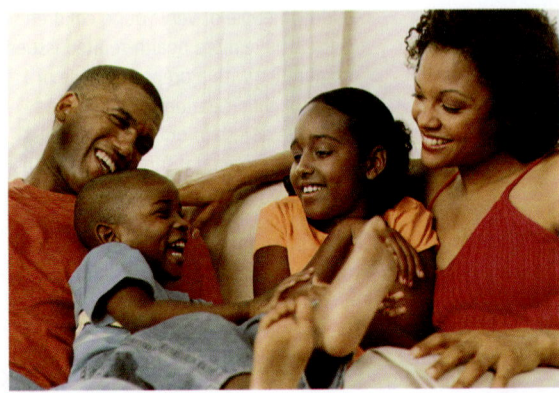

FIGURE 34-2 One of the three types of households cited by the Bureau of the Census is a married couple with children.

34 Assessing Communities   873

ASSESSMENT PROCEDURE	NORMAL FINDINGS	ABNORMAL FINDINGS
Obtain data to determine values and religious beliefs of the community. These data can be obtained from the local Chamber of Commerce, community directories, surveys, and personal observation and interviews. Each community's values are unique, rooted in tradition, and exist to meet the needs of the population. Religious beliefs and culture are closely related to the community's values (Fig. 34-3).	Healthy communities demonstrate an awareness and respect for different values and religions. There is a deliberate effort among various subgroups to communicate and to work together. Many communities form ministerial alliances, in which various denominations collaborate to meet the needs of the community. They may provide emergency shelters, operate soup kitchens or food pantries, and provide help for special populations. Certain religious beliefs directly affect health practices, such as use of family planning services.	Some communities exhibit conflict among subgroups. Different values, beliefs, and practices are seen as a threat to one group's own values and beliefs. An unhealthy community may fail to recognize the existence of cultural or religious differences and believe that all members of the community should conform to one set of values. In such communities, anyone who does not fit the accepted norm is "suspect." Such an atmosphere does not enhance the overall health status of the community, which makes it difficult or even impossible for members to collaborate on problem solving.

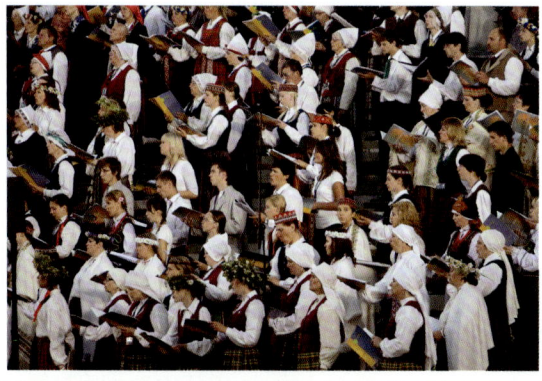

FIGURE 34-3 Community values and religious beliefs are unique and rooted in tradition.

Physical Environment

Identify geographic boundaries of the community. This information may be obtained from the library or local assessor's office.	Boundaries of a community should be clear, uncontested, and accepted by all members.	Boundaries may not always be clearly identified, and communities may not be able to resolve disputes without legal action. One community may seek to annex part of another because of access to certain resources, or a group or neighborhood may attempt to separate legally from the larger community because of ideologic differences, zoning regulations, or other issues. Disagreement about such issues may disrupt delivery of services.
Identify the neighborhood(s) that comprise the area. Note characteristics. Neighborhoods have specific populations and boundaries and may vary a great deal in culture, leadership, and ties to the larger community. They may be composed of certain ethnic groups, economic classes, or age groups.	Neighborhoods should be cohesive, with a sense of identity, yet have strong ties to the larger community.	Some neighborhoods may seek to isolate themselves from the larger community or may be resistant to others who wish to move into the neighborhood. In such situations, conflicts often arise and mistrust may be widespread.
Obtain housing information from census documents, local housing authority, and local realtors. A community should provide a variety of housing options.	A healthy community can provide enough safe, affordable housing to meet the needs of its members. Communities must seek to meet the needs of their homeless members as well. Due to partial recovery from the economic depression of recent years, the overall rate of "homelessness from 2013 to 2014 decreased by 2.3% and homelessness decreased among every major subpopulation:	A lack of adequate housing may be a serious problem in some communities. A shortage of safe, low-income housing contributes directly to the growing number of homeless individuals and families. Other communities may have a serious shortage of adequate rental property or special housing for the elderly or disabled. Inadequate housing contributes to various

Continued on following page

ASSESSMENT PROCEDURE	NORMAL FINDINGS	ABNORMAL FINDINGS
Physical Environment (Continued)		
	unsheltered persons (10%), families (2.7%), chronically homeless individuals (2.5%), and veterans (10.5%)" (National Alliance to End Homelessness, 2016, p. 1).	health problems related to safety, lead poisoning, and communicable diseases.
Determine climate and geographic terrain of the area. This information may be obtained from the local library, government agencies, and direct observation. Climate varies from region to region, as does geographic terrain. Both have a direct effect on the health of the community.	Healthy communities have the resources to deal with whatever problems climate and terrain present. Such problems include extreme cold or heat, floods, fires, blizzards, tornadoes, and earthquakes. Certain health problems may be more prevalent in particular geographic areas (e.g., West Nile virus, Hanta virus). Safety programs, civil defense and disaster plans, and health education programs should be in place.	Communities inadequately prepared to deal with disasters or health problems related to climate or terrain do not sufficiently meet the needs of their members. This may result in a higher incidence of the following problems: heat exhaustion, deaths due to overexposure to cold, myocardial infarctions related to shoveling snow, skin cancers, infectious diseases, and deaths and injuries related to other natural disasters.
Health and Social Services		
Determine the number of health care facilities and providers available to the community. Information about health services can be obtained from the Chamber of Commerce, local professional organizations, telephone directories, and from personal interviews and observations.	A healthy community provides adequate primary health care services (Fig. 34-4). These services include private and nonprofit facilities staffed with physicians, nurse practitioners, nurses, and ambulance paramedics who provide medical/surgical, obstetric/gynecologic, pediatric, emergency, and various diagnostic and preventive services. Specialty services, such as neonatal intensive care, should be easily accessible to the community. In addition to physicians and nurses,	Many communities (particularly rural ones) cannot provide needed services, especially in obstetric care. It is not unusual for a person to be 100 miles or more away from the nearest services. In addition, funding problems have caused many small rural hospitals to close, leaving residents miles away from any health care at all. Ambulance service also may be of concern for some communities. Accessibility may be limited because fewer health care providers

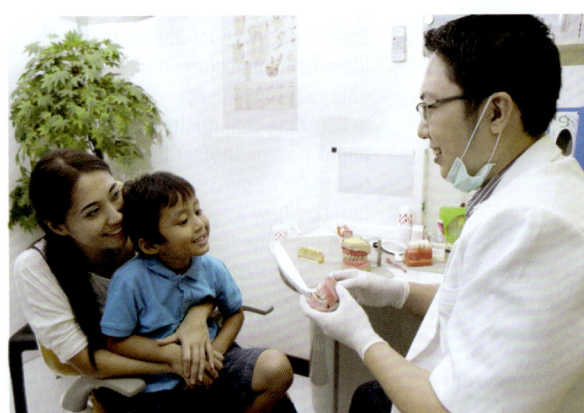

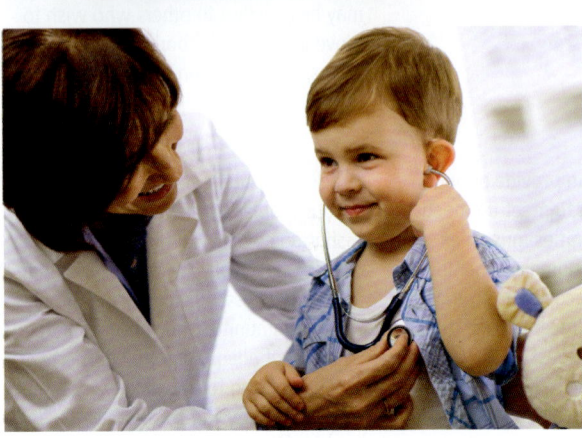

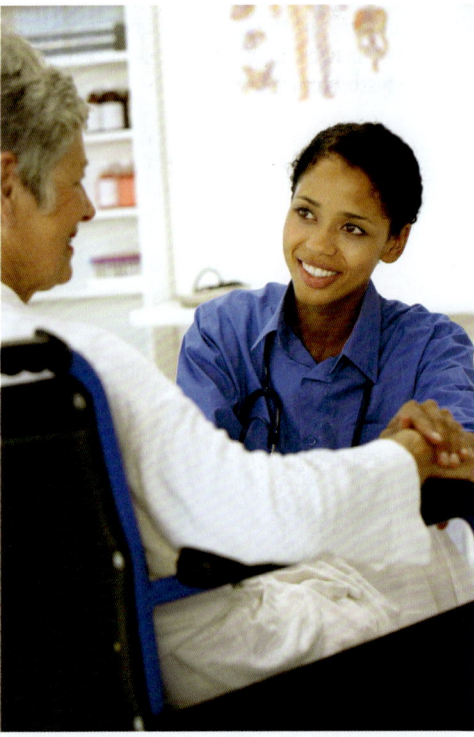

FIGURE 34-4 Healthy communities have access to adequate primary health care services.

ASSESSMENT PROCEDURE	NORMAL FINDINGS	ABNORMAL FINDINGS
	the health care delivery system should include dentists, physical therapists, and dietitians, among others. Facilities and providers should accept third-party reimbursement including insurance, workers' compensation, Medicare, and Medicaid.	are willing to accept some types of third-party reimbursement, especially Medicaid. The Zika virus spread from Africa, South America, and the Caribbean to the United States is expected to put stress on the U.S. health care system.
Obtain data concerning public health and home health services. This information can be obtained from local directories, the Chamber of Commerce, and personal interviews. Local public health agencies have the responsibility for protecting the health of the general population. Program objectives are related to primary prevention and early diagnosis, and are directed toward meeting health objectives of the federal program Healthy People 2020. Home health care is a fast-growing component of the health care system as hospital stays become briefer while the need for skilled care remains.	Local public health services are usually delivered through county or city health departments. Health promotion programs also may be offered through nonofficial agencies such as hospitals. Home health services may be provided through a number of different agencies such as a Visiting Nurses Association (VNA), official agencies, and free-standing proprietary agencies. Services provided include skilled nursing care, homemaker and home health aides, medical social services, nutritional consultation, and rehabilitation services (Fig. 34-5).	Many public health services are supported through local tax revenues. Therefore, small rural communities may not be able to provide the types of services needed, and limited access to these services may be another problem. Certain services may not be offered by home health agencies, and funding to cover visits for people who are not eligible for third-party reimbursement may be limited.

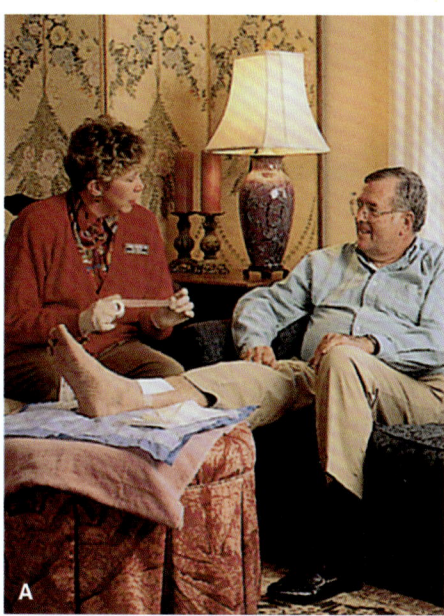
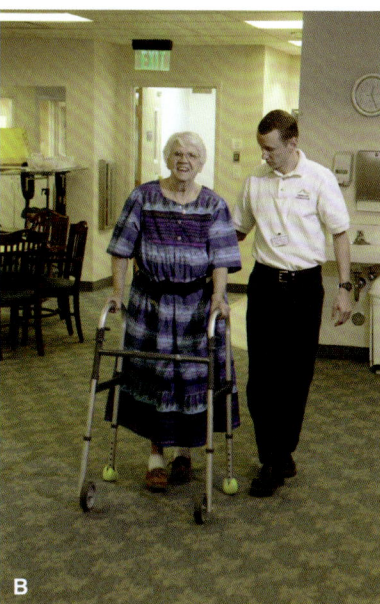

FIGURE 34-5 Healthy communities have adequate and available home health (**A**) and skilled nursing care (**B**), among other services.

Determine what level of social services is available in the community. Information may be obtained through local directories, the Chamber of Commerce, or personal interviews.	A community should provide agency social services—both public and voluntary—for people of all ages. Official agencies include mental health facilities and children and family services such as Medicaid, Medicare, and Aid to Families with Dependent Children. Other agencies may be substance-abuse treatment facilities, centers for abused women, hospices, and shelters for the homeless. Volunteer agencies (e.g., Meals on Wheels, Salvation Army, Red Cross) also offer community services (Fig. 34-6). Additional social programs may come from groups such as the YMCA and Parents Without Partners. Safe and certified childcare and eldercare facilities should also be available.	Lack of access to social service agencies may be an obstacle in urban areas. In addition, funding may limit the number of programs and people these agencies serve. Availability of programs may be limited in rural areas. For example, homeless shelters and shelters for abused women are nonexistent in many rural areas. Lack of transportation in rural areas may also make programs inaccessible. The cost of certain treatment programs can limit accessibility for those who are uninsured.

Continued on following page

ASSESSMENT PROCEDURE	NORMAL FINDINGS	ABNORMAL FINDINGS
Health and Social Services (Continued)		
Determine if long-term care services are available in the community. Long-term care services are those that meet the needs of elderly members, those with a chronic disabling illness, and those who have suffered disabilities due to accidents. Information can be obtained from local directories and the Chamber of Commerce.	A community should provide services for long-term care assistance in the home as well as extended care for those who can no longer function in their homes. For example, personal care assistance or a visiting nurse and skilled nursing and intermediate care facilities for those needing certain levels of nursing care should be available. Rehabilitation centers, boarding homes, continuing care, and retirement or assisted-living centers are other types of long-term care facilities (Fig. 34-7).	The capacity of available agencies may not meet the needs of a given community. Facilities that provide care for special concerns (e.g., Alzheimer disease) may not be available in all communities. Facilities in urban areas may be inaccessible because of cost. Rural areas, in general, are likely to have inadequate long-term care resources. This is especially true in areas such as respite care and personal care assistance in the home.

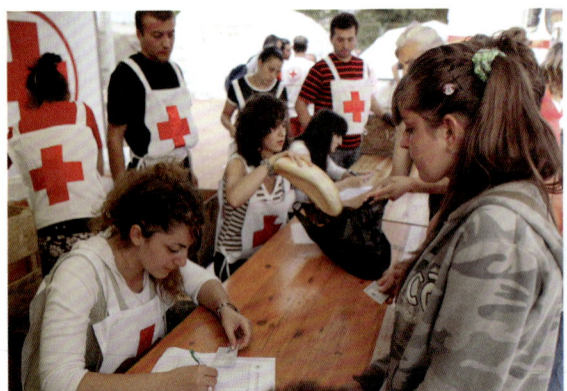

FIGURE 34-6 The Red Cross is a voluntary agency that provides full-scale community services in times of crisis (Courtesy of Kojoku/Shutterstock.com).

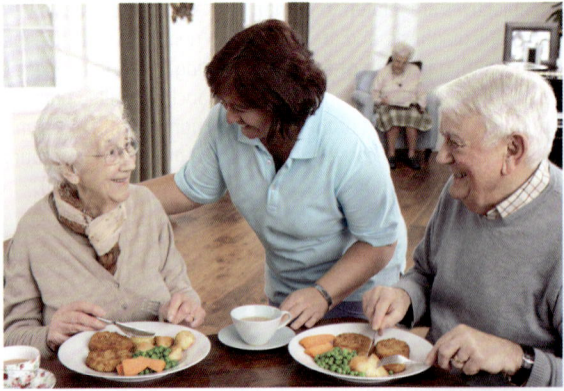

FIGURE 34-7 Residents gather for a meal at an assisted-living facility.

Gather community economic data. These data should include median household income, per capita income, percentage of households or individuals below the poverty level, percentage of people on public assistance, and unemployment statistics. In addition, collect data about local business and industry, types of occupations/jobs in which people are employed, and occupational health risks associated with certain occupations. Data can be collected from census records, Department of Labor, the Chamber of Commerce, and local and state unemployment offices.	Income has a direct relationship to the health of the residents of the community. The income of community members determines its tax base and, therefore, the ability of the community to provide needed services to its members. Businesses and other local employment opportunities are key factors in economic well-being. Businesses provide not only jobs but also goods and services such as groceries, pharmaceuticals, and clothing.	Economic instability in a community can lead to a number of health-related concerns. Poverty is associated with higher morbidity and mortality rates. High unemployment creates a stressful environment and a threat to the psychological well-being of the community. Occupationally related death and injuries cost the nation billions of dollars a year, with lung diseases and musculoskeletal injuries being the most frequent causes.
Gather information regarding fire, police, and environmental services in the community. This information can be obtained from local and regional police departments, fire departments, environmental agencies, and state health departments. Fire, police, and environmental services also are given the responsibility to protect the community from direct and indirect threats to its health and safety (Fig. 34-8). These services have both a direct and indirect relationship to a community's well-being in knowing that it is safe from a variety of threats.	Police should be equipped with personnel, equipment, and facilities to protect the community. Education programs such as Drug Abuse Resistance Education (DARE), property and personal identification programs, support programs such as Neighborhood Watch, and animal control programs may also be run by the police department. Number of firemen, equipment, response time, and education programs contribute to adequate fire protection services. Environmental protection includes a wide range of programs such as water and air quality; solid and hazardous waste disposal; sewage treatment; food/restaurant inspection; and monitoring of public swimming pools, motels, and other public facilities.	Violent crimes—such as homicide, rape, robbery, and assault—or increases in loss of life and property due to fires, may indicate that police and fire protection services are inadequate. This also contributes to a general sense of fear or uneasiness throughout the community and can lead to increased levels of stress and a loss of a sense of well-being. Poor environmental protection can result in repeated cases of illnesses, injuries, and even death. A number of health problems can be linked to the environment (e.g., waterborne illnesses and lead poisonings).

ASSESSMENT PROCEDURE	NORMAL FINDINGS	ABNORMAL FINDINGS
Determine transportation options available in the community. Obtain information from local businesses through interviews, from county and state highway departments, and direct observation.	The most common means of transportation in most communities is the private automobile. Other sources of transportation locally, in addition to walking, are taxis, buses, subways, and trains (Fig. 34-9). Long-distance transportation, in addition to automobiles, includes air, rail, and bus service. Roads, highways, and sidewalks should be kept in good repair, and communities should have adequate programs for snow and ice removal. Special transportation needs include school transportation and transportation for the elderly or disabled.	Lack of a private automobile is a particular problem in rural areas where public means of transportation are often nonexistent. Personal safety or cost may make public transportation inaccessible for many in urban areas. Inability to access health care services because of transportation difficulties is a particular problem for the elderly and for mothers with young children.

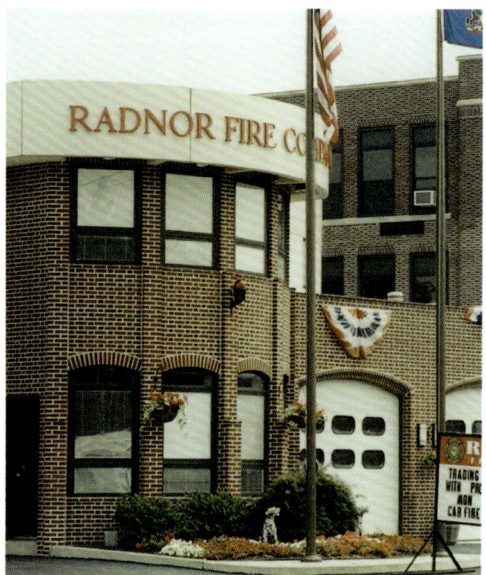

FIGURE 34-8 Adequate fire and police department protection are hallmarks of healthy communities.

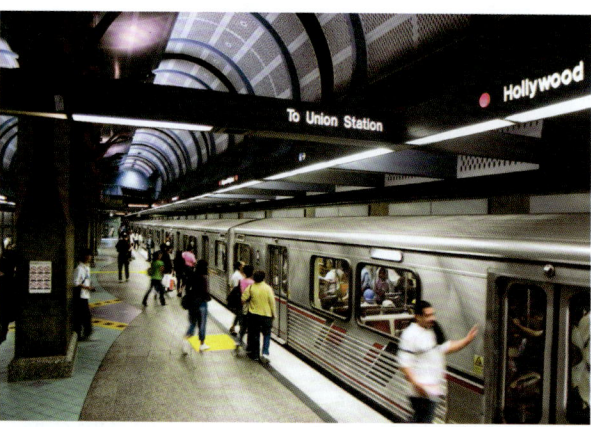

FIGURE 34-9 Access to transportation has a direct relationship to access to health care and other essential services.

Review levels of education, current school enrollment, and education resources in the community. Information may be obtained from census reports, local school districts, and state education agencies.	In general, the higher the community's education level, the healthier the community. Resources needed to meet community educational needs include preschool and early intervention programs, public or private elementary and secondary schools, and access to advanced education (Fig. 34-10). Adequate supply of qualified educators, up-to-date facilities and equipment, and programs that meet the needs of those with special needs are keys to a successful education system. Low absenteeism and higher-than-average scores on standardized achievement tests are indicators of effectiveness. Adult education, including general equivalency diploma (GED) classes, should be available. In addition, comprehensive school health programs directed by nurses, school meal programs, and after-school programs contribute to the health of a community. Public libraries are an important community supplement to the school system.	Funding for school systems is a growing problem for many communities, especially those in areas in which the economy is weak. Many school districts are supported in part by property taxes. In an area in which the tax base is low and unemployment is a problem, schools may struggle to maintain even minimum standards. As a result, many districts must cut equipment purchases, special programs, and extracurricular activities such as music and athletics. School violence is a growing problem for many communities. Another indication of problems in the school system is a high dropout rate and a low graduation rate. Availability of post–high school colleges or technical programs may be limited in rural areas. Access may be limited because of a lack of financial resources. Libraries often depend on local taxes. In times of economic difficulty, these facilities often face cutbacks.

Continued on following page

ASSESSMENT PROCEDURE	NORMAL FINDINGS	ABNORMAL FINDINGS

Health and Social Services (Continued)

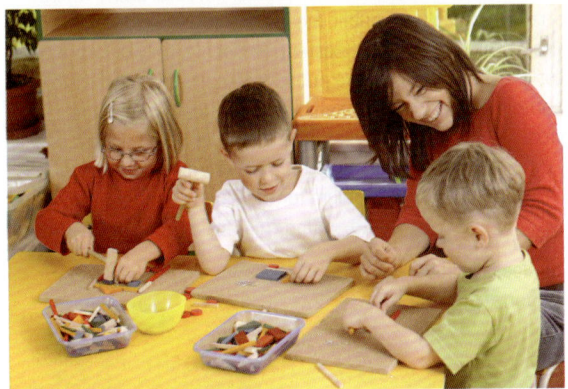
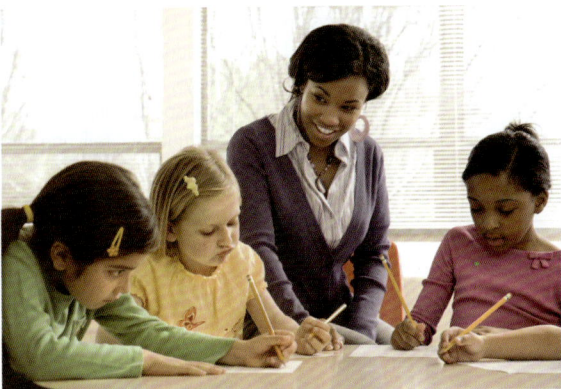
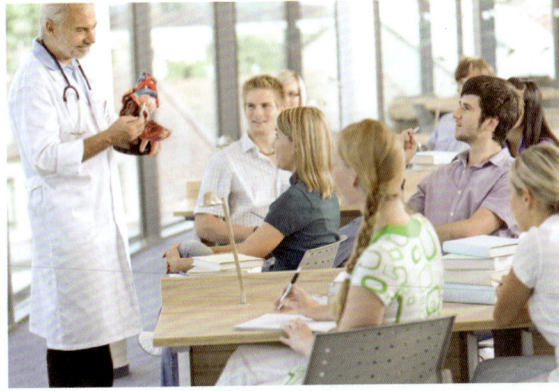

FIGURE 34-10 Preschool and elementary education lay the foundation for success in education (*top*). Schools at a higher level (community colleges and universities) offer the community significant opportunities for learning and vocational fulfillment (*bottom*).

Review the government and political structures of the community. Information may be obtained from local government agencies, local political organizations, and local directories. Government agencies are often directly involved in planning and implementing programs that affect the health of the community. In addition, the political system is responsible for health-related legislation. It is important to assess both the formal and informal power structures in the community.	The government of a community and its leaders should be responsible and accessible to the community. Members should participate in the governance of the community as evidenced by voter registration and percentage of registered voters who actually vote in elections. Open community meetings should be held to allow citizens a forum in which they may express their views. Political organizations should represent the differing views of the citizens; there should be an atmosphere of tolerance among the different groups.	If the government is not responsive to the views of the citizens, members of the community will become increasingly apathetic. As a result, the formal power structure becomes ineffective in meeting the needs of the community. Low voter turnout and little representation of groups with different views and interests may be indicative of an unresponsive or unrepresentative government.
Determine both the formal and informal means of communication in the community. Sources of information include the Chamber of Commerce, telephone book, and personal interviews and observations.	Open channels of communication are an important factor in maintaining the health of a community. Larger communities usually have many types of formal communication sources including local television and radio stations, local cable access, and one or more daily newspapers. Smaller communities usually have access to fewer television and radio stations, and newspapers are typically published weekly. Mail delivery may also be limited. However, online services are usually available in all communities. Informal communications include word of mouth; newsletters; bulletin board notices at community centers, stores, businesses, and churches; and fliers distributed by mail or door to door (Fig. 34-11).	Traditional means of communication may not be sufficient for some people in the community. Those who do not speak or understand English may not be able to obtain necessary information through either formal or informal means. Some people may not have access to a telephone or other means of communication. Elderly people and others who are isolated also may be at a disadvantage.

ASSESSMENT PROCEDURE	NORMAL FINDINGS	ABNORMAL FINDINGS

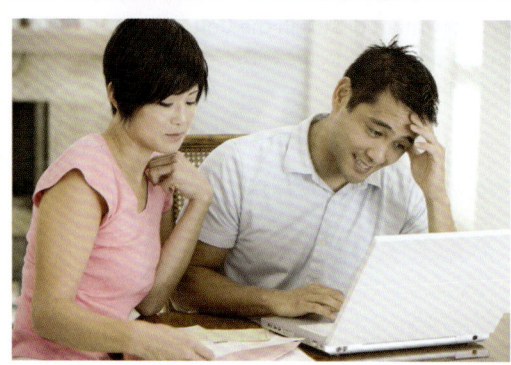 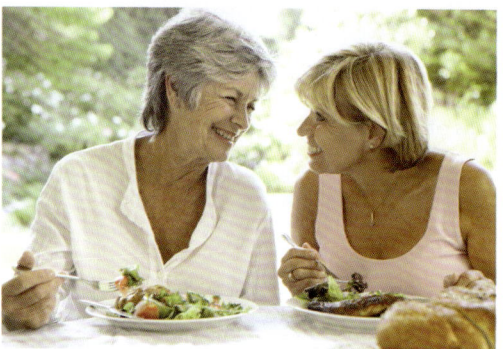

FIGURE 34-11 Communication: News travels over the airways (*left*) and by word of mouth (*right*).

Determine availability of community recreation and leisure programs for individuals and groups in all age ranges in the community. Information may be obtained from the Chamber of Commerce, park and recreation departments, churches, schools, businesses, and personal interview.	Schools in the area should have a regular program of physical education in which all students must participate. In addition, schools should provide equipment and programs for extracurricular activities, including both team and individual sports (e.g., tennis, softball), art, music, and foreign language programs, and other types of recreational programs. Churches may provide recreational programs, senior citizen dinners and outings, youth programs, church festivals, and special holiday activities. A comprehensive, community-based program is essential. Indoor or outdoor facilities (e.g., swimming pools, ball fields) should be available to all citizens, easily accessible, and kept in good repair. Organized activities for individuals and groups of all ages, genders, social status, and physical abilities should be available at minimal or no cost (Fig. 34-12).	Communities with a poor economic base or those with a large percentage of rural residents may not be able to provide adequate programs for recreation. Finding funds for building and maintaining recreational facilities is difficult; lack of transportation may seriously limit access. Social isolation may become a problem for people in these communities. In a community with no programs available for young people, gang activity and alcohol/drug abuse may develop. In communities in which activities such as water sports or snow sports are common, lack of programs related to safety issues could result in serious injury or even death.

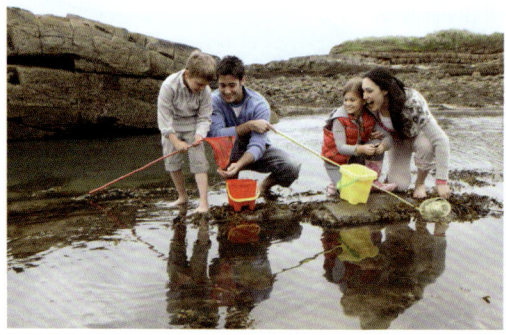 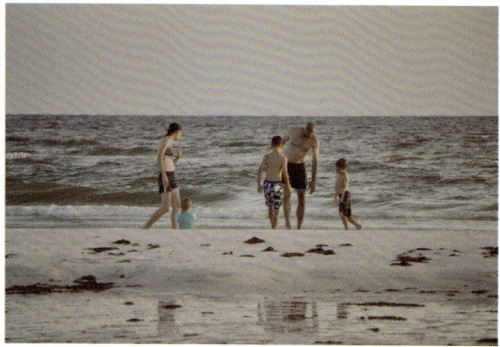

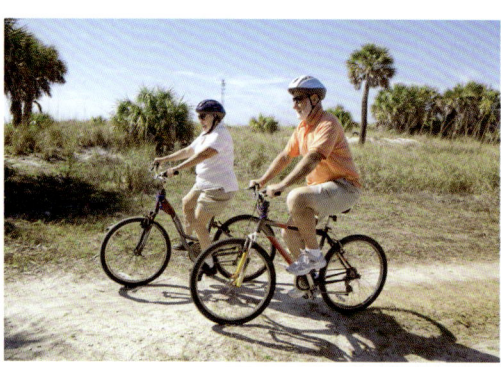

FIGURE 34-12 Recreational and leisure activities are directly related to a community's health status in that they connect people in the community and provide opportunities to socialize.

BOX 34-1 CAUSES OF NEONATAL AND INFANT MORTALITY FOR 2014—UNITED STATES

The following five leading causes of infant mortality accounted for about 57% of all infant deaths in the United States in 2014:
1. Birth defects
2. Preterm birth (birth before 37 weeks of gestation) and low birth weight
3. Maternal complications of pregnancy
4. Sudden infant death syndrome (SIDS)
5. Injuries (e.g., suffocation)

Centers for Disease Control and Prevention (CDC). (2016). Infant mortality. Available at http://www.cdc.gov/reproductivehealth/maternalinfanthealth/infantmortality.htm

BOX 34-2 CAUSES OF CHILDHOOD MORTALITY FOR 2014—UNITED STATES

AGES 1–4
1. Unintentional injuries
2. Congenital malformations, deformations, and chromosomal abnormalities
3. Homicide
4. Malignant neoplasms
5. Heart disease

AGES 5–9
1. Unintentional injuries
2. Malignant neoplasms
3. Congenital malformations, deformations, and chromosomal abnormalities
4. Homicide
5. Heart disease

AGES 10–14
1. Unintentional injury
2. Suicide
3. Malignant neoplasms
4. Congenital anomalies
5. Homicide

Centers for Disease Control and Prevention (CDC). (2016). Injury prevention & control: Data & statistics: Ten leading causes of death and injury—2014. Available at http://www.cdc.gov/injury/wisqars/leadingcauses.html

BOX 34-3 CAUSES OF TEEN AND ADULT MORTALITY FOR 2014—UNITED STATES

AGES 15–24
1. Unintentional injuries
2. Suicide
3. Homicide
4. Malignant neoplasms
5. Heart disease

AGES 25–34
1. Unintentional injuries
2. Suicide
3. Homicide
4. Malignant neoplasms
5. Heart disease

AGES 35–44
1. Unintentional injuries
2. Malignant neoplasms
3. Heart disease
4. Suicide
5. Homicide

AGES 45–54
1. Malignant neoplasms
2. Heart disease
3. Unintentional injuries
4. Suicide
5. Liver disease

AGES 55–64
1. Malignant neoplasms
2. Heart disease
3. Unintentional injuries
4. Chronic low respiratory disease
5. Diabetes mellitus

AGES 65+
1. Heart disease
2. Malignant neoplasms
3. Chronic low respiratory disease
4. Cerebrovascular disease
5. Alzheimer disease

Centers for Disease Control and Prevention (CDC). (2016). 10 leading causes of death by age group –2014. Available at http://www.cdc.gov/injury/images/lc-charts/leading_causes_of_death_age_group_2014_1050w760h.gif

CASE STUDY

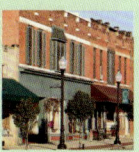

Assessment of the community reveals limited health resources available to the community. Several residents have expressed their concern about this to the nurse. The nurse explores this health concern using the COLDSPA mnemonic.

Mnemonic	Question	Data Provided
Character	Describe the sign or symptom (feeling, appearance, sound, smell, or taste if applicable).	"Our 50-bed skilled nursing facility is always full, and the nearest alternative is 25 miles away."
Onset	When did it begin?	"The facility was built 10 years ago and quickly filled up."
Location	Where is it? Does it radiate? Does it occur anywhere else?	N/A
Duration	How long does it last? Does it recur?	"This has put a strain on so many people and families over several years now."
Severity	How bad is it? or How much does it bother you?	"This puts many families under long-term stress if they have a family member who may need skilled care. They worry and then if the person has to go to another town, there is the worry about travel and travel expenses to see their loved one."
Pattern	What makes it better or worse?	"There is no change in pattern of worry, except that a committee has been formed that gives some hope for the future. But a few years ago, another committee did not make a difference."
Associated factors/ How it **A**ffects the client	What other symptoms occur with it? How does it affect you?	"Family members often have to stay home from work or give up work to care for an aging and sick relative. This puts an economic burden on the family and the whole community."

The nurse further assesses the community, starting with the history. Native American hunters and trappers first inhabited the area in and around Maple Grove. Later, German immigrants settled in the region and the lumber/logging industry became the economic base of the community. The town derived its name from the large stands of hardwood trees, especially maples, that grew in the area.

The nurse then explores the demographics. The total population for the town of Maple Grove as of the year 2010 was 2,352, a decrease of 13.6% from the 2010 census. Of the total number of residents, 56% are female and 26.3% are 65 years of age or older. Racial distribution includes 94.5% Caucasian, 3% African American, 1.3% Hispanic, and 1.2% other. Most residents aged 15 years and older are married (65.4%), 10.1% are either separated or divorced, 12.3% are single, and 12.2% are widowed. The leading cause of death in Maple Grove is cardiovascular disease. The German immigrants who originally settled the area brought with them their Lutheran faith; over 80% still practice that religion. There is also a small Baptist congregation in Maple Grove as well as small Methodist and Catholic churches.

The nurse notes that Maple Grove is situated in a very rural area and is bordered on the north by national forest land. The Cache River runs along its western border and an interstate highway lies 2 miles from the city limits on the east. The southern edge of the town is surrounded by farmland. Average temperature in January is 31.2°F, and in June 87.3°F.

The nurse assesses the health and social services. Maple Grove has no hospital; the nearest is 25 miles away and is an 85-bed, full-service facility. It is the only hospital in the county. A family practice physician and a nurse practitioner have an office in Maple Grove. The office is open 4 days a week. The county health department has a branch office in Maple Grove and offers immunizations, Special Supplemental Nutrition Program for Women, Infants, and Children (WIC), STI screening, family planning, and environmental services. A local VNA office offers home health services as well as hospice care. The nearest mental health center is approximately 25 miles away, as are many other services including county government offices. There is a 50-bed skilled nursing facility in Maple Grove operating at full capacity. A committee has been formed to examine ways in which the capacity of the facility could be increased.

The median household income for Maple Grove is $32,245, which is lower than the national average, and the median per capita income is $17,320, also below the national average. Of the nearly 2,400 people living in Maple Grove, 15.1% live below the poverty level (the national average is 12.7%). The single largest employer in the community is a minimum-security state correctional facility. Other areas of employment include forestry-related occupations, farming, and local businesses such as automobile sales, farm implement sales, grocery, and the like. The unemployment rate is 7.8%, which is higher than the state average.

Maple Grove maintains a small local police force of five full-time officers, two part-time officers, and one dispatcher/office worker. The community also receives services from the county sheriff's office and the state police. Maple Grove has a fire department with seven part-time firemen and a small group of volunteer firemen. There are no trained emergency medical personnel working with the fire department. The equipment is slightly outdated but still functional. Environmental services are provided through the county health department. The crime rate is relatively low, with the incidence of violent crime below the state average.

There is no public transportation in Maple Grove except for a small taxi service (one taxicab) and a van supported by the area Agency on Aging, which provides transportation for senior citizens. There is an interstate bus service available on a limited basis. The nearest airport is 70 miles away.

Maple Grove supports an elementary school and a high school, with a total of approximately 450 students in kindergarten through twelfth grade. There is no school nurse available. School administrators expressed some concern about this. Although health-related problems are referred to the local health department, schools have difficulty getting the required screenings completed and school immunization records are not up to date. The school principals also are concerned that there is no one available to care for injuries or illness when they occur. The high school provides a limited number of extracurricular activities including boys' and girls' basketball, baseball, softball, and track. The closest junior college is 30 miles away, and the nearest university is 55 miles from Maple Grove. There is a small library open in the afternoons and on Saturday. The community residents are proud of their library because it is entirely funded through contributions. They often hold chili suppers, raffles, and other fundraising events to support it.

Maple Grove has a mayor/city council form of government. The mayor was more than willing to meet with the nurse and invited her to attend the city council meeting on the first Monday of the month. Those members of the community with whom the nurse talked indicated that they felt comfortable with their elected officials and that they were free to voice concerns and opinions at any time. Both the Democratic and Republican parties are active in the town. The number of registered voters who voted in the last election was higher than the state average.

A radio station is located approximately 25 miles away, and the nearest television station is 50 miles from Maple Grove. The town has cable television service and a post office. A small local newspaper is published weekly. Dial-up and cable TV/Internet is available in some homes; fiber-optic cable access has not yet reached Maple Grove.

Maple Grove has a small city park equipped with playground equipment, three ball fields, and a picnic shelter. There are softball and baseball leagues for children ages 7 to 18 along with Boy Scout and Girl Scout troops. Other organized recreation activities, such as senior citizen programs, are offered through the churches.

Validating and Documenting Findings

Validate the community assessment data you have collected with community members and leaders (by asking additional questions, or comparing objective with subjective findings). This is necessary to verify that the data are reliable and accurate. Document the assessment data following the health care facility or agency policy.

CASE STUDY

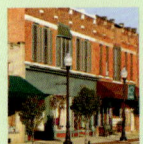

Think back to the case of Maple Grove. The nurse completes the following documentation.

History: Maple Grove (MG) first inhabited by Native American hunters. Then, German immigrants settled in the region and the lumber/logging industry became the economic base.

Demographics: Total population as of 2016 was 2352, a decrease of 13.6% from 2010 census. Residents: 56% are female and 26.3% are 65 years of age or older. Racial distribution: 94.5% Caucasian, 3% African American, 1.3% Hispanic, and 1.2% other. Of the population, 65.4% of those over 15 are married, 10.1% are either separated or divorced, 12.3% are single, and 12.2% are widowed. Leading cause of death is cardiovascular disease. Over 80% of residents practice Lutheran faith. MG also has small Baptist Methodist and Catholic churches.

Physical Environment: MG in a very rural area, bordered on the north by national forest land. The Cache River is on western border; interstate highway lies 2 miles from the city limits on the east. South is surrounded by farmland. Average temperature in January is 31.2°F, and in June 87.3°F.

Health and Social Services: MG has no hospital; the nearest is 25 miles away and is an 85-bed, full-service facility. It is the only hospital in the county. A family practice MD and an NP have an office in MG. It is open 4 days a week. County health department has a branch in MG and offers immunizations, Special Supplemental Nutrition Program for Women, Infants, and Children (WIC), STI screening, family planning, and environmental services. Local VNA office offers home health and hospice care. Mental health center is 25 miles away. MG has a 50-bed skilled nursing facility, operating at full capacity. A committee has been formed to examine ways in which the capacity of the facility could be increased.

Economics: Median household income is $32,245, median per capita income is $17,320 (both below the national average). 15.1% of population live below the poverty level. Largest employer in the community is a minimum-security state correctional facility. Other jobs include forestry-related occupations, farming, and local businesses such as automobile sales, farm implement sales, grocery, and the like. Unemployment rate is 7.8% (higher than the state average).

Safety: Small local police force of five full-time officers, two part-time officers, and one dispatcher/office worker. MG also receives services from the county sheriff's office and the state police. MG has a fire department with seven part-time firemen and a small group of volunteer firemen. No trained emergency medical personnel working. Equipment is outdated but functional. Environmental services are provided through the county health department. Crime rate is low, with the incidence of violent crime below the state average.

Transportation: No public transportation except for one taxicab and an Agency on Aging van, which provides transportation for senior citizens. Interstate bus service available on a limited basis. Nearest airport is 70 miles away.

Education: Elementary school and a high school, with a total of approximately 450 students. No school nurse available (school administrators expressed concern). Schools have difficulty getting the required screenings completed and school immunization records are not up to date. High school provides a limited number of extracurricular activities. Junior college is 30 miles away, university is 55 miles away. Small library funded by contributions open part-time.

Government: Mayor/city council form of government. The mayor cooperative. Community members indicate they are comfortable with their elected officials and free to voice concerns. Both the parties are active in the town. The number of registered voters who voted in the last election was higher than the state average.

Communication: A radio station is 25 miles away, and television station is 50 miles away. Cable television service and a post office available. A small local newspaper is published weekly. Dial-up and cable TV/Internet connections are available in some homes.

Recreation: Small city park equipped with playground, ball fields, and a picnic shelter. There are softball and baseball leagues for children ages 7 to 18 along with Boy Scout and Girl Scout troops. Other organized recreation activities, such as senior citizen programs, are offered through the churches.

ANALYSIS OF DATA: DIAGNOSTIC REASONING

After collecting subjective and objective data pertaining to community assessment, identify abnormal findings and community strengths. Then cluster the data to reveal any significant patterns or abnormalities. These data may then be used to make clinical judgments about the status of the community's health. The following sections provide possible conclusions that the nurse may make after assessing a community.

Selected Nursing Diagnoses

Following is a listing of selected nursing diagnoses (health promotion, risk, or actual) that may be identified when analyzing the cue clusters.

Health Promotion Diagnoses
- Readiness for Enhanced Community Coping

Risk Diagnoses
- Risk for Ineffective Community Coping related to low income and high unemployment
- Risk for Ineffective Community Protection

Actual Diagnoses
- Ineffective Community Coping related to generalized worry of inadequate community skilled-nursing facilities
- Ineffective Protection, Community related to lack of school nurse and availability of emergency care

Selected Collaborative Problems

After grouping the data, certain collaborative problems may become apparent. Remember that collaborative problems differ from nursing diagnoses in that they cannot be prevented or treated by nursing interventions alone. However, these physiologic complications of medical conditions can be detected and monitored by the nurse. In addition, the nurse can use physician- and nurse-prescribed interventions to minimize the complications of these problems. The nurse may also have to refer the client in such situations for further treatment of the problem. Following is a list of collaborative problems that may be identified when assessing a community. These problems are worded as Risk for Complications (RC), followed by the problem.
- RC: Post-traumatic stress disorder, community

Medical Problems

After grouping the data, the client's signs and symptoms may clearly require medical diagnosis and treatment. Referral to a primary care provider is necessary.

CASE STUDY

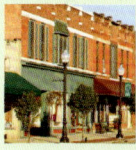

The nurse uses diagnostic reasoning to analyze the data collected on the Maple Grove community to arrive at the following possible conclusions.

Nursing Diagnoses
- Readiness for Enhanced Community Coping related to active voice of citizens and their concern to expand the community's skilled nursing facility by forming a committee
- Ineffective Community Coping related to a high level of poverty and unemployment rate
- Readiness for Enhanced Immunization Status related to not having a school nurse to assess for the currency of 450 student immunization records
- Deficient Community Health related to not having a hospital, mental health facility, or trained emergency personnel, with the nearest full-service hospital 25 miles away
- Risk for Ineffective Protection, Community related to low-income residents, a high unemployment rate, and a lack of availability of emergency care

To view an algorithm depicting the process for diagnostic reasoning in this case, go to thePoint.

Interdisciplinary Verbal Communication of Assessment Findings Using SBAR

SITUATION: Maple Grove (MG), is a small, rural Midwestern community, population 2,352 (a decrease of 13.6% from 2010 census). Median household and personal income are below the national averages, with 15.1% of population below poverty level. Unemployment rate 7.8%, which is higher than state average. MG does not have a hospital or trained emergency personnel, with the nearest full-service hospital 25 miles away. School of 450 students has no school nurse available and difficulty getting required screenings and immunization records up to date.

BACKGROUND: MG was first inhabited by Native American hunters, followed by German immigrants who settled the region with lumber/logging industry, the economic base, which has deteriorated over the years. Eighty percent of residents practice Lutheran faith. MG also has small Baptist, Methodist, and Catholic churches.

ASSESSMENT: Located in rural area 2 miles from the interstate with national forest on North side, Cache River on Western border; and farmland on the South. Average January temperature 31.2°F; June 87.3°F.

Residents: 56% female; 26.3% 65 years of age or older; 94.5% Caucasian, 3% African American, 1.3% Hispanic, and 1.2% other. 65.4% of those over 15 are married, 10.1% separated or divorced, 12.3% single, and 12.2% widowed. Leading cause of death is cardiovascular disease.

Family Practice MD and NP office open 4 days a week. County health department branch has WIC, STI screening, family planning, and environmental services. Local VNA office offers home health and hospice. Mental health center 25 miles away. Has a 50-bed skilled nursing facility operating at full capacity. Committee looking at ways to increase size of facility.

Largest employer is a minimum-security state correctional facility. Has small local police force and fire department but no trained emergency medical personnel. Equipment outdated, but functional. Has low crime rate.

One taxicab and an Agency on Aging van for senior citizens. Airport is 70 miles away.

Elementary and high school, with 450 students. Junior college is 30 miles away, university is 55 miles away. Small library funded by contributions open part-time.

Mayor/city council form of government cooperative. Active voice of community members, with large number of participating voters from both parties.

Radio and TV station 25 to 50 miles away with cable television service and a post office available. Small local newspaper published weekly. Small city park equipped with playground, ball fields, and a picnic shelter.

RECOMMENDATION: MG is ready for Enhanced Community status as demonstrated by its active citizens and their willingness to form a committee to expand the skilled nursing facility. Ineffective Community Coping related to a high level of poverty and unemployment rate. Has Readiness for Enhanced Immunization status related to not having a school nurse to assess for the currency of 450 student immunization records. There is deficient Community Health related to not having a hospital, mental health facility, or trained emergency personnel, with the nearest full-service hospital 25 miles away. The community at large is at Risk for Ineffective Protection related to low-income residents, a high unemployment rate and the lack of availability of emergency care. This information needs to be reported to the statewide public health initiative to work with health care providers to enhance safety and protection for the community.

Want to know more?

A wide variety of resources to enhance your learning and understanding of this book are available on thePoint. Visit thePoint to access:

NCLEX-Style Student Review Questions
Watch and Learn Videos
Concept in Action Animations
And more!

References and Selected Readings

Anderson, E., & McFarlane, J. (2015). *Community as partner* (7th ed.). Philadelphia, PA: Wolters Kluwer.

Centers for Disease Control and Prevention (CDC). (2012). *Community assessment for public health emergency response (CASPER) toolkit* (2nd ed.). Atlanta, GA: Centers for Disease Control and Prevention National Center for Environmental Health Division of Environmental Hazards and Health Effects Health Studies Branch. Available at https://www.cdc.gov/nceh/hsb/disaster/casper/docs/cleared_casper_toolkit.pdf

Centers for Disease Control and Prevention (CDC). (2016). Community assessment for public health emergency response (CASPER). Available at https://www.cdc.gov/nceh/hsb/disaster/casper/

Generations United. (2015). Multigenerational household information. Available at http://www.gu.org/OURWORK/Multigenerational/MultigenerationalHouseholdInformation.aspx

Maurer, F., & Smith, C. (2013). *Community/public health nursing practice* (5th ed.). St. Louis, MO: Elsevier/Saunders.

National Alliance to End Homelessness. (2016). The state of homelessness in American 2015. Available at http://www.endhomelessness.org/library/entry/the-state-of-homelessness-in-america-2015

Sociology Guide. (2011). Community. Available at http://www.sociologyguide.com/basic-concepts/Community.php

University of North Carolina Health Sciences Library. (2015). Finding information for a community health assessment. Available at http://guides.lib.unc.edu/CommunityHealhAssessment

U.S. Census Bureau. (2015a). Families and living arrangements. Available at http://www.census.gov/hhes/families/

U.S. Census Bureau. (2015b). FFF: Unmarried and single Americans Week of September 20–26, 2015. Available at https://www.census.gov/newsroom/facts-for-features/2015/cb15-ff19.html

Wang, W., Parker, K., & Taylor, P. (2013). Breadwinner moms. Available at http://www.pewsocialtrends.org/2013/05/29/breadwinner-moms/

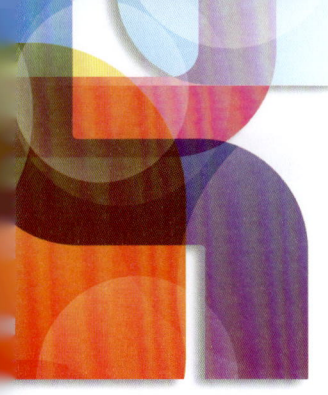

Appendix A
NURSING HISTORY GUIDE

This form is available on thePoint website for downloading or printing.

QUESTIONS	DOCUMENT YOUR FINDINGS
Biographic Data	
1. Name?	
2. Address?	
3. Phone?	
4. Birthdate?	
5. Provider history?	
6. Ethnicity?	
7. Educational level?	
8. Occupation?	
Current Symptoms	
1. History of present concern (COLDSPA)?	
Past History	
1. Birth problems?	
2. Childhood illnesses?	
3. Immunizations?	
4. Illnesses?	
5. Surgeries?	
6. Accidents?	
7. Pain?	
8. Allergies?	
Family History	
1. Family genogram?	
Review of Body Systems	
1. Skin, hair, nails?	
2. Ears?	
3. Mouth, throat, nose, sinuses?	
4. Thorax and lungs?	
5. Breasts and regional lymph nodes?	
6. Heart and neck vessels?	
7. Peripheral vascular?	
8. Abdomen?	
9. Male/female genitalia?	
10. Anus, rectum, and prostate?	
11. Musculoskeletal?	
12. Neurologic?	

Continued on following page

QUESTIONS	DOCUMENT YOUR FINDINGS
Lifestyle and Health Practices	
1. ADLs in a typical day?	
2. Diet for past 24 hours?	
3. Exercise regimen?	
4. Sleep patterns?	
5. Medications?	
6. Use of recreation drugs, alcohol, nicotine, or caffeine?	
7. Self-concept?	
8. Life stressors and coping strategies?	
9. Responsibilities and role at home and at work?	
10. Type of work and level of satisfaction?	
11. Finances?	
12. Educational plans?	
13. Social activities?	
14. Relationships with others?	
15. Values?	
16. Spirituality?	
17. Religious affiliations?	
18. Environment, residency, and neighborhood?	
Developmental Level	
1. Cognitive	
2. Moral	
3. Psychosocial	
4. Psychosexual	

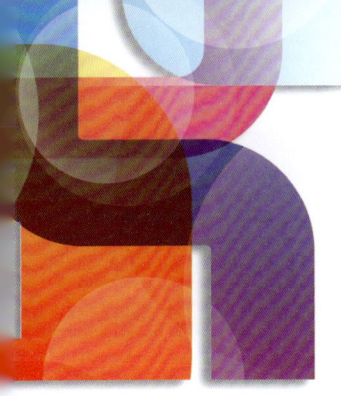

Appendix B
PHYSICAL ASSESSMENT GUIDE

This form is available on thePoint website for downloading or printing.

ASSESSMENT GUIDE	DOCUMENT YOUR FINDINGS
General Exam	
1. Gather all equipment needed for a head-to-toe exam. 2. Prepare client by explaining what you will be doing. 3. Observe appearance. 4. Assess vital signs. 5. Take body measurements. 6. Calculate ideal body weight, body mass index, waist-to-hip ratio, mid-arm muscle area and circumference. 7. Test vision.	☐ ☐
Mental Status and Substance Abuse	
1. Observe level of consciousness. 2. Observe posture and body movements. 3. Observe facial expressions. 4. Observe speech. 5. Observe mood, feelings, and expressions. 6. Observe thought processes and perceptions. 7. Assess cognitive abilities. 8. Give client a specimen cup if sample is needed, and ask client to empty bladder and change into gown. Ask client to sit on examination table.	☐
Skin	
1. Throughout examination, assess skin for color variations, texture, temperature, turgor, edema, and lesions. 2. Teach skin self-examination.	
Head	
1. Inspect and palpate head. 2. Note consistency, distribution, color of hair. 3. Observe face for symmetry, features, expressions, condition of skin. 4. Have client smile, frown, show teeth, blow out cheeks, raise eyebrows, and tightly close eyes (CN VII). 5. Test sensations of forehead, cheeks, and chin (CN V). 6. Palpate temporal arteries for elasticity and tenderness. 7. Palpate temporomandibular joint.	

Continued on following page

☐ indicates preparation for exam. No documentation needed.

ASSESSMENT GUIDE	DOCUMENT YOUR FINDINGS
Eyes	
1. Assess visual function.	
2. Inspect external eye.	
3. Test pupillary reaction to light.	
4. Test accommodation of pupils.	
5. Assess corneal reflex (CN VII facial).	
6. Use ophthalmoscope to inspect interior of eye.	
Ears	
1. Inspect auricle, tragus, and lobule.	
2. Palpate auricle and mastoid process.	
3. Use otoscope to inspect auditory canal.	
4. Use otoscope to inspect tympanic membrane.	
5. Test hearing.	
Nose	
1. Inspect external nose.	
2. Palpate external nose for tenderness.	
3. Check patency of airflow through nostrils.	
4. Occlude each nostril and ask client to smell for soap, coffee, or vanilla (CN I).	
5. Use otoscope to inspect internal nose.	
6. Transilluminate maxillary sinuses.	
Mouth	
1. Put on gloves.	☐
2. Inspect lips.	
3. Inspect teeth.	
4. Check gums and buccal mucosa.	
5. Inspect hard and soft palates.	
6. Observe uvula.	
7. Assess for gag reflex (CN X).	
8. Inspect tonsils.	
9. Inspect and palpate tongue.	
10. Assess tongue strength (CN IX and X).	
11. Check taste sensation (CN VII and IX).	
Neck	
1. Inspect appearance of neck.	
2. Test range of motion (ROM) of neck.	
3. Palpate preauricular, postauricular, occipital, tonsillar, submandibular, and submental nodes.	
4. Palpate trachea.	
5. Palpate thyroid gland.	
6. If enlarged, auscultate thyroid gland for bruits.	
7. Palpate and auscultate carotid arteries.	

☐ indicates preparation for exam. No documentation needed.

ASSESSMENT GUIDE	DOCUMENT YOUR FINDINGS
Musculoskeletal—Upper Extremities	
1. Inspect upper extremities. 2. Test shoulder shrug and ability to turn head against resistance (CN XI spinal). 3. Palpate arms. 4. Assess epitrochlear lymph nodes. 5. Test ROM of elbows. 6. Palpate brachial pulse. 7. Palpate ulnar and radial pulses. 8. Test ROM of wrist. 9. Inspect and palpate palms of hands. 10. Test ROM of fingers. 11. Use reflex hammer to test biceps, triceps, and brachioradialis reflexes. 12. Test rapid alternating movements of hands. 13. Test sensation in arms, hands, and fingers.	
Thorax	
1. Ask client to continue sitting with arms at sides and stand behind client. Untie gown to expose posterior chest. 2. Inspect scapulae and chest wall. 3. Note use of accessory muscles when breathing. 4. Palpate chest. 5. Evaluate chest expansion at T9 or T10. 6. Percuss at posterior intercostal spaces. 7. Determine diaphragmatic excursion. 8. Auscultate posterior chest. 9. Test for two-point discrimination on back. 10. Auscultate apex and left sternal border of heart during exhalation.	☐
Lungs	
1. Inspect chest. 2. Note quality and pattern of respirations. 3. Observe intercostal spaces. 4. Palpate anterior chest. 5. Percuss anterior chest. 6. Auscultate anterior chest. 7. Test skin mobility and turgor. 8. Ask client to fold gown to waist and sit with arms hanging freely.	☐
Breasts	
1. Inspect both breasts, areolas, and nipples. 2. Inspect for retractions and dimpling of nipples. 3. Palpate axillae.	
Lymph Nodes	
1. Inspect breast tissue. 2. Palpate breast tissue and axillae. 3. Assist client to supine position with the head elevated to 30 to 45 degrees. Stand on client's right side. 4. Evaluate jugular venous pressure. 5. Assist client to supine position (lower examination table).	☐ ☐

Continued on following page

☐ indicates preparation for exam. No documentation needed.

ASSESSMENT GUIDE	DOCUMENT YOUR FINDINGS
Breast—Malignancy	
1. Palpate breasts for masses and nipples for discharge.	
2. Teach breast self-examination.	
Heart	
1. Inspect and palpate for apical impulse.	
2. Palpate the apex, left sternal border, and base of the heart.	
3. Auscultate over aortic area, pulmonic area, Erb's point, tricuspid area, and apex.	
4. Auscultate apex of heart as client lies on left side.	
Abdomen	
1. Cover chest with gown and arrange draping to expose abdomen.	
2. Inspect abdomen.	
3. Auscultate abdomen.	
4. Percuss abdomen.	
5. Palpate abdomen.	
Musculoskeletal—Lower Extremities	
1. Observe muscles.	
2. Note hair distribution.	
3. Palpate joints of hips and test ROM.	
4. Palpate legs and feet.	
5. Palpate knees.	
6. Palpate ankles.	
7. Assess capillary refill.	
8. Test sensations (dull and sharp), two-point discrimination, reflexes, position sense, and vibratory sensation.	
9. Perform heel-to-shin test.	
10. Perform any special tests as warranted.	
11. Secure gown and assist client to standing position.	☐
Spine	
1. Observe for spinal curvatures and check for scoliosis.	
2. Observe gait.	
3. Observe tandem walk.	
4. Observe hopping on each leg.	
5. Perform Romberg's test.	
6. Perform finger-to-nose test.	
Genitalia—Female	
1. Have female client assume the lithotomy position. Apply gloves. Apply lubricant as appropriate.	☐
2. Inspect pubic hair.	
3. Inspect mons pubis, labia majora, and perineum.	
4. Inspect labia minora, clitoris, urethral meatus, and vaginal opening.	
5. Palpate Bartholin's glands, urethra, and Skene's glands.	
6. Inspect cervix.	
7. Inspect vagina.	
8. Obtain cytologic smears and culture.	
9. Palpate cervix.	
10. Palpate uterus.	
11. Palpate ovaries.	
12. Discard gloves and apply clean gloves and lubricant.	☐
13. Palpate rectovaginal septum.	

☐ indicates preparation for exam. No documentation needed.

ASSESSMENT GUIDE	DOCUMENT YOUR FINDINGS
Genitalia—Male	
1. Sit on a stool and have client stand and face you with gown raised. Apply gloves. 2. Inspect penis. 3. Palpate for urethral discharge. 4. Inspect scrotum. 5. Palpate both testes and epididymis. 6. Transilluminate scrotal contents. 7. Inspect for bulges in inguinal and femoral areas. 8. Palpate for scrotal hernia. 9. Palpate for inguinal hernia. 10. Teach testicular self-examination. 11. Inspect perineal area. 12. Inspect sacrococcygeal area. 13. Inspect for bulges or lesions as Valsalva maneuver is performed.	☐
Anus and Rectum	
1. Ask the client to remain standing and to bend over the exam table. Change gloves. 2. Palpate anus. 3. Palpate external sphincter. 4. Palpate rectum. 5. Palpate peritoneal cavity. 6. Palpate prostate. 7. Inspect stool.	☐

☐ indicates preparation for exam. No documentation needed.

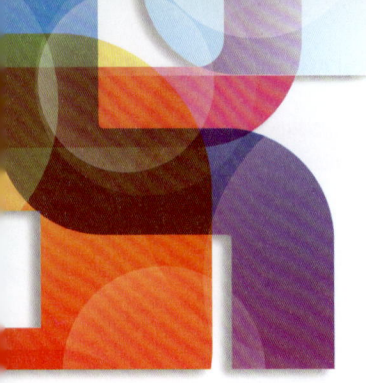

Appendix C
NANDA APPROVED NURSING DIAGNOSES 2015–2017

Domain 1: Health Promotion

Deficient diversional activity
Sedentary lifestyle
Frail elderly syndrome
Risk for frail elderly syndrome
Deficient community health
Risk-prone health behavior
Ineffective health maintenance
Ineffective health management
Readiness for enhanced health management
Ineffective family health management
Noncompliance
Ineffective protection

Domain 2: Nutrition

Insufficient breast milk
Ineffective breastfeeding
Interrupted breastfeeding
Readiness for enhanced breastfeeding
Ineffective infant feeding pattern
Imbalanced nutrition: less than body requirements
Readiness for enhanced nutrition
Obesity
Overweight
Risk for overweight
Impaired swallowing
None at present time
Risk for unstable blood glucose level
Neonatal jaundice
Risk for neonatal jaundice
Risk for impaired liver function
Risk for electrolyte imbalance
Readiness for enhanced fluid balance
Deficient fluid volume
Risk for deficient fluid volume
Excess fluid volume
Risk for imbalanced fluid volume

Domain 3: Elimination and Exchange

Impaired urinary elimination
Readiness for enhanced urinary elimination
Functional urinary incontinence
Overflow urinary incontinence
Reflex urinary incontinence
Stress urinary incontinence
Urge urinary incontinence
Risk for urge urinary incontinence
Urinary retention
Constipation
Risk for constipation
Chronic functional constipation
Risk for chronic functional constipation
Perceived constipation
Diarrhea
Dysfunctional gastrointestinal motility
Risk for dysfunctional gastrointestinal motility
Bowel incontinence
None at this time
Impaired gas exchange

Domain 4: Activity/Rest

Insomnia
Sleep deprivation
Readiness for enhanced sleep
Disturbed sleep pattern
Risk for disuse syndrome
Impaired bed mobility
Impaired physical mobility
Impaired wheelchair mobility
Impaired sitting
Impaired standing
Impaired transfer ability
Impaired walking
Fatigue
Wandering
Activity intolerance
Risk for activity intolerance
Ineffective breathing pattern
Decreased cardiac output
Risk for decreased cardiac output
Risk for impaired cardiovascular function
Risk for ineffective gastrointestinal perfusion
Risk for ineffective renal perfusion
Impaired spontaneous ventilation
Risk for decreased cardiac tissue perfusion
Risk for ineffective cerebral tissue perfusion
Ineffective peripheral tissue perfusion
Risk for ineffective peripheral tissue perfusion
Dysfunctional ventilatory weaning response

Impaired home maintenance
Bathing self-care deficit
Dressing self-care deficit
Feeding self-care deficit
Toileting self-care deficit
Readiness for enhanced self-care
Self-neglect

Domain 5: Perception/Cognition

Unilateral neglect
None at this time
Acute confusion
Risk for acute confusion
Chronic confusion
Labile emotional control
Ineffective impulse control
Deficient knowledge
Readiness for enhanced knowledge
Impaired memory
Readiness for enhanced communication
Impaired verbal communication

Domain 6: Self-Perception

Readiness for enhanced hope
Hopelessness
Risk for compromised human dignity
Disturbed personal identity
Risk for disturbed personal identity
Readiness for enhanced self-concept
Chronic low self-esteem
Risk for chronic low self-esteem
Situational low self-esteem
Risk for situational low self-esteem
Disturbed body image

Domain 7: Role Relationships

Caregiver role strain
Risk for caregiver role strain
Impaired parenting
Readiness for enhanced parenting
Risk for impaired parenting
Risk for impaired attachment
Dysfunctional family processes
Interrupted family processes
Readiness for enhanced family processes
Ineffective relationship
Readiness for enhanced relationship
Risk for ineffective relationship
Parental role conflict
Ineffective role performance
Impaired social interaction

Domain 8: Sexuality

None at present time
Sexual dysfunction
Ineffective sexuality pattern
Ineffective childbearing process
Readiness for enhanced childbearing process
Risk for ineffective childbearing process
Risk for disturbed maternal-fetal dyad

Domain 9: Coping/Stress Tolerance

Post-trauma syndrome
Risk for post-trauma syndrome
Rape-trauma syndrome
Relocation stress syndrome
Risk for relocation stress syndrome
Ineffective activity planning
Risk for ineffective activity planning
Anxiety
Defensive coping
Ineffective coping
Readiness for enhanced coping
Ineffective community coping
Readiness for enhanced community coping
Compromised family coping
Disabled family coping
Readiness for enhanced family coping
Death anxiety
Ineffective denial
Fear
Grieving
Complicated grieving
Risk for complicated grieving
Impaired mood regulation
Readiness for enhanced power
Powerlessness
Risk for powerlessness
Impaired resilience
Readiness for enhanced resilience
Risk for impaired resilience
Chronic sorrow
Stress overload
Decreased intracranial adaptive capacity
Autonomic dysreflexia
Risk for autonomic dysreflexia
Disorganized infant behavior
Readiness for enhanced organized infant behavior
Risk for disorganized infant behavior

Domain 10: Life Principles

None at this time
Readiness for enhanced spiritual well-being
Readiness for enhanced decision-making
Decisional conflict
Impaired emancipated decision-making
Readiness for enhanced emancipated decision-making
Risk for impaired emancipated decision-making
Moral distress
Impaired religiosity
Readiness for enhanced religiosity

Risk for impaired religiosity
Spiritual distress
Risk for spiritual distress

Domain 11: Safety/Protection

Risk for infection
Ineffective airway clearance
Risk for aspiration
Risk for bleeding
Risk for dry eye
Risk for falls
Risk for injury
Risk for corneal injury
Risk for perioperative positioning injury
Risk for thermal injury
Risk for urinary tract injury
Impaired dentition
Impaired oral mucous membrane
Risk for impaired oral mucous membrane
Risk for peripheral neurovascular dysfunction
Risk for pressure ulcer
Risk for shock
Impaired skin integrity
Risk for impaired skin integrity
Risk for sudden infant death syndrome
Risk for suffocation
Delayed surgical recovery
Risk for delayed surgical recovery
Impaired tissue integrity
Risk for impaired tissue integrity
Risk for trauma
Risk for vascular trauma
Risk for other-directed violence
Risk for self-directed violence
Self-mutilation
Risk for self-mutilation
Risk for suicide
Risk for contamination
Risk for poisoning
Risk for adverse reaction to iodinated contrast media
Risk for allergy response
Latex allergy response
Risk for latex allergy response
Risk for imbalanced body temperature
Hyperthermia
Hypothermia
Risk for hypothermia
Risk for perioperative hypothermia
Ineffective thermoregulation

Domain 12: Comfort

Impaired comfort
Readiness for enhanced comfort
Nausea
Acute pain
Chronic pain
Labor pain
Chronic pain syndrome
Impaired comfort
Readiness for enhanced comfort
Impaired comfort
Readiness for enhanced comfort
Risk for loneliness
Social isolation

Domain 13: Growth/Development

Risk for disproportionate growth
Risk for delayed development

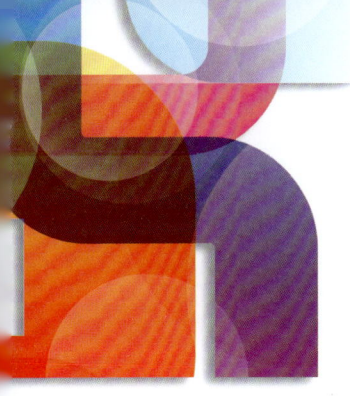

Appendix D
MANUAL OF COLLABORATIVE PROBLEMS

Risk for Complications of Cardiac/Vascular Dysfunction

RC of Bleeding
RC of Decreased Cardiac Output
RC of Arrhythmias
RC of Pulmonary Edema
RC of Deep Vein Thrombosis/Pulmonary Embolism
RC of Hypovolemia
RC of Compartment Syndrome
RC of Intra-Abdominal Hypertension

Risk for Complications of Respiratory Dysfunction

RC of Atelectasis, Pneumonia
RC of Hypoxemia

Risk for Complications of Metabolic/Immune/Hematopoietic Dysfunction

RC of Hypo/Hyperglycemia
RC of Negative Nitrogen Balance
RC of Electrolyte Imbalances
RC of Systemic Inflammatory Response Syndrome (SIRS)/Sepsis
RC of Metabolic or Respiratory Acidosis
RC of Metabolic or Respiratory Alkalosis
RC of Allergic Reaction
RC of Thrombocytopenia
RC of Opportunistic Infections
RC of Vaso-Occlusive/Sickling Crisis

Risk for Complications of Renal/Urinary Dysfunction

RC of Acute Urinary Retention
RC of Renal Calculi
RC of Renal Insufficiency

Risk for Complications of Neurologic/Sensory Dysfunction

Risk for Complications of Alcohol Withdrawal
Risk for Complications of Increased Intracranial Pressure
Risk for Complications of Seizures

Risk for Complications of Gastrointestinal/Hepatic/Biliary Dysfunction

RC of Paralytic Ileus
RC of GI Bleeding
RC of Hepatic Dysfunction
RC of Hyperbilirubinemia

Risks for Complications of Muscular/Skeletal Dysfunction

RC of Pathologic Fractures
RC of Joint Dislocation

Risks for Complications of Medication Therapy Adverse Effects

RC of Anticoagulant Therapy Adverse Effects
RC of Antianxiety Therapy Adverse Effects
RC of Adrenocorticosteroid Therapy Adverse Effects
RC of Antineoplastic Therapy Adverse Effects
RC of Anticonvulsant Therapy Adverse Effects
RC of Antidepressant Therapy Adverse Effects
RC of Antiarrhythmic Therapy Adverse Effects
RC of Antipsychotic Therapy Adverse Effects
RC of Antihypertensive Therapy Adverse Effects
RC of β-Adrenergic Blocker Therapy Adverse Effects
RC of Calcium Channel Blocker Therapy Adverse Effects
RC of Angiotensin-Converting Enzyme Inhibitor and Angiotensin Receptor Blocker Therapy Adverse Effects
RC of Diuretic Adverse Effects

Carpenito, L. J. [2017]. *Nursing Diagnosis: Application to Clinical Practice* [15th ed.]. Philadelphia: Wolters Kluwer.

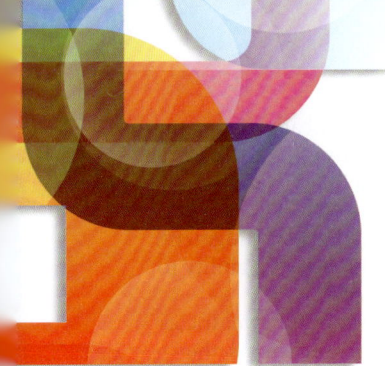

GLOSSARY

A

acculturation—the level of integration with and adoption of the cultural beliefs and behaviors by members of one cultural group living among members of another cultural group.
ADLs—activities of daily living
adrenarche—adrenocortical maturation, which occurs during puberty
adventitious breath sounds—abnormal breath sounds heard during auscultation of the lung fields; may include rales (crackles), rhonchi (wheezes), or pleural friction rubs
alopecia—hair loss
AMB—as manifested by
anatomic snuff box—triangular, depressed area on the dorsal radial side of the hand that lies over the scaphoid and trapezium carpal bones. The name comes from the practice of using this hollowed area to hold and sniff tobacco. This may be a tender point with scaphoid fractures of the hand.
anorexia—loss of appetite for food
anthropometer—a type of caliper used for measuring elbow breadth and other body parts
anthropometric measurements—measurements of the human body (e.g., height and weight, head circumference, waistline, percentage of body fat, and so forth)
anticholinergic effects—responses to anticholinergic medications, which inhibit the parasympathetic nervous system; in older adults, symptoms are associated with increased or decreased heart rate (depending on dosage), constipation, urinary retention, dilated pupils and vision problems, dry mouth, and drowsiness
anxiety—apprehensiveness related to an unknown source; occurs in different degrees
apical impulse—a normal visible pulsation in the area of the mid-clavicular line in the left fifth intercostal space; impulse can be seen in about half of the adult population
apnea—cessation of breathing
Argyll Robertson pupils—small, irregular pupils unresponsive to light
arthritis—inflammation of a joint
articulation—place of union or junction between two or more bones of the skeleton
atelectasis—collapse of a lung
atopic—allergic
atrial gallop—low-frequency heart sound known as S_4; occurs at the end of diastole when the atria contract and produced by vibrations from blood flowing rapidly into the ventricles after atrial contraction; S_4 has the rhythm of the word "Ten-nes-see" and may increase during inspiration
auscultation—assessment technique that uses a stethoscope to hear body sounds inaudible to the naked ear (e.g., heart sounds, movement of blood through the vessels, bowel sounds, and air moving through the respiratory tract)
AV—atrioventricular

B

BCP—birth control pills
benign breast disease—nonmalignant disease of the breast, such as fibrocystic breast disease
biologic variation—changes in physical status as a result of genetics and/or environment and/or the interaction of genetics and environment; human variation of a biologic and physiologic nature
Biot's respiration—breathing pattern marked by several short breaths followed by long, irregular periods of apnea; may be seen with increased intracranial pressure (IICP) or head trauma
bipolar disorder—mood disorder categorized as a psychosis and characterized by emotional ups and downs ranging from extreme depression to extreme elation
BP—blood pressure
bradycardia—heart rate less than 60 beats per minute
bradypnea—slow breathing pattern less than 10 breaths per minute
Braxton Hicks contractions—painless, irregular contractions of the uterus
Brudzinski's sign—flexion of the hips and knees in response to neck flexion; a sign of meningeal inflammation
bruit—abnormal sound; blowing, swishing, or murmuring sound caused by turbulent blood flow; heard during auscultation
bruxism—grinding the teeth
Buerger's disease—obliterative vascular disease marked by inflammation in small and medium-sized blood vessels.
bursa—small sac filled with synovial fluid that lubricates and cushions a joint

C

calcium—chemical element (Ca^{++}) that is a major component of bone structure and a necessary element for muscle contractions
CAM—The Confusion Assessment Method (CAM) is a two-part instrument to screen for overall cognitive impairment and to differentiate delirium or reversible confusion from other types of cognitive impairment.
capillary refill time—time it takes for reperfusion to occur after circulation has been stopped; test for capillary refill involves pressing on a fingernail firmly enough to stop circulation to the digit (signaled by blanching of the underlying tissue), releasing the pressure, and measuring the time it takes for color to return to the tissue; test is used to assess cardiac output

cardiac conduction—process of excitation initiated in the sinoatrial (SA) node, resulting in contraction of the heart muscle
cardiac cycle—cyclic filling and emptying of the heart
carotid artery—major coronary vessel that transports blood from the heart to the rest of the body
cataract—loss of transparency, or cloudiness in the crystalline lens of the eye
Cheyne-Stokes respiration—breathing pattern characterized by a period of apnea of 10 to 60 seconds, followed by increasing, then decreasing rate, followed by another period of apnea
chloasma—darkening of the skin on the face, known as the "mask of pregnancy"
chorionic villi sampling—test to detect birth defects
closed-ended question—question that can be answered with a yes, no, maybe, or other one- or two-word answers; typically used to clarify or specify information contributed in answers to open-ended questions; often begins with the words Are, Do, Did, Is, or Can.
clubbing—enlargement of fingertips and flattening of the angle between the fingernail and nailbed, as a result of heart and/or lung disease
CO—cardiac output
collaborative problems—physiologic complications that nurses monitor to detect their onset or changes in status
colonoscopy—internal examination and visualization of the colon performed by a physician with a colonoscope, a fiberoptic endoscope with a miniature camera attachment
compulsion—repetitive act that clients must perform and over which they have no control
crepitus—a crackling sound/tactile sensation due to air under the skin; may also be heard in joints
critical thinking—complex thought process that has many definitions; in this textbook, critical thinking is best described as a thinking process used to arrive at a conclusion about information that is available; necessary when trying to reason or analyze what a client's diagnosis is or is not; investigational process or inquiry used to examine data in order to arrive at a conclusion
culture—as defined by Purnell (2012), "the totality of socially transmitted behavioral patterns, arts, beliefs, values, customs, lifeways, and all other products of human work and thought characteristic of a population or people that guide their worldview and decision making"; all verbal and behavioral systems that transmit meaning
culture-bound syndrome—condition or state defined as an illness by a specific cultural group but not interpreted or perceived as an illness by other groups; may have a mental illness component or a spiritual cause
CVA—cerebrovascular accident, stroke
CVS—*see* chorionic villi sampling
cyanosis—bluish or gray coloring of the skin due to decreased amounts of hemoglobin in the blood, suggesting reduced oxygenation
cystocele—herniation of the urinary bladder through the vaginal wall

D

delirium—potentially reversible alteration in mental status that has developed over a short time and is characterized by a change in level of alertness

delusion—false feelings of self that are unreal; may be symptoms of psychotic disorders, delirium, or dementia
dementia—diagnostic category that includes multiple physical disorders characterized by slowly deteriorating memory and alterations in abstract thinking, judgment, and perception to the degree that the person's ability to perform everyday activities is affected
diastole—period when the heart relaxes and the ventricles fill with blood; in blood pressure measurements, the "bottom" value represents diastole
diastolic blood pressure—pressure between heartbeats (the pressure when the last sound is heard)
dimpling—indentation or retraction of subcutaneous tissue
direct percussion—direct tapping of a body part with one or two fingertips to elicit tenderness
documentation—committing findings in writing to the client's record
DRE—digital rectal examination
drug resistance—phenomenon that occurs when microorganisms develop a resistance to the effects of drug therapy, particularly antibiotic therapy
dyskinesia—incoordination marked by darting movements of the tongue and jerking movement of the arms and legs
dysphagia—difficulty swallowing solids or liquids
dystonia—abnormal muscle tone

E

ectopic pregnancy—pregnancy outside of the uterus; also called tubal pregnancy
ectropion—eversion of the lower eyelid
edema—accumulation of fluid in body tissues, which may cause swelling
ejection click—high-frequency heart sound auscultated just after S_1; produced by a diseased valve in mid-to-late systole
embryonic milk line—line formed during embryonic development; line starts in the axillary area, runs through the nipple, and extends down the abdomen on the outer side of the umbilicus down onto the upper, inner thigh; supernumerary breasts may occur along this line
entropion—inversion of the lower eyelid
epistaxis—nasal bleeding
erythema—redness due to capillary dilation
ethnicity—identification with a socially, culturally, and politically constructed group of people with common characteristics not shared by others with whom the group member comes in contact
ethnocentrism—perception that our worldview is the only acceptable truth and that our beliefs, values, and sanctioned behaviors are superior to all others
exophthalmos—protruding eyes
extrapyramidal tract—descending pathway of the nervous system outside of the pyramidal tract and responsible for conducting impulses to the muscles for maintaining muscle tone and body control
exudate—any fluid that has exuded out of tissues (e.g., pus)

F

fasciculations—fine tremors
fecal occult blood test (FOBT)—examination of a stool specimen to detect bleeding of unknown origin; also called guaiac smear test, guaiac smear, and stool occult blood test

fibroadenoma—abnormal formation of tissue or tumor of the glandular epithelium-forming fibrous tissue
fremitus—tactile vibration felt in neck and over the upper thorax from the transmission of vocal sounds from the airways to the surface of the chest wall
friction rub—auscultatory sound resulting from inflammation of the pericardial sac, as with pericarditis
fundus—uppermost part of a hollow organ such as uterus or stomach (gastric)

G

GCS—Glasgow Coma Scale, an instrument for evaluating level of consciousness
geriatric syndrome—symptoms that are common harbingers of disease and disability in a frail elderly person
graphesthesia—ability to identify letters and numbers and drawing by touch and without sight

H

heart murmur—sounds made by turbulent blood flow through the valves of the heart
hemorrhoids—varicose veins in the rectum
hepatomegaly—enlargement of the liver
heritage assessment—based on the concept of acculturation and how consistent the client's lifestyle is with the cultural group from which the client originates, or the traditional cultural habits of the client's family's culture.
HR—heart rate
hyperemesis gravidarum—severe and lengthy nausea with pregnancy

I

ICS—intercostal space
illusion—false interpretation of actual stimuli
indirect percussion—also known as mediate percussion; most common percussion method in which tapping elicits a tone that varies with the density of underlying structures (e.g., as density increases, the tone decreases)
induration—hardening
inframammary transverse ridge—firm compressed tissue that may be palpated below the mammary gland in the lower edges of the breasts, especially in large breasts; normal variation and not a tumor
inspection—physical examination technique using the senses (vision, smell, and hearing) to observe the condition of various body parts, including normal and abnormal findings
intercostal spaces—spaces between the ribs; the first intercostal space is directly below the first rib, the second intercostal space is below the second rib, and so forth

J

jaundice—yellowing of the skin, eye whites, or mucous membranes due to a deposit of bile pigments related to excess bilirubin in the blood; often seen in clients with liver or gallbladder disease, hemolysis, and some anemias
joint—place where two or more bones meet, providing a variety of ranges of motion; a joint may be classified as fibrous, cartilaginous, or synovial
jugular veins—major neck vessels that transport blood from the head and neck to the heart

K

keratin—protein that is the chief component of skin, hair, and nails
Kernig's sign—pain and resistance to extension of the knee in response to flexion of the leg at the hip and the knee; bilateral pain and resistance are signs of meningeal irritation
Korsakoff's syndrome—psychosis induced by excessive alcohol use and characterized by disorientation, amnesia, hallucinations, and confabulation
kyphosis—abnormally increased forward curvature of the upper spine

L

lanugo—fine, downy hairs that cover newborn's body
leading statement—statement made to elicit more information from the client; statements may begin with Explain, Describe, Tell, or Elaborate
lentigines—benign, spotty, brown skin discolorations, known as age spots or liver spots
lesion—abnormal change of tissue usually from injury or disease
leukoplakia—thick, white patches of cells that adhere to oral tissues; condition is precancerous
ligament—strong, dense band of fibrous connective tissue that joins the bones in synovial joints
linea nigra—dark line associated with pregnancy that extends from the umbilicus to the mons pubis
lordosis—exaggerated lumbar concavity often seen in pregnancy or obesity

M

macular degeneration—thinning or torn membrane in the center of the retina
mania—hyperexcitation; "manic" stage of manic–depressive disorder currently known as bipolar disorder
MCL—mid-clavicular line
McBurney's point/sign—point over the right side of the abdomen located one-third of the distance from the anterior superior iliac spine to the umbilicus; tenderness at McBurney's point is called McBurney's sign, which may indicate acute appendicitis
McMurray's test—test used to detect meniscal tears after a knee trauma; rotation and extension of the knee elicits a "click" when there is a torn meniscus.
melanin—pigment responsible for hair and skin color
menarche—first menstrual period
mucous plug—clump of mucus that seals the endocervical canal and prevents bacteria from ascending into the uterus
Murphy's sign—pain that occurs with inflammation of the gallbladder that is elicited by holding your fingers under the client's liver border while asking the client to take a deep breath; normally, no pain will occur

N

NANDA—North American Nursing Diagnosis Association
nonverbal communication—communication through body language including stance or posture, demeanor, facial expressions, and so forth
norms—learned behaviors that are perceived to be appropriate or inappropriate

NSR—normal sinus rhythm
nursing diagnosis—clinical judgment about individuals, family, or community responses to actual and potential health problems and life processes (North American Nursing Diagnosis Association, 2012–2014); provides the basis for selecting nursing interventions to achieve outcomes for which the nurse is accountable
nystagmus—rhythmic oscillation of the eyes

O

objective data—findings that are directly or indirectly observed through measurements; data can be physical characteristics (e.g., skin color, rashes, posture), body functions (e.g., heart rate, respiratory rate), appearance (e.g., dress, hygiene), behavior (e.g., mood, affect), measurements (e.g., blood pressure, temperature, height, weight), or the results of laboratory testing (e.g., platelet count, x-ray findings)
obsession—uncontrollable thought or thoughts that are unacceptable to client; characteristic of some neurotic disorders
obturator test/sign—test performed when one suspects appendicitis; when the test is positive, client has pain when the right leg is rotated internally and then externally, which may indicate a perforated appendix
open-ended question—question that cannot be answered with a yes, no, or maybe; usually requires a descriptive or explanatory answer; often begins with the words What, How, When, Where, or Who.
opening snap—extra heart sound occurring in early diastole and resulting from the opening of a stenotic or stiff mitral valve; often mistaken for a split S_2 or an S_3
orthopnea—difficulty breathing unless in a sitting or standing position; not uncommon in severe cardiac and pulmonary disease
orthostatic hypotension—drop in blood pressure when client arises from a sitting or lying position
osteoporosis—low bone density that occurs when bone-forming cells cannot keep pace with bone-destroying cells

P

PAD—peripheral artery disease
pallor—paleness, lack of color
palpation—examination technique in which the examiner uses the hands to touch and feel certain body characteristics, such as texture, temperature, mobility, shape, moisture, and motion
PAOD—peripheral arterial occlusive disease
paralytic strabismus—eyes deviate from normal position depending on the direction of gaze
parkinsonism—symptoms of Parkinson's disease that are secondary to another condition such as cerebral trauma, brain tumor, infection, or an adverse drug reaction
Parkinson's disease—chronic progressive degeneration of the brain's dopamine neuronal systems that is characterized by muscle rigidity, tremor, and slowed movements
PC—potential complication
percussion—tapping a body chamber with fingers to elicit the sounds from underlying organs and structures
perforator vein—vein that connects a superficial vein with a deep vein; also called communicator vein
PERRL—pupils equally reactive and responsive to light
pica—a craving for nonnutritional substances such as dirt or clay
pneumothorax—accumulation of air in the pleural space
point localization—ability to identify points touched on body without seeing the points touched
polyhydramnios—excessive amniotic fluid associated with multiple gestation or fetal abnormalities
postural hypotension—orthostatic hypotension characterized by dizziness or lightheadedness upon rising from a lying or sitting position
precordium—anterior surface of the body overlying the heart and great vessels
presbycusis—inability to hear high-frequency sounds or to discriminate a variety of simultaneous sounds caused by degeneration of the hair cells in the inner ear
presbyopia—farsightedness; person can see print and objects from farther away than considered normal
primary pain—original source of pain
proctosigmoidoscopy—internal examination and visualization of the sigmoid colon performed by a physician with a sigmoidoscope, a fiberoptic endoscope with miniature camera attachment
prodromal—precursor or early warning symptom of disease (e.g., aura before a migraine headache or seizure)
proprioception—sensory faculties mediated by sensory nerves located in tissues such as the muscles and tendons
prostatic hyperplasia—enlargement of the prostate gland
pruritus—itching
PSA—prostate-specific antigen
pseudodementia—depressive symptoms that are commonly mistaken in the elderly for a dementia
psoas test/sign—test performed by having the client lie on the side with knees extended, while passively extending the thigh, or asking the client to flex the thigh at the hip; movement causes abdominal pain with a positive psoas sign, which may indicate appendicitis, a psoas abscess, or other forms of retroperitoneal irritation.
pterygium—thickening of the bulbar conjunctiva that grows over the cornea and may interfere with vision
ptosis—drooping eyelids
ptyalism—excessive salivation
pulse amplitude—strength of the pulse
pyramidal tract—descending pathway of the nervous system; carries impulses that produce voluntary movements requiring skill and purpose

R

range of motion—natural distance and direction of movement of a joint
referral problem—problem that requires the attention or assistance of other health care professionals besides nurses
referred pain—pain perceived in an area that is not related to its original source (e.g., gallbladder pain may radiate to the right shoulder and pancreatic pain may radiate to the back)
reinforcement technique—presentation of a stimulus so as to modify a response; increasing of a reflex response by causing the person to perform a physical or mental task while the reflex is being tested
retraction—indentation
r/t—related to

Rovsing's sign—increased right lower quadrant pain that is elicited by palpation of the left lower quadrant of a client's abdomen; may indicate appendicitis.
ruga—wrinkle, or fold, of skin or mucous membrane

S

SA—sinoatrial
satiety—fullness, satisfaction commonly associated with meals
scleroderma—degenerative disease characterized by fibrosis and vascular abnormalities in the skin and internal organs
scoliosis—lateral curvature of the spine with an increase in convexity on the side that is curved
SLUMS—Saint Louis University Mental Status (SLUMS) Examination Tool to determine mild cognitive impairment and dementia
splenomegaly—enlargement of the spleen
stereognosis—ability to identify an object by touch rather than sight
sternal retraction—pulling in of sternum during respiration in a physiologic attempt to take in more oxygen; seen in hypoxia or air hunger
STI—sexually transmitted infection; also called sexually transmitted disease
stroke—also known as a CVA, cerebrovascular accident
subjective data—descriptive rather than measurable information; symptoms, sensations, feelings, perceptions, desires, preferences, beliefs, ideas, values, and personal information contributed by a client or other person and verifiable only by the client or other person
supernumerary nipple—more than two nipples
SV—stroke volume; the volume of blood pumped with each contraction of the heart
synovitis—inflammation of the synovial membrane, which surrounds the joint space and contains synovial fluid that lubricates the joint and enhances movement; characterized by painful movement of the joint
system—interacting whole formed of many parts
systole—cardiac phase during which the ventricles contract and eject blood into the pulmonary and circulatory systems
systolic blood pressure—pressure of the blood flow when the heart beats (the pressure when the first sound is heard)

T

tachycardia—heart rate exceeding 100 beats per minute
tachypnea—rapid, shallow breathing pattern exceeding 20 breaths per minute
temporal event—relating to a particular time of day or activity
tendon—strong, fibrous cord of connective tissue continuous with the fibers of a muscle; tendon attaches muscle to bone or cartilage
TENS—transcutaneous electrical nerve stimulation; treatment modality associated with muscle pain, particularly low back pain

thelarche—time during puberty when breasts develop in females
thrill—palpable vibration over the precordium or an artery; usually the result of stenosis or partial occlusion
TIA—transient ischemic attack; minor stroke, sometimes called mini-stroke
TMJ syndrome—temporomandibular joint problems; limited range of motion, swelling, tenderness, pain, or crepitation in the jaw area
torus palatinus—bony protuberance on the hard palate where the intermaxillary transverse palatine sutures join
trigger factors—factors (e.g., touch, pressure and/or chemical substances) that initiate or stimulate a response such as pain
turgor—normal skin tone, tension, and elasticity

U

uterine prolapse—protrusion of the cervix down through the vagina
UTI—urinary tract infection

V

validation—verification
values—learned beliefs about what is held to be good or bad
varicocele—varicose veins of the scrotum, which feels like a bag of worms upon palpation
venous hum—benign chest sound like roaring water caused by turbulence of blood in the jugular veins; common in children
ventricular gallop—another term for S_3, the third heart sound, which has low frequency and is often accentuated during inspiration; sound has rhythm of the word "Kentucky" and results from vibrations produced as blood hits the ventricular wall during filling
verbal communication—conversation with words, either spoken or written
viscera (solid, hollow)—internal organs; may consist of solid tissue (e.g., liver) or be hollow to fill with fluids or other substances (e.g., stomach or bladder)
visual field—what a person sees with one eye; field has four parts of quadrants: upper temporal, lower temporal, upper nasal, and lower nasal
vital signs—measurable signs of cardiopulmonary and thermoregulatory health status; signs include pulse rate, respiratory rate and character, blood pressure, and temperature (*Note:* Some experts do not consider temperature a vital sign)
voluntary guarding—person's willful attempt to protect body against pain by holding breath or tightening muscles

References

NANDA International. (2012). *Nursing diagnoses: Definitions and classification 2012–2014*. Oxford, UK: Wiley-Blackwell.
Purnell, L. (2012). *Transcultural health care: a culturally competent approach* (4th ed.). Philadelphia: F. A. Davis.

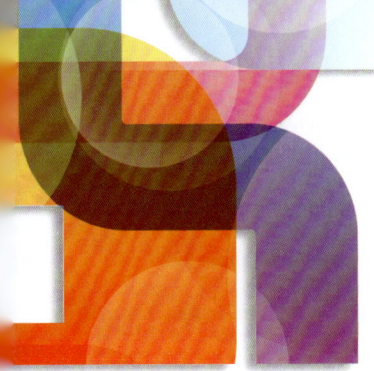

INDEX

Note: Page numbers followed by b indicate text in boxes; those followed by f indicate figures; and those followed by t indicate tables.

A

Abdomen
  auscultation of, 507b–508b
  contour of, 505b, 506f
  development of, 763
  distention of, 505b
  palpation, 513b–516b, 513f, 520b
  percussion, 508b–5012b, 509f–512f
  physical assessment of, 681b–682b, 681f, 682f
  quadrants, 492, 492f
  regions, 492, 492f
  scaphoid (sunken), 505b
  skin, 504b
  symmetry, 506b
  vascular structures, 495, 495f
Abdominal adhesions, 498b, 505b
Abdominal aortic aneurysm (AAA), 506b, 514b
  screening for, 507b
Abdominal assessment, 492–526
  abdominal pain, 499b–500b
  abdominal signs, 520b
  abnormal findings in
    abdominal bulges, 524b–525b
    abdominal distention, 523b–524b
    enlarged organs, 525b–526b
  case study, 502b, 520b–521b
  data analysis, 521
    collaborative problems, 522
    medical problems, 522
    nursing diagnoses, 521–522
  gastroesophageal reflex disease, 501b
  health history, 495–496
    abdominal pain, 499b–500b
    family history, 498b
    history of present health concern, 496b–498b
    lifestyle and health practices, 499b
    personal health history, 498b
  in older adults, 496b, 497b, 498b
  peptic ulcer disease, 500b–501b
  physical examination, 502–503
    abdominal girth (circumference), 519b
    appendicitis/peritoneal irritation, tests for, 517b–519b
    ascites, tests for, 516b–517b
    assessment, order for, 503
    cholecystitis, tests for, 519b
    client preparation, 503, 503f
    equipment for, 32t, 503
    general routine screening *vs.* focused specialty assessment, 504

  inspection, 504b–507b
  palpation, 520b
  ticklish client and, 503
  SBAR method, use of, 523
  structure and function in, 492
    abdominal quadrants, 492, 493b, 493f
    abdominal wall muscles, 492–493, 494f
    internal anatomy, 493–495, 494f, 495f
Abdominal girth, measurement of, 519b
Abdominal pain, 496b
  character of, 500b
  location of, 496b
  parietal pain, 499b
  referred pain, 496b, 499b
  types of, 499b
  visceral pain, 499b
Abdominal reflex, 595b, 596f
Abdominal viscera, 493–494, 494f
  hollow viscera, 495
  solid viscera, 494–495
Abdominal wall muscles, 492–493, 494f
Abortion, 698b, 699b
Absence seizure, 573b
Abuse
  adult (*See* Family violence)
  alcohol, 79b
  child
    consequences of, 164
    definition of, 163
  elder, 164
  family
    economic, 162
    physical, 162
    psychological, 162, 163b
    sexual, 162–163
Abuse assessment screen, 172b
Acanthosis nigricans, 258b, 258f, 424b
Acculturation, 183b
Achilles reflex, 594b, 594f
Acid reflux, 496b, 501b
Acquired immuno deficiency syndrome (AIDS), 222, 613b. *See also* Human immunodeficiency virus (HIV) infection
Acrocyanosis, 722, 724
Acromegaly
  head and neck findings in, 289, 301b
  physical appearance in, 128b, 140b
Actinic keratoses, 832b
Activities of daily living (ADLs), 4
  musculoskeletal system and, 534, 537b
  older adults and, 816

Actual nursing diagnoses, 63, 65
Acute angle-closure glaucoma (AACG), 312b
Acute rheumatic fever (ARF), 441b
Adam's apple. *See* Thyroid cartilage
Adipose tissue, 637
ADLs. *See* Activities of daily living
Adnexa, 639
Adnexal masses, 670b
Adolescents. *See also* Child and adolescent assessment
  athletic, 791b
  body piercing and tattoos in, 809b
  cognitive and language development in, 768
  growth pattern, 765
  Healthy People 2020 goals for, 788b
  interviewing, 777–779
  moral development in, 768
  motor development in, 766
  nutritional requirements, 771–772
  psychosexual development in, 770–771
  psychosocial development in, 769
  sensory perception in, 767
  sleep requirements, 774
  stressors in, 775t
  suicide assessment, 776b
Adrenocortical maturation, 761
Adventitious sounds, 398b, 402t
Afterload, 436
Age-related macular degeneration (AMD), prevention of, 313b–314b
AIDS. *See* Acquired immuno deficiency syndrome
Air trapping, 403t
Alcohol abuse, self-assessment for, 79b
Alcohol ingestion, 499b
Alcohol-related birth defects (ARBD), 702b
Alcohol Use Disorders Identification test (AUDIT), 76b–77b
Allen test, 477b, 477f
Alveolar sacs, 383, 384f
Alzheimer disease, 75b–76b
  culture and, 197
  SLUMS Mental Status Examination for, 91b
  vs. dementia, 93t
  warning signs of, 91b
American Academy of Ophthalmology (AAO), 5, 312b
American Academy of Pediatrics (AAP), 727
American Cancer Society (ACS), 5, 641

905

American College of Obstetricians and Gynecologists (ACOG), 697b
American Diabetic Association (ADA), 5
American Heart Association (AHA), 5
American Nurses Association, 1
American Speech-Language-Hearing Association, 344b
Amylase, 358
Anal canal, 607, 639
Anal crypts, 639
Anal fissure, 633b
Analgesia, 590b
Anal opening, 607, 639
Anal sex, 612b
Anal sphincter, 624b, 624f
Anal stage, 770
Anal verge. *See* Anal opening
Anatomic variation, 194
Anesthesia, 589b
Angina, 440b
Angle of Louis. *See* Sternal angle
Anisocoria, 334b
Ankle–brachial index (ABI), 483b–484b, 486b
Ankle-brachial pressure index (ABPI). *See* Ankle–brachial index (ABI)
Ankle clonus, 594b, 595f
Ankles and feet, 557b–559b
 inspection and palpation, 557b–558b, 558f
 range of motion of, 559b, 559f
 squeeze test, 558b, 558f
Ankylosing spondylitis, 563b
Annular skin lesions, 277b
Anorectal fistula, 623b, 633b
Anorectal junction, 607, 639
Anorexia nervosa, 128, 140b, 497b
Antacids, chronic use of, 498b
Anterior axillary line, 383, 383f
Anterior chamber, of eye
 inspection of, 326b
 structure and function of, 306, 306f
Anterior cord syndrome, 600b
Anthropometric measurements, 231–239, 236f, 237t
 body mass index, 224t, 233b–234b, 236f
 height, 232b, 233f
 ideal body weight, 233b
 ideal body weight percentage, 233b
 mid-arm circumference, 236b–237b
 mid-arm muscle circumference, 238b, 239t
 triceps skin fold thickness, 237b, 237f, 239t
 waist circumference, 234b, 235f, 236t
 waist-to-hip ratio, 235b, 235f
 weight measurement, 233b, 233f
Anti-inflammatory diet, 220–221
Antiretroviral treatment (ART), 613b
Anus and rectum, 639, 640f
 abnormalities of, 633b–634b
 inspection, 622b–623b, 656b–658b, 658f
 palpation, 623b–624b, 624f
 structure and function of, 607–608, 607f
Aorta, 431, 432f
Aortic aneurysm, 526b
Aortic regurgitation, murmur of, 461b–462b
Aortic stenosis, murmur of, 460b
Aortic valve, 433
Aortoiliac occlusion, 469b

Apgar score, 733t
Apical impulse, 448b
 palpation of, 449b, 449f
Apnea, sleep, 387b
Apocrine glands, 248, 248f
Appendicular skeleton, 528, 529f
Appetite
 changes in, 497b
 loss of, 497b
Aqueous humor, 306
Arcus senilis, 323f, 835b
Areola, 409
 inspection of, 420b
Argyll Robertson pupils, 582b
Arms
 inspection of, 474b, 475f
 measurements
  mid-arm circumference, 236b–237b, 236f, 237t
  triceps skin fold thickness, 237b, 237f, 239t
 palpation of, 475b–477b
 physical assessment of, 679b–680b, 679f, 680f
Arterial insufficiency, 488b
 testing for, 482b, 482f
Arterial pulse and pressure waves, 454b–455b, 463
 bigeminal pulse, 455b
 bisferiens pulse, 455b
 large, bounding pulse, 455b
 paradoxical pulse, 455b
 pulsus alternans, 455b
 small, weak pulse, 455b
Arterial ulcer, 489b
Arteries, 463–464, 464f, 465f
 of arm, 464, 465f
 of leg, 464, 465f
Arterioles, 305, 306f
Arteriovenous banking, 335b
Arteriovenous nicking, 335b
Arteriovenous tapering, 335b
Ascites, tests for, 516b–517b
Ascitic fluid, 524b
Aspirin, 470b
Assessment, 1. *See also* Health assessment
 by acute care nurse, 3, 3f
 by ambulatory care nurses, 3
 in critical care, 3
 emergency, 6–7, 6f
 focused or problem-oriented, 6
 by home health nurses, 3
 initial comprehensive, 5–6, 6f
 in nursing process, 3–8, 4t
  objective data collection, 8, 8f
  preparing for, 7, 7f
  subjective data collection, 7–8, 8f
  validation of data, 8, 9f
 ongoing or partial, 6, 6f
 by public health nurses, 3
Assessment forms
 focused or specialty area, 56, 57f
 frequent or ongoing, 52f–55f
  admission form, 51
  progress note, 56
 initial, 51, 51b
Assessment tools
 for family violence

abuse assessment screen in, 172b
 assessing a safety plan in, 177b
for mental status
 Alcohol Use Disorders Identification test, 76b–77b
 Confusion Assessment Method, 92b
 Glasgow Coma Scale, 90b
 SLUMS Mental Status Examination, 91b
for nutrition
 24-hour food recall, 225b
 nutrition history, 225, 226b
for pain
 FLACC Behavioral Scale, 151, 152b
 McCafferty Initial Pain Assessment Tool, 151, 153b
 Universal Pain Assessment Tool, 150, 151b
for skin
 Braden scale for pressure sore risk, 266b–268b
 PUSH tool for pressure ulcer healing, 268b
for spiritual and religious practices
 Brief Religious Coping Questionnaire, 210b
 Daily Spiritual Experiences Scale, 210b
 FICA Spiritual History Tool, 211b
 HOPE questions, 211b
 SPIRIT acronym, 209b
Assimilation, 183b
Asthma, 388b
 and gastroesophageal reflux disease, 388b
Ataxic respiration, 403t
Athetosis, 574b, 602b
Atria, 431
Atrial fibrillation, 457b
Atrial gallop, 436, 451b, 458b
Atrial kick, 435
Atrial systole, 435
Atrioventricular (AV) valves, 432
Atrophic vaginitis, 668b
Aura, 573b
Auricle
 inspection of, 347b
 palpation of, 348b
 structure of, 338
Auscultation, 42–43, 43b
Autonomic nervous system, 572
Aveoli, 383, 384f
AV node, 433
Axial skeleton, 528, 529f
Axillae, inspection and palpation, 424b
Axillary hair development, 763, 764
Axillary lymph nodes, 411, 411f
Axillary temperature, 130b, 130f
Azarcon, 781

B

Babinski response (reflex), 595b, 595f, 807b
 in children and adolescents, 807b
 in newborns and infants, 753b, 755b
Back pain
 during pregnancy, 695
 test for, 545b
Bacterial vaginosis, 669b
Balance, testing of, 587b, 587f
Balding, male pattern, 263b, 263f

Ballottement knee test, 556b, 556f
Barlow sign, 724
Barrel chest, 398b, 406b
Bartholin glands, 638
    palpation of, 652b, 653f
Basal cell carcinoma, 260b, 276b. *See also*
    Skin cancer
Beers Criteria for Potentially Inappropriate
    Medication (PIM) Use in Elderly,
    815
Beliefs, health care, 187–189
    blood products and transfusion in, 189
    causes of illness in, 189–190, 190f
    culture-based treatments in, 190, 192f
    culture-bound syndromes in, 191,
        191t–192t
    death rituals in, 190
    pain in, 193
    pregnancy and childbearing in, 190, 193
    traditional healers and practices in, 189t,
        192f
Bell palsy, 301b, 583b
Benign paroxysmal positional vertigo
    (BPPV), 340b
Benign prostatic hypertrophy (BPH), 612b,
    635b
    in older adults, 822b
Biceps reflex, 592b, 593f
Bicuspid (mitral) valve, 432
Bilateral transverse laceration, 661b
Bimanual palpation, 40, 41f
Biochemical variation, 194
Biologic theory, of violence, 162
Biot respiration, 403t
Birth control method, 611b
Blepharitis, 332f
Blood pressure
    in adults, 137
    assessment of, objective, 122f, 123b,
        133b, 134t, 135b
    in children, 791b, 791f
    classification of, 136t
    definition of, 122
    factors contributing to, 123b
    high (hypertension), 136t
    low (hypotension) orthostatic, 133b
    in older adults, 838b, 839f
Blood products, health care beliefs and, 193
Blood volume, effect of, on blood pressure,
    123b
Blue nailbeds, 794b
Blumberg sign, 517b, 520b
Body build (type), 231b, 231f
Body language, culture and, 187
Body mass index (BMI)
    adult, 222, 224t
    diabetes, hypertension, cardiovascular
        disease and, 236t
    measurement of, 233b–234b
Body surface variation, 194
Bone, 528, 529f
    density scans, 537b
    facial, 280
    formation, 764
    growth, 764
    pain, 532b, 535b
Borborygmus, 507b
Bouchard nodes, 552b, 564b

Boutonnière deformity, 564b
Bowel patterns, 642b–643b
    changes in, 497b–498b, 610b
Bowel sounds, 507b, 802b
    hyperactive, 507b
    hypoactive, 507b
Bowen's family system theory, 857, 859–860
    differentiation of self, 859–860
    triangles, 860
BPH. *See* Benign prostatic hypertrophy
BPPV. *See* Benign paroxysmal positional
    vertigo
Brachial artery, 464
Brachial pulse, 476b, 476f
Brachioradialis reflex, 593b, 593f
Bradycardia, 132b, 449b
Bradypnea, 403t
Brain gut axis, 499b
Brain stem, 569
Braxton Hick contractions, 694, 709b
Breast, 409, 410f
    benign breast disease, 423b, 429b
    cancerous tumors, 429b
    development of, 762
    dimpling of, 412b, 421b, 428b
    female, 409
        development of, 762, 762t
        fatty tissue, 411, 411f
        fibrous tissue, 411, 411f
        forward-leaning position for inspection,
            422b, 422f
        glandular tissue, 411, 411f
        inspection, 420b–422b, 420f–422f
        palpation, 422b–423b
    fibrocystic, 412b, 423b
    implants, 413b–414b
    lumps in, 412b
    male, 409
        inspection and palpation, 424b
    menstruation on, effect of, 413b
    in older adults, 412b, 420b, 422b, 841b
    pain and tenderness of, 412b
    palpation, 425
    peau d'orange, 420b, 428b
    physical assessment of, 681b, 681f
    quadrants of, 409, 410f
    retracted breast tissue, 428b
    sagging, 412b
Breastbone. *See* Sternum
Breast cancer
    BRCA mutations in, 414b
    client education, 416b
    dimpling of nipple and, 412b, 421b
    history of, 412b, 413b
    prevention of, 415b–416b
    risk assessment, 416b
    risk factors for, 412b–413b
    screening for, 414b, 415b
    types of, 415b
Breast(s) and lymphatic assessment,
    409–430
    abnormal findings
        on inspection of breast, 428b–429b
        on palpation of breast, 429b
    anatomic landmarks and position in
        thorax, 409, 410f
    data analysis, 426–427
        collaborative problems, 427

        medical problems, 427
        nursing diagnoses, 426–427
    health history, 411
        case study, 418b
        family history, 413b
        history of present health concern, 412b
        lifestyle and health practices,
            413b–414b
        personal health history, 412b–413b
    male *vs.* female breast, 409
    physical examination, 418–419
        assessment, key points for, 419
        axillae, 424b
        breast palpation, 425b
        breast self-examination, 424b
        case study, 426b
        client preparation, 419
        equipment, 419
        equipment for, 419
        female breasts, 420b–423b
        general routine screening *vs.* focused
            specialty assessment, 419b
        male breasts, 424b
        validating and documenting findings,
            426
    SBAR method, use of, 427
    structure and function in, 409
        external breast anatomy, 409–410, 410f
        internal breast anatomy, 411, 411f
        lymph nodes, 409, 411, 411f
        quadrants of breast, 409, 410f
Breast self-awareness, 413b
Breast self-examination (BSE), 413b, 416b,
    424b
    benefits and limitations of, 413b–414b
    steps of, 416b–417b
Breathing
    mechanics of, 385–386, 386f
    patterns, changes in, 385
Breath sounds, 800b
    adventitious, 398b, 402t
    diminished/absent, 397b
    normal, 397b, 402t
Brief Religious Coping Questionnaire, 210b
Brittle bone disease, 797b
Bronchi, 383, 384f
Bronchioles, 383
Bronchophony, 398b
Brown–Séquard syndrome, 586b, 600b
Brudzinski sign, 596b
Bruits, 507b
Brushfield spots, 797b
BSE. *See* Breast self-examination
Buccal mucosa, 368b, 368f
Buffalo hump, 833b
Bulbourethral galnds, 608
Bulge knee test, 555b, 555f
Bulla, 273b
Bundle of His, 433
Bunion, 557b. *See also* Hallux valgus
Bursae, 530
Butterfly rash, 259, 259f

C

Café-au-lait spot, 809b
CAGE Questionnaire, 78b, 82
Calf circumference, 478b, 478f

Calluses, 557b, 565b
Canal of Schlemm, 306
Cancer pain, 145, 146b
Candidal vaginitis (moniliasis), 668b
Canthus, 304
Capillaries, 466, 466f
Capillary refill testing, 265b, 265f
Capillary refill time, 475b
Carcinoma in situ (CIS), 647
Cardiac cycle, 433, 434–435, 434f
    diastole, 434–435
    systole, 435
Cardiac muscle cells, 433
Cardiac output (CO), 436
    effect of, on blood pressure, 123b
    and fatigue, 440b
Carotid arterial pulse, 439
Carotid arteries, 282, 436, 439f
    auscultation of, 447b, 447f
    palpation of, 448b, 448f
Carpal tunnel syndrome (CTS)
    and pregnancy, 695
    during pregnancy, 695
    tests for, 550b–551b, 550f, 551f
Cartilaginous joints, 530
Caruncle, 304
Casper toolkit, 871
Cataracts, 835b
    prevention of, 314b–315b
Cellular aging, 815
Centers for Disease Control and Prevention (CDC), 5, 33
    isolation precaution guidelines, 33, 34b–36b
Central cord syndrome, 600b
Central nervous system (CNS), 567–570
    brain, 567–569, 568f
        brain stem, 569
        cerebellum, 569
        cerebrum, 567, 568t
        diencephalon, 569
    neural pathways, 569–570, 570f
    spinal cord, 567, 569, 569f
Cerebellar ataxia, 603b
Cerebellar system examination, 579
Cerebellum, 569
Cerebral palsy, 587b
Cerebrovascular accident, 302b. *See also* Stroke
Cerebrovascular disease, culture and, 197
Cerebrum, 567, 568t
Cerumen, 338, 836b–837b
Cervical cancer, 647b
    client education, 647b
    risk assessment, 647b
    screening, 647b
Cervical erosion, 667b
Cervical eversion, 661b
Cervical intraepithelial neoplasia (CIN), 647
Cervical motion tenderness (CMT), 655
Cervical polyp, 667b
Cervical spine
    lateral bending, 544b, 544f
    range of motion of, 543b, 543f
    rotation, 544b, 544f
Cervical strain, 543
Cervical vertebrae
    inspection of, 292b
    structure and function of, 281, 282f
Cervix, 639
    abnormalities of, 667b–668b
        cancer of, 667b
        cyanosis of, 667b
    palpation, 655b
    stretches, 639
Chadwick sign, 694
Chalazion, 332f
Chancres, 619b
Cherry angiomas, 266b, 276b, 832b
Chest pain, 387b, 440b
    cardiac, 440b
    pleuritis and, 387b
Chest, physical assessment of, 680b–681b, 680f–681f
Cheyne-Stokes respiration, 403t
Chief complaint (CC), 21
Child abuse
    consequences of, 164
    definition of, 163
Child Abuse Prevention and Treatment Act (CAPTA), 163
Child and adolescent assessment, 761–812
    case study, 787b–788b, 810b, 811b
    data analysis, 811
        collaborative problems, 811
        medical problems, 811
        nursing diagnoses, 811
    growth and development in
        activity and exercise and, 772
        cognitive and language, 767–768
        coping and stress management, 775–776
        Healthy People 2020 on, 788b
        moral, 768
        motor, 765–766
        nutritional requirements and, 771–772
        physical, 761–765
        psychosexual, 769–771
        psychosocial, 769
        relationship and role development, 774
        self-esteem and self-concept development, 774–775, 775t
        sensory perception, 767
        sleep requirements and patterns, 772, 774
        socioeconomic situation and, 774
    nursing history in, 776–777
        abdomen, 785b
        anus and rectum, 786b
        biographic data in, 779b
        breasts and lymphatics, 784b
        ears, 783b
        eyes, 783b
        family history in, 781b–782b
        genitalia and sexuality, 785b–786b
        head and neck, 783b
        heart and neck vessels, 784b
        history of present concern in, 779b–780b
        interviewing in, 777–779
        lifestyle and health practices in, 782b
        mouth, throat, nose, and sinuses, 783b–784b
        musculoskeletal system, 787b
        neurologic system, 787b
        peripheral vascular system, 784b
        present health history in, 780b–781b
        review of systems in, 782b–787b
        skin, hair, nails, 782b–783b
        thorax and lungs, 784b
    physical examination in, 789
        abdomen, 801b–803b
        anus and rectum, 804b–805b
        breasts, 801b
        client preparation, 789
        developmental approaches to, 789, 789b
        developmental assessment, 790b
        ears, 798b–800b
        equipment for, 789
        eyes, 796b–798b
        female genitalia, 804b
        focused specialty assessment, 789
        general appearance and behavior, 790b
        head, neck, and cervical lymph nodes, 794b–795b
        heart, 801b
        male genitalia, 803b
        measurements in, 791b–792b
        mouth, throat, and sinuses, 795b–796b
        musculoskeletal, 805b–807b
        neurologic, 807b–808b
        skin, hair, and nails, 793b–794b
        thorax and lungs, 800b
        vital signs, 790b–791b
    SBAR method, use of, 811
    skin variations and, 808b–809b
    validating and documenting findings in, 809b
Childbearing, health care beliefs and, 190, 193
Childbearing women, 691–720
    assessment in, 697–720 (*See also* Pregnancy assessment)
    structure and function in, 691–695 (*See also* Pregnancy)
Children. *See also* Child and adolescent assessment
    blood pressure in, 791b, 791f
    coping mechanisms in, 775, 775t
    interview of
        for family violence, 171b
    obesity in, 771
    pain perception in, 148, 148b
    stressors in, 775, 775t
Cholecystitis, 519b
Chordae tendineae, 432
Chorea, 574b
Chorea choreiform, 602b
Choroid, 305, 306f
Chronic nonmalignant pain, 145
Chronic obstructive pulmonary disease (COPD), 389b–390b
    client education, 390b
    and dyspnea, 386b
    nutritional status in, 389b
    risk factors for, 390b
    screening for, 390b
    second-hand smoke and, 389b
Cilia, 383
Ciliary body, 305
Circular communication, 860
CLAS mandates, 184

Clavicles (collarbones), 381
Clitoris, 637
Closed-ended questions, 16
Clustered, skin lesions, 277b
Cluster headache, 299b–300b
Clustering data, 62
Cochlea, 339, 339f
Cognitive abilities, 88b–90b. *See also* Mental status
Cognitive development
　in child and adolescent, 767–768
　in newborns and infants, 726
　Piaget theory of, 102, 103t–104t
Coining, 190, 192f
Coitus, 637
Cold, herbal therapies for, 389b
COLDSPA (mnemonic), 21, 22b
Collaborative problems, 9
　definition of, 62
　vs. nursing diagnoses, 63f
Colon, 495
Colonoscopy, 644
Colorectal cancer (CRC), 611b, 648b
　client education, 648b
　risk assessment, 648b
　screening, 648b
Columbia Suicide Severity Rating Scale (CSSRS), 82, 88b
Columns of Morgagni, 607, 639
Communication
　body language and hand gestures in, 187
　cultural variations in, 17
　culture and, 186–187
　emotional variations in, 17–18, 19b
　examples of, 188b–189b
　eye contact and face positioning in, 187
　gerontologic variations in, 16–17, 17f
　during interview, 14–18
　nonverbal, 14–15
　　appearance, 14
　　attitude, 15
　　to avoid, 15b
　　demeanor, 14
　　facial expressions, 14
　　listening, 15
　　silence, 15
　play as, 777
　SBAR model of, 58, 58b
　silence in, 187
　techniques, 777–778
　touch in, 187
　verbal, 16
　　to avoid, 15b
　　closed-ended questions, 16
　　inferring information, 16
　　laundry list, 16
　　open-ended questions, 16
　　providing information, 16
　　rephrasing, 16
　　well-placed phrases, 16
Community
　boundaries of, 873b
　classification of, 870
　communication, means of, 878b, 879f
　definition of, 869–870
　education resources in, 877b, 878f
　geopolitical, 870

government and political structures of, 878b
　health services, 874b–875b
　housing options, 873b–874b
　long-term care services, 876b
　neighborhood, 873b
　recreation and leisure programs, 879b, 879f
　social programs, 875b
　transportation options, 877b
　values and religious beliefs, 873b, 873f
Community assessment, 869–884
　case study on, 869b, 881b–882b, 882b–883b, 883b–884b
　childhood mortality, causes of, 880b
　Community as Partner model, 870–871, 870f
　data analysis, 883
　　collaborative problems, 883
　　medical problems, 883
　　nursing diagnoses, 883
　general routine screening *vs.* focused specialty assessment, 871
　models of, 870–871
　neonatal and infant mortality, causes of, 880b
　procedure, 871
　　community history, 871b
　　demographic information, 871b–873b
　　health and social services, 874b–879b
　　physical environment, 873b–874b
　purpose of, 869
　SBAR method, use of, 884
　teen and adult mortality, causes of, 880b
　validating and documenting findings, 882
Community Assessment for Public Health Emergency Response (CASPER), 871
Compact bone, 528
Complementary and alternative medicine (CAM) therapies, for insomnia, 27b
Cone of light, 338
Cones, 305, 306f
Confluent skin lesions, 277b
Confusion Assessment Method (CAM), 92b, 818b
Conjunctiva
　inspection of, 321b
　structure and function of, 304
Conjunctivitis, 331f
Constipation, 497b–498b, 610b
Constricted arteriole, 335b
Cooing, 726
Cooper ligaments, 411
COPD. *See* Chronic obstructive pulmonary disease
Coping mechanisms, in children, 775, 775t
Copper wire arteriole, 335b
Cornea
　abnormalities of, 333b
　inspection of, 323b
　structure and function of, 305, 306f
Corneal reflex, testing of, 583b, 583f
Corns, 557b, 565b
Coronary artery disease, dyslipidemia and, 441b

Coronary heart disease
　client education, 443b
　prevention of, 442b–443b
　risk factors for, 443b
　screening for risk of, 443b
Corpus, 637, 639
Corpus callosum, 567
Corpus spongiosum, 605
Costal angle, 382
Costovertebral angle, 494, 495f
Cotton-wool patches, 326b, 336b
Cough, 387b–388b
　in evening, 387b
　in morning, 387b
　nonproductive, 388b
　and sputum, 388b
Cover test, 798b, 798f
Cowper's galnds, 608
Crabs, 618b
Crackles, 402b, 800b
Cranial nerves, 570, 571f, 571t, 579
　assessment of, 581b–586b
　CN I (olfactory), 581b, 581f
　CN II (optic), 581b
　CN III (oculomotor), 581b–582b
　CN IV (trochlear), 581b–582b
　CN IX (glossopharyngeal), 585b, 585f
　CN V (trigeminal), 582b–583b, 582f
　CN VI (abducens), 581b–582b
　CN VII (facial), 583b–584b, 584f
　CN VIII (acoustic/vestibulocochlear), 584b
　CN X (vagus), 585b, 585f
　CN XI (spinal accessory), 585b, 585f, 586f
　CN XII (hypoglossal), 585b
Cranium, 280, 281f
CRC. *See* Colorectal cancer
Cremasteric reflex, 595b, 596f, 606
Crepitus, 395b
Cricoid cartilage, 293b
Critical thinking, 9, 61, 61b
　in analysis of data, 61–67. *See also* Data analysis
Crura, 637
Crying, 726
Cryptorchidism, 620b, 631b
Cul-de-sac of Douglas, 639
Cullen sign, 505b
Cultural assessment, 182–200
　approach to providers in, 186–187, 188b–189b
　biologic variations in, 194–195
　case study on, 198b–199b
　concepts in, 182, 183f
　contexts for, 183
　diet and nutrition in, 193
　disease, illness, and health state in, 187, 196–197
　geographical and ethnic variations in, 195–197
　health care beliefs in, 187–193 (*See also* Beliefs, health care)
　heritage assessment *vs.*, 197
　national standards for care in, 184, 184b
　purposes of, 184–185
　scope of, 185
　spirituality in, 193
Cultural awareness, 182, 185f

Cultural competence, 182–183
Cultural diversity, 183b
Cultural imposition, 183b
Cultural knowledge, 184, 185f
Cultural relativism, 183b
Cultural skill, 180, 183f
Culture, 149t, 183b
   definition of, 181
   in pain perception, 148
   terms related to, 183b
Culture-based treatments, 190, 192f
Culture-bound syndromes, 191, 191t–192t
Cushing syndrome, 128b, 140b, 301b
Cutaneous horn, 266b
Cutaneous pain, 145
Cutaneous tag, 266b
Cuticle, 249, 249f
Cyanosis, 258b, 258f, 393b, 478b
Cystic fibrosis, 701b
Cystocele, 666b, 666f

D

Daily Spiritual Experiences Scale, 210b
Danger, self-assessment for, 176b
Darwin's tubercle, 348f
Data analysis, 8–9
   critical thinking in, 61, 61b
   definition of, 60
   diagnostic reasoning process in, 61–67
   pitfalls in, avoiding, 61–67, 66
   process of, 9–10
Data collection, 2, 4
   objective data, 8, 8f
   purpose of, 8
   subjective data, 7–8, 8f
Dead space, 383
Death rituals, 190
Decerebrate posture, 84b, 84f, 604b
Decorticate posture, 84b, 84f, 604b
Deep cervical chain nodes, palpation of, 296b
Deep palpation, 40, 41f
Deep retinal hemorrhages, 336b
Deep tendon reflexes, 592b
Deep vein thrombosis (DVT), 469b
   risk factors for, 469b
Degenerative joint disease (DJD), 845b, 845f
Dehydration, 222
Delirium
   hallucinations in, 93t
   vs. dementia, 93t
Dementia, 75b–76b
   vs. Alzheimer disease, 93t
   vs. delirium, 93t
Dental caries, 795b
Dentate line, 639
Denver Developmental Screening Test (DDST), 738b, 756b–757b, 765
Depression, in older adults, 818b, 824b
Dermis, 248–249, 248f
Development, 118–119
   analysis of data in, 119
   health assessment for, 104–119
   theories of
      Erikson's theory of psychosocial development, 100–102, 100t, 101f, 112b–114b, 113f

Freud's theory of psychosexual development, 98–104, 99t, 110b–112b, 112f
Kohlberg's theory of moral development, 102, 104, 105t, 116b–117b, 116f
Piaget theory of cognitive development, 102, 103t–104t, 114b–115b, 115f
Developmental variation, 194
Diabetic retinopathy, 836b, 851b
Diagnostic and Statistical Manual of Mental Disorders (DSM), 70
Diagnostic reasoning process, 61–67
   developing, 66
   pitfalls in, avoiding, 66
Diaphragm, 384, 385
Diarrhea, 498b, 610b
Diastasis recti, 506b, 525b, 802b
Diastasis recti abdominis, 693
Diastole, 434–435
Diastolic murmur, 461b–462b
Diencephalon, 569
Diet
   anti-inflammatory, 220–221
   culture and, 193
   low carbohydrate/high protein/fat vs. low fat, 219–220
   low glycemic index, 221
Dietary Reference Intake (DRI), 218
Diethylstilbestrol (DES), 647b
   malformations from exposure to, 668b
Differential disease susceptibility
   biochemical variation and, 194–195
Difficulty breathing. *See* Dyspnea
Difficulty swallowing, 574b
Diffuse episcleritis, 332f
Digital rectal exam (DRE), 611b, 649
Dimpling of breast, 428b
DINAMAP, 127, 127f
Discrete skin lesions, 277b
Dizziness, 440b, 573b
Documentation, data, 44–59
   assessment forms in, 51–56, 51b
      admission form, 51, 52f–55f
      case study on, 56–57
      focused or specialty area, 56, 57f
      initial, 51, 51b
      progress note, 51, 55f
   guidelines for, 50–51, 51b
   objective data in, 50
   purpose of, 45–47, 46b
   subjective data in, 48
Döderlein bacilli, 638
Doppler ultrasound, use of, 473b
Dorsal arch, 464
Dorsalis pedis artery, 464
Dorsalis pedis pulses, 481b, 481f
Dorsal recumbent position, 38b
Down syndrome, 794b, 795f, 796b, 805b
Dribbling, 609b
DRIVE4COPD questionnaire, 389b
Drooling, 723
Drooping of eyelid. *See* Ptosis
Dupuytren contracture, 552b
Dutasteride (Avodart), 612b
Dwarfism, 128b, 139b
Dysarthria, 574b
Dysdiadochokinesia, 588b

Dyslipidemia, 441b
Dyspareunia, 664
Dysphagia, 574b
   in older adults, 821b, 834b
Dysphasia, 574b
Dysplasia, 647
Dyspnea, 386b–387b, 440b
   COPD and, 386b
   in older adults, 387b
   onset of, 386b
   paroxysmal nocturnal, 387b, 440b
Dysrhythmias, in older adults, 841b

E

Earache, 340b
Ear assessment, 340–355
   abnormalities
      of external ear and ear canal, 347b–348b, 354b
      of tympanic membrane, 349b, 355b
   analysis of data, 353
   equipment for, 32t
   findings of, 353
   health history, nursing, 340–345
      case study on, 345
      family history, 341b
      history of present concern, 340b–341b
      lifestyle and health practices, 342b
      personal, 341b
   interdisciplinary verbal communication, 353
   physical examination, 346–351, 678b, 678f
   routine screening *vs.* focused specialty assessment, 347b
   validating and documenting findings, 351
Ear(s)
   external
      abnormalities of, 347b–348b
      physical examination of, 347b–348b, 347f
      structure and function of, 338, 339f
   internal
      physical examination of, 348b–349b
      structure and function of, 339, 339f
   middle, 338–339, 339f
   structure and function of, 338–339
Ecchymosis, 275b
Eccrine glands, 248, 248f
E chart. *See* Snellen chart
Ecomap, 857, 858f, 861
Economic abuse, family, 162–163
Ectocervix. *See* External os
Ectopic pregnancy, 670b, 699b
   sites of, 714f
Ectropion, 331f
Edema, in heart failure, 441b
Egophony, 398b
Ejaculatory duct, 606
Elasticity, arterial, 132b
Elbows
   inspection and palpation, 548b
   ranges of motion, 548b, 548f
Elder abuse, 814b
Electrocardiography (ECG), 433–434
   phases of, 434b
      PR interval, 434b
      P wave, 434b

QRS complex, 434b
QT interval, 434b
ST segment, 434b
U wave, 434b
Electronic health records (EHRs), 7, 46, 47f
Electronic medical records (EMRs), 46, 46f
Eleventh cranial nerve, 281, 281f
Emergency assessment, 6–7, 6f. *See also* Assessment
Emotional abuse, family, 161, 162b
Enculturation, 183b
Endocardium, 433
Endometriosis, 669b
Endometrium, 639
Entropion, 332f
Environmental irritants, 389b
Epicanthal folds, 797b
Epicardium, 433
Epidermis, 247–248, 248f
Epididymis, 606, 620b
Epididymitis, 610b, 631b
Epigastric hernia, 524b
Epispadias, 619b, 629b
Epitrochlear lymph nodes, 476b, 476f
Epitrochlear nodes, 468
Erectile dysfunction (ED), 469b, 610b
Erikson's theory of psychosocial development
  assessment of, 112b–114b, 113f
  theoretical aspects of, 100–102, 100t, 101f
Erythema, 259, 259f
Esotropia, 319b
Estimated calorie needs, by age, gender, and physical activity, 220t
Estrogen–progestin combination therapy (EPT), 641
Estrogen therapy (ET), 641
Ethmoidal sinuses, 359
Ethnic disease variation, 195
Ethnicity, 183b
Ethnocentrism, 183b
Eustachian tube, 339, 339f, 723
Evidence-based health promotion and disease prevention. *See* Health promotion and disease prevention, evidence-based
Exercise
  and colorectal cancer, 613b
  in health history, 26
  musculoskeletal changes and, 536b
  during pregnancy, 703b
Exophthalmos, 332f
Exostosis, 354b
Exotropia, 319b
Expected date of confinement (EDC), 699b
Expiration, 385, 386f
External auditory canal
  inspection of, 348b–349b
  structure and function of, 338, 339f
External genitalia, 637–638, 638f, 651b–652b, 652f
  abnormalities of, 665b–666b, 665f, 666f
External os, 639
External respiration, 385
External sphincter, 607, 639
Extraocular muscles
  abnormalities of, 330b–331b
  and eye movement, 305f

structure and function of, 304, 305f
Eye assessment, 307–336
  analysis of data, 328–329
  health history, nursing, 307–315
    case study, 311b
    family history, 309b
    history of present concern in, 308b
    lifestyle and health practices in, 310b
    personal, 308b–309b
  interdisciplinary verbal communication of, 328
  physical examination, 315–328
    case study, 327
  validating and documenting findings, 327–328
Eye contact, culture and, 187
Eye examination, equipment for, 32t
Eyelashes
  inspection of, 320b
  structure and function of, 304
Eyelid(s)
  abnormalities of, 320b, 332f
  foreign bodies in, 322b
  inflammation of, 323b
  inspection of, 320b, 322f
  structure and function of, 304
Eye movements, abnormal, 582b
Eye(s)
  anatomy of, 305–306, 306f
  external
    abnormalities of, 331f–332f
    evaluation of, 320b–324b
      consensual response in, 307, 307f, 324b
      inspection and palpation in, 320b–323b, 322f
      pupil accommodation in, 324b, 324f
      pupillary reaction to light in, 324b
    structure and function of, 304–305, 305f
  internal, 325b–326f
    abnormalities of, 333b–336b
    anterior chamber in, 326b
    fovea and macula in, 326b
    ophthalmoscopy in, 325b
    optic disc in, 325b, 325f
    retinal background, 326b
    retinal vessels in, 326b
  physical assessment of, 678b, 678f
  structure and function of, 304–307
    external structures, 304–305, 305f
    internal structures, 305–306
  vision and, 306–307
Eye tic, 601b
Eye trauma, 327b

F

Face
  bones of, 280, 281f
  inspection of, 290b
  physical assessment of, 677b, 677f
FACES Pain Rating Scale, 780b, 780f
Fallopian tubes, 639
Falls, in older adults, 819b–820b
Familial adenomatous polyposis (FAP), 648b
Family
  affective function, 857
  boundaries, 856

composition, 855
context of, 857
definition of, 853–854
expressive function, 857
extended, 856
external systems, 857
family caregiving, statistics on, 854b
function, 857
  Bowen's family system theory, 857, 859–860
  communication theory, 860
  systems theory, 857
health care function, 857
and illness, relationship between, 854
instrumental function, 857
life cycles, 857, 859b
power structure, 856
rank order and gender of family member, 855–856
socialization function, 857
structure, 855
  context, 857
  external structure, 856–857
  internal structure, 855–856
subsystems in, 856
Family assessment, 853–868
  case study, 865b, 866b
  data analysis, 866
    collaborative problems, 867
    medical problems, 867
    nursing diagnoses, 867
  ecomap in, 857, 858f
  family interview in, 860–861, 860b
    commendations, 861
    genograms and ecomaps, 861
    manners, 860–861
    therapeutic conversation, 861
  general routine screening *vs.* focused specialty assessment, 861
  genogram in, 855, 855f, 861
  models/frameworks for, 855
    Calgary Family Assessment Model, 855
    family development, 857
    family function, 857–860
    family structure, 855–857
    Friedman's Family Assessment Model, 855
  procedure
    family development, 863b
    family function, 863b–864b
    family structure, 861b–863b
  SBAR method, use of, 867–868
  terms related to, 853–854
  validating and documenting findings, 866b
Family attachment diagram, 856, 856f
Family health history, 23, 24f
Family systems theory, 162
Family violence, 161–174. *See also* Violence assessment
  assessment of, 167–179
  child abuse in, 163–164
  economic abuse in, 162
  elder mistreatment in, 164
  intimate partner, 163
  physical abuse in, 162
  psychological abuse in, 162, 163b
  sexual abuse in, 162–163
  theories of, 161–162

912 Index

FAS. *See* Fetal alcohol syndrome
Fasciculations, 574b, 586b
Fatigue
 cardiac output and, 440b
 during pregnancy, 703b
Fatty tissue, female breasts, 411, 411f
Fecal immunochemical test (FIT), 611b
Fecal incontinence, 610b
Fecal occult blood test (FOBT), 643
Feet, physical assessment of, 682b–683b, 682f, 683f
Female circumcision. *See* Female genital cutting (FGC)
Female genital cutting (FGC), 717b
Female genitalia examination, equipment for, 33t
Female genital mutilation. *See* Female genital cutting (FGC)
Feminist theory, of violence, 162
Femoral artery, 464
Femoral canal, 607
Femoral hernia, 622b, 632b
Femoral vein, 465
Fertility control, culture and, 193
Fetal alcohol spectrum disorders (FASD), 701b
Fetal alcohol syndrome (FAS), 701b, 794b
Fetal Doppler ultrasound device, 712b
Fetal heart rate, 712, 713f
Fetal heart rate, locations for auscultating, 717b
Fetoscope, 712b
Fibroadenomas, 423b, 429b
Fibrocystic breast changes, 412b, 423b
Fibromyalgia, 535b
Fibrous joints, 530
Fibrous tissue, female breasts, 411, 411f
FICA Spiritual History Tool, 211
Fimbriae, 639
Finasteride (Proscar), 612b
Fingers, physical assessment of, 679b–680b, 679f, 680f
Finger-to-nose test, 588b, 588f
First heart sound, 435
Fissure, 274b
FLACC Behavioral Scale, 151, 152b
Flat foot, 557b, 565b
Flatus, 524b
Flexible sigmoidoscopy, 611b
Floaters, 836b
Floating ribs, 382, 382f
Fluid requirement, for older adults, 821b
Fluid wave test, 517b, 517f
Focused assessment, 6. *See also* Assessment
Folliculitis, 263f
 of beard area, 262b
 of scalp, 262b, 263f
Footdrop (steppage) gait, 603b
Foreskin, penis, 619b
Fovea centralis
 inspection of, 326b
 structure and function of, 305–306, 306f
Frail elderly, 813. *See also* Older adults assessment
Freckles, 265b
Fremitus, 395b, 400b
Frenulum, 605, 637
Freud's theory of psychosexual development, 99t, 112f

 assessment of, 110b–112b
 theoretical aspects of, 98–100
Friction rubs, 508b
Frontal sinuses, 359
Functional incontinence, 829b
Functional status, in older adults, 816, 816b, 817b
Fundal height, measurement of, 710b, 710f
Fungal infection, skin, 260b

G

Gag reflex, 585b, 834b
Gait
 abnormal, 603b
 assessment of, 587b
 in older children, 806b
 during pregnancy, 695
 in toddlers, 806b
Galactorrhea
 causes of, 413b
 medication-induced, 413b
Gallbladder, 495
 cancer, 196
 enlarged, 526b
Ganglion, 564b
Gangrene, 478b
Gastroesophageal reflux disease (GERD), 501b
 asthma and, 388b
 client education, 501b
 indigestion in, 496b, 497b
 risk assessment, 501b
Gaze, 582b
Generalized seizures, 573b
General status assessment, 121–141
 abnormal findings in, 139b–140b
 assessment in, objective, 126–138
  client preparation in, 126
  diagnostic reasoning, 138
  equipment in, 126–127, 127f
  general impression, 128b
  validating and documenting findings, 137
  of vital signs, 129b–133b, 129f, 130f, 131f, 132f (*See also* Vital signs)
 assessment in, subjective
  case study, 126
  health history, 124–125
 structure and function in
  overall impression in, 121–122
  vital signs in, 122–124, 122f, 123f
General survey, 121
Genital herpes simplex, 666b, 666f
Genitalia
 development of, 763–764
 physical assessment of, 684b, 684f
Genitalia and rectum assessment, female, 637–670
 analysis of data in, 664
 health history in, nursing, 639–640
 hemorrhoids in, 646b
 physical examination in, 649–651, 650f
 routine screening, 651b
 structure and function of, 637–639
 tissue specimens for analysis, 659b–660b, 660f
 validating and documenting findings, 663

Genital stage, 770
Genital warts, 628b, 666b, 666f
Genogram, 855, 855f
Genu valgum, 555b, 806b, 806f
Genu varum, 555b, 806b, 806f
GERD. *See* Gastroesophageal reflux disease
Geriatric Depression Scale, 824b
Get up and go test, 844b, 845f
Gigantism, 128b, 139b
Gingival bleeding, 692
Glandular tissue, female breasts, 411, 411f
Glans, 637
Glans penis, cancer of, 628b
Glasgow Coma Scale (GCS), 90b
Glaucoma, 325, 334b, 835b, 850b
 culture and, 195
 prevention of, 312b–313b
 risk factors for, 312b
Gloves, use of, 34b, 36
Goniometer, 540
Gonorrhea, 619b
Goodell sign, 694
Gouty arthritis, 565b
Gowns, use of, 34b
Graphesthesia, 591b, 591f
Graves speculum, 659b
Gravida/para status, 698b
Greater vestibular glands, 638
Great saphenous vein, 465
Great vessels, 431
Greta, 781
Grey-Turner sign, 504b, 505b
Growth and development, 98–119, 106b–108b
 analysis of data in, 119
 health assessment in, 104–119
 health history in, nursing, 104
 theories of, 98–104
  Erikson's theory of psychosocial development, 100–102, 100t, 101f
  Freud's theory of psychosexual development, 98–100, 99t
  Kohlberg's theory of moral development, 102, 104, 105t
  Piaget theory of cognitive development, 102, 103t–104t
 validating and documenting findings in, 119–120
Growth charts, 791b
Guaiac stool test, 822b
Gynecomastia, 424b, 424f, 762, 784b, 801b

H

Hair
 loss, 250b, 263b
 male pattern balding, 263b, 263f
 patchy hair loss, 263, 264f
 structure and function of, 248f, 249
 terminal, 249
 vellus, 249
Hair assessment
 analysis of data in, 269–270
 equipment for, 32t
 history of present health concern in, 250b
 inspection in, 262b–264b, 262f, 263f, 264f
 lifestyle and health practices in, 252b–253b
 personal health history in, 251b

Hair follicle, 248f, 249
Half-and-half nails, 277b
Hallux valgus, 565b, 847b
Haloperidol (Haldol), galactorrhea and, 413b
Hammer toe, 565b
Handoff, 58
Hands
　and fingers
　　inspection and palpation, 552b
　　ranges of motion, 552b, 552f
　hygiene practices, 34b
　physical assessment of, 679b–680b, 679f, 680f
Hard exudate, 336b
Head. *See also* Head and neck assessment
　inspection of, 289b–290b, 290f
　palpation of, 290b
　physical assessment of, 677b, 677f
　structure and function of
　　cranium, 280, 281f
　　face, 280, 281f
　　lymph nodes, 282–283, 282f
　　muscles, 281
Headaches, 573b
　characteristics of, 299b–300b
　health history for, nursing, 284b
　from medicines, 285b
　types of, 299b–300b
Head and neck assessment, 283–302
　abnormal findings in, 299b–302b
　　headaches, 299b–300b
　　head and neck, 301b–302b
　analysis of data in, 297–298
　　collaborative problems, 298
　　medical problems, 298
　　nursing diagnoses, selected, 297–298
　focused specialty assessment, 289
　general routine screening, 289
　health history in, nursing, 283–288
　　altered thyroid function in, 287b
　　case study on, 286
　　family history, 285b
　　history of present concern, 283b–285b
　　lifestyle and health practices, 285b–286b
　　past health history, 285b
　　purpose and goals, 283
　　traumatic brain injury, 287b–288b
　interdisciplinary verbal communication of, 298
　physical examination in, 288–297
　　case study on, 297
　　client/patient preparation in, 288–289
　　cultural considerations in, 288, 289
　　equipment in, 32t, 289
　　of head and face, 289b–291b, 290f, 291f
　　of lymph nodes, 295b–296b, 295f, 296f
　　of neck, 291b–294b, 291f, 292f
　　validating and documenting findings in, 297
Head circumference (HC), 792b
Head-to-toe assessment, integrated, 672–690
　abbreviated, 689b–690b
　comprehensive health assessment in, 673–685
　　client preparation in, 673, 673f

　　data collection in, 673, 685
　　equipment in, 673, 674b–676b
　　physical assessment in, 676b–684b, 676f–684f
　documentation of, 685–690
　　case study on, 685–687
　　client's strengths in, 688
　　collaborative problems in, 688
　　diagnoses in, nursing, 688
　　physical assessment in, 687–688
Health assessment
　factors affecting, 10
　focus of, 4
　framework for, 4–5
　nurse's role in, 2–3
　　evolution of, 2b
　purpose of, 4
　steps of, 7
　types of, 5–7
Health Belief Model, 5
Health history, 18
　biographic data in, 18–19
　data from, 18
　family health history in, 23, 24f
　format summary for, 18, 20b
　history of present health concern in, 21, 22b
　importance of, 18
　lifestyle and health practices profile in, 25–29
　personal health history in, 21–22
　reasons for seeking health care in, 19, 21
　review of systems in, 23–25
Health Information Technology or Economic and Clinical Health (HITECH) Act, 45, 47
Health promotion and disease prevention, evidence-based
　age-related macular degeneration, 313b–314b
　breast cancer, 415b–416b
　cataracts, 314b–315b
　cervical cancer, 647b
　chronic obstructive pulmonary disease, 389b–390b
　colorectal cancer, 648b
　dementia and Alzheimer's disease, 75b–76b
　gastroesophageal reflex disease, 501b
　glaucoma, 312b–313b
　hearing loss, 343b–345b
　hemorrhoids, 646b
　HIV/AIDS, 613b–614b
　intimate partner violence, 167b–168b
　lung cancer, 390b–391b
　methicillin-resistant *Staphylococcus aureus* (MRSA), 253b
　models for, 5
　obesity, 223b
　older adults, 814b–815b
　oropharyngeal cancer, 360b
　peptic ulcer disease, 500b–501b
　peripheral artery disease, 471b
　pressure ulcers, 255b
　prostate cancer, 614b–615b
　sinusitis, 364b–365b
　skin cancer, 254b
　substance abuse, 78b–79b

　　traumatic brain injury, 287b–288b
　　Zika virus infection, 696b
Health Promotion Model, 5
Health promotion nursing diagnoses, 63, 65–66
Healthy People 2020, 647b, 648b, 691, 696b
Healthy People 2020, 5, 75b, 78b
Hearing, 339
　conductive, 339
　pathways of, 340f
　sensorineural, 339
　test for, 349b–351b
　　Rinne test, 350b, 350f
　　Romberg test, 351b
　　Weber test, 350b, 350f
　　whisper test, 349b–350b
Hearing acuity, 800b
Hearing loss, 352b
　age-related, 344b
　conductive, 343b
　culture and, 195
　mixed, 343b
　prevention of, 343b–345b
　recognizing, 343b
　sensorineural, 343b, 352b
　testing, 352b
　types of, 343b
Heart
　auscultation, 449b–452b
　chambers and valves, 431–433
　covering and walls, 433
　development of, 762–763
　electrical conduction of, 433–434, 433f
　inspection, 448b
　location and size of, 431, 432f
　palpation, 449b
　physical assessment of, 681b, 681f
Heart and neck vessel assessment, 431–462
　abnormal findings in
　　arterial pulse and pressure waves, 454b–455b
　　heart murmurs, 459b–462b
　　heart rhythms, 457b
　　heart sounds, extra, 457b–459b
　　ventricular impulses, 456b
　case study, 444b, 452b–453b, 454b
　data analysis, 453
　　collaborative problems, 453–454
　　medical problems, 454
　　nursing diagnoses, 453
　health history, 439
　　family history, 441b
　　history of present health concern, 440b–441b
　　lifestyle and health practices, 441b–442b
　　personal health history, 441b
　physical examination, 418–419
　　assessment, key points for, 445
　　client preparation, 445
　　equipment for, 445
　　general routine screening *vs.* focused specialty assessment, 446
　　heart, anterior chest, 448b–452b
　　neck vessels, 446b–448b
　　validating and documenting findings, 452

Heart and neck vessel assessment (*Continued*)
  SBAR method, use of, 454
  structure and function in, 431
    cardiac cycle, 434–435, 434f
    cardiac output, 436
    electrical conduction of heart, 433–434
    heart and great vessels, 431–433, 432f
    heart sounds, 435–436
    neck vessels, 436, 439, 439f
Heart and neck vessel examination, equipment for, 32t
Heart disease
  culture and, 196
  risk factors for, 441b–442b
  smoking and, 441b
Heart failure, 440b
  edema in, 441b
Heart murmurs, 459b
  characteristics
    intensity, 459b
    location, 460b
    pitch, 459b
    quality, 459b
    shape/pattern, 459b
    timing, 459b
    transmission, 460b
    ventilation and position, 460b
  diastolic, 461b
    aortic regurgitation, murmur of, 461b–462b
    mitral stenosis, murmur of, 462b
  midsystolic, 460b
    aortic stenosis, murmur of, 460b
    hypertrophic cardiomyopathy, murmur of, 461b
    innocent murmur, 460b
    physiologic murmur, 460b
    pulmonic stenosis, murmur of, 460b
  pansystolic, 461b
    mitral regurgitation, murmur of, 461b
    tricuspid regurgitation, murmur of, 461b
    ventricular septal defect, murmur of, 461b
Heart rate (HR), 436
Heart rhythm, changes in, 457b
Heart sounds, 435, 762
  auscultation of, 438b
  extra, 434f, 436, 457b–459b
    in both systole and diastole, 458b–459b
    during diastole, 458b
    during systole, 457b–459b
  first, 435–436
    variations in, 435b
  fourth, 458b
  murmurs, 436
  normal, 435–436
  second, 435, 436
    splitting of, 436
    variations in, 436b–437b
  third, 458b
Heberden nodes, 552b, 564b, 845b
Heel-to-shin test, 588b, 589f
Hegar sign, 669b
Height measurement
  in adults, 232b, 233f
  in children and adolescents, 791b–792b

Helicobacter pylori, 500b
Hemangioma, 809b
Hematocele, 620b
Hematoma, 275b
Hematuria, 609b
Hemoptysis, 388b
Hemorrhoids, 607, 607f, 646b, 695, 804b
  client education, 646b
  external, 633b
  risk assessment, 646b
Hepatomegaly, 510b, 525b
Hereditary nonpolyposis colorectal cancer (HNPCC), 648b
Heritage assessment, 197
Hernia, 506b
  femoral, 622b, 632b
  inguinal, 622b, 622f, 632b, 803b
  scrotal, 621b, 630b
  umbilical, 505b, 524b, 802b
Herpes progenitalis, 628b
Herpes zoster vesicles (shingles), 832b
Hierarchy of Pain Assessment, 150
HIPAA (Health Insurance Portability and Accountability Act), 13
Hips
  inspection and palpation, 553b
  range of motion of, 553b, 554f
Hirschberg test, 798b
Hirsutism, 263, 263b
Histamine-2 blockers, chronic use of, 498b
Histoplasmosis, 389b
Hooking technique, for liver palpation, 514b, 515f
HOPE questions, 211b
Hordeolum, 332f
Hormone-replacement therapy (HRT), 641
Hospital Infection Control Practices Advisory Committee (HICPAC), 33
  isolation precaution guidelines, 33, 34b–36b
Hot/cold theory, 189, 189t
Human immunodeficiency virus (HIV) infection
  client education, 614b
  prevention of, 613b–614b
  risk assessment, 614b
  screening for, 614b
Human papilloma virus (HPV), 647b
Human trafficking, 165–166
Huntington chorea, 587b
Hyaline cartilage, 383
Hydatidiform mole, 699b
Hydration, 218–219
  assessment of
    all settings, 238b
    inpatient, 238b
  dehydration in, 222
  overhydration in, 222
Hydrocele, 620b, 621b, 630b, 803b
Hymen, 638
Hyoid bone, 293b
Hypalgesia, 590b
Hyperalgesia, 590b
Hypercapnia, 385
Hyperesthesia, 590b
Hyperpigmentation, 692
Hyperpituitarism, 128b, 139b

Hypersensitivity test, 519b
Hypertension
  in African Americans, 449b
  follow-up of, 136t
Hyperthyroidism, 301b
  signs and symptoms of, 287b
Hypertrophic cardiomyopathy, murmur of, 461b
Hyperventilation, 403t
Hypesthesia, 589b
Hyphemia, 326b, 326f
Hypopyon, 326b, 326f
Hypospadias, 619b, 629b
Hypotension, orthostatic (postural), 133b
Hypothalamus, 569
Hypothyroidism, signs and symptoms of, 287b
Hypoventilation, 403t
Hypoxemia, 385

I

Ideal body weight (IBW), 233b, 233f
  percentage of, 233b
Illness causation, cultural beliefs on, 189–190, 190f
Imperforate anus, 804b
Incarcerated hernia, 621b
Incisional hernia, 525b
Incus, 338, 339f
Indigestion (pyrosis), 496b–497b
Inferior vena cava, 431
Inflammatory pain, 144
Inguinal area, 606–607, 607f
Inguinal canal, 607
Inguinal hernia, 622b, 622f, 632b, 803b
  direct, 632b
  indirect, 632b
Inguinal lymph nodes, 622b
Inner caruncle, 304
Innocent murmurs, 801b
Insomnia, 26, 27b
Inspection, 37
Inspiration, 385, 386f
Institute of Medicine, 3
Instrumental Activities of Daily Living (IADLs), 816, 817b
Integrated clinical practice, 3
Intention tremor, 602b
Intercostal space (ICS), 431
Intermittent claudication, 468b
Internal genitalia, 638–639, 638f, 653b–654b
Internal jugular veins, 282
Internal os, 639
Internal sphincter, 607, 639
International Osteoporosis Foundation (IOF) One-Minute Osteoporosis Risk Test, 537b
Intervertebral disc injuries, 575b
Interview, 12, 13f
  age-specific techniques, 778b
  children and adolescents, 777–779
  communication during, 14
    nonverbal, 14–15
    verbal, 16
  interpreter, use of, 17, 18b
  parental, 777, 777f

phases of, 12–13
  introductory phase, 13
  preintroductory phase, 13, 13f
  summary and closing, phase, 14
  working phase, 13–14
  rapport with client, 12, 13f
  special considerations during, 16–18
Intimate partner violence, 163, 167b–168b. *See also* Family violence
Intractable pain, 145
Intraductal papilloma, 423b
Involuntary reflex guarding, 513b
Iris
  inspection of, 323b
  irregularly shaped, 333b
  structure and function of, 305
Irritable bowel syndrome (IBS), 499b
Isometric contraction, 435
Itching and pain, 643b

J

Jaeger test, 316b
Jaundice, 258b, 258f
Joints, 530, 531f, 532b–534b
  ankle and foot, 534b
  cartilaginous, 530
  elbow, 532b
  fibrous, 530
  hip, 533b
  knee, 534b
  pain in, 535b
  ranges of motion, 530
  shoulder, 532b
  sternoclavicular, 532b
  synovial, 530, 531f
  temporomandibular, 532b
  vertebrae, 533b
  wrist, fingers, thumb, 533b
Jugular veins, 436, 439f
  external, 439
  internal, 439
Jugular venous pressure, 439, 446b, 447b, 447f
Jugular venous pulse, 439, 439f, 446b
Junctional contractions, 457b

K

Kaposi's sarcoma, in tongue, 371b, 378b
Katz Activities of Daily Living, 816, 816b, 819b
Keloids, 505b, 505f
Kernig sign, 596b
Kidneys, 494, 495f
  enlarged, 526b
  palpation, 516b, 516f
Kiesselbach area, 359
Knee-chest position, 39b
Knee jerk, 569
Knees
  ballottement test, 556b, 556f
  bulge test, 555b, 555f
  inspection and palpation, 555b–556b
  McMurray test, 556b, 557f
  range of motion of, 556b, 556f

Kohlberg's theory of moral development, 104, 105t, 116f
  assessment of, 116b–117b
  theoretical aspects, 102
Koilonychia, 278b, 794b
Koplik spots, 795b
Korotkoff's sounds, 134t
Kussmaul respiration, 403t
Kussmaul sign, 446b
Kwashiorkor, 237b, 243b
Kyphosis, 394b, 407b, 543b, 562b, 806b, 844b

L

Labia majora, 637
Labia minora, 637
Lacrimal apparatus
  inspection of, 323b
  palpation of, 323b, 323f
  structure and function of, 304, 305f
Lacrimal canals, 304, 305f
Lactiferous sinus, 411
Lactose intolerance, 536b
Lanugo, 723
Large intestine, 495
Laryngopharynx, 358
Latency period, 770
Lawton Scale for Instrumental Activities of Daily Living, 816, 817b, 819b
Laxatives, overuse of, 498b
Left atria, 431
Left main bronchus, 383
Left ventricle, 431–432
Leg
  arterial/venous insufficiency, testing for, 482b–485b, 482f
  dorsalis pedis pulses, 481b, 481f
  edema, 478b
  femoral pulses, 480b
  inspection of, 478b
  muscular atrophy, 478b
  palpation of, 479b
  physical assessment of, 682b–683b, 682f, 683f
  popliteal pulses, 480b, 480f
  posterior tibial pulses, 481b, 481f
  varicose veins in, 481b
Leg length, measurement of, 545b, 546f
Lens
  abnormalities of, 333b
  inspection of, 323b
  structure and function of, 305, 306f
Lentigines, 832b
Leopold maneuvers, 711b, 711f
Lesser vestibular glands, 638
Leukoplakia of tongue, 369b, 377b
Level of consciousness, 84b, 84f, 96b
  abnormal, 84f
Lifestyle and health practices profile
  activity level and exercise in, 26
  day description in, 25
  education and work in, 29
  environment in, 29
  in health history, 25–29
  nutrition and weight management in, 25–26
  relationships in, 28, 28f

  self-concept and self-care responsibilities in, 28
  sleep and rest in, 26, 26b, 27b
  social activities in, 28
  stress levels and coping styles in, 29
  substance use in, 26, 28
  values and belief system in, 28
Ligaments, 530
Lightening, 694
Light palpation, 40, 41f
Light touch sensation, testing of, 589b, 589f
Linea alba, 492
Linear, skin lesions, 277b
Lingual tonsils, 358
Lipomas, 423b
Lithotomy position, 40b
Liver, 494, 510b
  enlarged nodular, 525b
  hepatomegaly, 525b
  higher than normal, 525b
  lower than normal, 526b
  normal liver span, 510b, 510f
  palpation, 514b, 514f, 515f
  scratch test, 511b, 511f
Liver spots, 832b
Longitudinal ridging, nail, 276b
Lordosis, 543b, 562b
Lower respiratory system, 381
Low glycemic index diet, 221
Lumbar curvature, flattened, 543b, 562b
Lumbar hyperlordosis, 562b
Lumbar spine, range of motion of, 544b–544b, 544f, 545f
Lung cancer, 390b–391b
  client education, 391b
  culture and, 196
  risk factors for, 391b
  risk for, 388b
  screening for, 391b
Lungs, 383–384
  apex of, 383–384
  base of, 384
  development of, 762
  position of, 358f, 384
  structure and function of, 383–384
Lunula, 249, 249f
Lupus erythematosus, butterfly rash, 259, 259f
Lymphatic system, 466–468, 467f
Lymphedema, 474b, 490b
  edema with, 489b
  stages of, 485b
Lymph nodes, 409, 467–468, 468f
  axillary, 411, 411f
  of head and neck, 282–283, 282f
    assessment of, 295b–296b
    palpation of, 295b–296b, 295f, 296f
  inguinal, 622b
  shotty, 795b
Lynch syndrome, 648b

M

MAC. *See* Mid-arm circumference
Macrotia, 347b
Macula
  inspection of, 326b
  structure and function of, 305–306, 306f

Index

Macular degeneration, 836b, 851b
Macule, 273b
Magicoreligious, belief systems, 189, 190, 190f
Male genitalia and rectum assessment, 605–635
  abnormal findings in
    anus and rectum, 633b–634b
    inguinal and femoral hernias, 632b
    penis, 628b–629b
    prostate gland, 635b
    scrotum, 630b–632b
  case study, 616b, 626b, 627b
  data analysis, 626
    collaborative problems, 622
    medical problems, 622
    nursing diagnoses, 620–621
  health history, 608
    family history, 611
    history of present health concern, 609b–610b
    lifestyle and health practices, 611b–613b
    past health history, 610b–611b
  HIV/AIDS and, 613b–614b
  physical examination, 616–617
    anus and rectum, 622b–624b
    client preparation, 617
    equipment for, 33t, 617
    general routine screening *vs.* focused specialty assessment, 618
    inguinal area, 622b
    penis, 618b–619b, 618f, 619f
    physical assessment, 617
    positions for anorectal examination, 617f
    prostate gland, 625b
    scrotum, 620b–621b, 620f
    stool inspection, 625b
    validating and documenting findings, 626
  prostate cancer and, 614b–615b
  SBAR method, use of, 628
  structure and function in, 605
    anus and rectum, 607–608, 607f
    external genitalia, 605–606, 606f
    inguinal area, 606–607, 607f
    internal genitalia, 606, 606f
    penis, 605, 606f
    prostate gland, 608, 608f
    scrotum, 606
    spermatic cord, 606
    testes, 606, 606f
  testicular self-examination (TSE), 615b
Male pattern balding, 263b, 263f
Malleus, 338, 339f
Malnutrition, 221–222, 241b, 243b
Mammary ducts, 411
Mandible, 357
Manual compression test, 484b, 484f
Manubrium, 381
Marasmus, 237b, 243b
Marfan's syndrome, 128b, 140b
Mastectomy, 429b
Mastitis, 428b
McBurney point, 517b
McCafferty Initial Pain Assessment Tool, 151, 153b
McDonald's rule, 694
McMurray test, 556b, 557f

Median sulcus, 608, 608f
Mediastinum, 383, 431
Medical record, 7, 7f, 13
Medroxyprogesterone (Depo-Provera) injections
  and galactorrhea, 413b
Medulla oblongata, 569
Meibomian glands, 304
Melanoma, 260b, 276b. *See also* Skin cancer
Memory loss, 575b
Menarche, 640, 640b
Meningeal irritation/inflammation, tests for, 596b
Meningitis, 579
Menopause, 641b
  artificial/surgical, 641b
  cultural reflection, 641b
  delayed, 641b
  premature, 641b
Menstrual cycle, 640b
Mental status assessment, 71–96, 84f, 88b, 576, 579, 677b
  analysis of data in, 95
  assessment tools in, 90b–92b
    Alcohol Use Disorders Identification test, 76b–77b
    Confusion Assessment Method, 92b
    Glasgow Coma Scale, 90b
    SLUMS Mental Status Examination, 91b
  biographical data in, 71–74
  conceptual foundations, 70
  dementia *vs.* delirium in, 93t
  health history in, nursing, 71–75
    SAD PERSONS suicide risk assessment in, 81
  levels of consciousness in, 84b
    abnormal, 84f, 96b
  nursing diagnoses, selected, 95
  physical examination in, 82–91
    Alzheimer early signs in, 91b
    case study on, 91b
    client preparation in, 82
    validating and documenting findings in, 94–95
Metabolism, decrease in, 813, 815
Metatarsus varus, 805b
Methicillin-resistant *Staphylococcus aureus* (MRSA), 253b
Microaneurysms, 336b
Microcephaly, 289
Microtia, 347b, 354b
Mid-arm circumference (MAC), 236b–237b, 236f, 237t
Mid-arm muscle circumference (MAMC), 238b, 239t
Mid-axillary line, 383
Midclavicular line (MCL), 383, 383f, 431, 494
Midsternal line, 383, 383f
Midsystolic click, 458b
Midsystolic murmur, 460b–461b
Migraine headache, 299b–300b
Milia, 722, 742f
Milk cysts, 423b
Milk line, breast, 410, 410f
Mini Nutritional Assessment, 227
Minuchin, Salvador, 856
Miosis, 334b, 797b
Mitral regurgitation, murmur of, 461b

Mitral stenosis, murmur of, 462b
Mixed incontinence, 829b
Mobility, skin, 261–262, 261f
Modulation, of pain, 143, 144f
Molar pregnancy, 699b
Mole, 266b
Monocular blindness, 324b
Mons pubis, 637
Montgomery glands, 409
Moral development
  in child and adolescent, 768
  Kohlberg's theory of, 102, 104, 105t
  in newborn and infant, 726
Morning sickness, 497b
Moro (or startle) reflex, 755b
Mothers Against Drunk Driving (MADD), 870
Motor and cerebellar systems, 579, 586b–589f
Motor development, 765–766
Motor system examination, 579
Mouth
  abnormalities of, 377b–378b
  health history in, nursing, 361b
  physical examination of, 367b–372b
    buccal mucosa, 368b, 368f
    in head-to-toe assessment, 679b, 679f
    lips, 367
    teeth and gums, 367b–368b, 367f
    tongue, 369b–372b
  structure and function of, 357–358
Mouth, throat, nose, and sinus assessment
  abnormalities
    of mouth and throat, 377b–379b
    of nose, 379b
    tonsillitis, 379b
  analysis of data in, 375–376
  health history in, nursing, 359–365
  interdisciplinary verbal communication, 376
  physical examination, 366–375
    case study, 374b, 375b
    client/patient preparation in, 366
    equipment in, 32t, 366
    of mouth, 367b–372b
    of nose, 373b, 373f
    of sinuses, 374b, 374f
    validating and documenting findings in, 375
  routine screening *vs.* focused specialty assessment, 366b
Moxibustion, 190
Mucocutaneous junction, 639
Mucopurulent cervicitis, 667b
Multigenerational transmission process, 859
Multi-infarct dementia *vs.* delirium, 93t
Murmurs, 436, 451b
  auscultation of, 451b–452b
  innocent, 801b
Murphy sign, 520b, 526b
Muscle growth, 765
Muscle pain, 535b
Musculoskeletal system assessment, 528–566
  abnormal findings in
    feet and toes, 565b
    spinal curvatures, abnormal, 562b–563b
    upper extremities, 563b–564b

case study, 538b–539b, 559b, 560b, 561b
data analysis, 560
    collaborative problems, 561
    medical problems, 561
    nursing diagnoses, 560–561
health history, 534
    family history, 536b
    history of present health concern, 534b–535b
    lifestyle and health practices, 536b–537b
    personal health history, 535b
older adults and, 535b, 540b, 555b
osteoporosis, 537b–538b
Ottawa ankle rules, 559b
physical examination, 539
    ankles and feet, 557b–559b
    cervical, thoracic, and lumbar spine, 543b–546b
    client preparation, 539
    elbows, 548b
    equipment for, 32t, 540
    general routine screening *vs.* focused specialty assessment, 541
    guidelines for assessment, 540
    hands and fingers, 552b
    hips, 553b–554b
    knees, 555b–557b
    physical assessment, 540
    posture and gait, 541b
    shoulders, arms, and elbows, 546b–547b
    sternoclavicular joint, 542b
    temporomandibular joint, 542b
    validating and documenting findings, 559
    wrist, 549b–551b
SBAR method, use of, 561
structure and function in, 528
    bones, 528, 529f
    joints, 530, 531f, 532b–534b
    skeletal muscles, 528–530, 529b, 530f–531f
Musculoskeletal system, culture and, 197
Mydriasis, 334b, 797b
Myocardium, 433
Myoclonus, 574b
Myometrium, 639
Myopia (impaired far vision), 317b
MyPlate, 26
Myxedema, 302b

N

Nabothian (retention) cysts, 661b
Nail (s)
    clubbing, 264b
    structure and function of, 249, 249f
Nail assessment
    analysis of data in, 269–270
    history of present health concerning, 250b –252b
    inspection in, 264b
    lifestyle and health practices in, 252b
    personal health history in, 251b
    physical examination in, 265f
        abnormal findings, 277b–278b
        case study on, 257
        equipment in, 32t, 257
        palpation in, 264–265
    validating and documenting findings in, 269
Nailbeds, yellow, 794b
Nail pitting, in psoriasis, 255b, 277b
NANDA approved nursing diagnoses, 894–896
Nares, 359
Nasal cavity, 358f, 359
Nasal flaring, 393b
Nasolacrimal duct, 304, 305f, 359
Nasolacrimal sac, 304, 305f
Nasopharynx, 358
National Center for Chronic Disease Prevention and Health Promotion, 5
National Intimate Partner and Sexual Violence Survey (NISVS), 163
National standards for care, 184, 184b
Naturalistic belief systems, 189
Nausea and vomiting, 497b
Neck
    inspection of, 291b–292b
    movement, inspection of, 292b, 292f
    physical assessment of, 679b, 679f
    structure and function of, 281f
        blood vessels in, 282
        lymph nodes in, 282–283, 282f
        muscles and cervical vertebrae in, 281, 281f, 282f
        overview of, 280–281
        thyroid gland in, 281f, 282
Neck pain, 283b
Neck vessels, 436, 439, 439f
    auscultation, 447b, 447f
    inspection, 446b–447b
    palpation, 448b, 448f
4th nerve paralysis, 331b
6th nerve paralysis, 331b
Neuman's systems nursing theory model, 871
Neural pathways, 569–570, 570f
Neuro check, 579
Neurogenic anosmia, 581b
Neurologic system assessment, 567–604
    abnormal findings in
        gait, 603b
        motor and sensory findings in spinal cord injuries, 600b–601b
        muscle movements, 601b–602b
        postures in unconscious clients, 604b
    case study, 567b, 576b, 596b, 597b–598b, 599b
    cerebrovascular accident, 577b–578b
    data analysis, 598
        collaborative problems, 599
        medical problems, 599
        nursing diagnoses, 598–599
    health history, 572
        family history, 575b
        history of present health concern, 573b–575b
        lifestyle and health practices, 575b
        past health history, 575b
    in older adults, 575b, 584b, 586b, 587b, 592b
    physical examination, 576
    client preparation, 579
    cranial nerves, 581b–586b
    equipment for, 33t, 579
    general routine screening *vs.* focused specialty assessment, 580
    motor and cerebellar systems, 586b–589b
    physical assessment, 579
    reflexes, 593b–596b
    reflex hammer, use of, 580b
    sensory system, 589b–592b
    validating and documenting findings, 597, 597f
    SBAR method, use of, 599
    structure and function in, 567
        autonomic nervous system, 572
        central nervous system, 567–570
        cranial nerves, 570, 571f, 571t
        peripheral nervous system, 570–572
Neuropathic pain, 144
Newborn and infant assessment, 722–760
    analysis of data in, 759
    Apgar score, 733t
    biographical data, 728b
    case study, 732, 758–759
    cognitive and language development in, 726
    health history in, 727, 728b–729b
    initial physical assessment, 733, 733b–737b
    lifestyle and health practices, 729b
    moral development in, 726
    motor development in, 725, 725f
    nutritional requirements, 727
    physical development of, 722–724, 725f
        abdomen in, 724
        anus, rectum, and prostate in, 724
        breasts in, 724
        eyes and ears in, 723
        genitalia in, 724
        head and neck in, 723, 723f
        heart in, 724
        mouth, throat, nose, and sinus in, 723
        musculoskeletal system in, 724
        neurologic system in, 724
        peripheral vascular system in, 724
        skin, hair, and nails in, 722–723
        thorax and lungs in, 723–724
    physical examination, 732–733
    psychosexual development, 727
    psychosocial development, 726–727
    sensory perception development, 725–726
    sleep requirements and patterns, 727
    subsequent physical assessments, 733, 738b–753b
    validating and documenting findings, 758
Newborn reflexes, 754b
Nicotine, 575b
NIHL. *See* Noise-induced hearing loss
Nipples, 409
    discharge, 412b, 423b
    inspection of, 420b–421b
    palpation of, 423b, 423f
    retracted, 428b
Nociceptive pain, 144
Nocturia, 440b
Nodule, 273b

Index

Noise-induced hearing loss (NIHL), 344b
Nonjudgmental attitude, 15
North American Nursing Diagnosis Association, 9
Nose
   abnormalities of, 379b
   external, 359
   health history in, nursing, 361b–362b
   physical examination of, 373b, 373f, 678b, 678f
   structure and function of, 358f, 359
Nudge test, 541b
Numbness, 573b
Numeric Pain Intensity Scale (NPIS), 148
Numeric Rating Scale (NRS), 150, 151f
Nummular, skin lesions, 277b
Nursing
   definition of, 2
   health assessment in (See Assessment; Health assessment)
Nursing Diagnoses: Definitions and Classifications 2015-2017, 64
Nursing diagnosis, 5, 9. *See also* Data analysis
   actual, 63, 65
   assessment conclusions, 65t
   comparision of, 64t
   risk, 63, 66
   syndrome, 66
   wellness, 63, 65–66
Nursing history guide, 887–888
Nursing process
   assessment in, 3–8, 4t
   data analysis (nursing diagnosis), 8–10
   phases of, 4f, 4t
Nursing: Scope and Standards of Nursing Practice, 1–2
   Standard 1, 2
   Standard 2, 2
Nutrition, 211–212
   culture and, 193
   definition, 217
   essential nutrients in, 217–218
Nutritional assessment, 222–236
   analysis of data in, 240–243
   components of, 222
   health history in, nursing, 227, 227b–228b
   nutritional screening tools in
      24-hour food recall, 225b
      nutrition history, 226b
   physical examination in, 225–243
      abnormal findings, 243b
      anthropometric measurement, 231b–239b, 233f, 235f, 236f, 237f
      body build in, 231b, 231f
      client preparation in, 229–230
      equipment in, 230
      general status/appearance in, 231b
      hydration in, 238b
      laboratory tests in, 239, 241t
      nutritional disorders in, 232t
      validating and documenting findings in, 240
Nutritional disorders, evaluating, 232t
Nutritional guidelines, 219–222, 220t
   Controversies, in, 219–221
      anti-inflammatory diet, 220–221

Canada's food guides, 221
   low glycemic index diet, 221
Nutritional status, 216–243
   examination of, equipment for, 32t
   food safety in, 219
   health assessment in, 222–236
   hydration in, 218
   nutritional guidelines in, 219–222, 220t
   nutritional problems in, 221–222
      dehydration, 222
      malnutrition, 221–222
      overhydration, 222
      over nutrition and obesity, 222, 223b, 224t (*see also* Obesity)
   nutrition in, 216–217
Nutrition history, 226b
Nystagmus, 319b, 582b

O

Obesity, 128b, 140b, 222, 223b, 243, 523b
   assessment for, 131b
   body mass index in
      ideal adult, 224t
      measurement of, 233b–234b
   in children, 771
Objective data, 8, 8f, 9t, 31. *See also* Physical examination
Objective vertigo, 340b
Obstetric conjugate, 716b
Obturator sign, 519b, 519f, 520b
Occipital frontal circumference (OFC), 740b, 792b
Ocular fundus, 306f, 325f
Oedipal stage, 770
Office of Minority Health, standards for care of, 183–184, 184b
Older adults
   client education, 815b
   disease prevention in, 814b–815b
   Healthy People 2020 objectives for, 814b
   interviewing of, 16–17
   risk assessment in, 815b
   screening of, 814b–815b
Older adults assessment, 813–851
   abnormal findings in
      eye, age-related abnormalities of, 850b–851b
   case study, 829b–830b, 848b, 849b–850b
   challenges to, 813–816
      atypical presentation of illness, 815–816
      physiologic reserve, loss of, 813, 815
   data analysis, 848
      collaborative problems, 849
      medical problems, 849
      nursing diagnoses, 848–849
   delirium *vs.* dementia, 823b–824b
   Geriatric Depression Scale, 824b
   Geriatric Oral Health Assessment Index, 827b
   Mini Nutritional Assessment (MNA-SF), 826b
   nursing history in
      adapting interview techniques, 816
      biographical data, 816–817
      bowel elimination, 822b
      falls, 819b–820b

fatigue and dyspnea, 820b–821b
   functional ability, 819b
   functional status, 816
   history of present concern in, 818b
   mental status, 818b–819b
   nutrition and hydration, 821b, 827b–828b
   pain assessment, 822b–823b, 829b
   sexuality, 817–818
   urinary incontinence, 821b–822b, 828b–829b
physical examination
   abdomen, 842b
   anus, rectum, and prostate, 844b
   arteries and veins, 840b
   breasts, 841b
   client's height and weight, 831b
   ears and hearing, 836b–837b
   exercise tolerance, 839b
   eyes and vision, 835b–836b, 836f
   general routine screening *vs.* focused specialty assessment, 831
   genitalia, 842b–843b
   head and neck, 833b
   heart and blood vessels, 838b–841b, 839f
   heart sounds, 841b
   hydration status and muscle mass, 832b
   mouth and throat, 833b–834b
   musculoskeletal system, 844b–847b
   neurologic system, 847b
   nose and sinuses, 834b–835b
   pulses, 839b–840b
   sensory system, 847b
   skin and hair, 832b–833b
   thorax and lungs, 837b–838b
   validating and documenting findings, 848
physical examination in, 830
   client preparation, 830
   equipment for, 830–831
   modifications and techniques for, 831
SBAR method, use of, 850
Short Blessed Test, 824b–825b
SPICES (risk screening tools), 815, 815b
Ongoing assessment forms
   admission form, 51, 52f–55f
   progress note, 51, 55f, 56
Open-ended questions, 16, 779
Opening snaps (OSs), 451b, 458b
Ophthalmoscopy, 317b, 325b
Opportunistic infections (OIs), 613b
Optic atrophy, 325b, 334b
Optic chiasma, 306
Optic disc
   abnormalities of, 334b
   diameter of, 325b
   structure and function of, 305, 306f
Oral cavity, 357
Oral diseases, culture and, 195
Oral health, 821b
Oral stage, 727
Oral temperature, 130b, 130f
Orchitis, 631b
Oropharyngeal cancer, 360b
Oropharynx, 358
Orthopnea, 387b, 440b

Orthostatic edema, 478b
Orthostatic hypotension, 838b
Ortolani test, 724
Osteoarthritis, 556b, 564b
Osteoblasts, 528
Osteoclasts, 528
Osteoporosis
  client education, 538b
  culture and, 195
  older adults and, 535b
  prevention of, 537b–538b
  risk assessment, 538b
  risk factor for, 535b, 536b
  screening for, 538b
Otalgia, 340b
Otitis externa, 342b, 354b
  acute, 355b
Otitis media, 799b
Otoscope, 346b
Ottawa ankle rules, for x-ray referral, 559b
Outer caruncle, 304
Ovarian cancer, 670b
Ovarian cyst, 524b, 670b
Ovaries, 639, 655b, 655f
Overflow incontinence, 829b
Overhydration, 222
Overnutrition, 222, 223b, 224t
Over-the-counter (OTC) medications, 498b
Overweight, 222, 224t
Ovum, 639

P

Pacemaker of heart, 433
PAD. *See* Peripheral arterial disease (PAD)
Paget disease of breast, 420b, 428b
Pain
  assessment of, 142–159
  breast, 412b
  classification of, 144–145, 145b
    acute, 145, 147b
    cancer, 145, 146b
    chronic nonmalignant, 145
    cutaneous, 145
    deep somatic, 144
    inflammatory, 144
    intractable, 145
    neuropathic, 144
    nociceptive, 144
    phantom, 145
    radiating, 145
    referred, 145, 146f
    visceral, 145
  culture and, 189, 193
  definition of, 142
  management of, standards for, 142, 143b
  pathophysiology, 142–143, 144f, 145f
    modulation, 143, 144f
    transduction, 143, 144f
    transmission, 143, 144f, 145f
  perception of, 144f, 145
    culture on, 148–149, 148t
    developmental level on, 148, 148b
  physiologic responses to, 143–144
  seven dimensions of, 147, 147b
  structure and function of, 121–122
Pain assessment, 142–159
  analysis of data in, 158–159
  barriers to, 149, 149b
  health history in, nursing, 149–155
    case study on, 155
    client preparation in, 150
    family history in, 154b
    FLACC Behavioral Scale, 151, 152b
    Hierarchy of Pain Assessment in, 150
    history of present health concern in, 154b
    lifestyle and health practices in, 155b
    McCafferty Initial Pain Assessment Tool, 151, 153b
    Numeric Rating Scale in, 150, 150f
    personal health history in, 154b
    self-assessment in, 151, 152b
    tips for, 149b
    Universal Pain Assessment Tool in, 150, 151b
    Verbal Descriptor Scale in, 150, 151f
    Visual Analog Scale in, 150, 150f
  physical examination, 156–157
    general impression and vital signs in, 156b
    physical assessment in, 156
    validating and documenting findings in, 157
  psychosocial factors, 147
    culture in, 148, 149t
    developmental level in, 148, 148b
  standards for, 143
Pain scales, 780b, 780f
  FLACC Behavioral Scale, 151, 152b
  Hierarchy of Pain Assessment, 150
  McCafferty Initial Pain Assessment Tool, 151, 153b
  Numeric Pain Intensity Scale (NPIS), 148
  Numeric Rating Scale (NRS), 150, 151f
  Universal Pain Assessment Tool, 150, 151b
  Verbal Descriptor Scale (VDS), 150, 151f
  Visual Analog Scale (VAS), 150, 150f
Pain sensation, testing of, 589b, 589f
Palate, 357
Palatine tonsils, 358
Pale/cyanotic nails, 393b
Pallor, 258b, 478b
Palmar arches, 464, 465f
Palmar grasp reflex, 754b
Palpation, 37, 40
  bimanual, 40, 41f
  deep, 40, 41f
  light, 40, 41f
  moderate, 40
  parts of hand to be used for, 40t
Palpebral fissure, 304
Palpitations, 440b
Pancreas, 494
Pansystolic murmur, 461b
Papanicolaou smear (Pap test), 639, 659b
Papilledema, 325b, 334b, 581b
Papule, 273b
Paralytic strabismus, 331b, 582b
Paranasal sinuses, 357, 359, 359f
Paraphimosis, 619b, 629b
Paresthesia, 573b
Parietal pericardium, 433
Parietal peritoneum, 493
Parietal pleura, 384
Parkinson disease, 302b, 847b
Parkinsonian gait, 603b
Paronychia, 278b
Parotid glands, 280
Paroxysmal nocturnal dyspnea, 387b, 440b
Pars flaccida, 338
Pars tensa, 338
Partial assessment, 6, 6f. *See also* Assessment
Patch, skin, 273b
Patchy hair loss, 263b– 264b, 263f, 264f
Patellar reflex, 593b, 594f
Patent ductus arteriosus (PDA), 459b
Peau d'orange skin, breast, 420b, 428b
Pectinate line, 639
Pectus carinatum (pigeon chest), 398b, 407b
Pectus excavatum (funnel chest), 398b, 406b
Pederson speculum, 659b
Pediculosis pubis, 609b
Pelvic inflammatory disease (PID), 643b, 670b
Penis
  abnormalities of, 628b–629b
  inspection and palpation, 618b–619b, 618f, 619f
  structure and function of, 605, 606f
Pentoxifylline (Trental), 470b
Peptic ulcer disease, 500b–501b
  client education, 501b
  risk factors, 500b–501b
  symptoms, 500b
Percussion, 40
  blunt, 41, 42f
  direct, 40–41, 41f
  indirect, 41–42, 42f
  notes, 41, 42t
Perianal abscess, 623b, 633b
Perianal area, inspection of, 622b, 623f
Pericardial friction rub, 458b–459b
Pericardium, 433
Periosteum, 528
Peripheral arterial disease (PAD), 468b–469b
  client education, 471b
  prevention of, 471b
  risk assessment, 471b
  screening methods for, 471b
Peripheral arteries, 463
Peripheral edema, 469b, 489b
Peripheral nervous system, 570–572
  autonomic fibers, 570
  cranial nerves, 570, 571f, 571t
  somatic fibers, 570
  spinal nerves, 570, 572, 572f
Peripheral neuropathy, 575b
Peripheral vascular assessment, 463–490
  abnormal findings
    arterial insufficiency, 488b
    lymphedema, 490b
    necrotic great toe with blisters on toes and foot, 489b
    peripheral edema, 489b
    Raynaud disease, 489b
    superficial thrombophlebitis, 490b
    varicose veins, 490b
    venous insufficiency, 488b
  case study, 472b, 486b–487b
  data analysis, 487
    collaborative problems, 487

Peripheral vascular assessment (*Continued*)
  medical problems, 487
  nursing diagnoses, 487
 health history, 468
  family history, 470b
  history of present health concern, 468b–469b
  lifestyle and health practices, 470b
  personal health history, 469b
 physical examination, 472–473
  ankle–brachial index (ABI), 483b–484b, 483f, 486b
  arm, 474b–477b
  arterial/venous insufficiency, tests for, 482b–482b
  assessment, key points for, 473
  client preparation, 473
  equipment for, 32t, 473
  general routine screening *vs.* focused specialty assessment, 474
  legs, 478b–481b
  lymphedema, stages of, 485b
  manual compression test, 484b, 484f
  position change test, 482b, 482f
  pulse strength assessment, 485b
  Trendelenburg test, 485b
  validating and documenting findings, 486
 SBAR method, use of, 488
 structure and function related to, 463
  arteries, 463–464, 464f, 465f
  capillaries and fluid exchange, 466
  lymphatic system, 466–468, 467f, 468f
  veins, 464–466, 466f
Peripheral vascular resistance, effect of, on blood pressure, 123b
Peripheral venous disease (PVD), 469b
Peristaltic waves, 507b
Peritoneum, 493, 639
Periumbilical ecchymosis, 505b
Personal protective equipment (PPE), 34b
Pes planus. *See* Flat foot
Pes valgus, 557b
Pes varus, 557b
Petechiae, 275b
Phalen test, 550b–551b, 550f, 695
Phallic stage, 770
Phantom pain, 145
Pharyngeal tonsils, 358
Pharynx, 358
Phimosis, 619b, 629b
Phlebitis, 840b
Phoria, 319b, 331b
Phosphodiesterase-5 (PDE-5) inhibitors, 612b
Physical abuse, 162. *See also* Abuse
Physical assessment guide, 889–893
Physical development, of children and adolescents, 761–765
 abdomen, 763
 anus and rectum, 764
 breasts, 762
 ears, 761
 eyes, 761
 genitalia, 763–764, 763t, 764t
 growth patterns, 765
 head and neck, 761
 heart, 762–763

 mouth, nose, throat, and sinuses, 761–762
 musculoskeletal system, 764–765
 neurologic system, 765
 skin, hair, and nails, 761
 thorax and lungs, 762
Physical examination, 31
 client positioning during, 38b–40b
 equipment for, 31, 32t–33t
 isolation precaution guidelines, 33, 34b–36b
 older adult, considerations for, 40b
 preparation for, 31, 33
  approaching and preparing client in, 36–37
  physical setting and, 33
  preparing oneself in, 33, 34b–36b, 36
 techniques, 37
  auscultation, 42–43
  inspection, 37
  palpation, 37–38, 40
  percussion, 40–42
Physiologic cup, 305, 306f
Physiologic splitting, 450b
Piaget theory of cognitive development
 assessment of, 114b–115b, 115f
 theoretical aspects, 102, 103t–104t
Pica, 694
Piles. *See* Hemorrhoids
Pilonidal cyst, 623b, 634b
Pinna, 338
Pitting edema, 479b, 479f
Plantar fasciitis, 558b
Plantar grasp reflex, 754b
Plantar response, 595b, 595f
Plantar warts, 557b, 565b
Plaque, 273b
Play as communication, 777
Pleural friction rub, 402b
Pleural membranes, 384–385, 384f
Pleural space, 384–385
Pneumococcal vaccine (PCV13 or PCV23), 821b
POAG. *See* Primary open-angle glaucoma
Point of maximal impulse (PMI), 448b
Polycystic ovary syndrome (PCOS), 263b
Polydactyly, 805b
Polymyalgia rheumatica (PMR), 846b
Popliteal pulse, 464
Port-wine stain, 808b
Postauricular nodes, palpation of, 295b
Posterior axillary line, 383, 383f
Posterior cervical nodes, palpation of, 295b
Posterior chamber, of eye, 306, 306f
Posterior cord syndrome, 601b
Posterior tibial artery, 464
Posthysterectomy, 641
Postpartum depression, 700b
Postural tremor, 602b
Posture
 abnormal, in unconscious clients, 604b
 and back problems, 536b
 observation of, 541b
 during pregnancy, 695, 695f
Prayer, health and, 204, 204f
Preauricular nodes, palpation of, 295b
Precordium, 431, 432f
Pregnancy, 523b

 culture and, 192, 193
 structure and function in, 691–695
  of abdomen, 693–694, 694f
  of anus and rectum, 694–695
  of breasts, 692, 693f
  of ears and hearing, 692
  of genitalia, 694
  of heart, 692
  of mouth, throat, nose, and sinus, 692
  of musculoskeletal system, 695, 695f
  of neurologic system, 695
  of peripheral vascular system, 692–693
  of skin, hair, and nails, 692
  of thorax and lungs, 692
Pregnancy assessment, 697–720
 analysis of data in, 718–719
 health history in, nursing, 697
 physical examination in, 705–718
  of abdomen, 709b
  of anus and rectum, 715b–716b
  of breasts, 708b, 708f
  case study on, 718
  client preparation in, 705
  equipment in, 705
  of external genitalia, 713b
  of eyes and ears, 707b
  of fetal heart and heart rate, 712b
  of fetal position, 711b–712b, 711f–712f
  of fundal height, 710b, 710f
  of head and neck, 707b
  of heart, 708b
  of internal genitalia, 713b–714b
  of mouth, throat, and nose, 707b, 707f
  of musculoskeletal system, 715b
  palpation, 709b–710b, 709f–710f
  of peripheral vascular system, 709b
  of skin, hair, and nails, 706b–707b
  of thorax and lungs, 708b
  validating and documenting findings in, 718
  of vital signs, height, and weight, 706b, 706f
Prehn sign, 620b
Preload, 436
Premature atrial contractions, 457b
Premature ventricular contractions, 457b
Premenstrual syndrome (PMS), 640
Prepuce, 637
Presbycusis, 340b, 352b
Presbyopia (impaired near vision), 318b, 835b
Preschoolers. . *See also* Child and adolescent assessment
 cognitive and language development in, 767
 coping mechanisms in, 775t
 growth pattern, 765
 moral development in, 768
 motor development in, 766, 766f
 nutritional requirements, 771
 play characteristics, 773b
 psychosexual development in, 770
 psychosocial development in, 769
 sensory perception in, 767
 sleep requirements, 772, 774, 774f

Pressure ulcers (sores)
  assessment tools for
    Braden Scale for predicting risk, 266b–268b
    PUSH tool for healing, 268b
  inspection for, 260b
  stages of, 271b–272b
Pressure Ulcer Scale for Healing (PUSH), 268b
Presystole, 435
Preterm gestation, 698b
Primary open-angle glaucoma (POAG), 312b
Primary skin lesions, 273b–274b
Problem-oriented assessment, 6. *See also* Assessment
Prone position, 39b
Prostate cancer, 635b
  client education, 615b
  culture and, 197
  prevention of, 614b–615b
  risk factors for, 615b
  screening for, 614b–615b
Prostate gland
  abnormalities of, 635b
  palpation of, 625b
  structure and function of, 608, 608f
Prostate-specific antigen (PSA) test, 611b, 614b
Prostatitis, acute, 635b
Protodiastolic filling, 434
Pruritic urticarial papules and plaques of pregnancy (PUPPP), 692
Pseudoanemia, 692
Pseudodementia, 818b
Pseudostrabismus, 330b
Psoas sign, 518b, 518f, 520b
Psoriasis, nail pitting in, 255b, 277b
Psychological abuse, family, 162, 163b
Psychopathology theory, of violence, 162
Psychosexual development
  in child and adolescent, 769–771
  Freud's theory of, 98–100, 99t
  in newborn and infant, 727
Psychosocial development
  in child and adolescent, 769
  Erikson's theory of, 100–102, 100t, 101f
  in newborn and infant, 726–727
Pterygium, 835b
Ptosis, 331f, 581b, 581f, 797b
Ptyalism, 694
Pubertal rites, 619b
Puberty, 765
Pubic hair, 618b
  development of, 763–764, 763t, 764t
Pudendum. *See* Vulva
Pulmonary artery, 431
Pulmonary circulation, 431
Pulmonary valve, 433
Pulmonary vein, 431
Pulmonic ejection click, 458b
Pulmonic stenosis, murmur of, 460b
Pulse
  arterial (peripheral), 122
  assessment of, objective, 132b, 132f
  radial, 122
  rate of, 132b, 132f
Pulse amplitude, 132b, 485b
Pulse contour, 132b
Pulse deficit, 450b

Pulse pressure, 124, 454
Pulse rhythm, 132b
Puncta, 304, 305f
Pupil
  abnormalities of, 334b
  accommodation of, testing, 324b
  inspection of, 323b–324b
  structure and function of, 305, 306f
Pupillary light reflex, 307, 307f
Pupillary reaction, testing of, 835b, 836f
Pupils, abnormalities of, 582b
Purkinje fibers, 433
Pursed lip breathing, 393b
Pustule, 274b

Q
QUESTT principles
  pain in children, 148
Quick Inventory of Depressive Symptomatology, 79b–80b, 87

R
Radial artery, 464
Radial pulse, 122, 132f, 464, 475b
  rate of, 132b, 132f
Radiating pain, 145
Rapid response teams (RRTs), 58
Raynaud disease, 474b, 489b
Rebound tenderness, 517b–518b
Rectal ampulla, 639
Rectal cancer, 634b
Rectal polyps, 634b
Rectal prolapse, 633b
Rectal shelf, 634b
Rectal temperature, 131b
Rectocele, 666b, 666f
Rectouterine pouch, 608, 639
Rectovaginal examination, 656b, 656f
Rectovesical pouch, 608, 639
Rectum, 639, 640f
Rectus abdominis, 492
Red reflex, 798b
  abnormalities of, 325b
  inspection of, 325b, 325f
Referrals, 9
Referred pain, 145, 146f
Reflexes, 579
  testing of, 593b–596b
Reflex hammer, 580b
Regurgitation, 435
Reiter syndrome, 620f
Relaxin, 695
Religion, 182. *See also* Spirituality and religious practices
  characteristics of, 203b
  definition and scope of, 203, 203b, 203f
Religious Coping Questionnaire (RCOPE), 210b
Renal arterial stenosis (RAS), 507b
Respiration
  external, 385
  patterns, 403t
  purpose of, 385
  structure and function in, 121–122
  vital signs in, 132b–133b
Respiratory hygiene, 34b–35b

Resting pulse rate (RPR), 449b
Resting (static) tremors, 602b
Retinal background
  abnormalities of, 335b–336b
  inspection of, 326b
Retinal detachment, 851b
Retinal vessels
  abnormalities of, 335b–336b
  inspection of, 326b
  structure and function of, 305, 306f
Retracted nipple, 428b
Review of body systems (ROS), 673
Rheumatic carditis, 441b
Rheumatic heart disease (RHD), 441b
Rheumatoid arthritis
  acute, 563b
  chronic, 564b
  culture and, 197
RhoGAM, 699b
Ribs, 381–382, 382f
Right atria, 431
Right lymphatic duct, 467
Right main bronchus, 383
Right ventricle, 431
Rinne test, 584b
Risk for Complications (RC), 664
Risk nursing diagnoses, 63, 66
Rods, 305, 306f
Romberg test, 587b, 587f, 808b
Rooting reflex, 754b
Rovsing sign, 518f, 520b
Rugae, 638

S
SAD PERSONS suicide risk assessment, 81b, 88
Safety plan, assessing, 177b
Saint Louis University Mental Status (SLUMS), 818b
Saliva, 358
Salivary glands, 358, 358f
Saphenous vein, 465
Sarcopenia, 813, 821b
Sarcopenic obesity, 813, 821b
SBAR (Situation, Background, Assessment, Recommendation), 58, 58b
Scapular lines, 383
Scar
  abdomen, 505b
  skin, 266b, 274b
School-age children
  cognitive and language development in, 767–768, 768f
  coping mechanisms in, 775t
  growth pattern, 765
  moral development in, 768
  motor development in, 766, 766f
  nutritional requirements, 771
  play characteristics, 773b
  psychosexual development in, 770
  psychosocial development in, 769
  sensory perception in, 767
  sleep requirements, 774
School violence, 164–165
Scissors gait, 603b
Sclera, 305, 306f
Scleral jaundice, 332f

Scleroderma, 301b
Scoliosis, 407b, 562b, 563b, 806b
Scratch test, 511b, 511f
Scrotal hernia, 621b, 630b
Scrotal mass, 621b
Scrotum
    abnormalities of, 630b–632b
    inspection, 620b, 620f
    palpation, 620b–621, 621f
    structure and function of, 606
Sebaceous glands, 248–249, 248f, 637
Seborrheic keratoses, 266b, 832b
Sebum, 761
Secondary skin lesions, 274b
Second-hand smoke, 389b
Second heart sound, 435
Seizures, 573b
Self-assessment
    for danger, 176bf
    for pain, 151, 154b
    for skin, 255b
    for spiritual and religious practices
        Brief Religious Coping Questionnaire, 210b
        Daily Spiritual Experiences Scale, 210b
Self-concept, development of, 774–775, 775t
Semen, 606
Semicircular canals, 339, 339f
Semilunar valves, 433
Seminal vesicles, 608
Senile purpura, 832b
Sensory receptors, 339
Sensory system, assessment of, 589b–592b
Sentinel tag, 633b
Septum, 359
Severe acute respiratory syndrome (SARS), 388b
Sexual abuse
    family, 162–163
    physical examination for, 167
Sexual Assault Nurse Examiner (SANE), 173, 173b
Sexual dysfunction, 609b–610b, 642b
Sexuality, in older adults, 817–818
Sexually transmitted infections (STI), 609b, 610b–611b, 642b
    culture and, 197
Shifting dullness, test for, 516b–517b, 517f
Short Blessed Test, 824b–825b
Shortness of breath, 389b
Shoulder
    inspection and palpation, 546b
    range of motion of, 546b, 547f
Sigmoid colon, 607, 639
Sigmoidoscopy, 644b
Silence, culture and, 187
Silver wire arteriole, 335b
Sims' position, 38b
Sinoatrial (SA) node, 433
Sinus arrhythmia, 457b
Sinuses
    health history in, nursing, 361b–362b
    palpation of, 374, 374f
    percussion of, 374b
    physical examination of, 374b, 374f, 678b, 678f
    structure and function of, 359, 359f

Sinus headache, 299b–300b
Sinusitis
    culture and, 197
    prevention of, 364b–365b
Sitting position, 38b
Skeletal muscles, 528–530, 530f–531f
    movements, 528–530, 529b
Skene glands, 638
Skin
    in head-to-toe assessment, 677b, 677f
    structure and function of, 247–249, 248f
    types, 265b, 265t
    variation in, 265b–266b
Skin assessment, 241b–245b, 255f, 259b–260b, 271b–272b
    analysis of data in, 269–270
    family history in, 251b
    history of present health concern in, 249b–250b
    lifestyle and health practices in, 252b–253b
    personal health history, 251b
    physical examination in
        abnormal findings, 271b–278b
        Braden scale for pressure sore risk in, 266b–268b
        client preparation in, 257
        equipment in, 32t, 257
        inspection in, 258b–260b, 258f, 259f
        palpation in, 260b–262b, 261f
        PUSH tool for pressure ulcer healing in, 268b
        self-assessment in, 255b
        validating and documenting findings in, 269
    for pressure ulcers, 255b (See also Pressure ulcers (sores))
    for skin cancer, 254b, 276b
    variations, common
        in adults, 265b–266b
Skin cancer
    assessment for, 254b (See also Skin assessment)
    culture and, 195
    inspection for, 260b, 276b
    lesions in, 251b, 277b
Skin fold calipers, 230
Skin lesions
    cancerous, 260b, 276b
    configurations of, 277b
    inspection for, 259b– 260b
    primary, 273b–274b
    secondary, 274b
    vascular, 275b
Skin tags, 832b
Skull, anatomy of, 281f
Sleep apnea, 387b
Sleep, in health history, 26, 26b
Sleep Self-Assessment Quiz, 27b
SLUMS Mental Status Examination, 91b
Small intestine, 495
Small saphenous vein, 465
Small testes, 631b
Smoking
    cessation, 389b, 441b, 443b
    and heart disease, 441b
    and lung cancer, 391b
    and respiratory problems, 389b

Snare polypectomy, 634b
Snellen chart, 316b, 581b
Social learning theory, of violence, 162
Solar lentigines, 832b, 832f
Space, culture and, 187
Spastic hemiparesis, 603b
Specialty area assessment forms, 56, 57f
Spermatic cord, 606, 621b
    torsion of, 631b
Spermatocele, 632b
Sphenoidal sinuses, 359
Spider angioma, 275b, 504b
Spider nevi, 692
Spina bifida occulta, 794b
Spinal cord, 567, 569, 569f, 600b
Spinal nerves, 570, 572, 572f
SPIRIT acronym, 209b
Spiritual assessment, 203b, 208–216
    analysis of data in, 215–216
    approach in, 208
    characteristics of, 203b
    techniques in, 202–206
        Brief Religious Coping Questionnaire, 210b
        case study on, 214
        Daily Spiritual Experiences Scale, 210b
        FICA Spiritual History Tool, 211b
        formal, 209, 209b, 210b, 212b
        HOPE questions, 211b
        nonformal, 208, 210b
        sample format for, 209, 211b–213b
        SPIRIT acronym, 209b
        validating and documenting findings in, 214
Spiritual care, 203b
Spirituality
    characteristics of, 203b
    culture and, 193
    definition and scope of, 203, 203b, 203f
Spirituality and religious practices, 197–207
    health and, 201–207
    impact of, 204–205, 204f, 205f
    incorporation into care of, 205, 207, 207f
    major religions and, 206t–207t
    self-understanding of, 208
    spiritual assessment in, 203, 208–216 (See also Spiritual assessment)
    terms related to, 203
Spleen, 494
    enlarged, 526b
    palpation, 515b, 515f
    percussion of, 511b–512b
Splenomegaly, 511b, 526b
Spongy bone, 528
Sputum, 388b
    blood in, 388b
    color, 388b
Squamocolumnar junction, 639
Squamous cell carcinoma, 260b, 276b. See also Skin cancer
Squamous metaplasia, 661b
Squeeze test, 549b, 549f, 558b, 558f
Standing position, 39b
Stanford sleepiness scale, 26b
Stapes, 338, 339f
Steatorrhea, 610b
Stellate laceration, 661b

Stepping reflex, 755b
Stereognosis, 591b, 591f
Stereotyping, 183b
Sternal angle, 381
Sternoclavicular joint, inspection and palpation, 542b
Sternomastoid muscle, 281, 281f
Sternum, 381
Stethoscope, use of, 42–43, 43b
Stomach, 495
Stomach cancer, culture and, 196
Stomach growling, 507b
Stomatitis, 795b
Stool, 643b
    color of, 610b
    DNA test, 611b
    inspection of, 625b
    mucus in, 610b
Strabismus, 319b, 330b
Straight leg test, 545b, 546f
Stratum corneum, 247, 248f
Stratum germinativum, 247, 248f
Stratum granulosum, 247, 248f
Stratum lucidum, 247, 248f
Streptococcal pharyngitis, 378b
Stress incontinence, 828b
Stressors, in children, 775, 775t
Stretch marks. *See* Striae
Stretch reflex, 569
Striae, 265b
    abdomen, 505b
Stridor, 800b
Stroke
    client education, 578b
    hemorrhagic, 577b
    ischemic, 577b
    risk factors for, 578b
    signs and symptoms, 577b
    transcient ischemic attack, 577b
    warning signs of, 578b
Stroke volume (SV), 436
Subarachnoid space, 567
Subclavian veins, 467
Subconjunctival hemorrhage, 332f
Subculture, 183b
Subcutaneous tissue, 248f, 249
Subjective data, 7–8, 8f, 9t, 12. *See also* Interview
Subjective vertigo, 340b
Sublingual glands, 358
Submandibular glands, 280, 358
Submandibular nodes, palpation of, 295b, 295f
Substance abuse (use), 71f. *See also* Mental status assessment
    assessment for, 71–96
    definition of, 70
    in health history, 26, 28
Sucking reflex, 754b
Suicide, 88
    Modified SAD PERSONS suicide risk assessment, 81b
    past attempts at, 75b
    risks and signs, 776b
Summation gallop, 451b, 458b
Superficial cervical nodes, palpation of, 295b
Superficial inguinal nodes, 468

Superficial retinal hemorrhages, 336b
Superficial thrombophlebitis, 490b
Superior vena cava, 431
Supernumerary nipples, 410, 410f, 421b, 421f
Supine hypotensive syndrome, 695
Supine position, 38b
Supraclavicular nodes, palpation of, 296b, 296f
Suprasternal notch, 381
Suspensory ligaments, 411
Swan-neck deformity, 564b
Sweat glands, 248, 248f, 637
Swimmer's ear, 342b
Sympathetic nervous system, 572
Symphysis pubis, 637
Syndrome nursing diagnoses, 66
Synovial joints, 530, 531f
Syphilitic chancre, 628b
Systemic circulation, 431
Systole, 434, 435

T

Tachycardia, 132b, 440b, 449b
Tachypnea, 403t
Tactile discrimination, 591b, 591f
Tadalafil (Cialis), 612b
Tail of Spence, 409
Talipes equinovarus (clubfoot), 805b, 805f
Talipes varus, 805b
Tandem balance, 588b, 588f
Tanner's sexual maturity rating
    female breast development, 762t
    female pubic hair, 764t
    male genitalia and pubic hair, 763t
Tarsal plates, 304
Tay–Sachs disease, 701b
TBI. *See* Traumatic brain injury
Teeth, 358f
    crown, 358
    physical examination, 367b–368b, 367f
    root, 358
Telangiectasis, 275b
Temperature
    assessment of, objective, 129b–131b
        axillary, 130b, 130f
        oral, 130b, 130f
        rectal, 131b
        temporal artery, 131b, 131f
        tympanic, 129b, 129f
Temperature sensation, testing of, 590b
Temporal artery, 280
Temporal artery temperature, 131b, 131f
Temporomandibular joint (TMJ), 280, 532b
    dysfunction, 534b
    inspection and palpation, 542, 542b
    palpation of, 191f, 291
Tendons, 528
Tennis elbow, 548b
Tenosynovitis, 564b
Tension headache, 299b–300b
Terazosin (Hytrin), 612b
Terminal hair, 249
Testes, 620b, 803b
    absence of, 620b
    small, 631b
    structure and function of, 606, 606f

Testicular self-examination (TSE), 612b, 615b, 803b
Testicular tumor, 630b
Thenar atrophy, 564b
Therapeutic conversation, 861
Thoracic cage, 381
    anterior, 382f
    posterior, 382f
    ribs and thoracic vertebrae in, 381–382
    sternum and clavicles in, 381
    structure and function of, 381–383
    vertical reference lines in, 382–383, 383f
Thoracic cavity, 381, 383
    lungs in, 383–384
    mediastinum, 383
    pleural membranes, 384–385
    structure and function of, 383–385
    trachea and bronchi in, 383, 384f
Thoracic duct, 467
Thoracic vertebra, 382
Thorax, 381
    anterior
        auscultation, 400b–401b
        inspection, 398b–399b
        palpation, 399b–400b
        percussion, 400b
    posterior, 393b
        auscultation, 397b–398b
        inspection, 393b–394b
        palpation, 395b–396b
        percussion, 396b–397b
Thorax and lung assessment
    abnormal findings
        thoracic deformities and configurations, 406b–407b
    analysis of data in, 405
    data analysis
        case study on, 406
        collaborative problems, 405
        medical problems, 405
        nursing diagnoses, 405
    general routine screening *versus* focused specialty assessment, 393
    health history in, 386b–392b
        case study, 391–392
        family history, 388b–389b
        history of present health concern, 386b–388b
        lifestyle and health practices, 389b
        personal health history, 388b
    nursing diagnoses
        actual diagnoses, 405
        health promotion diagnoses, 405
        risk diagnoses, 405
    physical examination in, 392
        anterior thorax, 398b–401b
        case study, 403–404
        client preparation, 392
        equipment for, 32t, 392
        general inspection, 393b
        posterior thorax, 393b–398b
        validating and documenting findings, 404–405
    SBAR method, use of, 406
    structure and function, 381
        breathing mechanics in, 385
        thoracic cage, 381–383
        thoracic cavity, 383–385

Throat
    abnormalities of, 377b–379b
    health history in, nursing, 352b
    physical assessment of, 679b, 679f
    structure and function of, 358, 358f
Thrombophlebitis, 693
Thumb weakness, 551b
Thyroid cartilage, 281f, 282, 293b
Thyroid gland
    diffuse enlargement of, 291f
    palpation of, 293b–294b, 294f
    structure of, 282
Thyrotoxicosis. See Hyperthyroidism
Tibial torsion, 805b
Tics, 574b, 586b, 601b
Time, culture and, 186
Tineacapitis, 262b, 262f
Tinel sign, 551b, 551f, 695
TMJ. See Temporomandibular joint
Tobacco use, head and neck cancer and, 285b
Toddlers. . See also Child and adolescent assessment
    cognitive and language development in, 767
    coping mechanisms in, 775t
    growth pattern, 765
    moral development in, 768
    motor development in, 765, 766f
    nutritional requirements, 771
    play characteristics, 773b
    psychosexual development in, 770
    psychosocial development in, 769, 769f
    sensory perception in, 767
    sleep requirements, 772
Toeing in, 806b
Toeing out, 806b
Toes, physical assessment of, 682b–683b, 682f, 683f
Toilet training, 770, 770f
Tongue
    black hairy, 369b, 377b
    Candida albicans (thrush) in, 368b, 377b
    canker sore on, 370b
    carcinoma of, 377b
    fissured, 369f
    health history in, nursing, 361b
    in Kaposi's sarcoma, 371b, 378b
    leukoplakia of, 369b, 377b
    physical examination of, 369b–371b, 369f, 370f
    structure and function of, 358
    varicose veins on ventral surface of, 370b, 370f
    in vitamin B12 deficiency, 369b, 377b
Tonic neck reflex, 755b
Tonsillar nodes, palpation of, 295b, 295f
Tonsillitis, 379b
Tophi, 354b
Torsion of spermatic cord, 631b
Touch
    as communication tool, 778
    culture and, 187
Trabecular meshwork, 306
Trachea, 282, 383, 384f
    palpation of, 293b, 293f
Traditional healers and practices 189b, 192f
Transdermal contraceptives, 470b

Transduction, of pain, 143, 144f
Transfusion, health care beliefs and, 193
Transient ischemic attack (TIA), 577b
Transmission, of pain 143, 144f, 145f
Trapezius muscle, 281, 281f
Traumatic brain injury (TBI), 287b–288b
    culture and, 195
Tremors, 574b, 586b
    in older adults, 847b
Trendelenburg test, 485b
Triceps reflex, 593b, 593f
Triceps skin fold thickness (TSF), 237b, 237f, 239t, 676b
Trichomonas vaginitis (trichomoniasis), 668b
Tricuspid regurgitation, murmur of, 461b
Tricuspid valve, 432
Tripod position, 394b
Tropia, 319b, 330b
Trust versus mistrust, 726
TSE. See Testicular self-examination
TSF. See Triceps skin fold thickness (TSF)
Tumor, 273b
Tumor-related headache, 299b–300b
Tunica vaginalis, 606
Turbinates, 359
Turgor, skin, 261b, 261f
Turner syndrome, 232b
Two-point discrimination, 592b, 592f
Tympanic cavity, 338
Tympanic membrane, 799b
    inspection of, 349b
    structure and function of, 338, 339f
Tympanic temperature, 129b, 129f

U

Ulnar artery, 464
Ulnar pulse, 464, 475b
Umbilical hernia, 505b, 524b, 802b
Umbilicus, inspection of, 505b
Umbo, 338
Unilateral transverse laceration, 661b
Universal Pain Assessment Tool, 150, 151b
Urethral meatus, 638
Urethra, palpation of, 653b, 653f
Urethritis, 619b
Urge incontinence, 828b
Urinary bladder, 495
    palpation, 516b, 516f
Urinary incontinence, 609b, 828b–829b
    functional incontinence, 829b
    interventions for, 829b
    nursing assessment, 829b
    in older adults, 821b–822b
    overflow incontinence, 829b
    stress incontinence, 828b
    urge incontinence, 828b
Urinary meatus, 619b
Urinary tract infections (UTIs), 498b, 609b, 698b
Urinating, difficulty, 609b
Urination, 642b
Urine color, changes in, 609b
U.S. Department of Health and Human Services (USDHHS), 5, 650
U.S. Preventive Services Task Force (USPSTF), 5, 644b, 647

Uterine cancer, 669b
Uterine contractions, 709b–710b, 709f
Uterine enlargement, 669b
Uterine fibroids (myomas), 669b
Uterine glands, 639
Uterine prolapse, 666b, 666f
Uterus, 639
    palpate the, 655b, 655f
    position of, 662b
Uvula, 357

V

Vagina, 638
Vaginal discharge, 641b–642b
Vaginal infections, during pregnancy, 700b
Vaginal opening, abnormalities of, 665b–666b, 665f, 666f
Vaginal orifice, 638
Vaginal speculums, 659b
Vaginal wall, 638, 654b
Vaginitis, 668b–669b
Validation, data, 44–45
    methods of, 45
    purpose of, 45
Valves of Houston, 608, 639
Varicocele, 620b, 621b, 632b
Varicose veins, 469b, 490b, 840b
    culture and, 194
Vascular dementia vs. delirium, 93t
Vascular skin lesions, 275b
Vascular sounds, 507b–508b, 508f
Vas deferens, 606, 606f
Veins, 464–466, 466f
    deep veins, 465
    of legs, 466f
    perforator veins, 465, 466f
    superficial veins, 465
Vellus hair, 249
Venous hums, 459b, 508b
Venous insufficiency, 488b
Venous lakes, 832b
Venous stasis, 465
Ventricles, 431
Ventricular gallop, 436, 451b, 458b
Ventricular impulses, variations of, 456b
    accentuated apical impulse, 456b
    laterally displaced apical impulse, 456b
    lift, 456b
    thrill, 456b
Ventricular septal defect, murmur of, 461b
Venules, 305, 306f
Verbal communication, of data, 58, 58b, 58f
Verbal Descriptor Scale (VDS), 150, 151f
Vernix caseosa, 722
Verruca vulgaris, 557b
Vertebral line, 383
Vertebra prominens, 382
Vertical reference lines, 382–383, 383f
Vertigo, 341b
Vesicle, 273b
Vessel wall elasticity, effect of, on blood pressure, 123b
Vestibule, 339, 339f, 638
Vibratory sensation, testing of, 590b, 590f
Vibrissae, 359
Violence
    definition of, 161

domestic, 161
family, 160–174
  assessment of, 167–179
  child abuse in, 163–164
  economic abuse in, 162
  elder mistreatment in, 164
  intimate partner, 163
  physical abuse in, 162
  psychological abuse in, 162, 163b
  sexual abuse in, 162–163
  theories of, 161–162
human trafficking, 165–166
school, 164–165
war crimes, 166
Violence assessment, 167–179
  abuse assessment screen in, 172b
  analysis of data in, 178
  evidence-based guidelines on, 167b–168b
  health history in, nursing, 169–171
  physical examination in, 169–174
    assessing a safety plan in, 177b
    case study on, 172–173
    danger assessment in, 176b
    equipment in, 174
    patient preparation in, 173–174
    physical assessment in, 174
    SANE programs for, 173, 173b
    validating and documenting findings in, 178
  preparation for, 168
  universal screening in, 167
Viral hepatitis, 498b
Visceral pain, 145
Visceral peritoneum, 493
Visceral pleura, 384
Viscosity, effect of, on blood pressure, 123b
Vision
  binocular, 306, 307f
  double, 308b
  near, 305, 316b
  peripheral
    abnormalities of, 325b, 333b
    gross, 318b
    normal, 318b
    reduced, 318b
    testing of, 318b
  visual fields and pathways in, 306–307, 307f
  visual reflexes in, 307, 307f

Vision assessment, 317b–320b
  extraocular muscle function, 319b
  gross peripheral vision in, 318b
  Snellen (E) chart in, 316b
Vision charts, 316b–317b
Visual acuity, 316b
  distant, 317b, 318f
  near, 318b
  reduced, 307
  tests, 797b
Visual Analog Scale (VAS), 150, 150f
Visual fields
  defects of, 329f–330f
  for gross peripheral vision, 318b
  loss of, 581b
  structure and function of, 307, 307f
Visual impairment, culture and, 195
Visual pathways, 307, 307f
Visual perception, 306
Visual reflexes, 307, 307f
Vital signs
  assessment of, 32t, 129b–133b
  blood pressure, 122–123, 123b, 133b, 134t, 135b
  pain, 124, 133b
  pulse, 122, 132b, 132f
  respirations, 121–122, 132b–133b
  temperature, 122, 129b–131b, 129f, 130f
Vitamin B12 deficiency, and tongue, 369b, 377b
Vitamin D, 536b
Vitamin supplements, during pregnancy, 703b
Vitiligo, 265b, 273b
Vitreous chamber, 306, 306f
Voice–whisper test, 836b
Vomiting, 497b
Vulva, 637

W
Waddling, 695
Waist circumference, 234b, 235f, 236t
Waist-to-hip ratio, 235b, 235f
Walker's Cycle of Violence, 162
War crimes, 166

Warts
  genital, 628b
  plantar, 557b, 565b
Weakness, in older adults, 820b–821b
Weber test, 584b
Weight
  desirable, 224t, 233b
  ideal body, 233b, 233f
  measurement of, 233b, 233f, 792b
  during pregnancy, 697b, 697f
Wellness nursing diagnoses, 63, 65–66
Wharton ducts, 358
Wheal, 273b
Wheeze, 388b, 398b, 402b
  expiratory, 747b
  inspiratory, 747b
  in older adults, 838b
  sibilant, 402b
  sonorous, 402b
Whispered pectoriloquy, 398b
Worldview, 183b
Wrist
  anatomic snuffbox, 549b, 549f
  carpal tunnel syndrome, tests for, 550b–551b
  fracture, 549b
  inspection and palpation, 549b
  ranges of motion, 550b, 550f
  squeeze test, 549b, 549f
Wry neck
  in children and adolescents, 794b
  in infants, 744b

Y
Yellow nail syndrome, 278b
Yin-yang theory, 189, 189t, 192f
Yoga, health and, 204, 205f

Z
Zika virus infection, 696b, 697b
  client education, 696b
  risk assessment, 696b
  screening for, 696b
Zollinger–Ellison syndrome, 501b